Nursing Diagnosis Handbook

A Guide to Planning Care

Nursing Diagnosis Handbook

A Guide to Planning Care

Betty J. Ackley, MSN, EdS, RN
Gail B. Ladwig, MSN, RN, CHTP, HNC

fifth edition

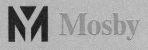

Mosby

A Harcourt Health Sciences Company

St. Louis   London   Philadelphia   Sydney   Toronto

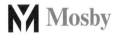

A Harcourt Health Sciences Company

Vice President and Publishing Director, Nursing: Sally Schrefer
Executive Editor: Barbara Nelson Cullen
Senior Developmental Editor: Cindi Anderson
Project Manager: Deborah L. Vogel
Production Editor: Kelley Barbarick
Design Manager: Bill Drone
Cover Designer: Judi Lang

FIFTH EDITION

Mosby, Inc.
A Harcourt Health Sciences Company
11830 Westline Industrial Drive
St. Louis, Missouri 63146

Printed in the United States of America

Library of Congress Cataloging in Publication Data
Nursing diagnosis handbook : a guide to planning care / [edited by] Betty J. Ackley, Gail B. Ladwig.—5th ed.
        p. ; cm.
     Includes bibliographical references and index.
     ISBN 0-323-01459-3 (alk. paper)
     1. Nursing diagnosis—Handbooks, manuals, etc.   2. Nursing care plans—Handbooks, manuals, etc.   I. Ackley, Betty J.   II. Ladwig, Gail B.
     [DNLM: 1. Nursing Diagnosis—Handbooks.   2. Patient Care Planning—Handbooks. WY 49 N9745 2002]
     RT48.6 .A35 2002
     610.73—dc21
                                                                        2001032703

01 02 03 04 05 CL/FF 9 8 7 6 5 4 3 2 1

To:

Dale Ackley, the greatest guy in the world, without whose support this book would have never happened; Dr. Dawn Ackley, who with Dale has been the joy of my life

Jerry Ladwig, my wonderful husband, who after 37 years is still supportive and patient—I couldn't have done it without him; my children and their spouses and my grandchildren—Jerry, Kathy Alexandra Elizabeth, and Benjamin; Chrissy, John, Sean, and Ciara; Jenny, Jim, Abby, and Katelyn; and Amy and Scott—the greatest family anyone could ever hope for

A special thank you to our nursing students who teach us every day and our nursing faculty colleagues—"friends are one of life's most precious gifts"

Contributors

Betty J. Ackley, MSN, EdS, RN
Professor of Nursing
Consultant in Online Learning
Jackson Community College
Jackson, Michigan

Donna Algase, PhD, RN, FAAN
Professor of Nursing
University of Michigan School of Nursing
Ann Arbor, Michigan

Jill M. Barnes, MS, RNCS
Family Nurse Practitioner
University of Michigan
Ann Arbor, Michigan

Brenda Emick-Herring, RN, MSN, CRRN
Admission Liaison for the Iowa Rehabilitation Network
Staff Development Specialist for Central Iowa Health
  System
Des Moines, Iowa

Roslyn Fine, MS, CCC, SLP
Preschool Speech Language Pathologist
Goshen Community Schools
Goshen, Indiana
First Step Provider: An Independent Contractor
Private Practitioner
State of Indiana Program

Terri Foster, BSN, CNOR
RN, Unit Educator, Surgery/PACU/CSP/Ortho
  Services
W.A. Foote Memorial Hospital
Jackson, Michigan

Judith R. Gentz, RN, CS, NP
Sole Proprietor
Nurse Practitioner Care
Grass Lake, Michigan

Mikel Gray, PhD, CUNP, CCCN, FAAN
Nurse Practitioner and Professor
Department of Urology and School of Nursing
University of Virginia
Charlottesville, Virginia

T. Heather Herdman, PhD, RN (BSN, MS)
Director of Research and Planning
St. Michaels Hospital and Rice Medical Center
Stevens Point, Wisconsin

Kimberly Hickey, MSN, RN
Clinical Nurse Specialist, Gerontology
University of Michigan Health System
Ann Arbor, Michigan

Diane Krasner, PhD, RN, CWOCN, CWS, FAAN
Wound Care Consultant and
Adjunct Associate Professor
Johns Hopkins University
School of Nursing
Baltimore, Maryland

Gail B. Ladwig, MSN, RN, CHTP, HNC
Associate Professor of Nursing
Consultant in Guided Imagery
Jackson Community College
Healing Touch Practitioner
Jackson, Michigan

Marcia LaHaie, MSN, RN, OCN
Hematology/Oncology Nurse Coordinator
Veterans Administration Ann Arbor Health Care
    Center
Ann Arbor, Michigan

Margaret Lunney, PhD, RN, CS
Professor of Nursing
The College of Staten Island
City University of New York
Staten Island, New York

Carroll A. Lutz, MA, BSN, RN
Associate Professor Emerita
Consultant in Nutrition
Jackson Community College
Jackson, Michigan

Leslie Lysaght, RN, MS, CS
Family Nurse Practitioner
Adult Asthma Program
Allegiance, LLC
Ann Arbor, Michigan

Mary Markle, MSN, RNC
Certified Family Nurse Practitioner
Center for Family Health
School Nurse
Northeast Elementary School
Jackson, Michigan

Margo McCaffery, MS, RN, FAAN
Consultant in the Nursing Care of Patients with Pain
Los Angeles, California

Vicki E. McClurg, MN, RN
Nurse Manager
Life Choices Pregnancy Clinic
Seattle, Washington

Pamela H. Mitchell, PhD, RN, CNRN, FAAN
Elizabeth S. Soule Distinguished Professor of Nursing
    and Health Promotion
Professor of Biobehavioral Nursing and Health
    Systems
Associate Dean for Research
University of Washington School of Nursing
Seattle, Washington

Chris Pasero, MS, RN
Pain Management Educator and Consultant
Rocklin, California

Linda L. Straight, MA, RN
Director of Education
Trillium Hospital
Albion, Michigan

Terry VandenBosch, MS, RN, CS
Research Specialist
Saint Joseph Mercy Health System
Ann Arbor, Michigan

Virginia R. Wall, RN, MN, IBCLC
Lactation Services Coordinator
University of Washington Medical Center
Seattle, Washington

Linda S. Williams, MSN, RN C, CS
Clinical Nurse Specialist
Jackson Community College
Staff Nurse, Preadmission Testing
W.A. Foote Memorial Hospital
Jackson, Michigan

Consultant in home care—contributor of home care interventions

Elizabeth L. Foster, MS, RN
Home Health Administrative Specialist
University Medical Center
Tucson, Arizona

Consultants in culturally competent nursing care

Debra Martinez, BSW
Youth Specialist
Maxie Training School
Whitmore Lake, Michigan

Marina Martinez-Kratz, RN, MS
Associate Professor of Nursing
Jackson Community College
Jackson, Michigan

Consultants in nursing research utilization—third edition

Ann F. Jacobson, PhD, RN
Assistant Professor
School of Nursing
Kent State University
Kent, Ohio

Elizabeth H. Winslow, PhD, RN, FAAN
Research Consultant
Presbyterian Hospital of Dallas
Dallas, Texas

Brenda J. Wagner, PhD, RN
Licensed Psychologist
Scottish Rite Children's Medical Center
Atlanta, Georgia

The authors would also like to thank the following individuals for their contributions to earlier editions:

Victoria L. Cole-Schonlau, DNSc, MPA, RN
Sandra Cunningham, MS, RN, CCRN, CS
Jane Maria Curtis, MSN, CAN, RN
Gwethalyn B. Edwards, MSN, RN
Pamela M. Emery, BS, RNFA, CNOR, RN
Nancy English, PhD, RN
Mary A. Fuerst-DeWys, BS, RN
J. Keith Hampton, MSN, RN, CS
Mary Henrikson, MN, RNC, ARNP
Kathie D. Hesnan, BSN, RN, CETN
Constance Hollman, MA, EdS
Leslie Kalbach, MN, RN, CETN
Helen Kelley, MSN, RN, CHTP, HNC, NP
Marty J. Martin, MSN, RN
Michelle Masta, RN, BSN

Cathy McClean, RN, BSN
Beverly Pickett, MA, BS, RN, CHTP, HNC
Nancee B. Radtke, MSN, RN
Judith S. Rizzo, MS, RN, CS
Pam B. Schweitzer, MS, RN, CS
Suzanne Skowronski, MSN, RN
Teepa Snow, MS, OTR-L, FAOTA
Martha A. Spies, MSN, RN
Kathy A. Stimac O'Brien, MSN, RN
Catherine Vincent, MSN, RN
Peggy A. Wetsch, RN, MSN, CNA
Fran Wistom, MSN, RN, CSW, CPN
Janet Woodruff, BSN, RN
Kathy Wyngarden, MSN, RN

Preface

Nursing Diagnosis Handbook: A Guide to Planning Care is a convenient reference to help the practicing nurse or nursing student make a nursing diagnosis and write a care plan with ease and confidence. This handbook helps nurses correlate nursing diagnoses with known information about clients on the basis of assessment findings, established medical or psychiatric diagnoses, and the current treatment plan.

Making a nursing diagnosis and planning care are complex processes that involve diagnostic reasoning and critical thinking skills. Nursing students and practicing nurses cannot possibly memorize the more than 1000 defining characteristics, related factors, and risk factors for the 157 diagnoses approved by the North American Nursing Diagnosis Association (NANDA). This book correlates suggested nursing diagnoses with what nurses know about clients and offers a care plan for each nursing diagnosis.

Section I, Nursing Diagnosis, the Nursing Process, and Evidence Based Nursing, explains how the nurse formulates a nursing diagnosis using assessment findings. In Section II, Guide to Nursing Diagnoses, the nurse can look up symptoms and problems and their suggested nursing diagnoses for more than 1200 client symptoms, medical and psychiatric diagnoses, diagnostic procedures, surgical interventions, and clinical states. In Section III, Guide to Planning Care, the nurse can find care plans for all nursing diagnoses suggested in Section II. In this edition, we have included the suggested nursing outcomes from the Nursing Outcomes Classification (NOC) and interventions from the Nursing Interventions Classification (NIC) by the Iowa Intervention Project, as well as a listing of all NOC outcomes labels and NIC intervention labels in appendixes C and D. We are excited about this work and believe it is a significant addition to the nursing process to further define nursing practice.

Nursing Diagnosis Handbook: A Guide to Planning Care Section II includes medical diagnoses and procedures because nurses find them useful for suggesting appropriate nursing diagnoses. For example, under the surgical procedure of **Mastectomy,** the nurse will find the nursing diagnosis **Disturbed Body image** related to (r/t) loss of sexually significant body part. The nurse needs to determine whether this suggested nursing diagnosis relates to the client based on the assessment of the client and the use of nursing diagnostic reasoning skills.

New special features of the fifth edition of Nursing Diagnosis Handbook: A Guide to Planning Care include the following:

- 7 new nursing diagnoses recently approved by NANDA
- The extensive changes made by NANDA in existing nursing diagnoses, including changes in names, definitions, defining characteristics, related factors, and risk factors
- The new Taxonomy II organizing framework from NANDA
- Suggested NOC outcomes for each nursing diagnosis, including the rating scale
- Suggested NIC interventions for each nursing diagnosis

- Information about Evidenced Based Nursing and rationales based as much as possible on evidence
- Culturally appropriate interventions added to care plans as relevant

MERLIN

- An associated MERLIN site that helps the student or nurse write a nursing care plan, including links to web sites for client education

The following features of *Nursing Diagnosis Handbook: A Guide to Planning Care* are included from the fourth edition:

- Suggested nursing diagnoses for more than 1200 clinical entities including signs and symptoms, medical diagnoses, surgeries, maternal-child disorders, mental health disorders, and geriatric disorders
- Rationales for nursing interventions that are based on nursing research and literature
- Nursing references identified for each care plan
- Major clinical practice guidelines of the Agency for Health Care Policy and Research (AHCPR) used in appropriate care plans
- A complete list of NOC outcomes in Appendix C
- A complete list of NIC interventions in Appendix D
- Nursing care plans that contain many holistic interventions
- Care plans for **Pain** written by national experts on pain, Margo McCaffery and Christine Pasero
- Care plans for **Skin integrity** written by national expert Dr. Diane Krasner
- Care plans for **Community** written by national expert Dr. Margaret Lunney
- Care plans for **Incontinence** written by national expert Dr. Mikel Gray
- Care plan for **Decreased Intracranial adaptive capacity** written by national expert Dr. Pamela Mitchell
- Care plan for **Wandering** written by national expert Dr. Donna Algase
- A format that facilitates analyzing signs and symptoms by the process already known by nurses, which is using defining characteristics of nursing diagnoses to make a diagnosis
- Use of NANDA terminology and approved diagnoses

- Inclusion of two additional nursing diagnoses, **Grieving** and **Impaired Comfort**
- An alphabetical format for Section II, Guide to Nursing Diagnoses, and Section III, Guide to Planning Care, which allows rapid access to information
- Nursing care plans for all nursing diagnoses listed in Section II
- Specific geriatric interventions in appropriate plans of care
- Specific client/family teaching interventions in each plan of care
- Information on culturally competent nursing care included where appropriate
- Inclusion of commonly used abbreviations (e.g., AIDS, MI, CHF) and cross-references to the complete term in Section II
- Contributions by leading nurse experts from throughout the United States who together represent all of the major nursing specialties and have extensive experience with nursing diagnoses and the nursing process

We acknowledge the work of NANDA, which is used extensively throughout this text. In some cases the authors and contributors have modified the NANDA work to increase ease of use. The original NANDA work can be found in *NANDA Nursing Diagnoses: Definitions and Classification 2001-2002*. Several contributors are the original authors of the nursing diagnoses established by NANDA. These contributors include the following:

Mary A. Fuerst-DeWys

Disorganized Infant behavior
Readiness for enhanced organized Infant behavior
Risk for disorganized Infant behavior

Dr. Nancy English

Impaired Environmental interpretation syndrome

Dr. Margaret Lunney

Effective Therapeutic regimen management
Ineffective community Coping
Ineffective Therapeutic regimen management
Ineffective community Therapeutic regimen management

Ineffective family Therapeutic regimen
   management
Readiness for enhanced community Coping

Vicki E. McClurg, Mary Henrikson, and Virginia R. Wall

Effective Breastfeeding
Ineffective Breastfeeding
Interrupted Breastfeeding

Dr. Pamela H. Mitchell

Decreased Intracranial adaptive capacity

Kathy Wyngarden

Risk for impaired parent/infant/child
   Attachment

Brenda Emick-Herring

Impaired bed Mobility
Impaired Transfer ability
Impaired Walking
Impaired wheelchair Mobility

We and the consultants and contributors trust that nurses will find this fifth edition of *Nursing Diagnosis Handbook: A Guide to Planning Care* a valuable tool that simplifies the process of diagnosing clients and planning for their care, thus allowing nurses more time to provide care that speeds each client's recovery.

ACKNOWLEDGMENTS
We would like to thank the following people at Mosby: Barbara Nelson Cullen, Executive Editor, who supported us with this fifth edition of the text with intelligence and kindness; Cindi Anderson, who was a continual support and constant source of wise advice; Amy DeSanto, who helped with the contributors; and a special thank you to Kelley Barbarick for production editing of this edition.

We acknowledge with gratitude the nursing students and graduates of Jackson Community College who made us think and shared a very special time with us; the nurses at W.A. Foote Memorial Hospital, Doctors Hospital, The Medical Care Facility in Jackson, Arbor Manor Care Center, Countryside Care Center, and Lifeways, as well as the professionals in Community Nursing Agencies who have helped us educate students and who have served as role models for excellence in nursing care; and finally, each other, for perseverance, patience, and friendship.

Care has been taken to confirm the accuracy of information presented in this book. The authors, editors, and publisher, however, cannot accept any responsibility for consequences resulting from errors or omissions of the information in this book and make no warranty, express or implied, with respect to its contents. The reader should use practices suggested in this book in accordance with agency policies and professional standards.

Web sites were accurate on the dates cited as retrieved. The World Wide Web is an unstable medium, and site addresses may change over time. The World Wide Web resources listed on the MERLIN site must be used cautiously because unsupported information about medical research and products can be rapidly disseminated on the Internet without the traditional process of peer review. This information is no substitute for clinical judgment and common sense.

Medical information available on the World Wide Web comes from many sources. Every effort has been made to ensure the accuracy of the information presented in this text.

Betty J. Ackley

Gail B. Ladwig

How to Use the Nursing Diagnosis Handbook: A Guide to Planning Care

ASSESS
Assess the client using the format provided by the clinical setting. Collect data including client's symptoms, clinical state, and known medical or psychiatric diagnoses.

DIAGNOSIS
Turn to Section II, Guide to Nursing Diagnoses, and locate the client's symptoms, clinical state, medical or psychiatric diagnoses, and anticipated or prescribed diagnostic studies or surgical interventions (listed in alphabetical order). Note suggestions for appropriate nursing diagnoses.

Use Section III, Guide to Planning Care, to evaluate each suggested nursing diagnosis and "related to" etiology statement. Section III is a listing of care plans according to NANDA, arranged alphabetically by diagnostic concept, for each nursing diagnosis referred to in Section II. Determine the appropriateness of each nursing diagnosis by comparing the Defining Characteristics and Risk Factors to the client data collected.

DETERMINE OUTCOMES
Use Section III, Guide to Planning Care, to find appropriate outcomes for the client. Use either the NOC outcomes with the associated rating scales, or Client Outcomes as desired.

PLAN INTERVENTIONS
Use Section III, Guide to Planning Care, to find appropriate interventions for the client. Use either the NIC interventions or Nursing Interventions as found in that section.

GIVE NURSING CARE
The nurse administers nursing care following the plan of care based on the interventions.

EVALUATE NURSING CARE
Evaluate nursing care administered using either the NOC outcomes or Client Outcomes. If the outcomes were not met, and the nursing interventions were not effective, it may be appropriate to reassess the client and determine if the appropriate nursing diagnoses were made.

DOCUMENT
Document all of the previous steps using the format provided in the clinical setting.

Contents

Section I

Nursing Diagnosis, the Nursing Process, and Evidence Based Nursing

The nursing process is an organizing framework for professional nursing practice. Components of the process include performing a nursing assessment, making nursing diagnoses, writing outcome/goal statements, determining appropriate nursing interventions, implementing care, and evaluating the nursing care that has been given. A new concept that has been added to this process is basing nursing practice on evidence or research. This is new concept is called Evidence Based Nursing (EBN). EBN uses the research of basic nursing interventions and incorporates theory, clinical decision-making, knowledge of nursing and the health care milieu, as well as cost effectiveness to forward nursing practice (Melnyk et al, 2000).

This book focuses on an essential part of the nursing process, the nursing diagnosis:

> A nursing diagnosis is a clinical judgment about individual, family, or community responses to actual or potential health problems or life processes. Nursing diagnoses provide the basis for selection of nursing interventions to achieve outcomes for which the nurse is accountable (NANDA, 1999).

The nursing diagnoses that are used throughout this book are taken from NANDA's Taxonomy II (NANDA, 2001). The complete nursing diagnosis list by NANDA's domains, classes, and diagnostic concepts is available in Appendix B.

ASSESSMENT

Before determining an appropriate nursing diagnosis, the nurse must perform a thorough holistic nursing assessment of the client. The nurse may use the assessment format adopted by the facility in which the practice is situated. Several organizational approaches to assessment are available, including Gordon's Functional Health Patterns and head-to-toe and body systems approaches. Regardless of the approach used, the nurse assesses for client symptoms to help formulate a nursing diagnosis.

To elicit as many symptoms as possible, the nurse uses open-ended rather than yes/no questions during the assessment. "Describe what you are feeling." "How long have you been feeling this way?" "When did the symptoms start?" "Describe the symptoms." These types of questions will encourage the client to give more information about his or her situation.

The nurse also obtains information via physical assessment and diagnostic test results. If the client is critically ill or unable to respond verbally, the nurse obtains most of the data from physical assessment and diagnostic test results, and possibly from the client's significant others. The nurse can use data from each of these sources to formulate a nursing diagnosis.

NURSING DIAGNOSIS STATEMENT

A working nursing diagnosis may have two or three parts. The two-part system consists of the nursing diagnosis and the "related to" statement. The three-part system consists of the nursing diagnosis, the "related to" statement, and the defining characteristics.

1. The nursing diagnosis—the label, a concise term or phrase that represents a pattern of related cues
2. "Related to" phrase (r/t) or etiology—related cause or contributor to the problem
3. Defining characteristics phrase—symptoms that the nurse identified in the assessment

Nursing Diagnosis

The first part of both the two-part and three-part system is the actual nursing diagnosis. The nurse makes a nursing diagnosis by categorizing symptoms identified in the assessment as common patterns of response to actual or potential health problems. After completing the assessment, the nurse makes a list of all identified symptoms. Similar symptoms are then put into clusters or groups.

For example, the following symptoms may be identified in the assessment of a client with an admitting medical diagnosis of COPD (chronic obstructive pulmonary disease): dyspnea and dysrhythmia with activity, verbal report of fatigue, and anxiety. Of these signs and symptoms, dyspnea and dysrhythmia with activity and verbal report of fatigue would be clustered or grouped together because they are similar. Using Section II: Guide to Nursing Diagnoses, the nurse can then look up dyspnea or dysrhythmia and find the nursing diagnosis **Activity intolerance** suggested for these symptoms.

To validate that the diagnosis **Activity intolerance** is appropriate for the client, the nurse then turns to Section III: Guide to Planning Care and reads through the definition of the nursing diagnosis **Activity intolerance.** When reading the definition, the nurse should ask if this definition describes what the nurse is observing with the client. If the appropriate nursing diagnosis has been selected, the definition should describe the condition that the nurse has observed.

The nurse then checks to see if the symptoms that were identified in the assessment are contained in the list of defining characteristics. To help verify the diagnoses made on the basis of client signs and symptoms, the nurse may look up the client's medical diagnosis in Section II: Guide to Nursing Diagnoses. For example, one of the nursing diagnoses listed under the medical diagnosis COPD is **Activity intolerance.**

The process of identifying significant symptoms, clustering or grouping them into logical patterns, and then choosing an appropriate nursing diagnosis involves diagnostic reasoning (critical thinking) skills that must be learned in the process of becoming a nurse. Our text serves as a tool to help the nurse in this process. It is here that you might pose a "clinical question" to incorporate the concept of EBN. *What are some of the ways to help a patient who has intolerance to activity? What does the literature say? What has helped this person in the past? How can the outcomes be measured using standards of practice for a patient with intolerance to activity?*

"Related To" Phrase or Etiology

The second part of the nursing diagnosis is the "related to" (r/t) phrase. This phrase states what may be causing or contributing to the nursing diagnosis, commonly referred to as the etiology. Pathophysiological and psychosocial changes, such as developmental age and cultural and environmental situations, may be causative or contributing factors.

Ideally the etiology, or cause, of the nursing diagnosis is something the nurse can treat. When this is the case, the diagnosis is identified as an independent nursing diagnosis. If medical intervention is also necessary, it might be identified as a collaborative diagnosis. A carefully written, individualized r/t statement enables the nurse to plan nursing interventions that will assist the client in accomplishing goals and returning to a state of optimum health.

For each suggested nursing diagnosis, the nurse should refer to the statements listed under the heading "Related Factors (r/t)" in Section III. These r/t factors may or may not be appropriate for the individual client. If they are not appropriate, the nurse should develop and write a r/t statement that is appropriate for the client.

Defining Characteristics Phrase

The defining characteristics phrase is the third part of the three-part diagnostic system. This part consists of the signs and symptoms that the nurse has gathered during the assessment phase. Signs and symptoms are labeled as defining characteristics in Section III: Guide to Planning Care. The phrase "as evidenced by" (aeb) may be used to connect the etiology (r/t) with the defining characteristics. The use of identifying defining characteristics is similar to the process the physician uses when making a medical diagnosis. For example, the physician who observes the following signs and symptoms—diminished inspiratory and expiratory capacity of the lungs, complaints of dyspnea on exertion, difficulty in inhaling and exhaling deeply, and sometimes-chronic cough—may make the medical diagnosis of COPD. The nurse uses the same process to identify the nursing diagnosis of **Activity intolerance.**

Writing a Nursing Diagnosis

1. Choose the label (nursing diagnosis), using the guidelines explained previously. A list of nursing diagnosis labels can be found in Section II of this text.
2. Write a "related to" phrase (etiology). These also can be found in Section II.
3. Write the defining characteristics (signs and symptoms). A list of the signs and symptoms associated with each nursing diagnosis can be found in Section III of this text.

Following are two examples of how to write a nursing diagnosis statement using this text.

A client with the medical diagnosis of COPD

Information from assessment: dyspnea and dysrhythmia with activity, verbal report of fatigue, and anxiety.

- Look up medical diagnosis **COPD** in Section II:

COPD (Chronic Obstructive Pulmonary Disease)
Activity intolerance (nursing diagnosis) definition: Insufficient physiological or psychological energy to endure or complete required or desired daily activities (definition from Section III)

- Look up **Activity intolerance** in Section III.
- Check defining characteristics: dyspnea and dysrhythmia with activity, verbal report of fatigue.
- Check related factors: imbalance between oxygen supply and demand.

With the preceding information, the nurse is able to make the following nursing diagnosis:

Activity intolerance r/t imbalance between oxygen supply-demand aeb fatigue, dysrhythmia, and dyspnea with activity.

Here is a second example of how to use this text.

A client with the symptom of sleep problems

Information from assessment: Client symptom, client statements about sleep: "It takes me about an hour to get to sleep and it is very hard to fall asleep. I feel like I can't do anything because I am so tired. My spouse passed away last month."

- Look up **Sleep** in Section II. Listed under the heading **Sleep Pattern Disorders** in Section II is the following information:

Sleep Pattern Disorders
Disturbed Sleep pattern (nursing diagnosis) definition: Time-limited disruption of sleep (natural, periodic suspension of consciousness) amount and quality (definition from Section III)

- Look up **Disturbed Sleep pattern** in Section III.
- Check defining characteristics for client statements about sleep: "It takes me about an hour to get to sleep and it is very hard to fall asleep; I feel like I can't do anything because I am so tired."
- Check related factors: grief, loss of sleep partner.

With the preceding information, the nurse is able to make the following nursing diagnosis:

> **Disturbed Sleep pattern** r/t grief, loss of sleep partner aeb client's statement: "It takes me about an hour to get to sleep and it is very hard to fall asleep; I feel like I can't do anything because I am so tired."

PLANNING

For most clients the nurse will make more than one nursing diagnosis. Therefore the next step in the nursing process is to determine the priority for care from the list of nursing diagnoses. The nurse can determine the highest priority nursing diagnoses by using Maslow's hierarchy of needs. In this hierarchy, priority is generally given to immediate problems that may be life threatening. For example, **Activity intolerance,** a *physiological need,* may be a higher priority than **Anxiety,** a *love and belonging need.* Refer to Appendix A: Nursing Diagnoses Arranged by Maslow's Hierarchy of Needs, for assistance in prioritizing nursing diagnoses.

Outcomes

After determining the appropriate priority of the nursing diagnoses, the nurse then develops outcomes. Outcomes are conceptualized as variable client states influenced by nursing intervention. Thus client outcomes represent patient states that vary and that can be measured and compared with a baseline over time (Johnson, Maas, Moorhead, 2000). If at all possible, the nurse involves the client in determining appropriate outcomes.

Development of appropriate outcomes can be done one of two ways: using Nursing Outcomes Classification (NOC) outcomes or writing an outcome statement, both of which are included in this book. If the nurse chooses to write an outcome statement, he or she will find suggested outcome statements for each nursing diagnosis in this text that can be used as written or modified as needed to meet the needs of the client.

Section III identifies appropriate NOC outcomes for each nursing diagnosis and includes suggested outcome statements. Appendix C includes a listing of suggested NOC outcome labels.

A nursing-sensitive patient outcome is a measurable patient or family state, behavior, or perception conceptualized as a variable, largely influenced by and sensitive to nursing interventions. To be measured, the outcome requires identification of a series of more specific indicators (Johnson, Maas, Moorehead, 2000). The use of NOC outcomes can be very helpful to the nurse because they contain a 5-point Likert-type rating scale that can be used to evaluate progress toward achieving the outcome. In this text the rating scale is listed, along with some of the more common indicators. As an example, the rating scale for the outcome Sleep is shown in Table I-1.

Because the NOC outcomes are very specific, they enhance the nursing process by helping the nurse to record change after interventions have been performed. The nurse can choose to have clients rate their own progress using the Likert-type rating scale. This involvement can help increase client motivation to progress toward outcomes.

TABLE I-1 NOC Outcome—Sleep

Definition: Extent and pattern of natural periodic suspension of consciousness during which the body is restored.

Sleep	Extremely Compromised 1	Substantially Compromised 2	Moderately Compromised 3	Mildly Compromised 4	Not Compromised 5
Hours of sleep	1	2	3	4	5
Observed hours of sleep	1	2	3	4	5
Sleep pattern	1	2	3	4	5
Sleep quality	1	2	3	4	5
Sleep quantity	1	2	3	4	5
Sleep efficiency (ratio of sleep time/total time trying)	1	2	3	4	5
Uninterrupted sleep	1	2	3	4	5
Sleep routine	1	2	3	4	5
Feelings of rejuvenation after sleep	1	2	3	4	5
Napping appropriate for age	1	2	3	4	5
Wakeful at appropriate times	1	2	3	4	5
EEG IER	1	2	3	4	5
EMG IER	1	2	3	4	5
EOG IER	1	2	3	4	5
Vital signs IER	1	2	3	4	5
Other (specify)	1	2	3	4	5

From Johnson M, Maas M, Moorhead S: *Nursing outcomes classification (NOC)*, ed 2, St Louis, 2000, Mosby.
EEG, Electroencephalogram; *IER*, in expected range; *EMG*, electromyogram; *EOG*, electro-oculogram.

After client outcomes are selected and discussed with a client, the nurse plans nursing care and establishes a means that will help the client to achieve the selected outcomes. The usual means are nursing interventions.

Interventions

Interventions are like road maps directing the best ways to provide nursing care. The more clearly a nurse writes an intervention, the easier it will be to complete the journey and arrive at the destination of successful client outcomes.

To increase the chance that the chosen interventions will be effective, nurses are now using Evidence Based Nursing (EBN), which is a set of interventions or guidelines that have been shown to be effective in helping clients. Development of EBN is

Strategies for Implementing Evidence Based Nursing Practice

1. Pose clinical questions—e.g., what is the best way to provide oral care for clients receiving chemotherapy?
2. Review and critique literature that is relevant from appropriate studies or systematic reviews in the area of the clinical question. Randomized clinical trials are generally the gold standard for producing the best evidence.
3. Develop practice guidelines utilizing the best evidence currently available.
4. Establish measurable outcomes that can be used to determine the effectiveness of the guidelines.
5. Measure the current outcomes based on existing practice so there is a "before" measurement to show that evidenced practice made a difference.
6. Implement the practice guidelines
7. Measure the proposed outcomes after the practice guidelines have been implemented.
8. Evaluate the effectiveness of the practice guidelines and determine where use should be continued, or revisions should be made in the guidelines.
9. Pose the next clinical question

Adapted from Melnyk BM et al: Evidenced-based practice: the past, the present, and recommendations for the millennium, *Pediatr Nurs* 26(1):79, 2000.

an ongoing process that should involve all nurses—determining the best methods of doing nursing interventions and providing nursing care. To implement EBN, nurses must work together and follow the strategies outlined in the box above.

This text includes EBN interventions whenever possible, along with references to research to validate their usefulness. This is an important part of EBN. It looks at standard protocol and determines if the protocol is effective based on gathered evidence.

Nurses can find evidence to guide their practice in many places. The British journal *Evidence Based Nursing* can be helpful, and the *Annual Review of Nursing Research* is very useful. Many nursing journals now publish practice guidelines based on reviews of nursing research that are helpful to the nurse heading in the direction of EBN.

There are multiple helpful web sites on evidence based care:

The Joanna Briggs Institute for Evidence Based Nursing and Midwifery. This site identifies areas in which nurses need summarized evidence on which to base their practice, facilitates systematic reviews of international research, undertakes multi-site randomized controlled clinical trials in areas in which research is needed, and prepares easy-to-read summaries of best practice in the form of Practice Information Sheets based on the results of systematic reviews. Web site: www.joannabriggs.edu.au

The University of York: Centre for Evidence-Based Nursing. This center works with nurse clinicians, researchers, educators, and managers to identify EBN through research and systematic reviews. Web site: www.york.ac.uk/depts/hstd/centres/evidence/ev-intro.htm

The Agency for Healthcare Research and Quality (AHRQ). The AHRQ has developed clinical guidelines for a number of conditions based on research. Also available are Evidence Based Practice Reports on specific topics. Web site: www.ahcpr.gov

The Cochrane Collaboration. This collaboration facilitates the creation, maintenance, and dissemination of more than 1000 reviews of the effects of health care in multiple conditions, working with researchers internationally. The Cochrane Collaboration is now medical in focus. Currently a nursing group is forming. Web site: www.cochrane.org

Netting the Evidence. A ScHARR Introduction to Evidence Based Practice on the Internet. An alphabetical list of over 150 web sites related to evidence based practice. Web site: www.shef.ac.uk/~scharr/ir/netting/

When using EBN it is vitally important that the clients' concerns and individual situations be taken under consideration (web site: www.ahcpr.gov). The nurse must always use critical thinking when applying EBN guidelines to any particular nursing situation. Each client is unique in his/her needs and capabilities. Prescriptive guidelines can be applied inappropriately, resulting in increased problems for the client (Mitchell, 1999). The goal is to provide the best care based on input from researchers, practitioners, and the recipients of care.

Section III supplies choices of interventions for each nursing diagnosis. The interventions are identified as independent (autonomous actions that are initiated by the nurse in response to a nursing diagnosis) or collaborative (actions that the nurse performs in collaboration with other health care professionals and that may require a physician's order and may be in response to both medical and nursing diagnoses). The nurse may choose the interventions appropriate for the client and individualize them accordingly or determine additional interventions. This text also contains several suggested Nursing Interventions Classification (NIC) interventions for each nursing diagnosis to help the reader see how NIC is used along with NOC and nursing diagnoses. The NIC interventions are a comprehensive, standardized classification of treatments that nurses perform. The classification includes both physiological and psychosocial interventions and covers all nursing specialties. A listing of NIC interventions is included in Appendix D. For more information about NIC interventions, the reader is referred to the NIC text, which is identified in the reference list (McCloskey, Bulechek, 2000).

Putting It All Together—Writing the Care Plan

The final planning phase is writing the actual care plan, including prioritized nursing diagnostic statements, outcomes, and interventions. To ensure continuity of care, the plan must be written and shared with all health care personnel caring for the client. This text provides rationales, most of which are research based, to validate that the interventions are appropriate and workable. Because it usually takes at least 1 year from the time a manuscript is accepted for publication for it to appear in print, we have provided many web sites as references for rationales and client/family teaching. In this time of rapid change in health care, we cannot wait a year for access to vital information. Today some material appears only in electronic form (Sparks, Rizzolo, 1998). Web sites for client/family teaching are available at the MERLIN web site.

IMPLEMENTATION

The implementation phase of the nursing process is the actual initiation of the nursing care plan. Client outcomes are achieved by the performance of the nursing interventions. During this phase the nurse continues to assess the client to determine whether the interventions are effective. An important part of this phase is documentation. The nurse should use the facility's tool for documentation and record the results of implementing nursing interventions. Documentation is also necessary for legal reasons because in a legal dispute, *if it wasn't charted, it wasn't done.*

EVALUATION

Although evaluation is listed as the last phase of the nursing process, it is actually an integral part of each phase and something the nurse does continually. When evaluation is performed as the last phase, the nurse refers to the client's outcomes and determines whether they were met. If the outcomes were not met, the nurse begins again with assessment and determines the reason they were not met. Were the outcomes attainable? Was the wrong nursing diagnosis made? Should the interventions be changed? At this point the nurse can look up any new symptoms or conditions that have been identified and adjust the care plan as needed. When using EBN, it is at this point that the nurse determines whether the practice that was followed was effective. Necessary revisions may be made at this time.

Many health care providers are using critical pathways to plan nursing care. The use of nursing diagnoses should be an integral part of any critical pathway to ensure that nursing care needs are being assessed and appropriate nursing interventions are planned and implemented.

The use of nursing diagnoses, NOC outcomes, and NIC interventions ensures that nurses are speaking a common language when taking care of client problems. This system also is easily computerized for simplified documentation and analysis of patterns of care. Nursing diagnosis is the essence of nursing, used to ensure that clients receive excellent, holistic nursing care.

REFERENCES Agency for Healthcare Research and Quality (AHRQ): *Evidence based practice outcomes and effectiveness*, retrieved from the World Wide Web Jan 9, 2001. Web site: www.ahcpr.gov/clinic/outcomix.htm

Elkan R, Blair M, Robinson JJ: Evidenced-based practice and health visiting: the need for theoretical underpinnings for evaluation, *J Adv Nurs* 31(6):1316-1323, 2000.

Johnson M, Maas M, Moorhead S: *Nursing outcomes classification (NOC)*, ed 2, St Louis, 2000, Mosby.

Mathieson A: Factors affecting the use of research in practice, *Prof Nurse* 15(6):406-407, 2000.

McCloskey JC, Bulechek GM: *Nursing interventions classification (NIC)*, ed 3, St Louis, 2000, Mosby.

Melnyk BM: Evidence-based practice: the past, the present, and recommendations for the millennium, *Pediatr Nurs* 26(1):79, 2000.

Mitchell GJ: Evidenced-based practice: critique and alternative view, *Nurs Sci Q* 12(1), 1999.

North American Nursing Diagnosis Association (NANDA): *Nursing diagnosis: definitions & classification, 1999-2000*, Philadelphia, 1999, The Association.

North American Nursing Diagnosis Association (NANDA): *Nursing diagnoses: definitions & classification, 2001-2002*, Philadelphia, 2001, The Association.

Sparks SM, Rizzolo MA: World Wide Web search tools, *Image J Nurs Sch* 30(2):167-171, 1998.

Section II

Guide to Nursing Diagnoses

A

Abdominal Distention

Acute **Pain** r/t retention of air, gastrointestinal secretions

Constipation r/t decreased activity, decreased fluid intake, pathological process

Delayed **Surgical** recovery r/t pain, nausea

Imbalanced **Nutrition**: less than body requirements r/t nausea, vomiting

Nausea r/t irritation to gastrointestinal tract

Abdominal Hysterectomy

See Hysterectomy

Abdominal Pain

Acute **Pain** r/t injury, pathological process

Imbalanced **Nutrition**: less than body requirements r/t unresolved pain

See cause of Abdominal Pain

Abdominal Perineal Resection

Risk for perioperative positioning **Injury** r/t prolonged surgery, lithotomy position

See Abdominal Surgery; Colostomy

Abdominal Surgery

Acute **Pain** r/t surgical procedure

Constipation r/t decreased activity, decreased fluid intake, anesthesia, narcotics

Imbalanced **Nutrition**: less than body requirements r/t high metabolic needs, decreased ability to digest food

Ineffective **Health** maintenance r/t deficit knowledge regarding self-care after surgery

Risk for ineffective **Tissue** perfusion: peripheral r/t immobility, abdominal surgery resulting in stasis of blood flow

Risk for **Infection** r/t invasive procedure

See Surgery

Abdominal Trauma

Deficient **Fluid** volume r/t hemorrhage

Disturbed **Body** image r/t scarring, change in body function, need for temporary colostomy

Ineffective **Breathing** pattern r/t abdominal distention, pain

Risk for **Infection** r/t possible perforation of abdominal structures

Abortion, Induced

Chronic **Sorrow** r/t loss of potential child

Compromised family **Coping** r/t unresolved feelings about decision

Health-seeking behaviors r/t desire to control fertility

Ineffective **Health** maintenance r/t deficit knowledge regarding self-care following abortion

Risk for delayed **Development** r/t unplanned or unwanted pregnancy

Risk for imbalanced **Fluid** volume r/t possible hemorrhage

Risk for **Infection** r/t open uterine blood vessels, dilated cervix

Risk for **Post-trauma** syndrome r/t psychological trauma of abortion

Risk for **Spiritual** distress r/t perceived moral implications of decision

Self-esteem disturbance r/t feelings of guilt

Spiritual distress r/t perceived moral implications of decision

Abortion, Spontaneous

Chronic **Sorrow** r/t loss of potential child

Disabled family **Coping** r/t unresolved feelings about loss

Disturbed **Body** image r/t perceived inability to carry pregnancy, produce child

Fear r/t implications for future pregnancies

Grieving r/t loss of fetus

Ineffective **Coping** r/t personal vulnerability

Ineffective **Health** maintenance r/t deficient knowledge regarding self-care following abortion

Interrupted **Family** processes r/t unmet expectations for pregnancy and childbirth

Pain r/t uterine contractions, surgical intervention

Risk for deficient **Fluid** volume r/t hemorrhage

Risk for **Infection** r/t septic or incomplete abortion of products of conception, open uterine blood vessels, dilated cervix

Risk for **Post-trauma** syndrome r/t psychological trauma of abortion

Risk for **Spiritual** distress r/t loss of fetus

Self-esteem disturbance r/t feelings of failure, guilt

Abruptio Placentae >36 weeks

Anxiety r/t unknown outcome, change in birth plans

Death **Anxiety** r/t unknown outcome, hemorrhage/pain

Fear r/t threat to well-being of self and fetus

Interrupted **Family** process r/t unmet expectations for pregnancy/childbirth

Ineffective **Health** maintenance r/t deficient knowledge regarding self-care with disorder

Impaired **Gas** exchange: placental r/t decreased utero-placental area

Pain r/t irritable uterus, hypertonic uterus

Risk for disproportionate **Growth** r/t uteroplacental insufficiency

Risk for deficient **Fluid** volume r/t hemorrhage

Risk for impaired **Tissue** integrity: maternal r/t possible uterine rupture

Risk for ineffective **Tissue** perfusion: fetal r/t uteroplacental insufficiency

Risk for **Infection** r/t partial separation of placenta

Abscess Formation

Ineffective **Health** maintenance r/t deficient knowledge regarding self-care with abscess

Ineffective **Protection** r/t inadequate nutrition, abnormal blood profile, drug therapy, treatment

Impaired **Tissue** integrity r/t altered circulation, nutritional deficit/excess

Abuse, Child

See Child Abuse

Abuse—Spouse, Parent, or Significant Other

Altered **Family** process: alcoholism r/t inadequate coping skills

Anxiety r/t threat to self-concept, situational crisis of abuse

Caregiver role strain r/t chronic illness, self-care deficits, lack of respite care, extent of caregiving required

Compromised family **Coping** r/t abusive patterns

Defensive **Coping** r/t low self-esteem

Disturbed **Sleep** pattern r/t psychological stress

Impaired verbal **Communication** r/t psychological barriers of fear

Post-trauma response r/t history of abuse

Powerlessness r/t lifestyle of helplessness

Risk for **Post-trauma** syndrome r/t inadequate social support

Risk for self-directed **Violence** r/t history of abuse

Self-esteem disturbance r/t negative family interactions

Accessory Muscle Use (to Breathe)

Ineffective **Breathing** pattern r/t neuromuscular impairment, pain, musculoskeletal impairment, perception/cognitive impairment, anxiety, decreased energy, fatigue

See Asthma; Bronchitis; COPD; Respiratory Infections, Acute Childhood

Accident Prone

Acute **Confusion** r/t altered level of consciousness

Adult **Failure** to thrive r/t fatigue

Ineffective **Coping** r/t personal vulnerability, situational crises

Risk for **Injury** r/t history of accidents

Achalasia

Impaired **Swallowing** r/t neuromuscular impairment

Ineffective **Coping** r/t chronic disease

Pain r/t stasis of food in esophagus

Risk for **Aspiration** r/t nocturnal regurgitation

Acidosis, Metabolic

Decreased **Cardiac** output r/t dysrhythmias from hyperkalemia

Disturbed **Thought** processes r/t central nervous system depression

Imbalanced **Nutrition:** less than body requirements r/t inability to ingest, absorb nutrients

Impaired **Memory** r/t electrolyte imbalance

Pain: headache r/t neuromuscular irritability

Risk for **Injury** r/t disorientation, weakness, stupor

Acidosis, Respiratory

Activity intolerance r/t imbalance between oxygen supply and demand

Disturbed **Thought** processes r/t central nervous system depression

Impaired **Gas** exchange r/t ventilation perfusion imbalance

Impaired **Memory** r/t hypoxia

Risk for decreased **Cardiac** output r/t dysrhythmias associated with respiratory acidosis

Acne Vulgaris

Disturbed **Body** image r/t biophysical changes associated with skin disorder

Impaired **Skin** integrity r/t hormonal changes (adolescence, menstrual cycle)

Ineffective management of **Therapeutic** regimen r/t deficient knowledge (medications, personal care, cause)

Acquired Immunodeficiency Syndrome

See AIDS

Acromegaly

Disturbed **Body** image r/t changes in body function and appearance

Risk for impaired **Mobility** r/t joint pain

Risk for ineffective **Airway** clearance r/t airway obstruction by enlarged tongue

A

Sexual dysfunction r/t changes in hormonal secretions

Activity Intolerance

Activity intolerance r/t bedrest/immobility, generalized weakness, sedentary lifestyle, imbalance between oxygen supply/demand, pain

Activity Intolerance, Potential to Develop

Risk for Activity intolerance r/t deconditioned status, presence of circulatory/respiratory problems, inexperience with activity

Acute Abdomen

Deficient Fluid volume r/t fluids trapped in bowel, inability to drink
Pain r/t pathological process
See cause of Acute Abdomen

Acute Alcohol Intoxication

Disturbed Thought processes r/t central nervous system depression
Dysfunctional Family processes: alcoholism r/t abuse of alcohol
Ineffective Breathing pattern r/t depression of the respiratory center
Risk for Aspiration r/t depressed reflexes with acute vomiting
Risk for Infection r/t impaired immune system from altered nutrition

Acute Back

Anxiety r/t situational crisis, back injury
Constipation r/t decreased activity
Impaired physical Mobility r/t pain
Ineffective Coping r/t situational crisis, back injury
Ineffective Health maintenance r/t deficient knowledge regarding self-care with painful back
Pain r/t back injury

Acute Confusion

Acute Confusion r/t being >60 years of age, dementia, alcohol abuse, drug abuse, delirium

Acute Respiratory Distress Syndrome

See ARDS

Adams-Stokes Syndrome

See Dysrhythmia

Addiction

See Alcoholism; Drug Abuse

Addison's Disease

Activity intolerance r/t weakness, fatigue
Disturbed Body image r/t increased skin pigmentation
Deficient Fluid volume r/t failure of regulatory mechanisms
Imbalanced Nutrition: less than body requirements r/t chronic illness
Ineffective Health maintenance r/t deficient knowledge
Risk for Injury r/t weakness

Adenoidectomy

Impaired Comfort r/t effects of anesthesia, nausea, vomiting
Ineffective Health maintenance r/t deficient knowledge of postoperative care
Ineffective Airway clearance r/t hesitation/reluctance to cough secondary to pain
Pain r/t surgical incision
Risk for Aspiration/suffocation r/t postoperative drainage, impaired swallowing
Risk for deficient Fluid volume r/t decreased intake secondary to painful swallowing, effects of anesthesia
Risk for imbalanced Nutrition: less than body requirements r/t hesitation/reluctance to swallow

Adhesions, Lysis of

See Abdominal Surgery

Adjustment Disorder

Anxiety r/t inability to cope with psychosocial stressor
Disturbed personal Identity r/t psychosocial stressor (specific to individual)
Impaired Adjustment r/t assault to self-esteem
Impaired Social interaction r/t absence of significant others or peers
Situational low Self-esteem r/t change in role function

Adjustment Impairment

Impaired Adjustment r/t disability requiring change in lifestyle, inadequate support systems, impaired cognition, sensory overload, assault to self-esteem, altered locus of control, incomplete grieving

Adolescent, Pregnant

Anxiety r/t situational and maturational crisis, pregnancy
Decisional Conflict: keeping child vs. giving up child vs. abortion r/t lack of experience with decision-

making, interference with decision-making, multiple or divergent sources of information, lack of support system

Delayed **Growth** and development r/t pregnancy

Disturbed **Body** image r/t pregnancy superimposed on developing body

Family **Coping**: disabling r/t highly ambivalent family relationships, chronically unresolved feelings of guilt, anger, despair

Fear r/t labor and delivery

Health-seeking behaviors r/t desire for optimal maternal and fetal outcome

Imbalanced **Nutrition**: less than body requirements r/t lack of knowledge of nutritional needs during pregnancy and as growing adolescent

Impaired **Social** interaction r/t self-concept disturbance

Ineffective **Coping** r/t situational and maturational crisis, personal vulnerability

Ineffective **Denial** r/t fear of consequences of pregnancy becoming known

Ineffective **Health** maintenance r/t deficient knowledge with denial of pregnancy, desire to keep pregnancy secret, fear

Ineffective **Role** performance r/t pregnancy

Interrupted **Family** processes r/t unmet expectations for adolescent, situational crisis

Noncompliance r/t denial of pregnancy

Risk for **Constipation** r/t hormone effect, inadequate fiber in diet

Risk for delayed **Development** r/t unplanned or unwanted pregnancy

Risk for urge urinary **Incontinence** r/t pressure on bladder by growing uterus

Situational low **Self-esteem** r/t feelings of shame and guilt about becoming/being pregnant

Adoption, Giving Child Up for

Chronic **Sorrow** r/t loss of relationship with child

Decisional **Conflict** r/t unclear personal values or beliefs, perceived threat to value system, support system deficit

Grieving r/t loss of child, loss of role of parent

Readiness for enhanced **Spiritual** well-being r/t harmony with self regarding final decision

Risk for **Post-trauma** syndrome r/t psychological trauma of relinquishment of child

Risk for **Spiritual** distress r/t perceived moral implications of decision

Adrenal Crisis

Deficient **Fluid** volume r/t insufficient ability to reabsorb water

Delayed **Surgical** recovery r/t inability to respond to stress

Ineffective **Protection** r/t inability to tolerate stress

See Addison's Disease; Shock

Advance Directives

Anticipatory **Grieving** r/t possible loss of self, significant other

Death **Anxiety** r/t planning for end-of-life health decisions

Decisional **Conflict** r/t unclear personal values or beliefs, perceived threat to value system, support system deficit

Readiness for enhanced **Spiritual** well-being r/t harmonious interconnectedness with self, others, higher power/God

Affective Disorders

Adult **Failure** to thrive r/t altered mood state

Chronic low **Self-esteem** r/t repeated unmet expectations

Chronic **Sorrow** r/t chronic mental illness

Constipation r/t inactivity, decreased fluid intake

Disturbed **Sleep** pattern r/t inactivity

Dysfunctional **Grieving** r/t lack of previous resolution of former grieving response

Fatigue r/t psychological demands

Hopelessness r/t feeling of abandonment, long-term stress

Ineffective **Coping** r/t dysfunctional grieving

Ineffective **Health** maintenance r/t lack of ability to make good judgments regarding ways to obtain help

Risk for **Loneliness** r/t pattern of social isolation, feelings of low self-esteem

Risk for self-directed **Violence** r/t panic state

Self-care deficit: specify r/t depression, cognitive impairment

Sexual dysfunction r/t loss of sexual desire

Social isolation r/t ineffective coping

See specific disorder: Depression; Dysthymic Disorder; Manic Disorder, Bipolar I

Aggressive Behavior

Fear r/t real or imagined threat to own well-being

Risk for **Violence**: self- or other-directed r/t antisocial character, battered woman, catatonic excitement, child abuse, manic excitement, organic brain syndrome, panic states, rage reactions, suicidal behavior, temporal lobe epilepsy, toxic reactions to medication

A

Aging

Adult **Failure** to thrive r/t depression, apathy, fatigue

Anticipatory **Grieving** r/t multiple losses, impending death

Chronic **Sorrow** r/t multiple losses

Death **Anxiety** r/t fear of unknown, loss of self, impact on significant others

Disturbed **Sensory** perception r/t aging process

Family **Coping** potential for growth r/t ability to gratify needs, address adaptive tasks

Functional urinary **Incontinence** r/t impaired vision, impaired cognition, neuromuscular limitations, altered environmental factors

Health-seeking behaviors r/t knowledge about medication, nutrition, exercise, coping strategies

Impaired **Dentition** r/t ineffective oral hygiene; barriers to self-care, professional care; nutritional deficits; dietary habits; selected prescription medications; chronic use of tobacco, coffee, tea, red wine; lack of knowledge regarding dental health

Impaired **Memory** r/t fluid and electrolyte imbalance, neurological disturbances, excessive environmental disturbances, anemia, acute or chronic hypoxia, decreased cardiac output

Ineffective management of **Therapeutic** regimen r/t deficient knowledge: medication, nutrition, exercise, coping strategies

Ineffective **Thermoregulation** r/t aging

Readiness for enhanced community **Coping** r/t providing social support and other resources identified as needed for elderly client

Readiness for enhanced **Spiritual** well-being r/t one's experience of life's meaning, harmony with self, others, higher power/God, environment

Risk for **Caregiver** role strain r/t inability to handle increasing needs of aging person

Risk for **Injury** r/t disturbed sensory perception

Risk for **Loneliness** r/t inadequate support system, role transition, health alterations, depression, fatigue

Sleep deprivation r/t aging-related sleep stage shifts

Agitation

Acute **Confusion** r/t side effects of medication, alcohol abuse or withdrawal, substance abuse or withdrawal, sensory deprivation, sensory overload

Sleep deprivation r/t sundowner's syndrome

Agoraphobia

Anxiety r/t real or perceived threat to physical integrity

Fear r/t leaving home, going out in public places

Ineffective **Coping** r/t inadequate support systems

Impaired **Social** interaction r/t disturbance in self-concept

Social isolation r/t altered thought process

Agranulocytosis

Delayed **Surgical** recovery r/t abnormal blood profile

Ineffective **Health** maintenance r/t deficient knowledge of protective measures to prevent infection

Ineffective **Protection** r/t abnormal blood profile

AICD (Automatic Implanted Cardioverter Defibrillator)

Preoperative

Anxiety r/t surgical procedure

Deficient **Knowledge** r/t purpose and function of AICD

Postoperative

Ineffective **Health** maintenance r/t deficient knowledge regarding self-care, care of internal cardiac defibrillator

Risk for decreased **Cardiac** output r/t possible dysrhythmia

Risk for **Infection** r/t invasive surgical procedure

See Coronary Artery Bypass Grafting

AIDS (Acquired Immunodeficiency Syndrome)

Anticipatory **Grieving**: family/parental r/t potential/impending death of loved one

Altered **Sexuality** pattern r/t possible transmission of disease

Anticipatory **Grieving**: individual r/t loss of physio-psychosocial well-being

Disturbed **Body** image r/t chronic contagious illness, cachexia

Caregiver role strain r/t unpredictable illness course, presence of situation stressors

Chronic **Pain** r/t tissue inflammation and destruction

Chronic **Sorrow** r/t living with long-term chronic illness

Death **Anxiety** r/t fear of premature death

Diarrhea r/t inflammatory bowel changes

Disturbed **Energy** field r/t chronic illness

Fatigue r/t disease process, stress, poor nutritional intake

Fear r/t powerlessness, threat to well-being

Hopelessness r/t deteriorating physical condition

Imbalanced **Nutrition**: less than body requirements r/t decreased ability to eat and absorb nutrients secondary to anorexia, nausea, diarrhea

Ineffective **Health** maintenance r/t deficient knowledge regarding transmission of infection, lack of exposure to information, misinterpretation of information

Ineffective **Protection** r/t risk for infection secondary to inadequate immune system

Interrupted **Family** processes r/t distress about diagnosis of human immunodeficiency virus (HIV) infection

Risk for deficient **Fluid** volume r/t diarrhea, vomiting, fever, bleeding

Risk for **Infection** r/t inadequate immune system

Risk for **Loneliness** r/t social isolation

Risk for disturbed **Thought** processes r/t infection in brain

Risk for impaired **Oral** mucous membranes r/t immunological deficit

Risk for impaired **Skin** integrity r/t immunological deficit, diarrhea

Risk for **Spiritual** distress r/t physical illness

Situational low **Self-esteem** r/t crisis of chronic contagious illness

Social isolation r/t self-concept disturbance, therapeutic isolation

Spiritual distress r/t challenged beliefs or moral system

See AIDS in Child; Cancer; Pneumonia

AIDS Dementia

Impaired **Environmental** interpretation syndrome r/t viral invasion of nervous system

See Dementia

AIDS in Child

Impaired **Parenting** r/t congenital acquisition of infection secondary to intravenous (IV) drug use, multiple sexual partners, history of contaminated blood transfusion

Risk for delayed **Development** r/t chronic illness

Risk for disproportionate **Growth** r/t chronic illness

See AIDS; Child with Chronic Condition; Hospitalized Child; Terminally Ill Child

Airway Obstruction/Secretions

Ineffective **Airway** clearance r/t decreased energy; fatigue; tracheobronchial infection, obstruction, secretions; perceptual/cognitive impairment; trauma; decreased force of cough because of aging

Alcohol Withdrawal

Acute **Confusion** r/t effects of alcohol withdrawal

Anxiety r/t situational crisis, withdrawal

Chronic low **Self-esteem** r/t repeated unmet expectations

Disturbed **Sensory** perception: visual, auditory, kinesthetic, tactile, olfactory r/t neurochemical imbalance in brain

Disturbed **Sleep** pattern r/t effect of depressants, alcohol withdrawal, anxiety

Disturbed **Thought** processes r/t potential delirium tremors

Dysfunctional **Family** processes: alcoholism r/t abuse of alcohol

Imbalanced **Nutrition:** less than body requirements r/t poor dietary habits

Ineffective **Coping** r/t personal vulnerability

Ineffective **Health** maintenance r/t deficient knowledge regarding chronic illness or effects of alcohol consumption

Risk for deficient **Fluid** volume r/t excessive diaphoresis, agitation, decreased fluid intake

Risk for **Violence** r/t substance withdrawal

Alcoholism

Acute **Confusion** r/t alcohol abuse

Anxiety r/t loss of control

Compromised/dysfunctional family **Coping** r/t codependency issues

Coping, defensive r/t alcoholism

Denial, ineffective r/t refusal to deny alcoholism

Disturbed **Sleep** pattern r/t irritability, nightmares, tremors

Imbalanced **Nutrition:** less than body requirements r/t anorexia

Impaired adjustment r/t lack of motivation to change behaviors

Impaired **Environmental** interpretation syndrome r/t neurological effects of chronic alcohol intake

Impaired **Home** maintenance r/t memory deficits, fatigue

Impaired **Memory** r/t alcohol abuse

Ineffective **Coping** r/t use of alcohol to cope with life events

Ineffective **Protection** r/t malnutrition, sleep deprivation

Interrupted **Family** process: alcoholism r/t alcohol abuse

Powerlessness r/t alcohol addiction

Risk for **Injury** r/t alteration in sensory/perceptual function

Risk for **Loneliness** r/t unacceptable social behavior

Risk for **Violence** r/t reactions to substances used, impulsive behavior, disorientation, impaired judgment

Self-esteem disturbance r/t failure at life events

Social isolation r/t unacceptable social behavior, values

A

Alcoholism, Altered Family Process

Altered **Family** process, alcoholism r/t abuse of alcohol, genetic predisposition, lack of problem-solving skills, inadequate coping skills, family history of alcoholism, resistance to treatment, biochemical influences, addictive personality

Alkalosis

See Metabolic Alkalosis

Allergies

Ineffective **Health** maintenance r/t deficient knowledge regarding allergies

Latex **Allergy** r/t hypersensitivity to natural rubber latex

Risk for latex **Allergy** r/t repeated exposure to products containing latex

Alopecia

Disturbed **Body** image r/t loss of hair, change in appearance

Altered Mental Status

See Acute Confusion; Chronic Confusion; Impaired Memory

Alzheimer Type Dementia

Adult **Failure** to thrive r/t difficulty in reasoning, judgment, memory, concentration

Disturbed **Thought** processes r/t chronic organic disorder

Caregiver role strain r/t duration and extent of caregiving required

Chronic **Confusion** r/t Alzheimer's disease

Compromised family **Coping** r/t interrupted family processes

Disturbed **Sleep** pattern r/t neurological impairment, daytime naps

Fear r/t loss of self

Hopelessness r/t deteriorating condition

Impaired **Environmental** interpretation syndrome r/t Alzheimer's disease

Impaired **Home** maintenance r/t impaired cognitive function, inadequate support systems

Impaired **Memory** r/t neurological disturbance

Impaired physical **Mobility** r/t severe neurological dysfunction

Ineffective **Health** maintenance r/t deficient knowledge of caregiver regarding appropriate care

Powerlessness r/t deteriorating condition

Risk for **Injury** r/t confusion

Risk for **Loneliness** r/t potential social isolation

Risk for other-directed **Violence** r/t frustration, fear, anger

Self-care deficit: specify r/t psychological-physiological impairment

Social isolation r/t fear of disclosure of memory loss

See Dementia

Amenorrhea

Imbalanced **Nutrition**: less than body requirements r/t inadequate food intake

Risk for **Sexual** dysfunction r/t altered body function

See Sexuality, Adolescent

Amnesia

Acute **Confusion** r/t alcohol abuse, delirium, dementia, drug abuse

Altered **Family** process: alcoholism r/t alcohol abuse, inadequate coping skills

Impaired **Memory** r/t excessive environmental disturbance, neurological disturbance

Post-trauma response r/t history of abuse, catastrophic illness, disaster, accident

Amniocentesis

Anxiety r/t threat to self and fetus, unknown future

Decisional **Conflict** r/t choice of treatment pending results of test

Risk for **Infection** r/t invasive procedure

Amnionitis

See Chorioamnionitis

Amniotic Membrane Rupture

See Premature Rupture of Membranes

Amputation

Chronic **Sorrow** r/t grief associated with loss of body part

Disturbed **Body** image r/t negative effects of amputation, response from others

Grieving r/t loss of body part, future lifestyle changes

Impaired physical **Mobility** r/t musculoskeletal impairment, limited movement

Impaired **Skin** integrity r/t poor healing, prosthesis rubbing

Ineffective **Health** maintenance r/t deficient knowledge of care of stump, rehabilitation

Ineffective **Tissue** perfusion: peripheral r/t impaired arterial circulation

Pain r/t surgery, phantom limb sensation

Risk for deficient **Fluid** volume: hemorrhage r/t vulnerable surgical site

Amyotrophic Lateral Sclerosis

Chronic **Sorrow** r/t chronic illness

Death **Anxiety** r/t impending progressive loss of function leading to death

Decisional **Conflict:** ventilator therapy r/t unclear personal values or beliefs, lack of relevant information

Impaired spontaneous **Ventilation** r/t weakness of muscles of respiration

Impaired **Swallowing** r/t weakness of muscles involved in swallowing

Impaired verbal **Communication** r/t weakness of muscles of speech, deficient knowledge of ways to compensate and alternative communication devices

Ineffective **Breathing** pattern r/t compromised muscles of respiration

Risk for **Aspiration** r/t impaired swallowing

Risk for **Spiritual** distress r/t chronic debilitating condition

See Neurological Disorders

Anal Fistula

See Hemorrhoidectomy

Anaphylactic Shock

Impaired spontaneous **Ventilation** r/t acute airway obstruction

Ineffective **Airway** clearance r/t laryngeal edema, bronchospasm

Latex **Allergy** response r/t no immune mechanism response

See Shock

Anasarca

Excess **Fluid** volume r/t excessive fluid intake, cardiac/renal dysfunction, loss of plasma proteins

Risk for impaired **Skin** integrity r/t impaired circulation to skin

See cause of Anasarca

Anemia

Anxiety r/t cause of disease

Delayed **Surgical** recovery r/t decreased oxygen supply to body, increased cardiac workload

Fatigue r/t decreased oxygen supply to the body, increased cardiac workload

Impaired **Memory** r/t anemia

Ineffective **Health** maintenance r/t deficient knowledge regarding nutritional and medical treatment of anemia

Ineffective **Protection** r/t bleeding disorder

Risk for **Injury** r/t alteration in peripheral sensory perception

Anemia in Pregnancy

Anxiety r/t concerns about health of self and fetus

Fatigue r/t decreased oxygen supply to the body, increased cardiac workload

Ineffective **Health** maintenance r/t deficient knowledge regarding nutrition in pregnancy

Risk for delayed **Development** r/t reduction in the oxygen-carrying capacity of blood

Risk for **Infection** r/t reduction in oxygen-carrying capacity of blood

Anemia, Sickle Cell

See Anemia; Sickle Cell Anemia/Crisis

Anencephaly

See Neurotube Defects

Aneurysm, Abdominal Surgery

Risk for deficient **Fluid** volume: hemorrhage r/t potential abnormal blood loss

Risk for ineffective **Tissue** perfusion: peripheral r/t impaired arterial circulation

Risk for **Infection** r/t invasive procedure

See Abdominal Surgery

Aneurysm, Cerebral

See Craniectomy/Craniotomy; Subarachnoid Hemorrhage (if aneurysm has ruptured)

Anger

Anxiety r/t situational crisis

Defensive **Coping** r/t inability to acknowledge responsibility for actions and results of actions

Fear r/t environmental stressor, hospitalization

Grieving r/t significant loss

Impaired **adjustment** r/t assault to self-esteem, disability requiring change in lifestyle, inadequate support system

Powerlessness r/t health care environment

Risk for **Post-trauma** syndrome r/t inadequate social support

Risk for **Violence** r/t history of violence, rage reaction

Angina Pectoris

Activity intolerance r/t acute pain, dysrhythmias

Altered **Sexuality** pattern r/t disease process, medications, loss of libido

Anxiety r/t situational crisis

Decreased **Cardiac** output r/t myocardial ischemia, medication effect, dysrhythmia

Grieving r/t pain, lifestyle changes

A

Ineffective **Coping** r/t personal vulnerability to situational crisis of new diagnosis, deteriorating health

Ineffective **Denial** r/t deficient knowledge (delays seeking help when symptoms occur)

Ineffective **Health** maintenance r/t deficient knowledge of care of angina condition

Pain r/t myocardial ischemia

Angiocardiography (Cardiac Catheterization)

See Cardiac Catheterization

Angioplasty, Coronary Balloon

Fear r/t possible outcome of interventional procedure

Ineffective **Health** maintenance r/t deficient knowledge regarding care following procedures, measures to limit coronary artery disease

Risk for ineffective **Tissue** perfusion: peripheral/cardiopulmonary r/t vasospasm, hematoma formation

Risk for decreased **Cardiac** output r/t ventricular ischemia, dysrhythmias

Risk for deficient **Fluid** volume r/t possible damage to coronary artery, hematoma formation, hemorrhage

Anomaly, Fetal/Newborn (Parent Dealing with)

Anxiety r/t threat to role functioning, situational crisis

Chronic **Sorrow** r/t loss of ideal child

Decisional **Conflict**: interventions for fetus/newborn r/t lack of relevant information, spiritual distress, threat to value system

Fear r/t real or imagined threat to baby, implications for future pregnancies, powerlessness

Hopelessness r/t long-term stress, deteriorating physical condition of child, lost spiritual belief

Deficient **Knowledge** r/t limited exposure to situation

Disabled family **Coping** r/t chronically unresolved feelings about loss of perfect baby

Ineffective **Coping** r/t personal vulnerability in situational crisis

Impaired **Parenting** r/t interruption of bonding process

Interrupted **Family** processes r/t unmet expectations for perfect baby, lack of adequate support systems

Parental role **Conflict** r/t separation from newborn, intimidation with invasive or restrictive modalities, specialized care center policies

Powerlessness r/t complication threatening fetus/newborn

Risk for dysfunctional **Grieving** r/t loss of perfect child

Risk for impaired **Parent**/infant/child attachment r/t ill infant who is unable to effectively initiate parental contact as result of altered behavioral organization

Risk for impaired **Parenting** r/t interruption of bonding process; unrealistic expectations for self, infant, or partner; perceived threat to own emotional survival; severe stress; lack of knowledge

Risk for **Spiritual** distress r/t lack of normal child to raise and carry on family name

Self-esteem disturbance r/t perceived inability to produce a perfect child

Spiritual distress r/t test of spiritual beliefs

Anorectal Abscess

Disturbed **Body** image r/t odor and drainage from rectal area

Pain r/t inflammation of perirectal area

Risk for **Constipation** r/t fear of painful elimination

Anorexia

Deficient **Fluid** volume r/t inability to drink

Delayed **Surgical** recovery r/t inadequate nutritional intake

Imbalanced **Nutrition**: less than body requirements r/t loss of appetite, nausea, vomiting

Anorexia Nervosa

Activity intolerance r/t fatigue, weakness

Altered patterns of **Sexuality** r/t loss of libido from malnutrition

Chronic low **Self-esteem** r/t repeated unmet expectations

Constipation r/t lack of adequate food, fluid intake

Disabled family **Coping** r/t highly ambivalent family relationships

Disturbed **Thought** processes r/t anorexia

Disturbed **Body** image r/t misconception of actual body appearance

Defensive **Coping** r/t psychological impairment, eating disorder

Diarrhea r/t laxative abuse

Imbalanced **Nutrition**: less than body requirements r/t inadequate food intake

Ineffective **Denial** r/t fear of consequences of therapy, possible weight gain

Ineffective family **Therapeutic** regimen management r/t family conflict, excessive demands on family associated with complexity of condition and treatment

Interrupted **Family** processes r/t situational crisis

Risk for **Infection** r/t malnutrition resulting in depressed immune system

Risk for **Spiritual** distress r/t low self-esteem

See Maturational Issues, Adolescent

Anosmia—Loss of Smell

Imbalanced **Nutrition**: less than body requirements r/t loss of appetite associated with loss of smell

Disturbed **Sensory** perception: olfactory r/t altered sensory reception, transmission, integration

Antepartum Period

See Pregnancy—Normal; Prenatal Care—Normal

Anterior Repair—Anterior Colporrhaphy

Risk for perioperative positioning **Injury**

Risk for urge urinary **Incontinence** r/t trauma to bladder

See Vaginal Hysterectomy

Anticoagulant Therapy

Anxiety r/t situational crisis

Ineffective **Health** maintenance r/t deficient knowledge regarding precautions to take with anticoagulant therapy

Ineffective **Protection** r/t altered clotting function from anticoagulant

Risk for deficient **Fluid** volume: hemorrhage r/t altered clotting mechanism

Antisocial Personality Disorder

Defensive **Coping** r/t excessive use of projection

Disturbed **Thought** processes r/t internal turmoil and conflict (intrusive thinking)

Hopelessness r/t abandonment

Impaired **Social** interaction r/t sociocultural conflict, chemical dependence, inability to form relationships

Ineffective **Coping** r/t frequently violating the norms and rules of society

Ineffective family **Therapeutic** regimen management r/t excessive demands on family

Risk for **Loneliness** r/t inability to interact appropriately with others

Risk for impaired **Parenting** r/t inability to function as parent or guardian, emotional instability

Risk for **Self-mutilation** r/t self-hatred, depersonalization

Risk for other-directed **Violence** r/t history of violence

Spiritual distress r/t separation from religious/cultural ties

Anuria

See Renal Failure

Anxiety

Anxiety r/t exposure to toxins, threat to or change in role status, unconscious conflict about essential goals and vaules of life, familial association/heredity, unmet needs, interpersonal transmission/contagion, situational/maturational crisis, threat of death, threat to or change in health status, threat to or change in interaction patterns, threat to or change in role function, threat to self-concept, unconscious conflict regarding essential values/goals of life, threat to or change in environment, stress, threat to or change in economic status, substance abuse

Anxiety Disorder

Anxiety r/t unmet security and safety needs

Death **Anxiety** r/t fears of unknown, powerlessness

Decisional **Conflict** r/t low self-esteem, fear of making a mistake

Defensive **Coping** r/t overwhelming feelings of dread

Disabled family **Coping** r/t ritualistic behavior, actions

Disturbed **Energy** field r/t hopelessness, helplessness, fear

Disturbed **Sleep** pattern r/t psychological impairment, emotional instability

Disturbed **Thought** processes r/t anxiety

Ineffective **Coping** r/t inability to express feelings appropriately

Ineffective **Denial** r/t overwhelming feelings of hopelessness, fear, threat to self

Powerlessness r/t lifestyle of helplessness

Risk for **Spiritual** distress r/t psychological distress

Self-care deficit r/t ritualistic behavior, activities

Sleep deprivation r/t prolonged psychological discomfort

Aortic Aneurysm Repair (Abdominal Surgery)

See Abdominal Surgery; Aneurysm, Abdominal Surgery

Aortic Valvular Stenosis

See Congenital Heart Disease/Cardiac Anomalies

Aphasia

Anxiety r/t situational crisis of aphasia

Impaired verbal **Communication** r/t decrease in circulation to brain

Ineffective **Coping** r/t loss of speech

Ineffective **Health** maintenance r/t deficient knowledge regarding information on aphasia and alternative communication techniques

Aplastic Anemia

Activity intolerance r/t imbalance between oxygen supply-demand

Anxiety r/t deficient knowledge of disease process and treatment

Delayed **Surgical** recovery r/t risk for infection

Risk for **Infection** r/t inadequate immune function

Apnea in Infancy

See Premature Infant; SIDS

Apneustic Respirations

Impaired **Breathing** pattern r/t perception/cognitive impairment, neurological impairment

See cause of Apneustic Respirations

Appendectomy

Deficient **Fluid** volume r/t fluid restriction, hypermetabolic state, nausea, vomiting

Ineffective **Health** maintenance r/t deficient knowledge regarding self-care following appendectomy

Pain r/t surgical incision

Risk for **Infection** r/t perforation/rupture of appendix, surgical incision, peritonitis

See Hospitalized Child; Surgery

Appendicitis

Deficient **Fluid** volume r/t anorexia, nausea, vomiting

Delayed **Surgical** recovery r/t risk for infection

Pain r/t inflammation

Risk for **Infection** r/t possible perforation of appendix

Apprehension

Anxiety r/t threat to self-concept, threat to health status, situational crisis

Death **Anxiety** r/t apprehension over loss of self, consequences to significant others

ARDS (Acute Respiratory Distress Syndrome)

Death **Anxiety** r/t seriousness of physical disease

Delayed **Surgical** recovery r/t complications associated with respiratory difficulty

Impaired **Gas** exchange r/t damage to alveolar-capillary membrane, change in lung compliance

Impaired spontaneous **Ventilation** r/t damage to alveolar capillary membrane

Ineffective **Airway** clearance r/t excessive tracheobronchial secretions

See Child with Chronic Condition; Ventilator Client

Arrhythmia

See Dysrhythmia

Arterial Insufficiency

Delayed **Surgical** recovery r/t ineffective tissue perfusion

Ineffective **Tissue** perfusion: peripheral r/t interruption of arterial flow

Arthritis

Activity intolerance r/t chronic pain, fatigue, weakness

Chronic **Pain** r/t progression of joint deterioration

Chronic **Sorrow** r/t presence of chronic condition

Disturbed **Body** image r/t ineffective coping with joint abnormalities

Impaired physical **Mobility** r/t musculoskeletal impairment

Ineffective **Health** maintenance r/t deficient knowledge regarding care of arthritis

Risk for **Spiritual** distress r/t presence of chronic condition

Self-care deficit: specify r/t pain, musculoskeletal impairment

See Rheumatoid Arthritis, Juvenile

Arthrocentesis

Pain r/t invasive procedure

Arthroplasty—Total Hip Replacement

Constipation r/t immobility

Impaired physical **Mobility** r/t decreased muscle strength, surgery

Impaired **Walking** r/t decreased muscle strength, surgery

Pain r/t tissue trauma associated with surgery

Risk for **Infection** r/t invasive surgery, foreign object in body, anesthesia, immobility with stasis of respiratory secretions

Risk for **Injury** r/t interruption of arterial blood flow, dislocation of prosthesis

Risk for perioperative positioning **Injury** r/t immobilization, muscle weakness

Risk for **Peripheral** neurovascular dysfunction r/t orthopedic surgery

See Surgery

Arthroscopy

Ineffective **Health** maintenance r/t deficient knowledge regarding procedure, postoperative restrictions

Ascites

Chronic **Pain** r/t altered body function

Delayed **Surgical** recovery r/t ineffective breathing pattern

Imbalanced **Nutrition:** less than body requirements r/t loss of appetite

Ineffective **Breathing** pattern r/t increased abdominal girth

Ineffective **Health** maintenance r/t deficient knowledge of care with condition of ascites

See cause of Ascites; Cancer; Cirrhosis

Asphyxia, Birth

Altered (cerebral) **Tissue** perfusion r/t poor placental perfusion or cord compression resulting in lack of oxygen to brain

Fear (parental) r/t concern over safety of infant

Impaired **Gas** exchange r/t poor placental perfusion, lack of initiation of breathing by newborn

Impaired spontaneous **Ventilation** r/t brain injury

Ineffective **Breathing** pattern r/t depression of breathing reflex secondary to anoxia

Risk for delayed **Development** r/t lack of oxygen to brain

Risk for disproportionate **Growth** r/t lack of oxygen to brain

Risk for **Injury** r/t lack of oxygen to brain

Risk for **Post-trauma** syndrome: parental r/t psychological trauma of sudden potential for loss of newborn

Aspiration, Danger of

Risk for **Aspiration** r/t reduced level of consciousness; depressed cough or gag reflexes; presence of tracheostomy or endotracheal tube; incomplete lower esophageal sphincter; presence of gastrointestinal tubes or tube feedings; medication administration; situations hindering elevation of upper body; increased intragastric pressure; increased gastric residual; decreased gastrointestinal motility; delayed gastric emptying; impaired swallowing; facial, oral, or neck surgery or trauma; wired jaws

Assault Victim

Post-trauma syndrome r/t assault

Rape-trauma syndrome r/t rape

Risk for **Post-trauma** syndrome r/t perception of event, inadequate social support, nonsupportive environment, diminished ego strength, duration of event

Risk for **Spiritual** distress r/t physical, psychological stress

Assaultive Client

Disturbed **Thought** process r/t use of hallucinogenic substance, psychological disorder

Ineffective **Coping** r/t lack of control of impulsive actions

Risk for **Injury** r/t confused thought process, impaired judgment

Risk for **Violence** r/t paranoid ideation

Asthma

Activity intolerance r/t fatigue, energy shift to meet muscle needs for breathing to overcome airway obstruction

Anxiety r/t inability to breathe effectively, fear of suffocation

Disturbed **Body** image r/t decreased participation in physical activities

Impaired **Home** maintenance r/t deficient knowledge regarding control of environmental triggers

Ineffective **Airway** clearance r/t tracheobronchial narrowing, excessive secretions

Ineffective **Breathing** pattern r/t anxiety

Ineffective **Coping** r/t personal vulnerability to situational crisis

Ineffective **Health** maintenance r/t deficient knowledge regarding physical triggers, medications, treatment of early warning signs

Sleep deprivation r/t ineffective breathing pattern

See Child with Chronic Condition; Hospitalized Child

Ataxia

Anxiety r/t change in health status

Disturbed **Body** image r/t staggering gait

Impaired physical **Mobility** r/t neuromuscular impairment

Risk for **Injury** r/t gait alteration

Atelectasis

Impaired **Gas** exchange r/t decreased alveolar-capillary surface

Ineffective **Breathing** pattern r/t loss of functional lung tissue, depression of respiratory function or hypoventilation because of pain

Athlete's Foot

Impaired **Skin** integrity r/t effects of fungal agent

Ineffective **Health** maintenance r/t deficient knowledge regarding treatment and prevention of athlete's foot

See Itching

Atrial Fibrillation

See Dysrhythmia

Atrial Septal Defect

See Congenital Heart Disease/Cardiac Anomalies

Attention Deficit Disorder

B

Disabled family **Coping** r/t significant person with chronically unexpressed feelings of guilt, anxiety, hostility, despair, etc.

Impaired **Adjustment** r/t intense emotional state

Risk for delayed **Development** r/t behavior disorders

Risk for impaired **Parenting** r/t lack of knowledge of factors contributing to child's behavior

Risk for **Loneliness** r/t social isolation

Risk for **Spiritual** distress r/t poor relationships

Self-esteem disturbance r/t difficulty in participating in expected activities

Social isolation r/t unacceptable social behavior

Autism

Compromised family **Coping** r/t parental guilt over etiology of disease, inability to accept or adapt to child's condition, inability to help child and other family members seek treatment

Delayed **Growth** and development r/t inability to develop relations with other human beings, inability to identify own body as separate from those of other people, inability to integrate concept of self

Disturbed personal **Identity** r/t inability to distinguish between self and environment, inability to identify own body as separate from those of other people, inability to integrate concept of self

Disturbed **Thought** processes r/t inability to perceive self or others, cognitive dissonance, perceptual dysfunction

Impaired **Social** interaction r/t communication barriers, inability to relate to others

Impaired verbal **Communication** r/t speech and language delays

Risk for delayed **Development** r/t autism

Risk for **Loneliness** r/t health alterations, cognition

Risk for **Self-mutilation** r/t autistic state

Risk for **Violence**: self- and other-directed r/t frequent destructive rages toward self or others secondary to extreme response to changes in routine, fear of harmless things

See Child with Chronic Condition; Mental Retardation

Automatic Implanted Cardioverter Defibrillator

See AICD

Autonomic Dysreflexia

Autonomic dysreflexia r/t bladder distention, bowel distention, noxious stimuli

Risk for **Autonomic** dysreflexia r/t bladder distention, bowel distention, noxious stimuli

Autonomic Hyperreflexia

See Autonomic Dysreflexia

B

Back Pain

Anxiety r/t situational crisis, back injury

Disturbed **Energy** field r/t chronic pain

Impaired physical **Mobility** r/t pain

Ineffective **Coping** r/t situational crisis, back injury

Ineffective **Health** maintenance r/t deficient knowledge regarding prevention of further injury, proper body mechanics

Pain r/t back injury

Risk for **Constipation** r/t decreased activity

Risk for **Disuse** syndrome r/t severe pain

Bacteremia

Ineffective **Protection** r/t compromised immune system

See Infection; Infection, Potential for

Barrel Chest

See Aging (if appropriate); COPD

Bathing/Hygiene Problems

Bathing/hygiene **Self-care** deficit r/t intolerance to activity, decreased strength and endurance, pain, discomfort, perceptual or cognitive impairment, neuromuscular impairment, musculoskeletal impairment, depression, severe anxiety

Impaired bed **Mobility** r/t chronic physically limiting condition

Battered Child Syndrome

Anxiety/Fear r/t threat of punishment for perceived wrongdoing

Chronic low **Self-esteem** r/t lack of positive feedback, excessive negative feedback

Chronic **Sorrow** r/t situational crises

Deficient **Diversional** activity r/t diminished/absent environmental or personal stimuli

Delayed **Growth** and development: regression vs. delayed r/t diminished/absent environmental stimuli, inadequate caretaking, inconsistent responsiveness by caretaker

Disturbed **Sleep** pattern r/t hypervigilance, anxiety

Dysfunctional **Family** process: alcoholism r/t inadequate coping skills

Imbalanced **Nutrition**: less than body requirements r/t inadequate caretaking

Impaired **Skin** integrity r/t altered nutritional state, physical abuse

Pain r/t physical injuries

Post-trauma syndrome r/t physical abuse, incest, rape, molestation

Risk for delayed **Development** r/t shaken baby, abuse

Risk for disproportionate **Growth** r/t abuse

Risk for **Poisoning** r/t inadequate safeguards, lack of proper safety precautions, accessibility of illicit substances secondary to impaired home maintenance

Risk for **Post-trauma** syndrome r/t physical abuse, incest, rape, molestation

Risk for **Self-mutilation** r/t feelings of rejection, dysfunctional family

Risk for **Suffocation/aspiration** r/t propped bottle, unattended child

Risk for **Trauma** r/t inadequate precautions, cognitive or emotional difficulties

Sleep deprivation r/t prolonged psychological discomfort

Social isolation: family imposed r/t fear of disclosure of family dysfunction and abuse

Battered Person

See Abuse—Spouse, Parent, or Significant Other

Bed Mobility, Impaired

Impaired bed **Mobility** r/t intolerance to activity, decreased strength and endurance, pain or discomfort, perceptual or cognitive impairment, neuromuscular impairment, musculoskeletal impairment, depression, severe anxiety

Bedbugs, Infestation

Impaired **Home** maintenance r/t deficient knowledge regarding prevention of bedbug infestation

Impaired **Skin** integrity r/t bites of bedbugs

See Itching

Bedrest, Prolonged

Deficient **Diversional** activity r/t prolonged bedrest

Disuse syndrome r/t prolonged immobility

Impaired bed **Mobility** r/t neuromuscular impairment

Risk for **Loneliness** r/t prolonged bedrest

Social isolation r/t prolonged bedrest

Bedsores

See Pressure Ulcer

Bedwetting

See Enuresis

Bell's Palsy

Disturbed **Body** image r/t loss of motor control on one side of face

Imbalanced **Nutrition**: less than body requirements r/t difficulty with chewing

Pain r/t inflammation of facial nerve

Risk for **Injury** (eye) r/t dysfunction of facial nerve

Benign Prostatic Hypertrophy

See BPH; Prostatic Hypertrophy

Bereavement

Chronic Sorrow r/t death of loved one, chronic illness, disability

Grieving r/t loss of significant person

Biliary Atresia

Anxiety/Fear r/t surgical intervention, possible liver transplantation

Imbalanced **Nutrition**: less than body requirements r/t decreased absorption of fat and fat-soluble vitamins, poor feeding

Impaired **Comfort** r/t pruritus, nausea

Risk for impaired **Skin** integrity r/t pruritus

Risk for ineffective **Breathing** pattern r/t enlarged liver, development of ascites

Risk for **Injury**: bleeding r/t vitamin K deficiency, altered clotting mechanisms

See Child with Chronic Condition; Cirrhosis (as complication); Hospitalized Child; Terminally Ill Child

Biliary Calculus

See Cholelithiasis

Biliary Obstruction

See Jaundice

Biopsy

Fear r/t outcome of biopsy

Ineffective **Health** maintenance r/t deficient knowledge regarding biopsy site, further needed health care

Bipolar Disorder I (Most Recent Episode, Depressed or Manic)

Chronic low **Self-esteem** r/t repeated unmet expectations

Disturbed **Energy** field r/t disharmony of mind, body, spirit

Dysfunctional **Grieving** r/t lack of previous resolution of former grieving response

Fatigue r/t psychological demands

Impaired **Adjustment** r/t low state of optimism

Ineffective **Coping** r/t dysfunctional grieving

B

Ineffective **Health** maintenance r/t lack of ability to make good judgments regarding ways to obtain help

Risk for **Loneliness** r/t stress, conflict

Risk for **Spiritual** distress r/t mental illness

Self-care deficit: specify r/t depression, cognitive impairment

Social isolation r/t ineffective coping

See Depression; Manic Disorder, Bipolar I

Birth Asphyxia

See Asphyxia, Birth

Birth Control

See Contraceptive Method

Bladder Cancer

Urinary retention r/t clots obstructing urethra

See Cancer; TURP

Bladder Distention

Risk for urge urinary **Incontinence** r/t small bladder capacity

Urge urinary **Incontinence** r/t overdistention of bladder

Urinary retention r/t high urethral pressure caused by weak detrusor, inhibition of reflex arc, blockage, strong sphincter

Bladder Training

Disturbed **Body** image r/t difficulty in maintaining control of urinary elimination

Functional **Incontinence** r/t altered environment; sensory, cognitive, mobility deficit

Ineffective **Health** maintenance r/t deficient knowledge regarding incontinence self-care

Stress urinary **Incontinence** r/t degenerative change in pelvic muscles and structural supports

Urge urinary **Incontinence** r/t decreased bladder capacity, increased urine concentration, overdistention of bladder

Bleeding Tendency

Ineffective **Protection** r/t abnormal blood profile, drug therapies

Risk for delayed **Surgical** recovery r/t bleeding tendency

Blepharoplasty

Disturbed **Body** image r/t effects of surgery

Ineffective **Health** maintenance r/t deficient knowledge regarding postoperative care of surgical area

Blindness

Disturbed **Sensory** perception: visual r/t altered sensory reception, transmission, integration

Impaired **Home** maintenance r/t decreased vision

Ineffective **Role** performance r/t alteration in health status (change in visual acuity)

Interrupted **Family** process r/t shift in health status of family member (change in visual acuity)

Risk for delayed **Development** r/t vision impairment

Risk for **Injury** r/t sensory dysfunction

Self-care deficit r/t inability to see to be able to perform activities of daily living

See Vision Impairment

Blood Disorder

Ineffective **Protection** r/t abnormal blood profile

See cause of Blood Disorder

Blood Pressure Alteration

See Hypertension; Hypotension

Blood Transfusion

Anxiety r/t possibility of harm from transfusion

See Anemia

Body Image Change

Disturbed **Body** image r/t psychosocial, biophysical, cognitive/perceptual, cultural, spiritual, developmental changes; illness; trauma or injury; surgery; illness treatment

Body Temperature, Altered

Risk for imbalanced **Body** temperature r/t extremes of age or weight, exposure to cold or hot environment, dehydration, change in activity, effects of medication, dysfunction of body temperature regulation center

Bone Marrow Biopsy

Fear r/t unknown outcome of results of biopsy

Ineffective **Health** maintenance r/t deficient knowledge of expectations following procedure, disease treatment following biopsy

Pain r/t bone marrow aspiration

See disease necessitating bone marrow biopsy (e.g., Leukemia)

Borderline Personality Disorder

Anxiety r/t perceived threat to self-concept

Disturbed **Thought** process r/t poor reality testing

Defensive **Coping** r/t difficulty with relationships, inability to accept blame for own behavior

Impaired **Judgment** r/t intense emotional state

Ineffective **Coping** r/t use of maladjusted defense mechanisms (e.g., projection, denial)

Ineffective family **Therapeutic** regimen management r/t manipulative behavior of client

Powerlessness r/t lifestyle of helplessness

Risk for **Caregiver** role strain r/t inability of care receiver to accept criticism, care receiver taking advantage of others to meet own needs or having unreasonable expectations

Risk for **Self-mutilation** r/t ineffective coping, feelings of self-hatred

Risk for **Spiritual** distress r/t poor relationships associated with behaviors attributed to borderline personality disorder

Risk for self-directed **Violence** r/t feelings of need to punish self, manipulative behavior

Social isolation r/t immature interests

Boredom

Deficient **Diversional** activity r/t environmental lack of diversional activity

Social isolation r/t altered state of wellness

Botulism

Deficient **Fluid** volume r/t profuse diarrhea

Ineffective **Health** maintenance r/t deficient knowledge regarding prevention of botulism, care following episode

Bowel Incontinence

Bowel incontinence r/t decreased awareness of need to defecate, loss of sphincter control, fecal impaction

Bowel Obstruction

Constipation r/t decreased motility, intestinal obstruction

Deficient **Fluid** volume r/t inadequate fluid volume intake, fluid loss in bowel

Imbalanced **Nutrition: less than body requirements** r/t nausea, vomiting

Pain r/t pressure from distended abdomen

Bowel Resection

See Abdominal Surgery

Bowel Sounds, Absent or Diminished

Constipation r/t decreased or absent peristalsis

Deficient **Fluid** volume r/t inability to ingest fluids, loss of fluids in bowel

Delayed **Surgical** recovery r/t inability to obtain adequate nutritional status

Bowel Sounds, Hyperactive

Diarrhea r/t increased gastrointestinal motility

Bowel Training

Bowel incontinence r/t loss of control of rectal sphincter

Ineffective **Health** maintenance r/t deficient knowledge regarding treatment of bowel incontinence

BPH (Benign Prostatic Hypertrophy)

Disturbed **Sleep** pattern r/t nocturia

Ineffective **Health** maintenance r/t deficient knowledge regarding self-care with prostatic hypertrophy

Risk for **Infection** r/t urinary residual postvoiding, bacterial invasion of bladder

Risk for urge urinary **Incontinence** r/t detrusor muscle instability with impaired contractility, involuntary sphincter relaxation

Urinary retention r/t obstruction

Bradycardia

Decreased **Cardiac** output r/t slow heart rate supplying inadequate amount of blood for body function

Ineffective **Health** maintenance r/t deficient knowledge of condition, effects of cardiac medications

Ineffective **Tissue** perfusion: cerebral r/t decreased cardiac output secondary to bradycardia

Risk for **Injury** r/t decreased cerebral tissue perfusion

Bradypnea

Ineffective **Breathing** pattern r/t neuromuscular impairment, pain, musculoskeletal impairment, perception/cognitive impairment, anxiety, fatigue/decreased energy, effects of drugs

See cause of Bradypnea

Brain Injury

See Intracranial Pressure, Increased

Brain Surgery

See Craniectomy/Craniotomy

Brain Tumor

Anticipatory **Grieving** r/t potential loss of physiosocial-psychosocial well-being

Decreased **Intracranial** adaptive capacity r/t presence of brain tumor

Disturbed **Sensory** perception: specify r/t tumor growth compressing brain tissue

Disturbed **Thought** processes r/t altered circulation, destruction of brain tissue

B

B

Fear r/t threat to well-being

Pain r/t neurological injury

Risk for Injury r/t sensory-perceptual alterations, weakness

See Cancer; Chemotherapy; Child with Chronic Condition; Craniectomy/Craniotomy; Hospitalized Child; Radiation Therapy; Terminally Ill Child

Braxton Hicks Contractions

Activity intolerance r/t increased perception of contractions with increased gestation

Anxiety r/t uncertainty about beginning labor

Fatigue r/t lack of sleep

Disturbed **Sleep** pattern r/t contractions when lying down

Ineffective **Sexuality** patterns r/t fear of contractions

Stress urinary **Incontinence** r/t increased pressure on bladder with contractions

Breast Biopsy

Ineffective **Health** maintenance r/t deficient knowledge regarding appropriate postoperative care of breasts

Fear r/t potential for diagnosis of cancer

Risk for Spiritual distress r/t fear of diagnosis of cancer

Breast Cancer

Chronic **Sorrow** r/t diagnosis of cancer, loss of body integrity

Death **Anxiety** r/t diagnosis of cancer

Fear r/t diagnosis of cancer

Ineffective **Coping** r/t treatment, prognosis

Risk for Spiritual distress r/t fear of diagnosis of cancer

Sexual dysfunction r/t loss of body part, partner's reaction to loss

See Cancer; Chemotherapy; Mastectomy; Radiation

Breast Lumps

Fear r/t potential for diagnosis of cancer

Ineffective **Health** maintenance r/t deficient knowledge regarding appropriate care of breasts

Breast Pumping

Anxiety r/t interrupted breastfeeding

Decisional **Conflict** r/t infant feeding method

Disturbed **Body** image r/t individual response to breastfeeding process

Ineffective **Health** maintenance r/t deficient knowledge regarding breast milk expression and storage

Risk for impaired Skin integrity r/t high suction

Risk for Infection r/t contaminated breast pump parts, incomplete emptying of breast

Breastfeeding, Effective

Effective **Breastfeeding** r/t basic breastfeeding knowledge, normal breast structure, normal infant oral structure, infant gestational age >34 weeks, support sources, maternal confidence

Breastfeeding, Ineffective

Ineffective **Breastfeeding** r/t prematurity, infant anomaly, maternal breast anomaly, previous breast surgery, previous history of breastfeeding failure, infant receiving supplemental feedings with artificial nipple, poor infant sucking reflex, nonsupportive partner/family, deficient knowledge, interruption in breastfeeding, maternal anxiety or ambivalence

See Painful Breasts—Sore Nipples; Painful Breasts—Engorgement

Breastfeeding, Interrupted

Interrupted **Breastfeeding** r/t maternal or infant illness, prematurity, maternal employment, contraindications to breastfeeding (e.g., drugs, true breast milk jaundice), need to abruptly wean infant

Breath Sounds, Decreased or Absent

See Atelectasis; Pneumothorax

Breathing Pattern Alteration

Ineffective **Breathing** pattern r/t neuromuscular impairment, pain, musculoskeletal impairment, perception/cognitive impairment, anxiety, decreased energy/fatigue

Breech Birth

Anxiety: maternal r/t threat to self, infant

Fear: maternal r/t danger to infant, self

Impaired **Gas** exchange: fetal r/t compressed umbilical cord

Ineffective cerebral **Tissue** perfusion r/t compressed umbilical cord

Risk for Aspiration: fetal r/t birth of body before head

Risk for delayed Development r/t compressed umbilical cord

Risk for impaired Tissue integrity: fetal r/t difficult birth

Risk for impaired Tissue integrity: maternal r/t difficult birth

Bronchitis

Anxiety r/t potential chronic condition
Health-seeking behavior r/t wish to stop smoking
Ineffective **Airway** clearance r/t excessive thickened mucus secretion
Ineffective **Health** maintenance r/t deficient knowledge regarding care of condition

Bronchopulmonary Dysplasia

Activity intolerance r/t imbalance between oxygen supply-demand
Excess Fluid volume r/t sodium and water retention
Imbalanced **Nutrition: less than body requirements** r/t poor feeding, increased caloric needs secondary to increased work of breathing
See Child with Chronic Condition; Hospitalized Child; Respiratory Conditions of the Neonate

Bronchoscopy

Risk for **Aspiration** r/t temporary loss of gag reflex
Risk for **Injury** r/t complication of pneumothorax, laryngeal edema, hemorrhage (if biopsy done)

Bruits, Carotid

Ineffective **Tissue** perfusion: cerebral r/t interruption of carotid blood flow
Risk for **Injury** r/t loss of motor, sensory, visual function

Bryant's Traction

See Traction and Casts

Buck's Traction

See Traction and Casts

Buerger's Disease

See Peripheral Vascular Disease

Bulimia

Chronic low **Self-esteem** r/t lack of positive feedback
Defensive **Coping** r/t eating disorder
Disturbance in **Body** image r/t misperception about actual appearance, body weight
Fear r/t food ingestion, weight gain
Imbalanced **Nutrition: less than body requirements** r/t induced vomiting
Ineffective family **Coping** r/t chronically unresolved feelings of guilt, anger, hostility
Noncompliance r/t negative feelings toward treatment regimen
Powerlessness r/t urge to purge self after eating
See Maturational Issues, Adolescent

Bunion

Ineffective **Health** maintenance r/t deficient knowledge regarding appropriate care of feet

Bunionectomy

Ineffective **Health** maintenance r/t deficient knowledge regarding postoperative care of feet
Impaired physical **Mobility** r/t sore foot
Impaired **Walking** r/t pain associated with surgery
Risk for **Infection** r/t surgical incision, advanced age

Burns

Anticipatory **Grieving** r/t loss of bodily function, loss of future hopes and plans
Anxiety/Fear r/t pain from treatments, possible permanent disfigurement
Disturbed **Body** image r/t altered physical appearance
Delayed **Surgical** recovery r/t ineffective tissue perfusion
Deficient **Diversional** activity r/t long-term hospitalization
Hypothermia r/t impaired skin integrity
Imbalanced **Nutrition: less than body requirements** r/t increased metabolic needs, anorexia, protein and fluid loss
Impaired **Skin** integrity r/t injury of skin
Ineffective **Tissue** perfusion: peripheral r/t circumferential burns, impaired arterial/venous circulation
Impaired physical **Mobility** r/t pain, musculoskeletal impairment, contracture formation
Pain r/t injury, treatments
Post-trauma response r/t life-threatening event
Risk for deficient **Fluid** volume r/t loss from skin surface, fluid shift
Risk for ineffective **Airway** clearance r/t potential tracheobronchial obstruction, edema
Risk for **Infection** r/t loss of intact skin, trauma, invasive sites
Risk for **Peripheral** neurovascular dysfunction r/t eschar formation with circumferential burn
Risk for **Post-trauma** syndrome r/t perception, duration of event that caused burns
See Hospitalized Child; Safety, Childhood

Bursitis

Impaired physical **Mobility** r/t inflammation in joint
Pain r/t inflammation in joint

Bypass Graft

See Coronary Artery Bypass Grafting

C

Cachexia

Adult **Failure** to thrive r/t imbalanced nutrition: less than body requirements

Imbalanced **Nutrition: less than body requirements** r/t inability to ingest food because of biological factors

Ineffective **Protection** r/t inadequate nutrition

Calcium Alteration

See Hypercalcemia; Hypocalcemia

Cancer

Activity intolerance r/t side effects of treatment, weakness from cancer

Anticipatory **Grieving** r/t potential loss of significant others, high risk for infertility

Chronic **Pain** r/t metastatic cancer

Chronic **Sorrow** r/t chronic illness of cancer

Compromised family **Coping** r/t prolonged disease or disability progression that exhausts supportive ability of significant others

Constipation r/t side effects of medication, altered nutrition, decreased activity

Death **Anxiety** r/t unresolved issues regarding dying

Decisional **Conflict** r/t selection of treatment choices, continuation/discontinuation of treatment, "do not resuscitate" decision

Disturbed **Body** image r/t side effects of treatment, cachexia

Disturbed **Sleep** pattern r/t anxiety, pain

Fear r/t serious threat to well-being

Hopelessness r/t loss of control, terminal illness

Imbalanced **Nutrition: less than body requirements** r/t loss of appetite, difficulty swallowing, side effects of chemotherapy, obstruction by tumor

Impaired physical **Mobility** r/t weakness, neuromusculoskeletal impairment, pain

Impaired **Skin** integrity r/t immunological deficit, immobility

Impaired **Oral** mucous membranes r/t chemotherapy, oral pH changes, decreased/altered oral flora

Ineffective **Denial** r/t dysfunctional grieving process

Ineffective **Health** maintenance r/t deficient knowledge regarding prescribed treatment

Ineffective **Protection** r/t cancer suppressing immune system

Ineffective **Role** performance r/t change in physical capacity, inability to resume prior role

Ineffective **Coping** r/t personal vulnerability in situational crisis, terminal illness

Readiness for enhanced **Spiritual** well-being r/t desire for harmony with self, others, higher power/God when faced with serious illness

Powerlessness r/t treatment, progression of disease

Risk for **Disuse** syndrome r/t severe pain, change in level of consciousness

Risk for impaired **Home** maintenance r/t lack of familiarity with community resources

Risk for **Infection** r/t inadequate immune system

Risk for **Injury** r/t bleeding secondary to bone marrow depression

Risk for **Spiritual** distress r/t physical illness of cancer

Self-care deficit: specify r/t pain, intolerance to activity, decreased strength

Social isolation r/t hospitalization, lifestyle changes

Spiritual distress r/t test of spiritual beliefs

See Chemotherapy; Child with Chronic Condition; Hospitalized Child; Terminally Ill Child

Candidiasis, Oral

Impaired **Oral** mucous membranes r/t overgrowth of infectious agent, depressed immune function

Ineffective **Health** maintenance r/t deficient knowledge regarding care of infected mouth

Capillary Refill Time, Prolonged

Impaired **Gas** exchange r/t ventilation perfusion imbalance

Ineffective **Tissue** perfusion: peripheral r/t interruption of arterial or venous flow

Risk for **Peripheral** neurovascular dysfunction r/t vascular obstruction

See Shock

Cardiac Catheterization

Anxiety/fear r/t invasive procedure, uncertainty of outcome of procedure

Impaired **Comfort** r/t postprocedure restrictions, invasive procedure

Ineffective **Health** maintenance r/t deficient knowledge regarding procedure, postprocedure care, treatment and prevention of coronary artery disease

Risk for decreased **Cardiac** output r/t ventricular ischemia, dysrhythmia

Risk for ineffective **Tissue** perfusion r/t impaired arterial or venous circulation

Risk for **Injury**: hematoma r/t invasive procedure

Risk for **Peripheral** neurovascular dysfunction r/t vascular obstruction

Cardiac Disorders

Decreased **Cardiac** output r/t cardiac disorder
See specific disorder

Cardiac Disorders in Pregnancy

Activity intolerance r/t cardiac pathophysiology, increased demand secondary to pregnancy, weakness, fatigue

Anxiety r/t unknown outcomes of pregnancy, family well-being

Compromised family **Coping** r/t prolonged hospitalization/maternal incapacitation that exhausts supportive capacity of significant others

Death **Anxiety** r/t potential danger of condition

Fatigue r/t metabolic demands, psychological-emotional demands

Fear r/t potential maternal effects, potential poor fetal/maternal outcome

Ineffective **Coping** r/t personal vulnerability

Ineffective **Health** maintenance r/t deficient knowledge regarding treatment, restrictions with cardiac disorder

Ineffective **Role** performance r/t changes in lifestyle, expectations secondary to disease process with superimposed pregnancy

Interrupted **Family** processes r/t hospitalization, maternal incapacitation, changes in role

Powerlessness r/t illness-related regimen

Risk for delayed **Development** r/t poor maternal oxygenation

Risk for disproportionate **Growth** r/t poor maternal oxygenation

Risk for excess **Fluid** volume r/t compromised regulatory mechanism with increased afterload, preload, circulating blood volume

Risk for imbalanced **Fluid** volume r/t sudden changes in circulation following delivery of placenta

Risk for impaired **Gas** exchange r/t pulmonary edema

Risk for ineffective fetal **Tissue** perfusion r/t poor maternal oxygenation

Risk for **Spiritual** distress r/t fear of diagnosis for self and infant

Situational low **Self-esteem** r/t situational crisis, pregnancy

Social isolation r/t limitations of activity, bedrest/hospitalization, separation from family and friends

Cardiac Dysrhythmia

See Dysrhythmia

Cardiac Output Decrease

Decreased **Cardiac** output r/t cardiac dysfunction

Cardiac Tamponade

Decreased **Cardiac** output r/t fluid in pericardial sac
See Pericarditis

Cardiogenic Shock

Decreased **Cardiac** output r/t decreased myocardial contractility, dysrhythmia
See Shock

Caregiver Role Strain

Caregiver role strain r/t pathophysiological factors, developmental factors, psychosocial factors, situational factors

Risk for **Caregiver** role strain r/t pathophysiological factors, developmental factors, psychosocial factors, situational factors

Carious Teeth

See Cavities in Teeth

Carotid Endarterectomy

Fear r/t surgery in vital area

Ineffective **Health** maintenance r/t deficient knowledge regarding postoperative care

Risk for ineffective **Airway** clearance r/t hematoma compressing trachea

Risk for ineffective **Tissue** perfusion: cerebral r/t hemorrhage, clot formation

Risk for **Injury** r/t possible hematoma formation

Carpal Tunnel Syndrome

Impaired physical **Mobility** r/t neuromuscular impairment

Pain r/t unrelieved pressure on median nerve

Self-care deficit: bathing/hygiene, dressing/grooming, feeding r/t pain

Carpopedal Spasm

See Hypocalcemia

Casts

Deficient **Diversional** activity r/t physical limitations from cast

Ineffective **Health** maintenance r/t deficient knowledge regarding cast care, personal care with cast

Impaired physical **Mobility** r/t limb immobilization

Impaired **Walking** r/t cast(s) on lower extremities, fracture of bones

Risk for impaired **Skin** integrity r/t unrelieved pressure on skin

Risk for **Peripheral** neurovascular dysfunction r/t mechanical compression from cast

C

Self-care deficit: bathing/hygiene, dressing/grooming, feeding r/t presence of cast(s) on upper extremities

Self-care deficit: toileting r/t presence of cast(s) on lower extremities

Cataract Extraction

Anxiety r/t threat of permanent vision loss, surgical procedure

Ineffective **Health** maintenance r/t deficient knowledge regarding postoperative restrictions

Risk for Injury r/t increased intraocular pressure, accommodation to new visual field

Disturbed **Sensory** perception: vision r/t edema from surgery

See Vision Impairment

Cataracts

Disturbed **Sensory** perception: vision r/t altered sensory input

See Vision Impairment

Catatonic Schizophrenia

Imbalanced **Nutrition: less than body requirements** r/t decrease in outside stimulation, loss of perception of hunger, resistance to instructions to eat

Impaired **Memory** r/t cognitive impairment

Impaired physical **Mobility** r/t cognitive impairment, maintenance of rigid posture, inappropriate/bizarre postures

Impaired verbal **Communication** r/t muteness

Social isolation r/t inability to communicate, immobility

See Schizophrenia

Catheterization, Urinary

Ineffective **Health** maintenance r/t deficient knowledge of normal sensation of catheter in place, care of catheter

Risk for Infection r/t invasive procedure

Cavities in Teeth

Impaired **Dentition** r/t ineffective oral hygiene, barriers to self-care, economic barriers to professional care, nutritional deficits, dietary habits

Ineffective **Health** maintenance r/t lack of knowledge regarding prevention of dental disease secondary to high-sugar diet, giving infants/toddlers with erupted teeth bottles of milk at bedtime, lack of fluoride treatments, inadequate or improper brushing of teeth

Cellulitis

Impaired **Skin** integrity r/t inflammatory process damaging skin

Ineffective **Tissue** perfusion: peripheral r/t edema

Pain r/t inflammatory changes in tissues from infection

Cellulitis, Periorbital

Disturbed **Sensory** perception: visual r/t decreased visual fields secondary to edema of eyelids

Hyperthermia r/t infectious process

Impaired **Skin** integrity r/t inflammation/infection of skin/tissues

Pain r/t edema and inflammation of skin/tissues

See Hospitalized Child

Central Line Insertion

Ineffective **Health** maintenance r/t deficient knowledge regarding precautions to take when central line in place

Risk for Infection r/t invasive procedure

Cerebral Aneurysm

See Craniectomy/Craniotomy; Intracranial Pressure, Increased; Subarachnoid Hemorrhage

Cerebral Palsy

Chronic **Sorrow** r/t presence of chronic disability

Deficient **Diversional** activity r/t physical impairments, limitations on ability to participate in recreational activities

Imbalanced **Nutrition: less than body requirements** r/t spasticity, feeding or swallowing difficulties

Impaired physical **Mobility** r/t spasticity, neuromuscular impairment/weakness

Impaired **Social** interaction r/t impaired communication skills, limited physical activity, perceived differences from peers

Impaired verbal **Communication** r/t impaired ability to articulate/speak words secondary to facial muscle involvement

Risk for delayed **Development** r/t chronic illness

Risk for disproportionate **Growth** r/t chronic illness

Risk for impaired **Parenting** r/t caring for child with overwhelming needs resulting from chronic change in health status

Risk for Injury/trauma r/t muscle weakness, inability to control spasticity

Risk for Spiritual distress r/t psychic and psychological stress associated with chronic illness

Self-care deficit: specify r/t neuromuscular impairments, sensory deficits

See Child with Chronic Condition

Cerebrovascular Accident

See CVA

Cervicitis

Ineffective **Health** maintenance r/t deficient knowledge regarding care and prevention of condition

Ineffective **Sexuality** pattern r/t abstinence during acute stage

Risk for **Infection** r/t spread of infection, recurrence of infection

Cesarean Delivery

Anxiety r/t unmet expectations for childbirth, unknown outcome of surgery

Disturbed **Body** image r/t surgery, unmet expectations for childbirth

Fear r/t perceived threat to own well-being

Impaired **Comfort:** nausea, vomiting, pruritus r/t side effects of systemic or epidural narcotics

Impaired physical **Mobility** r/t pain

Ineffective **Health** maintenance r/t deficient knowledge regarding postoperative care

Ineffective **Role** performance r/t unmet expectations for childbirth

Interrupted **Family** processes r/t unmet expectations for childbirth

Pain r/t surgical incision, decreased or absent peristalsis secondary to anesthesia, manipulation of abdominal organs during surgery, immobilization, restricted diet

Risk for **Aspiration** r/t positioning for general anesthesia

Risk for deficient **Fluid** volume r/t increased blood loss secondary to surgery

Risk for imbalanced **Fluid** volume r/t loss of blood

Risk for **Infection** r/t surgical incision, stasis of respiratory secretions secondary to general anesthesia

Risk for **Post-trauma** syndrome r/t emergency condition to save life of mother or baby

Risk for **Urinary** retention r/t regional anesthesia

Situational low **Self-esteem** r/t inability to deliver child vaginally

Chemical Dependence

See Alcoholism; Drug Abuse

Chemotherapy

Disturbed **Body** image r/t loss of weight, loss of hair

Death **Anxiety** r/t chemotherapy not accomplishing desired results

Delayed **Surgical** recovery r/t compromised immune system

Fatigue r/t disease process, anemia, drug effects

Imbalanced **Nutrition:** less than body requirements r/t side effects of chemotherapy

Impaired **Oral** mucous membranes r/t effects of chemotherapy

Ineffective **Health** maintenance r/t deficient knowledge regarding action, side effects, way to integrate chemotherapy into lifestyle

Ineffective **Protection** r/t suppressed immune system, decreased platelets

Nausea r/t effects of chemotherapy

Risk for deficient **Fluid** volume r/t vomiting, diarrhea

Risk for ineffective **Tissue** perfusion r/t anemia

Risk for **Infection** r/t immunosuppression

See Cancer

Chest Pain

Fear r/t potential threat of death

Pain r/t myocardial injury, ischemia

Risk for decreased **Cardiac** output r/t ventricular ischemia

See Angina Pectoris; MI

Chest Tubes

Impaired **Gas** exchange r/t decreased functional lung tissue

Ineffective **Breathing** pattern r/t asymmetrical lung expansion secondary to pain

Pain r/t presence of chest tubes, injury

Risk for **Injury** r/t presence of invasive chest tube

Cheyne-Stokes Respiration

Ineffective **Breathing** pattern r/t critical illness

See cause of Cheyne-Stokes Respiration

CHF (Congestive Heart Failure)

Activity intolerance r/t weakness, fatigue

Constipation r/t activity intolerance

Decreased **Cardiac** output r/t impaired cardiac function

Fatigue r/t disease process

Fear r/t threat to one's own well-being

Excess **Fluid** volume r/t impaired excretion of sodium and water

Impaired **Gas** exchange r/t excessive fluid in interstitial space of lungs, alveoli

Ineffective **Health** maintenance r/t deficient knowledge regarding care of disease

Powerlessness r/t illness-related regimen

See Child with Chronic Condition; Congenital Heart Disease/Cardiac Anomalies; Hospitalized Child

Chickenpox

See Communicable Diseases, Childhood

Child Abuse

Anxiety/fear r/t threat of punishment for perceived wrongdoing

Chronic low Self-esteem r/t lack of positive feedback, excessive negative feedback

Deficient Diversional activity r/t diminished or absent environmental/personal stimuli

Delayed Growth and development: regression vs. delayed r/t diminished/absent environmental stimuli, inadequate caretaking, inconsistent responsiveness by caretaker

Disturbed Sleep pattern r/t hypervigilance, anxiety

Imbalanced Nutrition: less than body requirements r/t inadequate caretaking

Impaired Parenting r/t psychological impairment, physical or emotional abuse of parent, substance abuse, unrealistic expectations of child

Impaired Skin integrity r/t altered nutritional state, physical abuse

Ineffective community Therapeutic regimen management r/t deficits in community regarding prevention of child abuse

Interrupted Family process: alcoholism r/t inadequate coping skills

Pain r/t physical injuries

Post-trauma response r/t physical abuse, incest, rape, molestation

Risk for delayed Development r/t shaken baby, abuse

Risk for disproportionate Growth r/t abuse

Risk for Poisoning r/t inadequate safeguards, lack of proper safety precautions, accessibility of illicit substances secondary to impaired home maintenance

Risk for Suffocation/aspiration r/t propped bottle, unattended child

Risk for Trauma r/t inadequate precautions, cognitive or emotional difficulties

Social isolation: family imposed r/t fear of disclosure of family dysfunction and abuse

Child Neglect

See Child Abuse; Failure to Thrive

Child with Chronic Condition

Activity intolerance r/t fatigue associated with chronic illness

Chronic low Self-esteem r/t actual or perceived differences; peer acceptance; decreased ability to participate in physical, school, and social activities

Chronic Pain r/t physical, biological, chemical, or psychological factors

Chronic Sorrow r/t developmental stages and missed opportunities or milestones that bring comparisons with social or personal norms, unending caregiving as reminder of loss

Compromised family Coping r/t prolonged overconcern for child; distortion of reality regarding child's health problem, including extreme denial about its existence or severity

Impaired Home maintenance r/t overtaxed family members (e.g., exhausted, anxious)

Decisional Conflict r/t treatment options, conflicting values

Deficient Diversional activity r/t immobility, monotonous environment, frequent/lengthy treatments, reluctance to participate, self-imposed social isolation

Deficient Knowledge: readiness for enhanced **Health maintenance** r/t knowledge/skill acquisition regarding health practices, acceptance of limitations, promotion of maximal potential of child, self-actualization of rest of family

Delayed Growth and development r/t regression or lack of progression toward developmental milestones secondary to frequent or prolonged hospitalization, inadequate or inappropriate stimulation, cerebral insult, chronic illness, effects of physical disability, prescribed dependence

Disabled family Coping r/t prolonged disease or disability progression that exhausts supportive capacity of significant people

Disturbed Sleep pattern: child or parent r/t time-intensive treatments, exacerbation of condition, 24-hour care needs

Hopelessness: child r/t prolonged activity restriction, long-term stress, lack of involvement in or passively allowing care secondary to parental overprotection

Imbalanced Nutrition: more than body requirements r/t effects of steroid medications on appetite

Impaired Social interaction r/t developmental lag/delay, perceived differences

Imbalanced Nutrition: less than body requirements r/t anorexia, fatigue secondary to physical exertion

Ineffective Coping: child r/t situational or maturational crises

Ineffective Health maintenance r/t exhausting family resources (finances, physical energy, support systems)

Ineffective Sexuality patterns: parental r/t disrupted relationship with sexual partner

Interrupted Family processes r/t intermittent situational crisis of illness, disease, hospitalization

Parental role Conflict r/t separation from child as a result of chronic illness, home care of child with special needs, interruptions of family life resulting from home care regimen

Powerlessness: child r/t health care environment, illness-related regimen, lifestyle of learned helplessness

Readiness for enhanced family Coping r/t impact of crisis on family values, priorities, goals, or relationships; changes in family choices to optimize wellness

Risk for delayed Development r/t chronic illness

Risk for disproportionate Growth r/t chronic illness

Risk for impaired Parenting r/t impaired/disrupted bonding, caring for child with perceived overwhelming care needs

Risk for Infection r/t debilitating physical condition

Risk for Noncompliance r/t complex or prolonged home care regimens; expressed intent to not comply secondary to value systems, health beliefs, cultural/religious practices

Social isolation: family r/t actual or perceived social stigmatization, complex care requirements

Childbirth

See Labor—Normal; Postpartum, Normal Care

Chills

Hyperthermia r/t infectious process

Chlamydia Infection

See STD (Sexually Transmitted Disease)

Choking/Coughing with Feeding

Impaired Swallowing r/t neuromuscular impairment

Risk for Aspiration r/t depressed cough and gag reflexes

Cholasma

Disturbed Body image r/t change in skin color

Cholecystectomy

Imbalanced Nutrition: less than body requirements r/t high metabolic needs, decreased ability to digest fatty foods

Ineffective Health maintenance r/t deficient knowledge regarding postoperative care

Pain r/t recent surgery

Risk for deficient Fluid volume r/t restricted intake, nausea, vomiting

Risk for ineffective Breathing pattern r/t proximity of incision to lungs resulting in pain with deep breathing

See Abdominal Surgery

Cholelithiasis

Imbalanced Nutrition: less than body requirements r/t anorexia, nausea, vomiting

Ineffective Health maintenance r/t deficient knowledge regarding care of disease

Pain r/t obstruction of bile flow, inflammation in gallbladder

Chorioamnionitis

Anticipatory Grieving r/t guilt about potential loss of ideal pregnancy and birth

Anxiety r/t threat to self and infant

Hyperthermia r/t infectious process

Risk for delayed Growth and development r/t risk of preterm birth

Risk for Infection transmission from mother to fetus r/t infection in fetal environment

Situational low Self-esteem r/t guilt about threat to infant's health

Chronic Lymphocytic Leukemia

See Leukemia

Chronic Obstructive Pulmonary Disease

See COPD

Chronic Pain

See Pain, Chronic

Chronic Renal Failure

See Renal Failure

Chvostek's Sign

See Hypocalcemia

Circumcision

Ineffective Health maintenance r/t deficient knowledge (parental) regarding care of surgical area

Pain r/t surgical intervention

Risk for deficient Fluid volume r/t hemorrhage

Risk for Infection r/t surgical wound

Cirrhosis

Chronic low Self-esteem r/t chronic illness

Chronic Pain r/t liver enlargement

Chronic Sorrow r/t presence of chronic illness

Diarrhea r/t dietary changes, medications

Disturbed Thought processes r/t chronic organic disorder with increased ammonia levels, substance abuse

Fatigue r/t malnutrition

Imbalanced Nutrition: less than body requirements r/t loss of appetite, nausea, vomiting

C

Ineffective **Health** maintenance r/t deficient knowledge regarding correlation between lifestyle habits and disease process

Ineffective management of **Therapeutic** regimen r/t denial of severity of illness

Ineffective **Protection** r/t risk of impaired blood coagulation, bleeding from portal hypertension

Nausea r/t irritation to gastrointestinal system

Risk for deficient **Fluid** volume: hemorrhage r/t abnormal bleeding from esophagus

Risk for **Injury** r/t substance intoxication, potential delirium tremors

Risk for impaired **Oral** mucous membranes r/t altered nutrition

Risk for impaired **Skin** integrity r/t altered nutritional state, altered metabolic state

Cleft Lip/Cleft Palate

Chronic **Sorrow** r/t loss of perfect child, birth of child with congenital defect

Fear: parental r/t special care needs, surgery

Grieving r/t loss of perfect child, birth of child with congenital defect

Imbalanced **Nutrition:** less than body requirements r/t inability to feed with normal techniques

Impaired **Oral** mucous membranes r/t surgical correction

Impaired physical **Mobility** r/t imposed restricted activity, use of elbow restraints

Impaired **Skin** integrity r/t incomplete joining of lip, palate ridges

Impaired verbal **Communication** r/t inadequate palate function, possible hearing loss from infected eustachian tubes

Ineffective **Airway** clearance r/t common feeding and breathing passage, postoperative laryngeal, incisional edema

Ineffective **Breastfeeding** r/t infant anomaly

Ineffective **Health** maintenance r/t lack of parental knowledge regarding feeding techniques, wound care, use of elbow restraints

Ineffective **Infant** feeding pattern r/t cleft lip, cleft palate

Pain r/t surgical correction, elbow restraints

Risk for **Aspiration** r/t common feeding and breathing passage

Risk for deficient **Fluid** volume r/t inability to take liquids in usual manner

Risk for delayed **Development** r/t inadequate nutrition resulting from difficulty feeding

Risk for disproportionate **Growth** r/t inability to feed with normal techniques

Risk for disturbed **Body** image r/t disfigurement, speech impediment

Risk for **Infection** r/t invasive procedure, disruption of eustachian tube development, aspiration

Clotting Disorder

Anxiety/Fear r/t threat to well-being

Ineffective **Health** maintenance r/t deficient knowledge regarding treatment of disorder

Ineffective **Protection** r/t clotting disorder

Risk for deficient **Fluid** volume r/t uncontrolled bleeding

See Anticoagulant Therapy; DIC; Hemophilia

Coarctation of Aorta

See Congenital Heart Disease/Cardiac Anomalies

Cocaine Abuse

Disturbed **Thought** processes r/t excessive stimulation of nervous system by cocaine

Ineffective **Breathing** pattern r/t drug effect on respiratory center

Ineffective **Coping** r/t inability to deal with life stresses

See Substance Abuse

Cocaine Baby

See Crack Baby

Codependency

Caregiver role strain r/t codependency

Decisional **Conflict** r/t support system deficit

Denial r/t unmet self-needs

Impaired verbal **Communication** r/t psychological barriers

Ineffective **Coping** r/t inadequate support systems

Powerlessness r/t lifestyle of helplessness

Cognitive Deficit

Disturbed **Thought** processes r/t neurological impairment

Cold, Viral

Impaired **Comfort:** sore throat, aching, nasal discomfort r/t viral infection

Ineffective **Health** maintenance r/t deficient knowledge regarding care of viral condition, prevention of further infections

Colectomy

Constipation r/t decreased activity, decreased fluid intake

Imbalanced **Nutrition:** less than body requirements r/t high metabolic needs, decreased ability to ingest/digest food

Ineffective **Health** maintenance r/t deficient knowl-
edge regarding procedure, postoperative care
Pain r/t recent surgery
Risk for **Infection** r/t invasive procedure
See Abdominal Surgery

Colitis

Deficient **Fluid** volume r/t frequent stools
Diarrhea r/t inflammation in colon
Pain r/t inflammation in colon
See Crohn's Disease; Inflammatory Bowel Syndrome; Ul-
cerative Colitis

Collagen Disease

See specific disease (e.g., Lupus Erythematosus; Rheumatoid Arthritis, Juvenile)

Colostomy

Disturbed **Body** image r/t presence of stoma, daily
care of fecal material
Ineffective **Health** maintenance r/t deficient knowledge regarding care of stoma, integrating colostomy care into lifestyle
Risk for altered **Sexuality** pattern r/t altered body image, self-concept
Risk for **Constipation**/diarrhea r/t inappropriate diet
Risk for impaired **Skin** integrity r/t irritation from
bowel contents
Risk for **Social** isolation r/t anxiety about appearance
of stoma and possible leakage

Colporrhaphy, Anterior

See Vaginal Hysterectomy

Coma

Death **Anxiety**: significant others r/t unknown out-
come of coma state
Disturbed **Thought** processes r/t neurological
changes
Ineffective family **Therapeutic** regimen management
r/t complexity of therapeutic regimen
Interrupted **Family** processes r/t illness/disability of
family member
Risk for **Aspiration** r/t impaired swallowing, loss of
cough/gag reflex
Risk for **Disuse** syndrome r/t altered level of consciousness impairing mobility
Risk for impaired **Skin** integrity r/t immobility
Risk for impaired **Oral** mucous membranes r/t dry
mouth
Risk for **Injury** r/t potential seizure activity
Risk for **Spiritual** distress: significant others r/t loss of
ability to relate to loved one, unknown outcome
of coma

Self-care deficit: specify r/t neuromuscular impairment
Total urinary **Incontinence** r/t neurological dysfunction
See cause of Coma

Comfort, Loss of

Impaired **Comfort** r/t injury agent

Communicable Diseases, Childhood (Measles, Mumps, Rubella, Chickenpox, Scabies, Lice, Impetigo)

Deficient **Diversional** activity r/t imposed isolation
from peers, disruption in usual play activities,
fatigue, activity intolerance
Impaired **Comfort** r/t hyperthermia secondary to
infectious disease process, pruritus secondary to
skin rash or subdermal organisms
Ineffective **Health** maintenance r/t nonadherence to
appropriate immunization schedules, lack of
prevention of transmission of infection
Pain r/t impaired skin integrity, edema
Risk for **Infection**: transmission to others r/t contagious organisms
See Meningitis/Encephalitis; Respiratory Infections, Acute
Childhood; Reye's Syndrome

Communication Problems

Impaired verbal **Communication** r/t decrease in circulation to brain, brain tumor, physical barrier
(e.g., tracheostomy, intubation), anatomical defect, impaired hearing, cleft palate, psychological barriers (e.g., psychosis, lack of stimuli), cultural difference, developmentally related or age-
related factors, side effects of medication, environmental barriers, absence of significant others,
altered perceptions, lack of information, stress,
alteration of self-esteem or self-concept, physiological conditions, alteration of central nervous
system, weakening of musculoskeletal system,
emotional conditions

Community Coping

Ineffective community **Coping** r/t natural or manmade disasters; ineffective or nonexistent community systems (e.g., lack of emergency medical, transportation, or disaster planning systems),
deficits in community social support services and
resources, inadequate resources for problem solving
Readiness for enhanced community **Coping** r/t community sense of power to manage stressors, social supports available, resources available for
problem solving

C

Community Management of Therapeutic Regimen

Ineffective community **Therapeutic** regimen management r/t inadequate community resources

Compartment Syndrome

Fear r/t possible loss of limb, damage to limb
Ineffective **Tissue** perfusion: peripheral r/t increased pressure within compartment
Pain r/t pressure in compromised body part

Compulsion

See Obsessive-Compulsive Disorder

Conduction Disorders (Cardiac)

See Dysrhythmia

Confusion, Acute

Acute **Confusion** r/t >60 years of age, alcohol abuse, delirium, dementia, drug abuse
Adult **Failure** to thrive r/t confusion
Impaired **Memory** r/t fluid and electrolyte imbalance, neurological disturbances, excessive environmental disturbances, anemia, acute or chronic hypoxia, decreased cardiac output

Confusion, Chronic

Adult **Failure** to thrive r/t confusion
Chronic **Confusion** r/t Alzheimer's disease, Korsakoff's psychosis, multiinfarct dementia, cerebrovascular accident, head injury
Disturbed **Thought** processes r/t organic mental disorder, disruption of cerebral arterial blood flow, chemical imbalance, intoxication
Impaired **Memory** r/t fluid and electrolyte imbalance, neurological disturbances, excessive environmental disturbances, anemia, acute or chronic hypoxia, decreased cardiac output

Congenital Heart Disease/Cardiac Anomalies

Acyanotic

Patent ductus arteriosus, atrial/ventricular septal defect, pulmonary stenosis, endocardial cushion defect, aortic valvular stenosis, coarctation of aorta

Cyanotic

Tetralogy of Fallot, tricuspid atresia, transposition of great vessels, truncus arteriosus, total anomalous pulmonary venous return, hypoplastic left lung

Activity intolerance r/t fatigue, generalized weakness, lack of adequate oxygenation
Decreased **Cardiac** output r/t cardiac dysfunction
Delayed **Growth** and development r/t inadequate oxygen and nutrients to tissues

Excess **Fluid** volume r/t cardiac defect, side effects of medication
Imbalanced **Nutrition:** less than body requirements r/t fatigue, generalized weakness, inability of infant to suck and feed, increased caloric requirements
Impaired **Gas** exchange r/t cardiac defect, pulmonary congestion
Ineffective **Breathing** pattern r/t pulmonary vascular disease
Interrupted **Family** processes r/t ill child
Risk for deficient **Fluid** volume r/t side effects of diuretics
Risk for delayed **Development** r/t inadequate oxygen and nutrients to tissues
Risk for disproportionate **Growth** r/t inadequate oxygen and nutrients to tissues
Risk for disorganized **Infant** behavior r/t invasive procedures
Risk for ineffective **Thermoregulation** r/t neonatal age
Risk for **Poisoning** r/t potential toxicity of cardiac medications
See Child with Chronic Illness; Hospitalized Child

Congestive Heart Failure

See CHF

Conjunctivitis

Disturbed **Sensory** perception r/t change in visual acuity resulting from inflammation
Pain r/t inflammatory process
Risk for **Injury** r/t change in visual acuity

Consciousness, Altered Level of

Acute **Confusion** r/t alcohol abuse, delirium, dementia, drug abuse
Adult **Failure** to thrive r/t altered level of consciousness
Chronic **Confusion** r/t multiinfarct dementia, Korsakoff's psychosis, head injury, Alzheimer's disease, cerebrovascular accident
Decreased **Intracranial** adaptive capacity r/t brain injury
Disturbed **Thought** processes r/t neurological changes
Impaired **Memory** r/t neurological disturbances
Ineffective **Tissue** perfusion: cerebral r/t increased intracranial pressure, decreased cerebral perfusion
Risk for **Aspiration** r/t impaired swallowing, loss of cough/gag reflex
Risk for **Disuse** syndrome r/t impaired mobility resulting from altered level of consciousness
Risk for impaired **Oral** mucous membranes r/t dry mouth

Risk for impaired **Skin** integrity r/t immobility

Self-care deficit: specify r/t neuromuscular impairment

Total urinary **Incontinence** r/t neurological dysfunction

See cause of Altered Level of Consciousness

Constipation

Constipation r/t decreased fluid intake, decreased intake of foods containing bulk, inactivity, immobility, deficient knowledge of appropriate bowel routine, lack of privacy for defecation

Constipation, Perceived

Perceived **Constipation** r/t cultural or family health beliefs, faulty appraisal, impaired thought processes

Constipation, Risk for

Risk for **Constipation** r/t functional factors impeding defecation, inappropriate diet, psychological factors, physical factors, medications

Continent Ileostomy (Kock Pouch)

Imbalanced **Nutrition**: less than body requirements r/t malabsorption

Ineffective **Health** maintenance r/t deficient knowledge regarding postoperative care

Ineffective **Coping** r/t stress of disease, exacerbations caused by stress

Risk for **Injury** r/t failure of valve, stomal cyanosis, intestinal obstruction

See Abdominal Surgery

Contraceptive Method

Decisional **Conflict**: method of contraception r/t unclear personal values or beliefs, lack of experience or interference with decision-making, lack of relevant information, support system deficit

Health-seeking behavior r/t requesting information about available and appropriate birth control methods

Ineffective **Sexuality** patterns r/t fear of pregnancy

Conversion Disorder

Anxiety r/t unresolved conflict

Disturbed personal **Identity** r/t overwhelming stress

Hopelessness r/t long-term stress

Impaired **Adjustment** r/t multiple stressors

Impaired physical **Mobility** r/t physical conversion symptom

Impaired **Social** interaction r/t altered thought process

Ineffective **Coping** r/t personal vulnerability

Ineffective **Role** performance r/t physical conversion system

Powerlessness r/t lifestyle of helplessness

Risk for **Injury** r/t physical conversion symptom

Self-esteem disturbance r/t unsatisfactory or inadequate interpersonal relationships

Convulsions

Anxiety r/t concern over controlling convulsions

Impaired **Memory** r/t neurological disturbance

Ineffective **Health** maintenance r/t deficient knowledge regarding need for medication and care during seizure activity

Risk for **Aspiration** r/t impaired swallowing

Risk for delayed **Development** r/t seizures

Risk for **Injury** r/t seizure activity

Risk for disturbed **Thought** processes r/t seizure activity

See Seizure Disorders

COPD (Chronic Obstructive Pulmonary Disease)

Activity intolerance r/t imbalance between oxygen supply-demand

Altered **Family** process r/t role changes

Anxiety r/t breathlessness, change in health status

Chronic low **Self-esteem** r/t chronic illness

Chronic **Sorrow** r/t presence of chronic illness

Death **Anxiety** r/t seriousness of medical condition, difficulty being able to "catch breath," feeling of suffocation

Health-seeking behavior r/t wish to stop smoking

Imbalanced **Nutrition**: less than body requirements r/t decreased intake because of dyspnea, unpleasant taste in mouth left by medications

Impaired **Gas** exchange r/t ventilation-perfusion inequality

Impaired **Social** interaction r/t social isolation secondary to oxygen use, activity intolerance

Ineffective **Airway** clearance r/t bronchoconstriction, increased mucus, ineffective cough, infection

Ineffective **Health** maintenance r/t deficient knowledge regarding care of disease

Noncompliance r/t reluctance to accept responsibility for changing detrimental health practices

Powerlessness r/t progressive nature of disease

Risk for **Infection** r/t stasis of respiratory secretions

Self-care deficit: specify r/t fatigue secondary to increased work of breathing

Sleep deprivation r/t breathing difficulties when lying down

C

Coping Problems

Defensive **Coping** r/t superior attitude toward others, difficulty establishing or maintaining relationships, hostile laughter or ridicule of others, difficulty in reality-testing perceptions, lack of follow-through or participation in treatment or therapy

Ineffective **Coping** r/t gender differences in coping strategies, inadequate level of confidence in ability to cope, uncertainty, inadequate social support created by characteristics of relationships, inadequate level of perception of control, inadequate resources available, high degree of threat, disturbance in pattern of tension release, inadequate opportunity to prepare for stressor, inability to conserve adaptive energies, disturbance in appraisal of threat

See Community Coping; Family Problems

Corneal Reflex, Absent

Risk for **Injury** r/t accidental corneal abrasion, drying of cornea

Coronary Artery Bypass Grafting

Decreased **Cardiac** output r/t dysrhythmia, depressed cardiac function, increased systemic vascular resistance

Deficient **Fluid** volume r/t intraoperative fluid loss, use of diuretics in surgery

Fear r/t outcome of surgical procedure

Ineffective **Health** maintenance r/t deficient knowledge regarding postprocedure care, lifestyle adjustment after surgery

Pain r/t traumatic surgery

Risk for perioperative positioning **Injury** r/t hypothermia, extended supine position

Costovertebral Angle Tenderness

See Kidney Stone; Pyelonephritis

Cough, Effective/Ineffective

Ineffective **Airway** clearance r/t decreased energy, fatigue, normal aging changes

See Bronchitis; COPD; Pulmonary Edema

Crack Abuse

See Cocaine Abuse

Crack Baby

Delayed **Growth** and development r/t effects of maternal use of drugs, neurological impairment, decreased attentiveness to environmental stimuli

Diarrhea r/t effects of withdrawal, increased peristalsis secondary to hyperirritability

Disorganized **Infant** behavior r/t prematurity, pain, lack of attachment

Disturbed **Sensory** perception: specify r/t hypersensitivity to environmental stimuli

Disturbed **Sleep** pattern r/t hyperirritability, hypersensitivity to environmental stimuli

Imbalanced **Nutrition: less than body requirements** r/t feeding problems; uncoordinated/ineffective suck and swallow; effects of diarrhea, vomiting, colic

Impaired **Parenting** r/t impaired/lack of attachment behaviors, inadequate support systems

Ineffective **Protection** r/t effects of maternal substance abuse

Ineffective **Airway** clearance r/t pooling of secretions secondary to lack of adequate cough reflex

Ineffective **Infant** feeding r/t prematurity, neurological impairment

Risk for delayed **Development** r/t substance abuse

Risk for disproportionate **Growth** r/t substance use/abuse

Risk for **Infection** (skin, meningeal, respiratory) r/t effects of withdrawal

Crackles in Lungs, Coarse

Ineffective **Airway** clearance r/t excessive secretions in airways, ineffective cough

See cause of Coarse Crackles

Crackles in Lungs, Fine

Ineffective **Breathing** pattern r/t fatigue, surgery, decreased energy

See Bronchitis or Pneumonia (if from pulmonary infection); CHF (cardiac in origin); Infection

Craniectomy/Craniotomy

Adult **Failure** to thrive r/t altered cerebral tissue perfusion

Decreased **Intracranial** adaptive capacity r/t brain injury, intracranial hypertension

Fear r/t threat to well-being

Impaired **Memory** r/t neurological surgery

Ineffective **Tissue** perfusion: cerebral r/t cerebral edema, decreased cerebral perfusion, increased intracranial pressure

Pain r/t recent surgery, headache

Risk for disturbed **Thought** processes r/t neurophysiological changes

Risk for **Injury** r/t potential confusion

See Coma (if relevant)

C

Crepitation, Subcutaneous

See Pneumothorax

Creutzfeldt-Jakob Disease (CJD)

Acute **Pain** r/t neck (nuchal) rigidity, inflammation of meninges, headache, kinesthetic

Decreased **Intracranial** adaptive capacity r/t sustained increase in intracranial pressure (10 to 15 mm Hg)

Delayed **Growth** and development r/t brain damage secondary to infectious process, increased intracranial pressure

Disturbed **Sensory** perception: hearing r/t central nervous system infection, ear infection

Disturbed **Sensory** perception: kinesthetic r/t central nervous system infection

Disturbed **Thought** processes r/t inflammation of brain, fever

Excess **Fluid** volume r/t increased intracranial pressure, syndrome of inappropriate secretion of antidiuretic hormone (SIADH)

Impaired **Comfort** r/t central nervous system inflammation

Impaired **Comfort**: photophobia r/t increased sensitivity to external stimuli secondary to central nervous system inflammation

Impaired physical **Mobility** r/t neuromuscular or central nervous system insult

Ineffective **Airway** clearance r/t seizure activity

Ineffective **Tissue** perfusion: cerebral r/t inflamed cerebral tissues and meninges, increased intracranial pressure

Risk for **Aspiration** r/t seizure activity

Risk for **Falls** r/t neuromuscular dysfunction

Risk for **Injury** r/t seizure activity

Crisis

Anticipatory **Grieving** r/t potential significant loss

Anxiety r/t threat to or change in environment, health status, interaction patterns, situation, self-concept, or role-functioning; threat of death of self or significant other

Compromised family **Coping** r/t situational or developmental crisis

Death **Anxiety** r/t feelings of hopelessness associated with crisis

Disturbed **Energy** field r/t disharmony caused by crisis

Fear r/t crisis situation

Ineffective **Coping** r/t situational or maturational crisis

Risk for **Spiritual** distress r/t physical or psychological stress, natural disasters, situational losses, maturational losses

Situational low **Self-esteem** r/t perception of inability to handle crisis

Spiritual distress r/t intense suffering

Crohn's Disease

Anxiety r/t change in health status

Diarrhea r/t inflammatory process

Imbalanced **Nutrition**: less than body requirements r/t diarrhea, altered ability to digest and absorb food

Ineffective **Coping** r/t repeated episodes of diarrhea

Ineffective **Health** maintenance r/t deficient knowledge regarding management of disease

Pain r/t increased peristalsis

Powerlessness r/t chronic disease

Risk for deficient **Fluid** volume r/t abnormal fluid loss with diarrhea

Croup

See Respiratory Infections, Acute Childhood

Cryosurgery for Retinal Detachment

See Retinal Detachment

Cushing's Syndrome

Activity intolerance r/t fatigue, weakness

Disturbed **Body** image r/t change in appearance from disease process

Excess **Fluid** volume r/t failure of regulatory mechanisms

Ineffective **Health** maintenance r/t deficient knowledge regarding needed care

Risk for **Infection** r/t suppression of immune system secondary to increased cortisol

Risk for **Injury** r/t decreased muscle strength, osteoporosis

Sexual dysfunction r/t loss of libido

CVA (Cerebrovascular Accident)

Adult **Failure** to thrive r/t neurophysiological changes

Anxiety r/t situational crisis, change in physical or emotional condition

Ineffective **Health** maintenance r/t deficient knowledge regarding self-care following CVA

Interrupted **Family** process r/t illness, disability of family member

Caregiver role strain r/t cognitive problems of care receiver, need for significant home care

Chronic **Confusion** r/t neurological changes

Constipation r/t decreased activity

C

Disturbed **Body** image r/t chronic illness, paralysis

Disturbed **Sensory** perception: visual, tactile, kinesthetic r/t neurological deficit

Disturbed **Thought** processes r/t neurophysiological changes

Grieving r/t loss of health

Impaired **Home** maintenance r/t neurological disease affecting ability to perform activities of daily living (ADLs)

Impaired **Memory** r/t neurological disturbances

Impaired physical **Mobility** r/t loss of balance and coordination

Impaired **Social** interaction r/t limited physical mobility, limited ability to communicate

Impaired **Swallowing** r/t neuromuscular dysfunction

Impaired **Transfer** ability r/t limited physical mobility

Impaired verbal **Communication** r/t pressure damage, decreased circulation to brain in speech center informational sources

Impaired **Walking** r/t loss of balance and coordination

Ineffective **Coping** r/t disability

Risk for **Aspiration** r/t impaired swallowing, loss of gag reflex

Risk for **Disuse** syndrome r/t paralysis

Risk for impaired **Skin** integrity r/t immobility

Reflex **Incontinence** r/t loss of feeling to void

Risk for **Injury** r/t disturbed sensory perception

Self-care deficit: specify r/t decreased strength and endurance, paralysis

Total urinary **Incontinence** r/t neurological dysfunction

Unilateral **Neglect** r/t disturbed perception from neurological damage

Cyanosis, Central with Cyanosis of Oral Mucous Membranes

Impaired **Gas** exchange r/t alveolar-capillary membrane changes

Cyanosis, Peripheral with Cyanosis of Nailbeds

Ineffective **Tissue** perfusion r/t interruption of arterial flow, severe vasoconstriction, cold temperatures

Risk for **Peripheral** neurovascular dysfunction r/t condition causing disruption in circulation

Cystic Fibrosis

Activity intolerance r/t imbalance between oxygen supply-demand

Anxiety r/t dyspnea, oxygen deprivation

Disturbed **Body** image r/t changes in physical appearance, treatment of chronic lung disease (clubbing, barrel chest, home oxygen therapy)

Chronic **Sorrow** r/t presence of chronic disease

Imbalanced **Nutrition:** less than body requirements r/t anorexia; decreased absorption of nutrients, fat; increased work of breathing

Impaired **Gas** exchange r/t ventilation-perfusion imbalance

Impaired **Home** maintenance r/t extensive daily treatment, medications necessary for health, mist/oxygen tents

Ineffective **Airway** clearance r/t increased production of thick mucus

Risk for delayed **Development** r/t chronic illness

Risk for **Caregiver** role strain r/t illness severity of care receiver, unpredictable course of illness

Risk for disproportionate **Growth** r/t chronic illness

Risk for deficient **Fluid** volume r/t decreased fluid intake, increased work of breathing

Risk for **Infection** r/t thick, tenacious mucus; harboring of bacterial organisms; debilitated state

Risk for **Spiritual** distress r/t presence of chronic disease

See Child with Chronic Condition; Hospitalized Child; Terminally Ill Child

Cystitis

Impaired **Urinary** elimination: frequency r/t urinary tract infection

Ineffective **Health** maintenance r/t deficient knowledge regarding methods to treat and prevent urinary tract infections

Pain: dysuria r/t inflammatory process in bladder

Risk for urge urinary **Incontinence** r/t infection in bladder

Cystocele

Ineffective **Health** maintenance r/t deficient knowledge regarding personal care, Kegel exercises to strengthen perineal muscles

Risk for urge urinary **Incontinence** r/t lack of bladder support

Stress urinary **Incontinence** r/t prolapsed bladder

Urge urinary **Incontinence** r/t prolapsed bladder

Cystoscopy

Ineffective **Health** maintenance r/t deficient knowledge regarding postoperative care

Risk for **Infection** r/t invasive procedure

Urinary retention r/t edema in urethra obstructing flow of urine

D

Deafness

Disturbed **Sensory** perception: auditory r/t alteration in sensory reception, transmission, integration

Impaired verbal **Communication** r/t impaired hearing

Risk for delayed **Development** r/t impaired hearing

Risk for **Injury** r/t alteration in sensory perception

Death, Oncoming

Anticipatory **Grieving** r/t loss of significant other

Compromised family **Coping** r/t client's inability to provide support to family

Death **Anxiety** r/t unresolved issues surrounding dying

Fear r/t threat of death

Ineffective **Coping** r/t personal vulnerability

Powerlessness r/t effects of illness, oncoming death

Readiness for enhanced **Spiritual** well-being r/t desire of client and family to be in harmony with each other and higher power/God

Social isolation r/t altered state of wellness

Spiritual distress r/t intense suffering

See Terminally Ill Child

Decisions, Difficulty Making

Decisional **Conflict** r/t support system deficit, perceived threat to value system, multiple or divergent sources of information, lack of relevant information, unclear personal values/beliefs

Decubitus Ulcer

See Pressure Ulcer

Deep Vein Thrombosis

See DVT

Defensive Behavior

Defensive **Coping** r/t nonacceptance of blame, denial of problems or weakness

Ineffective **Denial** r/t inability to face situation realistically

Dehiscence, Abdominal

Delayed **Surgical** recovery r/t altered circulation, malnutrition, opening in incision

Fear r/t threat of death, severe dysfunction

Impaired **Skin** integrity r/t altered circulation, malnutrition, opening in incision

Impaired **Tissue** integrity r/t exposure of abdominal contents to external environment

Pain r/t stretching of abdominal wall

Risk for imbalanced **Fluid** volume r/t altered circulation associated with opening of wound and exposure of abdominal contents

Risk for **Infection** r/t loss of skin integrity

Dehydration

Deficient **Fluid** volume r/t active fluid volume loss

Impaired **Oral** mucous membranes r/t decreased salivation, fluid deficit

Ineffective **Health** maintenance r/t deficient knowledge regarding treatment and prevention of dehydration

See cause of Dehydration

Delirium

Acute **Confusion** r/t effects of medication, response to hospitalization, alcohol abuse, substance abuse, sensory deprivation or overload

Adult **Failure** to thrive r/t delirium

Disturbed **Thought** processes r/t head trauma, altered metabolic state, substance abuse, sleep deprivation, sensory deprivation or overload

Impaired **Memory** r/t delirium

Risk for **Injury** r/t altered level of consciousness

Sleep deprivation r/t nightmares

Delirium Tremens (DT)

See Alcohol Withdrawal

Delivery

See Labor—Normal

Delusions

Acute **Confusion** r/t alcohol abuse, delirium, dementia, drug abuse

Adult **Failure** to thrive r/t delusional state

Anxiety r/t content of intrusive thoughts

Disturbed **Thought** processes r/t mental disorder

Impaired verbal **Communication** r/t psychological impairment, delusional thinking

Ineffective **Coping** r/t distortion and insecurity of life events

Risk for **Violence** directed at self or others r/t delusional thinking

Dementia

Adult **Failure** to thrive r/t depression, apathy

Altered **Family** process r/t disability of family member

Chronic **Confusion** r/t neurological dysfunction

D

Chronic **Sorrow** r/t chronic mental illness

Disturbed **Sleep** pattern r/t neurological impairment, naps during the day

Imbalanced **Nutrition: less than body requirements** r/t psychological impairment

Impaired **Environmental** interpretation syndrome r/t dementia

Impaired **Home** maintenance r/t inadequate support system

Impaired physical **Mobility** r/t neuromuscular impairment

Risk for **Caregiver** role strain r/t number of caregiving tasks, duration of caregiving required

Risk for impaired **Skin** integrity r/t altered nutritional status, immobility

Risk for **Injury** r/t confusion, decreased muscle coordination

Self-care deficit: specify r/t psychological or neuromuscular impairment

Total urinary **Incontinence** r/t neuromuscular impairment

Denial of Health Status

Ineffective **Denial** r/t lack of perception about health status effects of illness

Ineffective management of **Therapeutic** regimen r/t denial of seriousness of health situation

Dental Caries

Impaired **Dentition** r/t ineffective oral hygiene, barriers to self-care, economic barriers to professional care, nutritional deficits, dietary habits

Ineffective **Health** maintenance r/t lack of knowledge regarding prevention of dental disease secondary to high-sugar diet, giving infants or toddlers with erupted teeth bottles of milk at bedtime, lack of fluoride treatments, inadequate or improper brushing of teeth

Dentition Problems

See Dental Caries

Depression (Major Depressive Disorder)

Adult **Failure** to thrive r/t depression

Chronic low **Self-esteem** r/t repeated unmet expectations

Chronic **Sorrow** r/t unresolved grief

Constipation r/t inactivity, decreased fluid intake

Death **Anxiety** r/t feelings of lack of self-worth

Disturbed **Sleep** pattern r/t inactivity

Dysfunctional **Grieving** r/t lack of previous resolution of former grieving response

Disturbed **Energy** field r/t disharmony

Fatigue r/t psychological demands

Hopelessness r/t feeling of abandonment, long-term stress

Impaired **Environmental** interpretation syndrome r/t severe mental functional impairment

Ineffective **Coping** r/t dysfunctional grieving

Ineffective **Health** maintenance r/t lack of ability to make good judgments regarding ways to obtain help

Powerlessness r/t pattern of helplessness

Risk for self-directed **Violence** r/t panic state

Self-care deficit: specify r/t depression, cognitive impairment

Sexual dysfunction r/t loss of sexual desire

Social isolation r/t ineffective coping

Dermatitis

Anxiety r/t situational crisis imposed by illness

Impaired **Comfort: pruritus** r/t inflammation of skin

Impaired **Skin** integrity r/t side effect of medication, allergic reaction

Ineffective **Health** maintenance r/t deficient knowledge regarding methods to decrease inflammation

Despondency

Hopelessness r/t long-term stress

See Depression

Destructive Behavior toward Others

Impaired adjustment r/t intense emotional state

Ineffective **Coping** r/t situational crises, maturational crises, personal vulnerability

Risk for other-directed **Violence** r/t history of violence, neurological impairment, cognitive impairment, history of childhood abuse, history of witnessing family violence, cruelty to animals, firesetting, history of alcohol/drug abuse, pathological intoxication, psychotic symptomatology, motor vehicle offenses, impulsivity, availability or possession of weapon, body language

Developmental Concerns

Prenatal

Risk for delayed **Development** r/t maternal age <15 or >35 years; substance abuse; infections; genetic or endocrine disorders; unplanned or unwanted pregnancy; lack of, late, poor prenatal care; inadequate nutrition; illiteracy; poverty

Individual

Risk for delayed **Development** r/t prematurity, seizures, congenital or genetic disorders, positive drug screening test, brain damage (e.g., hemorrhage in postnatal period, shaken baby, abuse, accident), vision impairment, hearing impairment or frequent otitis media, chronic illness, technology dependence, failure to thrive, inadequate nutrition, foster or adopted child, lead poisoning, chemotherapy, radiation therapy, natural disaster, behavior disorders, substance abuse

Environmental

Risk for delayed **Development** r/t poverty, violence

Caregiver

Risk for delayed **Development** r/t abuse, mental illness, mental retardation or severe learning disability

Diabetes in Pregnancy

See Gestational Diabetes

Diabetes Insipidus

Deficient **Fluid** volume r/t inability to conserve fluid

Ineffective **Health** maintenance r/t deficient knowledge regarding care of disease, importance of medications

Diabetes Mellitus

Adult **Failure** to thrive r/t undetected disease process

Disturbed **Sensory** perception r/t ineffective tissue perfusion

Imbalanced **Nutrition: less than body requirements** r/t inability to use glucose (type I [insulin-dependent] diabetes)

Imbalanced **Nutrition: more than body requirements** r/t excessive intake of nutrients (type II diabetes)

Ineffective **Health** maintenance r/t deficient knowledge regarding care of diabetic condition

Ineffective management of **Therapeutic** regimen r/t complexity of therapeutic regimen

Ineffective **Tissue** perfusion: peripheral r/t impaired arterial circulation

Noncompliance r/t restrictive lifestyle; changes in diet, medication, exercise

Powerlessness r/t perceived lack of personal control

Risk for disturbed **Thought** processes r/t hypoglycemia, hyperglycemia

Risk for impaired **Skin** integrity r/t loss of pain perception in extremities

Risk for **Infection** r/t hyperglycemia, impaired healing, circulatory changes

Risk for **Injury:** hypoglycemia or hyperglycemia r/t failure to consume adequate calories, failure to take insulin

Sexual dysfunction r/t neuropathy associated with disease

Diabetes Mellitus, Juvenile (IDDM Type I)

Disturbed **Body** image r/t imposed deviations from biophysical and psychosocial norm, perceived differences from peers

Imbalanced **Nutrition: less than body requirements** r/t inability of body to adequately metabolize and use glucose and nutrients, increased caloric needs of child to promote growth and physical activity participation with peers

Impaired **adjustment** r/t inability to participate in normal childhood activities

Ineffective **Health** maintenance r/t parental/child deficient knowledge regarding dietary management, medication administration, physical activity, and interaction between the three; daily changes in diet, medications, activity associated with child's growth spurts and needs; need to instruct other caregivers and teachers regarding signs and symptoms of hypoglycemia or hyperglycemia and treatment

Pain r/t insulin injections, peripheral blood glucose testing

Risk for delayed **Development** r/t chronic illness

Risk for disproportionate **Growth** r/t chronic illness

Risk for **Noncompliance** r/t disturbed body image, impaired adjustment secondary to adolescent maturational crises

See Diabetes Mellitus; Child with Chronic Illness; Hospitalized Child

Diabetic Coma

Deficient **Fluid** volume r/t hyperglycemia resulting in polyuria

Disturbed **Thought** processes r/t hyperglycemia, presence of excessive metabolic acids

Ineffective management of **Therapeutic** regimen r/t lack of understanding of preventive measures, adequate blood sugar control

Risk for **Infection** r/t hyperglycemia, changes in vascular system

See Diabetes Mellitus

Diabetic Ketoacidosis

See Ketoacidosis

Diabetic Retinopathy

Disturbed **Sensory** perception r/t change in sensory reception

Grieving r/t loss of vision

D

Ineffective **Health** maintenance r/t deficient knowledge regarding preserving vision with treatment if possible, use of low vision aids

See Vision Impairment

Dialysis

See Hemodialysis; Peritoneal Dialysis

Diaphoresis

Impaired **Comfort** r/t excessive sweating

Diaphragmatic Hernia

See Hiatus Hernia

Diarrhea

Diarrhea r/t infection, change in diet, gastrointestinal disorders, stress, medication effect, impaction

DIC (Disseminated Intravascular Coagulation)

Fear r/t threat to well-being
Deficient **Fluid** volume: hemorrhage r/t depletion of clotting factors
Ineffective **Protection** r/t abnormal clotting mechanism
Risk for ineffective **Tissue** perfusion: peripheral r/t hypovolemia from profuse bleeding, formation of microemboli in vascular system

Digitalis Toxicity

Decreased **Cardiac** output r/t drug toxicity affecting cardiac rhythm, rate
Ineffective management of **Therapeutic** regimen r/t deficient knowledge regarding action, appropriate method of administration of digitalis

Dilation and Curettage (D & C)

Ineffective **Health** maintenance r/t deficient knowledge regarding postoperative self-care
Pain r/t uterine contractions
Risk for deficient **Fluid** volume: hemorrhage r/t excessive blood loss during or after procedure
Risk for ineffective **Sexuality** patterns r/t painful coitus, fear associated with surgery on genital area
Risk for **Infection** r/t surgical procedure

Discharge Planning

Deficient **Knowledge** r/t lack of exposure to information for home care
Impaired **Home** maintenance r/t family member's disease or injury interfering with home maintenance
Ineffective **Health** maintenance r/t lack of material sources

Discomforts of Pregnancy

Acute **Pain**: leg cramps r/t nerve compression, calcium/phosphorus/potassium imbalance
Constipation r/t decreased gastrointestinal tract motility, pressure from enlarged uterus, supplementary iron
Disturbed **Body** image r/t pregnancy-induced body changes
Disturbed **Sleep** pattern r/t psychological stress, fetal movement, muscular cramping, urinary frequency, shortness of breath
Fatigue r/t hormonal, metabolic, body changes
Headache r/t vascular and hormonal changes
Hemorrhoids r/t enlarged uterus, constipation, pelvic venous stasis, decreased gastrointestinal tract motility
Impaired **Comfort** r/t hormonal changes (nausea, ptyalism, leukorrhea, urinary frequency), enlarged uterus (shortness of breath, abdominal distention, pruritus, reduced bladder capacity), increased vascularization (nasal stuffiness, varicosities)
Nausea r/t hormone effect
Risk for **Constipation** r/t decreased intestinal motility, inadequate fiber in diet
Risk for **Injury** r/t faintness and/or syncope secondary to vasomotor lability or postural hypotension, venous stasis in lower extremities
Risk for urge urinary **Incontinence** r/t hormone effect, pressure on bladder from growing uterus
Stress urinary **Incontinence** r/t enlarged uterus, fetal movement

Dissecting Aneurysm

Fear r/t threat to well-being
See Abdominal Surgery; Aneurysm

Disseminated Intravascular Coagulation

See DIC

Dissociative Disorder (Not Otherwise Specified)

Anxiety r/t psychosocial stress
Disturbance in **Self-concept** r/t childhood trauma, childhood abuse
Disturbed personal **Identity** r/t inability to distinguish self caused by multiple personality disorder, depersonalization, disturbance in memory
Disturbed **Sensory** perception: kinesthetic r/t underdeveloped ego
Disturbed **Thought** processes r/t repressed anxiety
Impaired **Memory** r/t altered state of consciousness
Ineffective **Coping** r/t personal vulnerability in crisis of accurate self-perception

Distress

Anxiety r/t situational crises, maturational crises

Death **Anxiety** r/t denial of one's own immortality or impending death

Disturbed **Energy** field r/t disruption in flow of energy as result of pain, depression, fatigue, anxiety, stress

Disuse Syndrome, Potential to Develop

Risk for **Disuse** syndrome r/t paralysis, mechanical immobilization, prescribed immobilization, severe pain, altered level of consciousness

Diversional Activity, Lack of

Deficient **Diversional** activity r/t environmental lack of diversional activity as in frequent hospitalizations, lengthy treatments

Diverticulitis

Constipation r/t dietary deficiency of fiber and roughage

Diarrhea r/t increased intestinal motility secondary to inflammation

Deficient **Knowledge** r/t diet needed to control disease, medication regimen

Imbalanced **Nutrition: less than body requirements** r/t loss of appetite

Pain r/t inflammation of bowel

Risk for deficient **Fluid** volume r/t diarrhea

Dizziness

Decreased **Cardiac** output r/t dysfunctional electrical conduction

Impaired physical **Mobility** r/t dizziness

Ineffective **Tissue** perfusion: cerebral r/t interruption of cerebral arterial blood flow

Risk for **Injury** r/t difficulty maintaining balance

Down Syndrome

See Child with Chronic Illness; Mental Retardation

Dress Self (Inability to)

Dressing/grooming **Self-care** deficit r/t intolerance to activity, decreased strength and endurance, pain, discomfort, perceptual or cognitive impairment, neuromuscular impairment, musculoskeletal impairment, depression, severe anxiety

Dribbling of Urine

Stress urinary **Incontinence** r/t degenerative changes in pelvic muscles and structural supports

Drooling

Impaired **Swallowing** r/t neuromuscular impairment, mechanical obstruction

Risk for **Aspiration** r/t impaired swallowing

Drug Abuse

Anxiety r/t threat to self-concept, lack of control of drug use

Disturbed **Sensory** perception: specify r/t substance intoxication

Disturbed **Sleep** pattern r/t effects of medications

Disturbed **Thought** process r/t mind-altering effects of drugs

Imbalanced **Nutrition: less than body requirements** r/t poor eating habits

Impaired adjustment r/t failure to intend to change behavior

Impaired **Social** interaction r/t disturbed thought processes from drug abuse

Ineffective **Coping** r/t situational crisis

Noncompliance r/t denial of illness

Powerlessness r/t feeling unable to change patterns of abuse

Risk for **Injury** r/t hallucinations, drug effects

Risk for **Violence** r/t poor impulse control

Sexual dysfunction r/t actions and side effects of drug abuse

Sleep deprivation r/t prolonged psychological discomfort

Spiritual distress r/t separation from religious, cultural ties

Drug Withdrawal

Acute **Confusion** r/t effects of substance withdrawal

Anxiety r/t physiological withdrawal

Disturbed **Sensory** perception: specify r/t substance intoxication

Disturbed **Sleep** pattern r/t effects of medications

Imbalanced **Nutrition: less than body requirements** r/t poor eating habits

Ineffective **Coping** r/t situational crisis, withdrawal

Noncompliance r/t denial of illness

Risk for **Injury** r/t hallucinations

Risk for **Violence** r/t poor impulse control

See Drug Abuse

DTs (Delirium Tremens)

See Alcohol Withdrawal

DVT (Deep Vein Thrombosis)

Constipation r/t inactivity, bedrest

Delayed **Surgical** recovery r/t impaired physical mobility

D

Impaired physical **Mobility** r/t pain in extremity, forced bedrest

Ineffective **Health** maintenance r/t deficient knowledge regarding self-care needs, treatment regimen, outcome

Ineffective **Tissue** perfusion: peripheral r/t interruption of venous blood flow

Pain r/t vascular inflammation, edema

See Anticoagulant Therapy

Dying Client

See Terminally Ill Adult

Dysfunctional Eating Pattern

Imbalanced **Nutrition:** less than body requirements r/t psychological factors

Risk for imbalanced **Nutrition:** more than body requirements r/t observed use of food as reward or comfort measure

See Anorexia Nervosa; Bulimia

Dysfunctional Family Unit

See Family Problems

Dysfunctional Grieving

Dysfunctional **Grieving** r/t actual or perceived loss

Dysfunctional Ventilatory Weaning

Dysfunctional **Ventilatory** weaning response r/t physical, psychological, situational factors

Dysmenorrhea

Ineffective **Health** maintenance r/t deficient knowledge regarding prevention and treatment of painful menstruation

Nausea r/t prostaglandin effect

Pain r/t cramping from hormonal effects

Dyspareunia

Sexual dysfunction r/t lack of lubrication during intercourse, alteration in reproductive organ function

Dyspepsia

Anxiety r/t pressures of personal role

Ineffective **Health** maintenance r/t deficient knowledge regarding treatment of disease

Pain r/t gastrointestinal disease, consumption of irritating foods

Dysphagia

Impaired **Swallowing** r/t neuromuscular impairment

Risk for **Aspiration** r/t loss of gag or cough reflex

Dysphasia

Impaired **Social** interaction r/t difficulty in communicating

Impaired verbal **Communication** r/t decrease in circulation to brain

Dyspnea

Activity intolerance r/t imbalance between oxygen supply-demand

Anxiety r/t ineffective breathing pattern

Disturbed **Sleep** pattern r/t difficulty breathing, positioning required for effective breathing

Fear r/t threat to state of well-being, potential death

Impaired **Gas** exchange r/t alveolar-capillary damage

Ineffective **Airway** clearance r/t decreased energy, fatigue

Ineffective **Breathing** pattern r/t decreased lung expansion, neurological impairment affecting respiratory center, extreme anxiety

Sleep deprivation r/t ineffective breathing pattern

Dysrhythmia

Activity intolerance r/t decreased cardiac output

Anxiety/fear r/t threat of death, change in health status

Decreased **Cardiac** output r/t altered electrical conduction

Ineffective **Health** maintenance r/t deficient knowledge regarding self-care with disease

Ineffective **Tissue** perfusion: cerebral r/t interruption of cerebral arterial flow secondary to decreased cardiac output

Dysthymic Disorder

Altered **Sexual** pattern r/t loss of sexual desire

Chronic low **Self-esteem** r/t repeated unmet expectations

Disturbed **Sleep** pattern r/t anxious thoughts

Ineffective **Coping** r/t impaired social interaction

Ineffective **Health** maintenance r/t inability to make good judgments regarding ways to obtain help

Social isolation r/t ineffective coping

See Depression

Dystocia

Anxiety r/t difficult labor, deficient knowledge regarding normal labor pattern

Fatigue r/t prolonged labor

Grieving r/t loss of ideal labor experience

Ineffective **Coping** r/t situational crisis

Pain r/t difficult labor, medical interventions

Powerlessness r/t perceived inability to control outcome of labor

Risk for deficient **Fluid** volume r/t hemorrhage secondary to uterine atony

Risk for delayed **Development** r/t difficult labor and birth

Risk for disproportionate **Growth** r/t difficult labor and birth

Risk for ineffective **Tissue** perfusion: cerebral (fetal) r/t difficult labor and birth

Risk for impaired **Tissue** integrity: maternal and fetal r/t difficult labor

Risk for **Infection** r/t prolonged rupture of membranes

Risk for **Post-trauma** syndrome r/t sudden emergency during delivery of infant

Situational low **Self-esteem** r/t perceived inability to have normal labor and delivery

Dysuria

Impaired **Urinary** elimination r/t urinary tract infection

Risk for urge urinary **Incontinence** r/t detrusor hyperreflexia from cystitis, urethritis

E

Ear Surgery

Disturbed **Sensory** perception: hearing r/t invasive surgery of ears, dressings

Ineffective **Health** maintenance r/t deficient knowledge regarding postoperative restrictions, expectations, care

Pain r/t edema in ears from surgery

Risk for delayed **Development** r/t hearing impairment

Risk for **Injury** r/t dizziness from excessive stimuli to vestibular apparatus

See Hospitalized Child

Earache

Disturbed **Sensory** perception: auditory r/t altered sensory reception, transmission, integration

Pain r/t trauma, edema

Eating Disorder

See Anorexia Nervosa; Bulimia; Obesity

Eclampsia

Fear r/t threat of well-being to self and fetus

Interrupted **Family** processes r/t unmet expectations for pregnancy and childbirth

Risk for altered fetal **Tissue** perfusion r/t uteroplacental insufficiency

Risk for **Aspiration** r/t seizure activity

Risk for delayed **Development** r/t uteroplacental insufficiency

Risk for excess **Fluid** volume r/t decreased urine output secondary to renal dysfunction

Risk for imbalanced **Fluid** volume r/t retained fluid, decreased renal activity

Risk for disproportionate **Growth** r/t uteroplacental insufficiency

Risk for **Injury**: maternal r/t seizure activity

ECT (Electroconvulsive Therapy)

Decisional **Conflict** r/t lack of relevant information

Fear r/t real or imagined threat to well-being

Impaired **Memory** r/t effects of treatment

See Depression

Ectopic Pregnancy

Chronic **Sorrow** r/t loss of pregnancy, potential loss of fertility

Deficient **Fluid** volume r/t loss of blood

Disturbed **Body** image r/t negative feelings about body and reproductive functioning

Death **Anxiety** r/t emergency condition, hemorrhage

Fear r/t threat to self, surgery, implications for future pregnancy

Ineffective **Role** performance r/t loss of pregnancy

Pain r/t stretching or rupture of implantation site

Risk for ineffective **Coping** r/t loss of pregnancy

Risk for **Infection** r/t traumatized tissue, blood loss

Risk for interrupted **Family** processes r/t situational crisis

Risk for **Spiritual** distress r/t grief process

Situational low **Self-esteem** r/t loss of pregnancy, inability to carry pregnancy to term

Eczema

Disturbed **Body** image r/t change in appearance from inflamed skin

Ineffective **Health** maintenance r/t deficient knowledge regarding how to decrease inflammation and prevent further outbreaks

Impaired **Skin** integrity r/t side effect of medication, allergic reaction

Pain: pruritus r/t inflammation of skin

Edema

Excess **Fluid** volume r/t excessive fluid intake, cardiac dysfunction, renal dysfunction, loss of plasma proteins

Ineffective **Health** maintenance r/t deficient knowledge regarding treatment of edema

Risk for impaired **Skin** integrity r/t impaired circulation, fragility of skin
See cause of Edema

Elderly

See Aging

Elderly Abuse

See Abuse—Spouse, Parent, or Significant Other

Electroconvulsive Therapy

See ECT

E

Emaciated Person

Adult **Failure** to thrive r/t imbalanced nutrition: less than body requirements
Imbalanced **Nutrition:** less than body requirements r/t inability to ingest food, digest food, absorb nutrients because of biological, psychological, economic factors

Embolectomy

Fear r/t threat of great bodily harm from embolus
Risk for deficient **Fluid** volume: hemorrhage r/t postoperative complication, surgical area
Risk for **Peripheral** neurovascular dysfunction r/t decreased circulation to extremity
See Surgery—Postoperative Care

Emboli

See Pulmonary Embolism

Emesis

Nausea r/t chemotherapy, irritation of gastrointestinal system, stimulation of neuropharmacologic mechanisms
See Vomiting

Emotional Problems

See Coping Problems

Empathy

Health-seeking behaviors r/t desire to attain maximum level of health
Readiness for enhanced community **Coping** r/t social supports, being available for problem solving
Readiness for enhanced family **Coping** r/t basic needs met, desire to move to higher level of health
Readiness for enhanced **Spiritual** well-being r/t desire to establish interconnectedness through spirituality

Emphysema

See COPD

Emptiness

Chronic **Sorrow** r/t unresolved grief
Social isolation r/t inability to engage in satisfying personal relationships
Spiritual distress r/t separation from religious/cultural ties

Encephalitis

See Meningitis/Encephalitis

Endocardial Cushion Defect

See Congenital Heart Disease/Cardiac Anomalies

Endocarditis

Activity intolerance r/t reduced cardiac reserve, prescribed bedrest
Acute **Pain** r/t biological injury, inflammation
Decreased **Cardiac** output r/t inflammation of lining of heart and change in structure of valve leaflets, increased myocardial workload
Ineffective **Health** maintenance r/t deficient knowledge regarding treatment of disease, preventive measures against further incidence of disease
Ineffective **Tissue** perfusion: cardiopulmonary/peripheral r/t high risk for development of emboli
Risk for imbalanced **Nutrition:** less than body requirements r/t fever, hypermetabolic state associated with fever

Endometriosis

Anticipatory **Grieving** r/t possible infertility
Ineffective **Health** maintenance r/t deficient knowledge about disease condition, medications, other treatments
Nausea r/t prostaglandin effect
Pain r/t onset of menses with distention of endometrial tissue
Sexual dysfunction r/t painful coitus

Endometritis

Anxiety r/t prolonged hospitalization, fear of unknown
Hyperthermia r/t infectious process
Ineffective **Health** maintenance r/t deficient knowledge regarding condition, treatment, antibiotic regimen
Pain r/t infectious process in reproductive tract

Enuresis

Ineffective **Health** maintenance r/t unachieved developmental task, neuromuscular immaturity, diseases of urinary system, infections or illnesses such as diabetes mellitus or insipidus, regression in developmental stage secondary to hospitalization or stress, parental deficient knowledge regarding involuntary urination at night after age 6, fluid intake at bedtime, lack of control during sound sleep, male gender

See Toilet Training

Environmental Interpretation Problems

Adult **Failure** to thrive r/t impaired environmental interpretation syndrome

Chronic **Confusion** r/t impaired environmental interpretation syndrome

Disturbed **Thought** processes r/t lack of orientation to person, place, time, circumstances

Impaired **Environmental** interpretation syndrome r/t dementia, Parkinson's disease, Huntington's disease, depression, alcoholism

Impaired **Memory** r/t environmental disturbances

Risk for **Injury** r/t lack of orientation to person, place, time, circumstances

Epididymitis

Anxiety r/t situational crisis, pain, threat to future fertility

Ineffective **Health** maintenance r/t deficient knowledge regarding treatment for pain and infection

Ineffective **Sexuality** patterns r/t edema of epididymis and testes

Pain r/t inflammation in scrotal sac

Epiglottitis

See Respiratory Infections, Acute Childhood

Epilepsy

Anxiety r/t threat to role functioning

Ineffective **Health** maintenance r/t deficient knowledge regarding seizures and seizure control

Impaired **Memory** r/t seizure activity

Ineffective **Therapeutic** regimen management r/t deficient knowledge regarding seizure control

Risk for **Aspiration** r/t impaired swallowing, excessive secretions

Risk for delayed **Development** r/t seizure disorder

Risk for disturbed **Thought** processes r/t excessive, uncontrolled neurological stimuli

Risk for **Injury** r/t environmental factors during seizure

See Seizure Disorders

Episiotomy

Anxiety r/t fear of pain

Disturbed **Body** image r/t fear of resuming sexual relations

Impaired physical **Mobility** r/t pain, swelling, tissue trauma

Impaired **Skin** integrity r/t perineal incision

Pain r/t tissue trauma

Risk for **Infection** r/t tissue trauma

Sexual dysfunction r/t altered body structure, tissue trauma

Epistaxis

Fear r/t large amount of blood loss

Risk for deficient **Fluid** volume r/t excessive fluid loss

Epstein-Barr Virus

See Mononucleosis

Esophageal Varices

Deficient **Fluid** volume: hemorrhage r/t portal hypertension, distended variceal vessels that can easily rupture

Fear r/t threat of death

See Cirrhosis

Esophagitis

Ineffective **Health** maintenance r/t deficient knowledge regarding treatment of disease

Pain r/t inflammation of esophagus

ETOH Withdrawal

See Alcohol Withdrawal

Evisceration

See Dehiscence

Exposure to Hot or Cold Environment

Risk for **Imbalanced** body temperature r/t exposure

External Fixation

Disturbed **Body** image r/t trauma, change to affected part

Risk for **Infection** r/t pressure of pins on skin surface

See Fracture

Eye Surgery

Anxiety r/t possible loss of vision

Disturbed **Sensory** perception: visual r/t surgical procedure

Ineffective **Health** maintenance r/t deficient knowledge regarding postoperative activity, medications, eye care

Risk for **Injury** r/t impaired vision

Self-care deficit r/t impaired vision

See Hospitalized Child; Vision Impairment

E

F

Failure to Thrive, Adult

Adult **Failure** to thrive r/t depression, apathy, fatigue

Failure to Thrive, Nonorganic

Chronic low **Self-esteem**: parental r/t feelings of inadequacy, support system deficiencies, inadequate role model

Delayed **Growth** and development r/t parental deficient knowledge, lack of stimulation, nutritional deficit, long-term hospitalization

Disorganized **Infant** behavior r/t lack of boundaries

Disturbed **Sleep** pattern r/t inconsistency of caretaker, lack of quiet environment

Imbalanced **Nutrition: less than body requirements** r/t inadequate type/amounts of food for infant, inappropriate feeding techniques

Impaired **Parenting** r/t lack of parenting skills, inadequate role modeling

Risk for delayed **Development** r/t failure to thrive

Risk for disproportionate **Growth** r/t failure to thrive

Risk for impaired **Parent/infant attachment** r/t inability of parents to meet infant's needs

Social isolation r/t limited support systems, self-imposed situation

Falls, Risk for

Risk for **Falls** r/t history of falls, physiological factors, cognitive impairment, medication effect, unsafe environment, young child or older adult

Family Problems

Compromised family **Coping** r/t inadequate or incorrect information or understanding by primary person, temporary preoccupation by significant person who is trying to manage emotional conflicts and personal suffering and is unable to perceive or act effectively in regard to client's needs, temporary family disorganization and role changes, other situational or developmental crises the significant person may be facing, little support provided by client for primary person, prolonged disease or disability progression that exhausts supportive capacity of significant people

Disabled family **Coping** r/t significant person with chronically unexpressed feelings such as guilt, anxiety, hostility, despair; dissonant discrepancy of coping styles for dealing with adaptive tasks by significant person and client or among significant people; highly ambivalent family relationships; arbitrary handling of family's resistance to treatment, which tends to solidify defensiveness as it fails to deal adequately with underlying anxiety

Ineffective family **Therapeutic** regimen management r/t complexity of health care system, complexity of therapeutic regimen, decisional conflicts, economic difficulties, excessive demands made on individual or family, family conflict

Interrupted **Family** processes r/t situation transition and/or crises, developmental transition and/or crises

Readiness for enhanced family **Coping** r/t needs sufficiently gratified, adaptive tasks effectively addressed to enable goals of self-actualization to surface

Fatigue

Disturbed **Energy** field r/t disharmony

Fatigue r/t decreased or increased metabolic energy production, overwhelming psychological or emotional demands, increased energy requirements to perform ADLs, excessive social and/or role demands, states of discomfort, altered body chemistry

Fear

Death **Anxiety** r/t fear of death

Fear r/t identifiable physical or psychological threat to person

Febrile Seizures

See Seizure Disorders, Childhood

Fecal Impaction

See Impaction of Stool

Fecal Incontinence

Bowel incontinence r/t neurological impairment, gastrointestinal disorders, anorectal trauma

Feeding Problems—Newborn

Ineffective **Breastfeeding** r/t prematurity, infant anomaly, maternal breast anomaly, previous breast surgery, previous history of breastfeeding failure, infant receiving supplemental feedings with artificial nipple, poor infant sucking reflex, nonsupportive partner and family, deficient knowledge, maternal anxiety or ambivalence

Ineffective **Infant** feeding pattern r/t prematurity, neurological impairment or delay, oral hypersensitivity, prolonged NPO

Interrupted **Breastfeeding** r/t maternal or infant illness, prematurity, maternal employment, contraindications to breastfeeding, need to abruptly wean infant

Risk for delayed **Development** r/t inadequate nutrition

Risk for disproportionate **Growth** r/t feeding problems

Risk for imbalanced **Fluid** volume r/t inability to take in adequate amount of fluids

Femoral Popliteal Bypass

Anxiety r/t threat to or change in health status

Pain r/t surgical trauma, edema in surgical area

Risk for deficient **Fluid** volume: hemorrhage r/t abnormal blood loss

Risk for ineffective **Tissue** perfusion: peripheral r/t impaired arterial circulation

Risk for **Infection** r/t invasive procedure

Risk for peripheral **Neurovascular** dysfunction r/t vascular surgery, emboli

Fetal Alcohol Syndrome

See Infant of Substance-Abusing Mother

Fetal Distress/Nonreassuring Fetal Heart Rate Pattern

Fear r/t threat to fetus

Ineffective **Tissue** perfusion: fetal r/t interruption of umbilical cord blood flow

Ineffective **Tissue** perfusion: placental r/t small or old placenta, interference with gas exchange transplacentally

Fever

Hyperthermia r/t infectious process, damage to hypothalamus, exposure to hot environment, medications, anesthesia, inability or decreased ability to perspire

Ineffective **Thermoregulation** r/t fluctuating environmental temperature, trauma, illness

Fibrocystic Breast Disease

See Breast Lumps

Filthy Home Environment

Impaired **Home** maintenance r/t individual or family member disease or injury, insufficient family organization or planning, impaired cognitive or emotional functioning, lack of knowledge, economic factors

Financial Crisis in the Home Environment

Impaired **Home** maintenance r/t insufficient finances

Fistulectomy

See Hemorrhoidectomy (same nursing care)

Flail Chest

Anxiety r/t difficulty breathing

Impaired spontaneous **Ventilation** r/t paradoxical respirations

Ineffective **Breathing** pattern r/t chest trauma

Flashbacks

Post-trauma syndrome r/t catastrophic event

Risk for **Post-trauma** syndrome r/t occupation (e.g., police, fire, rescue, corrections, emergency room staff, mental health), exaggerated sense of responsibility, perception of event, survivor's role in event, displacement from home, inadequate social support, nonsupportive environment, diminished ego strength, duration of event

Flat Affect

Adult **Failure** to thrive r/t apathy

Hopelessness r/t prolonged activity restriction creating isolation, failing or deteriorating physiological condition, long-term stress, abandonment, lost belief in transcendent values or higher power/God

Risk for **Loneliness** r/t social isolation, lack of interest in surroundings

See Dysthymic Disorder

Fluid Volume Deficit

Deficient **Fluid** volume r/t active fluid loss, failure of regulatory mechanisms

Fluid Volume Excess

Excess **Fluid** volume r/t compromised regulatory mechanism, excess sodium intake

Fluid Volume Imbalance, Risk for

Delayed **Surgical** recovery r/t fluid volume imbalance

Risk for imbalanced **Fluid** volume r/t major invasive surgeries

Foreign Body Aspiration

Impaired **Home** maintenance r/t insufficient family organization or planning, lack of resources or support systems, inability to maintain orderly and clean surroundings

Ineffective **Airway** clearance r/t obstruction of airway

F

Ineffective **Health** maintenance r/t parental deficient knowledge regarding small toys, pieces of toys, nuts, balloons

Risk for **Suffocation** r/t inhalation of small object

See Safety, Childhood

Formula Feeding

Decisional **Conflict**: maternal r/t multiple or divergent sources of information, values conflict, support system deficit

Grieving: maternal r/t loss of desired breastfeeding experience

Ineffective **Health** maintenance r/t maternal deficient knowledge regarding formula feeding

Risk for imbalanced **Nutrition**: more than body requirements r/t composition of formula and bottle feeding, overuse of food for reward or comfort measures

Risk for **Constipation**: infant r/t iron-fortified formula

Risk for **Infection**: infant r/t lack of passive maternal immunity, supine feeding position

Fracture

Deficient **Diversional** activity r/t immobility

Impaired physical **Mobility** r/t limb immobilization

Impaired **Walking** r/t limb immobility

Ineffective **Health** maintenance r/t deficient knowledge regarding care of fracture

Pain r/t muscle spasm, edema, trauma

Risk for impaired **Skin** integrity r/t immobility, presence of cast

Risk for ineffective **Tissue** perfusion r/t immobility, presence of cast

Risk for **Peripheral** neurovascular dysfunction r/t mechanical compression, treatment of fracture

Fractured Hip

See Hip Fracture

Frequency of Urination

Impaired **Urinary** elimination r/t anatomical obstruction, sensory-motor impairment, urinary tract infection

Risk for urge urinary **Incontinence** r/t effects of medications, caffeine, alcohol

Stress urinary **Incontinence** r/t degenerative change in pelvic muscles and structural support

Urge urinary **Incontinence** r/t decreased bladder capacity, irritation of bladder stretch receptors causing spasm, alcohol, caffeine, increased fluids, increased urine concentration, overdistended bladder

Urinary retention r/t high urethral pressure caused by weak detrusor, inhibition of reflex arc, strong sphincter, blockage

Frostbite

Impaired **Skin** integrity r/t freezing of skin

Pain r/t decreased circulation from prolonged exposure to cold

See Hypothermia

Frothy Sputum

See CHF; Pulmonary Edema; Seizure Disorders

Fusion, Lumbar

Anxiety r/t fear of surgical procedure, possible recurring problems

Impaired physical **Mobility** r/t limitations from surgical procedure, presence of brace

Ineffective **Health** maintenance r/t deficient knowledge regarding postoperative mobility restrictions, body mechanics

Pain r/t discomfort at bone donor site

Risk for **Injury** r/t improper body mechanics

Risk for perioperative positioning **Injury** r/t immobilization

G

Gag Reflex, Depressed or Absent

Impaired **Swallowing** r/t neuromuscular impairment

Risk for **Aspiration** r/t depressed cough/gag reflex

Gallop Rhythm

Decreased **Cardiac** output r/t decreased contractility of heart

Gallstones

See Cholelithiasis

Gangrene

Delayed **Surgical** recovery r/t obstruction of arterial flow

Fear r/t possible loss of extremity

Ineffective **Tissue** perfusion: peripheral r/t obstruction of arterial flow

Gas Exchange, Impaired

Impaired **Gas** exchange r/t ventilation-perfusion imbalance

Gastric Surgery

Risk for **Injury** r/t inadvertent insertion of nasogastric tube through gastric incision line
See Abdominal Surgery

Gastric Ulcer

See Ulcer, Peptic

Gastritis

Imbalanced **Nutrition: less than body requirements** r/t vomiting, inadequate intestinal absorption of nutrients, restricted dietary regimen
Pain r/t inflammation of gastric mucosa
Risk for deficient **Fluid** volume r/t excessive loss from gastrointestinal tract secondary to vomiting, decreased intake

Gastroenteritis

Diarrhea r/t infectious process involving intestinal tract
Deficient **Fluid** volume r/t excessive loss from gastrointestinal tract secondary to diarrhea, vomiting
Imbalanced **Nutrition: less than body requirements** r/t vomiting, inadequate intestinal absorption of nutrients, restricted dietary intake
Ineffective **Health** maintenance r/t deficient knowledge regarding treatment of disease
Nausea r/t irritation to gastrointestinal system
Pain r/t increased peristalsis causing cramping
See Gastroenteritis—Child

Gastroenteritis—Child

Impaired **Skin** integrity: diaper rash r/t acidic excretions on perineal tissues
Ineffective **Health** maintenance r/t lack of parental knowledge regarding fluid and dietary changes
Risk for delayed **Development** r/t inadequate nutrition
See Gastroenteritis; Hospitalized Child

Gastroesophageal Reflux

Anxiety/fear: parental r/t possible need for surgical intervention (Nissen fundoplication, gastrostomy tube)
Deficient **Fluid** volume r/t persistent vomiting
Imbalanced **Nutrition: less than body requirements** r/t poor feeding, vomiting
Ineffective **Airway** clearance r/t reflux of gastric contents into esophagus and tracheal or bronchial tree
Ineffective **Health** maintenance r/t deficient knowledge regarding antireflux regimen (e.g., positioning, oral or enteral feeding techniques, medications), possible home apnea monitoring

Pain r/t irritation of esophagus from gastric acids
Risk for **Aspiration** r/t entry of gastric contents in tracheal or bronchial tree
Risk for impaired **Parenting** r/t disruption in bonding secondary to irritable or inconsolable infant
See Child with Chronic Condition; Hospitalized Child

Gastrointestinal Hemorrhage

See GI Bleed

Gastroschisis/Omphalocele

Anticipatory **Grieving** r/t threatened loss of infant, loss of perfect birth or infant secondary to serious medical condition
Impaired **Gas** exchange r/t effects of anesthesia, subsequent atelectasis
Ineffective **Airway** clearance r/t complications of anesthetic effects
Risk for deficient **Fluid** volume r/t inability to feed secondary to condition, subsequent electrolyte imbalance
Risk for **Infection** r/t disrupted skin integrity with exposure of abdominal contents
Risk for **Injury** r/t disrupted skin integrity, ineffective protection
See Hospitalized Child; Premature Infant

Gastrostomy

Risk for impaired **Skin** integrity r/t presence of gastric contents on skin
See Tube Feeding

Genital Herpes

See Herpes Simplex

Genital Warts

See STD

Gestational Diabetes (Diabetes in Pregnancy)

Anxiety r/t threat to self and/or fetus
Impaired fetal **Nutrition: more than body requirements** r/t excessive glucose uptake
Impaired maternal **Nutrition: less than body requirements** r/t decreased insulin production and glucose uptake in cells
Ineffective **Health** maintenance: maternal r/t deficient knowledge regarding care of diabetic condition in pregnancy
Powerlessness r/t lack of control over outcome of pregnancy
Risk for delayed **Development:** fetal r/t endocrine disorder of mother
Risk for disproportionate **Growth:** fetal r/t endocrine disorder of mother

G

Risk for impaired **Tissue** integrity: fetal r/t macrosomia, congenital defects, birth injury

Risk for impaired **Tissue** integrity: maternal r/t delivery of large infant

See Diabetes Mellitus

GI Bleed (Gastrointestinal Bleeding)

Deficient **Fluid** volume r/t gastrointestinal bleeding

Fatigue r/t loss of circulating blood volume, decreased ability to transport oxygen

Fear r/t threat to well-being, potential death

Imbalanced **Nutrition**: less than body requirements r/t nausea, vomiting

Pain r/t irritated mucosa from acid secretion

Risk for ineffective **Coping** r/t personal vulnerability in crisis, bleeding, hospitalization

Gingivitis

Impaired **Dentition** r/t ineffective oral hygiene, barriers to self-care

Impaired **Oral** mucous membrane r/t ineffective oral hygiene

Glaucoma

Disturbed **Sensory** perception: visual r/t increased intraocular pressure

See Vision Impairment

Glomerulonephritis

Acute **Pain** r/t edema of kidney

Excess **Fluid** volume r/t renal impairment

Imbalanced **Nutrition**: less than body requirements r/t anorexia, restrictive diet

Ineffective **Health** maintenance r/t deficient knowledge regarding care of disease

Gonorrhea

Ineffective **Health** maintenance r/t deficient knowledge regarding treatment and prevention of disease

Pain r/t inflammation of reproductive organs

Risk for **Infection** r/t spread of organism throughout reproductive organs

See STD

Gout

Impaired physical **Mobility** r/t musculoskeletal impairment

Ineffective **Health** maintenance r/t deficient knowledge regarding medications and home care

Pain r/t inflammation of affected joint

Grand Mal Seizure

See Seizure Disorders

Grandiosity

Defensive **Coping** r/t inaccurate perception of self and abilities

Graves' Disease

See Hyperthyroidism

Grieving

Anticipatory **Grieving** r/t anticipated significant loss

Chronic **Sorrow** r/t unresolved grief

Dysfunctional **Grieving** r/t actual or perceived significant loss

Grieving r/t actual significant loss; change in life status, style, or function

Groom Self (Inability to)

Dressing/grooming **Self-care** deficit r/t intolerance to activity, decreased strength and endurance pain, discomfort, perceptual or cognitive impairment, neuromuscular impairment, musculoskeletal impairment, depression, severe anxiety

Growth and Development Lag

Delayed **Growth** and development r/t inadequate caretaking, indifference, inconsistent responsiveness, multiple caretakers, separation from significant others, environmental and stimulation deficiencies, effects of physical disability, prescribed dependence

Prenatal

Risk for disproportionate **Growth** r/t congenital/genetic disorders, maternal nutrition, multiple gestation, teratogen exposure, substance use/abuse

Individual

Risk for disproportionate **Growth** r/t infection, prematurity, malnutrition, organic and inorganic factors, caregiver and/or individual maladaptive feeding behaviors, anorexia, insatiable appetite, infection, chronic illness, substance abuse

Environmental

Risk for disproportionate **Growth** r/t deprivation, teratogen, lead poisoning, poverty, violence, natural disasters

See Developmental Concerns

Guillain-Barré Syndrome

Impaired spontaneous **Ventilation** r/t weak respiration muscles

See Neurological Disorders

G

Guilt

Anticipatory **Grieving** r/t potential loss of significant person, animal, prized material possession

Chronic **Sorrow** r/t unresolved grieving

Dysfunctional **Grieving** r/t actual loss of significant person, animal, prized material possession

Readiness for enhanced **Spiritual** well-being r/t desire to be in harmony with self, others, higher power/God

Risk for **Post-trauma** response r/t exaggerated sense of responsibility for traumatic event

Self-esteem disturbance r/t unmet expectations of self

H

Hair Loss

Disturbed **Body** image r/t psychological reaction to loss of hair

Imbalanced **Nutrition: less than body requirements** r/t inability to ingest food because of biological, psychological, economic factors

Halitosis

Impaired **Dentition** r/t ineffective oral hygiene

Impaired **Oral** mucous membranes r/t ineffective oral hygiene

Hallucinations

Acute **Confusion** r/t alcohol abuse, delirium, dementia, drug abuse

Adult **Failure** to thrive r/t altered mental status

Anxiety r/t threat to self-concept

Disturbed **Thought** processes r/t inability to control bizarre thoughts

Ineffective **Coping** r/t distortion and insecurity of life events

Risk for **Self-mutilation** r/t command hallucinations

Risk for self- or other-directed **Violence** r/t catatonic excitement, manic excitement, rage/panic reactions, response to violent internal stimuli

Head Injury

Acute **Confusion** r/t brain injury

Disturbed **Thought** processes r/t pressure damage to brain

Disturbed **Sensory** perception r/t pressure damage to sensory centers in brain

Decreased **Intracranial** adaptive capacity r/t brain injury

Ineffective **Breathing** pattern r/t pressure damage to breathing center in brain stem

Ineffective **Tissue** perfusion: cerebral r/t effects of increased intracranial pressure

See Neurological Disorders

Headache

Acute **Pain:** headache r/t lack of knowledge of pain control techniques or methods to prevent headaches

Disturbed **Energy field** r/t disharmony

Ineffective management of **Therapeutic** regimen r/t lack of knowledge, identification and elimination of aggravating factors

Health Maintenance Problems

Ineffective **Health** maintenance r/t significant alteration in communication skills, lack of ability to make deliberate and thoughtful judgments, perceptual or cognitive impairment, ineffective coping, dysfunctional grieving, unachieved developmental tasks, ineffective family coping, disabling spiritual distress, lack of material resources

Health-Seeking Person

Health-seeking behavior r/t expressed desire for increased control of own personal health

Hearing Impairment

Disturbed **Sensory** perception: auditory r/t altered state of auditory system

Impaired verbal **Communication** r/t inability to hear own voice

Social isolation r/t difficulty with communication

Heart Failure

See CHF

Heart Surgery

See Coronary Artery Bypass Grafting

Heartburn

Ineffective **Health** maintenance r/t deficient knowledge regarding information about factors that cause esophageal reflex

Nausea r/t gastrointestinal irritation

Pain: heartburn r/t gastroesophageal reflux

Risk for imbalanced **Nutrition: less than body requirements** r/t pain after eating

Heat Stroke

Deficient **Fluid** volume r/t profuse diaphoresis

Disturbed **Thought** processes r/t hyperthermia, increased oxygen needs

Hyperthermia r/t vigorous activity, hot environment

H

Helplessness

Chronic **Sorrow** r/t unresolved grief

Hopelessness r/t prolonged activity restriction creating isolation, failing or deteriorating physiological condition, long-term stress, abandonment, lost belief in transcendent values or higher power/God

Powerlessness r/t lifestyle of helplessness

Hematemesis

See GI Bleed

Hematological Disorder

Ineffective **Protection** r/t abnormal blood profile
See cause of Hematological Disorder

Hematuria

Risk for deficient **Fluid** volume r/t excessive loss of blood through urinary system

Hemianopia

Anxiety r/t change in vision

Disturbed **Sensory** perception r/t altered sensory reception, transmission, integration

Risk for **Injury** r/t disturbed sensory perception

Unilateral **Neglect** r/t effects of disturbed perceptual abilities

Hemiplegia

Anxiety r/t change in health status

Disturbed **Body** image r/t functional loss of one side of body

Impaired physical **Mobility** r/t loss of neurological control of involved extremities

Impaired **Transfer** ability r/t partial paralysis

Impaired **Walking** r/t loss of neurological control of involved extremities

Risk for impaired **Skin** integrity r/t alteration in sensation, immobility

Risk for **Injury** r/t impaired mobility

Risk for unilateral **Neglect** r/t neurological impairment; loss of sensation, vision, movement

Self-care deficit: specify r/t neuromuscular impairment

Unilateral **Neglect** r/t effects of disturbed perceptual abilities
See CVA

Hemodialysis

Excess **Fluid** volume r/t renal disease with minimal urine output

Ineffective **Health** maintenance r/t deficient knowledge regarding hemodialysis procedure, restrictions, blood access care

Ineffective **Coping** r/t situational crisis

Interrupted **Family** processes r/t changes in role responsibilities as a result of therapy regimen

Noncompliance: dietary restrictions r/t denial of chronic illness

Powerlessness r/t treatment regimen

Risk for **Caregiver** role strain r/t complexity of care receiver treatment

Risk for deficient **Fluid** volume r/t excessive removal of fluid during dialysis

Risk for **Infection** r/t exposure to blood products, risk for developing hepatitis B or C

Risk for **Injury: clotting of blood access** r/t abnormal surface for blood flow
See Renal Failure; Renal Failure, Acute/Chronic—Child

Hemodynamic Monitoring

Risk for **Infection** r/t invasive procedure

Risk for **Injury** r/t inadvertent wedging of catheter, dislodgement of catheter, disconnection of catheter with embolism

Hemolytic Uremic Syndrome

Deficient **Fluid** volume r/t vomiting, diarrhea

Impaired **Comfort: nausea/vomiting** r/t effects of uremia

Risk for impaired **Skin** integrity r/t diarrhea

Risk for **Injury** r/t decreased platelet count, seizure activity
See Hospitalized Child; Renal Failure, Acute/Chronic—Child

Hemophilia

Fear r/t high risk for AIDS secondary to contaminated blood products

Impaired physical **Mobility** r/t pain from acute bleeds, imposed activity restrictions

Ineffective **Health** maintenance r/t knowledge and skill acquisition regarding home administration of intravenous clotting factors, protection from injury

Ineffective **Protection** r/t deficient clotting factors

Pain r/t bleeding into body tissues

Risk for **Injury** r/t deficient clotting factors, child's developmental level, age-appropriate play, inappropriate use of toys or sports equipment
See Child with Chronic Condition; Hospitalized Child; Maturational Issues, Adolescent

Hemoptysis

Fear r/t serious threat to well-being

Risk for deficient **Fluid** volume r/t excessive loss of blood

Risk for ineffective **Airway** clearance r/t obstruction of airway with blood and mucus

Hemorrhage

Fear r/t threat to well-being
Deficient Fluid volume r/t massive blood loss
See cause of Hemorrhage; Hypovolemic Shock

Hemorrhoidectomy

Anxiety r/t embarrassment, need for privacy
Constipation r/t fear of pain with defecation
Ineffective **Health** maintenance r/t deficient knowledge regarding pain relief, use of stool softeners, dietary changes
Pain r/t surgical procedure
Risk for deficient **Fluid** volume: hemorrhage r/t inadequate clotting
Urinary retention r/t pain, anesthetic effect

Hemorrhoids

Constipation r/t painful defecation, poor bowel habits
Impaired **Comfort:** pruritus r/t inflammation of hemorrhoids
Ineffective **Health** maintenance r/t deficient knowledge regarding care of condition

Hemothorax

Deficient Fluid volume r/t blood in pleural space
See Pneumothorax

Hepatitis

Activity intolerance r/t weakness or fatigue secondary to infection
Acute Pain r/t edema of liver, bile irritating skin
Deficient Diversional activity r/t isolation
Fatigue r/t infectious process, altered body chemistry
Imbalanced **Nutrition: less than body requirements** r/t anorexia, impaired use of proteins and carbohydrates
Ineffective **Health** maintenance r/t deficient knowledge regarding disease process and home management
Risk for deficient **Fluid** volume r/t excessive loss of fluids via vomiting and diarrhea
Social isolation r/t treatment-imposed isolation

Hernia

See Hiatus Hernia; Inguinal Hernia Repair

Herniated Disk

See Low Back Pain

Herniorrhaphy

See Inguinal Hernia Repair

Herpes in Pregnancy

Fear r/t threat to fetus, impending surgery
Impaired **Urinary** elimination r/t pain with urination
Ineffective **Health** maintenance r/t deficient knowledge regarding treatment of disease, protection of fetus
Impaired **Tissue** integrity r/t active herpes lesion
Pain r/t active herpes lesion
Risk for **Infection** transmission r/t transplacental transfer during primary herpes, exposure to active herpes during birth process
Situational low **Self-esteem** r/t threat to fetus secondary to disease process

Herpes Simplex I

Impaired **Dentition** r/t impaired oral mucous membranes
Impaired **Oral** mucous membranes r/t inflammatory changes in mouth

Herpes Simplex II

Acute Pain r/t active herpes lesion
Impaired **Urinary** elimination r/t pain with urination
Impaired **Tissue** integrity r/t active herpes lesion
Ineffective **Health** maintenance r/t deficient knowledge regarding treatment, prevention of spread of disease
Sexual dysfunction r/t disease process
Situational low **Self-esteem** r/t expressions of shame or guilt

Herpes Zoster

See Shingles

HHNC

See Hyperosmolar Hyperglycemic Nonketotic Coma

Hiatus Hernia

Imbalanced **Nutrition: less than body requirements** r/t pain after eating
Ineffective **Health** maintenance r/t deficient knowledge regarding care of disease
Nausea r/t effects of gastric contents in esophagus
Pain: heartburn r/t gastroesophageal reflux

Hip Fracture

Acute Confusion r/t sensory overload, sensory deprivation, medication side effects
Acute Pain r/t injury, surgical procedure
Constipation r/t immobility, narcotics, anesthesia

H

Fear r/t outcome of treatment, future mobility, present helplessness

Impaired physical **Mobility** r/t surgical incision, temporary absence of weight bearing

Impaired **Transfer** ability r/t immobilization of hip

Impaired **Walking** r/t temporary absence of weight bearing

Powerlessness r/t health care environment

Risk for deficient **Fluid** volume: hemorrhage r/t postoperative complication, surgical blood loss

Risk for impaired **Skin** integrity r/t immobility

Risk for **Infection** r/t invasive procedure

Risk for **Injury** r/t dislodged prosthesis, unsteadiness when ambulating

Risk for perioperative positioning **Injury** r/t immobilization, muscle weakness, emaciation

Self-care deficit: specify r/t musculoskeletal impairment

Hip Replacement

See Total Joint Replacement

Hirschsprung's Disease

Acute **Pain** r/t distended colon, incisional postoperative pain

Constipation: bowel obstruction r/t inhibited peristalsis secondary to congenital absence of parasympathetic ganglion cells in distal colon

Grieving r/t loss of perfect child, birth of child with congenital defect even though child expected to be normal within 2 years

Imbalanced **Nutrition**: less than body requirements r/t anorexia, pain from distended colon

Impaired **Skin** integrity r/t stoma, potential skin care problems associated with stoma

Ineffective **Health** maintenance r/t parental deficient knowledge regarding temporary stoma care, dietary management, treatment for constipation or diarrhea

See Hospitalized Child

Hirsutism

Disturbed **Body** image r/t excessive hair

Hitting Behavior

Acute **Confusion** r/t dementia, alcohol abuse, drug abuse, delirium

Impaired adjustment r/t intense emotional state

Ineffective **Coping** r/t situational crises, maturational crises, personal vulnerability

Risk for other-directed **Violence** r/t history of violence, neurological impairment, cognitive impairment, history of childhood abuse, history of witnessing family violence, cruelty to animals, firesetting, history of alcohol/drug abuse, pathological intoxication, psychotic symptomatology, motor vehicle offenses, impulsivity, availability or possession of weapon, body language

HIV (Human Immunodeficiency Virus)

Fear r/t possible death

Ineffective **Protection** r/t depressed immune system

See AIDS

Hodgkin's Disease

See Anemia; Cancer

Home Maintenance Problems

Impaired **Home** maintenance r/t individual or family member disease or injury, insufficient family organization or planning, insufficient finances, unfamiliarity with neighborhood resources, impaired cognitive or emotional functioning, lack of knowledge, lack of role modeling, inadequate support systems

Homelessness

Impaired **Home** maintenance r/t impaired cognitive or emotional functioning, inadequate support system, insufficient finances

Powerlessness r/t interpersonal interactions

Risk for **Trauma** r/t being in high-crime neighborhood

Hopelessness

Chronic **Sorrow** r/t unresolved grief

Hopelessness r/t prolonged activity restriction creating isolation, failing or deteriorating physiological condition, long-term stress, abandonment, lost belief in transcendent values or higher power/God

Powerlessness r/t lifestyle of helplessness

Hospitalized Child

Activity intolerance r/t fatigue associated with acute illness

Anxiety: separation (child) r/t familiar surroundings and separation from family and friends

Compromised family **Coping** r/t possible prolonged hospitalization that exhausts supportive capacity of significant people

Deficient **Diversional** activity r/t immobility, monotonous environment, frequent or lengthy treatments, reluctance to participate, therapeutic isolation, separation from peers

Delayed **Growth** and development r/t regression or lack of progression toward developmental milestones secondary to frequent or prolonged hospitalization, inadequate or inappropriate stimulation, cerebral insult, chronic illness, effects of physical disability, prescribed dependence

Disturbed **Sleep** pattern: child or parent r/t 24-hour care needs of hospitalization

Fear r/t deficient knowledge or maturational level with fear of unknown, mutilation, painful procedures, surgery

Hopelessness: child r/t prolonged activity restriction, uncertain prognosis

Ineffective **Coping**: parent r/t possible guilt regarding hospitalization of child, parental inadequacies

Interrupted **Family** processes r/t situational crisis of illness, disease, hospitalization

Pain r/t treatments, diagnostic or therapeutic procedures

Powerlessness: child r/t health care environment, illness-related regimen

Readiness for enhanced family **Coping** r/t impact of crisis on family values, priorities, goals, relationships in family

Risk for altered parent/child **Attachment** r/t separation

Risk for delayed **Growth** and development: regression r/t disruption of normal routine, unfamiliar environment or caregivers, developmental vulnerability of young children

Risk for imbalanced **Nutrition**: less than body requirements r/t anorexia, absence of familiar foods, cultural preferences

Risk for **Injury** r/t unfamiliar environment, developmental age, lack of parental knowledge regarding safety (e.g., side rails, IV site/pole)

Hostile Behavior

Risk for self- or other-directed **Violence** r/t antisocial personality disorder

HTN (Hypertension)

Disturbed **Energy** field r/t pain, discomfort

Imbalanced **Nutrition**: more than body requirements r/t lack of knowledge of relationship between diet and disease process

Ineffective **Health** maintenance r/t deficient knowledge regarding treatment and control of disease process

Noncompliance r/t side effects of treatments, lack of understanding regarding importance of controlling hypertension

Human Immunodeficiency Virus

See AIDS; HIV

Hydrocele

Altered **Sexuality** pattern r/t recent surgery on area of scrotum

Pain r/t severely enlarged hydrocele

Hydrocephalus

Decisional **Conflict**: cerebral ventricles r/t unclear or conflicting values regarding selection of treatment modality

Delayed **Growth** and development r/t sequelae of increased intracranial pressure

Excess **Fluid** volume: cerebral ventricles r/t compromised regulatory mechanism

Imbalanced **Nutrition**: less than body requirements r/t inadequate intake secondary to anorexia, nausea, vomiting; feeding difficulties

Impaired **Skin** (tissue) integrity r/t impaired physical mobility, mechanical irritation

Ineffective **Tissue** perfusion: cerebral r/t interrupted flow, hypervolemia of cerebral ventricles

Interrupted **Family** processes r/t situational crisis

Risk for delayed **Development** r/t sequelae of increased intracranial pressure

Risk for disproportionate **Growth** r/t sequelae of increased intracranial pressure

Risk for **Infection** r/t sequelae of invasive procedure (shunt placement)

See Child with Chronic Condition; Hospitalized Child; Mental Retardation (if appropriate); Premature Infant

Hygiene, Inability to Provide Own

Adult **Failure** to thrive r/t depression, apathy as evidenced by inability to perform self-care

Bathing/hygiene **Self-care** deficit r/t intolerance to activity, decreased strength and endurance, pain, discomfort, perceptual or cognitive impairment, neuromuscular impairment, musculoskeletal impairment, depression, severe anxiety

Hyperactive Syndrome

Compromised family **Coping** r/t unsuccessful strategies to control excessive activity, behaviors, frustration, anger

Decisional **Conflict** r/t multiple or divergent sources of information regarding education, nutrition, medication regimens; willingness to change own food habits; limited resources

Impaired **Social** interaction r/t impulsive and overactive behaviors, concomitant emotional difficulties, distractibility and excitability

H

Ineffective Role performance: parent r/t stressors associated with dealing with hyperactive child, perceived or projected blame for causes of child's behavior, unmet needs for support or care, lack of energy to provide for those needs

Parental role Conflict: when siblings present r/t increased attention toward hyperactive child

Risk for delayed Development r/t behavior disorders

Risk for impaired Parenting r/t disruptive or uncontrollable behaviors of child

Risk for Violence: parent or child r/t frustration with disruptive behavior, anger, unsuccessful relationship(s)

Self-esteem disturbance/chronic low Self-esteem r/t inability to achieve socially acceptable behaviors; frustration; frequent reprimands, punishment, or scoldings secondary to uncontrolled activity and behaviors; mood fluctuations and restlessness; inability to succeed academically; lack of peer support

Hyperalimentation

See TPN

Hyperbilirubinemia

Anxiety: parents r/t threat to infant, unknown future

Disturbed Sensory perception: visual (infant) r/t use of eye patches for protection of eyes during phototherapy

Imbalanced Nutrition: less than body requirements (infant) r/t disinterest in feeding because of jaundice-related lethargy

Parental role Conflict r/t interruption of family life because of care regimen

Risk for Imbalanced body temperature: infant r/t phototherapy

Risk for disproportionate Growth: infant r/t disinterest in feeding because of jaundice-related lethargy

Risk for Injury: infant r/t kernicterus, phototherapy lights

Hypercalcemia

Decreased Cardiac output r/t bradydysrhythmia

Disturbed Thought processes r/t elevated calcium levels that cause paranoia, decreased level of consciousness

Imbalanced Nutrition: less than body requirements r/t gastrointestinal manifestations of hypercalcemia (nausea, anorexia, ileus)

Impaired physical Mobility r/t decreased tone in smooth and striated muscle

Risk for Trauma r/t risk for fractures

Hypercapnia

Fear r/t difficulty breathing

Impaired Gas exchange r/t ventilation perfusion imbalance

Hyperemesis Gravidarum

Anxiety r/t threat to self and infant, hospitalization

Deficient Fluid volume r/t vomiting

Imbalanced Nutrition: less than body requirements r/t vomiting

Impaired Home maintenance r/t chronic nausea, inability to function

Nausea r/t hormonal changes of pregnancy

Powerlessness r/t health care regimen

Social isolation r/t hospitalization

Hyperglycemia

Ineffective management of Therapeutic regimen r/t complexity of therapeutic regimen, decisional conflicts, economic difficulties, nonsupportive family, insufficient cues to action, deficient knowledge, mistrust, lack of acknowledgement of seriousness of condition

See Diabetes Mellitus

Hyperkalemia

Risk for Activity intolerance r/t muscle weakness

Risk for decreased Cardiac output r/t possible dysrhythmia

Risk for excess Fluid volume r/t untreated renal failure

Hypernatremia

Risk for deficient Fluid volume r/t abnormal water loss, inadequate water intake

Hyperosmolar Hyperglycemic Nonketotic Coma (HHNC)

Deficient Fluid volume r/t polyuria, inadequate fluid intake

Disturbed Thought processes r/t dehydration, electrolyte imbalance

Risk for Injury: seizures r/t hyperosmolar state, electrolyte imbalance

See Diabetes

Hypersensitivity to Slight Criticism

Defensive Coping r/t situational crisis, psychological impairment, substance abuse

Hypertension

Imbalanced **Nutrition**: more than body requirements r/t lack of knowledge of relationship between diet and disease process

Ineffective **Health** maintenance r/t deficient knowledge regarding treatment and control of disease process

Noncompliance r/t side effects of treatment

Hyperthermia

Hyperthermia r/t exposure to hot environment, vigorous activity, medications, anesthesia, inappropriate clothing, increased metabolic rate, illness, trauma, dehydration, inability or decreased ability to perspire

Hyperthyroidism

Activity intolerance r/t increased oxygen demands from increased metabolic rate

Anxiety r/t increased stimulation, loss of control

Diarrhea r/t increased gastric motility

Disturbed **Sleep** pattern r/t anxiety, excessive sympathetic discharge

Imbalanced **Nutrition**: less than body requirements r/t increased metabolic rate, increased gastrointestinal activity

Ineffective **Health** maintenance r/t deficient knowledge regarding medications, methods of coping with stress

Risk for **Injury**: eye damage r/t exophthalmos

Hyperventilation

Ineffective **Breathing** pattern r/t anxiety, acid-base imbalance

Hypocalcemia

Activity intolerance r/t neuromuscular irritability

Imbalanced **Nutrition**: less than body requirements r/t effects of vitamin D deficiency, renal failure, malabsorption, laxative use

Ineffective **Breathing** pattern r/t laryngospasm

Hypoglycemia

Disturbed **Thought** processes r/t insufficient blood glucose to brain

Imbalanced **Nutrition**: less than body requirements r/t imbalance of glucose and insulin level

Ineffective **Health** maintenance r/t deficient knowledge regarding disease process, self-care

See Diabetes

Hypokalemia

Activity intolerance r/t muscle weakness

Decreased **Cardiac** output r/t possible dysrhythmia from electrolyte imbalance

Hypomania

Disturbed **Sleep** pattern r/t psychological stimulus

See Manic Disorder

Hyponatremia

Disturbed **Thought** processes r/t electrolyte imbalance

Excess **Fluid** volume r/t excessive intake of hypotonic fluids

Risk for **Injury** r/t seizures, new onset of confusion

Hypoplastic Left Lung

See Congenital Heart Disease/Cardiac Anomalies

Hypotension

Decreased **Cardiac** output r/t decreased preload, decreased contractility

Disturbed **Thought** processes r/t decreased oxygen supply to brain

Ineffective **Tissue** perfusion: cardiopulmonary/peripheral r/t hypovolemia, decreased contractility, decreased afterload

Risk for deficient **Fluid** volume r/t excessive fluid loss

See cause of Hypotension

Hypothermia

Hypothermia r/t exposure to cold environment, illness, trauma, damage to hypothalamus, malnutrition, aging

Hypothyroidism

Activity intolerance r/t muscular stiffness, shortness of breath on exertion

Constipation r/t decreased gastric motility

Disturbed **Thought** processes r/t altered metabolic process

Imbalanced **Nutrition**: more than body requirements r/t decreased metabolic process

Impaired **Gas** exchange r/t possible respiratory depression

Impaired **Skin** integrity r/t edema, dry or scaly skin

Ineffective **Health** maintenance r/t deficient knowledge regarding disease process and self-care

Hypovolemic Shock

See Shock

H

Hypoxia

Acute **Confusion** r/t decreased oxygen supply to brain

Disturbed **Thought** processes r/t decreased oxygen supply to brain

Fear r/t breathlessness

Impaired **Gas** exchange r/t altered oxygen supply, inability to transport oxygen

Impaired **Memory** r/t hypoxia

Ineffective **Airway** clearance r/t decreased energy and fatigue, increased secretions

Hysterectomy

Acute **Pain** r/t surgical injury

Anticipatory **Grieving** r/t change in body image, loss of reproductive status

Constipation r/t opioids, anesthesia, bowel manipulation during surgery

Ineffective **Coping** r/t situational crisis of surgery

Ineffective **Health** maintenance r/t deficient knowledge regarding precautions and self-care following surgery

Risk for **Constipation** r/t narcotics, anesthesia, bowel manipulation during surgery

Risk for deficient **Fluid** volume r/t abnormal blood loss, hemorrhage

Risk for ineffective **Tissue** perfusion r/t thromboembolism

Risk for urge urinary **Incontinence** r/t edema in area, anesthesia, narcotics, pain

Risk for **Urinary** retention r/t edema in area, anesthesia, opioids, pain

Sexual dysfunction r/t disturbance in self-concept

See Surgery

I

IBS (Irritable Bowel Syndrome)

Chronic **Pain** r/t spasms, increased motility of bowel

Constipation r/t low-residue diet, stress

Diarrhea r/t increased motility of intestines associated with stress

Ineffective **Health** maintenance r/t deficient knowledge regarding self-care with IBS

Ineffective management of **Therapeutic** regimen r/t deficient knowledge, powerlessness

IDDM (Insulin-Dependent Diabetes)

See Diabetes Mellitus

Identity Disturbance

Disturbed personal **Identity** r/t situational crisis, psychological impairment, chronic illness, pain

Idiopathic Thrombocytopenic Purpura

See ITP

Ileal Conduit

Altered **Sexuality** pattern r/t altered body function and structure

Deficient **Knowledge** r/t care of stoma

Disturbed **Body** image r/t presence of stoma

Ineffective management of **Therapeutic** regimen r/t new skills required to care for appliance and self

Risk for impaired **Skin** integrity r/t difficulty obtaining tight seal of appliance

Social isolation r/t alteration in physical appearance, fear of accidental spill of ostomy contents

Ileostomy

Altered **Sexuality** pattern r/t altered body function and structure

Chronic **Sorrow** r/t physical changes associated with presence of stoma

Constipation/diarrhea r/t dietary changes, change in intestinal motility

Deficient **Knowledge** r/t limited practice of stoma care, dietary modifications

Disturbed **Body** image r/t presence of stoma

Ineffective management of **Therapeutic** regimen r/t new skills required to care for appliance and self

Risk for impaired **Skin** integrity r/t difficulty obtaining tight seal of appliance, caustic drainage

Social isolation r/t alteration in physical appearance, fear of accidental spill of ostomy contents

Ileus

Acute **Pain** r/t pressure, abdominal distention

Constipation r/t decreased gastric motility

Deficient **Fluid** volume r/t loss of fluids from vomiting, fluids trapped in bowel

Nausea r/t gastrointestinal irritation

Immobility

Adult **Failure** to thrive r/t limited physical mobility

Constipation r/t immobility

Disturbed **Thought** process r/t sensory deprivation from immobility

Disuse syndrome r/t immobilization

Impaired physical **Mobility** r/t medically imposed bedrest

Impaired **Transfer** r/t limited physical mobility

Impaired **Walking** r/t limited physical mobility

Ineffective **Breathing** pattern r/t inability to deep breathe in supine position

Ineffective **Tissue** perfusion: peripheral r/t interruption of venous flow

Powerlessness r/t forced immobility from health care environment

Risk for impaired Skin integrity r/t pressure on immobile parts, shearing forces when moving

Immunosuppression

Ineffective Protection r/t medications/treatments suppressing immune system function

Risk for Infection r/t immunosuppression

Impaction of Stool

Constipation r/t decreased fluid intake, less than adequate amounts of fiber and bulk-forming foods in diet, immobility

Imperforate Anus

Anxiety r/t ability to care for newborn

Deficient Knowledge r/t home care for newborn

Impaired Skin integrity r/t pruritus

Risk for impaired Skin integrity r/t presence of stool at surgical repair site

Impetigo

Ineffective Health maintenance r/t parental deficient knowledge regarding care of impetigo

See Communicable Diseases, Childhood

Impotence

Self-esteem disturbance r/t physiological crisis, inability to practice usual sexual activity

Sexual dysfunction r/t altered body function

Inactivity

Impaired physical Mobility r/t intolerance to activity, decreased strength and endurance, depression, severe anxiety, musculoskeletal impairment, perceptual or cognitive impairment, neuromuscular impairment, pain, discomfort

Risk for Constipation r/t insufficient physical activity

Incompetent Cervix

See Premature Dilation of the Cervix

Incontinence of Stool

Bowel incontinence r/t decreased awareness of need to defecate, loss of sphincter control

Deficient Knowledge r/t lack of information on normal bowel elimination

Disturbed Body image r/t inability to control elimination of stool

Risk for impaired Skin integrity r/t presence of stool

Situational low Self-esteem r/t inability to control elimination of stool

Toileting Self-care deficit r/t toileting needs

Incontinence of Urine

Functional Incontinence r/t altered environment; sensory, cognitive, or mobility deficits

Reflex Incontinence r/t neurological impairment

Risk for impaired Skin integrity r/t presence of urine

Risk for urge urinary Incontinence r/t effects of alcohol, caffeine, decreased bladder capacity, irritation of bladder stretch receptors causing spasm, increased urine concentration, overdistention of bladder

Self-care deficit: toileting r/t toileting needs

Situational low Self-esteem r/t inability to control passage of urine

Stress urinary Incontinence r/t degenerative change in pelvic muscles and structural supports associated with increased age, high intraabdominal pressure (e.g., from obesity, gravid uterus), incompetent bladder outlet, overdistention between voidings, weak pelvic muscles and structural supports

Total urinary Incontinence r/t neuropathy preventing transmission of reflex indicating bladder fullness, neurological dysfunction causing triggering of micturition at unpredictable times, independent contraction of detrusor reflex resulting from surgery, trauma or disease affecting spinal cord nerves, anatomical fistula

Urge urinary Incontinence r/t decreased bladder capacity (i.e., history of pelvic inflammatory disease, abdominal surgeries, indwelling urinary catheter), irritation of bladder stretch receptors causing spasm (e.g., bladder infection), alcohol, caffeine, increased fluids, increased urine concentration, overdistention of bladder

Indigestion

Impaired Comfort r/t burning, bloating, heaviness, unpleasant sensations experienced when eating

Imbalanced Nutrition: less than body requirements r/t discomfort when eating

Nausea r/t gastrointestinal irritation

Induction of Labor

Anxiety r/t medical interventions

Decisional Conflict r/t perceived threat to idealized birth

Ineffective Coping r/t situational crisis of medical intervention in birthing process

Risk for imbalanced Fluid volume r/t intravenous fluid therapy

I

Risk for **Injury:** maternal and fetal r/t hypertonic uterus, potential prematurity of newborn

Self-esteem disturbance r/t inability to carry out normal labor

Infant Apnea

See Premature Infant; Respiratory Conditions of the Neonate; SIDS

Infant Behavior

Disorganized **Infant** behavior r/t pain, oral/motor problems, feeding intolerance, environmental overstimulation, lack of containment/boundaries, prematurity, invasive/painful procedures

Readiness for enhanced organized **Infant** behavior r/t prematurity, pain

Risk for disorganized **Infant** behavior r/t pain, oral/motor problems, environmental overstimulation, lack of containment/boundaries

Infant of Diabetic Mother

Deficient **Fluid** volume r/t increased urinary excretion and osmotic diuresis

Delayed **Growth** and development r/t prolonged and severe postnatal hypoglycemia

Imbalanced **Nutrition:** less than body requirements r/t hypotonia, lethargy, poor sucking, postnatal metabolic changes from hyperglycemia to hypoglycemia and hyperinsulinism

Risk for decreased **Cardiac** output r/t increased incidence of cardiomegaly

Risk for delayed **Development** r/t prolonged and severe postnatal hypoglycemia

Risk for disproportionate **Growth** r/t prolonged and severe postnatal hypoglycemia

Risk for impaired **Gas** exchange r/t increased incidence of cardiomegaly, prematurity

See Premature Infant; Respiratory Conditions of Neonate

Infant Feeding Pattern, Ineffective

Ineffective **Infant** feeding pattern r/t prematurity, neurological impairment or delay, oral hypersensitivity, prolonged NPO

Risk for imbalanced **Fluid** volume r/t intravenous fluid therapy, inadequate intake or absorption of fluids, regurgitation

Infant of Substance-Abusing Mother (Fetal Alcohol Syndrome, Crack Baby, Other Drug Withdrawal Infants)

Delayed **Growth** and development r/t effects of maternal use of drugs, effects of neurological impairment, decreased attentiveness to environmental stimuli or inadequate stimuli

Diarrhea r/t effects of withdrawal, increased peristalsis secondary to hyperirritability

Disturbed **Sensory** perception r/t hypersensitivity to environmental stimuli

Disturbed **Sleep** pattern r/t hyperirritability/hypersensitivity to environmental stimuli

Imbalanced **Nutrition:** less than body requirements r/t feeding problems; uncoordinated or ineffective suck and swallow; effects of diarrhea, vomiting, or colic associated with maternal substance abuse

Impaired **Parenting** r/t impaired or absent attachment behaviors, inadequate support systems

Ineffective **Airway** clearance r/t pooling of secretions secondary to lack of adequate cough reflex, effects of viral or bacterial lower airway infection secondary to altered protective state

Ineffective **Infant** feeding pattern r/t uncoordinated or ineffective sucking reflex

Ineffective **Protection** r/t effects of maternal substance abuse

Interrupted **Breastfeeding** r/t use of drugs or alcohol by mother

Risk for delayed **Development** r/t substance abuse

Risk for disproportionate **Growth** r/t substance abuse

Risk for **Infection:** skin, meningeal, respiratory r/t effects of withdrawal

See Cerebral Palsy; Failure to Thrive, Nonorganic; Hospitalized Child; Hyperactive Syndrome; SIDS

Infantile Spasms

See Seizure Disorders, Childhood

Infection

Hyperthermia r/t increased metabolic rate

Ineffective **Protection** r/t inadequate nutrition, abnormal blood profiles, drug therapies, treatments

Infection, Potential for

Risk for **Infection** r/t inadequate primary defenses (e.g., broken skin, traumatized tissue, decrease in ciliary action, stasis of body fluids, change in pH secretions, altered peristalsis), inadequate secondary defenses (e.g., decreased hemoglobin, leukopenia suppressed inflammatory response), immunosuppression, inadequate acquired immunity, tissue destruction and increased environmental exposure, chronic disease, invasive procedures, malnutrition, pharmaceutical agents, trauma, rupture of amniotic membranes, insufficient knowledge to avoid exposure to pathogens

Infertility

Chronic **Sorrow** r/t inability to conceive a child
Ineffective **Therapeutic** regimen management r/t deficient knowledge about infertility
Powerlessness r/t infertility
Risk for **Powerlessness** r/t inability to conceive a child

Inflammatory Bowel Disease (Child and Adult)

Acute **Pain** r/t abdominal cramping and anal irritation
Deficient **Fluid** volume r/t frequent and loose stools
Diarrhea r/t effects of inflammatory changes of the bowel
Imbalanced **Nutrition:** less than body requirements r/t anorexia, decreased absorption of nutrients from gastrointestinal tract
Impaired **Skin** integrity r/t frequent stools, development of anal fissures
Ineffective **Coping** r/t repeated episodes of diarrhea
Social isolation r/t diarrhea
See Child with Chronic Condition; Crohn's Disease; Hospitalized Child; Maturational Issues, Adolescent

Influenza

Acute **Pain** r/t inflammatory changes in joints
Deficient **Fluid** volume r/t inadequate fluid intake
Hyperthermia r/t infectious process
Ineffective **Health** maintenance r/t deficient knowledge regarding self-care
Ineffective **Therapeutic** regimen management r/t lack of knowledge regarding preventive immunizations

Inguinal Hernia Repair

Acute **Pain** r/t surgical procedure
Impaired physical **Mobility** r/t pain at surgical site and fear of causing hernia to "break open"
Risk for **Infection** r/t surgical procedure
Urinary retention r/t possible edema at surgical site

Injury

Risk for **Falls** r/t orthostatic hypertension, impaired physical mobility, diminished mental status
Risk for **Injury** r/t environmental conditions interacting with client's adaptive and defensive resources

Insomnia

Anxiety r/t actual or perceived loss of sleep
Disturbed **Sleep** pattern r/t sensory alterations, internal factors, external factors

Sleep deprivation r/t sustained inadequate sleep hygiene, prolonged use of pharmacologic agents, aging-related sleep stage shifts

Insulin Shock

See Hypoglycemia

Intermittent Claudication

Acute **Pain** r/t decreased circulation to extremities with activity
Deficient **Knowledge** r/t lack of knowledge of cause and treatment of peripheral vascular diseases
Ineffective **Tissue** perfusion: peripheral r/t interruption of arterial flow
Risk for **Injury** r/t tissue hypoxia
Risk for **Peripheral** neurovascular dysfunction r/t disruption in arterial flow
See Peripheral Vascular Disease

Internal Cardioverter Defibrillator

See AICD

Internal Fixation

Impaired **Walking** r/t repair of fracture
Risk for **Infection** r/t traumatized tissue, broken skin
See Fracture

Interstitial Cystitis

Acute **Pain** r/t inflammatory process
Impaired **Urinary** elimination r/t inflammation of bladder
Risk for **Infection** r/t suppressed inflammatory response
Risk for urge urinary **Incontinence** r/t effects of alcohol, caffeine, decreased bladder capacity, irritation of bladder stretch receptors causing spasm, increased urine concentration, overdistention of bladder

Intervertebral Disk Excision

See Laminectomy

Intestinal Obstruction

See Ileus

Intoxication

Acute **Confusion** r/t alcohol abuse
Anxiety r/t loss of control of actions
Disturbed **Thought** processes r/t effect of substance on central nervous system
Ineffective **Coping** r/t use of mind-altering substances as a means of coping

I

Risk for **Falls** r/t diminished mental status

Risk for other-directed **Violence** r/t inability to control thoughts and actions

Disturbed **Sensory** perception r/t neurochemical imbalance in brain

Intraaortic Balloon Counterpulsation

Anxiety r/t device providing cardiovascular assistance

Compromised family **Coping** r/t seriousness of significant other's medical condition

Decreased **Cardiac** output r/t failing heart needing counterpulsation

Impaired physical **Mobility** r/t restriction of movement because of mechanical device

Risk for **Peripheral** neurovascular dysfunction r/t vascular obstruction of balloon catheter, thrombus formation, emboli, edema

Intracranial Pressure, Increased

Acute **Confusion** r/t increased intracranial pressure

Adult **Failure** to thrive r/t undetected changes from increased intracranial pressure

Decreased **Intracranial** adaptive capacity r/t sustained increase in intracranial pressure (10 to 15 mm Hg)

Disturbed **Thought** processes r/t pressure damage to brain

Ineffective **Tissue** perfusion: cerebral r/t effects of increased intracranial pressure

Ineffective **Breathing** pattern r/t pressure damage to breathing center in brain stem

Disturbed **Sensory** perception r/t pressure damage to sensory centers in brain

See cause of Increased Intracranial Pressure

Intrauterine Growth Retardation

Anxiety: maternal r/t threat to fetus

Delayed **Growth** and development r/t insufficient supply of oxygen and nutrients

Imbalanced **Nutrition:** less than body requirements r/t insufficient placenta

Impaired **Gas** exchange r/t insufficient placental perfusion

Ineffective **Coping:** maternal r/t situational crisis, threat to fetus

Risk for delayed **Development** r/t insufficient supply of oxygen and nutrients

Risk for disproportionate **Growth** r/t insufficient supply of oxygen and nutrients

Risk for **Injury** r/t insufficient supply of oxygen and nutrients

Risk for **Powerlessness** r/t unknown outcome of fetus

Situational low **Self-esteem:** maternal r/t guilt about threat to fetus

Intubation—Endotracheal or Nasogastric

Disturbed **Body** image r/t altered appearance with mechanical devices

Imbalanced **Nutrition:** less than body requirements r/t inability to ingest food resulting from presence of tubes

Impaired **Oral** mucous membrane r/t presence of tubes

Impaired verbal **Communication** r/t endotracheal tube

Irregular Pulse

See Dysrhythmia

Irritable Bowel Syndrome

See IBS

Isolation

Adult **Failure** to thrive r/t depression

Risk for **Loneliness** r/t lack of affection, physical isolation, cathectic deprivation, social isolation

Risk for situational low **Self-esteem** r/t decreased power, control over environment

Social isolation r/t factors contributing to absence of satisfying personal relationships, such as delay in accomplishing developmental tasks, immature interests, alterations in mental status, unacceptable social behavior, unacceptable social values, altered state of wellness, inadequate personal resources, inability to engage in satisfying personal relationships

Itching

Impaired **Comfort** r/t irritation of the skin

Risk for **Infection** r/t potential break in skin

ITP (Idiopathic Thrombocytopenic Purpura)

Deficient **Diversional** activity r/t activity restrictions, safety precautions

Impaired **Home** health maintenance r/t parental lack of ability to follow through with safety precautions secondary to child's developmental stage (active toddler)

Ineffective **Protection** r/t decreased platelet count

Risk for **Injury** r/t decreased platelet count, developmental level, age-appropriate play

See Hospitalized Child

J

Jaundice

Disturbed **Thought** processes r/t toxic blood metabolites

Impaired **Comfort:** pruritus r/t toxic metabolites excreted in the skin

Risk for impaired **Skin** integrity r/t pruritus, itching
See Cirrhosis

Jaw Surgery

Acute **Pain** r/t surgical procedure

Imbalanced **Nutrition: less than body requirements** r/t jaws wired closed

Deficient **Knowledge** r/t emergency care for wired jaws (e.g., cutting bands and wires), oral care

Impaired **Swallowing** r/t edema from surgery

Risk for **Aspiration** r/t wired jaws

Jittery

Anxiety r/t unconscious conflict about essential values and goals, threat to or change in health status

Death **Anxiety** r/t unresolved issues relating to end of life

Risk for **Post-trauma** syndrome r/t occupation, survivor's role in event, inadequate social support

Jock Itch

Ineffective **Therapeutic** regimen management r/t prevention and treatment
See Itching

Joint Replacement

Risk for **Peripheral** neurovascular dysfunction r/t orthopedic surgery
See Total Joint Replacement

JRA (Juvenile Rheumatoid Arthritis)

See Rheumatoid Arthritis, Juvenile

K

Kaposi's Sarcoma

See AIDS

Kawasaki Syndrome (Formerly Called "Mucocutaneous Lymph Node Syndrome")

Acute **Pain** r/t enlarged lymph nodes; erythematous skin rash that progresses to desquamation, peeling, and denuding of skin

Anxiety: parental r/t progression of disease, complications of arthritis and cardiac involvement

Hyperthermia r/t inflammatory disease process

Imbalanced **Nutrition: less than body requirements** r/t impaired oral mucous membrane

Impaired **Oral** mucous membrane r/t inflamed mouth and pharynx; swollen lips that become dry, cracked, and fissured

Impaired **Skin** integrity r/t inflammatory skin changes
See Hospitalized Child

Kegel Exercise

Health-seeking behavior r/t desire for information to relieve incontinence

Risk for urge urinary **Incontinence** r/t effects of alcohol, caffeine, decreased bladder capacity, irritation of bladder stretch receptors causing spasm, increased urine concentration, overdistention of bladder

Stress urinary **Incontinence** r/t degenerative change in pelvic muscles

Urge urinary **Incontinence** r/t decreased bladder capacity

Ketoacidosis

Deficient **Fluid** volume r/t excess excretion of urine, nausea, vomiting, increased respiration

Imbalanced **Nutrition: less than body requirements** r/t body's inability to use nutrients

Impaired **Memory** r/t fluid and electrolyte imbalance

Ineffective **Therapeutic** regimen management r/t denial of illness, lack of understanding of preventive measures and adequate blood sugar control

Noncompliance: diabetic regimen r/t ineffective coping with chronic disease

Risk for **Powerlessness** r/t illness-related regimen
See Diabetes Mellitus

Kidney Failure

See Renal Failure

Kidney Stone

Acute **Pain** r/t obstruction from renal calculi

Deficient **Knowledge** r/t fluid requirements and dietary restrictions

Impaired **Urinary** elimination: urgency and frequency r/t anatomical obstruction, irritation caused by stone

Risk for deficient **Fluid** volume r/t nausea, vomiting

Risk for **Infection** r/t obstruction of urinary tract with stasis of urine

 K

Knee Replacement

See Total Joint Replacement

Deficient Knowledge

Deficient **Knowledge** r/t lack of exposure, lack of recall, information misinterpretation, cognitive limitation, lack of interest in learning, unfamiliarity with information resources

Ineffective **Health** maintenance r/t lack of or significant alteration in communication skills (written, verbal, and/or gestural)

Kock Pouch

See Continent Ileostomy

Korsakoff's Syndrome

Acute **Confusion** r/t alcohol abuse

Impaired **Memory** r/t neurological changes

Risk for imbalanced **Nutrition: less than body requirements** r/t lack of adequate balanced intake

Risk for **Falls** r/t cognitive impairment

Risk for **Injury** r/t sensory dysfunction, lack of coordination when ambulating

L

Labor, Induction of

See Induction of Labor

Labor, Normal

Acute **Pain** r/t uterine contractions, stretching of cervix and birth canal

Anxiety r/t fear of the unknown, situational crisis

Death **Anxiety** r/t threat of maternal mortality

Deficient **Knowledge** r/t lack of preparation for labor

Fatigue r/t childbirth

Health-seeking behaviors r/t healthy outcome of pregnancy, prenatal care, and childbirth education

Impaired **Tissue** integrity r/t passage of infant through birth canal, episiotomy

Risk for deficient **Fluid** volume r/t excessive loss of blood

Risk for **Infection** r/t multiple vaginal examinations, tissue trauma, prolonged rupture of membranes

Risk for **Injury:** fetal r/t hypoxia

Risk for **Post-trauma** syndrome r/t trauma or violence associated with labor pains, birth process, medical/surgical interventions, history of sexual abuse

Risk for **Powerlessness** r/t labor process

Laminectomy

Acute **Pain** r/t localized inflammation and edema

Anxiety r/t change in health status, surgical procedure

Deficient **Knowledge** r/t appropriate postoperative and postdischarge activities

Impaired physical **Mobility** r/t neuromuscular impairment

Risk for impaired **Tissue** perfusion r/t edema, hemorrhage, or embolism

Risk for perioperative positioning **Injury** r/t prone position

Disturbed **Sensory** perception: tactile r/t possible edema or nerve injury

Urinary retention r/t competing sensory impulses, effects of narcotics/anesthesia

See Scoliosis; Surgery

Laparotomy

See Abdominal Surgery

Laparoscopic Laser Cholecystectomy

See Cholecystectomy; Laser Surgery

Laryngectomy

Anticipatory **Grieving** r/t loss of voice, fear of death

Chronic **Sorrow** r/t change in body image

Death **Anxiety** r/t unknown results of surgery

Disturbed **Body** image r/t change in body structure and function

Interrupted **Family** processes r/t surgery, serious condition of family member, difficulty communicating

Imbalanced **Nutrition: less than body requirements** r/t absence of oral feeding, difficulty swallowing, increased need for fluids

Impaired **Oral** mucous membrane r/t absence of oral feeding

Impaired **Swallowing** r/t edema, laryngectomy tube

Impaired verbal **Communication** r/t removal of larynx

Ineffective **Airway** clearance r/t surgical removal of glottis, decreased humidification of air

Ineffective **Health** maintenance r/t deficient knowledge regarding self-care with laryngectomy

Risk for **Infection** r/t invasive procedure, surgery

Risk for **Powerlessness** r/t chronic illness, change in communication

Risk for situational low **Self-esteem** r/t disturbed body image

Laser Surgery

Acute **Pain** r/t heat from laser

Constipation r/t laser intervention in vulval and perianal areas

Deficient **Knowledge** r/t preoperative and postoperative care associated with laser procedure

Risk for **Infection** r/t delayed heating reaction of tissue exposed to laser

Risk for **Injury** r/t accidental exposure to laser beam

Latex Allergy

Latex **Allergy** r/t hypersensitivity to natural latex rubber

Risk for latex **Allergy** response r/t multiple surgical procedures, especially from infancy (e.g., spina bifida); allergies to bananas, avocados, tropical fruits, kiwi, chestnuts; professions with daily exposure to latex (e.g., medicine, nursing, dentistry); conditions needing continuous or intermittent catheterization; history of reactions to latex (e.g., balloons, condoms, gloves); allergies to poinsettia plants; history of allergies and asthma

Laxative Abuse

Perceived **Constipation** r/t health belief, faulty appraisal, impaired thought processes

Lens Implant

See Cataract Extraction

Lethargy/Listlessness

Adult **Failure** to thrive r/t apathy

Disturbed **Sleep** pattern r/t internal or external stressors

Fatigue r/t decreased metabolic energy production

Ineffective **Tissue** perfusion: cerebral r/t lack of oxygen supply to brain

See cause of Lethargy/Listlessness

Leukemia

Ineffective **Protection** r/t abnormal blood profile

Risk for deficient **Fluid** volume r/t nausea, vomiting, bleeding, side effects of treatment

Risk for **Infection** r/t ineffective immune system

See Cancer; Chemotherapy

Leukopenia

Risk for **Infection** r/t low white blood cell count

Level of Consciousness, Decreased

See Confusion

Lice

See Communicable Diseases, Childhood

Limb Reattachment Procedures

Anticipatory **Grieving** r/t unknown outcome of reattachment procedure

Anxiety r/t unknown outcome of reattachment procedure, use and appearance of limb

Disturbed **Body** image r/t unpredictability of function and appearance of reattached body part

Risk for deficient **Fluid** volume: hemorrhage r/t severed vessels

Risk for perioperative positioning **Injury** r/t immobilization

Risk for **Peripheral** neurovascular dysfunction r/t trauma, orthopedic and neurovascular surgery, compression of nerves and blood vessels

Risk for **Powerlessness** r/t unknown outcome of procedure

See Surgery, Postoperative Care

Liver Biopsy

Anxiety r/t procedure and results

Risk for deficient **Fluid** volume r/t hemorrhage from biopsy site

Risk for **Powerlessness** r/t inability to control outcome of procedure

Liver Disease

See Cirrhosis; Hepatitis

Living Will

See Advanced Directives

Lobectomy

See Thoracotomy

Loneliness

Risk for **Loneliness** r/t lack of affection, physical isolation, cathectic deprivation, social isolation

Risk for situational low **Self-esteem** r/t failure, rejection

Loose Stools

Diarrhea r/t increased gastric motility

See cause of Loose Stools

Low Back Pain

Chronic **Pain** r/t degenerative processes, musculotendinous strain, injury, inflammation, congenital deformities

Ineffective **Health** maintenance r/t deficient knowledge regarding self-care with back pain

Impaired physical **Mobility** r/t back pain

L

Risk for **Powerlessness** r/t living with chronic pain

Urinary retention r/t possible spinal cord compression

Lumbar Puncture

Acute **Pain:** headache r/t possible loss of cerebrospinal fluid

Anxiety r/t invasive procedure and unknown results

Deficient **Knowledge** r/t information about procedure

Risk for **Infection** r/t invasive procedure

Lung Cancer

See Cancer; Thoracotomy

Lupus Erythematosus

Acute **Pain** r/t inflammatory process

Chronic **Sorrow** r/t presence of chronic illness

Disturbed **Body** image r/t change in skin, rash, lesions, ulcers, mottled erythema

Fatigue r/t increased metabolic requirements

Ineffective **Health** maintenance r/t deficient knowledge regarding medication, diet, and activity

Powerlessness r/t unpredictability of course of disease

Risk for impaired **Skin** integrity r/t chronic inflammation, edema, altered circulation

Spiritual distress r/t chronicity of disease, unknown etiology

Lyme Disease

Acute **Pain** r/t inflammation of joints, urticaria, rash

Deficient **Knowledge** r/t lack of information concerning disease, prevention, and treatment

Fatigue r/t increased energy requirements

Risk for decreased **Cardiac** output r/t dysrhythmia

Risk for **Powerlessness** r/t possible chronic condition

Lymphedema

Disturbed **Body** image r/t change in appearance of body part with edema

Excess **Fluid** volume r/t compromised regulatory system; inflammation, obstruction, or removal of lymph glands

Deficient **Knowledge** r/t management of condition

Risk for situational low **Self-esteem** r/t disturbed body image

Lymphoma

See Cancer

M

Mad Cow Disease

See Creutzfeldt-Jakob Disease (CJD)

Magnetic Resonance Imaging

See MRI

Major Depressive Disorder

See Depression

Malabsorption Syndrome

Deficient **Knowledge** r/t lack of information about diet and nutrition

Diarrhea r/t lactose intolerance, gluten sensitivity, resection of small bowel

Imbalanced **Nutrition:** less than body requirements r/t inability of body to absorb nutrients because of biological factors

Risk for deficient **Fluid** volume r/t diarrhea

Maladaptive Behavior

See Crisis; Post-Trauma Syndrome; Risk for Post-Trauma Syndrome; Suicide Attempt

Malnutrition

Adult **Failure** to thrive r/t undetected malnutrition

Deficient **Knowledge** r/t misinformation about normal nutrition, social isolation, lack of food preparation facilities

Imbalanced **Nutrition:** less than body requirements r/t inability to ingest food, digest food, or absorb nutrients because of biological, psychological, or economic factors; institutionalization (i.e., lack of menu choices)

Ineffective **Protection** r/t inadequate nutrition

Ineffective **Therapeutic** regimen management r/t economic difficulties

Risk for **Powerlessness** r/t possible inability to provide adequate nutrition

Manic Disorder, Bipolar I

Anxiety r/t change in role function

Deficient **Fluid** volume r/t decreased intake

Disturbed **Thought** processes r/t mania

Disturbed **Sleep** pattern r/t constant anxious thoughts

Imbalanced **Nutrition:** less than body requirements r/t lack of time and motivation to eat, constant movement

Impaired **Home** maintenance r/t altered psychological state, inability to concentrate

Ineffective **Coping** r/t situational crisis

Ineffective **Denial** r/t fear of inability to control behavior

Ineffective **Role** performance r/t impaired social interactions

Interrupted **Family** processes r/t family member's illness

Ineffective **Therapeutic** regimen management r/t lack of social supports

Ineffective **Therapeutic** regimen management: families r/t unpredictability of client, excessive demands on family, chronicity of condition

Noncompliance r/t denial of illness

Risk for **Caregiver** role strain r/t unpredictability of condition, mood swings

Risk for **Powerlessness** r/t inability to control changes in mood

Risk for self- or other-directed **Violence** r/t hallucinations, delusions

Risk for **Suicide** r/t bipolar disorder

Sleep deprivation r/t hyperagitated state

Manipulative Behavior

Defensive **Coping** r/t superior attitude toward others

Impaired **Social** interaction r/t self-concept disturbance

Ineffective **Coping** r/t inappropriate use of defense mechanisms

Risk for **Loneliness** r/t inability to interact appropriately with others

Risk for **Self-mutilation** r/t inability to cope with increased psychological or physiological tension in healthy manner

Risk for situational low **Self-esteem** r/t history of learned helplessness

Self-mutilation r/t use of manipulation to obtain nurturing relationship with others

Marasmus

See Failure to Thrive, Nonorganic

Marshall-Marchetti-Krantz Operation

Preoperative

Stress urinary **Incontinence** r/t weak pelvic muscles and pelvic supports

Postoperative

Acute **Pain** r/t manipulation of organs, surgical incision

Deficient **Knowledge** r/t lack of exposure to information regarding care after surgery and at home

Risk for **Infection** r/t presence of urinary catheter

Urinary retention r/t swelling of urinary meatus

Mastectomy

Acute **Pain** r/t surgical procedure

Disturbed **Body** image r/t loss of sexually significant body part

Chronic **Sorrow** r/t disturbed body image, unknown long-term health status

Death **Anxiety** r/t threat of mortality associated with breast cancer

Deficient **Knowledge** r/t self-care activities

Fear r/t change in body image, prognosis

Nausea r/t chemotherapy

Risk for impaired physical **Mobility** r/t nerve or muscle damage, pin

Risk for **Post-trauma** syndrome r/t associated with loss of body part, surgical wounds.

Risk for **Powerlessness** r/t fear of unknown outcome of procedure

Sexual dysfunction r/t change in body image, fear of loss of femininity

See Cancer; Surgery

Mastitis

Acute **Pain** r/t infectious disease process, swelling of breast tissue

Anxiety r/t threat to self, concern over safety of milk for infant

Deficient **Knowledge** r/t antibiotic regimen, comfort measures

Ineffective **Breastfeeding** r/t breast pain, conflicting advice from health care providers

Ineffective **Role** performance r/t change in capacity to function in expected role

Maternal Infection

Ineffective **Protection** r/t invasive procedures, traumatized tissue, stress of recent childbirth

See Postpartum Normal Care

Maturational Issues, Adolescent

Deficient **Knowledge**: potential for enhanced health maintenance r/t information misinterpretation, lack of education regarding age-related factors

Impaired **Social** interaction r/t ineffective, unsuccessful, or dysfunctional interaction with peers

Ineffective **Coping** r/t maturational crises

Interrupted **Family** processes r/t developmental crises of adolescence secondary to challenge of parental authority and values, situational crises secondary to change in parental marital status

Risk for **Injury/Trauma** r/t thrill-seeking behaviors

Risk for situational low **Self-esteem** r/t developmental changes

M

Social isolation r/t perceived alteration in physical appearance, social values not accepted by dominant peer group

See Sexuality, Adolescent; Substance Abuse (if relevant)

Measles (Rubeola)

See Communicable Diseases, Childhood

Meconium Aspiration

See Respiratory Conditions of Neonate

Melanoma

Acute **Pain** r/t surgical incision

Disturbed **Body** image r/t altered pigmentation, surgical incision

Fear r/t threat to well-being

Ineffective **Health** maintenance r/t deficient knowledge regarding self-care and treatment of melanoma

See Cancer

Melena

Fear r/t presence of blood in feces

Risk for deficient **Fluid** volume r/t hemorrhage

See GI Bleed

Memory Deficit

Impaired **Memory** r/t acute or chronic hypoxia, anemia, decreased cardiac output, fluid and electrolyte imbalance, neurological disturbance, excessive environmental disturbances

Meningitis/Encephalitis

Acute **Pain** r/t neck (nuchal) rigidity, inflammation of meninges, headache

Decreased **Intracranial** adaptive capacity r/t sustained increase in intracranial pressure (10 to 15 mm Hg ICP)

Delayed **Growth** and development r/t brain damage secondary to infectious process, increased intracranial pressure

Disturbed **Sensory** perception: hearing r/t central nervous system infection, ear infection

Disturbed **Sensory** perception: kinesthetic r/t central nervous system infection

Disturbed **Sensory** perception: visual r/t photophobia secondary to central nervous system infection

Disturbed **Thought** processes r/t inflammation of brain, fever

Excess **Fluid** volume r/t increased intracranial pressure, syndrome of inappropriate secretion of antidiuretic hormone (SIADH)

Impaired **Comfort** r/t central nervous system inflammation

Impaired **Comfort**: photophobia r/t increased sensitivity to external stimuli secondary to central nervous system inflammation

Impaired **Mobility** r/t neuromuscular or central nervous system insult

Ineffective **Airway** clearance r/t seizure activity

Ineffective **Tissue** perfusion: cerebral r/t inflamed cerebral tissues and meninges, increased intracranial pressure

Risk for **Aspiration** r/t seizure activity

Risk for **Injury** r/t seizure activity

Risk for **Falls** r/t neuromuscular dysfunction

See Hospitalized Child

Meningocele

See Neurotube Defects

Menopause

Effective **Therapeutic** regimen management r/t verbalized desire to manage menopause

Ineffective **Sexuality** patterns r/t altered body structure, lack of physiological lubrication, lack of knowledge of artificial lubrication

Health-seeking behavior r/t menopause, therapies associated with change in hormonal levels

Impaired **Memory** r/t change in hormonal levels

Ineffective **Thermoregulation** r/t changes in hormonal levels

Readiness for enhanced **Spiritual** well-being r/t desire for harmony of mind, body, and spirit

Risk for imbalanced **Nutrition**: more than body requirements r/t change in metabolic rate caused by fluctuating hormone levels

Risk for **Powerlessness** r/t changes associated with menopause

Risk for situational low **Self-esteem** r/t developmental changes: menopause

Risk for urge urinary **Incontinence** r/t changes in hormonal levels affecting bladder function

Menorrhagia

Fear r/t loss of large amounts of blood

Risk for deficient **Fluid** volume r/t excessive loss of menstrual blood

Mental Illness

Chronic **Sorrow** r/t presence of mental illness

Compromised family **Coping** r/t lack of available support from client

Defensive **Coping** r/t psychological impairment, substance abuse

Disabled family **Coping** r/t chronically unexpressed feelings of guilt, anxiety, hostility, or despair

Disturbed **Thought** processes r/t head injury, mental disorder, personality disorder, organic mental disorder, substance abuse, severe interpersonal conflict, sleep deprivation, sensory deprivation or overload, impaired cerebral perfusion

Ineffective community **Therapeutic** regimen management r/t inadequate services to care for mentally ill clients, lack of information regarding how to access services

Ineffective **Coping** r/t situational crisis, coping with mental illness

Ineffective **Denial** r/t refusal to acknowledge abuse problem, fear of the social stigma of disease

Ineffective **Therapeutic** regimen management: families r/t chronicity of condition, unpredictability of client, unknown prognosis

Risk for **Loneliness** r/t social isolation

Risk for **Powerlessness** r/t lifestyle of helplessness

Mental Retardation

Chronic low **Self-esteem** r/t perceived differences

Delayed **Growth** and development r/t cognitive or perceptual impairment, developmental delay

Grieving r/t loss of perfect child, birth of child with congenital defect or subsequent head injury

Impaired **Home** maintenance r/t insufficient support systems

Impaired **Social** interaction r/t developmental lag or delay, perceived differences

Impaired **Swallowing** r/t neuromuscular impairment

Impaired verbal **Communication** r/t developmental delay

Interrupted **Family** processes r/t crisis of diagnosis and situational transition

Parental role **Conflict** r/t home care of child with special needs

Readiness for enhanced family **Coping** r/t adaptation and acceptance of child's condition and needs

Risk for delayed **Development** r/t cognitive or perceptual impairment

Risk for disproportionate **Growth** r/t mental retardation

Risk for **Self-mutilation** r/t separation anxiety, depersonalization

Self-care deficit: bathing/hygiene, dressing/grooming, feeding, toileting r/t perceptual or cognitive impairment

Self-mutilation r/t inability to express tension verbally

See Child with Chronic Condition; Safety, Childhood

Metabolic Acidosis

See Ketoacidosis

Metabolic Alkalosis

Deficient **Fluid** volume r/t fluid volume loss, vomiting, gastric suctioning, failure of regulatory mechanisms

MI (Myocardial Infarction)

Acute **Pain** r/t myocardial tissue damage from inadequate blood supply

Anxiety r/t threat of death, possible change in role status

Constipation r/t decreased peristalsis from decreased physical activity, medication effect, change in diet

Death **Anxiety** r/t seriousness of medical condition

Decreased **Cardiac** output r/t ventricular damage, ischemia, dysrhythmias

Fear r/t threat to well-being

Ineffective **Health** maintenance r/t deficient knowledge regarding self-care and treatment

Ineffective **Sexuality** patterns r/t fear of chest pain, possibility of heart damage

Ineffective **Denial** r/t fear, deficient knowledge about heart disease

Ineffective family **Coping** r/t spouse or significant other's fear of partner loss

Interrupted **Family** processes r/t crisis, role change

Risk for **Powerlessness** r/t acute illness

Risk for **Spiritual** distress r/t physical illness: MI

Situational low **Self-esteem** r/t crisis of MI

Midlife Crisis

Ineffective **Coping** r/t inability to deal with changes associated with aging

Readiness for enhanced **Spiritual** well-being r/t desire to find purpose and meaning to life

Powerlessness r/t lack of control over life situation

Spiritual distress r/t questioning belief/value system

Migraine Headache

Acute **Pain**: headache r/t vasodilation of cerebral and extracerebral vessels

Disturbed **Energy** field r/t pain, disruption of normal flow of energy

Ineffective **Health** maintenance r/t deficient knowledge regarding prevention and treatment of headaches

M

Miscarriage

See Pregnancy Loss

Mitral Stenosis

Activity intolerance r/t imbalance between oxygen supply and demand

Anxiety r/t possible worsening of symptoms, activity intolerance, fatigue

Decreased **Cardiac** output r/t incompetent heart valves, abnormal forward or backward blood flow, flow into a dilated chamber, flow through an abnormal passage between chambers

Ineffective **Health** maintenance r/t deficient knowledge regarding self-care with disorder

Fatigue r/t reduced cardiac output

Mitral Valve Prolapse

Acute **Pain** r/t mitral valve regurgitation

Anxiety r/t symptoms of condition: palpitations, chest pain

Fatigue r/t abnormal catecholamine regulation, decreased intravascular volume

Fear r/t lack of knowledge about mitral valve prolapse, feelings of having a heart attack

Ineffective **Health** maintenance r/t deficient knowledge regarding methods to relieve pain and treat dysrhythmia and shortness of breath, need for prophylactic antibiotics before invasive procedures

Ineffective **Tissue** perfusion: cerebral r/t postural hypotension

Risk for **Infection** r/t invasive procedures

Risk for **Powerlessness** r/t unpredictability of onset of symptoms

Mobility, Impaired Physical

Impaired physical **Mobility** r/t intolerance to activity, decreased strength and endurance, pain, discomfort, perceptual or cognitive impairment, neuromuscular impairment, musculoskeletal impairment, depression, severe anxiety

Risk for **Falls** r/t impaired physical mobility

Modified Radical Mastectomy

Decisional **Conflict** r/t treatment of choice

See Mastectomy

Mononucleosis

Activity intolerance r/t generalized weakness

Acute **Pain** r/t enlargement of lymph nodes, irritation of oropharyngeal cavity

Hyperthermia r/t infectious process

Fatigue r/t disease state, stress

Impaired **Swallowing** r/t irritation of oropharyngeal cavity

Ineffective **Health** maintenance r/t deficient knowledge concerning transmission and treatment of disease

Risk for **Injury** r/t possible rupture of spleen

Mood Disorders

Caregiver role strain r/t symptoms associated with disorder of care receiver

Impaired **Adjustment** r/t hopelessness, altered locus of control

Risk for situational low **Self-esteem** r/t unpredictable changes in mood

Social isolation r/t alterations in mental status

See specific disorder: Depression; Dysthymic Disorder; Hypomania; Manic Disorder

Moon Face

Disturbed **Body** image r/t change in appearance from disease and medication

Risk for situational low **Self-esteem** r/t change in body image

See Cushing's Syndrome

Moral/Ethical Dilemmas

Decisional **Conflict** r/t questioning personal values and belief which alter decision

Risk for **Powerlessness** r/t lack of knowledge to make a decision

Risk for **Spiritual** distress r/t moral or ethical crisis

Mottling of Peripheral Skin

Ineffective **Tissue** perfusion: peripheral r/t interruption of arterial flow, decreased circulating blood volume

Mouth Lesions

See Mucous Membranes, Impaired Oral

MRI (Magnetic Resonance Imaging)

Anxiety r/t fear of being in closed spaces

Deficient **Knowledge** r/t preparation for examination, contraindications to test, especially presence of any metal in body

Mucocutaneous Lymph Node Syndrome

See Kawasaki Syndrome

Mucous Membranes, Impaired Oral

Impaired **Oral** mucous membrane r/t pathological conditions—oral cavity (radiation to head or neck), dehydration, chemical trauma (e.g., acidic foods, drugs, noxious agents, alcohol), mechanical trauma (e.g., ill-fitting dentures, braces, endotracheal or nasogastric tubes, surgery in oral cavity), NPO for more than 24 hours, ineffective oral hygiene, mouth breathing, malnutrition, infection, lack of or decreased salivation, medication

Multiinfarct Dementia

See Dementia

Multiple Gestation

Anxiety r/t uncertain outcome of pregnancy

Death **Anxiety** r/t maternal complications associated with multiple gestation

Deficient **Knowledge** r/t caring for more than one infant

Fatigue r/t physiological demands of a multifetal pregnancy and/or care of more than one infant

Imbalanced **Nutrition:** less than body requirements r/t physiological demands of a multifetal pregnancy

Impaired **Home** maintenance r/t fatigue

Impaired physical **Mobility** r/t increased uterine size

Impaired **Transfer** ability r/t enlarged uterus

Risk for **Constipation** r/t enlarged uterus

Risk for delayed **Development:** fetus r/t multiple gestation

Risk for disproportionate **Growth:** fetus r/t multiple gestation

Risk for ineffective **Breastfeeding** r/t lack of support, physical demands of feeding more than one infant

Disturbed **Sleep** pattern r/t discomforts of multiple gestation or care of infants

Stress urinary **Incontinence** r/t increased pelvic pressure

Multiple Personality Disorder (Dissociative Identity Disorder)

Anxiety r/t loss of control of behavior and feelings

Chronic low **Self-esteem** r/t inability to deal with life events, history of abuse

Defensive **Coping** r/t unresolved past traumatic events, severe anxiety

Disturbed **Body** image r/t feelings of powerlessness with personality changes

Disturbed personal **Identity** r/t severe child abuse

Hopelessness r/t long-term stress

Ineffective **Coping** r/t history of abuse

Risk for **Self-mutilation** r/t need to act out to relieve stress

See Dissociative Disorder

Multiple Sclerosis (MS)

Chronic **Sorrow** r/t loss of physical ability

Disturbed **Energy** field r/t disruption in energy flow resulting from disharmony between mind and body

Disuse syndrome r/t physical immobility

Impaired physical **Mobility** r/t neuromuscular impairment

Ineffective **Airway** clearance r/t decreased energy/fatigue

Powerlessness r/t progressive nature of disease

Readiness for enhanced **Spiritual** well-being r/t struggling with chronic debilitating condition

Risk for imbalanced **Nutrition:** less than body requirements r/t impaired swallowing, depression

Risk for **Injury** r/t altered mobility, sensory dysfunction

Risk for **Powerlessness** r/t chronic illness

Self-care deficit: specify r/t neuromuscular impairment

Disturbed **Sensory** perception: specify r/t pathology in sensory tracts

Sexual dysfunction r/t biopsychosocial alteration of sexuality

Spiritual distress r/t perceived hopelessness of diagnosis

Urinary retention r/t inhibition of the reflex arc

See Neurological Disorders

Mumps

See Communicable Diseases, Childhood

Murmurs

Decreased **Cardiac** output r/t incompetent heart valves, abnormal forward or backward blood flow, flow into a dilated chamber, flow through an abnormal passage between chambers

Muscular Atrophy/Weakness

Risk for **Disuse** syndrome r/t impaired physical mobility

Risk for **Falls** r/t impaired physical mobility

Muscular Dystrophy (MD)

Activity intolerance r/t fatigue

Constipation r/t immobility

Decreased **Cardiac** output r/t effects of congestive heart failure

Fatigue r/t increased energy requirements to perform activities of daily living

Imbalanced **Nutrition:** less than body requirements r/t impaired swallowing or chewing

M

Imbalanced **Nutrition:** more than body requirements r/t inactivity

Impaired **Mobility** r/t muscle weakness and development of contractures

Impaired **Transfer** ability r/t muscle weakness

Impaired **Walking** r/t muscle weakness

Ineffective **Airway** clearance r/t muscle weakness and decreased ability to cough

Risk for **Aspiration** r/t impaired swallowing

Risk for **Disuse** syndrome r/t complications of immobility

Risk for **Falls** r/t muscle weakness

Risk for impaired **Gas** exchange r/t ineffective airway clearance and ineffective breathing pattern secondary to muscle weakness

Risk for impaired **Skin** integrity r/t immobility, braces, or adaptive devices

Risk for ineffective **Breathing** pattern r/t muscle weakness

Risk for **Infection** r/t pooling of pulmonary secretions secondary to immobility and muscle weakness

Risk for **Injury** r/t muscle weakness and unsteady gait

Risk for **Powerlessness** r/t chronic condition

Risk for situational low **Self-esteem** r/t presence of chronic condition

Self-care deficits: feeding, bathing, dressing, toileting r/t muscle weakness and fatigue

See Child with Chronic Condition; Hospitalized Child; Terminally Ill Child

MVA (Motor Vehicle Accident)

See Fracture; Head Injury; Injury; Pneumothorax

Myasthenia Gravis

Fatigue r/t paresthesia, aching muscles

Imbalanced **Nutrition:** less than body requirements r/t difficulty eating and swallowing

Impaired physical **Mobility** r/t defective transmission of nerve impulses at the neuromuscular junction

Impaired **Swallowing** r/t neuromuscular impairment

Ineffective **Airway** clearance r/t decreased ability to cough and swallow

Ineffective **Therapeutic** regimen management r/t lack of knowledge of treatment, uncertainty of outcome

Interrupted **Family** processes r/t crisis of dealing with diagnosis

Risk for **Caregiver** role strain r/t severity of illness of client

See Neurological Disorders

Mycoplasma Pneumonia

See Pneumonia

Myelocele

See Neurotube Defects

Myelogram, Contrast

Acute **Pain** r/t irritation of nerve roots

Risk for deficient **Fluid** volume r/t possible dehydration, loss of cerebrospinal fluid

Risk for ineffective **Tissue** perfusion: cerebral r/t hypotension, loss of cerebrospinal fluid

Urinary retention r/t pressure on spinal nerve roots

Myelomeningocele

See Neurotube Defects

Myocardial Infarction

See MI

Myocarditis

Activity intolerance r/t reduced cardiac reserve and prescribed bedrest

Decreased **Cardiac** output r/t impaired contractility of ventricles

Deficient **Knowledge** r/t treatment of disease

See CHF (if appropriate)

Myringotomy

Acute **Pain** r/t surgical procedure

Ineffective **Health** maintenance r/t deficient knowledge regarding self-care following surgery

Fear r/t hospitalization, surgical procedure

Risk for **Infection** r/t invasive procedure

Disturbed **Sensory** perception r/t possible hearing impairment

Myxedema

See Hypothyroidism

N

Narcissistic Personality Disorder

Decisional **Conflict** r/t lack of realistic problem-solving skills

Defensive **Coping** r/t grandiose sense of self

Impaired **Social** interaction r/t self-concept disturbance

Risk for **Loneliness** r/t inability to interact appropriately with others

Risk for **Self-mutilation** r/t inadequate coping

Narcolepsy

Anxiety r/t fear of lack of control over falling asleep

Disturbed **Sleep** pattern r/t uncontrollable desire to sleep

Risk for **Trauma** r/t falling asleep during potentially dangerous activity

Narcotic Use

Risk for **Constipation** r/t effects of opioids on peristalsis

See Substance Abuse (if relevant)

Nasogastric Suction

Impaired **Comfort** r/t presence of nasogastric tube

Impaired **Oral** mucous membrane r/t presence of nasogastric tube

Risk for deficient **Fluid** volume r/t loss of gastrointestinal fluids without adequate replacement

Nausea

Nausea r/t chemotherapy, postsurgical anesthesia, irritation to the gastrointestinal system, stimulation of neuropharmacologic mechanisms

Near-Drowning

Anticipatory/dysfunctional **Grieving** r/t potential death of child, unknown sequelae, guilt about accident

Aspiration r/t aspiration of fluid into the lungs

Fear: parental r/t possible death of child, possible permanent and debilitating sequelae

Hypothermia r/t central nervous system injury, prolonged submersion in cold water

Impaired **Gas** exchange r/t laryngospasm, holding breath, aspiration

Ineffective **Airway** clearance r/t aspiration, impaired gas exchange

Ineffective **Health** maintenance r/t parental deficient knowledge regarding safety measures appropriate for age

Readiness for enhanced **Spiritual** well-being r/t struggle with survival of life-threatening situation

Risk for delayed **Development** and disproportionate growth r/t hypoxemia, cerebral anoxia

Risk for **Infection** r/t aspiration, invasive monitoring

See Child with Chronic Condition; Hospitalized Child; Safety, Childhood; Terminally Ill Child/Death of Child

Neck Vein Distention

Decreased **Cardiac** output r/t decreased contractility of heart and resulting increased preload

Excess **Fluid** volume r/t excess fluid intake, compromised regulatory mechanisms

See CHF

Necrotizing Enterocolitis (NEC)

Deficient **Fluid** volume r/t vomiting, gastrointestinal bleeding

Imbalanced **Nutrition: less than body requirements** r/t decreased ability to absorb nutrients, decreased perfusion to gastrointestinal tract

Ineffective **Breathing** pattern r/t abdominal distention, hypoxia

Ineffective **Tissue** perfusion: gastrointestinal r/t shunting of blood away from mesenteric circulation and toward vital organs secondary to perinatal stress, hypoxia

Risk for **Infection** r/t bacterial invasion of gastrointestinal tract, invasive procedures

See Hospitalized Child; Premature Infant

Negative Feelings about Self

Chronic low **Self-esteem** r/t long-standing negative self-evaluation

Self-esteem disturbance r/t inappropriate learned negative feelings about self

Neglect, Unilateral

See Unilateral Neglect of One Side of Body

Neglectful Care of Family Member

Caregiver role strain r/t care demands of family member, lack of social or financial support

Deficient **Knowledge** r/t care needs

Disabled family **Coping** r/t highly ambivalent family relationships, lack of respite care

Ineffective community **Therapeutic** regimen management r/t deficits in community for support of caregivers, detection of client neglect

Interrupted **Family** processes r/t situational transition or crisis

Neoplasm

Fear r/t possible malignancy

See Cancer

Nephrectomy

Acute **Pain** r/t incisional discomfort

Anxiety r/t surgical recovery, prognosis

Constipation r/t lack of return of peristalsis

Impaired **Urinary** elimination r/t loss of kidney

N

Ineffective **Breathing** pattern r/t location of surgical incision

Risk for deficient **Fluid** volume r/t vascular losses, decreased intake

Risk for **Infection** r/t invasive procedure, lack of deep breathing because of location of surgical incision

Nephrostomy, Percutaneous

Acute **Pain** r/t invasive procedure

Impaired **Urinary** elimination r/t nephrostomy tube

Risk for **Infection** r/t invasive procedure

Nephrotic Syndrome

Activity intolerance r/t generalized edema

Disturbed **Body** image r/t edematous appearance and side effects of steroid therapy

Excess **Fluid** volume r/t edema secondary to oncotic fluid shift resulting from serum protein loss and renal retention of salt and water

Impaired **Comfort** r/t edema

Imbalanced **Nutrition**: less than body requirements r/t anorexia, protein loss

Imbalanced **Nutrition**: more than body requirements r/t increased appetite secondary to steroid therapy

Risk for impaired **Skin** integrity r/t edema

Risk for **Infection** r/t altered immune mechanisms secondary to disease and effects of steroids

Risk for **Noncompliance** r/t side effects of home steroid therapy

Social **Isolation** r/t edematous appearance

See Child with Chronic Condition; Hospitalized Child

Nerve Entrapment

See Carpal Tunnel Syndrome

Neuritis

Activity intolerance r/t pain with movement

Acute **Pain** r/t stimulation of affected nerve endings, inflammation of sensory nerves

Ineffective **Health** maintenance r/t deficient knowledge regarding self-care with neuritis

Neurogenic Bladder

Reflex **Incontinence** r/t neurological impairment

Urinary retention r/t interruption in the lateral spinal tracts

Neurological Disorders

Acute **Confusion** r/t dementia, alcohol abuse, drug abuse, delirium

Anticipatory **Grieving** r/t loss of usual body functioning

Imbalanced **Nutrition**: less than body requirements r/t impaired swallowing, depression, difficulty feeding self

Impaired **Home** maintenance r/t client's or family member's disease

Impaired **Memory** r/t neurological disturbance

Impaired physical **Mobility** r/t neuromuscular impairment

Impaired **Swallowing** r/t neuromuscular dysfunction

Ineffective **Airway** clearance r/t perceptual or cognitive impairment, decreased energy, fatigue

Ineffective **Coping** r/t disability requiring change in lifestyle

Interrupted **Family** processes r/t situational crisis, illness, or disability of family member

Powerlessness r/t progressive nature of disease

Risk for **Disuse** syndrome r/t physical immobility, neuromuscular dysfunction

Risk for impaired **Skin** integrity r/t altered sensation, altered mental status, paralysis

Risk for **Injury** r/t altered mobility, sensory dysfunction, cognitive impairment

Self-care deficit: specify r/t neuromuscular dysfunction

Sexual dysfunction r/t biopsychosocial alteration of sexuality

Social isolation r/t altered state of wellness

Wandering r/t cognitive impairment

Neurotube Defects (Meningocele, Myelomeningocele, Spina Bifida, Anencephaly)

Chronic low **Self-esteem** r/t perceived differences, decreased ability to participate in physical and social activities at school

Constipation r/t immobility or less than adequate mobility

Delayed **Growth** and development r/t physical impairments, possible cognitive impairment

Grieving r/t loss of perfect child, birth of child with congenital defect

Impaired **Mobility** r/t neuromuscular impairment

Impaired **Skin** integrity r/t incontinence

Readiness for enhanced family **Coping** r/t effective adaptive response by family members

Reflex **Incontinence** r/t neurogenic impairment

Risk for delayed **Development** r/t chronic illness

Risk for disproportionate **Growth** r/t chronic illness

Risk for imbalanced **Nutrition**: more than body requirements r/t diminished, limited, or impaired physical activity

Risk for impaired **Skin** integrity: lower extremities r/t decreased sensory perception

Risk for latex **Allergy** r/t multiple exposures to latex products

Risk for **Powerlessness** r/t debilitating disease

Disturbed **Sensory** perception: visual r/t altered reception secondary to strabismus

Total urinary **Incontinence** r/t neurogenic impairment

Urge urinary **Incontinence** r/t neurogenic impairment

See Child with Chronic Condition; Premature Infant

Newborn, Normal

Effective **Breastfeeding** r/t normal oral structure and gestational age >34 weeks

Ineffective **Protection** r/t immature immune system

Ineffective **Thermoregulation** r/t immaturity of neuroendocrine system

Readiness for enhanced organized **Infant** behavior r/t appropriate environmental stimuli

Risk for **Infection** r/t open umbilical stump

Risk for **Injury** r/t immaturity, need for caretaking

Newborn, Postmature

Hypothermia r/t depleted stores of subcutaneous fat

Impaired **Skin** integrity r/t cracked and peeling skin secondary to decreased vernix

Risk for ineffective **Airway** clearance r/t meconium aspiration

Risk for **Injury** r/t hypoglycemia secondary to depleted glycogen stores

Newborn, Small for Gestational Age (SGA)

Imbalanced **Nutrition:** less than body requirements r/t history of placental insufficiency

Ineffective **Thermoregulation** r/t decreased brown fat, subcutaneous fat

Risk for delayed **Development** r/t history of placental insufficiency

Risk for disproportionate **Growth** r/t history of placental insufficiency

Risk for **Injury** r/t hypoglycemia, perinatal asphyxia, meconium aspiration

Nicotine Addiction

Ineffective **Health** maintenance r/t lack of ability to make a judgment about smoking cessation

Powerlessness r/t perceived lack of control over ability to give up nicotine

NIDDM (Non–Insulin-Dependent Diabetes Mellitus)

Health-seeking behaviors r/t desiring information on exercise and diet to manage diabetes

See Diabetes Mellitus

Nightmares

Disturbed **Energy** field r/t disharmony of body and mind

Post-trauma response r/t disaster, war, epidemic, rape, assault, torture, catastrophic illness or accident

Rape-trauma syndrome: compound reaction/silent reaction r/t forced violent sexual penetration against the victim's will and consent

Nipple Soreness

Acute **Pain** r/t injury to nipples

See Painful Breasts—Sore Nipples

Nocturia

Impaired **Urinary** elimination r/t sensory motor impairment, urinary tract infection

Risk for **Powerlessness** r/t to inability to control nighttime voidings

Total **Urinary** incontinence r/t neuropathy preventing transmission of reflex indicating bladder fullness, neurological dysfunction causing triggering of micturition at unpredictable times, independent contraction of detrusor reflex as result of surgery, trauma or disease affecting spinal cord nerves, anatomical fistula

Urge urinary **Incontinence** r/t decreased bladder capacity, irritation of bladder stretch receptors causing spasm, alcohol, caffeine, increased fluids, increased urine concentration, overdistention of bladder

Nocturnal Paroxysmal Dyspnea

See PND

Noncompliance

Noncompliance r/t client value system, health beliefs, cultural influences, spiritual values, client-provider relationships, deficient knowledge

Non–Insulin-Dependent Diabetes Mellitus (NIDDM)

See Diabetes Mellitus

Nutrition, Imbalanced

Imbalanced **Nutrition:** risk for more than body requirements r/t obesity in parents, use of food as reward or comfort measure, dysfunctional eating

N

pattern, eating in response to cues other than hunger

Imbalanced **Nutrition: less than body requirements** r/t inability to ingest or digest food or absorb nutrients because of biological, psychological, economic factors

Imbalanced **Nutrition: more than body requirements** r/t excessive intake in relation to metabolic need

O

Obesity

Disturbed **Body** image r/t eating disorder, excess weight

Chronic low **Self-esteem** r/t ineffective coping, overeating

Imbalanced **Nutrition: more than body requirements** r/t caloric intake exceeding energy expenditure

Obsessive-Compulsive Disorder

Anxiety r/t threat to self-concept, unmet needs

Decisional **Conflict** r/t inability to make a decision for fear of reprisal

Disabled family **Coping** r/t family process being disrupted by client's ritualistic activities

Disturbed **Thought** processes r/t persistent thoughts, ideas, impulses that seem irrelevant and will not relent

Ineffective **Coping** r/t expression of feelings in an unacceptable way, ritualistic behavior

Powerlessness r/t unrelenting repetitive thoughts to perform irrational activities

Risk for situational low **Self-esteem** r/t inability to control repetitive thoughts and actions

Obstruction, Bowel

See Bowel Obstruction

Older Adult

See Aging

Oligohydramnios

Anxiety: maternal r/t fear of unknown, threat to fetus

Risk for **Injury:** fetal r/t decreased umbilical cord blood flow secondary to compression

Oliguria

Deficient **Fluid** volume r/t active fluid loss, failure of regulatory mechanism

See Cardiac Output Decrease; Renal Failure; Shock

Omphalocele

See Gastroschisis/Omphalocele

Onychomycosis

See Ringworm of Nails

Oophorectomy

Risk for ineffective **Sexuality** patterns r/t altered body function

See Surgery

Open Reduction of Fracture with Internal Fixation (Femur)

Anxiety r/t outcome of corrective procedure

Impaired physical **Mobility** r/t postoperative position, abduction of leg, avoidance of acute flexion

Powerlessness r/t loss of control, unanticipated change in lifestyle

Risk for perioperative positioning **Injury** r/t immobilization

Risk for **Peripheral** neurovascular dysfunction r/t mechanical compression, orthopedic surgery, immobilization

See Surgery, Postoperative Care

Opiate Use

Risk for **Constipation** r/t effects of opiates on peristalsis.

See Drug Abuse

Opportunistic Infection

Risk for **Infection** r/t abnormal blood profiles

Delayed **Surgical** recovery r/t abnormal blood profiles, impaired healing

See AIDS

Oral Mucous Membrane, Impaired

Impaired **Oral** mucous membrane r/t pathological conditions—oral cavity (radiation to head or neck), dehydration, chemical trauma (e.g., acidic foods, drugs, noxious agents, alcohol), mechanical trauma (e.g., ill-fitting dentures, braces, endotracheal and nasogastric tubes, surgery in oral cavity), NPO for more than 24 hours, ineffective oral hygiene, mouth breathing, malnutrition, infection, lack of or decreased salivation, medication

Organic Mental Disorders

Adult **Failure** to thrive r/t undetected organic mental disorder

Impaired **Social** interaction r/t disturbed thought processes

Risk for **Injury** r/t disorientation to time, place, person

See Dementia

Orthopedic Traction

Impaired **Social** interaction r/t limited physical mobility

Impaired **Transfer** ability r/t limited physical mobility

Ineffective **Role** performance r/t limited physical mobility

See Traction and Casts

Orthopnea

Decreased **Cardiac** output r/t inability of heart to meet demands of body

Ineffective **Breathing** pattern r/t inability to breathe with head of bed flat

Orthostatic Hypotension

See Dizziness

Osteoarthritis

Activity intolerance r/t pain after exercise or use of joint

Impaired **Transfer** ability r/t pain

Acute **Pain** r/t movement

See Arthritis

Osteomyelitis

Acute **Pain** r/t inflammation in affected extremity

Deficient **Diversional** activity r/t prolonged immobilization, hospitalization

Fear: parental r/t concern regarding possible growth plate damage secondary to infection, concern that infection may become chronic

Hyperthermia r/t infectious process

Impaired physical **Mobility** r/t imposed immobility secondary to infected area

Ineffective **Health** maintenance r/t continued immobility at home, possible extensive casts, continued antibiotics

Risk for **Constipation** r/t immobility

Risk for impaired **Skin** integrity r/t irritation from splint/cast

Risk for spread of **Infection** r/t inadequate primary and secondary defenses

See Hospitalized Child

Osteoporosis

Acute **Pain** r/t fracture, muscle spasms

Deficient **Knowledge** r/t diet, exercise, need to abstain from alcohol and nicotine

Effective **Therapeutic** regimen management: individual r/t appropriate choices for diet and exercise to prevent and manage condition

Imbalanced **Nutrition:** less than body requirements r/t inadequate intake of calcium and vitamin D

Impaired physical **Mobility** r/t pain, skeletal changes

Risk for **Injury:** fracture r/t lack of activity, risk of falling resulting from environmental hazards, neuromuscular disorders, diminished senses, cardiovascular responses, responses to drugs

Risk for **Powerlessness** r/t debilitating disease

Ostomy

See Child with Chronic Condition; Colostomy; Ileal Conduit; Ileostomy

Otitis Media

Acute **Pain** r/t inflammation, infectious process

Risk for delayed **Development** r/t frequent otitis media

Risk for **Infection** r/t eustachian tube obstruction, traumatic eardrum perforation, infectious disease process

Disturbed **Sensory** perception: auditory r/t incomplete resolution of otitis media, presence of excess drainage in middle ear

Ovarian Carcinoma

Death **Anxiety** r/t unknown outcome, possible poor prognosis

Fear r/t unknown outcome, possible poor prognosis

Ineffective **Health** maintenance r/t deficient knowledge regarding self-care, treatment of condition

See Chemotherapy; Hysterectomy; Radiation Therapy

P

Pacemaker

Acute **Pain** r/t surgical procedure

Anxiety r/t change in health status, presence of pacemaker

Death **Anxiety** r/t worry over possible malfunction of pacemaker

Deficient **Knowledge** r/t self-care program, when to seek medical attention

Risk for decreased **Cardiac** output r/t malfunction of pacemaker

Risk for **Infection** r/t invasive procedure, presence of foreign body (catheter and generator)

Risk for **Powerlessness** r/t presence of electronic device to stimulate heart

Paget's Disease

Chronic **Sorrow** r/t chronic condition with altered body image

Deficient **Knowledge** r/t appropriate diet of high protein and high calcium, mild exercise

Disturbed **Body** image r/t possible enlarged head, bowed tibias, kyphosis

Risk for **Trauma**: fracture r/t excessive bone destruction

Pain, Acute

Acute **Pain** r/t injury agents (biological, chemical, physical, psychological)

Disturbed **Energy** field r/t unbalanced energy field

Pain, Chronic

Chronic **Pain** r/t chronic physical or psychosocial disability

Painful Breasts—Engorgement

Acute **Pain** r/t distention of breast tissue

Ineffective **Role** performance r/t change in physical capacity to assume role of breast-feeding mother

Impaired **Tissue** integrity r/t excessive fluid in breast tissues

Risk for ineffective **Breastfeeding** r/t pain, infant's inability to latch on to engorged breast

Risk for **Infection** r/t milk stasis

Painful Breasts—Sore Nipples

Acute **Pain** r/t cracked nipples

Impaired **Skin** integrity r/t mechanical factors involved in suckling, breastfeeding management

Ineffective **Role** performance r/t change in physical capacity to assume role of breastfeeding mother

Ineffective **Breastfeeding** r/t pain

Risk for **Infection** r/t break in skin

Pallor of Extremities

Ineffective **Tissue** perfusion: peripheral r/t interruption of vascular flow

Pancreatic Cancer

Anticipatory **Grieving** r/t shortened life span

Death **Anxiety** r/t possible poor prognosis of disease process

Deficient **Knowledge** r/t disease-induced diabetes, home management

Fear r/t poor prognosis of the disease

Ineffective family **Coping** r/t poor prognosis

Spiritual distress r/t poor prognosis

See Cancer; Radiation Therapy; Surgery

Pancreatitis

Acute **Pain** r/t irritation and edema of the inflamed pancreas

Chronic **Sorrow** r/t chronic illness

Diarrhea r/t decrease in pancreatic secretions resulting in steatorrhea

Deficient **Fluid** volume r/t vomiting, decreased fluid intake, fever, diaphoresis, fluid shifts

Imbalanced **Nutrition**: less than body requirements r/t inadequate dietary intake, increased nutritional needs secondary to acute illness, increased metabolic needs caused by increased body temperature

Ineffective **Breathing** pattern r/t splinting from severe pain

Ineffective **Denial** r/t ineffective coping, alcohol use

Ineffective **Health** maintenance r/t deficient knowledge concerning diet, alcohol use, medication

Nausea r/t irritation of gastrointestinal system

Panic Disorder

Anxiety r/t situational crisis

Ineffective **Coping** r/t personal vulnerability

Post-trauma syndrome r/t previous catastrophic event

Risk for **Loneliness** r/t inability to socially interact because of fear of losing control

Risk for **Powerlessness** r/t ineffective coping skills

Risk for **Post-trauma** syndrome r/t perception of the event, diminished ego strength

Social isolation r/t fear of lack of control

Paralysis

Acute **Pain** r/t prolonged immobility

Chronic **Sorrow** r/t loss of physical mobility

Constipation r/t effects of spinal cord disruption, inadequate fiber in diet

Disturbed **Body** image r/t biophysical changes, loss of movement, immobility

Disuse syndrome r/t paralysis

Impaired **Home** maintenance r/t physical disability

Impaired physical **Mobility** r/t neuromuscular impairment

Impaired **Transfer** ability r/t paralysis

Ineffective **Health** maintenance r/t deficient knowledge regarding self-care with paralysis

Powerlessness r/t illness-related regimen

Reflex **Incontinence** r/t neurological impairment

Risk for impaired **Skin** integrity r/t altered circulation, altered sensation, immobility

Risk for **Injury** r/t altered mobility, sensory dysfunction

P

Risk for **Falls** r/t to paralysis

Risk for **Post-trauma** syndrome r/t event causing paralysis

Risk for situational low **Self-esteem** r/t change in body image and function

Self-care deficit: specify r/t neuromuscular impairment

Sexual dysfunction r/t loss of sensation, biopsychosocial alteration

See Child with Chronic Condition; Hemiplegia; Hospitalized Child; Neurotube Defects; Spinal Cord Injury

Paralytic Ileus

Acute **Pain** r/t pressure, abdominal distention

Constipation r/t decreased gastric motility

Deficient **Fluid** volume r/t loss of fluids from vomiting, retention of fluid in bowel

Impaired **Oral** mucous membrane r/t presence of nasogastric tube

Nausea r/t gastrointestinal irritation

Paranoid Personality Disorder

Anxiety r/t uncontrollable intrusive, suspicious thoughts

Chronic low **Self-esteem** r/t inability to trust others

Impaired **Adjustment** r/t intense emotional state

Disturbed personal **Identity** r/t difficulty with reality testing

Disturbed **Thought** processes r/t psychological conflicts

Risk for **Loneliness** r/t social isolation

Risk for **Post-trauma** syndrome r/t exaggerated sense of responsibility

Risk for other-directed **Violence** r/t being suspicious of others and others' actions

Risk for **Suicide** r/t psychiatric illness

Disturbed **Sensory** perception: specify r/t psychological dysfunction, suspicious thoughts

Social **Isolation** r/t inappropriate social skills

Paraplegia

See Spinal Cord Injury

Parathyroidectomy

Anxiety r/t surgery

Risk for impaired verbal **Communication** r/t possible laryngeal damage, edema

Risk for ineffective **Airway** clearance r/t edema or hematoma formation, airway obstruction

Risk for **Infection** r/t surgical procedure

See Hypocalcemia

Parent Attachment

Chronic **Sorrow** r/t difficult parent-child relationship

Risk for impaired parent/infant/child **Attachment** r/t inability of parents to meet personal needs; anxiety associated with parental role; substance abuse; premature infant; ill infant/child who is unable to effectively initiate parental contact as a result of altered behavioral organization, separation, physical barriers, or lack of privacy

Risk for **Spiritual** distress r/t altered relationships

Parental Role Conflict

Chronic **Sorrow** r/t difficult parent-child relationship

Parental role **Conflict** r/t separation from child because of chronic illness, intimidation with invasive or restrictive modalities (e.g., isolation, intubation), specialized care center policies, home care of a child with special needs (e.g., apnea monitoring, postural drainage, hyperalimentation), change in marital status, interruptions of family life because of home care regimen (e.g., treatments, caregivers, lack of respite)

Risk for **Spiritual** distress r/t altered relationships

Parenting, Impaired

Chronic **Sorrow** r/t difficult parent-child relationship

Impaired **Parenting** r/t lack of available role model; ineffective role model; physical and psychosocial abuse of nurturing figure; lack of support between and from significant other(s); unmet social, emotional, or maturational needs of parenting figures; interruption in bonding process (e.g., maternal, paternal, other); unrealistic expectations for self, infant, partner; physical illness; presence of stress (e.g., financial, legal, recent crisis, cultural, move); lack of knowledge; limited cognitive functioning; lack of role identity; lack or inappropriate response of child to relationship; multiple pregnancies

Risk for **Spiritual** distress r/t altered relationships

Parenting, Risk for Impaired

Chronic **Sorrow** r/t difficult parent-child relationship

Risk for impaired **Parenting** r/t lack of available role model; ineffective role model; physical and psychosocial abuse of nurturing figure; lack of support between or from significant other(s); unmet social, emotional, or maturational needs of parenting figures; interruption in bonding process (e.g., maternal, paternal, other); unrealistic

P

expectations for self, infant, partner; physical illness; presence of stress (e.g., financial, legal, recent crisis, cultural move); lack of knowledge; limited cognitive functioning; lack of role identity; lack of inappropriate response of child to relationship; multiple pregnancies

Risk for **Spiritual** distress r/t altered relationships

Paresthesia

Risk for **Injury** r/t inability to feel temperature changes, pain

Disturbed **Sensory** perception: tactile r/t altered sensory reception, transmission, integration

Parkinson's Disease

Chronic **Sorrow** r/t loss of physical capacity

Constipation r/t weakness of defecation muscles, lack of exercise, inadequate fluid intake, decreased autonomic nervous system activity

Imbalanced **Nutrition:** less than body requirements r/t tremor, slowness in eating, difficulty in chewing and swallowing

Impaired verbal **Communication** r/t decreased speech volume, slowness of speech, impaired facial muscles

Risk for **Injury** r/t tremors, slow reactions, altered gait

See Neurological Disorders

Paroxysmal Nocturnal Dyspnea

See PND

Patent Ductus Arteriosus (PDA)

See Congenital Heart Disease/Cardiac Anomalies

Patient-Controlled Analgesia

See PCA

Patient Education

Deficient **Knowledge** r/t lack of exposure to information, information misinterpretation, unfamiliarity with information resources

Effective **Therapeutic** regimen management r/t verbalized desire to manage illness, prevent complications

Health-seeking behaviors r/t expressed or observed desire to seek a higher level of wellness, control of health practices

Readiness for enhanced **Spiritual** well-being r/t desire to reach harmony with self, others, higher power/God

PCA (Patient-Controlled Analgesia)

Deficient **Knowledge** r/t self-care of pain control

Effective **Therapeutic** regimen management r/t ability to manage pain with appropriate use of patient-controlled analgesia

Impaired **Comfort:** pruritus, nausea, vomiting r/t side effects of medication

Risk for **Injury** r/t possible complications associated with PCA

Pelvic Inflammatory Disease

See PID

Penile Prosthesis

Health-seeking behavior r/t information regarding use and care of prosthesis

Ineffective **Sexuality** pattern r/t use of penile prosthesis

Risk for **Infection** r/t invasive surgical procedure

Risk for situational low **Self-esteem** r/t altered sexuality pattern

Peptic Ulcer

See Ulcer

Percutaneous Transluminal Coronary Angioplasty (PTCA)

See Angioplasty, Coronary Balloon

Pericardial Friction Rub

Acute **Pain** r/t inflammation, effusion

Decreased **Cardiac** output r/t inflammation in pericardial sac, fluid accumulation compressing heart

Delayed **Surgical** recovery r/t complications associated with cardiac problems

Pericarditis

Activity intolerance r/t reduced cardiac reserve, prescribed bedrest

Acute **Pain** r/t biological injury, inflammation

Delayed **Surgical** recovery r/t complications associated with cardiac problems

Deficient **Knowledge** r/t unfamiliarity with information sources

Ineffective **Tissue** perfusion: cardiopulmonary/peripheral r/t risk for development of emboli

Risk for decreased **Cardiac** output r/t inflammation in pericardial sac, fluid accumulation compressing heart function

Risk for imbalanced **Nutrition:** less than body requirements r/t fever, hypermetabolic state associated with fever

P

Risk for decreased **Cardiac** output r/t inflammation in pericardial sac, fluid accumulation compressing heart function

Perioperative Positioning

Risk for perioperative positioning **Injury** r/t disorientation; immobilization; muscle weakness; sensory/perceptual disturbances resulting from anesthesia, obesity, emaciation, edema

Peripheral Neurovascular Dysfunction, Risk for

Risk for **Peripheral** neurovascular dysfunction r/t fractures, mechanical compression, orthopedic surgery, trauma, immobilization, burns, vascular obstruction

Peripheral Vascular Disease

Activity intolerance r/t imbalance between peripheral oxygen supply and demand

Chronic **Pain**: intermittent claudication r/t ischemia

Ineffective **Health** maintenance r/t deficient knowledge regarding self-care and treatment of disease

Ineffective **Tissue** perfusion: peripheral r/t interruption of vascular flow

Risk for impaired **Skin** integrity r/t altered circulation or sensation

Risk for **Falls** r/t altered mobility

Risk for **Injury** r/t tissue hypoxia, altered mobility, altered sensation

Risk for **Peripheral** neurovascular dysfunction r/t possible vascular obstruction

Peritoneal Dialysis

Acute **Pain** r/t instillation of dialysate, temperature of dialysate

Chronic **Sorrow** r/t chronic disability

Deficient **Knowledge** r/t treatment procedure, self-care with peritoneal dialysis

Impaired **Home** maintenance r/t complex home treatment of client

Risk for **Fluid** volume excess r/t retention of dialysate

Risk for ineffective **Breathing** pattern r/t pressure from dialysate

Risk for ineffective **Coping** r/t disability requiring change in lifestyle

Risk for **Infection**: peritoneal r/t invasive procedure, presence of catheter, dialysate

Risk for **Powerlessness** r/t chronic condition and care involved

See Child with Chronic Condition; Hospitalized Child; Renal Failure; Renal Failure, Acute/Chronic—Child

Peritonitis

Acute **Pain** r/t inflammation, stimulation of somatic nerves

Constipation r/t decreased oral intake, decrease of peristalsis

Deficient **Fluid** volume r/t retention of fluid in bowel with loss of circulating blood volume

Imbalanced **Nutrition**: less than body requirements r/t nausea, vomiting

Ineffective **Breathing** pattern r/t pain, increased abdominal pressure

Nausea r/t gastrointestinal irritation

Persistent Fetal Circulation

See Congenital Heart Disease/Cardiac Anomalies

Personal Identity Problems

Disturbed personal **Identity** r/t situational crisis, psychological impairment, chronic illness, pain

Personality Disorder

Chronic low **Self-esteem** r/t inability to set and achieve goals

Compromised family **Coping** r/t inability of client to provide positive feedback to family, chronicity exhausting family

Decisional **Conflict** r/t low self-esteem, feelings that choices will always be wrong

Disturbed personal **Identity** r/t lack of consistent positive self-image

Impaired **Adjustment** r/t ambivalent behavior toward others, testing of others' loyalty

Impaired **Social** interaction r/t knowledge or skill deficit regarding ways to interact effectively with others, self-concept disturbances

Risk for **Loneliness** r/t inability to interact appropriately with others

Risk for situational low **Self-esteem** r/t history of learned helplessness

Risk for **Self-mutilation** r/t disturbed interpersonal relationships, borderline personality disorders

Spiritual distress r/t lack of identifiable values, lack of meaning to life

See Antisocial Personality Disorder; Borderline Personality Disorder

Pertussis (Whooping Cough)

See Respiratory Infections, Acute Childhood

Petechiae

See Clotting Disorder

Pharyngitis

See Sore Throat

P

Pheochromocytoma

Anxiety r/t symptoms from increased catecholamines-headache, palpitations, sweating, nervousness, nausea, vomiting, syncope

Disturbed **Sleep** pattern r/t high levels of catecholamines

Ineffective **Health** maintenance r/t deficient Knowledge regarding treatment and self-care

Nausea r/t increased catecholamines

Risk for Ineffective **Tissue** perfusion: cardiopulmonary and renal r/t episodes of hypertension

See Surgery

Phobia (Specific)

Anxiety r/t inability to control emotions when dreaded object or situation is encountered

Fear r/t presence or anticipation of specific object or situation

Ineffective **Coping** r/t transfer of fears from self to dreaded object situation

Powerlessness r/t anxiety about encountering unknown or known entity

Risk for **Post-trauma** syndrome r/t exposure to dreaded object or situation

Risk for **Powerlessness** r/t inadequate coping patterns

Risk for situational low **Self-esteem** r/t decreased power/control over fears

See Anxiety; Panic Disorder

Photosensitivity

Ineffective **Health** maintenance r/t deficient knowledge regarding medications inducing photosensitivity

Risk for impaired **Skin** integrity r/t exposure to sun

Physical Abuse

See Abuse

P

PID (Pelvic Inflammatory Disease)

Acute **Pain** r/t biological injury; inflammation, edema, congestion of pelvic tissues

Ineffective **Health** maintenance r/t deficient knowledge regarding self-care, treatment of disease

Ineffective **Sexuality** patterns r/t medically imposed abstinence from sexual activities until acute infection subsides, change in reproductive potential

Risk for **Infection** r/t insufficient knowledge to avoid exposure to pathogens; proper hygiene, nutrition, other health habits

Risk for urge urinary **Incontinence** r/t inflammation, edema, congestion of pelvic tissues

See Maturational Issues, Adolescent

PIH (Pregnancy-Induced Hypertension/Preeclampsia)

Anxiety r/t fear of the unknown, threat to self and infant, change in role functioning

Death **Anxiety** r/t threat of preeclampsia

Deficient **Diversional** activity r/t bedrest

Deficient **Knowledge** r/t lack of experience with situation

Excess **Fluid** volume r/t decreased renal function

Impaired **Parenting** r/t bedrest

Impaired **Home** maintenance r/t bedrest

Impaired physical **Mobility** r/t medically prescribed limitations

Interrupted **Family** processes r/t situational crisis

Ineffective **Role** performance r/t change in physical capacity to assume role of pregnant woman or resume other roles

Impaired **Social** interaction r/t imposed bedrest

Powerlessness r/t complication threatening pregnancy, medically prescribed limitations

Risk for imbalanced **Fluid** volume r/t hypertension, altered renal function

Risk for **Injury**: fetal r/t decreased uteroplacental perfusion, seizures

Risk for **Injury**: maternal r/t vasospasm, high blood pressure

Situational low **Self-esteem** r/t loss of idealized pregnancy

Piloerection

Hypothermia r/t exposure to cold environment

Placenta Previa

Death **Anxiety** r/t threat of mortality associated with bleeding

Deficient **Diversional** activity r/t long-term hospitalization

Disturbed **Body** image r/t negative feelings about body and reproductive ability, feelings of helplessness

Fear r/t threat to self and fetus, unknown future

Impaired **Home** maintenance r/t maternal bed rest, hospitalization

Impaired physical **Mobility** r/t medical protocol, maternal bed rest

Ineffective **Coping** r/t threat to self and fetus

Ineffective **Role** performance r/t maternal bed rest, hospitalization

Ineffective **Tissue** perfusion: placental r/t dilation of cervix, loss of placental implantation site

Interrupted **Family** processes r/t maternal bed rest, hospitalization

Risk for **Constipation** r/t bed rest, pregnancy

Risk for deficient **Fluid** volume r/t maternal blood loss

Risk for imbalanced **Fluid** volume r/t maternal blood loss

Risk for impaired **Parenting** r/t maternal bed rest, hospitalization

Risk for **Injury**: fetal and maternal r/t threat to uteroplacental perfusion, hemorrhage

Risk for **Powerlessness** r/t complications of pregnancy and unknown outcome

Situational low **Self-esteem** r/t situational crisis

Spiritual distress r/t inability to participate in usual religious rituals, situational crisis

Pleural Effusion

Acute **Pain** r/t inflammation, fluid accumulation

Excess **Fluid** volume r/t compromised regulatory mechanisms; heart, liver, or kidney failure

Hyperthermia r/t increased metabolic rate secondary to infection

Ineffective **Breathing** pattern r/t pain

Pleural Friction Rub

Acute **Pain** r/t inflammation, fluid accumulation

Ineffective **Breathing** pattern r/t pain

See cause of Pleural Friction Rub

Pleurisy

Acute **Pain** r/t pressure on pleural nerve endings associated with fluid accumulation or inflammation

Ineffective **Breathing** pattern r/t pain

Risk for impaired **Gas** exchange r/t ventilation perfusion imbalance

Risk for impaired physical **Mobility** r/t activity intolerance, inability to "catch breath"

Risk for ineffective **Airway** clearance r/t increased secretions, ineffective cough because of pain

PMS (Premenstrual Tension Syndrome)

Acute **Pain** r/t hormonal stimulation of gastrointestinal structures

Deficient **Knowledge** r/t methods to deal with and prevent syndrome

Excess **Fluid** volume r/t alterations of hormonal levels inducing fluid retention

Effective **Therapeutic** regimen management: individual r/t desire for information to manage and prevent symptoms

Fatigue r/t hormonal changes

Risk for **Powerlessness** r/t lack of knowledge and ability to deal with symptoms

PND (Paroxysmal Nocturnal Dyspnea)

Anxiety r/t inability to breathe during sleep

Decreased **Cardiac** output r/t failure of the left ventricle

Disturbed **Sleep** pattern r/t suffocating feeling from fluid in lungs on awakening from sleep

Ineffective **Breathing** pattern r/t increase in carbon dioxide levels, decrease in oxygen levels

Risk for **Powerlessness** r/t inability to control nocturnal dyspnea

Sleep deprivation r/t inability to breathe during sleep

Pneumonia

Activity intolerance r/t imbalance between oxygen supply and demand

Deficient **Knowledge** r/t risk factors predisposing person to pneumonia, treatment

Hyperthermia r/t dehydration, increased metabolic rate, illness

Impaired **Oral** mucous membrane r/t dry mouth from mouth breathing, decreased fluid intake

Imbalanced **Nutrition: less than body requirements** r/t loss of appetite

Impaired **Gas** exchange r/t decreased functional lung tissue

Ineffective **Health** maintenance r/t deficient knowledge regarding self-care and treatment of disease

Ineffective **Airway** clearance r/t inflammation and presence of secretions

Risk for deficient **Fluid** volume r/t inadequate intake of fluids

See Respiratory Infections, Acute Childhood (for child)

Pneumothorax

Acute **Pain** r/t recent injury, coughing, deep breathing

Fear r/t threat to own well-being, difficulty breathing

Impaired **Gas** exchange r/t ventilation-perfusion imbalance

Risk for **Injury** r/t possible complications associated with closed chest drainage system

Poisoning, Risk for

Internal

Risk for **Poisoning** r/t reduced vision, verbalization of occupational settings without adequate safeguards, lack of safety or drug education, lack of proper precaution, cognitive or emotional difficulties, insufficient finances

P

External

Risk for **Poisoning** r/t large supplies of drugs in house, medicine stored in unlocked cabinets accessible to children or confused persons, dangerous products placed or stored within the reach of children or confused persons, availability of illicit drugs potentially contaminated by poisonous additives, flaking or peeling paint or plaster in presence of young children, chemical contamination of food and water, unprotected contact with heavy metals or chemicals, paint or lacquer used in poorly ventilated areas or without effective protection, presence of poisonous vegetation, presence of atmospheric pollutants

Polydipsia

See Diabetes Mellitus

Polyphagia

See Diabetes Mellitus

Polyuria

See Diabetes Mellitus

Postoperative Care

See Surgery, Postoperative

Postpartum, Normal Care

Acute **Pain** r/t episiotomy, lacerations, bruising, breast engorgement, headache, sore nipples, epidural or IV site, hemorrhoids

Anxiety r/t change in role functioning, parenting

Constipation r/t hormonal effects on smooth muscles, fear of straining with defecation, effects of anesthesia

Deficient **Knowledge: infant care** r/t lack of preparation for parenting

Disturbed **Sleep** pattern r/t care of infant

Effective **Breastfeeding** r/t basic breastfeeding knowledge, support of partner and health care provider

Fatigue r/t childbirth, new responsibilities of parenting, body changes

Health-seeking behaviors r/t postpartum recovery and adaptation

Impaired **Skin** integrity r/t episiotomy, lacerations

Ineffective **Role** performance r/t new responsibilities of parenting

Impaired **Urinary** elimination r/t effects of anesthesia, tissue trauma

Ineffective **Breastfeeding** r/t lack of knowledge, lack of support, lack of motivation

Readiness for enhanced family **Coping** r/t adaptation to new family member

Risk for Impaired **Parenting** r/t lack of role models, deficient knowledge

Risk for **Constipation** r/t hormonal effects on smooth muscles, fear of straining with defecation, effects of anesthesia

Risk for imbalanced **Fluid** volume r/t shift in blood volume, edema

Risk for **Infection** r/t tissue trauma, blood loss

Risk for **Post-trauma** syndrome r/t trauma or violence associated with labor and birth process, medical/surgical interventions, history of sexual abuse

Risk for urge urinary **Incontinence** r/t effects of anesthesia or tissue trauma

Sexual dysfunction r/t fear of pain or pregnancy

Postpartum Blues

Anxiety r/t new responsibilities of parenting

Deficient **Knowledge** r/t lifestyle changes

Disturbed **Body** image r/t normal postpartum recovery

Disturbed **Sleep** pattern r/t new responsibilities of parenting

Chronic **Sorrow** r/t loss of ideal postpartum experience or ideal parent-infant relationship

Fatigue r/t childbirth, postpartum state

Impaired **Adjustment** r/t lack of support systems

Impaired **Parenting** r/t hormone-induced depression

Impaired **Home** maintenance r/t fatigue, care of newborn

Impaired **Social** interaction r/t change in role functioning

Ineffective **Coping** r/t hormonal changes, maturational crisis

Ineffective **Role** performance r/t new responsibilities of parenting

Risk for **Post-trauma** syndrome r/t trauma or violence associated with labor and birth process, medical/surgical interventions, history of sexual abuse

Risk for situational low **Self-esteem** r/t decreased power over feelings of sadness

Risk for **Spiritual** distress r/t altered relationships, social isolation

Sexual dysfunction r/t fear of another pregnancy, postpartum pain, lochia flow

Postpartum Hemorrhage

Activity intolerance r/t anemia from loss of blood

Acute **Pain** r/t nursing and medical interventions to control bleeding

Death **Anxiety** r/t threat of mortality associated with bleeding

P

Decreased **Cardiac** output r/t hypovolemia

Deficient **Fluid** volume r/t uterine atony, loss of blood

Deficient **Knowledge** r/t lack of exposure to situation

Disturbed **Body** image r/t loss of ideal childbirth

Fear r/t threat to self, unknown future

Ineffective **Tissue** perfusion r/t hypovolemia

Impaired **Home** maintenance r/t lack of stamina

Interrupted **Breastfeeding** r/t separation from infant for medical treatment

Risk for Impaired **Parenting** r/t weakened maternal condition

Risk for imbalanced **Fluid** volume r/t maternal blood loss

Risk for **Infection** r/t loss of blood, depressed immunity

Risk for **Powerlessness** r/t acute illness

Post-Trauma Syndrome

Post-trauma syndrome r/t events outside the range of the usual human experience; physical and psychosocial abuse; tragic occurrence involving multiple deaths; sudden destruction of one's home or community; natural or produced disasters; wars; being held as a prisoner of war or criminal victimization (torture); epidemics; serious accidents; rape; assault; witnessing mutilation, violent death, or other horrors; serious threat or injury to self or loved ones; industrial and motor vehicle accidents; catastrophic illnesses or accidents; military combat

Post-Traumatic Stress Disorder

Disturbed **Thought** processes r/t sense of reliving the experience (flashbacks)

Anxiety r/t exposure to internal or external cues that symbolize or resemble an aspect of the traumatic event

Death **Anxiety** r/t psychological stress associated with traumatic event

Disturbed **Energy** field r/t disharmony of mind, body, spirit

Disturbed **Sleep** pattern r/t recurring nightmares

Ineffective **Breathing** pattern r/t hyperventilation associated with anxiety

Ineffective **Coping** r/t extreme anxiety

Post-trauma syndrome r/t exposure to a traumatic event

Readiness for enhanced **Spiritual** well-being r/t desire for harmony after stressful event

Risk for self- or other-directed **Violence** r/t fear of self or others

Risk for **Powerlessness** r/t flashbacks, reliving event

Disturbed **Sensory** perception r/t psychological stress

Sleep deprivation r/t nightmares associated with traumatic event

Spiritual distress r/t feelings of detachment or estrangement from others

Potassium, Increase/Decrease

See Hyperkalemia/Hypokalemia

Powerlessness

Powerlessness r/t health care environment, illness-related regimen, interpersonal interaction, lifestyle of helplessness

Risk for **Powerlessness** r/t chronic or acute illness, acute injury or progressive debilitating disease process, aging, dying, lack of knowledge of illness or health care style, lifestyle of dependency with inadequate coping patterns, absence of integrality, decreased self-esteem, low or unstable body image

Preeclampsia

See PIH

Pregnancy–Cardiac Disorders

See Cardiac Disorders in Pregnancy

Pregnancy-Induced Hypertension/Preeclampsia

See PIH

Pregnancy Loss

Acute **Pain** r/t surgical intervention

Anxiety r/t threat to role functioning, health status, situational crisis

Chronic **Sorrow** r/t loss of a fetus or child

Compromised family **Coping** r/t lack of support by significant other because of personal suffering

Ineffective **Coping** r/t situational crisis

Ineffective **Role** performance r/t inability to assume parenting role

Ineffective **Sexuality** patterns r/t self-esteem disturbance resulting from pregnancy loss and anxiety about future pregnancies

Readiness for enhanced **Spiritual** well-being r/t desire for acceptance of loss

Risk for ineffective **Sexuality** patterns r/t self-esteem disturbance, anxiety, grief

Risk for dysfunctional **Grieving** r/t loss of pregnancy

Risk for deficient **Fluid** volume r/t blood loss

Risk for **Infection** r/t retained products of conception

Risk for **Powerlessness** r/t situational crisis

Risk for **Spiritual** distress r/t intense suffering

Spiritual distress r/t intense suffering

P

Pregnancy—Normal

Deficient **Knowledge** r/t primiparity

Disturbed **Body** image r/t altered body function and appearance

Disturbed **Sleep** pattern r/t sleep deprivation secondary to uncomfortable pregnant state

Imbalanced **Nutrition: less than body requirements** r/t growing fetus, nausea

Imbalanced **Nutrition: more than body requirements** r/t deficient knowledge regarding nutritional needs of pregnancy

Interrupted **Family** processes r/t developmental transition of pregnancy

Readiness for enhanced family **Coping** r/t satisfying partner relationship, attention to gratification of needs, effective adaptation to developmental tasks of pregnancy

Fear r/t labor and delivery

Health-seeking behaviors r/t desire to promote optimal fetal and maternal health

Ineffective **Coping** r/t personal vulnerability, situational crisis

Nausea r/t hormonal changes of pregnancy

Sexual dysfunction r/t altered body function, self-concept, body image with pregnancy

See Discomforts of Pregnancy

Premature Dilation of the Cervix (Incompetent Cervix)

Ineffective **Role** performance r/t inability to continue usual patterns of responsibility

Anticipatory **Grieving** r/t potential loss of infant

Deficient **Diversional** activity r/t bed rest

Deficient **Knowledge** r/t treatment regimen, prognosis for pregnancy

Fear r/t potential loss of infant

Impaired physical **Mobility** r/t imposed bed rest to prevent preterm birth

Impaired **Social** interaction r/t bed rest

Ineffective **Coping** r/t bed rest, threat to fetus

Powerlessness r/t inability to control outcome of pregnancy

Risk for **Infection** r/t invasive procedures to prevent preterm birth

Risk for **Injury: fetal** r/t preterm birth, use of anesthetics

Risk for **Injury: maternal** r/t surgical procedures to prevent preterm birth (e.g., cerclage)

Risk for **Spiritual** distress r/t physical/psychological stress

Sexual dysfunction r/t fear of harm to fetus

Situational low **Self-esteem** r/t inability to complete normal pregnancy

Premature Infant (Child)

Delayed **Growth** and development: developmental lag r/t prematurity, environmental and stimulation deficiencies, multiple caretakers

Imbalanced **Nutrition: less than body requirements** r/t delayed or understimulated rooting reflex, easy fatigue during feeding, diminished endurance

Disorganized **Infant** behavior r/t prematurity

Disturbed **Sleep** pattern r/t noisy and noxious intensive care environment

Impaired **Gas** exchange r/t effects of cardiopulmonary insufficiency

Impaired **Swallowing** r/t decreased or absent gag reflex, fatigue

Ineffective **Thermoregulation** r/t large body surface/weight ratio, immaturity of thermal regulation, state of prematurity

Readiness for enhanced organized **Infant** behavior r/t prematurity

Risk for delayed **Development** r/t prematurity

Risk for disproportionate **Growth** r/t prematurity

Risk for **Infection** r/t inadequate, immature, or undeveloped acquired immune response

Risk for **Injury** r/t prolonged mechanical ventilation, retrolental fibroplasia (RLF) secondary to 100% oxygen environment

Disturbed **Sensory** perception r/t noxious stimuli, noisy environment

Premature Infant (Parent)

Anticipatory **Grieving** r/t loss of perfect child possibly leading to dysfunctional grieving

Chronic **Sorrow** r/t threat of loss of a child, prolonged hospitalization

Compromised family **Coping** r/t disrupted family roles and disorganization, prolonged condition exhausting supportive capacity of significant persons

Decisional **Conflict** r/t support system deficit, multiple sources of information

Dysfunctional **Grieving** (prolonged) r/t unresolved conflicts

Ineffective **Breastfeeding** r/t disrupted establishment of effective pattern secondary to prematurity or insufficient opportunities

Parental role **Conflict** r/t expressed concerns, expressed inability to care for child's physical, emotional, or developmental needs

Risk for impaired parent/infant/child **Attachment** r/t separation, physical barriers, lack of privacy

Risk for **Powerlessness** r/t inability to control situation

P

Risk for **Spiritual** distress r/t challenged belief or value systems regarding moral or ethical implications of treatment plans

Spiritual distress r/t challenged belief or value systems regarding moral or ethical implications of treatment plans

See Child with Chronic Condition; Hospitalized Child

Premature Rupture of Membranes

Anticipatory **Grieving** r/t potential loss of infant

Anxiety r/t threat to infant's health status

Disturbed **Body** image r/t inability to carry pregnancy to term

Ineffective **Coping** r/t situational crisis

Risk for **Infection** r/t rupture of membranes

Risk for **Injury**: fetal r/t risk of premature birth

Situational low **Self-esteem** r/t inability to carry pregnancy to term

Premenstrual Tension Syndrome

See PMS

Prenatal Care–Normal

Anxiety r/t unknown future, threat to self secondary to pain of labor

Constipation r/t decreased gastrointestinal motility secondary to hormonal stimulation

Deficient **Knowledge** r/t lack of experience with pregnancy and care

Disturbed **Sleep** pattern r/t discomforts of pregnancy and fetal activity

Fatigue r/t increased energy demands

Health-seeking behaviors r/t consistent prenatal care and education

Imbalanced **Nutrition**: less than body requirements r/t nausea from normal hormonal changes

Impaired **Urinary** elimination r/t frequency caused by increased pelvic pressure and hormonal stimulation

Ineffective **Breathing** pattern r/t increased intrathoracic pressure and decreased energy secondary to enlarged uterus

Interrupted **Family** processes r/t developmental transition

Readiness for enhanced **Spiritual** well-being r/t oncoming new role as parent

Risk for **Activity** intolerance r/t enlarged abdomen, increased cardiac workload

Risk for **Constipation** r/t decreased gastrointestinal motility secondary to hormonal stimulation

Risk for **Injury**: maternal r/t change in balance and center of gravity secondary to enlarged abdomen

Risk for **Sexual** dysfunction r/t enlarged abdomen, fear of harm to infant

Prenatal Testing

Acute **Pain** r/t invasive procedures

Anxiety r/t unknown outcome, delayed test results

Health-seeking behaviors r/t desire to have information regarding prenatal testing

Risk for **Infection** r/t invasive procedures during amniocentesis or chorionic villi sampling

Risk for **Injury**: fetal r/t invasive procedures

Preoperative Teaching

Health-seeking behaviors r/t preoperative regimens, postoperative precautions, expectations of role of client during preoperative or postoperative time

See Surgery, Preoperative Care

Pressure Ulcer

Acute **Pain** r/t tissue destruction, exposure of nerves

Imbalanced **Nutrition**: less than body requirements r/t limited access to food, inability to absorb nutrients because of biological factors, anorexia

Impaired bed **Mobility** r/t intolerance to activity, pain, cognitive impairment, depression, severe anxiety

Impaired **Skin** integrity: stage I or II pressure ulcer r/t physical immobility, mechanical factors, altered circulation, skin irritants

Impaired **Tissue** integrity: stage III or IV pressure ulcer r/t altered circulation, impaired physical mobility

Risk for **Infection** r/t physical immobility, mechanical factors (shearing forces, pressure, restraint, altered circulation, skin irritants)

Total urinary **Incontinence** r/t neurological dysfunction

Preterm Labor

Anticipatory **Grieving** r/t loss of idealized pregnancy, potential loss of fetus

Anxiety r/t threat to fetus, change in role functioning, change in environment and interaction patterns, use of tocolytic drugs

Deficient **Diversional** activity r/t long-term hospitalization

Disturbed **Sleep** pattern r/t change in usual pattern secondary to contractions, hospitalization, treatment regimen

Impaired **Home** maintenance r/t medical restrictions

Impaired physical **Mobility** r/t medically imposed restrictions

Impaired **Social** interaction r/t prolonged bedrest or hospitalization

Ineffective **Coping** r/t situational crisis, preterm labor

P

Ineffective **Role** performance r/t inability to carry out normal roles secondary to bedrest or hospitalization, change in expected course of pregnancy

Risk for **Injury**: fetal r/t premature birth, immature body systems

Risk for **Injury**: maternal r/t use of tocolytic drugs

Risk for **Powerlessness** r/t lack of control over preterm labor

Sexual dysfunction r/t actual or perceived limitation imposed by preterm labor and/or prescribed treatment, separation from partner because of hospitalization

Situational low **Self-esteem** r/t threatened ability to carry pregnancy to term

Problem-Solving Ability

Defensive **Coping** r/t situational crisis

Impaired **Adjustment** r/t altered locus of control

Ineffective **Coping** r/t situational crisis

Readiness for enhanced **Spiritual** well-being r/t desire to draw on inner strength and find meaning and purpose to life

Projection

Anxiety r/t threat to self-concept

Chronic low **Self-esteem** r/t failure

Defensive **Coping** r/t inability to acknowledge that own behavior may be a problem, blaming others

Impaired **Social** interaction r/t self-concept disturbance, confrontational communication style

Risk for **Loneliness** r/t blaming others for problems

Risk for **Post-trauma** syndrome r/t diminished ego strength

Prolapsed Umbilical Cord

Ineffective **Tissue** perfusion: fetal r/t interruption in umbilical blood flow

Fear r/t threat to fetus, impending surgery

Risk for **Injury**: fetal r/t cord compression, ineffective tissue perfusion

Risk for **Injury**: maternal r/t emergency surgery

Prolonged Gestation

Anxiety r/t potential change in birthing plans, need for increased medical intervention, unknown outcome for fetus

Defensive **Coping** r/t underlying feeling of inadequacy regarding ability to give birth normally

Imbalanced **Nutrition**: less than body requirements (fetal) r/t aging of placenta

Powerlessness r/t perceived lack of control over outcome of pregnancy

Situational low **Self-esteem** r/t perceived inadequacy of body functioning

Prostatectomy

See TURP

Prostatic Hypertrophy

Disturbed **Sleep** pattern r/t nocturia

Ineffective **Health** maintenance r/t deficient knowledge regarding self-care and prevention of complications

Risk for **Infection** r/t urinary residual post voiding, bacterial invasion of bladder

Risk for urge urinary **Incontinence** r/t small bladder capacity

Urinary retention r/t obstruction

Prostatitis

Ineffective **Health** maintenance r/t deficient knowledge regarding treatment

Ineffective **Protection** r/t depressed immune system

Risk for urge **Incontinence** r/t irritation of bladder

Protection, Altered

Ineffective **Protection** r/t extremes of age, inadequate nutrition, alcohol abuse, abnormal blood profiles (leukopenia, thrombocytopenia, anemia, coagulation), drug therapies (antineoplastic, corticosteroid, immune, anticoagulant, thrombolytic), treatments (surgery, radiation), diseases (e.g., cancer, immune disorders)

Pruritus

Deficient **Knowledge** r/t methods to treat and prevent itching

Impaired **Comfort**: pruritus r/t inflammation in tissues

Risk for impaired **Skin** integrity r/t scratching from pruritus

Psoriasis

Disturbed **Body** image r/t lesions on body

Ineffective **Health** maintenance r/t deficient knowledge regarding treatment modalities

Impaired **Skin** integrity r/t lesions on body

Powerlessness r/t lack of control over condition with frequent exacerbations and remissions

Psychosis

Anxiety r/t unconscious conflict with reality

Chronic **Sorrow** r/t chronic mental illness

Disturbed **Sleep** pattern r/t sensory alterations contributing to fear and anxiety

Disturbed **Thought** processes r/t inaccurate interpretations of environment

Fear r/t altered contact with reality

Imbalanced **Nutrition**: less than body requirements r/t lack of awareness of hunger, disinterest toward food

Impaired **Home** maintenance r/t impaired cognitive or emotional functioning, inadequate support systems

Impaired **Social** interaction r/t impaired communication patterns, self-concept disturbance, disturbed thought processes

Impaired verbal **Communication** r/t psychosis, inaccurate perceptions, hallucinations, delusions

Ineffective **Coping** r/t inadequate support systems, unrealistic perceptions, disturbed thought processes, impaired communication

Ineffective **Health** maintenance r/t cognitive impairment, ineffective individual and family coping

Interrupted **Family** processes r/t inability to express feelings, impaired communication

Risk for **Post-trauma** syndrome r/t diminished ego strength

Risk for self- or other-directed **Violence** r/t lack of trust, panic, hallucinations, delusional thinking

Risk for **Suicide** r/t psychiatric illness/disorder

Self-care deficit r/t loss of contact with reality, impairment of perception

Self-esteem disturbance r/t excessive use of defense mechanisms (e.g., projection, denial, rationalization)

Social **Isolation** r/t lack of trust, regression, delusional thinking, repressed fears

See Schizophrenia

PTCA (Percutaneous Transluminal Coronary Angioplasty)

See Angioplasty

Pulmonary Edema

Anxiety r/t fear of suffocation

Ineffective **Health** maintenance r/t deficient knowledge regarding treatment regimen

Impaired **Gas** exchange r/t extravasation of extravascular fluid in lung tissues and alveoli

Ineffective **Breathing** pattern r/t presence of tracheobronchial secretions

Sleep deprivation r/t inability to breathe

See CHF

Pulmonary Embolism

Acute **Pain** r/t biological injury, lack of oxygen to cells

Deficient **Knowledge** r/t activities to prevent embolism, self-care after diagnosis of embolism

Delayed **Surgical** recovery r/t complications associated with respiratory difficulty

Fear r/t severe pain, possible death

Impaired **Gas** exchange r/t altered blood flow to alveoli secondary to lodged embolus

Ineffective **Tissue** perfusion: pulmonary r/t interruption of pulmonary blood flow secondary to lodged embolus

Risk for altered **Cardiac** output r/t right ventricular failure secondary to obstructed pulmonary artery

See Anticoagulant Therapy

Pulmonary Stenosis

See Congenital Heart Disease/Cardiac Anomalies

Pulse Deficit

Decreased **Cardiac** output r/t dysrhythmia

See Dysrhythmia

Pulse Oximetry

See Hypoxia

Pulse Pressure, Increased

See Intracranial Pressure, Increased

Pulse Pressure, Narrowed

See Shock

Pulses, Absent or Diminished Peripheral

Ineffective **Tissue** perfusion: peripheral r/t interruption of arterial flow

Risk for **Peripheral** neurovascular dysfunction r/t fractures, mechanical compression, orthopedic surgery trauma, immobilization, burns, vascular obstruction

See Cause of Absent or Diminished Peripheral Pulses

Purpura

See Clotting Disorder

Pyelonephritis

Acute **Pain** r/t inflammation and irritation of urinary tract

Disturbed **Sleep** pattern r/t urinary frequency

Impaired **Comfort** r/t chills and fever

Ineffective **Health** maintenance r/t deficient knowledge regarding self-care, treatment of disease, prevention of further urinary tract infections

Impaired **Urinary** elimination r/t irritation of urinary tract

Risk for urge urinary **Incontinence** r/t irritation of urinary tract

P

Pyloric Stenosis

Acute **Pain** r/t surgical incision
Deficient **Fluid** volume r/t vomiting, dehydration
Ineffective **Health** maintenance r/t parental deficient knowledge regarding home care feeding regimen, wound care
Imbalanced **Nutrition:** less than body requirements r/t vomiting secondary to pyloric sphincter obstruction
See Hospitalized Child

Q

Quadriplegia

Anticipatory **Grieving** r/t loss of normal lifestyle, severity of disability
Impaired **Transfer** ability r/t quadriplegia
Impaired wheelchair **Mobility** r/t quadriplegia
Ineffective **Breathing** pattern r/t inability to use intercostal muscles
Risk for **Autonomic** dysreflexia r/t bladder distention, bowel distention, skin irritation, lack of client and caregiver knowledge
See Spinal Cord Injury

R

Rabies

Acute **Pain** r/t multiple immunization injections
Health-seeking behaviors r/t prophylactic immunization of domestic animals, avoidance of contact with wild animals
Hopelessness r/t poor prognosis
Ineffective **Health** maintenance r/t deficient knowledge regarding care of wound, isolation and observation of infected animal

Radiation Therapy

Activity intolerance r/t fatigue from possible anemia
Deficient **Knowledge** r/t what to expect with radiation therapy
Diarrhea r/t irradiation effects
Disturbed **Body** image r/t change in appearance, hair loss
Imbalanced **Nutrition:** less than body requirements r/t anorexia, nausea, vomiting, irradiation of areas of pharynx and esophagus
Impaired **Oral** mucous membrane r/t irradiation effects
Ineffective **Protection** r/t suppression of bone marrow
Nausea r/t side effects of radiation

Risk for impaired **Skin** integrity r/t irradiation effects
Risk for **Powerlessness** r/t medical treatment and possible side effects
Risk for **Spiritual** distress r/t radiation treatment, prognosis

Radical Neck Dissection

See Laryngectomy

Rage

Risk for other-directed **Violence** r/t panic state, manic excitement, organic brain syndrome
Risk for **Self-mutilation** r/t command hallucinations
Risk for **Suicide** r/t desire to kill oneself

Rape-Trauma Syndrome

Chronic **Sorrow** r/t forced loss of virginity
Rape-trauma syndrome r/t forced, violent sexual penetration against victim's will and consent
Rape-trauma syndrome: compound reaction r/t forced and violent sexual penetration against victim's will and consent, activation of previous health disruptions (e.g., physical illness, psychiatric illness, substance abuse)
Rape-trauma syndrome: silent reaction r/t forced and violent sexual penetration against victim's will and consent, demonstration of repression of incident
Risk for **Post-trauma** syndrome r/t trauma or violence associated with rape
Risk for **Powerlessness** r/t inability to control thoughts about incident
Risk for **Spiritual** distress r/t forced loss of virginity

Rash

Impaired **Comfort:** pruritus r/t inflammation in skin
Impaired **Skin** integrity r/t mechanical trauma
Risk for **Infection** r/t traumatized tissue, broken skin
Risk for latex **Allergy** r/t multiple surgical procedures, allergies to products associated with latex allergy, professions with daily associations with latex, history of reactions to latex

Rationalization

Defensive **Coping** r/t situational crisis, inability to accept blame for consequences of own behavior
Ineffective **Denial** r/t fear of consequences, actual or perceived loss
Readiness for enhanced **Spiritual** well-being r/t possibility of seeking harmony with self, others, higher power/God
Risk for **Post-trauma** syndrome r/t survivor's role in event

R

Rats, Rodents in the Home

Impaired **Home** maintenance r/t lack of knowledge, insufficient finances

Raynaud's Disease

Ineffective **Tissue** perfusion: peripheral r/t transient reduction of blood flow
Deficient **Knowledge** r/t lack of information about disease process, possible complications, self-care needs regarding disease process and medication

RDS (Respiratory Distress Syndrome)

See Respiratory Conditions of Neonate

Rectal Fullness

Constipation r/t decreased activity level, decreased fluid intake, inadequate fiber in diet, decreased peristalsis, side effects from antidepressant or antipsychotic therapy
Risk for **Constipation** r/t habitual denial/ignoring of urge to defecate

Rectal Pain/Bleeding

Acute **Pain** r/t pressure of defecation
Constipation r/t pain on defecation
Deficient **Knowledge** r/t possible causes of rectal bleeding, pain, treatment modalities
Risk for deficient **Fluid** volume: bleeding r/t untreated rectal bleeding

Rectal Surgery

See Hemorrhoidectomy

Rectocele Repair

Acute **Pain** r/t surgical procedure
Constipation r/t painful defecation
Ineffective **Health** maintenance r/t deficient knowledge of postoperative care of surgical site, dietary measures, exercise to prevent constipation
Risk for **Infection** r/t surgical procedure, possible contamination of site with feces
Risk for urge urinary **Incontinence** r/t edema from surgery
Urinary retention r/t edema from surgery

Reflex Incontinence

Reflex **Incontinence** r/t neurological impairment

Regression

Anxiety r/t threat to or change in health status
Defensive **Coping** r/t denial of obvious problems, weaknesses
Ineffective **Role** performance r/t powerlessness over health status

Powerlessness r/t health care environment
See Hospitalized Child; Separation Anxiety

Regretful

Anxiety r/t situational or maturational crises
Death **Anxiety** r/t feelings of not having accomplished goals in life
Risk for **Spiritual** distress r/t inability to forgive

Rehabilitation

Impaired **Comfort** r/t difficulty in performing rehabilitation tasks
Impaired physical **Mobility** r/t injury, surgery, psychosocial condition warranting rehabilitation
Ineffective **Coping** r/t loss of normal function
Self-care deficit r/t impaired physical mobility

Relaxation Techniques

Anxiety r/t disturbed energy field
Health-seeking behaviors r/t requesting information about ways to relieve stress
Readiness for enhanced **Spiritual** well-being r/t seeking comfort from higher power

Religious Concern

Readiness for enhanced **Spiritual** well-being r/t desire for increased spirituality
Risk for **Spiritual** distress r/t physical or psychological stress
Spiritual distress r/t separation from religious or cultural ties

Relocation Stress Syndrome

Relocation stress syndrome r/t past, concurrent, and recent losses; losses involved with decision to move; feeling of powerlessness; lack of adequate support system; little or no preparation for the impending move; moderate to high degree of environmental change; history and types of previous transfers; impaired psychosocial health status; decreased physical health status; advanced age
Risk for **Relocation** stress syndrome (see Relocation stress syndrome)

Renal Failure

Activity intolerance r/t effects of anemia, congestive heart failure
Chronic **Sorrow** r/t chronic illness
Death **Anxiety** r/t unknown outcome of disease
Decreased **Cardiac** output r/t effects of congestive heart failure, elevated potassium levels interfering with conduction system

Excess **Fluid** volume r/t decreased urine output, sodium retention, inappropriate fluid intake

Fatigue r/t effects of chronic uremia and anemia

Impaired **Comfort:** pruritus r/t effects of uremia

Imbalanced **Nutrition:** less than body requirements r/t anorexia, nausea, vomiting, altered taste sensation, dietary restrictions

Impaired **Oral** mucous membrane r/t irritation from nitrogenous waste products

Impaired **Urinary** elimination r/t effects of disease, need for dialysis

Ineffective **Coping** r/t depression secondary to chronic disease

Risk for impaired **Oral** mucous membrane r/t dehydration, effects of uremia

Risk for **Infection** r/t altered immune functioning

Risk for **Injury** r/t bone changes, neuropathy, muscle weakness

Risk for **Noncompliance** r/t complex medical therapy

Risk for **Powerlessness** r/t chronic illness

Spiritual distress r/t dealing with chronic illness

Renal Failure, Acute/Chronic–Child

Disturbed **Body** image r/t growth retardation, bone changes, visibility of dialysis access devices (shunt, fistula), edema

Deficient **Diversional** activity r/t immobility during dialysis

See Child with Chronic Illness; Hospitalized Child; Renal Failure

Renal Failure, Nonoliguric

Anxiety r/t change in health status

Risk for deficient **Fluid** volume r/t loss of large volumes of urine

See Renal Failure

Renal Transplantation, Donor

Decisional **Conflict** r/t harvesting of kidney from traumatized donor

Readiness for enhanced family **Coping** r/t decision to allow organ donation

Readiness for enhanced **Spirituality** r/t inner peace resulting from allowance of organ donation

Spiritual distress r/t anticipatory grieving from loss of significant person

See Nephrectomy

Renal Transplantation, Recipient

Anxiety r/t possible rejection, procedure

Deficient **Knowledge** r/t specific nutritional needs, possible paralytic ileus, fluid or sodium restrictions

Impaired **Urinary** elimination r/t possible impaired renal function

Ineffective **Protection** r/t immunosuppression therapy

Impaired **Health** maintenance r/t long-term home treatment after transplantation, diet, signs of rejection, use of medications

Risk for **Infection** r/t use of immunosuppressive therapy to control rejection

Spiritual distress r/t obtaining transplanted kidney from someone's traumatic loss

Respiratory Acidosis

See Acidosis, Respiratory

Respiratory Conditions of the Neonate (Respiratory Distress Syndrome [RDS], Meconium Aspiration, Diaphragmatic Hernia)

Fatigue r/t increased energy requirements and metabolic demands

Impaired **Gas** exchange r/t decreased surfactant, immature lung tissue

Ineffective **Airway** clearance r/t sequelae of attempts to breathe in utero resulting in meconium aspiration

Ineffective **Breathing** pattern r/t prolonged ventilator dependence

Risk for **Infection** r/t tissue destruction or irritation secondary to aspiration of meconium fluid

See Bronchopulmonary Dysplasia; Hospitalized Child; Premature Infant

Respiratory Distress

See Dyspnea

Respiratory Distress Syndrome (RDS)

See Respiratory Conditions of Neonate

Respiratory Infections, Acute Childhood (Croup, Epiglottitis, Pertussis, Pneumonia, Respiratory Syncytial Virus)

Activity intolerance r/t generalized weakness, dyspnea, fatigue, poor oxygenation

Anxiety/fear r/t oxygen deprivation, difficulty breathing

Deficient **Fluid** volume r/t insensible losses (fever, diaphoresis), inadequate oral fluid intake

Hyperthermia r/t infectious process

Imbalanced **Nutrition:** less than body requirements r/t anorexia, fatigue, generalized weakness, poor sucking and breathing coordination, dyspnea

Impaired **Gas** exchange r/t insufficient oxygenation secondary to inflammation or edema of epiglottis, larynx, bronchial passages

R

Ineffective **Airway** clearance r/t excess tracheobronchial secretions

Ineffective **Breathing** pattern r/t inflamed bronchial passages, coughing

Risk for **Aspiration** r/t inability to coordinate breathing, coughing, sucking

Risk for **Infection**: transmission to others r/t virulent infectious organisms

Risk for **Injury** (to pregnant others) r/t exposure to aerosolized medications (e.g., ribavirin, pentamidine), resultant potential fetal toxicity

Risk for **Suffocation** r/t inflammation of larynx, epiglottis

See Hospitalized Child

Respiratory Syncytial Virus

See Respiratory Infections, Acute Childhood

Retching

Imbalanced **Nutrition**: less than body requirements r/t inability to ingest food

Nausea r/t chemotherapy, postsurgical anesthesia, irritation to gastrointestinal system, stimulation of neuropharmacologic mechanisms

Retinal Detachment

Anxiety r/t change in vision, threat of loss of vision

Deficient **Knowledge** r/t symptoms, need for early intervention to prevent permanent damage

Risk for Impaired **Home** maintenance r/t postoperative care, activity limitations, care of affected eye

Disturbed **Sensory** perception: visual r/t changes in vision, sudden flashes of light, floating spots, blurring of vision

See Vision Impairment

Reye's Syndrome

Anticipatory **Grieving** r/t uncertain prognosis and sequelae

Compromised family **Coping** r/t acute situational crisis

Deficient **Fluid** volume r/t vomiting, hyperventilation

Disturbed **Thought** processes r/t degenerative changes in fatty brain tissue

Excess **Fluid** volume: cerebral r/t cerebral edema

Ineffective **Health** maintenance r/t deficient knowledge regarding use of salicylates during viral illness of child

Imbalanced **Nutrition**: less than body requirements r/t effects of liver dysfunction, vomiting

Impaired **Gas** exchange r/t hyperventilation, sequelae of increased intracranial pressure

Impaired **Skin** integrity r/t effects of decorticate or decerebrate posturing, seizure activity

Ineffective **Breathing** pattern r/t neuromuscular impairment

Risk for **Injury** r/t combative behavior, seizure activity

Disturbed **Sensory** perception r/t cerebral edema

Situational low **Self-esteem**: family r/t negative perceptions of self, perceived inability to manage family situation, expressions of guilt

See Hospitalized Child

Rh Factor Incompatibility

Anxiety r/t unknown outcome of pregnancy

Health-seeking behaviors r/t prenatal care, compliance with diagnostic and treatment regimen

Deficient **Knowledge** r/t treatment regimen from lack of experience with situation

Powerlessness r/t perceived lack of control over outcome of pregnancy

Risk for fetal **Injury** r/t intrauterine destruction of red blood cells, transfusions

Rheumatic Fever

See Endocarditis

Rheumatoid Arthritis, Juvenile (JRA)

Acute **Pain** r/t swollen or inflamed joints, restricted movement, physical therapy

Delayed **Growth** and development r/t effects of physical disability, chronic illness

Fatigue r/t chronic inflammatory disease

Impaired physical **Mobility** r/t pain, restricted joint movement

Risk for impaired **Skin** integrity r/t splints, adaptive devices

Risk for **Injury** r/t impaired physical mobility, splints, adaptive devices, increased bleeding potential secondary to antiinflammatory medications

Risk for situational low **Self-esteem** r/t disturbed in body image

Self-care deficits: feeding, bathing/hygiene, dressing/grooming, toileting r/t restricted joint movement, pain

See Child with Chronic Condition; Hospitalized Child

Rib Fracture

Acute **Pain** r/t movement, deep breathing

Ineffective **Breathing** pattern r/t fractured ribs

See Ventilator Client (if relevant)

R

Ridicule of Others

Defensive **Coping** r/t situational crisis, psychological impairment, substance abuse

Risk for **Post-trauma** syndrome r/t perception of the event

Ringworm of Body

Impaired **Skin** integrity r/t presence of macules associated with fungus

Ineffective **Therapeutic** regimen management r/t deficient knowledge of prevention, treatment

See Itching

Ringworm of Nails

Disturbed **Body** image r/t appearance of nails, removed nails

Ineffective **Therapeutic** regimen management r/t deficient knowledge of prevention, treatment

Ringworm of Scalp

Disturbed **Body** image r/t possible hair loss (alopecia)

Ineffective **Therapeutic** regimen management r/t deficient knowledge of prevention, treatment

See Itching

Roaches, Invasion of Home with

Impaired **Home** maintenance r/t lack of knowledge, insufficient finances

Role Performance, Altered

Ineffective **Role** performance r/t inability to perform role as anticipated

RSV (Respiratory Syncytial Virus)

See Respiratory Infection, Acute Childhood

Rubella

See Communicable Diseases, Childhood

Rubor of Extremities

Ineffective **Tissue** perfusion: peripheral r/t interruption of arterial flow

See Peripheral Vascular Disease

S

Sadness

Dysfunctional **Grieving** r/t actual or perceived loss

Readiness for enhanced **Spiritual** well-being r/t desire for harmony following actual or perceived loss

Risk for **Powerlessness** r/t actual or perceived loss

Risk for **Spiritual** distress r/t loss of loved one

Spiritual distress r/t intense suffering

Safety, Childhood

Deficient **Knowledge:** potential for enhanced health maintenance r/t parental knowledge and skill acquisition regarding appropriate safety measures

Health-seeking behaviors: enhanced parenting r/t adequate support systems, appropriate requests for help, desire and request for safety information, requests for information or assistance regarding parenting skills

Risk for altered **Health** maintenance r/t parental deficient knowledge regarding appropriate safety needs per developmental stage, childproofing house, infant and child car restraints, water safety, teaching of child the way to avoid molestation

Risk for impaired **Parenting** r/t lack of available and effective role model, lack of knowledge, misinformation from other family members (old wives' tales)

Risk for **Aspiration** and/or suffocation r/t pillow or propped bottle placed in infant's crib; sides of playpen/crib being wide enough for child to get head through; child left in car with engine running; enclosed areas; plastic bags or small objects used as toys; toys with small, breakaway parts; refrigerators or freezers with doors accessible as play areas; child left unattended in or near bathtub, pool, spa; low clotheslines; electric garage doors without automatic stop/reopen; pacifier hung around infant's neck; food not cut into small, bite-size, age-appropriate pieces; balloons, hot dogs, nuts, or popcorn given to infant or young child (especially <1 year of age); use of baby powder

Risk for **Injury/Trauma** r/t developmental age, altered home maintenance management (house not childproofed), impaired parenting, hot liquids within child's reach, no infant or child car restraints, no gate at top of stairs, lack of immunization, no fences or pool or spa covers, child left unattended in car with closed windows in hot weather, firearms loaded and within child's reach

Risk for **Poisoning** r/t use of lead-based paint, presence of asbestos or radon gas, drugs not locked in cabinet, household products left in accessible area (bleach, detergent, drain cleaners, household cleaners), alcohol and perfume within reach of child, presence of poisonous plants, atmospheric pollutants

Salmonella

See Gastroenteritis

Salpingectomy

Anticipatory **Grieving** r/t possible loss due to tubal pregnancy

Decisional **Conflict** r/t sterilization procedure

Risk for impaired **Urinary** elimination r/t trauma to ureter during surgery

See Hysterectomy; Surgery

Sarcoidosis

Acute **Pain** r/t possible disease affecting joints

Anxiety r/t change in health status

Impaired **Gas** exchange r/t ventilation-perfusion imbalance

Ineffective **Health** maintenance r/t deficient knowledge regarding home care and medication regimen

Risk for decreased **Cardiac** output r/t dysrhythmias

SBE (Self Breast Examination)

Health-seeking behaviors r/t desire to have information about self breast examination

Scabies

See Communicable Diseases, Childhood

Scared

Anxiety r/t threat of death, threat to or change in health status

Death **Anxiety** r/t unresolved issues surrounding end of life decisions

Fear r/t hospitalization, real or imagined threat to own well-being

Schizophrenia

Anxiety r/t unconscious conflict with reality

Chronic **Sorrow** r/t chronic mental illness

Deficient **Diversional** activity r/t social isolation, possible regression

Disturbed **Sleep** pattern r/t sensory alterations contributing to fear and anxiety

Disturbed **Thought** processes r/t inaccurate interpretations of environment

Fear r/t altered contact with reality

Imbalanced **Nutrition: less than body requirements** r/t fear of eating, unaware of hunger, disinterest toward food

Impaired **Home** maintenance r/t impaired cognitive or emotional functioning, insufficient finances, inadequate support systems

Impaired **Social** interaction r/t impaired communication patterns, self-concept disturbance, disturbed thought processes

Impaired verbal **Communication** r/t psychosis, disorientation, inaccurate perception, hallucinations, delusions

Ineffective **Coping** r/t inadequate support systems, unrealistic perceptions, inadequate coping skills, disturbed thought processes, impaired communication

Ineffective **Health** maintenance r/t cognitive impairment, ineffective individual and family coping, lack of material resources

Ineffective **Therapeutic** regimen management: families r/t chronicity and unpredictability of condition

Interrupted **Family** processes r/t inability to express feelings, impaired communication

Risk for **Caregiver** role strain r/t bizarre behavior of client, chronicity of condition

Risk for **Loneliness** r/t inability to interact socially

Risk for **Post-trauma** syndrome r/t diminished ego strength

Risk for **Powerlessness** r/t intrusive, distorted thinking

Risk for self- and other-directed **Violence** r/t lack of trust, panic, hallucinations, delusional thinking

Risk for **Suicide** r/t psychiatric illness

Self-care deficit r/t loss of contact with reality, impairment of perception

Self-esteem disturbance r/t excessive use of defense mechanisms (e.g., projection, denial, rationalization)

Sleep deprivation r/t intrusive thoughts, nightmares

Social isolation r/t lack of trust, regression, delusional thinking, repressed fears

Scoliosis

Acute **Pain** r/t musculoskeletal restrictions, surgery, reambulation with cast or spinal rod

Chronic **Sorrow** r/t chronic disability

Disturbed **Body** image r/t use of therapeutic braces, postsurgery scars, restricted physical activity

Impaired **Adjustment** r/t lack of developmental maturity to comprehend long-term consequences of noncompliance with treatment procedures

Impaired **Gas** exchange r/t restricted lung expansion secondary to severe presurgery curvature of spine, immobilization

Impaired physical **Mobility** r/t restricted movement, dyspnea secondary to severe curvature of spine

Impaired **Skin** integrity r/t braces, casts, surgical correction

Ineffective **Breathing** pattern r/t restricted lung expansion secondary to severe curvature of spine

Ineffective **Health** maintenance r/t deficient knowledge regarding treatment modalities, restrictions, home care, postoperative activities

Risk for **Infection** r/t surgical incision

Risk for perioperative positioning **Injury** r/t prone position

See Hospitalized Child; Maturational Issues, Adolescent

Sedentary Lifestyle

Activity intolerance r/t sedentary lifestyle

Seizure Disorders, Adult

Acute **Confusion** r/t postseizure state

Impaired **Memory** r/t seizure activity

Ineffective **Health** maintenance r/t lack of knowledge regarding anticonvulsive therapy

Risk for disturbed **Thought** processes r/t effects of anticonvulsant medications

Risk for **Falls** r/t uncontrolled seizure activity

Risk for ineffective **Airway** clearance r/t accumulation of secretions during seizure

Risk for **Injury** r/t uncontrolled movements during seizure, falls, drowsiness secondary to anticonvulsants

Risk for **Powerlessness** r/t possible seizure

Social isolation r/t unpredictability of seizures, community-imposed stigma

See Epilepsy

Seizure Disorders, Childhood (Epilepsy, Febrile Seizures, Infantile Spasms)

Ineffective **Health** maintenance r/t lack of knowledge regarding anticonvulsive therapy, fever reduction (febrile seizures)

Risk for delayed **Development** and disproportionate growth r/t effects of seizure disorder, parental overprotection

Risk for disturbed **Thought** processes r/t effects of anticonvulsant medications

Risk for **Falls** r/t possible seizure

Risk for ineffective **Airway** clearance r/t accumulation of secretions during seizure

Risk for **Injury** r/t uncontrolled movements during seizure, falls, drowsiness secondary to anticonvulsants

Social isolation r/t unpredictability of seizures, community-imposed stigma

See Epilepsy

Self Breast Examination

See SBE

Self-Care Deficit, Bathing/Hygiene

Bathing/hygiene **Self-care** deficit r/t intolerance to activity, decreased strength and endurance, pain, discomfort, perceptual or cognitive impairment, neuromuscular impairment, musculoskeletal impairment, depression, severe anxiety

Self-Care Deficit, Dressing/Grooming

Dressing/grooming **Self-care** deficit r/t intolerance to activity, decreased strength and endurance, pain, discomfort, perceptual or cognitive impairment, neuromuscular impairment, musculoskeletal impairment, depression, severe anxiety

Self-Care Deficit, Feeding

Feeding **Self-care** deficit: r/t intolerance to activity, decreased strength and endurance, pain, discomfort, perceptual or cognitive impairment, neuromuscular impairment, musculoskeletal impairment, depression, severe anxiety

Self-Care Deficit, Toileting

Toileting **Self-care** deficit r/t impaired transfer ability, impaired mobility status, intolerance to activity, decreased strength and endurance, pain, discomfort, perceptual or cognitive impairment, neuromuscular impairment, musculoskeletal impairment, depression, severe anxiety

Self-Destructive Behavior

Post-trauma response r/t unresolved feelings from traumatic event

Risk for **Self-mutilation** r/t feelings of depression, rejection, self-hatred, depersonalization; command hallucinations

Risk for self-directed **Violence** r/t panic state, history of child abuse, toxic reaction to medication

Risk for **Suicide** r/t history of self-destructive behavior

Self-Esteem, Chronic Low

Chronic low **Self-esteem** r/t long-standing negative self-evaluation

Self-Esteem, Situational Low

Situational low **Self-esteem** r/t developmental crisis, disturbed body image, functional impairment, loss, social role changes, lack of recognition/rewards, behavior inconsistent with values, failures/rejections

S

Risk for situational low **Self-esteem** r/t self-esteem disturbance

Self-esteem disturbance r/t inappropriate and learned negative feelings about self

Self-Mutilation, Risk for

Risk for **Self-mutilation** r/t inability to cope with increased psychological or physiological tension in a healthy manner; feelings of depression, rejection, self-hatred, separation anxiety, guilt, depersonalization; fluctuating emotions; command hallucinations; need for sensory stimuli; parental emotional deprivation; dysfunctional family

Self-mutilation r/t psychotic state (command hallucinations); inability to express tension verbally; childhood sexual abuse; violence between parental figures; family divorce; family alcoholism; family history of self-destructive behaviors; adolescence; peers who self-mutilate; isolation from peers; perfectionism; substance abuse; eating disorders; sexual identity crisis; low or unstable self-esteem; low or unstable body image; labile behavior (mood swings); history of inability to plan solutions or see long-term consequences; use of manipulation to obtain nurturing relationship with others; chaotic/disturbed interpersonal relationships; emotional disturbance; battered child; feels threatened with actual or potential loss of significant relationship (e.g., loss of parent/parental relationship); experiences dissociation or depersonalization; mounting tension that is intolerable; impulsivity; inadequate coping; irresistible urge to cut/damage self; needs quick reduction of stress; childhood illness or surgery; foster, group, or institutional care; incarceration; character disorder; borderline personality disorder; developmental delay or autism; history of self-injurious behavior; feelings of depression, rejection, self-hatred, separation anxiety, guilt, depersonalization; poor parent-adolescent communication; lack of family confidant.

Senile Dementia

See Dementia

Sensory/Perceptual Alterations

Disturbed **Sensory** perceptions: visual, auditory, kinesthetic, gustatory, tactile, olfactory r/t altered, excessive, or insufficient environmental stimuli; altered sensory reception, transmission, and/or integration; endogenous (electrolyte) or exogenous (e.g., drugs) chemical alterations; psychological stress

Separation Anxiety

Ineffective **Coping** r/t maturational and situational crises, vulnerability secondary to developmental age, hospitalization, separation from family and familiar surroundings, multiple caregivers

See Hospitalized Child

Sepsis—Child

Delayed **Surgical** recovery r/t presence of infection

Impaired **Comfort**: increased sensitivity to environmental stimuli r/t disturbed sensory perceptions: visual, auditory, kinesthetic

Imbalanced **Nutrition**: less than body requirements r/t anorexia, generalized weakness, poor sucking reflex

Ineffective **Tissue** perfusion: cardiopulmonary, peripheral r/t arterial or venous blood flow exchange problems, septic shock

Ineffective **Thermoregulation** r/t infectious process, septic shock

Risk for impaired **Skin** integrity r/t desquamation secondary to disseminated intravascular coagulation (DIC)

See Hospitalized Child; Premature Infant

Septicemia

Deficient **Fluid** volume r/t vasodilation of peripheral vessels, leaking of capillaries

Imbalanced **Nutrition**: less than body requirements r/t anorexia, generalized weakness

Ineffective **Tissue** perfusion r/t decreased systemic vascular resistance

See Sepsis—Child; Shock; Shock, Septic

Sexual Dysfunction

Chronic **Sorrow** r/t loss of ideal sexual experience, altered relationships

Sexual dysfunction r/t biopsychosocial alteration of sexuality, ineffectual or absent role models, physical abuse or harmful relationships, vulnerability, conflicting values, lack of privacy, lack of significant others, altered body structure or function (pregnancy, recent childbirth, drug use, surgery, anomalies, disease process, trauma, radiation), misinformation or lack of knowledge

Sexuality, Adolescent

Decisional **Conflict**: sexual activity r/t undefined personal values or beliefs, multiple or divergent sources of information, lack of relevant information

Deficient **Knowledge**: potential for enhanced health maintenance r/t multiple or divergent sources of

S

information or lack of relevant information regarding sexual transmission of disease, contraception, prevention of toxic shock syndrome

Disturbed **Body** image r/t anxiety secondary to unachieved developmental milestone (puberty) or deficient knowledge regarding reproductive maturation as manifested by amenorrhea or expressed concerns regarding lack of growth of secondary sex characteristics

Risk for **Rape-trauma** syndrome r/t date rape, campus rape, insufficient knowledge regarding self-protection mechanisms

See Maturational Issues, Adolescent

Sexuality Patterns, Ineffective

Ineffective **Sexuality** patterns r/t knowledge or skill deficit regarding alternative responses to health-related transitions, altered body function or structure, illness or medical problems, lack of privacy, lack of significant other, ineffective or absent role models, fear of pregnancy or acquiring a sexually transmitted disease, impaired relationship with a significant other

Sexually Transmitted Disease

See STD

Shakiness

Anxiety r/t situational or maturational crisis, threat of death

Shame

Self-esteem disturbance r/t inability to deal with past traumatic events, blaming of self for events not under one's control

Shingles

Acute **Pain** r/t vesicular eruption along the nerves

Ineffective **Protection** r/t abnormal blood profiles

Risk for **Infection** r/t tissue destruction

Social isolation r/t altered state of wellness, contagiousness of disease

See Itching

Shivering

Hypothermia r/t exposure to cool environment

Shock

Fear r/t serious threat to health status

Ineffective **Tissue** perfusion: cardiopulmonary, peripheral r/t arterial/venous blood flow exchange problems

Risk for **Injury** r/t prolonged shock resulting in multiple organ failure, death

See Shock, Cardiogenic; Shock, Hypovolemic; Shock, Septic

Shock, Cardiogenic

Decreased **Cardiac** output r/t decreased myocardial contractility, dysrhythmia

See Shock

Shock, Hypovolemic

Deficient **Fluid** volume r/t abnormal loss of fluid

See Shock

Shock, Septic

Deficient **Fluid** volume r/t abnormal loss of fluid through capillaries, pooling of blood in peripheral circulation

Ineffective **Protection** r/t inadequately functioning immune system

See Sepsis, Child; Septicemia; Shock

Shoulder Repair

Risk for perioperative positioning **Injury** r/t immobility

Self-care deficit: bathing/hygiene, dressing/grooming, feeding r/t immobilization of affected shoulder

See Surgery; Total Joint Replacement

Sickle Cell Anemia/Crisis

Activity intolerance r/t fatigue, effects of chronic anemia

Acute **Pain** r/t viscous blood, tissue hypoxia

Deficient **Fluid** volume r/t decreased intake, increased fluid requirements during sickle cell crisis, decreased ability of kidneys to concentrate urine

Impaired physical **Mobility** r/t pain, fatigue

Risk for ineffective **Tissue** perfusion: renal, cerebral, cardiac, gastrointestinal, peripheral r/t effects of red cell sickling, infarction of tissues

Risk for **Infection** r/t alterations in splenic function

See Child with Chronic Condition; Hospitalized Child

SIDS

Anticipatory **Grieving** r/t potential loss of infant

Anxiety/Fear: parental r/t life-threatening event

Deficient **Knowledge:** potential for enhanced health maintenance r/t knowledge or skill acquisition of CPR and home apnea monitoring

Disturbed **Sleep** pattern: parental/infant r/t home apnea monitoring

Interrupted **Family** processes r/t stress secondary to special care needs of infant with apnea

S

Risk for **Powerlessness** r/t unanticipated life-threatening event
See Terminally Ill Child/Death of Child

Situational Crisis

Ineffective **Coping** r/t situational crisis
Interrupted **Family** processes r/t situational crisis
Readiness for enhanced **Spiritual** well-being r/t desire for harmony following crisis

Skin Cancer

Impaired **Skin** integrity r/t abnormal cell growth in skin, treatment of skin cancer
Ineffective **Health** maintenance r/t deficient knowledge regarding self-care with skin cancer

Skin Disorders

External

Impaired **Skin** integrity r/t hyperthermia, hypothermia, chemical substances, mechanical factors (shearing forces, pressure, restraint), radiation, physical immobilization, humidity

Internal

Impaired **Skin** integrity r/t medication, altered nutritional state (obesity, emaciation), altered metabolic state, altered circulation, altered sensation, altered pigmentation, skeletal prominence, developmental factors, immunological deficit, alterations in turgor (change in elasticity)

Skin Integrity, Risk for Impaired

Risk for impaired **Skin** integrity r/t internal or external factors that are potentially harmful to skin

Skin Turgor, Change in Elasticity

Deficient **Fluid** volume r/t active fluid loss (NOTE: decreased skin turgor can be a normal finding in the elderly)

Sleep Apnea

See PND

Sleep Deprivation

Disturbed **Sensory** perception r/t lack of sleep
Fatigue r/t lack of sleep
Sleep deprivation r/t prolonged physical discomfort; prolonged psychological discomfort; sustained inadequate sleep hygiene; prolonged use of pharmacological or dietary antisoporifics; aging-related sleep stage shifts; sustained circadian asynchrony; inadequate daytime activity; sustained environmental stimulation; sustained unfamiliar or uncomfortable sleep environment; non–sleep-inducing parenting practices; sleep

apnea; periodic limb movement (e.g., restless leg syndrome, nocturnal myoclonus); sundowner's syndrome; narcolepsy; idiopathic central nervous system hypersomnolence; sleep walking; sleep terror; sleep-related enuresis; nightmares; familial sleep paralysis; sleep-related painful erections; dementia

Sleep Pattern Disorders

Sleep pattern disorders r/t sensory alterations, internal factors (illness, psychological stress), external factors (environmental changes, social cues)

Sleep Pattern, Disturbed—Parent/Child

Disturbed **Sleep** pattern: child r/t anxiety or apprehension secondary to parental deprivation (see Suspected Child Abuse and Neglect), fear, night terrors, enuresis, inconsistent parental responses to child's requests to alter bedtime rules, frequent nighttime awakening, inability to wean from parents' bed, hypervigilance
Disturbed **Sleep** pattern: parent r/t time-intensive home treatments, increased caretaker demands

Slurring of Speech

Impaired verbal **Communication** r/t decrease in circulation to brain, brain tumor, anatomical defect, cleft palate
Situational low **Self-esteem** r/t speech impairment

Small Bowel Resection

See Abdominal Surgery

Smell, Loss of

Adult **Failure** to thrive r/t imbalanced nutrition: less than body requirements associated with loss of smell
Disturbed **Sensory** perception: olfactory r/t altered sensory reception, transmission, or integration

Smoking Behavior

Altered **Health** maintenance r/t denial of effects of smoking, lack of effective support for smoking withdrawal

Social Interaction, Impaired

Social interaction: impaired r/t knowledge or skill deficit regarding ways to enhance mutuality, communication barriers, self-concept disturbance, absence of available significant others or peers, limited physical mobility, therapeutic isolation, sociocultural dissonance, environmental barriers, disturbed thought processes

S

Social Isolation

Social isolation r/t factors contributing to absence of satisfying personal relationships, such as delay in accomplishing developmental tasks, immature interests, alterations in physical appearance, alterations in mental status, unaccepted social behavior, unaccepted social values, altered state of wellness, inadequate personal resources, inability to engage in satisfying personal relationships, fear

Sociopath

See Antisocial Personality Disorder

Sodium, Decrease/Increase

See Hyponatremia/Hypernatremia

Somatoform Disorder

Anxiety r/t unresolved conflicts channeled into physical complaints or conditions
Chronic **Pain** r/t unexpressed anger, multiple physical disorders, depression
Ineffective **Coping** r/t lack of insight into underlying conflicts

Sore Nipples: Breastfeeding

Ineffective **Breastfeeding** r/t deficient knowledge regarding correct feeding procedure
See Painful Breasts—Sore Nipples

Sore Throat

Acute **Pain** r/t inflammation, irritation, dryness
Deficient **Knowledge** r/t treatment, relief of discomfort
Impaired **Oral** mucous membrane r/t inflammation or infection of oral cavity
Impaired **Swallowing** r/t irritation of oropharyngeal cavity

Sorrow

Anticipatory **Grieving** r/t impending loss of significant person or object
Chronic **Sorrow** r/t unresolved grief
Grieving r/t loss of significant person, object, or role
Readiness for enhanced **Spiritual** well-being r/t desire to find purpose and meaning of loss

Speech Disorders

Anxiety r/t difficulty with communication
Impaired verbal **Communication** r/t anatomical defect, cleft palate, psychological barriers, decrease in circulation to brain

Spina Bifida

Risk for latex **Allergy** response r/t multiple exposures to latex products
See Neurotube Defects

Spinal Cord Injury

Chronic **Sorrow** r/t immobility, change in body function
Constipation r/t immobility, loss of sensation
Deficient **Diversional** activity r/t long-term hospitalization, frequent lengthy treatments
Disturbed **Body** image r/t change in body function
Dysfunctional **Grieving** r/t loss of usual body function
Fear r/t powerlessness over loss of body function
Impaired **Home** maintenance r/t change in health status, insufficient family planning or finances, deficient knowledge, inadequate support systems
Impaired physical **Mobility** r/t neuromuscular impairment
Ineffective **Health** maintenance r/t deficient knowledge regarding self-care with spinal cord injury
Reflex **Incontinence** r/t spinal cord lesion interfering with conduction of cerebral messages
Risk for **Disuse** syndrome r/t paralysis
Risk for **Autonomic** dysreflexia r/t bladder or bowel distention, skin irritation, deficient knowledge of patient and caregiver
Risk for impaired **Skin** integrity r/t immobility, paralysis
Risk for ineffective **Breathing** pattern r/t neuromuscular impairment
Risk for **Infection** r/t chronic disease, stasis of body fluids
Risk for **Loneliness** r/t physical immobility
Risk for **Powerlessness** r/t loss of function
Self-care deficit r/t neuromuscular impairment
Sexual dysfunction r/t altered body function
Urinary retention r/t inhibition of reflex arc
See Child with Chronic Condition; Hospitalized Child; Neurotube Defects

Spiritual Distress

Risk for **Spiritual** distress r/t energy-consuming anxiety, low self-esteem, mental illness, physical illness, blocks to self-love, poor relationships, physical or psychological stress, substance abuse, loss of loved one, natural disasters, situational losses, maturational losses, inability to forgive
Spiritual distress r/t separation from religious or cultural ties, challenged belief and value system resulting from moral or ethical implications of therapy or from intense suffering

S

Spiritual Well-Being

Readiness for enhanced **Spiritual** well-being r/t desire for harmonious interconnectedness, desire to find purpose and meaning to life

Splenectomy

See Abdominal Surgery

Stapedectomy

Acute **Pain** r/t headache
Disturbed **Sensory** perception: auditory r/t hearing loss caused by edema from surgery
Risk for **Infection** r/t invasive procedure
Risk for **Falls** r/t dizziness
Risk for **Injury:** falls r/t dizziness

Stasis Ulcer

Impaired **Tissue** integrity r/t chronic venous congestion
See Varicose Veins

STD (Sexually Transmitted Disease)

Acute **Pain** r/t biological or psychological injury
Ineffective **Health** maintenance r/t deficient knowledge regarding transmission, symptoms, and treatment of sexually transmitted disease
Ineffective **Sexuality** patterns r/t illness, altered body function
Fear r/t altered body function, risk for social isolation, fear of incurable illness
Risk for **Infection**/spread of infection r/t lack of knowledge concerning transmission of disease
Social isolation r/t fear of contracting or spreading disease
See Maturational Issues, Adolescent

Stertorous Respirations

Ineffective **Airway** clearance r/t pharyngeal obstruction

Stillbirth

See Pregnancy Loss

Stoma

See Ostomy

Stomatitis

Impaired **Oral** mucous membrane r/t pathological conditions of oral cavity

Stone, Kidney

See Kidney Stone

Stool, Hard/Dry

Constipation r/t inadequate fluid intake, inadequate fiber intake, decreased activity level, decreased gastric motility

Straining with Defecation

Constipation r/t less than adequate fluid intake, less than adequate dietary intake
Risk for decreased **Cardiac** output r/t vagal stimulation with dysrhythmia secondary to Valsalva's maneuver

Stress

Anxiety r/t feelings of helplessness, feelings of being threatened
Disturbed **Energy** field r/t low energy level, feelings of hopelessness
Fear r/t powerlessness over feelings
Ineffective **Coping** r/t ineffective use of problem-solving process, feelings of apprehension or helplessness
Readiness for enhanced **Spiritual** well-being r/t desire for harmony and peace in stressful situation
Risk for **Post-trauma** syndrome r/t perception of event, survivor's role in event
Self-esteem disturbance r/t inability to deal with life events

Stress Urinary Incontinence

Risk for urge urinary **Incontinence** r/t involuntary sphincter relaxation
Stress urinary **Incontinence** r/t degenerative change in pelvic muscles
See Incontinence of Urine

Stridor

Ineffective **Airway** clearance r/t obstruction, tracheobronchial infection, trauma

Stroke

See CVA

Stuttering

Anxiety r/t impaired verbal communication
Impaired verbal **Communication** r/t anxiety, psychological problems

Subarachnoid Hemorrhage

Acute **Pain:** headache r/t irritation of meninges from blood, increased intracranial pressure
Ineffective **Tissue** perfusion: cerebral r/t bleeding from cerebral vessel
See Intracranial Pressure, Increased

S

Substance Abuse

Anxiety r/t loss of control

Compromised/dysfunctional family **Coping** r/t codependency issues

Defensive **Coping** r/t substance abuse

Disturbed **Sleep** pattern r/t irritability, nightmares, tremors

Dysfunctional **Family** processes: alcohol r/t inadequate coping skills

Imbalanced **Nutrition**: less than body requirements r/t anorexia

Ineffective **Protection** r/t malnutrition, sleep deprivation

Ineffective **Denial** r/t refusal to acknowledge substance abuse problem

Ineffective **Coping** r/t use of substances to cope with life events

Powerlessness r/t substance addiction

Risk for impaired parent/infant/child **Attachment** r/t substance abuse

Risk for **Injury** r/t alteration in sensory perception

Risk for self- or other-directed **Violence** r/t reactions to substances used, impulsive behavior, disorientation, impaired judgment

Risk for **Suicide** r/t substance abuse

Self-esteem disturbance r/t failure at life events

Social isolation r/t unacceptable social behavior or values

See Maturational Issues, Adolescent

Substance Abuse, Adolescent

See Alcohol Withdrawal; Maturational Issues, Adolescent; Substance Abuse

Substance Abuse in Pregnancy

Altered **Health** maintenance r/t addiction

Defensive **Coping** r/t denial of situation, differing value system

Deficient **Knowledge** r/t lack of exposure to information regarding effects of substance abuse in pregnancy

Noncompliance r/t differing value system, cultural influences, addiction

Risk for fetal **Injury** r/t effects of drugs on fetal growth and development

Risk for impaired **Parenting** r/t lack of ability to meet infant's needs

Risk for **Infection** r/t intravenous drug use, lifestyle

Risk for maternal **Injury** r/t drug use

See Substance Abuse

Sucking Reflex

Effective **Breastfeeding** r/t regular and sustained suckling and swallowing at breast

Sudden Infant Death Syndrome, Near Miss (Infant Apnea)

See SIDS

Suffocation, Risk for

Internal

Risk for **Suffocation** r/t reduced olfactory sensation, reduced motor abilities, lack of safety education, lack of safety precautions, cognitive or emotional difficulties, disease or injury process

External

Risk for **Suffocation** r/t pillow or propped bottle placed in infant's crib; vehicle running in closed garage; child playing with plastic bags; child inserting small objects into mouth or nose; accessible discarded or unused refrigerators or freezers with doors; child left unattended in or near bathtub, pool, spa; low clotheslines; pacifier hung around infant's neck; large mouthfuls of food

Suicide Attempt

Hopelessness r/t perceived or actual loss, substance abuse, low self-concept, inadequate support systems

Ineffective **Coping** r/t anger, dysfunctional grieving

Post-trauma response r/t history of traumatic events, abuse, rape, incest, war, torture

Readiness for enhanced **Spiritual** well-being r/t desire for harmony and inner strength to help redefine purpose for life

Risk for **Post-trauma** syndrome r/t survivor's role in suicide attempt

Risk for **Suicide** r/t history of prior attempt, impulsiveness, gun purchase, medication stockpile, suicide threats, family history of suicide, physical illness, hopelessness, social isolation

Self-esteem disturbance r/t guilt, inability to trust, feelings of worthlessness or rejection

Social isolation r/t inability to engage in satisfying personal relationships

Spiritual distress r/t hopelessness, despair

Support System

Readiness for enhanced family **Coping** r/t ability to adapt to tasks associated with care, support of significant other during health crisis

Suppression of Labor

See Preterm Labor; Tocolytic Therapy

Surgery, Perioperative Care

Risk for imbalanced **Fluid** volume r/t surgery

Risk for perioperative positioning **Injury** r/t predisposing condition, prolonged surgery

Surgery, Postoperative Care

Activity intolerance r/t pain, surgical procedure

Acute **Pain** r/t inflammation or injury in surgical area

Anxiety r/t change in health status, hospital environment

Deficient **Knowledge** r/t postoperative expectations, lifestyle changes

Imbalanced **Nutrition: less than body requirements** r/t anorexia, nausea, vomiting, decreased peristalsis

Nausea r/t manipulation of gastrointestinal tract, postsurgical anesthesia

Risk for ineffective **Tissue** perfusion: peripheral r/t hypovolemia, circulatory stasis, obesity, prolonged immobility, decreased coughing, decreased deep breathing

Risk for **Constipation** r/t decreased activity, decreased food or fluid intake, anesthesia, pain medication

Risk for deficient **Fluid** volume r/t hypermetabolic state, fluid loss during surgery, presence of indwelling tubes

Risk for ineffective **Breathing** pattern r/t pain, location of incision, effects of anesthesia/narcotics

Risk for **Infection** r/t invasive procedure, pain, anesthesia, location of incision, weakened cough as a result of aging

Urinary retention r/t anesthesia, pain, fear, unfamiliar surroundings, client's position

Surgery, Preoperative Care

Anxiety r/t threat to or change in health status, situational crisis, fear of the unknown

Deficient **Knowledge** r/t preoperative procedures, postoperative expectations

Disturbed **Sleep** pattern r/t anxiety about upcoming surgery

Suspected Child Abuse and Neglect (SCAN)—Child

Acute **Pain** r/t physical injuries

Anxiety/Fear: child r/t threat of punishment for perceived wrongdoing

Chronic low **Self-esteem** r/t lack of positive feedback, excessive negative feedback

Deficient **Diversional** activity r/t diminished or absent environmental or personal stimuli

Delayed **Growth** and development: regression vs. delayed r/t diminished or absent environmental stimuli, inadequate caretaking, inconsistent responsiveness by caretaker

Disturbed **Sleep** pattern r/t hypervigilance, anxiety

Impaired **Skin** integrity r/t altered nutritional state, physical abuse

Imbalanced **Nutrition: less than body requirements** r/t inadequate caretaking

Post-trauma response r/t physical abuse, incest, rape, molestation

Readiness for enhanced community **Coping** r/t obtaining resources to prevent child abuse, neglect

Rape-trauma syndrome: compound/silent reaction r/t altered lifestyle secondary to abuse, changes in residence

Risk for **Poisoning** r/t inadequate safeguards, lack of proper safety precautions, accessibility of illicit substances secondary to impaired home maintenance

Risk for **Suffocation: secondary to aspiration** r/t propped bottle, unattended child

Risk for **Trauma** r/t inadequate precautions, cognitive or emotional difficulties

Social isolation: family-imposed r/t fear of disclosure of family dysfunction and abuse

See Hospitalized Child; Maturational Issues, Adolescent

Suspected Child Abuse and Neglect (SCAN)—Parent

Chronic low **Self-esteem** r/t lack of successful parenting experiences

Disabled family **Coping** r/t dysfunctional family, underdeveloped nurturing parental role, lack of parental support systems or role models

Dysfunctional **Family** processes: alcoholism r/t inadequate coping skills

Impaired **Home** maintenance r/t disorganization, parental dysfunction, neglect of safe and nurturing environment

Impaired **Parenting** r/t unrealistic expectations of child; lack of effective role model; unmet social, emotional, or maturational needs of parents; interruption in bonding process

Ineffective **Health** maintenance r/t deficient knowledge of parenting skills secondary to unachieved developmental tasks

Powerlessness r/t inability to perform parental role responsibilities

Risk for **Violence** toward child r/t inadequate coping mechanisms, unresolved stressors, unachieved maturational level by parent

Suspicion

Impaired **Social** interaction r/t disturbed thought processes, paranoid delusions, hallucinations

Powerlessness r/t repetitive paranoid thinking

Risk for self- or other-directed **Violence** r/t inability to trust

S

Swallowing Difficulties

Impaired **Swallowing** r/t neuromuscular impairment (e.g., decreased or absent gag reflex, decreased strength or excursion of muscles involved in mastication), perceptual impairment, facial paralysis, mechanical obstruction (e.g., edema, tracheostomy tube, tumor), fatigue, limited awareness, reddened or irritated oropharyngeal cavity, improper feeding or positioning

Syncope

Anxiety r/t fear of falling
Decreased **Cardiac** output r/t dysrhythmia
Impaired physical **Mobility** r/t fear of falling
Ineffective **Tissue** perfusion: cerebral r/t interruption of blood flow
Risk for **Falls** r/t syncope
Risk for **Injury** r/t altered sensory perception, transient loss of consciousness, risk for falls
Social isolation r/t fear of falling

Syphilis

See STD

Systemic Lupus Erythematosus

See Lupus Erythematosus

T

T & A (Tonsillectomy and Adenoidectomy)

Acute **Pain** r/t surgical incision
Deficient **Knowledge:** potential for enhanced health maintenance r/t insufficient knowledge regarding postoperative nutritional and rest requirements, signs and symptoms of complications, positioning
Impaired **Comfort** r/t effects of anesthesia (nausea and vomiting)
Ineffective **Airway** clearance r/t hesitation or reluctance to cough secondary to pain
Risk for imbalanced **Nutrition:** less than body requirements r/t hesitation or reluctance to swallow
Risk for **Aspiration/Suffocation** r/t postoperative drainage and impaired swallowing
Risk for deficient **Fluid** volume r/t decreased intake secondary to painful swallowing, effects of anesthesia (nausea, vomiting), hemorrhage

Tachycardia

See Dysrhythmia

Tachypnea

Ineffective **Breathing** pattern r/t pain, anxiety
See cause of Tachypnea

Taste Abnormality

Adult **Failure** to thrive r/t imbalanced nutrition: less than body requirements associated with taste abnormality
Disturbed **Sensory** perception: gustatory r/t medication side effects; altered sensory reception, transmission, integration; aging changes

TBI (Traumatic Brain Injury)

Acute **Confusion** r/t brain injury
Chronic **Sorrow** r/t change in person's health status and functional ability
Decreased **Intracranial** adaptive capacity r/t brain injury
Disturbed **Thought** processes r/t pressure damage to brain
Interrupted **Family** processes r/t traumatic injury to family member
Ineffective **Tissue** perfusion: cerebral r/t effects of increased intracranial pressure
Ineffective **Breathing** pattern r/t pressure damage to breathing center in brain stem
Risk for **Post-trauma** syndrome r/t perception of event causing traumatic brain injury
Disturbed **Sensory** perception: specify r/t pressure damage to sensory centers in brain

Temperature, Decreased

Hypothermia r/t exposure to cold environment

Temperature, Increased

Hyperthermia r/t dehydration, illness, trauma

Temperature Regulation, Impaired

Ineffective **Thermoregulation** r/t trauma, illness

Tension

Anxiety r/t threat to or change in health status, situational crisis
Disturbed **Energy** field r/t change in health status, discouragement, pain

Terminally Ill Adult

Anticipatory **Grieving** r/t loss of self or significant other
Compromised family **Coping** r/t inability to discuss impending death
Death **Anxiety** r/t unresolved issues relating to death and dying

Decisional **Conflict** r/t planning for advance directives

Disturbed **Energy** field r/t impending disharmony of mind, body, spirit

Readiness for enhanced **Spiritual** well-being r/t desire to achieve harmony of mind, body, spirit

Risk for **Spiritual** distress r/t impending death

Spiritual distress r/t suffering before death

Terminally Ill Child–Adolescent

Disturbed **Body** image r/t effects of terminal disease, already critical feelings of group identity and self-image

Impaired **Social** interaction/social isolation r/t forced separation from peers

Ineffective **Coping** r/t inability to establish personal and peer identity secondary to threat of being different or not being, inability to achieve maturational tasks

See Child with Chronic Condition; Hospitalized Child

Terminally Ill Child–Infant/Toddler

Ineffective **Coping** r/t separation from parents and familiar environment secondary to inability to grasp external meaning of death

Terminally Ill Child–Preschool Child

Fear r/t perceived punishment, bodily harm, feelings of guilt secondary to magical thinking (i.e., believing that thoughts cause events)

Terminally Ill Child–School-Age Child/Preadolescent

Fear r/t perceived punishment, body mutilation, feelings of guilt

Terminally Ill Child/Death of Child–Parent

Anticipatory **Grieving** r/t possible, expected, or imminent death of child

Compromised family **Coping** r/t inability or unwillingness to discuss impending death and feelings with child or to support child through terminal stages of illness

Decisional **Conflict** r/t continuation or discontinuation of treatment, "do not resuscitate" decision, ethical issues regarding organ donation

Interrupted **Family** processes r/t situational crisis

Impaired **Parenting** r/t risk for overprotection of surviving siblings

Readiness for enhanced family **Coping** r/t impact of crisis on family values, priorities, goals, or relationships; expressed interest or desire to attach meaning to child's life and death

Grieving r/t death of child

Hopelessness r/t overwhelming stresses secondary to terminal illness

Impaired **Social** interaction r/t dysfunctional grieving

Ineffective **Denial** r/t dysfunctional grieving

Powerlessness r/t inability to alter course of events

Risk for dysfunctional **Grieving** r/t prolonged, unresolved, obstructed progression through stages of grief and mourning

Disturbed **Sleep** pattern r/t grieving process

Social isolation: imposed by others r/t feelings of inadequacy in providing support to grieving parents

Social isolation: self-imposed r/t unresolved grief, perceived inadequate parenting skills

Spiritual distress r/t sudden and unexpected death, prolonged suffering before death, questioning the death of youth, questioning the meaning of one's own existence

Tetralogy of Fallot

See Congenital Heart Disease/Cardiac Anomalies

Therapeutic Regimen, Effective Management

Effective **Therapeutic** regimen management r/t adequate ability to manage needed health care

Therapeutic Regimen, Ineffective Management of: Families

Ineffective family **Therapeutic** regimen management r/t complexity of health care system, complexity of therapeutic regimen, decisional conflicts, economic difficulties, excessive demands on individual or family, family conflict

Therapeutic Regimen, Ineffective Management

Ineffective **Therapeutic** regimen management r/t complexity of health care system; complexity of therapeutic regimen; decisional conflicts; economic difficulties; excessive demands made on individual or family; family conflict; family patterns of health care; inadequate number and types of cues to action; deficient knowledge; mistrust of regimen or health care personnel; perceived seriousness, susceptibility, barriers, or benefits; powerlessness; social support deficits

Therapeutic Touch

Disturbed **Energy** field r/t low energy levels, disturbance in energy fields, pain, depression, fatigue

Thermoregulation, Ineffective

Ineffective **Thermoregulation** r/t trauma, illness, immaturity, aging, fluctuating environmental temperature

T

Thoracotomy

Activity intolerance r/t pain, imbalance between oxygen supply and demand, presence of chest tubes

Acute **Pain** r/t surgical procedure, coughing, deep breathing

Deficient **Knowledge** r/t self-care, effective breathing exercises, pain relief

Ineffective **Airway** clearance r/t drowsiness, pain with breathing and coughing

Ineffective **Breathing** pattern r/t decreased energy, fatigue, pain

Risk for **Infection** r/t invasive procedure

Risk for **Injury** r/t disruption of closed-chest drainage system

Risk for perioperative positioning **Injury** r/t lateral positioning, immobility

Thought Disorders

Disturbed **Thought** processes r/t disruption in cognitive thinking, processing

See Schizophrenia

Thought Processes, Disturbed

Disturbed **Thought** processes r/t head injury, mental disorder, personality disorder, organic mental disorder, substance abuse, severe interpersonal conflict, sleep deprivation, sensory deprivation or overload, impaired cerebral perfusion

Thrombocytopenic Purpura

See ITP

Thrombophlebitis

Acute **Pain** r/t vascular inflammation, edema

Constipation r/t inactivity, bedrest

Deficient **Diversional** activity r/t bedrest

Deficient **Knowledge** r/t pathophysiology of condition, self-care needs, treatment regimen and outcome

Delayed **Surgical** recovery r/t complication associated with inactivity

Impaired physical **Mobility** r/t pain in extremity, forced bedrest

Ineffective **Tissue** perfusion: peripheral r/t interruption of venous blood flow

Risk for **Injury** r/t possible embolus

See Anticoagulant Therapy

Thyroidectomy

Risk for altered verbal **Communication** r/t edema, pain, vocal cord of laryngeal nerve damage

Risk for ineffective **Airway** clearance r/t edema or hematoma formation, airway obstruction

Risk for **Injury** r/t possible parathyroid damage or removal

See Surgery

TIA (Transient Ischemic Attack)

Acute **Confusion** r/t hypoxia

Health-seeking behaviors r/t obtaining knowledge regarding treatment, prevention of inadequate oxygenation

Ineffective **Tissue** perfusion: cerebral r/t lack of adequate oxygen supply to brain

Risk for decreased **Cardiac** output r/t dysrhythmia contributing to inadequate oxygen supply to brain

Risk for **Falls** r/t hypoxia

Risk for **Injury** r/t possible syncope

See Syncope

Tinea Capitis

See Ringworm of Scalp

Tinea Corporis

See Ringworm of Body

Tinea Cruris

See Jock Itch

Tinea Pedis

See Athlete's Foot

Tinea Unguium (Onychomycosis)

See Ringworm of Nails

Tinnitus

Ineffective **Health** maintenance r/t deficient knowledge regarding self-care with tinnitus

Disturbed **Sensory** perception: auditory r/t altered sensory reception, transmission, integration

Tissue Damage—Corneal, Integumentary, or Subcutaneous

Impaired **Tissue** integrity r/t altered circulation, nutritional deficit or excess, fluid deficit or excess, deficient knowledge, impaired physical mobility, chemical irritants (including body excretions, secretions, medications), thermal irritants (temperature extremes), mechanical irritants (pressure, shear, friction), radiation irritants (including therapeutic radiation)

Tissue Perfusion, Decreased

Ineffective **Tissue** perfusion r/t arterial or venous interruption of flow, exchange problems, hypovolemia, hypervolemia

T

Tocolytic Therapy

Ineffective **Health** maintenance r/t deficient knowledge regarding management of preterm labor, treatment regimen

Risk for **Fluid** volume excess r/t effects of tocolytic drugs

See Preterm Labor

Toilet Training

Health-seeking behaviors: bladder/bowel training r/t achievement of developmental milestone secondary to enhanced parenting skills

Toileting Problems

Impaired **Transfer** ability r/t neuromuscular deficits

Self-care deficit: toileting r/t impaired transfer ability, impaired mobility status, intolerance of activity, neuromuscular impairment, cognitive impairment

Tonsillectomy and Adenoidectomy

See T & A

Toothache

Impaired **Dentition** r/t ineffective oral hygiene, barriers to self-care, economic barriers to professional care, nutritional deficits, lack of knowledge regarding dental health

Total Anomalous Pulmonary Venous Return

See Congenital Heart Disease/Cardiac Anomalies

Total Urinary Incontinence

Total urinary **Incontinence** r/t neuropathy, neurological dysfunction, compromised contraction of detrusor reflex, anatomical incontinence (fistula)

Total Joint Replacement—Total Hip/Total Knee

Acute **Pain** r/t possible edema, physical injury, surgery

Deficient **Knowledge** r/t self-care, treatment regimen, outcomes

Disturbed **Body** image r/t large scar, presence of prosthesis

Impaired physical **Mobility** r/t musculoskeletal impairment, surgery, prosthesis

Risk for **Infection** r/t invasive procedure, anesthesia, immobility

Risk for **Injury**: neurovascular r/t altered peripheral tissue perfusion, altered mobility, prosthesis

Total Parenteral Nutrition

See TPN

Toxemia

See PIH

TPN (Total Parenteral Nutrition)

Imbalanced **Nutrition**: less than body requirements r/t inability to ingest or digest food or absorb nutrients as a result of biological or psychological factors

Risk for **Fluid** volume excess r/t rapid administration of TPN

Risk for **Infection** r/t concentrated glucose solution, invasive administration of fluids

Tracheoesophageal Fistula

Imbalanced **Nutrition**: less than body requirements r/t difficulties in swallowing

Ineffective **Airway** clearance r/t aspiration of feeding secondary to inability to swallow

Risk for **Aspiration** r/t common passage of air and food

See Respiratory Conditions of the Neonate; Hospitalized Child

Tracheostomy

Acute **Pain** r/t edema, surgical procedure

Anxiety r/t impaired verbal communication, ineffective airway clearance

Deficient **Knowledge** r/t self-care, home maintenance management

Disturbed **Body** image r/t abnormal opening in neck

Impaired verbal **Communication** r/t presence of mechanical airway

Risk for **Aspiration** r/t presence of tracheostomy

Risk for ineffective **Airway** clearance r/t increased secretions, mucus plugs

Risk for **Infection** r/t invasive procedure, pooling of secretions

Traction and Casts

Acute **Pain** r/t immobility, injury, or disease

Constipation r/t immobility

Deficient **Diversional** activity r/t immobility

Impaired physical **Mobility** r/t imposed restrictions on activity secondary to bone or joint disease injury

Impaired **Transfer** ability r/t presence of traction, casts

Risk for **Disuse** syndrome r/t mechanical immobilization

Risk for impaired **Skin** integrity r/t contact of traction or cast with skin

Risk for **Peripheral** neurovascular dysfunction r/t mechanical compression

T

Self-care deficit: feeding, dressing/grooming, bathing/hygiene, toileting r/t degree of impaired physical mobility, body area affected by traction or cast

Transfer Ability

Impaired **Transfer** ability r/t intolerant of activity, decreased strength and endurance, pain or discomfort, perceptual or cognitive impairment, neuromuscular impairment, musculoskeletal impairment, depression, severe anxiety

Transient Ischemic Attack

See TIA

Transposition of Great Vessels

See Congenital Heart Disease/Cardiac Anomalies

Transurethral Resection of the Prostate

See TURP

Trauma in Pregnancy

Acute **Pain** r/t trauma

Anxiety r/t threat to self or fetus, unknown outcome

Deficient **Knowledge** r/t lack of exposure to situation

Impaired **Skin** integrity r/t trauma

Risk for fetal **Injury** r/t premature separation of placenta

Risk for deficient **Fluid** volume r/t blood loss

Risk for **Infection** r/t traumatized tissue

Trauma, Risk for

Internal

Risk for **Trauma** r/t weakness, poor vision, balancing difficulties, reduced temperature and/or tactile sensation, reduced large or small muscle coordination, reduced hand-eye coordination, lack of safety education, lack of safety precautions, insufficient finances to purchase safety equipment or effect repairs, cognitive or emotional difficulties, history of previous trauma

External

Risk for **Trauma** r/t slippery floors or walkways, unanchored rugs, bathtub without hand grip or antislip equipment, use of unsteady ladders or chairs, entering unlighted rooms, unsturdy or absent stair rails, unanchored electrical wires, litter or liquid spills on floors or stairways, high beds, children playing at top of ungated stairs, obstructed passageways, unsafe window protection in home with young children, inappropriate call-for-aid mechanisms for client on bedrest, pot handles facing toward front of stove, bathing in very hot water, unsupervised bathing of young children, potentially ignitable gas leaks, delayed lighting of gas burner or oven, experimenting with chemicals or gasoline, unscreened fires or heaters, wearing plastic apron or flowing clothes around open flame, children playing with dangerous objects (e.g., matches, candles, cigarettes), inadequately stored combustible items or corrosives, highly flammable children's toys or clothing, overloaded fuse box, contact with rapidly moving objects (e.g., machinery, industrial belts, pulleys), sliding on coarse bed linen or struggling within bed restraints, faulty electrical plugs, frayed wires, defective appliances, contact with acids or alkalis, playing with fireworks or gunpowder, contact with intense cold, overexposure to sun or radiotherapy, misuse of sun lamps, use of cracked dishware or glasses, knives stored uncovered, guns or ammunition stored unlocked, large icicles hanging from the roof, exposure to dangerous machinery, children playing with sharp-edged toys, high-crime neighborhoods and vulnerable clients, driving a mechanically unsafe vehicle, driving after consuming alcoholic beverages or drugs, driving at excessive speeds, driving without necessary visual aids, children riding in the front seat of a vehicle, smoking in bed or near oxygen, overloaded electrical outlets, grease waste collected on stoves, use of thin or worn potholders, misuse of necessary headgear for motorized cyclists, young children carried on adult bicycles, unsafe road or road-crossing conditions, playing or working near vehicle pathways, nonuse or misuse of seat restraints

Traumatic Brain Injury (TBI)

See TBI; Intracranial Pressure, Increased

Traumatic Event

Post-trauma syndrome r/t previously experienced trauma

Trembling of Hands

Anxiety/Fear r/t threat to or change in health status, threat of death, situational crisis

Tricuspid Atresia

See Congenital Heart Disease/Cardiac Anomalies

Trigeminal Neuralgia

Acute **Pain** r/t irritation of trigeminal nerve

Imbalanced **Nutrition**: less than body requirements r/t pain when chewing

Ineffective **Therapeutic** regimen management r/t deficient knowledge regarding prevention of stimuli that trigger pain

Risk for **Injury** (eye) r/t possible decreased corneal sensation

Truncus Arteriosus

See Congenital Heart Disease/Cardiac Anomalies

TSE (Testicular Self-Examination)

Health-seeking behavior r/t procedure for doing testicular self-examinations

Tube Feeding

Risk for Imbalanced **Nutrition**: less than body requirements r/t intolerance to tube feeding, inadequate calorie replacement to meet metabolic needs

Risk for **Aspiration** r/t improperly administered feeding, improper placement of tube, improper positioning of client during and after feeding, excessive residual feeding or lack of digestion, altered gag reflex

Risk for deficient **Fluid** volume r/t inadequate water administration with concentrated feeding

TURP (Transurethral Resection of the Prostate)

Acute **Pain** r/t incision, irritation from catheter, bladder spasms, kidney infection

Deficient **Knowledge** r/t postoperative self-care, home maintenance management

Risk for deficient **Fluid** volume r/t fluid loss, possible bleeding

Risk for **Infection** r/t invasive procedure, route for bacteria entry

Risk for **Urinary** retention r/t obstruction of urethra or catheter with clots

Risk for urge urinary **Incontinence** r/t edema from surgical procedure

U

Ulcer, Peptic or Duodenal

Acute **Pain** r/t irritated mucosa from acid secretion

Fatigue r/t loss of blood, chronic illness

Ineffective **Health** maintenance r/t lack of knowledge regarding health practices to prevent ulcer formation

Nausea r/t gastrointestinal irritation

See GI Bleed

Ulcerative Colitis

See Inflammatory Bowel Disease

Ulcers, Stasis

See Stasis Ulcers

Unilateral Neglect of One Side of Body

Unilateral **Neglect** r/t effects of disturbed perceptual abilities (e.g., hemianopsia), one-sided blindness, neurological illness or trauma

Unsanitary Living Conditions

Impaired **Home** maintenance r/t impaired cognitive or emotional functioning, lack of knowledge, insufficient finances

Urgency to Urinate

Risk for urge urinary **Incontinence** r/t effects of alcohol, caffeine, decreased bladder capacity, irritation of bladder stretch receptors causing spasm, increased urine concentration, overdistention of bladder

Urge urinary **Incontinence** r/t decreased bladder capacity, irritation of bladder stretch receptors causing spasm, alcohol, caffeine, increased fluids, increased urine concentration, overdistention of bladder

Urinary Diversion

See Ileal Conduit

Urinary Elimination, Altered

Impaired **Urinary** elimination r/t anatomical obstruction, sensory motor impairment, urinary tract infection

Urinary Incontinence

See Incontinence of Urine

Urinary Retention

Urinary retention r/t high urethral pressure caused by weak detrusor, inhibition of reflex arc, strong sphincter, blockage

Urinary Tract Infection

See UTI

Urolithiasis

See Kidney Stone

Uterine Atony in Labor

See Dystocia

Uterine Atony in Postpartum

See Postpartum Hemorrhage

Uterine Bleeding

See Hemorrhage; Postpartum Hemorrhage; Shock

UTI (Urinary Tract Infection)

Acute **Pain:** dysuria r/t inflammatory process in bladder

Impaired **Urinary** elimination: frequency r/t urinary tract infection

Ineffective **Health** maintenance r/t deficient knowledge regarding methods to treat and prevent UTIs

Risk for urge urinary **Incontinence** r/t hyperreflexia from cystitis

V

Vaginal Hysterectomy

Risk for **Infection** r/t surgical site

Risk for **Perioperative** positioning injury r/t lithotomy position

Risk for urge urinary **Incontinence** r/t edema, congestion of pelvic tissues

Urinary retention r/t edema at surgical site

See Hysterectomy

Vaginitis

Acute **Pain:** pruritus r/t inflamed tissues, edema

Ineffective **Health** maintenance r/t deficient knowledge regarding self-care with vaginitis

Ineffective **Sexuality** patterns r/t abstinence during acute stage, pain

Risk for **Infection** r/t spread of infection, risk of reinfection

Vagotomy

See Abdominal Surgery

Value System Conflict

Readiness for enhanced **Spiritual** well-being r/t desire for harmony with self, others, higher power/God

Spiritual distress r/t challenged value system

Varicose Veins

Chronic **Pain** r/t impaired circulation

Ineffective **Health** maintenance r/t deficient knowledge regarding health care practices, prevention, treatment regimen

Ineffective **Tissue** perfusion: peripheral r/t venous stasis

Risk for impaired **Skin** integrity r/t altered peripheral tissue perfusion

Vascular Dementia (formerly called "Multiinfarct Dementia")

See Dementia

Vascular Obstruction—Peripheral

Acute **Pain** r/t vascular obstruction

Anxiety r/t lack of circulation to body part

Ineffective **Tissue** perfusion: peripheral r/t interruption of circulatory flow

Risk for **Peripheral** neurovascular dysfunction r/t vascular obstruction

Venereal Disease

See STD

Ventilation, Inability to Sustain Spontaneous

Impaired spontaneous **Ventilation** r/t metabolic factors, respiratory muscle fatigue

Ventilator Client

Dysfunctional **Ventilatory** weaning response r/t psychological, situational, and physiological factors

Fear r/t inability to breathe on own, difficulty communicating

Impaired **Gas** exchange r/t ventilation-perfusion imbalance

Impaired verbal **Communication** r/t presence of endotracheal tube, decreased mentation

Impaired spontaneous **Ventilation** r/t metabolic factors, respiratory muscle fatigue

Ineffective **Airway** clearance r/t increased secretions, decreased cough and gag reflex

Ineffective **Breathing** pattern r/t decreased energy and fatigue secondary to possible altered nutrition: less than body requirements

Powerlessness r/t health treatment regimen

Risk for **Infection** r/t presence of endotracheal tube, pooled secretions

Risk for latex **Allergy** r/t repeated exposure to latex products

Social isolation r/t impaired mobility, ventilator dependence

See Child with Chronic Condition; Hospitalized Child; Respiratory Conditions of the Neonate

Ventilatory, Dysfunctional Weaning Response (DVWR)

Dysfunctional **Ventilatory** weaning response r/t perceived inefficacy about the ability to wean, powerlessness, decreased motivation, adverse environment, inadequate social support, inadequate

V

nutrition, sleep pattern disturbance, uncontrolled pain, ineffective airway clearance

Vertigo

Ineffective **Tissue** perfusion: cerebral r/t decreased blood supply to brain
Risk for **Falls** r/t vertigo
Risk for **Injury** r/t disturbed sensory perception
Disturbed **Sensory** perception: kinesthetic r/t altered sensory reception, transmission, integration; medications

Violent Behavior

Risk for other-directed **Violence** r/t body language, history of violence against others, history of violent antisocial behavior, history of violence, indirect, neurological impairment, cognitive impairment, history of childhood abuse, history of witnessing family violence, cruelty to animals, firesetting, prenatal/perinatal complications and abnormalities, history of drug/alcohol abuse, pathological intoxication, psychotic symptomatology, motor vehicle offenses, suicidal behavior, impulsivity, availability/possession of weapon(s)
Risk for self-directed **Violence** r/t suicidal ideation, suicidal plan, history of multiple suicide attempts, behavioral clues of suicide, verbal clues of suicide, emotional status, mental health, physical health, unemployment, ages 15-19, age >45, marital status, occupation, conflictual interpersonal relationships, family background, sexual orientation, personal resources, social resources, engage in autoerotic sexual acts

Vision Impairment

Disturbed **Sensory** perception r/t altered sensory reception associated with impaired vision
Fear r/t loss of sight
Risk for **Injury** r/t disturbed sensory perception
Self-care deficit: specify r/t perceptual impairment
Social isolation r/t altered state of wellness, inability to see
See Blindness

Vomiting

Nausea r/t chemotherapy, postsurgical anesthesia, irritation to the gastrointestinal system, stimulation of neuropharmacologic mechanisms
Risk for deficient **Fluid** volume r/t decreased intake, loss of fluids with vomiting
Risk for imbalanced **Nutrition**: less than body requirements r/t inability to ingest food

W

Walking Impairment

Impaired **Walking** r/t intolerance to activity, decreased strength and endurance, pain or discomfort, perceptual or cognitive impairment, neuromuscular impairment, musculoskeletal impairment, depression, severe anxiety, lower extremity amputation

Wandering

Wandering r/t cognitive impairment, specifically memory and recall deficits, disorientation, poor visuoconstructive (or visuospatial) ability, language (primarily expressive) defects; cortical atrophy; premorbid behavior (e.g., outgoing, sociable personality; premorbid dementia); separation from familiar people and places; sedation; emotional state, especially frustration, anxiety, boredom, or depression (agitation); overstimulating/under stimulating social or physical environment; physiological state or need (e.g., hunger/thirst, pain, urination, constipation); time of day

Weakness

Fatigue r/t decreased or increased metabolic energy production
Risk for **Falls** r/t weakness

Weight Gain

Imbalanced **Nutrition**: more than body requirements r/t excessive intake in relation to metabolic need

Weight Loss

Imbalanced **Nutrition**: less than body requirements r/t inability to ingest food because of biological, psychological, economic factors

Wellness-Seeking Behavior

Health-seeking behavior r/t expressed desire for increased control of health practice

Wheelchair Use Problems

Impaired wheelchair **Mobility** r/t intolerance to activity, decreased strength and endurance, pain or discomfort, perceptual or cognitive impairment, neuromuscular impairment, musculoskeletal impairment, depression, severe anxiety, amputation

Wheezing

Ineffective **Airway** clearance r/t tracheobronchial obstructions, secretions

Withdrawal from Alcohol

See Alcohol Withdrawal

Withdrawal from Drugs

See Drug Withdrawal

Wound Debridement

Acute **Pain** r/t debridement of wound

Impaired **Tissue** integrity r/t debridement, open wound

Risk for **Infection** r/t open wound, presence of bacteria

Wound Dehiscence, Evisceration

Fear r/t client fear of body parts falling out, surgical procedure not going as planned

Imbalanced **Nutrition: less than body requirements** r/t inability to digest nutrients, need for increased protein for healing

Risk for delayed **Surgical** recovery r/t separation of wound, exposure of abdominal contents

Risk for deficient **Fluid** volume r/t inability to ingest nutrients, obstruction, fluid loss

Risk for **Injury** r/t exposed abdominal contents

Wound Infection

Disturbed **Body** image r/t dysfunctional open wound

Imbalanced **Nutrition: less than body requirements** r/t biological factors, infection, hyperthermia

Hyperthermia r/t increased metabolic rate, illness, infection

Impaired **Tissue** integrity r/t wound, presence of infection

Risk for delayed **Surgical** recovery r/t presence of infection

Risk for deficient **Fluid** volume r/t increased metabolic rate

Risk for **Infection: spread of** r/t imbalanced nutrition: less than body requirements

Guide to Planning Care

Activity intolerance

Linda L. Straight

 Definition Insufficient physiological or psychological energy to endure or complete required or desired daily activities

Defining Characteristics

Verbal report of fatigue or weakness, abnormal heart rate or blood pressure response to activity, exertional discomfort or dyspnea, electrocardiographic changes reflecting dysrhythmias or ischemia

Related Factors (r/t)

Bed rest or immobility; generalized weakness; sedentary lifestyle; imbalance between oxygen supply and demand

NOC **Outcomes (Nursing Outcomes Classification)**

Suggested NOC Labels

Endurance; Energy Conservation; Activity Tolerance; Self-Care: Activities of Daily Living (ADLs)

> **Example NOC Outcome**
> Demonstrates **Endurance** as evidenced by the following indicators: Performance of usual routine/Activity/Rested appearance/Blood oxygen level within normal limits/Expresses feelings about loss/Verbalizes acceptance of loss/Describes meaning of the loss or death/Reports decreased preoccupation with loss/Expresses positive expectations about the future (Rate each indicator of **Endurance:** 1 = extremely compromised, 2 = substantially compromised, 3 = moderately compromised, 4 = mildly compromised, 5 = not compromised [see Section I])

Client Outcomes

- Participates in prescribed physical activity with appropriate increases in heart rate, blood pressure, and breathing rate; maintains monitor patterns (rhythm and ST segment) within normal limits
- States symptoms of adverse effects of exercise and reports onset of symptoms immediately
- Maintains normal skin color and skin is warm and dry with activity
- Verbalizes an understanding of the need to gradually increase activity based on testing, tolerance, and symptoms
- Expresses an understanding of the need to balance rest and activity
- Demonstrates increased activity tolerance

NIC **Interventions (Nursing Interventions Classification)**

Suggested NIC Labels

Energy Management; Activity Therapy

> **Example NIC Interventions—Energy Management**
> - Monitor cardiorespiratory response to activity
> - Monitor location and nature of discomfort or pain during movement/activity

• = Independent; ▲ = Collaborative

Nursing Interventions and Rationales

- Determine cause of activity intolerance (see Related Factors) and determine whether cause is physical, psychological, or motivational.
  Determining the cause of a disease can help direct appropriate interventions.
- ▲ Assess client daily for appropriateness of activity and bed rest orders.
  Inappropriate prolonged bed rest orders may contribute to activity intolerance. A review of 39 studies on bed rest resulting from 15 disorders demonstrated that bed rest for treatment of medical conditions is associated with worse outcomes than early mobilization (Allen, Glasziou, Del Mar, 1999).
- Minimize cardiovascular deconditioning by positioning clients as close to the upright position as possible several times daily.
  The hazards of bed rest in the elderly are multiple, serious, quick to develop, and slow to reverse. Deconditioning of the cardiovascular system occurs within days and involves fluid shifts, fluid loss, decreased cardiac output, decreased peak oxygen uptake, and increased resting heart rate (Resnick, 1998).
- ▲ If appropriate, gradually increase activity, allowing client to assist with positioning, transferring, and self-care as possible. Progress from sitting in bed to dangling, to chair sitting, to standing, to ambulation.
  Increasing activity helps to maintain muscle strength, tone, and endurance. Allowing the client to participate decreases the perception of the client as incapable and frail (Eliopoulous, 1997).
- Ensure that clients change position slowly. Consider using a chair-bed (stretcher-chair) for clients who cannot get out of bed. Monitor for symptoms of activity intolerance.
  Bed rest in the supine position results in loss of plasma volume, which contributes to postural hypotension and syncope (Creditor, 1994).
- When getting clients up, observe for symptoms of intolerance such as nausea, pallor, dizziness, visual dimming, and impaired consciousness, as well as changes in vital signs.
  Heart rate and blood pressure responses to orthostasis vary widely. Vital sign changes by themselves should not define orthostatic intolerance (Winslow, Lane, Woods, 1995).
- Perform range-of-motion exercises if client is unable to tolerate activity.
  Inactivity rapidly contributes to muscle shortening and changes in periarticular and cartilaginous joint structure. These factors contribute to contracture and limitation of motion (Creditor, 1994).
- ▲ Refer client to physical therapy to help increase activity levels and strength.
- Monitor and record client's ability to tolerate activity: note pulse rate, blood pressure, monitor pattern, dyspnea, use of accessory muscles, and skin color before and after activity. If the following signs and symptoms of cardiac decompensation develop, activity should be stopped immediately (ACSM, 1995):
  - Excessive fatigue
  - Lightheadedness, confusion, ataxia, pallor, cyanosis, dyspnea, nausea, or any peripheral circulatory insufficiency
  - Onset of angina with exercise
  - Palpitations
  - Dysrhythmia (symptomatic supraventricular tachycardia, ventricular tachycardia, exercise-induced left bundle block, second- or third-degree atrioventricular block, frequent premature ventricular contractions)

- **= Independent; ▲ = Collaborative**

- Exercise hypotension (drop in systolic blood pressure of more than 10 mm Hg from baseline blood pressure despite an increase in workload, when accompanied by other evidence of ischemia)
- Excessive rise in blood pressure (systolic >220 mm Hg or diastolic >110 mm Hg); NOTE: these are upper limits; activity may be stopped before reaching these values
- Inappropriate bradycardia (drop in heart rate greater than 10 beats/min) with no change or increase in workload
- Increased heart rate above the prescribed limit

▲ Instruct client to stop activity immediately and report to physician if experiencing the following symptoms: new or worsened intensity or increased frequency of discomfort; tightness or pressure in chest, back, neck, jaw, shoulders, and/or arms; palpitations; dizziness; weakness; unusual and extreme fatigue; excessive air hunger.
These are common symptoms of angina and are caused by a temporary insufficiency of coronary blood supply. Symptoms typically last for minutes as opposed to momentary twinges. If symptoms last longer than 5 to 10 minutes, the client should be evaluated by a physician (McGoon, 1993). The client should be evaluated before resuming activity (Thompson, 1988).

• Allow for periods of rest before and after planned exertion periods such as meals, baths, treatments, and physical activity.
Rest periods decrease oxygen consumption (Prizant-Weston, Castiglia, 1992).

• Observe and document skin integrity several times a day.
Activity intolerance may lead to pressure ulcers. Mechanical pressure, moisture, friction, and shearing forces all predispose to their development (Resnick, 1998).

• Assess urinary incontinence related to functional ability. Assess independent ability to get to the toilet and remove and adjust clothing.
The loss of functional ability that accompanies disease often leads to continence problems. The cause may not be the person's bladder instability but his or her ability to get to the toilet quickly (Nazarko, 1997).

• Assess for constipation.
Impaired mobility is associated with increased risk of bowel dysfunction, including constipation. Constipation increases the risk of urinary tract infection and urge incontinence (Nazarko, 1997).

▲ Consider dietitian referral to assess nutritional needs related to activity intolerance.
Severe malnutrition can lead to activity intolerance. Dietitians can recommend dietary changes that can improve the client's health status (Peckenpaugh, Poleman, 1999).

▲ Refer the cardiac client to cardiac rehabilitation for assistance in developing safe exercise guidelines based on testing and medications.
Cardiac rehabilitation exercise training improves objective measures of exercise tolerance in both men and women, including elderly patients with coronary heart disease and heart failure. This functional improvement occurs without significant cardiovascular complications or other adverse outcomes (Wenger et al, 1995).

▲ Ensure that the chronic pulmonary client has oxygen saturation testing with exercise. Use supplemental oxygen to keep oxygen saturation 90% or above or as prescribed with activity.
Supplemental oxygen increases circulatory oxygen levels and improves activity tolerance (Petty, Finigan, 1968; Casaburi, Petty, 1993).

• = **Independent;** ▲ = **Collaborative**

- Monitor a chronic obstructive pulmonary disease (COPD) client's response to activity by observing for symptoms of respiratory intolerance such as increased dyspnea, loss of ability to control breathing rhythmically, use of accessory muscles, and skin tone changes such as pallor and cyanosis.
- Instruct and assist COPD clients in using conscious controlled breathing techniques such as pursing their lips and diaphragmatic breathing.
  Training clients with COPD to slow their respiratory rate with a prolonged exhalation (with or without pursed lips) helps control dyspnea and results in improved ventilation, increased tidal volume, decreased respiratory rate, and a reduced alveolar-arterial oxygen difference. This breathing pattern not only helps relieve dyspnea but can improve the ability to exercise and carry out ADLs (Mueller, Petty, Filley, 1970; Casaburi, Petty, 1993).
- Provide emotional support and encouragement to client to gradually increase activity.
  Fear of breathlessness, pain, or falling may decrease willingness to increase activity.
- ▲ Refer the COPD client to a pulmonary rehabilitation program.
  Pulmonary rehabilitation has been shown to improve exercise capacity, walking ability, and sense of well-being (Fishman, 1994).
- ▲ Observe for pain before activity. If possible, treat pain before activity, and ensure that client is not heavily sedated.
  Pain restricts the client from achieving a maximal activity level and is often exacerbated by movement.
- ▲ Obtain any necessary assistive devices or equipment needed before ambulating client (e.g., walkers, canes, crutches, portable oxygen).
  Assistive devices can increase mobility by helping the client overcome limitations.
- Use a walking belt when ambulating a client who is unsteady.
  With a walking belt the client can walk independently, but the nurse can provide support if the client's knees buckle.
- Work with client to set mutual goals that increase activity levels.

Geriatric

- Slow the pace of care. Allow client extra time to carry out activities.
- Encourage families to help/allow elder to be independent in whatever activities possible. Sometimes families believe they are assisting by allowing clients to be sedentary.
  Encouraging activity not only enhances good functioning of the body's systems but also promotes a sense of worth by providing an opportunity for productivity (Eliopoulous, 1997).
- When mobilizing the elderly client, watch for orthostatic hypotension accompanied by dizziness and fainting.
  Orthostatic hypotension is common in the elderly as a result of cardiovascular changes, chronic diseases, and medication effects (Mobily, Kelley, 1991).

Home Care Interventions

- ▲ Begin discharge planning as soon as possible with case manager or social worker to assess need for home support systems and the need for community or home health services.
- ▲ Assess the home environment for factors that precipitate decreased activity tolerance: presence of allergens such as dust, smoke, and those associated with pets; temperature; energy-intensive activity patterns; and furniture placement. Refer to occupational therapy if needed to assist the client in restructuring the home and activity of daily living patterns.

• = Independent; ▲ = Collaborative

Clients and families often estimate energy requirements inaccurately during hospitalization because of the availability of support.

- Teach the client/family the importance of and methods for setting priorities for activities, especially those having a high energy demand (e.g., home/family events).
- Provide client/family with resources such as senior centers, exercise classes, educational and recreational programs, and volunteer opportunities that can aid in promoting socialization and appropriate activity.
  Social isolation can contribute to activity intolerance.
- Discuss the importance of sexual activity as part of daily living. Instruct the client in adaptive techniques to conserve energy during sexual interactions.
  Families may make unsafe choices for sexual activity or place added stress on themselves trying to cope with this issue without proper support or teaching.
- Instruct the client and family in the importance of maintaining proper nutrition and rest for energy conservation and rehabilitation.
- ▲ Refer to medical social services as necessary to assist the family in adjusting to major changes in patterns of living.
- ▲ Assess the need for long-term supports for optimal activity tolerance of priority activities (e.g., assistive devices, oxygen, medication, catheters, massage), especially for hospice patients. Evaluate intermittently.
  Assessments ensure the safety and appropriate use of these supports.
- ▲ Refer to home health aide services to support the client and family through changing levels of activity tolerance. Introduce aide support early. Instruct the aide to promote independence in activity as tolerated.
  Providing unnecessary assistance with transfers and bathing activities may promote dependence and a loss of mobility (Mobily, Kelley, 1991).
- Be aware of increased risk of bone fracture even after muscle strength is normalized, especially in osteopenic-prone individuals such as estrogen-deficient women and the elderly.
  Reduction in weight bearing muscle activity during bed rest invariably produces significant changes in calcium balance and, in weeks, changes in bone mass (Bloomfield, 1997)
- Allow terminally ill clients and their families to guide care.
  Control by the client or family promotes effective coping.
- ▲ Provide increased attention to comfort and dignity of the terminally ill client in care planning. For example, oxygen may be more valuable as a support to the client's psychological comfort than as a booster of oxygen saturation.

Client/Family Teaching

- Instruct client on rationale and techniques for avoiding activity intolerance.
- Teach client to use controlled breathing techniques with activity.
- Teach client the importance and method of coughing, clearing secretions.
- Instruct client in the use of relaxation techniques during activity.
- Help client with energy conservation and work simplification techniques in ADLs.
- Teach client the importance of proper nutrition.
- Describe to client the symptoms of activity intolerance, including which symptoms to report to the physician.
- Explain to client how to use assistive devices or medications before or during activity.
- Help client set up an activity log to record exercise and exercise tolerance.

• = **Independent;** ▲ = **Collaborative**

REFERENCES   Allen C, Glasziou P, Del Mar C: Bed rest: a potentially harmful treatment needing more careful evaluation, *Lancet* 354(9186):1229-1233, 1999.

American College of Sports Medicine: *Guidelines for exercise testing and prescription,* ed 5, Baltimore, 1995, Williams & Wilkins.

Bloomfield SA: Changes in musculoskeletal structure and function with prolonged bed rest, *Med Sci Sports Exerc* 29(2):197-206, 1997.

Casaburi R, Petty T: *Principles and practice of pulmonary rehabilitation,* Philadelphia, 1993, WB Saunders.

Creditor M: Hazards of hospitalization of the elderly, *Ann Intern Med* 118(3):219-223, 1994.

Eliopoulous C: *Gerontological nursing,* ed 4, Philadelphia, 1997, JB Lippincott.

Fishman AP: Pulmonary rehabilitation research, *Am J Respir Crit Care Med* 149(3 Pt 1):825-833, 1994.

McGoon M: *Mayo Clinic heart book,* New York, 1993, William Morrow.

Mobily PR, Kelley LS: Iatrogenesis in the elderly: factors of immobility, *J Gerontol Nurs* 17(9):5-11, 1991.

Mueller RE, Petty TL, Filley GF: Ventilation and arterial blood gas changes induced by pursed lips breathing, *J Appl Physiol* 28(6):784-789, 1970.

Nazarko L: The whole story: continence in people with dementia, *Nurs Times* 93(43):63-68, 1997.

Peckenpaugh N, Poleman C: *Nutrition essentials and diet therapy,* ed 8, Philadelphia, 1999, WB Saunders.

Petty TL, Finigan MM: Clinical evaluation of prolonged ambulatory oxygen therapy in chronic airway obstruction, *Am J Med* 45(2):242-252, 1968.

Prizant-Weston M, Castiglia K: Hemodynamic regulation. In Bulechek GM, McCloskey JC, editors: *Nursing interventions: essential nursing treatments,* Philadelphia, 1992, WB Saunders.

Resnick N: Geriatric medicine. In Tierney L Jr, McPhee S, Papadakis M, editors: *Current medical diagnosis and treatment,* ed 37, Stamford, Conn, 1998, Appleton & Lange.

Thompson P: The safety of exercise testing and participation. In Blair SN et al, editors: *Resource manual for guidelines for exercise testing and prescriptions,* Philadelphia, 1988, Lea & Febiger.

Wenger NK et al: Cardiac rehabilitation clinical practice guideline No 17, ACPHR No 96-0672, Rockville, Md, 1995, U.S. Department of Health and Human Services, Public Health Service, Agency for Health Care and Policy and Research and the National Heart, Lung, and Blood Institute.

Winslow EH, Lane LD, Woods RJ: Dangling: a review of relevant physiology, research, and practice, *Heart Lung* 24(4):263-272, 1995.

Risk for Activity intolerance

NANDA   **Definition** At risk for experiencing insufficient physiological or psychological energy to endure or complete required or desired daily activities

Risk Factors

History of intolerance to activity; deconditioned status; presence of circulatory or respiratory problems; inexperience with activity

Related Factors (r/t)

See Risk Factors

NOC   **Outcomes (Nursing Outcomes Classification)**
Suggested NOC Labels
Endurance; Energy Conservation; Activity Tolerance

• = Independent; ▲ = Collaborative

Example NOC Outcome

Demonstrates **Endurance** as evidenced by the following indicators: Performance of usual routine/Activity/Rested appearance/Blood oxygen level within normal limits/Expresses feelings about loss/Verbalizes acceptance of loss/Describes meaning of the loss or death/Reports decreased preoccupation with loss/Expresses positive expectations about the future (Rate each indicator of **Endurance:** 1 = extremely compromised, 2 = substantially compromised, 3 = moderately compromised, 4 = mildly compromised, 5 = not compromised [see Section I])

NIC   Interventions (Nursing Interventions Classification)

Suggested NIC Labels

Energy Management; Exercise Promotion: Strength Training; Activity Therapy

Example NIC Interventions—Energy Management
- Monitor cardiorespiratory response to activity
- Monitor location and nature of discomfort or pain during movement/activity

Client Outcomes, Nursing Interventions and Rationales, Client/Family Teaching

See care plan for **Activity intolerance.**

WEB SITES FOR EDUCATION

 See the MERLIN web site for World Wide Web resources for client education.

Impaired Adjustment

Gail B. Ladwig and Jill M. Barnes

NANDA   Definition   Inability to modify lifestyle/behavior in a manner consistent with a change in health status

Defining Characteristics

Denial of health status change; failure to achieve optimal sense of control; failure to take actions that would prevent further health problems; demonstration of nonacceptance of health status change

Related Factors (r/t)

Low state of optimism; intense emotional state; negative attitude toward health behavior; failure to intend to change behavior; multiple stressors; absence of social support for changed beliefs and practices; disability or health status change requiring change in lifestyle; lack of motivation to change behaviors

NOC   Outcomes (Nursing Outcomes Classification)

Suggested NOC Labels

Acceptance: Health Status; Coping; Grief Resolution; Health Seeking Behavior; Participation: Health Care Decisions; Psychosocial Adjustment: Life Change; Treatment Behavior: Illness or Injury

• = Independent; ▲ = Collaborative

Example NOC Outcome
Demonstrates **Acceptance: Health Status** as evidenced by the following indicators:
Peacefulness/Relinquishment of previous concept of health/Expressed reactions to
health status/Recognition of reality of health situation/Coping with health status
(Rate each indicator of **Acceptance: Health Status:** 1 = none, 2 = limited, 3 =
moderate, 4 = substantial, 5 = extensive [see Section I])

Client Outcomes

- States acceptance of change in health status
- Lists behaviors needed to adjust to change in health status and to maintain control
- States personal goals for dealing with change in health status and means to prevent further health problems
- Experiences a period of grief that is proportional to the actual or perceived effect of the loss

 ## Interventions (Nursing Interventions Classification)

Suggested NIC Labels
Coping Enhancement

Example NIC Interventions—Coping Enhancement
- Assist the client with developing an objective appraisal of the event
- Explore with the client previous methods of dealing with life problems

Nursing Interventions and Rationales

- Assess client's perception about the illness/event. Ask client to state feelings related to the change in health status.
  Two important determinants of threat are the strength of the commitments being endangered and the individual's belief in his or her ability to control the situation (Godfrey, Knight, Partridge, 1996). A clinician's ability to understand a client's perceptions of the impact of the illness is crucial to the clinician's ability to be therapeutic. Knowledge of a patient's perceptions about chronic illness will help nurses intervene sensitively and effectively (Yuen-Juen, 1995). Negative appraisals of events such as divorce significantly alter the ability to adjust to the event (Mazur et al, 1999).
- Assess patient and family for the presence of additional stressors (e.g., financial difficulty, health of other family members, occupational changes).
  Additional stressors have been found to hinder the client's adjustment (Grootenhuis, Last, 1997).
- Assess the client's feelings about whether change in health status is personally being dealt with effectively.
  Identification of the usual coping mechanisms is vital and may provide information on other coping styles that can be introduced to promote effective adaptation (Anderson, Maksud, 1994). Nurses must understand how each client perceives personal coping with stressful experiences associated with a chronic illness (Downe-Wamboldt, Melanson, 1995).
- Assess for negative affect and internalization of problems.
  Maladjustment is often manifested in these ways (Kotchick et al, 1997).

• = **Independent;** ▲ = **Collaborative**

- Assess the socioeconomic status of all patients.
  Patients of low socioeconomic status have been found to have more difficulty with adjustment in social functioning, mental health, pain, fatigue, and physical fitness than patients of high socioeconomic status (Sykes et al, 1999).
- Allow client adequate time to express feelings about the change in health status.
  To promote adaptation, verbalization of feelings following a traumatic event should be encouraged (Anderson, Maksud, 1994). Although the client cannot be pushed into coping with the change in health status (Johnson, 1994), verbalization of feelings leads to acceptance and understanding of changes.
- Help client work through the stages of grief. Denial is usually the initial response. Acknowledge that grief takes time, and give client permission to grieve; accept crying.
  Acceptance of feelings conveys empathy and promotes movement toward adjustment.
- Recognize that denial may be adaptive at certain stages of a threatening encounter.
  This is true both when denial of implication may preserve hope and optimism and therefore be psychologically beneficial and during the early stages of a crisis when the situation cannot be faced in its entirety (Godfrey, Knight, Partridge, 1996).
- Discuss resources (e.g., client's support system) that have worked previously when dealing with changes in lifestyle or health status.
  Effective use of social support can directly affect a patient's ability to adjust to new situations (Godfrey, Knight, Partridge, 1996).
- ▲ Refer to community resources. Provide general and contact information for ease of use.
  Social support theory suggests that people respond to stressful circumstances better when they have the support of family, friends, helping professionals, or organizations (Abbott et al, 1997).
- Use open-ended questions to allow the client free expression (e.g., "Tell me about your last hospitalization" or "How does this time compare?").
  Open-ended questions allow the client to be more actively involved in the exchange.
- Discuss client's current goals. If appropriate, have client list goals so that they can be referred to and steps can be taken to accomplish them.
  Social production function (SPF) basically asserts that people produce their own well-being by trying to optimize achievement of universal human goals (Ormel et al, 1997).
- List client activities that may require assistance and those that can be performed independently.
  This list gives the client permission to ask for help and informs the client that outside resources are available.
- Allow client choices in daily care, particularly choices that result from the change in health status.
  To perceive ownership of change, the client needs to value the proposed change, feel able to carry it out, and accept responsibility for it (Fleury, 1991).
- Allow client time to adjust to new situations. Introduce new material gradually to prevent overload. Ask for frequent feedback.
  The stress of changes in health care can be overwhelming. New material takes longer to learn and absorb, thus clarification of information and frequent repetition may be necessary.
- Give client positive feedback for accomplishments, no matter how small.
  A degree of optimism and encouragement must be provided to maintain the morale of the individual (Godfrey, Knight, Partridge, 1996). Empathic communication has been shown to be therapeutic and health promoting (Wells-Federman et al, 1995).

• = Independent; ▲ = Collaborative

- Manipulate the environment to decrease stress; allow the client to display personal items that have meaning.
  Personalization of the new environment can lead to better adjustment to that environment (Armor, 1996).
- Maintain consistency and continuity in daily schedule. When possible, provide the same caregiver.
  Continuity with the clinicians providing care will allow for a better atmosphere to assist the patient and family through this physical state (Anderson, Maksud, 1994).
- Foster communication between the patient/family and medical staff.
  People often rely on medical personnel for an understanding of the condition (Grootenhuis, Last, 1997).

Geriatric

- Assess for signs of depression resulting from illness-associated changes.
  The elderly are at risk of depression when living with a chronic illness (Badger, 1993).
- Monitor client for agitation.
  The elderly often use agitation to express an inability to accept change.

Multicultural

- Assess for the influence of cultural beliefs, norms, and values on the client's ability to modify health behavior.
  What the client considers normal and abnormal health behavior may be based on cultural perceptions (Leininger, 1996).
- Discuss with the client those aspects of their health behavior/lifestyle that will remain unchanged by their health status.
  Aspects of the client's life that are meaningful and valuable to them should be understood and preserved without change (Leininger, 1996).
- Negotiate with the client regarding the aspects of health behavior which will need to be modified.
  Give and take with the client will lead to culturally congruent care (Leininger, 1996).
- Assess the role of fatalism on the client's ability to modify health behavior
  Fatalistic perspectives, which involve the belief that you cannot control your own fate, may influence health behaviors in some African-American and Latino populations (Phillips, Cohen, Moses, 1999; Harmon, Castro, Coe, 1996).
- Validate the client's feelings regarding the impact of health status on current lifestyle.
  Validation lets the client know that the nurse has heard and understands what was said, thus promoting the nurse-client relationship (Stuart, Laraia, 2001; Giger, Davidhizar, 1995).

Home Care Interventions

- ▲ Include a spiritual assessment in overall assessment of client and family resources.
- ▲ Refer to medical social services to facilitate the listed interventions and support client care goals.
  Support for transition to the home setting can facilitate acceptance of the changes required to maintain the client in the home setting.
- Assess affective climate within family and family support system.
  Positive family affective climate and family support have been found to enhance social adjustment (Langfitt et al, 1999).
- ▲ Observe for signs of caregiver stress on an ongoing basis. Refer to necessary support services.
  Caregiver stress may increase as time progresses.

- **= Independent; ▲ = Collaborative**

▲ Refer client to counselor or therapist for follow-up care.
Arranging for referral assists the client with working with the system, and resource use helps to develop problem solving and coping skills (Feeley, Gottlieb, 1998). Clients who maintained contacts with counselors or therapists achieved greater levels of success in managing their original problems (Di Donato, Schaffer, 1994).

▲ Initiate community referrals as needed (e.g., grief counseling, self-help groups).
Community support services can assist in the adaptation process (Godfrey, Knight, Partridge, 1996). Motivation, sharing of experiences, camaraderie with and support from peers, and the feeling of not being alone have been identified as advantages of group learning (Payne, 1993). Social support is both essential for an individual to develop a sense of belonging and known to buffer the individual from the psychological effects of adverse life events (Godfrey, Knight, Partridge, 1996). Support groups can provide families with a close setting that allows for minor problems and fears to be resolved readily (Herranz, Gavilan, 1999).

Client/Family Teaching

• Teach client to maintain a positive outlook by listing current strengths.
The use of optimistic coping strategies is positively related to psychological well-being (Downe-Wamboldt, Melanson, 1995).

• Teach clients and family relaxation techniques (controlled breathing, guided imagery) and help them practice.
Relaxation techniques, desensitization, and guided imagery can help clients to cope, increase their control, and allay anxiety (Narsavage, 1997). Teaching and guiding client in positive self-care techniques empowers the client (Wells-Federman et al, 1995).

• Instruct client to keep a journal documenting positive ways of coping with the current health change.
Diaries can facilitate pattern identification and support a client's sense of control (Narsavage, 1997). By documenting daily experiences, clients are better able to take an active role in treatment (Burham, 1995).

• Allow client to proceed at own pace in learning; provide time for return demonstrations (e.g., self-injection of insulin). Use clear and distinct language free of medical jargon and meaningless values.
Everyone learns at a different pace, and some clients need frequent repetition. A comfortable teaching atmosphere both allows for openness and comfort when delivering disturbing information and facilitates trust (Hopkins, 1994).

• Involve significant others in planning and teaching.
The support of significant others facilitates desired changes. Through positive reinforcement and an expression of congruency in behavioral change, significant others often serve as powerful external motivators (Fleury, 1991).

• If long-term deficits are expected, inform the family as soon as possible.
Having all the facts early on promotes acceptance and results in decreased anxiety (Hilton, 1994).

• Teach families intervention techniques for family members such as setting limits, communicating acceptable behavior, and having time-outs.
If there are deficits related to the changed health, there may be anger and agitation; these interventions are effective in those situations (Hilton, 1994).

• = Independent; ▲ = Collaborative

- Educate and prepare families regarding the appearance of the patient and the environment before initial exposure.

  Appearance and unfamiliar environment may be a source of distress leading to maladjustment (Doering, Dracup, Moser, 1999).

WEB SITES FOR EDUCATION

MERLIN See the MERLIN web site for World Wide Web resources for client education.

REFERENCES   Abbott DA et al: The influence of a big brothers program on the adjustment of boys in single-parent families, *J Psychol* 131(2):143-156, 1997.

Anderson RC, Maksud DP: Psychologic adjustments to reconstructive surgery, *Nurs Clin North Am* 29(4):711-724, 1994.

Armor JM: Degree of personalization as a cue in the assessment of adjustment to congregate housing by rural elders, *Geriatr Nurs* 17(2):79-80, 1996 (research brief).

Badger T: Physical health impairment and depression among older adults, *Image J Nurs Sch* 25:325, 1993.

Burham M: Health diaries in nursing research and practice, *Image J Nurs Sch* 27(2):147, 1995.

Di Donato BA, Schaffer VL: The importance of outcome data in brain injury rehabilitation, *Rehabil Nurs* 19:219, 1994.

Doering LV, Dracup K, Moser D: Comparison of psychosocial adjustment of mothers and fathers of high-risk infants in the neonatal intensive care unit, *J Perinatol* 19(2):132-137, 1999.

Downe-Wamboldt B, Melanson P: Emotions, coping and psychological well-being in elderly people with arthritis, *West J Nurs Res* 7:250, 1995.

Feeley N, Gottlieb LN: Classification systems for health concerns, nursing strategies, and client outcomes: nursing practice with families who have a child with a chronic illness, *Can J Nurs Res* 30(1):45-59, 1998.

Fleury D: Empowering potential: a theory of wellness motivation, *Nurs Res* 40:286-291, 1991.

Giger JN, Davidhizar RE: *Transcultural nursing*, ed 2, St Louis, 1995, Mosby.

Godfrey H, Knight RG, Partridge F: Emotional adjustment following traumatic brain injury—a stress appraisal coping formulation, *J Head Trauma Rehab* 11(6):29-40, 1996.

Grootenhuis MA, Last BF: Adjustment and coping by parents of children with cancer: a review of the literature, *Support Care Cancer* 5(6):466-484, 1997.

Harmon MP, Castro FG, Coe K: Acculturation and cervical cancer: knowledge, beliefs, and behaviors of Hispanic women, *Women Health* 24(3):37-57, 1996.

Herranz J, Gavilan J: Psychosocial adjustment after laryngeal cancer surgery, *Ann Otol Rhinol Laryngol* 108(10):990-997, 1999.

Hilton T: Behavioral and cognitive sequelae of head trauma, *Orthop Nurse* 13:22, 1994.

Hopkins A: The trauma nurse's role with families in crisis, *Crit Care Nurse* 14:35, 1994.

Johnson J: Caring for the woman who's had a mastectomy, *Am J Nurs* 94:25, 1994.

Kotchick BA et al: The role of parental and extrafamilial social support in the psychosocial adjustment of children with a chronically ill father, *Behav Modif* 21(4):409-432, 1997.

Langfitt JT et al: Family interactions as targets for intervention to improve social adjustment after epilepsy surgery, *Epilepsia* 40(6):735-744, 1999.

Leininger MM: *Transcultural nursing: theories, research and practices*, ed 2, Hilliard, Ohio, 1996, McGraw-Hill.

Mazur E et al: Cognitive moderators of children's adjustment to stressful divorce events: the role of negative cognitive errors and positive illusions, *Child Dev* 70(1):231-245, 1999.

Narsavage GL: Promoting function in clients with chronic lung disease by increasing their perception of control, *Holistic Nurs Pract* 12(1):17-26, 1997.

Ormel J et al: Quality of life and social production functions: a framework for understanding health effects, *Soc Sci Med* 45(7):1051-1063, 1997.

Payne J: The contribution of group learning to the rehabilitation of spinal cord injured adults, *Rehabil Nurs* 18:375, 1993.

Phillips JM, Cohen MZ, Moses G: Breast cancer screening and African American women: fear, fatalism, and silence, *Oncol Nurs Forum* 26(3):561-571, 1999.

Stuart GW, Laraia MT: Therapeutic nurse-patient relationship. In Stuart GW, Laraia MT, editors: *Principles and practice of psychiatric nursing*, St Louis, 2001, Mosby, p 30.

• = **Independent;** ▲ = **Collaborative**

Sykes DH et al: Socioeconomic status, social environment, depression and postdischarge adjustment of the cardiac patient, *J Psychosom Res* 46(1):83-98, 1999.

Wells-Federman C et al: The mind-body connection: the psychophysiology of many traditional nursing interventions, *Clin Nurse Spec* 9:59, 1995.

Yuen-Juen H: The impact of chronic illness on patients, *Rehabil Nurs* 20:221, 1995.

Ineffective Airway clearance

Betty J. Ackley

NANDA   **Definition** Inability to clear secretions or obstructions from the respiratory tract to maintain a clear airway

Defining Characteristics

Dyspnea; diminished breath sounds; orthopnea; adventitious breath sounds (crackles, wheezes); cough, ineffective or absent; sputum production; cyanosis; difficulty vocalizing; wide-eyed; changes in respiratory rate and rhythm; restlessness

Related Factors (r/t)

Environmental Smoking; smoke inhalation; second-hand smoke

Obstructed airway

Airway spasm; retained secretions; excessive mucus; presence of artificial airway; foreign body in airway; secretions in bronchi; exudate in alveoli

Physiological Neuromuscular dysfunction; hyperplasia of bronchial walls; chronic obstructive pulmonary disease; infection; asthma; allergic airways

NOC   **Outcomes (Nursing Outcomes Classification)**

Suggested NOC Labels

Respiratory Status: Ventilation; Respiratory Status: Airway Patency; Respiratory Status: Gas Exchange; Aspiration Control

> **Example NOC Outcome**
> Maintains **Respiratory Status: Ventilation** as evidenced by the following indicators: Respiratory rate IER*/Moves sputum out of airway/Adventitious breath sounds not present/SOB not present/Auscultated breath sounds IER/Auscultated vocalization IER/Chest x-ray findings IER (Rate each indicator of **Respiratory Status: Ventilation:** 1 = extremely compromised, 2 = substantially compromised, 3 = moderately compromised, 4 = mildly compromised, 5 = not compromised [see Section I])

*In Expected Range

Client Outcomes

- Demonstrates effective coughing and clear breath sounds; is free of cyanosis and dyspnea
- Maintains a patent airway at all times
- Relates methods to enhance secretion removal
- Relates the significance of changes in sputum to include color, character, amount, and odor
- Identifies and avoids specific factors that inhibit effective airway clearance

• = Independent; ▲ = Collaborative

NIC **Interventions (Nursing Interventions Classification)**

Suggested NIC Labels

Airway Management; Airway Suctioning; Cough Enhancement

Example NIC Interventions—Airway Management
- Instruct how to cough effectively
- Auscultate breath sounds, noting areas of decreased or absent ventilation and presence of adventitious sounds

Nursing Interventions and Rationales

- Auscultate breath sounds q _____ h(rs).

   Breath sounds are normally clear or scattered fine crackles at bases, which clear with deep breathing. The presence of coarse crackles during late inspiration indicates fluid in the airway; wheezing indicates an airway obstruction.

- Monitor respiratory patterns, including rate, depth, and effort.

   A normal respiratory rate for an adult without dyspnea is 12 to 16. With secretions in the airway, the respiratory rate will increase.

▲ Monitor blood gas values and pulse oxygen saturation levels as available.

   Normal blood gas values are a PO_2 of 80 to 100 mm Hg and a PCO_2 of 35 to 45 mm Hg. An oxygen saturation of less than 90% indicates problems with oxygenation. Hypoxemia can result from ventilation-perfusion mismatches secondary to respiratory secretions.

- Position client to optimize respiration (e.g., head of bed elevated 45 degrees and repositioned at least every 2 hours).

   An upright position allows for maximal air exchange and lung expansion; lying flat causes abdominal organs to shift toward the chest, which crowds the lungs and makes it more difficult to breathe. Studies have shown that in mechanically ventilated clients receiving enteral feedings, there is a decreased incidence of nosocomial pneumonia if the client is positioned at a 45-degree semirecumbent position as opposed to a supine position (Torres et al, 1992; Drakulovic et al, 1999).

- If the client has unilateral lung disease, alternate a semi-Fowler's position with a lateral position (with a 10- to 15-degree elevation and "good lung down") for 60 to 90 minutes. This method is contraindicated for a client with a pulmonary abscess or hemorrhage or with interstitial emphysema.

   Gravity and hydrostatic pressure allow the dependent lung to become better ventilated and perfused, which increases oxygenation (Yeaw, 1992; Smith-Sims, 2001).

- Help client to deep breathe and perform controlled coughing. Have client inhale deeply, hold breath for several seconds, and cough two to three times with mouth open while tightening the upper abdominal muscles.

   This technique can help increase sputum clearance and decrease cough spasms (Celli, 1998). Controlled coughing uses the diaphragmatic muscles, making the cough more forceful and effective.

- If the client has COPD, consider helping the client use the "huff cough." The client does a series of coughs while saying the word "huff."

   This technique prevents the glottis from closing during the cough and is effective in clearing secretions in the central airways (Lewis, Heitkemper, Dirksen, 1999).

▲ Encourage client to use incentive spirometer.

• = **Independent;** ▲ = **Collaborative**

The incentive spirometer is an effective tool that can help prevent atelectasis and retention of bronchial secretions (Peruzzi, Smith, 1995).

- Assist with clearing secretions from pharynx by offering tissues and gentle suction of the oral pharynx if necessary. Do not do nasotracheal suctioning.
  It is preferable for the client to cough up secretions. In the debilitated client, gentle suctioning of the posterior pharynx may stimulate coughing and help remove secretions; nasotracheal suctioning is dangerous because the nurse is unable to hyperoxygenate before, during, and after to maintain adequate oxygenation (Peruzzi, Smith, 1995).
- Observe sputum, noting color, odor, and volume.
  Normal sputum is clear or gray and minimal; abnormal sputum is green, yellow, or bloody; malodorous; and often copious.
- When suctioning an endotracheal tube or tracheostomy tube for a client on a ventilator, do the following:
  - Hyperoxygenate before, between, and after endotracheal suction sessions.
    Nursing research has demonstrated that the client should be hyperoxygenated during suctioning (Winslow, 1993a).
  - Use a closed, in-line suction system.
    The closed, in-line suction system is associated with a decrease in nosocomial pneumonia (Deppe et al, 1990; Johnson et al, 1994; Mathews, Mathews, 2000), reduced suction-induced hypoxemia, and fewer physiological disturbances (including decreased development of dysrhythmia) and often saves money (Carroll, 1998).
  - Avoid saline instillation during suctioning.
    Saline instillation before suctioning has an adverse effect on oxygen saturation (Ackerman, Mick, 1998; Winslow, 1993b; Raymond, 1995).
- Document results of coughing and suctioning, particularly client tolerance and secretion characteristics such as color, odor, and volume.
- Provide oral care every 4 hours.
  Oral care freshens the mouth after respiratory secretions have been expectorated. Research is promising on the use of chlorhexidine oral rinses after oral care to reduce bacteria, and possibly reduce the incidence of nosocomial pneumonia (Kollef, 1999).
- Encourage activity and ambulation as tolerated. If unable to ambulate client, turn client from side to side at least every 2 hours.
  Body movement helps mobilize secretions. The supine position and immobility have been shown to predispose postoperative clients to pneumonia (Brooks-Brunn, 1995). See interventions for **Impaired Gas exchange** *for further information on positioning a respiratory client.*
- Encourage increased fluid intake of up to 3000 ml/day within cardiac or renal reserve.
  Fluids help minimize mucosal drying and maximize ciliary action to move secretions (Carroll, 1994). Some clients cannot tolerate increased fluids because of underlying disease.
- ▲ Administer oxygen as ordered.
  Oxygen has been shown to correct hypoxemia, which can be caused by retained respiratory secretions.
- ▲ Administer medications such as bronchodilators or inhaled steroids as ordered. Watch for side effects such as tachycardia or anxiety with bronchodilators, inflamed pharynx with inhaled steroids.
  Bronchodilators decrease airway resistance secondary to bronchoconstriction.

• = **Independent**; ▲ = **Collaborative**

▲ Provide postural drainage, percussion, and vibration as ordered.
Chest physical therapy helps mobilize bronchial secretions; it should be used only when pre-scribed because it can cause harm if client has underlying conditions such as cardiac disease or increased intracranial pressure (Peruzzi, Smith, 1995).

▲ Refer for physical therapy or respiratory therapy for further treatment.

Geriatric

• Encourage ambulation as tolerated without causing exhaustion.
Immobility is often harmful to the elderly because it decreases ventilation and increases stasis of secretions, leading to atelectasis or pneumonia (Hoyt, 1992; Tempkin, Tempkin, Goodman, 1997).

• Actively encourage the elderly to deep breathe and cough.
Cough reflexes are blunted and coughing is decreased in the elderly (Sparrow, Weiss, 1988).

• Ensure adequate hydration within cardiac and renal reserves.
The elderly are prone to dehydration and therefore more viscous secretions because they frequently use diuretics or laxatives and forget to drink adequate amounts of water (Hoyt, 1992).

Home Care Interventions

• Assess home environment for factors that exacerbate airway clearance problems (e.g., presence of allergens, lack of adequate humidity in air, stressful family relationships).

• Limit client exposure to persons with upper respiratory infections.

▲ Provide/teach percussion and postural drainage per physician orders. Teach adaptive breathing techniques.
Adaptive breathing, percussion, and postural drainage loosen secretions and allow more effective oxygenation.

• Determine client compliance with medical regimen.

▲ Teach client when and how to use inhalant or nebulizer treatments at home.

▲ Teach client/family importance of maintaining regimen and having prn drugs easily accessible at all times.
Success in avoiding emergency or institutional care may rest solely on medication compli-ance or availability.

▲ Identify an emergency plan, including criteria for use.
Ineffective airway clearance can be life threatening.

▲ Refer for home health aide services for assist with ADLs.
Clients with decreased oxygenation and copious respiratory secretions are often unable to maintain energy for ADLs.

▲ Assess family for role changes and coping skills. Refer to medical social services as necessary.
Clients with decreased oxygenation are unable to maintain role activities and therefore experience frustration and anger, which may pose a threat to family integrity.

• Provide family with support for care of a client with a chronic or terminal illness.
Severe compromise to respiratory function creates fear in clients and caregivers. Fear in-hibits effective coping.

Client/Family Teaching

• Teach importance of not smoking. Be aggressive in approach, ask to set a date for smoking cessation, and recommend nicotine replacement therapy (nicotine patch or gum). Refer to smoking cessation programs, and encourage clients who relapse to keep trying to quit.

• = Independent; ▲ = Collaborative

All health care clinicians should be aggressive in helping smokers quit (AHCPR Guidelines, 1996).

▲ Teach client how to use a flutter clearance device if ordered, which vibrates to loosen mucus and gives positive pressure to keep airways open.
This device has been shown to effectively decrease mucous viscosity and elasticity (App et al, 1998), increase amount of sputum expectorated (Langenderfer, 1998; Bellone et al, 2000), and increase peak expiratory flow rate (Burioka et al, 1998).

▲ Teach client how to use peak expiratory flow rate (PEFR) meter if ordered and when to seek medical attention if PEFR reading drops. Also teach how to use metered dose inhalers and self-administer inhaled corticosteroids following precautions to decrease side effects (Owen, 1999).

• Teach client how to deep breathe and cough effectively. Teach how to use the ELTGOL method—an airway clearance method that uses lateral posture and different lung volumes to control expiratory flow of air to avoid airway compression.
Controlled coughing uses the diaphragmatic muscles, making the cough more forceful and effective. The ELTGOL method was shown to be more effective in secretion removal in chronic bronchitis than postural drainage (Bellone et al, 2000).

• Teach client/family to identify and avoid specific factors that exacerbate ineffective airway clearance, including known allergens and especially smoking (if relevant) or exposure to second-hand smoke.

• Educate client and family about the significance of changes in sputum characteristics, including color, character, amount, and odor.
With this knowledge the client and family can identify early the signs of infection and seek treatment before acute illness occurs.

▲ Teach client/family need to take antibiotics until prescription has run out.
Taking the entire course of antibiotics helps to eradicate bacterial infection, which decreases lingering, chronic infection.

WEB SITES FOR EDUCATION

MERLIN   See the MERLIN web site for World Wide Web resources for client education.

REFERENCES   Ackerman MH, Mick DJ: Instillation of normal saline before suctioning in patients with pulmonary infections: a prospective randomized controlled trial, *Am J Crit Care* 7(4):261-266, 1998.

Agency for Health Care Policy and Research: *Smoking cessation, clinical practice guideline,* Washington, DC, 1996, U.S. Government Printing Office.

App EM et al: Sputum rheology changes in cystic fibrosis lung disease following two different types of physiotherapy: flutter vs autogenic drainage, *Chest* 114(1):171-177, 1998.

Bellone A et al: Chest physical therapy in patients with acute exacerbation of chronic bronchitis: effectiveness of three modes, *Arch Phys Med Rehabil* 81(5):558-560, 2000.

Brooks-Brunn JA: Postoperative atelectasis and pneumonia: risk factors, *Am J Crit Care* 4(5):340-349, 1995.

Burioka N et al: Clinical efficacy of the FLUTTER device for airway mucus clearance in patients with diffuse panbronchiolitis, *Respirology* 3(3):183-186, 1998.

Carroll P: Safe suctioning prn, *RN* 57(5):32, 1994.

Carroll P: Spotting the difference in respiratory care, *RN* 96(6):26-30, 1998.

Celli BR: Pulmonary rehabilitation for COPD, *Postgrad Med* 103(4):159-176, 1998.

Deppe SA et al: Incidence of colonization, nosocomial pneumonia, and mortality in critically ill patients using a Trach Care closed-suction system: prospective, randomized study, *Crit Care Med* 18:1389, 1990.

Drakulovic MB et al: Supine body position as a risk factor for nosocomial pneumonia in mechanically ventilated patients: a randomised trial, *Lancet* 354(9193):1851-1858, 1999.

• = Independent; ▲ = Collaborative

Hoyt MM: Impaired gas exchange in the elderly, *Geriatr Nurs* 13:262, 1992.

Johnson KL et al: Closed versus open endotracheal suctioning: costs and physiologic consequences, *Crit Care Med* 22(4):658-665, 1994.

Kollef MH: Epidemiology and risk factors for nosocomial pneumonia, *Clin Chest Med* 20(3):653-670, 1999.

Langenderfer B: Alternatives to percussion and postural drainage: a review of mucus clearance therapies, *J Cardiopulm Rehab* 18(4):283-289, 1998.

Lewis SM, Heitkemper MM, Dirksen SR: *Medical-surgical nursing,* ed 5, St Louis, 1999, Mosby.

Mathews PJ, Mathews LM: Reducing the risks of ventilator-associated infections, *Dimens Crit Care Nurs* 19(1):17-20, 2000.

Owen CL: New directions in asthma management, *Am J Nurs* 99(3):27-34, 1999.

Peruzzi WT, Smith B: Bronchial hygiene therapy, *Crit Care Clin* 11(1):79-94, 1995.

Raymond SJ: Normal saline instillation before suctioning: helpful or harmful? a review of the literature, *Am J Crit Care* 4(4):267-271, 1995.

Smith-Sims K: Hospital-acquired pneumonia, *Am J Nurs* 101(1), 2001.

Sparrow D, Weiss S: Pulmonary system. In Rose JW, Besdine RS, editors: *Geriatric medicine,* Boston, 1988, Little, Brown.

Tempkin T, Tempkin A, Goodman H: Geriatric rehabilitation, *Nurse Pract Forum* 8(2):59-63, 1997.

Torres A et al: Pulmonary aspiration of gastric contents in patients receiving mechanical ventilation: the effect of body position, *Ann Intern Med* 116:540-543, 1992.

Winslow EH: Open-and-closed debate on hyperoxygenation: working smart, *Am J Nurs* 13:16, 1993a.

Winslow EH: Save the saline, *Am J Nurs* 13:16, 1993b.

Yeaw P: Good lung down, *Am J Nurs* 92:27, 1992.

Latex Allergy response

Gail B. Ladwig

NANDA   **Definition** An allergic response to natural latex rubber products

Defining Characteristics

Type I reactions: Immediate reactions (<1 hour) to latex proteins (can be life threatening); contact urticaria progressing to generalized symptoms; edema of the lips, tongue, uvula, and/or throat; shortness of breath; tightness in chest; wheezing; bronchospasm leading to respiratory arrest; hypotension; syncope; cardiac arrest
May also include: orofacial characteristics: edema of sclera or eyelids, erythema and/or itching of the eyes, tearing of the eyes, nasal congestion, itching and/or erythema, rhinorrhea, facial erythema, facial itching; gastrointestinal characteristics: abdominal pain, nausea; generalized characteristics: flushing, general discomfort, generalized edema, increasing complaint of total body warmth, restlessness
Type IV reactions: delayed onset: eczema; irritation; reaction to additives causes discomfort (e.g., thiurams, carbamates); redness; delayed onset (hours)
Irritant reactions: erythema; chapped or cracked skin; blisters

Related Factors (r/t)

No immune mechanism response

NOC   ## Outcomes (Nursing Outcomes Classification)

Suggested NOC Labels

Immune Hypersensitivity Control; Symptom Severity; Tissue Integrity: Skin and Mucous Membranes

• = **Independent;** ▲ = **Collaborative**

Example NOC Outcome
Demonstrates **Immune Hypersensitivity Control,** as evidenced by the following indicators: Respiratory, cardiac, gastrointestinal, renal and neurological function status IER*/Free of allergic reactions (Rate each indicator of **Immune Hypersensitivity Control:** 1 = not controlled, 2 = slightly controlled, 3 = moderately controlled, 4 = well controlled, 5 = very well controlled [see Section I])

*In Expected Range

Client Outcomes

- Identifies presence of latex allergy
- Lists history of risk factors
- Identifies type of reaction
- States reasons not to use or to have anyone use latex products
- Experiences a latex-free environment for all health care procedures
- Avoids areas where there is powder from latex gloves
- States the importance of wearing a Medic-Alert bracelet and wears one

 ## Interventions (Nursing Interventions Classification)
Suggested NIC Labels
Allergy Management; Latex Precautions

Example NIC Interventions—Latex Precautions
- Question client or appropriate other about history of systemic reaction to natural rubber latex (e.g., facial or scleral edema, tearing eyes, urticaria, rhinitis, and wheezing)
- Place an allergy band on client

Nursing Interventions and Rationales

- Take a careful history of clients at risk: health care workers, rubber industry workers, clients with neural tube defects, and atopic individuals (hayfever, asthma, atopic eczema). ·
  Individuals at highest risk of development of IgE-mediated latex allergy are either atopic, highly exposed to latex, or both (Kelly, Walsh-Kelly, 1998). Early recognition of sensitization to natural latex rubber is crucial to prevent the occurrence of life-threatening reactions in sensitized health care providers and their clients (Tarlo, 1998). Allergic reactions to natural rubber latex have increased during the past 10 years, especially in the many health care workers who have high exposure to latex allergens both by direct skin contact and by inhalation of latex particles from powdered gloves (Nielsen et al, 2000)
- If IgE-mediated latex allergy is suspected, question the client about food allergies to chestnuts, avocados, bananas, kiwis, and other tropical fruits.
  Clients with IgE-mediated allergy may have cross-reactivity with food allergens such as bananas, kiwis, and other tropical fruits (Kelly, Walsh-Kelly, 1998). Class I chitinases have been identified as the major panallergens in fruits associated with the latex-fruit syndrome, such as avocado, banana, and chestnut (Sanchez-Monge et al, 2000).
- Question the client about associated symptoms of itching, swelling, and redness after contact with rubber products such as rubber gloves, balloons, and barrier contraceptives, or swelling of the tongue and lips after dental examinations.

• = Independent; ▲ = Collaborative

Products Containing Latex

Emergency Equipment
Blood pressure cuffs
Stethoscopes
Disposable gloves
Oral and nasal airways
Endotracheal tubes
Tourniquets
Intravenous tubing
Syringes
Electrode pads
Personal Protective Equipment
Gloves
Surgical masks
Goggles
Respirators
Rubber aprons
Office Supplies
Rubber bands
Erasers
Hospital Supplies
Anesthesia masks

Catheters
Wound drains
Injection ports
Rubber tops of multidose vials
Dental dams
Household Objects
Automobile tires
Motorcycle and bicycle handgrips
Carpeting
Swimming goggles
Racquet handles
Shoe soles
Expandable fabric (waistbands)
Dishwashing gloves
Hot water bottles
Condoms
Diaphragms
Balloons
Pacifiers
Baby bottle nipples

From National Institute for Occupational Safety and Health: *NOSH alert: preventing allergic reactions to natural rubber latex in the workplace,* DHHS (NIOSH) Pub. No. 97-135, June 1997 (www.cdc.gov/niosh/latexalt.html).

A client's history can suggest the likelihood of his or her developing a reaction to latex; the itching and swelling mentioned are reliable indicators of significant sensitivity to latex (Dakin, Yentis, 1998).

- Materials and items that contain latex must be identified, and latex-free alternatives must be found. A wide variety of products contain latex: medical supplies, personal protective equipment, and numerous household objects (Evangelisto, 1998).
- All latex-sensitive clients (e.g., those who experience reddened, irritated areas under Band-Aid adhesive) are treated as if they have a latex allergy.
  According to the Centers for Disease Control (CDC) guidelines, all latex-sensitive clients are treated as if they have a latex allergy (Harrau, 1998).
- See the box above for examples of products that may contain latex.
- ▲ Five principles for management of latex-allergic clients: (1) recognize the problem, (2) avoid exposure to latex, (3) inform the surgeons and operating room nurses, (4) be prepared to treat anaphylaxis, (5) be vigilant postoperatively and arrange follow-up care. *Reactions may be prevented by providing a latex-free environment (Kantor, Smith, Kalhan, 1999). Medical personnel must stay abreast of new data and product information*

• = **Independent**; ▲ = **Collaborative**

to provide up-to-date care for patients, as well as protection for themselves (Floyd, 2000). Latex aeroallergen is primarily generated by active glove use; carpeting and fabric uphol-stery can serve as important aeroallergen repositories. Site-wide substitution of nonpow-dered latex gloves eliminates detectable latex aeroallergen (Charous, Schuenemann, Swanson, 2000).

▲ Anaphylaxis from latex allergy is a medical emergency and must be treated differ-ently than anaphylaxis from other causes.
   Clients with latex-induced anaphylaxis must be placed in a latex-free environment (Kelly, Walsh-Kelly, 1998).

• Do not open or use powdered latex gloves in the client's room. At times it is neces-sary to convert the whole building to a latex-free environment to prevent inhalation of symptoms of IgE-mediated allergy.
   Most inhalation allergen exposure derives from protein bound to the cornstarch donning powder on gloves. Transfer of this allergen to other products or even the air duct of build-ings where gloves are used may result in exposure and clinical symptoms of rhinoconjuncti-vitis, throat irritation, airway edema, and asthma (Kelly, Walsh-Kelly, 1998). Gloves are the single most important piece of equipment responsible for triggering a reaction to latex. Starch or modified starch gloves are the worst culprits (Dakin, Yentis, 1998).

Home Care Interventions

• Assess the home environment for presence of natural latex products (e.g., balloons, condoms, gloves, and products of related allergies, such as bananas, avocados, and poinsettia plants).
   Identification and/or removal of allergy stimulants decreases allergic response risk.

▲ At onset of care, assess client history and current status of latex allergy response. Seek medical care as necessary.
   Immediate identification of allergic response promotes prompt treatment and decreases risk of severe response.

• Do not use latex products in caregiving.

• Assist client in identifying and obtaining alternatives to latex products.
   Preventing exposure to latex is the key to managing and preventing this allergy. Provid-ing a safe environment for patients with latex allergy is the responsibility of all health care professionals (Baumann, 1999).

Client/Family Teaching

• Provide written information about latex allergy and sensitivity.
   Education of the public is necessary and has been provided by the development of a latex allergy pamphlet, which contains an explanation of symptoms and risk factors for latex allergy (Harrau, 1998).

• Instruct clients to inform health care professionals if they have a latex allergy, par-ticularly if they are scheduled for surgery.
   To prevent problems associated with exposure to products containing latex, it is essential that clients with latex allergy are identified (Dakin, Yentis, 1998).

• Teach clients what products contain natural rubber latex and to avoid direct contact with all latex products and foods that trigger allergic reactions.
   Once latex allergy has developed, the client is at risk for anaphylaxis and needs to be in-formed as to what products contain latex (Tarlo, 1998; Department of Health and Human Services, 1999). This allergy is potentially preventable for both the patient and nurse (Gritter, 1999).

• = Independent; ▲ = Collaborative

- Teach client to avoid areas where powdered latex gloves are used, as well as where latex balloons are inflated or deflated.
  Exposure can lead to an anaphylactic reaction (Tarlo, 1998).
- Instruct clients with latex allergy to wear a Medic-Alert bracelet that identifies them as such.
  Identification of clients with latex allergy is critical for preventing problems and for early intervention with appropriate treatment if an exposure occurs (Kelly, Walsh-Kelly, 1998).
- ▲ Instruct client to carry an autoinjectable epinephrine syringe if at risk for anaphylactic episode.
  An autoinjectable epinephrine syringe should be prescribed to sensitized clients who are at risk for an anaphylactic episode with accidental latex exposure (Tarlo, 1998).

WEB SITES FOR EDUCATION

Merlin See the MERLIN web site for World Wide Web resources for client education.

REFERENCES   Baumann NH: Latex allergy: an orthopaedic case presentation and considerations in patient care, *Orthop Nurs* 18(3):15-20, 1999.

Charous BL, Schuenemann PJ, Swanson MC: Passive dispersion of latex aeroallergen in a health care facility, *Ann Allergy Asthma Immunol* 85(4):285-290, 2000.

Dakin J, Yentis S: Latex allergy: a strategy for management, *Anesthesia* 53:774-781, 1998.

Department of Health and Human Services: (NIOSH) Publication No 97-135, retrieved February 6, 1999, from the World Wide Web. Web site: www.cdc.gov/niosh/latexalt.html.

Evangelisto M: Making the choice: can you go 'latex free'? *Todays Surg Nurse* 20(1):40-44, 1998.

Floyd PT: Latex allergy update, *J Perianesth Nurs* 15(1):26-30, 2000.

Gritter M: Latex allergy: prevention is the key, *Intraven Nurs* 22(5), 1999.

Harrau B: Managing latex allergy patients, *Nurs Manage* 29(10):48N, 48P, 1998.

Kantor G, Smith M, Kalhan S: Cleveland Clinic Foundation management of latex-allergic patients—the five principles, retrieved February 6, 1999, from the World Wide Web. Web site: www.anes.ccf.org:8080/pilot/latex/5MINUTE.HTM.

Kelly K, Walsh-Kelly C: Latex allergy: a patient and health care system emergency, *Ann Emerg Med* 32:725, 1998.

Nielsen PS et al: Assessment of IgE allergen specificity among latex-allergic health care workers: review of IgE-binding components of various latex extracts, *Ann Allergy Asthma Immunol* 85(6 Pt 1), 2000.

Sanchez-Monge R et al: Class I chitinases, the panallergens responsible for the latex-fruit syndrome, are induced by ethylene treatment and inactivated by heating, *J Allergy Clin Immunol* 106(1 Pt 1), 2000.

Tarlo S: Latex allergy: a problem for both health care professionals and patients, *Ostomy Wound Manage* 44(8):80-88 (discussion pp 81-83), 1998.

Risk for latex Allergy response

Gail B. Ladwig

NANDA   **Definition** At risk for allergic response to natural latex rubber products

Risk Factors

Multiple surgical procedures, especially from infancy (e.g., spina bifida); allergies to bananas, avocados, tropical fruits, kiwis, chestnuts; professions with daily exposure to

• = Independent; ▲ = Collaborative

latex (e.g., medicine, nursing, dentistry); conditions needing continuous or intermittent catheterization; history of reactions to latex (e.g., balloons, condoms, gloves); allergies to poinsettia plants; history of allergies and asthma

NOC **Outcomes (Nursing Outcomes Classification)**

Suggested NOC Labels

Immune Hypersensitivity Control; Knowledge: Health Behaviors; Risk Control; Risk Detection; Tissue Integrity: Skin and Mucous Membranes

> **Example NOC Outcome**
>
> Demonstrates **Immune Hypersensitivity Control,** as evidenced by the following indicators: Respiratory, cardiac, gastrointestinal, renal and neurological function status IER*/Free of allergic reactions (Rate each indicator of **Immune Hypersensitivity Control:** 1 = not controlled, 2 = slightly controlled, 3 = moderately controlled, 4 = well controlled, 5 = very well controlled [see Section I])

*In Expected Range

Client Outcomes

- States risk factors for latex allergy
- Requests latex-free environment
- Demonstrates knowledge of plan to treat latex allergic reaction

NIC **Interventions (Nursing Interventions Classification)**

Suggested NIC Labels

Allergy Management; Latex Precautions

> **Example NIC Interventions—Latex Precautions**
> - Question client or appropriate other about history of systemic reaction to natural rubber latex (e.g., facial or scleral edema, tearing eyes, urticaria, rhinitis, and wheezing)
> - Place an allergy band on client

Nursing Interventions and Rationales

- Clients at high risk need to be identified, such as those with exposure to frequent bladder catheterizations, occupational exposure to latex, past history of atopy (hayfever, asthma, dermatitis, or food allergy to fruits such as bananas, avocados, papaya, chestnut, or kiwi); those with a history of anaphylaxis of uncertain etiology, especially if associated with surgery; health care workers; and females exposed to barrier contraceptives and routine examinations during gynecological and obstetric procedures.
  Health care professionals, hospital patients, and rubber industry workers have noted a marked increase in allergic reactions to natural rubber latex in the last 10 years (Puopolo, Stephens, 2000). Recent studies have shown that allergy to natural rubber latex is significantly associated with hypersensitivity to certain foods, including avocados, chestnuts, papayas, kiwis, and bananas (Chen et al, 1998). A latex-directed history is the primary method of identifying latex sensitivity, although both skin and serum testing are available and are increasingly accurate (Birmingham, Suresh, 1999).
- ▲ Clients with spina bifida are a high-risk group for latex allergy and should remain latex-free from the first day of life.

• = Independent; ▲ = Collaborative

Results indicate that an atopic disposition, a large number of operations, and the presence of a shunt system increase the risk of becoming not only sensitized but also allergic to latex (Niggemann et al, 1998).

- Children who are on home ventilation should be assessed for latex allergy.
  This study showed a high incidence of latex allergy in children on home ventilation. All children on home ventilation should be screened for latex allergy to prevent untoward reactions from exposure to latex (Nakamura, Ferdman, Keens, Davidson-Ward, 2000).
- Assess for latex allergy in workers who are exposed to the use of "natural" cosmetics in the work setting.
  History of a woman who had eight episodes of angioedema over 2 years: precipitating events included wearing starch powdered natural rubber latex gloves, eating a banana, and packaging banana hair conditioner on a production line of a company manufacturing a range of "natural" cosmetics (Smith, Wakelin, White, 1998).
- See care plan for **Latex Allergy response.**

Home Care Interventions

- ▲ Ensure that client has medical plan if response develops.
  Prompt treatment decreases potential severity of response.
- See care plan for **Latex Allergy response.** Note client history and environmental assessment.

Client/Family Teaching

- ▲ Clients who have had symptoms of latex allergy or who suspect they are allergic to latex should tell their employer and contact their institution's occupational health services.
  Occupational health services can arrange testing by an allergist. If an allergy is present, measures to protect the client's well-being in the workplace should be instituted (Sibbald, Fryer, 1998).
- ▲ Provide written information about latex allergy and sensitivity.
  Education of the public is necessary and has been provided by the development of a latex allergy pamphlet, which contains an explanation of symptoms and risk factors for latex allergy (Harrau, 1998).
- If the client has a suspected allergy to foods associated with latex allergy, instruct the patient to heat the suspected foods.
  The allergenic activity of plant class I chitinases seems to be lost by heating (Sanchez-Monge et al, 2000).
- Health care workers should avoid the use of latex gloves and seek an alternative glove such as one made from nitrile.
  Preliminary reports of primary preventive strategies suggest that avoidance of high-protein, powdered gloves in health care facilities can be cost-effective and is associated with a decline in sensitized workers (Tarlo, 2001). Nitrile examination gloves offer better protection than latex types when handling lipid-soluble substances and chemicals (Russell-Fell, 2000).

REFERENCES   Birmingham PK, Suresh S: Latex allergy in children: diagnosis and management, *Indian J Pediatr* 66(5):717-724, 1999.
Chen Z et al: Identification of hevein (Hev b 6.02) in Hevea latex as a major cross-reacting allergen with avocado fruit in patients with latex allergy, *J Allergy Clin Immunol* 102(3):351-352, 1998.
Harrau B: Managing latex allergy patients, *Nurs Manage* 29(10):48N, 48P, 1998.

• = Independent; ▲ = Collaborative

Nakamura CT et al: Latex allergy in children on home ventilation, *Chest* 118(4):1000-1003, 2000.

Niggemann B, et al: Latex provocation tests in patients with spina bifida: who is at risk of becoming symptomatic? *J Allergy Clin Immunol* 102(4 part 1):665-670, 1998.

Puopolo R, Stephens A: Tackling latex allergy with a product database, *Can Nurse* 96(4):25-28, 2000.

Russell-Fell RW: Avoiding problems: evidence-based selection of medical gloves, *Br J Nurs* 9(3):144-146, 2000.

Sanchez-Monge R et al: Class I chitinases, the panallergens responsible for the latex-fruit syndrome, are induced by ethylene treatment and inactivated by heating, *J Allergy Clin Immunol* 106(1 Pt 1):190-195, 2000.

Sibbald R, Fryer P: Latex allergy, an institutional approach, questionnaire and information for health care workers, *Ostomy Wound Manage* 44(9):88-91, 1998.

Smith H, Wakelin S, White I: Banana hair conditioner and natural rubber latex allergy, *Contact Dermatitis* 39:202, 1998.

Tarlo SM: Natural rubber latex allergy and asthma, *Curr Opin Pulm Med* 7(1), 2001.

Anxiety

Pam B. Schweitzer and Gail B. Ladwig

NANDA   **Definition**   A vague, uneasy feeling of discomfort or dread accompanied by an autonomic response, with the source often nonspecific or unknown to the individual; a feeling of apprehension caused by anticipation of danger. Anxiety is an altering signal that warns of impending danger and enables the individual to take measures to deal with threat.

Defining Characteristics

Behavioral   Diminished productivity; scanning and vigilance; poor eye contact; restlessness; glancing about; extraneous movement (e.g., foot shuffling, hand/arm movements); expressed concerns resulting from change in life events; insomnia; fidgeting

Affective   Regretful; irritability; anguish; scared; jittery; overexcited; painful and persistent increased helplessness; rattled; uncertainty; increased wariness; focus on self; feelings of inadequacy; fearful; distressed; apprehension; anxious

Physiological   Voice quivering

Objective   Trembling/hand tremors; insomnia

Subjective   Shakiness; worried; regretful

Physiological-sympathetic

Increased pulse; increased blood pressure; increased tension; cardiovascular excitation; heart pounding; superficial vasoconstriction; respiratory difficulties; increased respiration; increased perspiration; facial flushing; facial tension; pupil dilation; anorexia; dry mouth; weakness; increased reflexes; twitching

Physiological-parasympathetic

Decreased pulse; decreased blood pressure; abdominal pain; nausea; diarrhea; urinary urgency; urinary hesitancy; urinary frequency; tingling in extremities; fatigue; faintness; sleep disturbance

Cognitive   Blocking of thoughts; confusion; preoccupation; forgetfulness; rumination; impaired attention; decreased perceptual field; fear of nonspecific consequences; tendency to blame others; difficulty concentrating; diminished ability to problem solve; diminished learning ability; awareness of physiological symptoms

• = Independent; ▲ = Collaborative

Related Factors (r/t)

Unconscious conflict regarding essential values or life goals; threat to self-concept; threat of death; threat to or change in health status, environment, interaction patterns; situational or maturational crises; interpersonal transmission of contagion; unmet needs

NOC   Outcomes (Nursing Outcomes Classification)

Suggested NOC Labels

Anxiety Control; Aggression Control; Coping; Impulse Control

> **Example NOC Outcome**
> Demonstrates **Anxiety Control** as evidenced by the following indicators: Eliminates precursors of anxiety/Reports absence of physical manifestations of anxiety/Controls anxiety response (Rate each indicator of **Anxiety Control:** 1 = never demonstrated, 2 = rarely demonstrated, 3 = sometimes demonstrated, 4 = often demonstrated, 5 = consistently demonstrated [see Section I])

Client Outcomes

- Identifies and verbalizes symptoms of anxiety
- Identifies, verbalizes, and demonstrates techniques to control anxiety
- Verbalizes absence of or decrease in subjective distress
- Has vital signs that reflect baseline or decreased sympathetic stimulation
- Has posture, facial expressions, gestures, and activity levels that reflect decreased distress
- Demonstrates improved concentration and accuracy of thoughts
- Identifies and verbalizes anxiety precipitants, conflicts, and threats
- Demonstrates return of basic problem-solving skills
- Demonstrates increased external focus
- Demonstrates some ability to reassure self

NIC   Interventions (Nursing Interventions Classification)

Suggested NIC Labels

Anxiety Reduction

> **Example NIC Interventions—Anxiety Reduction**
> - Use a calm, reassuring approach
> - Explain all procedures, including sensations likely to be experienced

Nursing Interventions and Rationales

- Assess client's level of anxiety and physical reactions to anxiety (e.g., tachycardia, tachypnea, nonverbal expressions of anxiety). Validate observations by asking client, "Are you feeling anxious now?"
  Anxiety is a highly individualized, normal physical and psychological response to internal or external life events (Badger, 1994).
- Use presence, touch (with permission), verbalization, and demeanor to remind clients that they are not alone and to encourage expression or clarification of needs, concerns, unknowns, and questions.
  Being supportive and approachable encourages communication (Olson, Sneed, 1995).
- Accept client's defenses; do not confront, argue, or debate.
  If defenses are not threatened, the client may feel safe enough to look at behavior (Rose, Conn, Rodeman, 1994).

• = Independent; ▲ = Collaborative

- Allow and reinforce client's personal reaction to or expression of pain, discomfort, or threats to well-being (e.g., talking, crying, walking, other physical or nonverbal expressions).
  Talking or otherwise expressing feelings sometimes reduces anxiety (Johnson, 1972).
- Help client identify precipitants of anxiety that may indicate interventions.
  Gaining insight enables the client to reevaluate the threat or identify new ways to deal with it (Damrosch, 1991).
- If the situational response is rational, use empathy to encourage client to interpret the anxiety symptoms as normal.
  Anxiety is a normal response to actual or perceived danger (Peplau, 1963).
- If irrational thoughts or fears are present, offer client accurate information and encourage him or her to talk about the meaning of the events contributing to the anxiety.
  This study shows that during diagnosis and management of cancer, highlighting the importance of the meaning of events to an individual is an important factor in helping clients to identify what makes them anxious. Acknowledgment of this meaning may help to reduce anxiety (Stark, House, 2000).
- Encourage the client to use positive self-talk such as "Anxiety won't kill me," "I can do this one step at a time," "Right now I need to breathe and stretch," "I don't have to be perfect."
  Cognitive therapies focus on changing behaviors and feelings by changing thoughts. Replacing negative self-statements with positive self-statements helps to decrease anxiety (Fishel, 1998).
- Avoid excessive reassurance; this may reinforce undue worry.
  Reassurance is not helpful for the anxious individual (Garvin, Huston, Baker, 1992).
- Intervene when possible to remove sources of anxiety.
  Anxiety is a normal response to actual or perceived danger; if the threat is removed, the response will stop.
- Explain all activities, procedures, and issues that involve the client; use nonmedical terms and calm, slow speech. Do this in advance of procedures when possible, and validate client's understanding.
  With preadmission patient education, patients experience less anxiety and emotional distress and have increased coping skills because they know what to expect (Review, 2000). Uncertainty and lack of predictability contribute to anxiety (Garvin, Huston, Baker, 1992).
- Explore coping skills previously used by client to relieve anxiety; reinforce these skills and explore other outlets.
  Methods of coping with anxiety that have been successful in the past are likely to be helpful again. Listening to clients and helping them to sort through their fears and expectations encourages them to take charge of their lives (Fishel, 1998).
- Provide backrubs for clients to decrease anxiety.
  In one study the dependent variable, anxiety, was measured prior to back massage, immediately following, and 10 minutes later on four consecutive evenings. There was a statistically significant difference in the mean anxiety (STAI) score between the back massage group and the no intervention group (Fraser, Kerr, 1993). In a discussion of the results of a systematic review of 22 articles examining the effect of massage on relaxation, comfort, and sleep, the most consistent effect of massage was reduction in anxiety. Out of 10 original research studies, 8 reported that massage significantly decreased anxiety or perception of tension (Richards, Gibson, Overton-McCoy, 2000).

• = Independent; ▲ = Collaborative

- Provide massage before procedures to decrease anxiety.

  In one study parents performed massage on their hospitalized preschoolers and school-age children before venous puncture. The results obtained indicate that massage had a significant effect on nonverbal reactions, especially those related to muscular relaxation (Garcia, Horta, Farias, 1997).

- Use therapeutic touch and healing touch techniques.

  Various techniques that involve intention to heal, laying on of hands, clearing the energy field surrounding the body, and transfer of healing energy from the environment through the healer to the subject can reduce anxiety (Fishel, 1998). In a recent study, anxiety was significantly reduced in a therapeutic touch placebo condition. Healing touch may be one of the most useful nursing interventions available to reduce anxiety (Gagne, Toye in Fishel, 1998).

- Provide clients with a means to listen to music of their choice. Provide a quiet place and encourage clients to listen for 20 minutes.

  Music is a simple, inexpensive, esthetically pleasing means of alleviating anxiety. When allowed to participate in decision-making regarding their care, patients can regain a partial sense of control. As patient advocates, nurses should take advantage of the therapeutic effect of music by incorporating it into their plan of care (Evans, Rubio, 1994). Immediately and 1 hour after listening to music for 20 minutes in a quiet environment, reductions in heart rate, respiratory rate, and myocardial oxygen demand were significantly greater in the experimental group of patients with myocardial infarction than in the control group (White, 1999).

- For the client experiencing preoperative anxiety, provide music of their choice for listening.

  A study indicates that music combined with preoperative instruction can be more beneficial than preoperative instruction alone for reducing the anxiety of ambulatory surgery patients. Patients who listened to their choice of music before surgery in addition to receiving preoperative instruction had significantly lower heart rates than patients in the control group who received only preoperative instruction (Augustin, Hains, 1996).

- Animal-assisted therapy (AAT) can be incorporated into the care of perioperative patients.

  A study of perioperative clients has shown that interacting with animals reduces blood pressure and cholesterol, decreases anxiety, and improves a person's sense of well-being (Miller, Ingram, 2000).

- Rule out withdrawal from alcohol, sedatives, or smoking as the cause of anxiety.

  Withdrawal from these substances is characterized by anxiety (Badger, 1994).

- Identify and limit, discontinue, or be aware of the use of any stimulants such as caffeine, nicotine, theophylline, terbutaline sulfate, amphetamines, and cocaine.

  Many substances cause or potentiate anxiety symptoms.

Geriatric

- ▲ Monitor client for depression. Use appropriate interventions and referrals.

  Anxiety often accompanies or masks depression in elderly adults.

- Provide a protective and safe environment. Use consistent caregivers and maintain the accustomed environmental structure.

  Elderly clients tend to have more perceptual impairments and adapt to changes with more difficulty than younger clients, especially during illness (Halm, Alpen, 1993).

- ▲ Observe for adverse changes if antianxiety drugs are taken.

  Age renders clients more sensitive to both the clinical and toxic effects of many agents.

• = Independent; ▲ = Collaborative

- Provide a quiet environment with diversion.
  Excessive noise increases anxiety; involvement in a quiet activity can be soothing to the elderly.

Multicultural

- Assess for the presence of culture-bound anxiety states.
  The context in which anxiety is experienced, its meaning, and responses to it are culturally mediated. The following culture-bound syndromes are related to anxiety: Susto—Latin America, Nervios—Latin America, Dhat—Asia, Koro—Southeast Asia, Kayak angst—Eskimo, Taijin kyousho—Japan, Nervous breakdown—African Americans (Kavanagh, 1999; Charron, 1998).
- Assess for the influence of cultural beliefs, norms, and values on the client's perspective of a stressful situation.
  What the client considers stressful may be based on cultural perceptions (Leininger, 1996).
- In the culturally diverse client identify how anxiety is manifested.
  Anxiety is manifested differently from culture to culture through cognitive to somatic symptoms (Charron, 1998).
- Acknowledge that value conflicts from acculturation stresses may contribute to increased anxiety.
  Challenges to traditional beliefs and values are anxiety provoking (Charron, 1998).

Client/Family Teaching

- Teach client and family the symptoms of anxiety.
  If client and family can identify anxious responses, they can intervene earlier than otherwise (Reider, 1994). Information is empowering and reduces anxiety (Fishel, 1998).
- Because intensive care unit (ICU) stays are increasingly shorter, provide *written* teaching information that is readily available to clients when they are transferred out.
  Time constraints have become a barrier to effective teaching. A pamphlet (available in Spanish and English) has been developed to ease the move for patients, families, and critical care and medical nurses from a medical ICU (MICU) to a general floor. Reading this pamphlet has helped to reduce symptoms of anxiety (Maillet, Pata, Grossman, 1993).
- Help client to define anxiety levels (from "easily tolerated" to "intolerable") and select appropriate interventions.
  Mild anxiety enhances learning and adaptation, but moderate to severe anxiety may impede or immobilize progress (Peplau, 1963).
- ▲ Consider referral for the prescription of antianxiety medications for clients who have panic disorder (PD) associated with anxiety.
  PD may be treated with drugs, psychosocial intervention, or both. In a recent study, the combination of imipramine and cognitive-behavioral therapy appeared to confer limited advantage acutely but more substantial advantage by the end of maintenance (Barlow et al, 2000).
- Teach client techniques to self-manage anxiety.
  Mental health interventions during hospitalization should emphasize teaching patients to manage their own anxiety instead of directly intervening to reduce current levels of anxiety (Rose, Conn, Rodeman, 1994).
- Teach client to identify and use distraction or diversion tactics when possible.
  Early interruption of the anxious response prevents escalation.
- Teach client to allow anxious thoughts and feelings to be present until they dissipate.
  Allowing and even devoting time and energy to a thought, purposefully and repetitively, reduces associated anxiety (Beck, Emery, 1985).

• = Independent; ▲ = Collaborative

- Teach progressive muscle relaxation techniques.
  In one study, a significant reduction in anxiety level was obtained by using progressive muscle relaxation interventions (Weber, 1996).
- Teach relaxation breathing for occasional use: client should breathe in through nose, fill slowly from abdomen upward while thinking "re," and then breathe out through mouth, from chest downward, and think "lax."
  Anxiety management training effectively treats both specific and generalized anxiety (Fishel, 1998).
- Teach client to visualize or fantasize about the absence of anxiety or pain, successful experience of the situation, resolution of conflict, or outcome of procedure.
  Use of guided imagery has been useful for reducing anxiety (Weber, 1996).
- Teach relationship between a healthy physical and emotional lifestyle and a realistic mental attitude.
  Health and well-being are influenced by how well-defined and met needs are in areas of safety, diet, exercise, sleep, work, pleasure, and social belonging. Exercise is an excellent means of decreasing anxiety (Fishel, 1998). Results of cross-sectional and longitudinal studies seem to indicate that aerobic exercise training has antidepressant and anxiolytic effects and protects against harmful consequences of stress (Salmon, 2001).
- ▲ Teach use of appropriate community resources in emergency situations (e.g., suicidal thoughts), such as hotlines, emergency rooms, law enforcement, and judicial systems.
  The method of suicide prevention found to be most effective is a systematic, direct-screening procedure that has a high potential for institutionalization (Shaffer, Craft, 1999).
- ▲ Encourage use of appropriate community resources: family, friends, neighbors, self-help and support groups, volunteer agencies, churches, clubs and centers for recreation, and other persons with similar interests.
  One of the most reassuring elements of care includes access to the family (Fishel, 1998). Vicarious experience provided through dyadic support is effective in helping patients undergoing cardiac surgery to cope with surgical anxiety and in improving self-efficacy expectations and self-reported activity after surgery (Parent, Fortin, 2000).
- Provide family members with information to help them to distinguish between a panic attack and serious physical illness symptoms. Instruct family members to consult a health care professional if they have questions.
  Education on managing anxiety disorders must include family members because they are the ones usually called upon to take the client for emergency care. Family members can be expert informants because of their familiarity with the client's history and symptoms (Fishel, 1998).

WEB SITES FOR EDUCATION

MERLIN See the MERLIN web site for World Wide Web resources for client education.

REFERENCES   Augustin P, Hains AA: Effect of music on ambulatory surgery patients' preoperative anxiety, *AORN J* 63(4):750, 753-758, 1996.

Badger JM: Calming the anxious patient, *Am J Nurs* 94:46, 1994.

Barlow DH et al: Cognitive-behavioral therapy, imipramine, or their combination for panic disorder: a randomized controlled trial, *JAMA* 283(19):2529-2936, 2000.

Beck AT, Emery G: *Anxiety disorders and phobias: a cognitive perspective,* New York, 1985, Basic Books.

Charron HS: Anxiety disorders. In Varcarolis EM, editor: *Foundations of psychiatric mental health nursing,* ed 3, Philadelphia, 1998, WB Saunders.

• = Independent; ▲ = Collaborative

Damrosch S: General strategies for motivating people to change their behavior, *Nurs Clin North Am* 26:833, 1991.

Evans MM, Rubio PA: Music: a diversionary therapy, *Todays OR Nurse* 16(4):17-22, 1994.

Fishel A: Nursing management of anxiety and panic, *Nurs Clin North Am* 33(1):135-149, 1998.

Fraser J, Kerr JR: Psychophysiological effects of back massage on elderly institutionalized patients, *J Adv Nurs* 18(2):238-245, 1993.

Gagne D, Toye FC, in Fishel A: Nursing management of anxiety and panic, *Nurs Clin North Am* 33(1):135-149, 1998.

Garcia RM, Horta AL, Farias F: The effect of massage before venipuncture on the reaction of pre-school and school children, *Rev Esc Enferm USP* 31(1):119-128, 1997.

Garvin BJ, Huston GP, Baker CF: Information used by nurses to prepare patients for a stressful event, *Appl Nurs Res* 5:158, 1992.

Halm MA, Alpen MA: The impact of technology on patients and families, *Nurs Clin North Am* 28:443, 1993.

Johnson J: Effects of structuring patients' expectations on their reactions to threatening events, *Nurs Res* 21(6):499-504, 1972.

Kavanagh KH: The role of cultural diversity in mental health nursing. In Fontaine KL, Fletcher JS, editors: *Mental health nursing,* ed 4, Menlo Park, Calif, 1999, Addison Wesley.

Leininger MM: *Transcultural nursing: theories, research and practices,* ed 2, Hilliard, Ohio, 1996, McGraw-Hill.

Maillet RJ, Pata I, Grossman S: A strategy for decreasing anxiety of ICU transfer patients and their families, *Nurs Connect* 6(4):5-8, 1993.

Miller J, Ingram L: Perioperative nursing and animal-assisted therapy, *AORN J* 72(3):477-483, 2000.

Olson M, Sneed N: Anxiety and therapeutic touch, *Issues Mental Health Nurs* 16:97, 1995.

Parent N, Fortin F: A randomized, controlled trial of vicarious experience through peer support for male first-time cardiac surgery patients: impact on anxiety, self-efficacy expectation, and self-reported activity, *Heart Lung* 29(6):389-400, 2000.

Peplau H: A working definition of anxiety. In Burd S, Marshall M, editors: *Some clinical approaches to psychiatric nursing,* New York, 1963, Macmillan.

Reider JA: Anxiety during critical illness of a family member, *Dimen Crit Care Nurs* 13:272, 1994.

Review: A practical guide to improving patient outcomes, *Orthop Nurs* 19(suppl):22-28, 2000.

Richards KC, Gibson R, Overton-McCoy AL: Effects of massage in acute and critical care, *AACN Clin Issues,* 11(1):77-96, 2000.

Rose SK, Conn VS, Rodeman BJ: Anxiety and self-care following myocardial infarction, *Issues Ment Health Nurs* 15(4):433-443, 1994.

Salmon P: Effects of physical exercise on anxiety, depression, and sensitivity to stress: a unifying theory, *Clin Psychol Rev* 21(1):33-61, 2001.

Shaffer D, Craft L: Methods of adolescent suicide prevention, *J Clin Psychiatry* 60(suppl 2):70-74, 1999; discussion 60(suppl 2):75-76, 113-116, 1999.

Stark DP, House A: Anxiety in cancer patients, *Br J Cancer* 83(10):1261-1267, 2000.

Weber S: The effects of relaxation exercises on anxiety levels in psychiatric inpatients, *J Holist Nurs* 14(3):196-205, 1996.

White J: Effects of relaxing music on cardiac autonomic balance and anxiety after acute myocardial infarction, *Am J Crit Care* 8(4):220-230, 1999.

Death Anxiety

Gail B. Ladwig

NANDA **Definition** The apprehensions, worry, or fear related to death or dying

Defining Characteristics

Worrying about impact of one's own death on significant others; powerless over issues related to dying; fear of loss of physical and/or mental abilities when dying; anticipated

• = **Independent;** ▲ = **Collaborative**

pain related to dying; deep sadness; fear of process of dying; concerns of overworking caregiver as terminal illness incapacitates self; concern about meeting one's creator or feeling doubtful about existence of God or higher being; total loss of control over any aspect of one's own death; negative death images or unpleasant thoughts about any event related to death or dying; fear of delayed demise; fear of premature death because it prevents accomplishment of important life goals; worrying about being the cause of others' grief and suffering; fear of leaving family alone after death; fear of developing a terminal illness; denial of one's own mortality or impending death

Related Factors (r/t)

To be developed—refer to Defining Characteristics

NOC   Outcomes (Nursing Outcomes Classification)

Suggested NOC Labels

Dignified Dying; Fear Control; Health Beliefs: Perceived Threat

Example NOC Outcome

Demonstrates **Dignified Dying** as evidenced by the following indicators: Expresses readiness for death/Resolves important issues and concerns/Shares feelings about dying/Discusses spiritual concerns (Rate each indicator of **Dignified Dying**: 1 = not at all, 2 = slightly, 3 = moderately, 4 = substantially, 5 = extensively [see Section I])

Client Outcomes

- State concerns about impact of death on others
- Expresses feelings associated with dying
- Seeks help in dealing with feelings
- Discusses concerns about God or higher being
- Discusses realistic goals
- Uses prayer or other religious practice for comfort

NIC   Interventions (Nursing Interventions Classification)

Suggested NIC Labels

Dying Care; Spiritual Support; Grief Work Facilitation

Example NIC Interventions—Dying Care

- Communicate willingness to discuss death
- Support client and family through stages of grief

Nursing Interventions and Rationales

- Assess the psychosocial maturity of the individual. Erikson's scale of task accomplishment may be used.
  A study using the framework of Erikson indicates that the higher the ego integrity, the lower the death anxiety (Fishman, 1992). As psychosocial maturity and age increase, death anxiety decreases. Findings have shown that psychosocial maturity is a better predictor of death anxiety than age (Rasmussen, Brems, 1996).
- Assist clients to identify with their culture and its values.
  The process of identification with one's culture is identified as a coping mechanism that may protect the individual from increased death anxiety (Tomer, Eliason, 1996).

• = Independent; ▲ = Collaborative

- Assess clients for pain and provide pain relief measures.
  Over a 14-month period, telephone interviews were conducted with 475 family infor-mants who had been involved in caring for a patient in the last month of life. Barriers to optimal care of the dying remain, despite a generally positive overall profile. These barriers include level of pain and management of pain (Tolle et al, 2000).
- Assist clients with life planning: consider and redefine main life goals, focus on areas of strength and/or goals that will provide satisfaction, adopt realistic goals and recognize those that are impossible to achieve.
  Life planning processes affect self-esteem and self-concept. By changing unrealistic goals, the individual may be able to reduce the amount of future-related regret that the prospect of a not-too-distant death may produce (Tomer, Eliason, 1996).
- Assist clients with life review and reminiscence.
  Life reviewing can foster the integration of past conflicts. It can improve ego integrity and life satisfaction, lower depression, and reduce stress (Tomer, Eliason, 1996).
- Provide music of a client's choosing.
  Music therapy is a nonpharmacological nursing intervention that may be used to promote relaxation (Chlan, 2000).
- Provide social support for families receiving CPR training to save the life of a family member at risk for sudden death.
  Findings support tailoring family CPR training so that instruction does not result in negative psychological states in patients. The findings also illustrate the efficacy of a simple intervention that combines CPR training with social support (Dracup et al, 1997).
- Encourage clients to pray.
  Participants in one study stated their belief that God listened to their prayers and an-swered them when they were seeking comfort. It was this reassurance that gave them the strength to face uncertainty and possible death (Hawley, Irurita, 1998).

Geriatric

- Carefully assess older adults for issues regarding death anxiety.
  Results from literature review indicate that lower ego integrity, more physical problems, and more psychological problems are predictive of higher levels of death anxiety in elderly people (Fortner, Neimeyer, 1999).
- Provide back massage for clients who have anxiety regarding issues such as death.
  Back massage used on elderly residents in a long-term care facility reduced anxiety levels (Fraser, Kerr, 1993).
  Refer to care plan **Anticipatory Grieving.**

Home Care Interventions

- Identify times and places when anxiety is greatest. Provide for psychological support at those times using such strategies as personal contact, telephone contact, diversion-ary activities, or therapeutic self.
  Anxiety may be related to earlier events associated with home setting or daily patterns that created pain and now serve as triggers.
- Support religious beliefs; encourage client to participate in services and activities of choice.
  Belief in a supreme being/higher power provides a feeling of ever-present help.
- ▲ Refer to medical social services or mental health services, including support groups as ap-propriate (e.g., anticipatory grieving groups from hospice, visiting volunteers of hospice).
  Referral to specialty groups may be a key part of the nursing plan.

• = **Independent;** ▲ = **Collaborative**

- Encourage client to verbalize feelings to family/caregivers, counselors, and self.
  Expression of feelings relieves fear burden and allows examination and validation of feelings.
- Assist client in making contact with death-related planning organizations, if appropriate, such as the Cremation Society and funeral homes.
  Planning and direct action (contracting for after-death care) often relieves anxiety and provides the client with a measure of control.
- With client, create a memento book reflecting life achievements. Leave in home for regular review by client.
- With client/caregivers, establish realistic life goals for anticipated lifespan of self or others. Create manageable, tangible steps that client can refer to and use to measure activity.
  Memento books and written life goals are tangible milestones related to life and death. They provide comfort, reassurance, hope, and direction for the client and more definition for client/caregiver expectations.

Client/Family Teaching

- Promote more effective communication to family members engaged in the caregiving role. Encourage them to talk to their loved one about areas of concern.
  One study investigated both the content and avoidance of communication between 84 spousal and filial caregivers and care receivers. The study findings indicate that both caregivers and care receivers avoid discussing issues of concern. Nurses working with families are well placed to promote more effective communication (Edwards, Forster, 1999).
- Allow family members to be physically close to their dying loved one, giving them permission, instruction, and opportunities to touch. Keep family members informed.
  Tertiary care centers are criticized for not providing a peaceful death experience. A qualitative study was undertaken to ascertain suggestions family members (N = 29) (Pierce, 1999). The suggestions mentioned came out of this study.
- To increase clients' knowledge about end-of-life issues, teach them and their family members about options for care such as advance directives.
  A survey of 1000 patients suggests that greater public knowledge about end-of-life care is needed, and advance care planning must be preceded by education about options (Silveira et al, 2000).

WEB SITES FOR EDUCATION

MERLIN See the MERLIN web site for World Wide Web resources for client education.

REFERENCES   Chlan LL: Music therapy as a nursing intervention for patients supported by mechanical ventilation, *AACN Clin Issues* 11(1):128-138, 2000.

Dracup K et al: The psychological consequences of cardiopulmonary resuscitation training for family members of patients at risk for sudden death, *Am J Public Health* 87(9):1434-1439, 1997.

Edwards H, Forster E: Avoidance of issues in family care giving, *Contemp Nurse* 8(2):5-13, 1999.

Fishman S: Relationships among an older adult's life review, ego integrity, and death anxiety, *Int Psychogeriatr* 4(suppl 2):267-277, 1992.

Fortner BV, Neimeyer RA: Death anxiety in older adults: a quantitative review, *Death Stud* 23(5):387-411, 1999.

Fraser J, Kerr JR: Psychophysiological effects of back massage on elderly institutionalized patients, *J Adv Nurs* 18(2):238-245, 1993.

• = **Independent**; ▲ = **Collaborative**

Hawley G, Irurita V: Seeking comfort through prayer, *Int J Nurs Pract* 4(1):9-18, 1998.

Pierce SF: Improving end-of-life care: gathering suggestions from family members, *Nurs Forum* 34(2):5-14, 1999.

Rasmussen CA, Brems C: The relationship of death anxiety with age and psychosocial maturity, *J Psychol* 130(2):141-144, 1996.

Silveira MJ et al: Patients' knowledge of options at the end of life: ignorance in the face of death, *JAMA* 284(19):2483-2488, 2000.

Tolle SW et al: Family reports of barriers to optimal care of the dying, *Nurs Res* 49(6):310-317, 2000.

Tomer A, Eliason G: Toward a comprehensive model of death anxiety, *Death Stud* 20:343-365, 1996.

Risk for Aspiration

Betty J. Ackley

Definition   At risk for entry of gastrointestinal secretions, oropharyngeal secretions, solids, or fluids into the tracheobronchial passages

Risk Factors

Increased intragastric pressure; tube feedings; situations hindering elevation of upper body; reduced level of consciousness; presence of tracheostomy or endotracheal tube; medication administration; wired jaws; increased gastric residual; incomplete lower esophageal sphincter; impaired swallowing; gastrointestinal tubes; facial, oral, or neck surgery or trauma; depressed cough and gag reflexes; decreased gastrointestinal motility; delayed gastric emptying

NOC   Outcomes (Nursing Outcomes Classification)

Suggested NOC Labels

Respiratory Status: Ventilation; Aspiration Control; Swallowing Status

> **Example NOC Outcome**
> Maintains **Respiratory Status: Ventilation** as evidenced by the following indicators: Respiratory rate IER*/Moves sputum out of airway/Adventitious breath sounds not present/SOB not present/Auscultated breath sounds IER/Auscultated vocalization IER/Chest x-ray findings IER (Rate each indicator of **Respiratory Status: Ventilation:** 1 = extremely compromised, 2 = substantially compromised, 3 = moderately compromised, 4 = mildly compromised, 5 = not compromised [see Section I])

*In Expected Range

Client Outcomes

- Swallows and digests oral, nasogastric, or gastric feeding without aspiration
- Maintains patent airway and clear lung sounds

NIC   Interventions (Nursing Interventions Classification)

Suggested NIC Labels

Aspiration Precautions

> **Example NIC Interventions—Aspiration Precautions**
> - Monitor level of consciousness, cough reflex, gag reflex, and swallowing ability
> - Check NG or gastrostomy residual before feeding

• = Independent; ▲ = Collaborative

Nursing Interventions and Rationales

- Monitor respiratory rate, depth, and effort. Note any signs of aspiration such as dyspnea, cough, cyanosis, wheezing, or fever.
  Signs of aspiration should be detected as soon as possible to prevent further aspiration and to initiate treatment that can be lifesaving. Because of laryngeal pooling and residue in clients with dysphagia, silent aspiration (i.e., not manifested by choking or coughing) may occur.
- Auscultate lung sounds frequently and before and after feedings; note any new onset of crackles or wheezing.
- Take vital signs q _____ h(rs).
- Before initiating oral feeding, check client's gag reflex and ability to swallow by feeling the laryngeal prominence as the client attempts to swallow.
  It is important to check client's ability to swallow before feeding. A client can aspirate even with an intact gag reflex (Baker, 1993).
- When feeding client, watch for signs of impaired swallowing or aspiration, including coughing, choking, spitting food, or excessive drooling. If client is having problems swallowing, see Nursing Interventions for **Impaired Swallowing.**
- ▲ Have suction machine available when feeding high-risk clients. If aspiration does occur, suction immediately.
  A client with aspiration needs immediate suctioning and will need further lifesaving interventions such as intubation (Fater, 1995).
- Keep head of bed elevated when feeding and for at least a half hour afterward.
  Maintaining a sitting position after meals may help decrease aspiration pneumonia in the elderly (Sasaki et al, 1997).
- ▲ Note presence of any nausea, vomiting, or diarrhea. Treat nausea promptly with antiemetics.
- Listen to bowel sounds qh, noting if they are decreased, absent, or hyperactive.
  Decreased or absent bowel sounds can indicate an ileus with possible vomiting and aspiration; increased high-pitched bowel sounds can indicate mechanical bowel obstruction with possible vomiting and aspiration.
- Note new onset of abdominal distention or increased rigidity of abdomen.
  Abdominal distention or rigidity can be associated with paralytic or mechanical obstruction and an increased likelihood of vomiting and aspiration.
- ▲ If client has a tracheostomy, ask for referral to speech pathologist for swallowing studies before attempting to feed. After evaluation, decision should be made to either have cuff inflated or deflated when client eats.
  The presence of a tracheostomy tube increases the incidence of aspiration (Elpern, Jacobs, Bone, 1993). For some clients, inflating the cuff may help decrease aspiration; for others the inflated cuff will interfere with swallowing. This decision should be made following swallowing studies for the safety of the client's airway (Murray, Brzozowski, 1998).
- Feed client only during formal rest periods from restraints.
- If client shows symptoms of nausea and vomiting, position on side.
- If client needs to be fed, feed slowly and allow adequate time for chewing and swallowing.

Enteral feedings

- ▲ Check to make sure initial feeding tube placement was confirmed by x-ray, especially if a small-bore feeding tube is used. If unable to use x-ray for verification, check the

• = Independent; ▲ = Collaborative

pH of the aspirate. If pH reading is 4 or less, tube is probably in the stomach. Also check bilirubin level of aspirate if possible.

X-ray verification of placement remains the gold standard for determining safe placement of feeding tubes (Metheny et al, 1998; Rakel et al, 1994). Small-bore feeding tubes have been inadvertently placed in the respiratory tract, and clients did not demonstrate any signs of respiratory distress (Metheney et al, 1990a; Fater, 1995). Use of pH and bilirubin measurement has been found to be predictive of correct placement of feeding tubes, both gastric and intestinal. Bilirubin testing is done using urinary bilirubin test strip and a developed visual bilirubin scale (Metheny, Smith, Stewart, 2000).

• Keep nasogastric tube securely taped. Use pink tape to secure the tube.
Use of pink tape as opposed to clear tape or butterfly tape increases the length of time a tube stays taped (Burns et al, 1995).

• Determine placement of feeding tube before each feeding or every 4 hours if client is on continuous feeding. Check pH of aspirate and note characteristic appearance of aspirate; do not rely on air insufflation method.
The auscultatory air insufflation method is often not reliable for differentiating between gastric or respiratory placement (Metheney et al, 1990b). Testing the pH generally predicts feeding tube position in the gastrointestinal tract, especially if combined with identification of appearance of aspirate (Metheny et al, 1993, 1998).

• Check for gastric residual every 4 hours during continuous feedings or before feedings; if residual is >100 ml for gastrostomy feedings or >200 ml for nasogastric tube feedings (McClave et al, 1992), hold feedings following institutional protocol.
Increased intragastric pressure from retained feeding can result in regurgitation and aspiration, but holding feeding unnecessarily can also result in an inadequate caloric intake (Edwards, Metheny, 2000).

▲ If ordered by physician, put several drops of blue or green food coloring in tube feeding to help indicate aspiration. In addition, test the glucose in tracheobronchial secretions to detect aspiration of enteral feedings.
Colored secretions suctioned or coughed from the respiratory tract indicate aspiration (Ackerman, 1993; Fater, 1995). However, this technique is not reliable and use of a multiple-use bottle may result in contamination of feedings and spread bacteria (Fellows et al, 2000). Tracheobronchial secretions that test positive for glucose can indicate aspiration of enteral feedings (Metheny, St John, Clouse, 1998).

• During enteral feedings, position client with head of bed elevated 30 to 40 degrees; maintain for 30 to 45 minutes after feeding.
Keeping client's head elevated helps keep food in stomach and decreases incidence of aspiration (Fater, 1995; Sasaki et al, 1997). A study of mechanically ventilated clients receiving enteral feedings demonstrated a decreased incidence of nosocomial pneumonia if the client was positioned at a 45-degree semirecumbent position as opposed to a supine position (Drakulovic et al, 1999).

• Stop continual feeding temporarily when turning or moving client.
When turning or moving a client, it is difficult to keep the head elevated to prevent regurgitation and possible aspiration.

Geriatric

• Carefully check elderly client's gag reflex and ability to swallow before feeding.
Laryngeal nerve endings are reduced in the elderly, which diminishes the gag reflex (Close, Woodson, 1989).

• = Independent; ▲ = Collaborative

- Watch for signs of aspiration pneumonia in the elderly with cerebrovascular accidents, even if there are no apparent signs of difficulty swallowing or of aspiration. *Bedside evaluation for swallowing and aspiration can be inaccurate; silent aspiration can occur in this population (Smithard et al, 1998).*
- ▲ Use central nervous system depressants cautiously; elderly clients may have an increased incidence of aspiration with altered levels of consciousness. *Elderly clients have altered metabolism, distribution, and excretion of drugs. Some medications can interfere with the swallowing reflex.*

Home Care Interventions

- For clients at high risk for aspiration, obtain complete information from the discharging institution regarding institutional management. *Continuity of care can prevent unnecessary stress for the client and family and can facilitate successful management in the home setting.*
- Assess the client and family for willingness and cognitive ability to learn and cope with swallowing, feeding, and related disorders. *Food and feeding habits may be strongly tied to family cultural values. Acknowledgment and/or adjustment to cultural values can facilitate compliance and successful family coping.*
- Establish emergency and contingency plans for care of client. *Clinical safety of client between visits is a primary goal of home care nursing (Stanhope, Lancaster, 1996).*
- ▲ Have a speech and occupational therapist assess client's swallowing ability and other physiological factors and recommend strategies for working with client in the home (e.g., pureeing foods served to client; providing adaptive equipment for independence in eating). *Successful strategies allow the client to remain part of the family.*
- Assess caregiver understanding and reinforce teaching regarding positioning and assessment of the client for possible aspiration.
- ▲ Obtain suction equipment for the home as necessary.
- ▲ Teach caregivers safe, effective use of suctioning devices. Inform client and family that only individuals instructed in suctioning should perform the procedure.

Client/Family Teaching

- Teach client and family signs of aspiration and precautions to prevent aspiration.
- Teach client and family how to safely administer tube feeding.

WEB SITES FOR EDUCATION

Merlin See the MERLIN web site for World Wide Web resources for client education.

REFERENCES   Ackerman MI: Ask the experts, *Crit Care Nurse* 13:103, 1993.
Baker DM: Assessment and management of impairments in swallowing, *Nurs Clin North Am* 28:793, 1993.
Burns SM et al: Comparison of nasogastric tube securing methods and tube types in medical intensive care patients, *Am J Crit Care* 4:198, 1995.
Close LG, Woodson GE: Common upper airway disorders in the elderly and their management, *Geriatrics* 44:67, 1989.
Drakulovic MB et al: Supine body position as a risk factor for nosocomial pneumonia in mechanically ventilated patients: a randomised trial, *Lancet* 354(9193):1851-1858, 1999.

• = **Independent;** ▲ = **Collaborative**

Edwards SJ, Metheny NA: Measurement of gastric residual volume: state of the science, *MedSurg Nursing* 9(3):125-128, 2000.

Elpern EH, Jacobs ER, Bone RC: Incidence of aspiration in tracheally intubated adults, *Heart Lung* 16:527, 1993.

Fater KH: Determining nasoenteral feeding tube placement, *Medsurg Nurs* 4:27, 1995.

Fellows LS et al: Evidence-based practice for enteral feedings: aspiration prevention strategies, bedside detection, and practice change, *Medsurg Nurs* 9(1):27-31, 2000.

McClave SA et al: Use of residual volume as a marker for enteral feeding intolerance: prospective blinded comparison with physical examination and radiographic findings, *JPEN J Parenter Enteral Nutr* 16(2):99-105, 1992.

Metheny N et al: Detection of inadvertent respiratory placement of small-bore feeding tubes: a report of 10 cases, *Heart Lung* 19(6):631-638, 1990a.

Metheny N et al: Effectiveness of the auscultatory method in predicting feeding tube location, *Nurs Res* 39(5):262-267, 1990b.

Metheny N et al: Effectiveness of pH measurements in predicting feeding tube placement: an update, *Nurs Res* 42(6):324-331, 1993.

Metheny N et al: Visual characteristics of aspirates from feeding tubes as a method for predicting tube location, *Nurs Res* 43(5):282-287, 1994.

Metheny NA, St John RE, Clouse RE: Measurement of glucose in tracheobronchial secretions to detect aspiration of enteral feedings, *Heart Lung* 27(5):285-292, 1998.

Metheny NA, Smith L, Stewart BJ: Development of a reliable and valid bedside test for bilirubin and its utility for improving prediction of feeding tube location. *Nurs Res* 49(6):302-309, 2000.

Metheny NA et al: pH, color and feeding tubes, *RN* 1(1):25-27, 1998.

Murray KA, Brzozowski LA: Swallowing in patients with tracheotomies, *AACN Clin Issues* 9(3):416-426, 1998.

Rakel BA et al: Nasogastric and nasointestinal feeding tube placement: an integrative review of research, *AACN Clin Issues Crit Care Nurs* 5(2):194-206, 1994.

Sasaki H et al: New strategies for aspiration pneumonia, *Intern Med* 36(12):851-855, 1997.

Smithard et al: Can bedside assessment reliably exclude aspiration following acute stroke? *Age Ageing* 27(2):99-106, 1998.

Stanhope M, Lancaster J, editors: *Community health nursing: promoting health of aggregates, families, and individuals,* ed 4, St Louis, 1996, Mosby.

Risk for impaired parent/infant/child Attachment

T. Heather Herdman, Kathy Wyngarden, Mary A. Fuerst-DeWys, and Gail B. Ladwig

 Definition Disruption of the interactive process between parent/significant other and infant/child that fosters the development of a protective and nurturing reciprocal relationship

Risk Factors

Physical barriers; anxiety associated with the parent role; substance abuse; premature infant, ill infant/child who is unable to effectively initiate parental contact as a result of altered behavioral organization; lack of privacy; inability of parents to meet personal needs; separation

NOC   **Outcomes (Nursing Outcomes Classification)**

Suggested NOC Labels

Parent-Infant Attachment; Parenting; Child Development: 2 Months, 4 Months, 6 Months, 12 Months, 2 Years, 3 Years, 4 Years, 5 Years; Caregiver Adaptation to Patient

• = **Independent;** ▲ = **Collaborative**

Institutionalization; Parenting: Social Safety; Safety Behavior: Home Physical Environment; Family Environment: Internal; Coping

> **Example NOC Outcome**
> Demonstrates appropriate **Child Development: 2 Months** as evidenced by: Coos and vocalizes/Shows interest in visual stimuli/Shows interest in auditory stimuli/Smiles/Shows pleasure in interactions, especially with parent(s) (Rate each indicator with regard to delay from expected range: 1 = extreme delay, 2 = substantial delay, 3 = moderate delay, 4 = mild delay, 5 = no delay [see Section I])

Client Outcomes

- Infant/child development appropriate for age
- Parent(s) able to participate in caregiving for infant/child
- Parent(s) visit nursery/hospital unit
- Parent(s) respond to infant/child cues
- Parent(s) eliminate controllable environmental hazards
- Parent(s) use community and other resources as appropriate

NIC   Interventions (Nursing Interventions Classification)

Suggested NIC Labels

Attachment Promotion; Attachment Process; Parent Education: Infant; Developmental Enhancement: Child; Parenting Promotion; Role Enhancement; Coping Enhancement; Developmental Care; Environmental Management: Attachment Process; Family Integrity Promotion

> **Example NIC Interventions—Attachment Promotion**
> - Provide opportunity for parent(s) to see, hold, and examine newborn immediately after birth
> - Demonstrate ways to touch infant confined to isolette
> - Discuss infant behavioral characteristics with parent(s)

Nursing Interventions and Rationales

Family interventions

- Establish a trusting relationship with the parents.
  If trust is established with family members, they are more likely to openly share the real difficulties of integrating therapeutic regimens with family processes (Clemen-Stone, McGuire, Eigsti, 1998).
- Assist parents in recognizing behaviors used by infant/child to communicate avoidance/stress and approach/engagement.
  Understanding infant behaviors gives meaning to these behaviors and provides parents with a guideline for choosing their own behaviors (Oehler, Hannan, Catlett, 1993). Providing nursing interventions that focus on supporting positive appraisal and promoting knowledge of infant crying promotes later adaptive functioning of parents (Elliott, Drummond, Barnard, 1996).
- Support parents' ability to alleviate infant's/child's distress.
  When parents respond quickly to alleviate stress, the child is more likely to calm down than to be spoiled. In this way parents are building a foundation for security and trust. Assist parents in recognizing how their own interactions affect their infant/child (Hedlund, 1986).

• = Independent; ▲ = Collaborative

- If necessary, allow parents to verbalize their fears of "ghosts in the nursery" that may influence attachment to their infant/child.
  Ghosts in the nursery are parents' early memories of painful experiences (e.g., unanswered cries, feeling abandoned, being abused) and are real and powerful. "Hearing a mother's cries" is necessary to help her "hear her child's cries," an important aspect of therapeutic healing (Frailberg, Adelson, Shapiro, 1975).
- Listen to the parents' stories to understand their struggle to attach.
  Acknowledge the parents' point of view and stories as worthy of respect; important truths can be learned, such as what they think and how they feel about themselves and their infant (Trout, 1987). One study indicated that health care providers may recommend storytelling as the central mechanism of interactions in support groups that help participants to cope with daily anxieties of living (Dickerson, Posluszny, Kennedy, 2000).
- Assist parents with recognizing how their infant/child learns through the senses (e.g., visual, auditory, tactile/kinesthetic) and with strategies that can be used, such as timing, intensity, imitation, repetition, to initiate interactions.
  By recognizing infant likes and dislikes based on their behavioral responses to stimuli, parents can generate their own strategies regarding which stimuli are most effective (McCollum, Stayton, 1985).
- Guide parents in adapting to infant/child cues and changing needs.
  Premature infants respond more positively to less intense maternal stimulation (Lozoff et al, 1977).
- Nurture parents so that they in turn can nurture their infant/child.
  Offer a safe, nonjudgmental environment in which parents can express their feelings. If parents are unable to focus on infant, nurse should focus on parents' feelings (Zabielski, 1994). Acknowledge and support the strengths of the infant/child, parent, and family (Goodfriend, 1993).
- Provide child development guidance and peer support.
  The unrealistic expectations of parents regarding infant/child abilities can negatively influence the parent-child relationship. Offer another parent as peer support (Lindsay et al, 1993).
- Attend to both the parents and infant/child in an effort to strengthen the early developing attachment relationship.
  Identifying the infant's/child's strengths and limitations can provide parents with more information regarding how they can encourage optimal growth and development (Denehy, 1992).
- Encourage parents of hospitalized infants to "personalize" their infant by bringing in baby clothes, pictures of themselves, toys, and tapes of their voices.
  These actions help parents claim the infant as their own.
- Encourage skin-to-skin experience for parents and infants as appropriate.
  Parents who participate in bonding and skin-to-skin activities are less likely to reject their infant (Hamelin, Ramachandran, 1993). The mothers studied perceived skin-to-skin contact with their very immature infants as a positive and helpful intervention. Skin-to-skin contact took place regularly and for increasing periods (Bauer, Uhrig, Versmold, 1999).
- Encourage parents and caregivers to massage their infants and children.
  One study demonstrated that massage therapy on infants and children with various medical conditions resulted in lower anxiety and stress hormones and improved clinical

• = Independent; ▲ = Collaborative

course. Having grandparent volunteers and parents provide the therapy enhances their own wellness and provides a cost-effective treatment for the infants/children (Field, 1995).

- Assist parents in developing new caregiving practice competencies and/or revising and extending old ones.
  Caregiving competencies foster a child's development. A caregiving practice is a patterned and customary act of giving care that involves activities addressed to a child's physical, physiological, psychological needs and includes functions concerned with health needs. Five domains of caregiving activities have been identified: (1) being with the baby, (2) knowing the baby as a person, (3) giving care to the baby, (4) communicating and engaging with others about needs (infant and parental), (5) problem solving/decision-making/learning (Pridham et al, 1998).

- Plan ways for parents to interact with/assist with caregiving for their infant/child.
  Research has shown that the most stressful aspect of parental role alteration is the feeling of helplessness in not being able to protect or help the infant/child during hospitalization/institutionalization. Finding ways to help parents feel important as parents and allowing touching/holding as soon as possible are important interventions in strengthening the attachment process (Miles, Funk, Kasper, 1991).

Infant interventions

- Provide lyrical, soothing music in the nursery.
  The results from one study suggest that soothing music may be a feasible intervention to help newborns demonstrate fewer high-arousal states and less state lability (Kaminski, Hall, 1996).

- Protect and enhance infant's interactive capacities through organization of the environment.
  Minimizing meaningless, unpatterned stimuli (noise, light, procedures, etc.) enhances depth and duration of sleep, which allows infants to retain more energy for use during interaction with parents. Well-regulated sleep and wake states contributes to a more satsifying parent-child interaction (Goldson, 1992).

- Provide therapeutic touch for children with anxiety.
  In one study the therapeutic touch (TT) intervention resulted in lower overall mean anxiety scores, whereas the mimic TT did not. These findings provide preliminary support for the use of TT in reducing the anxiety level of children with HIV infection (Ireland, 1998).

Multicultural

- Discuss cultural norms with families in order to provide care that is appropriate for enhancing attachment with the infant/child.
  Misinterpretation of parenting behaviors can occur when the nurse and parent are from different cultures. It is inappropriate to pressure parents to relate to the infant/child in a way that is culturally unacceptable/abnormal for the family (Coffman, 1992). This limits family choice and sets up a tense environment rather than a trusting, supportive one.

- Encourage a reciprocal attachment process.
  Parents who develop a sensitivity to their infant's/child's communication patterns and behavioral cues will respond appropriately to the infant's/child's desire for increased interaction; the infant may then attempt to obtain the parent's attention. This encourages a process of mutual feedback that enhances the attachment process (Goulet et al, 1998).

• = **Independent**; ▲ = **Collaborative**

REFERENCES Bauer K, Uhrig C, Versmold H: How do mothers experience skin contact with their very immature (gestational age 27-30 weeks), only days old premature infants? *Geburtshilfe Neonatol* 203(6), 1999 (article in German).

Clemen-Stone S, McGuire SL, Eigsti DG: *Comprehensive community health nursing: family aggregate and community practice,* ed 5, St Louis, 1998, Mosby.

Coffman S: Parent and infant attachment: review of nursing research 1981-1990, *Pediatr Nurs* 18(4):421-425, 1992.

Denehy J: Interventions related to parent-infant attachment, *Nurs Intervent* 27:425, 1992.

Dickerson SS, Posluszny M, Kennedy MC: Help seeking in a support group for recipients of implantable cardioverter defibrillators and their support persons, *Heart Lung* (2), 2000.

Elliott M, Drummond J, Barnard K: Subjective appraisal of infant crying, *Clin Nurs Res* 5(2):37-50, 1996.

Field T: Massage therapy for infants and children, *J Dev Behav Pediatr* 16(2):105-111, 1995.

Frailberg S, Adelson E, Shapiro V: Ghosts in the nursery: a psychoanalytic approach to the problems of impaired infant-mother relationships, *J Am Acad Child Psychiatry* 14:387, 1975.

Goldson, E: The neonatal intensive care unit: premature infants and parents, *Infants Young Children,* 4(3):31-42, 1992.

Goodfriend MS: Treatment of attachment disorders of infancy in a neonatal intensive care unit, *Pediatrics* 91:139, 1993.

Goulet C et al: A concept analysis of parent-infant attachment, *J Adv Nurs* 28(5):1071-1081, 1998.

Hamelin K, Ramachandran C: Kangaroo care, *Can Nurse* 89:15, 1993.

Hedlund R: Fostering positive social interactions between parents and infants, *Teaching Exceptional Children* p 43, 1986.

Ireland M: Therapeutic touch with HIV-infected children: a pilot study, *J Assoc Nurses AIDS Care* 9(4):68-77, 1998.

Kaminski J, Hall W: The effect of soothing music on neonatal behavioral states in the hospital newborn nursery, *Neonatal Netw* 15(1):45-54, 1996.

Lindsay JK et al: Creative caring in the NJCO parent to parent support, *Neonatal Netw* 12:37, 1993.

Lozoff B, et al: The mother-newborn relationship: limits of adaptability, *J Pediatr* 91:1, 1977.

McCollum J, Stayton V: Infant/parent interaction: studies and intervention guidelines based on the SIAI model, *J Div Early Childhood* 9:123, 1985.

Miles S, Funk S, Kasper M: The neonatal intensive care unit environment: sources of stress for parents, *AACN Clin Issues* 2(2):346-354, 1991.

Oehler J, Hannan T, Catlett A: Maternal views of preterm infants' responsiveness to social interaction, *Neonatal Netw* 12:67, 1993.

Pridham K et al: Guided participation and development of caregiving competencies for families of low birth-weight babies, *J Adv Nurs* 28(5):948-958, 1998.

Trout M: *Working papers on process in infant mental health assessment and intervention,* Champaign, Ill, 1987, The Infant-Parent Institute.

Zabielski M: Recognition of maternal identity in preterm and fullterm mothers, *Matern Child Nurs J* 22:2, 1994.

Autonomic dysreflexia

Betty J. Ackley

NANDA   **Definition** Life-threatening, uninhibited sympathetic response of the nervous system to a noxious stimulus after a spinal cord injury at T7 or above

• = Independent; ▲ = Collaborative

Defining Characteristics

Pallor (below the injury); paroxysmal hypertension (sudden, periodic elevated blood pressure where systolic pressure is >140 mm Hg and diastolic is >90 mm Hg); red splotches on skin (above the injury); bradycardia or tachycardia (pulse rate of <60 or >100 bpm); diaphoresis above the injury; headache (diffuse pain in different parts of the head, not confined to any nerve distribution area); blurred vision; chest pain; chilling; conjunctival congestion; Horner's syndrome (contraction of pupil on one side, partial ptosis of the eyelid, recession of eyeball into the head, occasional loss of sweating over the affected side of the face); metallic taste in mouth; nasal congestion; paresthesia; pilomotor reflex (gooseflesh formation when skin is cooled)

Related Factors (r/t)

Bladder distention; bowel distention; skin irritation; lack of client and caregiver knowledge

NOC   Outcomes (Nursing Outcomes Classification)

Suggested NOC Labels

Neurological Status; Neurological Status: Autonomic; Vital Signs Status

> **Example NOC Outcome**
> Demonstrates **Neurological Status: Autonomic** as evidenced by the following indicators: Systolic BP WNL*/Diastolic BP WNL/Heart rate WNL/Perspiration pattern/Goose bumps when appropriate/Pupil size/Peripheral tissue perfusion (Rate each indicator of **Neurological Status: Autonomic:** 1 = extremely compromised, 2 = substantially compromised, 3 = moderately compromised, 4 = mildly compromised, 5 = not compromised [see Section I])

*Within Normal Limits

Client Outcomes/Goals

- Maintains normal vital signs
- Remains free of dysreflexia symptoms
- Explains symptoms, prevention, and treatment of dysreflexia

NIC   Interventions (Nursing Interventions Classification)

Suggested NIC Labels

Dysreflexia Management

> **Example NIC Interventions—Dysreflexia Management**
> - Identify and minimize stimuli that may precipitate dysreflexia
> - Monitor for signs and symptoms of autonomic dysreflexia

Nursing Interventions and Rationales

- Monitor client for symptoms of dysreflexia. See Defining Characteristics.
- ▲ Observe with physician the cause of dysreflexia (e.g., distended bladder, impaction, pressure ulcer, urinary calculi, bladder infection, acute condition in the abdomen, penile pressure, ingrown toenail, or other source of noxious stimuli).
  Noxious stimuli cause an uncontrolled sympathetic nervous system response (Bergman, Yarkony, Stiens, 1997; Curt et al, 1997; Kavchak-Keyes, 2000).
- Use the following interventions to prevent dysreflexia:
  - Ensure that drainage from Foley catheter is good and that bladder is not distended.

• = Independent; ▲ = Collaborative

- Ensure a regular pattern of defecation to prevent fecal impaction.
  Bladder distention and bowel impaction are the most common causes of dysreflexia (Bergman, Yarkony, Stiens, 1997; Karlsson, 1999).
- Frequently change position of client to relieve pressure and prevent the formation of pressure ulcers.
- ▲ If ordered, apply an anesthetic agent to any wound below level of injury before performing wound care.

▲ If symptoms of dysreflexia are present, place client in high Fowler's position, remove all support hoses or binders, and immediately determine the identity of the noxious stimuli causing the response. If BP cannot be decreased within 1 minute, notify the physcian STAT (Karlsson, 1999).

These steps promote venous pooling, decrease venous return, and decrease blood pressure. A large number of different stimuli can cause dysreflexia (Adsit, Bishop, 1995). The client should be rapidly evaluated by both the physician and nurse to find the possible cause (Kavchak-Keyes, 2000).

- To determine the stimulus for dysreflexia:
  - ▲ First, assess bladder function. Check for distention, and if present catheterize using an anesthetic jelly as a lubricant. Don't use valsalva maneuver or Crede' method to empty the bladder. Ensure existing catheter patency (Travers, 1999).
  - ▲ Second, assess bowel function. Numb the bowel area with a topical anesthetic as ordered, and once agent is effective (5 minutes), check for impaction (Travers, 1999).
  - • Third, assess the skin looking for any points of pressure (Travers, 1999).

  The stimulus for dysreflexia is most commonly bladder distention, then bowel impaction, then pressure on the skin (Travers, 1999).

▲ Initiate antihypertensive therapy as soon as ordered.
  A severely elevated blood pressure needs to be decreased for client safety (Kavchak-Keyes, 2000).

▲ Be careful not to increase noxious sensory stimuli. If numbing agent is ordered, use it on anus and 1 inch of rectum before attempting to remove a fecal impaction. Also spray pressure ulcer with it. If necessary to replace an obstructed catheter, use an anesthetic jelly as ordered.

Increased noxious sensory stimuli can exacerbate the abnormal response and worsen the client's prognosis (Travers, 1999).

- Monitor vital signs every 3 to 5 minutes during acute event; continue to monitor vital signs after event is resolved.

It is possible for the client to develop rebound hypotension after the acute event because of the use of antihypertensive medications, or symptoms of dysreflexia may reoccur (Travers, 1999).

▲ Watch for complications of dysreflexia, including signs of cerebral hemorrhage, seizures, myocardial infarction, or intraocular hemorrhage.

Extremely high blood pressure can cause rupture of cerebral vessels, myocardial damage, and bleeding within the eye (Wirtz, LaFavor, Ang, 1996).

- Acurately and completely record any incidences of dysreflexia; especially note the precipitating stimuli.

It is imperative to determine both the causes of the condition and whether the condition is persistent, requiring the client to take medications routinely to prevent repeat incidences (Kavchak-Keyes, 2000).

• = Independent; ▲ = Collaborative

▲ Because episodes can reoccur, notify all health care team members of the possibility of a dysreflexia episode.
All health care personnel working with the client should be aware of the condition because symptoms could begin while the client is away from the nursing unit (Travers, 1999).

Home Care Interventions

• Instruct client with any known proclivity toward dysreflexia to wear a Medic-Alert bracelet and carry a Medic-Alert wallet card when not in a safe environment (i.e., not with someone who knows client has the condition and can respond appropriately).
Autonomic dysreflexia is life-threatening response (Kavchak-Keyes, 2000).

▲ Establish an emergency plan: obtain physician orders for medications to be used in situations in which first aid does not work (e.g., nifedipine, nitroglycerin ointment) (Wirtz, LaFavor, Ang, 1996).
Medication administered immediately can reverse early stage dysreflexia. Dysreflexia that is not recognized and treated can result in death (Tepper, 1997).

• If orders have not been obtained or client does not have medications, use emergency medical services.

▲ If episode of dysreflexia is resolved, monitor blood pressure every 30 to 60 minutes for next 4 to 5 hours or admit to institution for observation.
After an episode of autonomic dysreflexia, it is not uncommon for a second episode or rebound to occur (Hammond et al, 1989).

Client/Family Teaching

• Teach recognition of the earliest symptoms of dysreflexia, the actions that should be taken when they occur, and the need to summon help immediately. Give client a written card that contains this information.
The client must know the symptoms and treatment well enough to instruct people in his or her environment how to relieve the symptoms (Kavchak-Keyes, 2000).

• Teach steps to prevent dysreflexia episodes: care of bladder, bowel, and skin and prevention of other forms of noxious stimuli (i.e., not wearing clothing that is too tight).
Dysreflexia can occur anytime after discharge (Spoltore, O'Brien, 1995). Prevention of dysreflexia is the most effective treatment (Nolan, 1994).

WEB SITES FOR EDUCATION
MERLIN See the MERLIN web site for World Wide Web resources for client education.

REFERENCES   Adsit PA, Bishop C: Autonomic dysreflexia: let it be a surprise, *Orthop Nurs* 14(3):17, 1995.
Bergman SB, Yarkony RM, Stiens SA: Spinal cord injury rehabilitation: medical complications, *Arch Phys Med Rehabil* 78(3 suppl):S53, 1997.
Curt A et al: Assessment of autonomic dysreflexia in patients with spinal cord injury, *J Neurol Neurosurg Psychiatry* 62(5):473, 1997.
Hammond M et al, editors: *Yes you can: a guide to self-care for persons with spinal cord injury*, 1989, Paralyzed Veterans of America.
Karlsson AK: Autonomic dysreflexia, *Spinal Cord* 37(6):383-391, 1999.
Kavchak-Keyes MA: Autonomic hyperreflexia, *Rehabil Nurs* 25(1):31-35, 2000.

• = **Independent;** ▲ = **Collaborative**

Nolan S: Current trends in the management of acute spinal cord injury, *Crit Care Nurs* 17(1):64, 1994.

Spoltore TA, O'Brien AM: Rehabilitation of the spinal cord injured patient, *Orthop Nurs* 14(3):7-14, 1995.

Tepper K: Management of autonomic dysreflexia in a home care setting, *Clin Excel Nurse Practition* 1(3):163-166, 1997.

Travers PL: Autonomic dysreflexia: a clinical rehabilitation problem, *Rehabil Nurs* 24(1):19-23, 1999.

Wirtz KM, LaFavor KM, Ang R: Managing chronic spinal cord injury: issues in critical care, *Crit Care Nurse* 16(4):24, 1996.

Risk for Autonomic dysreflexia

Betty J. Ackley

NANDA   **Definition**   At risk for life-threatening, uninhibited response of the sympathetic nervous system; post–spinal shock; in an individual with spinal cord injury or lesion at T6 or above (has been demonstrated in patients with injuries at T7 or T8)

Defining Characteristics (Risk Factors)

An injury/lesion at T6 or above *and* at least one of the following noxious stimuli:

Neurological stimuli
Painful/irritating stimuli below the level of injury

Urological stimuli
Bladder distention; detrusor sphincter dyssynergia; bladder spasms; instrumentation or surgery; epididymitis; urethritis; urinary tract infection; calculi; cystitis; catheterization

Gastrointestinal stimuli
Bowel distention; fecal impaction; digital stimulation; suppositories; hemorrhoids; difficult passage of feces; constipation; enemas; GI system pathology; gastric ulcers; esophageal reflux; gallstones

Reproductive stimuli
Menstruation; sexual intercourse; pregnancy; labor and delivery; ovarian cyst; ejaculation

Regulatory stimuli
Temperature fluctuations; extreme environmental temperatures

Musculoskeletal-integumentary stimuli
Cutaneous stimulations (e.g., pressure ulcer, ingrown toenail, dressings, burns, rash); heterotrophic bone; pressure over bony prominences or genitalia; spasm; fractures; range-of-motion exercises; wounds; sunburns

Situational stimuli
Positioning; drug reactions (e.g., decongestants, sympathomimetics, vasoconstrictors, narcotic withdrawal); constrictive clothing (e.g., straps, stockings, shoes); surgical procedures

Cardiac/pulmonary problems
Pulmonary emboli; deep vein thrombosis

NOC   **Outcomes (Nursing Outcomes Classification)**

Suggested NOC Labels
Neurological Status; Neurological Status: Autonomic; Vital Signs Status

 = Independent; ▲ = Collaborative

> **Example NOC Outcome**
> Demonstrates appropriate **Neurological Status: Autonomic** as evidenced by the following indicators: Systolic BP WNL*/Diastolic BP WNL/Heart rate WNL/ Perspiration pattern/Goose bumps when appropriate/Pupil size/Peripheral tissue perfusion (Rate each indicator with regard to **Neurological Status: Autonomic:** 1 = extremely compromised, 2 = substantially compromised, 3 = moderately compromised, 4 = mildly compromised, 5 = not compromised [see Section I])

*Within Normal Limits

NIC   **Interventions (Nursing Interventions Classification)**
Suggested NIC Labels
Dysreflexia Management

> **Example NIC Interventions—Dysreflexia Management**
> - Identify and minimize stimuli that may precipitate dysreflexia
> - Monitor for signs and symptoms of autonomic dysreflexia

Client Outcomes, Nursing Interventions and Rationales, Web Sites for Education
Refer to care plan for **Autonomic dysreflexia.**

Disturbed Body image

Gail B. Ladwig

NANDA   **Definition** Confusion in mental picture of one's physical self

Defining Characteristics

Nonverbal response to actual or perceived change in structure and/or function; verbalization of feelings that reflect an altered view of one's body in appearance, structure, or function; verbalization of perceptions that reflect an altered view of one's body in appearance, structure, or function; behaviors of avoidance, monitoring, or acknowledgment of one's body

Objective   Missing body part; actual change in structure or function; avoidance of looking at or touching body part; intentional or unintentional hiding or overexposure of body part; trauma to nonfunctioning part; change in social involvement; change in ability to estimate spatial relationship of body to environment

Subjective   Change in lifestyle; fear of rejection or reaction by others; focus on past strength, function, or appearance; negative feelings about body; feelings of helplessness, hopelessness, or powerlessness; preoccupation with change or loss; emphasis on remaining strengths and heightened achievement; extension of body boundary to incorporate environmental objects; personalization of part or loss by name; depersonalization of part or loss by impersonal pronouns; refusal to verify actual change

Related Factors (r/t)

Psychosocial, biophysical, cognitive/perceptual, cultural, spiritual, or developmental changes; illness; trauma or injury; surgery; illness treatment

• = Independent; ▲ = Collaborative

NOC   **Outcomes (Nursing Outcomes Classification)**
Suggested NOC Labels
Body Image; Child Development: 2 Years; Child Development: 3 Years; Child Development: 4 Years; Child Development: 5 Years; Child Development: Middle Childhood (6-11 Years); Child Development: Adolescence (12-17 Years); Distorted Thought Control; Grief Resolution; Psychosocial Adjustment: Life Change; Self-Esteem

Example NOC Outcome
Demonstrates **Body Image** as evidenced by the following indicators: Congruence between body reality, body ideal, and body presentation/Satisfaction with body appearance/Adjustment to changes in physical appearance (Rate each indicator of **Body Image:** 1 = never positive, 2 = rarely positive, 3 = sometimes positive, 4 = often positive, 5 = consistantly positive [see Section I])

Client Outcomes
- States or demonstrates acceptance of change or loss and an ability to adjust to lifestyle change
- Calls body part or loss by appropriate name
- Looks at and touches changed or missing body part
- Cares for changed or nonfunctioning part without inflicting trauma
- Returns to previous social involvement
- Correctly estimates relationship of body to environment

NIC   **Interventions (Nursing Interventions Classification)**
Suggested NIC Labels
Body Image Enhancement

Example NIC Interventions—Body Image Enhancement
- Determine client's body image expectations based on developmental stage
- Assist client to identify activities that will enhance appearance

Nursing Interventions and Rationales
- Use a tool such as the Body Image Instrument (BII) to identify clients who have concerns about changes in body image.
  The five BII subscales—General Appearance, Body Competence, Others' Reaction to Appearance, Value of Appearance, and Body Parts—exhibited moderate to high internal reliability and concurrent validity (Kopel et al, 1998).
- Observe client's usual coping mechanisms during times of extreme stress and reinforce their use in the current crisis.
  Clients are in shock during acute phase, and their own value system must be considered. Clients deal better with change over time (Price, 1992).
- Acknowledge denial, anger, or depression as normal feelings when adjusting to changes in body and lifestyle.
  Changes in body image cause anxiety. People in this situation use a variety of unconscious coping mechanisms to deal with their altered body image (ABI). Defense mechanisms are normal, unless they are used so much that they interfere with rather than improve self-esteem (MacGinley, 1993).

• = Independent; ▲ = Collaborative

- Identify clients at risk for body image disturbance (e.g., body builders, cancer survivors).

  The results of one study suggest that male body builders are at risk for body image disturbance and the associated psychological characteristics that have been commonly reported among eating disorder patients. These psychological characteristics also appear to predict steroid use in this group of males. Steroid users reported an elevated drive to put on muscle mass in the form of bulk (Blouin, Goldfield, 1995).

- Clients should not be rushed into sharing their feelings.

  Feelings associated with complicated and emotionally powerful issues involving an altered body image take time to work through and express (Johnson, 1994).

- Do not ask clients to explore feelings unless they have indicated a need to do so.

  Patients reported keeping their feelings to themselves as a frequently used coping strategy (Zacharias, Gilig, Foxall, 1994).

- Explore strengths and resources with client. Discuss possible changes in weight and hair loss; select a wig before hair loss occurs.

  Emphasizing strengths promotes a positive self-image. Planning for an event such as hair loss helps to decrease the anxiety associated with a sudden change in appearance.

- Encourage client to purchase clothes that are attractive and that deemphasize their disability.

  Individuals with osteoporosis are not usually disabled but may perceive themselves as unattractive and experience social isolation as a result of ill-fitting clothes that accentuate the physical changes (Sedlak, Doheny, 2000).

- Allow client and others gradual exposure to the body change. Begin by having the client touch the affected area; then use a mirror to look at it. Go to a hospital shop with a nurse or support person and discuss feelings associated with the reaction of others to the body change.

  Part of the rehabilitation process is graded exposure—the client moves from a protected to an unprotected environment with the support of the nurse (MacGinley, 1993).

- Encourage client to discuss interpersonal and social conflicts that may arise.

  A good perception of body image is best achieved within a supportive social framework. Clients with an active social support network are likely to make better progress (Price, 1990). Changes in physical appearance and function associated with disease processes (and sometimes treatment) need to be integrated into the interaction that occurs between patients and lay caregivers (Price, 2000).

- Encourage client to make own decisions, participate in plan of care, and accept both inadequacies and strengths.

  It is important for clients to be involved in their own care. If they have received information about their altered body image, treatment, and rehabilitation, they will be able to make their own choices. Consequently they will be more likely to come to terms with and adapt to their ABI (Price, 1986). Healthy adaptation to body image exists when the person is able to maximize ability despite disability (Samonds, Cammermeyer, 1989).

- Help client accept help from others; provide a list of appropriate community resources (e.g., Reach to Recovery, Ostomy Association).

  Motivation, sharing of experiences, camaraderie with and support from peers, and knowledge of not being alone have been identified as advantages of group learning (Payne, 1993).

• = **Independent;** ▲ = **Collaborative**

- Help client describe self-ideal, identify self-criticisms, and be accepting of self.
  The perception of self-image involves knowing the self and what is important and valued. Disability causes individuals to live as changed human beings whether they are willing to or not (Pohl, Winland-Brown, 1992).
- Encourage client to write a narrative description of their changes.
  An analysis based on the grounded theory method revealed that one's experience of coping or adjustment to a disability is represented as narratives about himself or herself. Each person with traumatic brain injury (TBI) reconstructed certain self-narratives when coping with their changed self-images and daily lives (Nochi, 2000).
- Avoid looks of distaste when caring for clients who have had disfiguring surgery or injuries. Provide privacy; care should be completed without unnecessary exposure.
  Nurses must be aware of their nonverbal behavior; clients often become acutely aware of nurses' feelings as a result of the nurses' facial expressions, tone of voice, touch, or other behaviors (MacGinley, 1993).
- Encourage client to continue same personal care routine that was followed before the change in body image. It is preferable that this care be completed in the bathroom and not in bed.
  This routine gives the client privacy and also prevents the client from settling into an "invalid" role. Research has shown that women who resume familiar routines and habits heal better and suffer less depression than those who settle into the role of patient (Johnson, 1994).

Geriatric

- Focus on remaining abilities. Have client make a list of strengths.
  Results from unstructured interviews with women aged 61 to 92 regarding their perceptions and feelings about their aging bodies suggest that women exhibit the internalization of ageist beauty norms, even as they assert that health is more important to them than physical attractiveness and comment on the "naturalness" of the aging process (Hurd, 2000). Motivation and self-worth are increased in the elderly by highlighting their capabilities. Even a severely disabled client is usually capable of accomplishing some tasks. Normal changes in body image occur as a result of the aging process (MacGinley, 1993).

Multicultural

- Assess for the influence of cultural beliefs, norms, and values on the client's body image.
  The client's body image may be based on cultural perceptions, as well as influences from the larger social context (Leininger, 1996).
- Validate the client's feelings with regard to the impact of health status on disturbances in body image.
  Validation lets the client know that the nurse has heard and understands what was said and promotes the nurse-client relationship (Stuart, Laraia, 2001; Giger, Davidhizar, 1995).
- Acknowledge that body image disturbances can affect all individuals regardless of culture, race, or ethnicity.
  Body image disturbances are pervasive across western cultures and appear to increase in other cultures with acculturation to western ideals.

Home Care Interventions

- Assess client's stage of grieving or acceptance of body change upon return to home setting. Include the future role of sexuality in the psychological assessment of acceptance as appropriate.

• = **Independent;** ▲ = **Collaborative**

- Assess family/caregiver level of acceptance of client's body changes.
- Be accepting of changes in all interactions with client and family/caregivers. *Acceptance promotes trust.*
- Help client to see new or changing roles in family. Point out ways in which the community can help support client and family strengths.
- ▲ Refer to medical social services for level of acceptance and possible financial impact of changes.
  Clients and caregivers may see the nurse's visit as being solely involved with physiological issues such as dressing, especially under managed care systems. Social worker visits can support the client or caregivers with dedicated time and can help the nurse be supportive and adapt interventions to promote acceptance. The nurse or social worker can introduce or reinforce use of community resources.
- Teach all aspects of care. Involve client and caregivers in self-care as soon as possible. Do this in stages if client still has difficulty looking at or touching changed body part.
  The quicker the involvement in self-care, the greater the chances for permanent acceptance and positive self-esteem.
- ▲ Teach family and client complications of medical condition and when to contact physician.
- ▲ Refer to occupational therapy if necessary to evaluate home setting for safety and adaptive equipment and to assist client with return to normal activities.
  The quicker the reinvolvement in daily living activities and self-care, the greater the chances for permanent acceptance and positive self-esteem.
- ▲ If appropriate, provide home health aide support to help the client and family through activities of daily living (ADLs) transition.
- ▲ Refer to physical therapy if necessary to build range-of-joint-motion (ROJM) flexibility and strength, prevent contractures, assist with transfer/ambulation safety, or obtain use of a prosthetic device in the home setting.
- Assess for and promote good nutrition and sleep patterns. Adapt nutrition to specific physiological situations (e.g., client with ostomy).
  Good nutrition and sleep patterns promote faster healing and better coping.
- ▲ Assist family with obtaining needed supplies.
  Cost of ostomy supplies and adaptive equipment can be an added stressor for the client. Community resources can assist.

Client/Family Teaching

- Teach appropriate care of surgical site (e.g., mastectomy site, amputation site, ostomy site).
  Patient teaching by ET nurses may alleviate problems associated with altered body image in relation to the presence of an ostomy (Tomaselli, Jenks, Morin, 1991).
- ▲ Inform client of available community support groups; offer to make initial phone call.
  Motivation, sharing of experiences, camaraderie with and support from peers, and knowledge of not being alone have been identified as advantages of group learning (Payne, 1993).
- ▲ Refer client to counseling for help adjusting to body change.
  Counseling is important for a client who is trying to create a new body ideal or work through a grief process (Price, 1990).

- **= Independent;** ▲ **= Collaborative**

- Provide printed material and didactic information for significant others.
  Some significant others prefer to receive didactic material rather than vent their feelings as a way of showing support (Northouse, Peters-Golden, 1993).
- Encourage significant others to offer support.
  Social support from significant others enhances both emotional and physical health (Badger, 1990).
- Direct social support as follows: instruct regarding practical care (bandaging), encourage appraisal support (listening), encourage self-esteem support (favorable comparisons between client's and other's appearance), and encourage sense of belonging (assist with socializing).
  The preceding are four categories of support recognized in the body-image care model. Clients with an active social support network are likely to make better progress than those without support (Price, 1990).
- ▲ Refer to an interdisciplinary team clients with ostomies who are having difficulty with personal acceptance, personal and social body-image disruption, sexual concerns, reduced self-care skills, and the management of surgical complications.
  Many clinical studies have found patients with ostomies to be a group facing multiple adjustment demands. One of these demands is coping with a significant change in body image. At the Medical College of Wisconsin, a team approach has been initiated; the ET nurse, the psychologist, and the surgeon deal with body image concerns together. The multidisciplinary approach has been demonstrated to be successful in facilitating adaptation to an altered body image (Walsh et al, 1995).

WEB SITES FOR EDUCATION

MERLIN   See the MERLIN web site for World Wide Web resources for client education.

REFERENCES   Badger V: Men with cardiovascular disease and their spouses: coping, health and marital adjustment, *Arch Psychiatr Nurs* 4:319, 1990.

Blouin AG, Goldfield GS: Body image and steroid use in male bodybuilders, *Int J Eat Disord* 18(2):159-165, 1995.

Giger JN, Davidhizar RE: *Transcultural nursing*, ed 2, St Louis, 1995, Mosby.

Hurd LC: Older women's body image and embodied experience: an exploration, *J Women Aging* 12(3-4):77-97, 2000.

Johnson J: Caring for the woman who's had a mastectomy, *Am J Nurs* 94:25, 1994.

Kopel SJ et al: Brief report: assessment of body image in survivors of childhood cancer, *J Pediatr Psychol* 23(2):141-147, 1998.

Leininger MM: *Transcultural nursing: theories, research and practices*, ed 2, Hilliard, Ohio, 1996, McGraw-Hill.

MacGinley K: Nursing care of the patient with altered body image, *Br J Nurs* 2:1098, 1993.

Nochi M: Reconstructing self-narratives in coping with traumatic brain injury, *Soc Sci Med* 51(12):1795-1804, 2000.

Northouse L, Peters-Golden H: Cancer and the family: strategies to assist spouses, *Semin Oncol Nurs* 9:74, 1993.

Payne J: The contribution of group learning to the rehabilitation of spinal cord injured adults, *Rehabil Nurs* 18:375, 1993.

Pohl C, Winland-Brown J: The meaning of disability in a caring environment, *J Nurs Adm* 22:29, 1992.

Price B: Keeping up appearances, *Nurs Times* 82:58, 1986.

Price B: A model for body-image care, *J Adv Nurs* 15:585, 1990.

Price B: Living with altered body image: the classic patient experience, *Br J Nurs* 25:641, 1992.

Price B: Altered body image: managing social encounters, *Int J Palliat Nurs* 6(4):179-185, 2000.

Samonds R, Cammermeyer M: Perceptions of body image in subjects with multiple sclerosis: a pilot study, *J Neurosci Nurs* 21:190, 1989.

Sedlak CA, Doheny MO: Fashion tips for women with osteoporosis, *Orthop Nurs* 19(5):31-35, 2000.

• = **Independent;** ▲ = **Collaborative**

Stuart GW, Laraia MT: Therapeutic nurse-patient relationship. In Stuart GW, Laraia MT, editors: *Principles and practice of psychiatric nursing,* St Louis, 2001, Mosby, p 30.

Tomaselli N, Jenks J, Morin K: Body image in patients with stomas: a critical review of the literature, *J ET Nurs* 18:95, 99, 1991.

Walsh BA et al: Multidisciplinary management of altered body image in the patient with an ostomy, *J Wound Ostomy Continence Nurs* 22(5):227-236, 1995.

Zacharias DR, Gilig CA, Foxall MJ: Quality of life and coping in patients with gynecologic cancer and their spouses, *Oncol Nurs Forum* 21:1699, 1994.

Risk for imbalanced Body temperature

Sandra K. Cunningham and Betty J. Ackley

NANDA   **Definition**   At risk for failure to maintain body temperature within a normal range

Risk Factors

Altered metabolic rate; extremes of age or weight; exposure to cool/cold or hot/warm environments; dehydration; inactivity or vigorous activity; medications that cause vaso-constriction or vasodilatation; sedation; clothing inappropriate for environmental tem-perature; illness or trauma that affects body temperature regulation

Related Factors (r/t)

See Risk Factors

NOC   **Outcomes (Nursing Outcomes Classification)**

Suggested NOC Labels

Thermoregulation; Thermoregulation: Neonate

> **Example NOC Outcome**
> Accomplishes **Thermoregulation** as evidenced by the following indicators: Body tem-perature WNL*/Skin temperature IER†/Skin color changes not present/Hydration adequate/Reported thermal comfort (Rate each indicator of **Thermoregulation:** 1 = extremely compromised, 2 = substantially compromised, 3 = moderately compro-mised, 4 = mildly compromised, 5 = not compromised [see Section I])

*Within Normal Limits
†In Expected Range

Client Outcomes

- Maintains temperature within normal range of 97° to 99° F in the adult
- Explains measures needed to maintain normal temperature
- Identifies symptoms of hypothermia or hyperthermia

NIC   **Interventions (Nursing Interventions Classification)**

Suggested NIC Labels

Temperature Regulation; Temperature Regulation: Intraoperative; Vital Signs Monitoring

> **Example NIC Interventions—Temperature Regulation**
> - Institute a continuous core temperature monitoring device as appropriate
> - Promote adequate fluid and nutritional intake

• = Independent; ▲ = Collaborative

Nursing Interventions and Rationales

- Monitor temperature q _____ h(rs) or use continuous temperature monitoring as appropriate.
  Normal adult temperature is usually identified at 98.6° F (37° C), but in actuality the normal temperature fluctuates throughout the day. In the early morning it may be as low as 96.4° F (35.8° C) and in the late afternoon or evening as high as 99.1° F (37.3° C) (Bates, 1998). Disease, injury, or pharmacological agents may impair regulation of body temperature (Holtzclaw, 1993; Dennison, 1995).
- Take vital signs q _____ h(rs), noting changes associated with hypothermia: first, increased blood pressure, pulse, and respirations; then, decreased values as hypothermia progresses (Edwards, 1999).
- Note changes in vital signs associated with hyperthermia: rapid, bounding pulse; increased respiratory rate; and decreased blood pressure with orthostatic hypotension present (Worfolk, 2000).
  Consistent monitoring promotes prevention and early intervention in clients with altered cardiopulmonary status associated with hypothermia or hyperthermia.
- Monitor client for signs of hypothermia (e.g., shivering, cool skin, piloerection, pallor, slow capillary refill, cyanotic nailbeds, decreased mentation, dysrhythmias) (Edwards, 1999).
- Monitor client for signs of hyperthermia (e.g., headache, nausea and vomiting, weakness, absence of sweating, delirium, and coma) (Worfolk, 2000).
  Monitoring for defining characteristics of hypothermia and hyperthermia allows for prevention and/or early intervention.
- Maintain a consistent room temperature (72° F).
  A consistent temperature limits environmental effects on thermoregulation.
- Promote adequate nutrition and hydration.
  These measures help maintain a normal body temperature.
- Adjust clothing to facilitate passive warming or cooling as appropriate.
  This will help maintain a normal body temperature.
- See Nursing Interventions and Rationales for **Hypothermia** or **Hyperthermia** as appropriate.

Geriatric

- Do not allow geriatric clients to become chilled. Keep covered when giving a bath or doing a procedure. Offer socks to wear when in bed.
  Older adults have a decreased ability to adapt to temperature extremes and need protection from extreme environmental temperatures. Older adults have a higher threshold of central temperature for sweating, diminished or absent sweating, impaired warmth or cold perception, impaired shiver response, diminished thermogenesis, abnormal peripheral blood flow response to warmth or cold, and compromised cardiovascular reserve (Robbins, 1989; Florez-Duquet, McDonald, 1998; Ballester, Harchelroad, 1999).
- ▲ Assess medication profile for potential risk of drug-related altered body temperature.
  Anesthetics, barbiturates, salicylates, nonsteroidal antiinflammatory drugs (NSAIDs), diuretics, antihistamines, anticholinergics, beta-blockers, and thyroid hormones have been linked to altered body temperatures (Haskell et al, 1997).

• = **Independent**; ▲ = **Collaborative**

Pediatric

- Recognize that pediatric clients have a decreased ability to adapt to temperature extremes. Take the following actions to maintain body temperature in the infant/child:
  - Keep the head covered.
  - Use blankets to keep the client warm.
  - Keep client covered during procedures, transport, and diagnostic testing.
  - Maintain a consistent room temperature of 72° F.

  These measures can help prevent hypothermia, which is highly possible, especially in the pediatric trauma client (Bernardo, Henker, 1999) The combination of a relatively large body surface area, small body-fluid volume, less well-developed temperature control mechanisms, and a small amount of protective body fat limits the pediatric client's ability to maintain normal temperatures (Henderson, 1990; Roncoli, Medoff-Cooper, 1992; Noerr, 1997).

Home Care Interventions

- Prevention of Hypothermia in Cold Weather
  - Avoid prolonged exposure outside. Wear a hat and gloves. Wool or fleece clothing can help to maintain body heat.
  - Keep room temperature at 68° to 72° F.
  - ▲ Ensure adequate source of heat; refer to social services if client is low income and heat could be turned off.
  - Help elderly client determine a warm environment they can go to for safety in cold weather if his or her home environment is no longer warm.
- Prevention of Hyperthermia in Hot Weather
  - Encourage client to wear lightweight cotton clothing. Help elderly remove their usual sweaters.
  - Ensure that client drinks adequate amounts of fluids (2000 ml/day), avoiding caffeine and alcohol.

    Adequate fluids are needed during hot weather to replace fluids lost from sweating. Fluids containing caffeine and alcohol can serve as a diuretic and decrease fluid volume in the body.
  - ▲ Help client obtain a fan to increase evaporation, or an air conditioner as needed, using social services if needed.
  - Take the temperature of the elderly in hot weather.

    The elderly may not be able to tell that they are hot because of decreased sensation (Worfolk, 2000).
  - Help elderly client determine a cool environment they can go to for safety in hot weather.

Client/Family Teaching

- Teach client and family the signs of hypothermia and hyperthermia and the appropriate actions they should take if either condition develops.

  Adequate teaching improves compliance and reduces anxiety.
- Teach client and family proper method for taking temperature.

  Optimal placement of the appropriate device is essential for accurate monitoring.
- Teach to avoid alcohol and medications that depress cerebral function.

  When the client is sedated or under the influence of alcohol, mentation is depressed, resulting in decreased activities to maintain an adequate body temperature.

• = Independent; ▲ = Collaborative

REFERENCES   Ballester JM, Harchelroad FP: Hypothermia: an easy-to-miss, dangerous disorder in winter weather, *Geriatrics* 54(2):51, 1999.

Bates B, Bickley LS, Hoekelman RA: *A guide to physical examination and history taking,* ed 7, Philadelphia, 1998, JB Lippincott.

Bernardo LM, Henker R: Thermoregulation in pediatric trama: an overview, *Int J Trauma Nurs* 5(3):101-105, 1999.

Dennison D: Thermal regulation of patients during the perioperative period, *AORN J* 61:827, 1995.

Edwards SL: Hypothermia, *Professional Nurse* 14(4):253-258, 1999.

Florez-Duquet M, McDonald RB: Cold-induced thermoregulation and biological aging, *Physiol Rev* 78(2):339, 1998.

Haskell RM et al: Hypothermia, *AACN Clin Issues* 8(3):368, 1997.

Henderson DP: Pediatric update: hypothermia and the pediatric patient, *J Emerg Nurs* 16:411, 1990.

Holtzclaw BJ: Monitoring body temperature, *AACN Clin Issues Crit Care Nurs* 4:44, 1993.

Noerr B: Keeping the newborn warm: understanding thermoregulation, *Mother Baby J* 2(5):6, 1997.

Robbins AS: Hypothermia and heat stroke: protecting the elderly patient, *Geriatrics* 44(1):73-77, 80, 1989.

Roncoli M, Medoff-Cooper B: Thermoregulation in low-birth-weight infants, *NAACOG Clin Issues* 3:25, 1992.

Worfolk JB: Heat waves: their impact on the health of elders, *Geratr Nurs* 21(2):70-77, 2000.

Bowel incontinence

Mikel Gray

NANDA   **Definition**   Change in normal bowel habits characterized by involuntary passage of stool

Defining Characteristics

Constant dribbling of soft stool, fecal odor; inability to delay defecation; rectal urgency; self-report of inability to feel rectal fullness or presence of stool in bowel; fecal staining of underclothing; recognizes rectal fullness but reports inability to expel formed stool; inattention to urge to defecate; inability to recognize urge to defecate, red perianal skin

Related Factors (r/t)

Change in stool consistency (diarrhea, constipation, fecal impaction); abnormal motility (metabolic disorders, inflammatory bowel disease, infectious disease, drug induced motility disorders, food intolerance); defects in rectal vault function (low rectal compliance from ischemia, fibrosis, radiation, infectious proctitis, Hirschprung's disease, local or infiltrating neoplasm, severe rectocele); sphincter dysfunction (obstetric or traumatic induced incompetence, fistula or abscess, prolapse, third degree hemorrhoids, pseudo-dyssynergia of the pelvic muscles); neurological disorders impacting gastrointestinal motility, rectal vault function and sphincter function (cerebrovascular accident, spinal injury, traumatic brain injury, central nervous system tumor, advanced stage dementia, encephalopathy, profound mental retardation, multiple sclerosis, myelodysplasia and related neural tube defects, gastroparesis of diabetes mellitus, heavy metal poisoning, chronic alcoholism, infectious or autoimmune neurological disorders, myasthenia gravis)

• = Independent; ▲ = Collaborative

NOC   **Outcomes (Nursing Outcomes Classification)**
Suggested NOC Labels
Bowel Continence; Bowel Elimination

Example NOC Outcome
Accomplishes **Bowel Continence** as evidenced by the following indicators: Predict-able evacuation of stool/Maintains control of passage of stool/Regular evacuation of stool at least q 3 days (Rate each indicator of **Bowel Continence:** 1 = never dem-onstrated, 2 = rarely demonstrated, 3 = sometimes demonstrated, 4 = often dem-onstrated, 5 = consistently demonstrated [see Section I])

Client Outcomes

- Regular, complete evacuation of fecal contents from the rectal vault (pattern may vary from every day to every 3 to 5 days) (Roig et al, 1993)
- Defecates soft-formed stool
- Decreased or absence of bowel incontinence incidences
- Intact skin in the perianal/perineal area
- Demonstrates the ability to isolate, contract, and relax pelvic muscles (when inconti-nence related to sphincter incompetence, pseudodyssynergia)
  Increases pelvic muscle strength (when incontinence related to sphincter incompetence)

NIC   **Interventions (Nursing Interventions Classification)**
Suggested NIC Labels
Bowel Incontinence Care; Bowel Training; Bowel Incontinence Care: Encopresis

Example NIC Interventions—Bowel Incontinence Care
- Determine physical or psychological cause of fecal incontinence
- Instruct client/family to record fecal output, as appropriate

Nursing Interventions and Rationales

- In a reasonably private setting, directly question any client at risk about the presence of fecal incontinence. If the client reports altered bowel elimination patterns, prob-lems with bowel control or "uncontrollable diarrhea," complete a focused nursing history including previous and present bowel elimination routines, dietary history, frequency and volume of uncontrolled stool loss, and aggravating and alleviating factors.
  Unless questioned directly, patients are unlikely to report the presence of fecal incontinence (Schultz, Dickey, Skoner, 1997). The nursing history determines the patterns of stool elimination to characterize involuntary stool loss and the likely etiology of the incontinence (Norton, Chelvanaygam, 2000).
- ▲ Complete a focused physical assessment including inspection of perineal skin, pelvic muscle strength assessment, digital examination of the rectum for presence of impac-tion and anal sphincter strength, and evaluation of functional status (mobility, dex-terity, visual acuity).
  A focused physical examination helps determine the severity of fecal leakage and its likely etiology. A functional assessment provides information concerning the impact of functional status on stool elimination patterns and incontinence (Gray, Burns, 1996).

• = Independent; ▲ = Collaborative

▲ Complete an assessment of cognitive function.
Dementia, acute confusion, and mental retardation are risk factors for fecal incontinence (O'Donnel et al, 1992; Norton, Chelvanaygam, 2000).

• Document patterns of stool elimination and incontinent episodes via a bowel record, including frequency of bowel movements, stool consistency, frequency and severity of incontinent episodes, precipitating factors, and dietary and fluid intake.
This document is used to confirm the verbal history (Resnick et al, 1994) and to assist in determining the likely etiology of stool incontinence. It also serves as a baseline to evaluate treatment efficacy (Norton, Chelvanaygam, 2000).

▲ Identify the probable causes of fecal incontinence.
Fecal incontinence is frequently multifactorial; therefore identification of the probable etiology of fecal incontinence is necessary to select a treatment plan likely to control or eliminate the condition (Norton, Chelvanaygam, 2000).

• Improve access to toileting:
  ▪ Identify usual toileting patterns among persons in the acute care or long term care facility and plan opportunities for toileting accordingly.
  ▪ Provide assistance with toileting for patients with limited access or impaired functional status (e.g., mobility, dexterity, access).
  ▪ Institute a prompted toileting program for persons with impaired cognitive status (e.g., retardation, dementia).
  ▪ Provide adequate privacy for toileting.
  ▪ Respond promptly to requests for assistance with toileting.
Acute or transient fecal incontinence frequently occurs in the acute care or long term care facility because of inadequate access to toileting facilities, insufficient assistance with toileting, or inadequate privacy when attempting to toilet (Gray, Burns, 1996; Ouslander, Snelle, 1995).

• For the client with intermittent episodes of fecal incontinence related to acute changes in stool consistency, begin a bowel reeducation program consisting of:
  ▲ Cleansing the bowel of impacted stool if indicated.
  ▪ Normalizing stool consistency by adequate intake of fluids (30 ml/kg of body weight/day) and dietary or supplemental fiber.
  ▪ Establishing a regular routine of fecal elimination based on established patterns of bowel elimination (patterns established before onset of incontinence).
Bowel reeducation is designed to reestablish normal defecation patterns and to normalize stool consistency to reduce or eliminate the risk of recurring fecal incontinence associated with changes in stool consistency (Doughty, 1996).

• Begin a prompted defecation program for the adult with dementia, mental retardation, or related learning disabilities.
Prompted urine and fecal elimination programs have been shown to reduce or eliminate incontinence in the long term care facility and community settings (Doughty, 1996; Ouslander, Snelle, 1995; Smith et al, 1994).

• Begin a scheduled stimulation defecation program, including the following steps, for persons with neurological conditions causing fecal incontinence:
  ▪ Before beginning the program, cleanse the bowel of impacted fecal material.
  ▪ Implement strategies to normalize stool consistency, including adequate intake of fluid and fiber and avoidance of foods associated with diarrhea.

• = Independent; ▲ = Collaborative

- Whenever feasible, determine a regular schedule for bowel elimination (typically every day or every other day) based on previous patterns of bowel elimination.
▲ Provide a stimulus before assisting the patient to a position on the toilet. Digital stimulation, stimulating suppository, "mini-enema," or pulsed evacuation enema may be used.

The scheduled, stimulated defecation program relies on consistency of stool and a mechanical or chemical stimulus to produce a bolus contraction of the rectum with evacuation of fecal material (Doughty, 1996; Dunn, Galka, 1994; King, Currie, Wright, 1994; Munchiando, Kendall, 1993).

▲ Begin a pelvic floor reeducation or muscle exercise program for persons with sphincter incompetence or pseudodyssynergia of the pelvic muscles, or refer persons with fecal incontinence related to sphincter dysfunction to a nurse specialist or other therapist with clinical expertise in these techniques of care.

Pelvic muscle reeducation, including biofeedback, pelvic muscle exercise, and/or pelvic muscle relaxation techniques, is a safe and effective treatment for selected persons with fecal incontinence related to sphincter or pelvic floor muscle dysfunction (Arhan et al, 1994; Enck et al, 1994; Keck et al, 1994; McIntosh et al, 1993).

• Begin a pelvic muscle biofeedback program among patients with urgency to defecate and fecal incontinence related to recurrent diarrhea.

Pelvic muscle reeducation, including biofeedback, can reduce uncontrolled loss of stool among persons who experience urgency and diarrhea as provacative factors for fecal incontinence (Chiarioni et al, 1993). Reducing the incidence of diarrhea can help to reduce bowel incontinence (Bliss et al, 2000).

• Cleanse the perineal and perianal skin following each episode of fecal incontinence. When incontinence is frequent, use an incontinence cleansing product specifically designed for this purpose.

Frequent cleaning with soap and water may compromise perianal skin integrity and enhance the irritation produced by fecal leakage (Byers et al, 1995; Lyder et al, 1992).

• Apply mineral oil or a petroleum based ointment to the perianal skin when frequent episodes of fecal incontinence occur.

These products form a moisture and chemical barrier to the perianal skin that may prevent or reduce the severity of compromised skin integrity with severe fecal incontinence (Fiers, Thayer, 2000).

• Assist the patient to select and apply a containment device for occasional episodes of fecal incontinence.

A fecal containment device will prevent soiling of clothing and reduce odors in the patient with uncontrolled stool loss (Fiers, Thayer, 2000).

• Teach the caregivers of the patient with frequent episodes of fecal incontinence and limited mobility to regularly monitor the sacrum and perineal area for pressure ulcerations.

Limited mobility, particularly when combined with fecal incontinence, increases the risk of pressure ulceration. Routine cleansing, pressure reduction techniques, and management of fecal and urinary incontinence reduces this risk (Johanson, Irizarry, Doughty, 1997; Schnelle et al, 1997).

▲ Consult the physician concerning the use of an anal continence plug for the patient with frequent stool loss and teach the patient its application.

• = **Independent;** ▲ = **Collaborative**

The anal continence plug is a device that can reduce or eliminate persistent liquid or solid stool incontinence in selected patients (Blair et al, 1992).

- Apply a fecal pouch to the patient with frequent stool loss, particularly when fecal incontinence produces altered perianal skin integrity.
  Fecal pouches contain stool loss, reduce odor, and protect the perianal skin from chemical irritation resulting from contact with stool (Fiers, Thayer, 2000).
▲ Consult the physician concerning the use of a rectal tube for the patient with severe fecal incontinence.
  A large-sized French indwelling catheter has been used for fecal containment when incontinence is severe and perianal skin integrity significantly compromised (Birdsall, 1986). The safety of this technique remains unknown (Doughty, Broadwell-Jackson, 1993).

Geriatric

- Evaluate elderly client for established or acute fecal incontinence when client enters the acute or long term care facility; intervene as indicated.
  The rate of fecal incontinence among patients in acute care facilities is as high as 3%; in long term care facilities the rate is as high as 50% (Egan, Plymad, Thomas, 1983; Leigh, Turnberg, 1982).
- Evaluate cognitive status in the elderly person with a NEECHAM confusion scale (Neelan et al, 1992). To identify acute cognitive changes, use a Folstein Mini-Mental Status Examination (MMSE) (Folstein, Folstein, 1975) or other tool as indicated.
  Acute or established dementia increases the risk of fecal incontinence among elderly persons.

Home Care Interventions

- Assess and teach a bowel management program to support continence.
- Provide clothing that is nonrestrictive, can be manipulated easily for toileting, and can be changed with ease.
  Avoidance of complicated maneuvers increases the chance of success in toileting programs and decreases the client's risk for embarrassing incontinent episodes.
- Assist the family in arranging care in a way that allows the client to participate in family or favorite activities without embarrassment.
  Careful planning can both help client retain dignity and maintain integrity of family patterns.
▲ If the client is limited to bed (or bed and chair), provide a commode or bedpan that can be easily accessed. If necessary, refer the client to physical therapy services to learn side transfers and to build strength for transfers.
▲ If the client is frequently incontinent, refer for home health aide services to assist with hygiene and skin care.

Client/Family Teaching

- Teach the client and family to perform a bowel reeducation program; scheduled, stimulated program; or other strategies to manage fecal incontinence.
- Teach the client and family about common dietary sources of fiber, as well as supplemental fiber or bulking agents as indicated.
▲ Refer the family to support services to assist with in-home management of fecal incontinence as indicated.
- Teach nursing colleagues and nonprofessional care providers the importance of providing toileting opportunities and adequate privacy for the patient in an acute or long term care facility.
  NOTE: Refer to care plans for **Diarrhea** and **Constipation** for detailed management of these related conditions.

• = **Independent;** ▲ = **Collaborative**

REFERENCES   Arhan P et al: Biofeedback reeducation of fecal incontinence in children, *Int J Colorectal Dis* 9:128-133, 1994.

Birdsall C: Would you put a Foley in the rectum? *Am J Nurs* 9:1050, 1986.

Blair GK et al: The bowel management tube: an effective means for controlling fecal incontinence, *J Pediatr Surg* 27(10):1269-1272, 1992.

Bliss DA et al: Fecal incontinence in hosptialized patients who are acutely ill, *Nurs Res* 49(2):101-107, 2000.

Byers PH et al: Effects of incontinence care cleansing regimens on skin integrity, *J Wound Ostomy Continence Nurs* 22:187-192, 1995.

Chiarioni G et al: Liquid stool incontinence with severe urgency: anorectal function and effective biofeedback treatment, *Gut* 34:1576-1580, 1993.

Doughty DB: A physiologic approach to bowel training, *J Wound Ostomy Continence Nurs* 23:46-56, 1996.

Doughty DB, Broadwell-Jackson D: *Gastrointestinal disorders,* St Louis, 1993, Mosby.

Dunn KL, Galka ML: A comparison of the effectiveness of Therevac SB and bisacodyl suppositories in SCI patients' bowel programs, *Rehabil Nurs* 19:334-338, 1994.

Egan M, Plymad K, Thomas T: Incontinence in patients in two district general hospitals, *Nurs Times* 79:22, 1983.

Enck P et al: Long term efficacy of biofeedback for fecal incontinence, *Dis Colon Rectum* 37:997-1001, 1994.

Fiers S, Thayer D: Management of intractable incontinence. In Doughty DB, editor: *Urinary and fecal incontinence: nursing management,* St Louis, 2000, Mosby, pp 183-207.

Folstein MF, Folstein EF, McHugh P: Mini mental state: a practical method of grading the cognitive status of the patient for the clinician, *J Psychiatr Rev* 12:189-198, 1975.

Gray ML, Burns SM: Continence management, *Crit Care Nurs Clin North Am* 8:29-38, 1996.

Johanson JF, Irizarry F, Doughty A: Risk factors for fecal incontinence in a nursing home population, *J Clin Gastroenterol* 24:156-160, 1997.

Keck JO et al: Biofeedback training is useful in fecal incontinence but disappointing in constipation, *Dis Colon Rectum* 37:1271-1276, 1994.

King JC, Currie DM, Wright E: Bowel training in spina bifida: importance of education, patient compliance, age, and anal reflexes, *Arch Phys Med Rehabil* 75:243-247, 1994.

Leigh RJ, Turnberg LA: Faecal incontinence: the unvoiced symptom, *Lancet* 1:1349-1351, 1982.

Lyder CH et al: Structured skin care regimen to prevent perineal dermatitis in the elderly, *J ET Nurs* 19:12-16, 1992.

McIntosh LJ et al: Pelvic floor rehabilitation in the treatment of incontinence, *J Reprod Med* 38:662-666, 1993.

Munchiando JF, Kendall K: Comparison of the effectiveness of two bowel programs for CVA patients, *Rehabil Nurs* 18:168-172, 1993.

Neelan VJ et al: Use of the NEECHAM confusion scale to assess acute confusional states of hospitalized older patients. In Funk SG et al, editors: Key aspects of elder care: managing falls, incontinence and cognitive impairment, New York, 1992, Springer.

Norton C, Chelvanayagam S: A nursing assessment tool for adult with fecal incontinence. *J Wound Ostomy Continence Nurs* 27: 279, 2000.

O'Donnell BF et al: Incontinence and troublesome behaviors predict institutionalization in dementia, *J Geriatr Psychiatry Neurol* 5:45-52, 1992.

Ouslander JG, Schnelle JF: Predictors of successful prompted voiding among incontinent nursing home residents, *JAMA* 273:1366, 1995.

Resnick NM et al: Short term viability of self report of incontinence in older persons, *J Am Geriatr Soc* 42:202-207, 1994.

Roig Vila JV et al: The defecation habits in a normal working population, *Rev Esp Enferm Dig* 84:224-230, 1993.

Schnelle JF et al: Skin disorders and moisture in incontinent nursing home residents: intervention implications, J Am Geriatr Soc 45:1182-1188, 1997.

Schultz A, Dickey G, Skoner M: Self-report of incontinence in acute care, *Urol Nurs* 17:23-28, 1997.

Smith LJ et al: A behavioral approach to retraining bowel function after long-standing constipation and fecal impaction in people with learning disabilities, *Dev Med Child Neurol* 36:41-49, 1994.

• = **Independent;** ▲ = **Collaborative**

Effective Breastfeeding

Vicki E. McClurg and Virginia R. Wall

NANDA   **Definition** Mother-infant dyad exhibits adequate proficiency and satisfaction with the breastfeeding process

Defining Characteristics

Effective mother/infant communication patterns; regular and sustained suckling/swallowing at the breast; appropriate infant weight pattern for age; infant content after feeding; mother able to position infant at breast to promote a successful latch-on response; signs and/or symptoms of oxytocin release; adequate infant elimination patterns for age; eagerneess of infant to nurse; maternal verbalization of satisfaction with the breastfeeding process and response

Related Factors (r/t)

Basic breastfeeding knowledge/normal breast structure/normal infant oral structure/infant gestational age >34 weeks/support sources (e.g., encouraging partner, history of positive breastfeeding experiences among relatives and friends, access to support groups such as La Leche League)/maternal confidence

NOC   **Outcomes (Nursing Outcomes Classification)**

Suggested NOC Labels

Breastfeeding Establishment: Infant; Breastfeeding Establishment: Maternal; Breastfeeding Maintenance

> ### Example NOC Outcome
> Accomplishes **Breastfeeding Establishment: Infant** as evidenced by the following indicators: Proper alignment and latch-on/Proper areolar grasp/Proper areolar compression/Correct suck and tongue placement/Swallowing a minimum of 5 to 10 minutes per breast/minimum, eight feedings per day/Six or more urinations per day/Age-appropriate weight gain (Rate each indicator of **Breastfeeding Establishment: Infant:** 1 = not adequate, 2 = slightly adequate, 3 = moderately adequate, 4 = substantially adequate, 5 = Totally adequate [see Section I])

Client Outcomes

- Maintains effective breastfeeding
- Maintains normal growth patterns (infant)
- Verbalizes satisfaction with breastfeeding process (mother)

NIC   **Interventions (Nursing Interventions Classification)**

Suggested NIC Labels

Breastfeeding Assistance

> ### Example NIC Interventions—Breastfeeding Assistance
> - Discuss with parents an estimate of effort and length of time they would like to put toward breastfeeding
> - Provide early mother/infant contact opportunity to breastfeed within 2 hours after birth

• = Independent; ▲ = Collaborative

Nursing Interventions and Rationales

- Assess knowledge regarding basic breastfeeding.

  Support and teaching must be individualized to the client's level of understanding. Women prepare to breastfeed by acquiring information. This exposure to a variety of sources of information is an important predictor of breastfeeding duration (Duffy, Percival, Kershaw, 1997; Trado, Hughes, 1996; Susin et al, 1999; Zimmerman 1999).

- Assess breast and nipple structure.

  Normal nipple and breast structure or early detection and treatment of abnormalities is important for successful breastfeeding (Wilson-Clay, 1996).

- Provide continuous emotional and physical support during labor, and assist client with first attachment at breast within first hour after birth.

  Support during labor is related to increased rates of breastfeeding initiation, decreased symptoms of depression, improved self-esteem, exclusive breastfeeding, and increased sensitivity of the mother to her child's needs. During the quiet-alert state in the first hour following birth, the infant is most likely to latch on successfully. Early breastfeeding has a positive effect on lactation performance. A successful first feeding boosts maternal confidence (Janken et al, 1999; Scott, Klaus, Klaus, 1999).

- Assess client's knowledge of prevention and treatment of common breastfeeding problems.

  Common problems that can lead to early termination of breastfeeding are mainly preventable or can be overcome with assistance and support (Lavergne, 1997; Cox, Turnbull, 1998).

- Monitor breastfeeding process.

  The nurse's presence and involvement allows for early detection of difficulties and fosters success (Pugh, Milligan, 1998).

- Encourage rooming-in and breastfeeding on demand.

  Rooming-in and breastfeeding on demand are positively associated with breastfeeding success (American Academy of Pediatrics, 1997; Janken et al, 1999).

- Encourage frequent and unlimited suckling times.

  Frequent and unlimited breastfeeding are positively associated with breastfeeding success (Janken et al, 1999).

- Evaluate adequacy of infant intake.

  Infant intake can be measured by objective criteria such as number and quality of feedings, infant elimination, and weight gain appropriate for age (Neifert, 1998).

- Avoid supplemental bottle feedings.

  Supplemental feedings can interfere with the infant's desire to breastfeed, increases the risk of allergies, and conveys the subtle message that the mother's breast milk is not adequate. The longer and more exclusively a mother breastfeeds, the greater the health benefits to both her and her infant (American Academy of Pediatrics, 1997; Chezem, Friesen, 1998; Righard, 1998; Janken et al, 1999).

- Assess support person network.

  Social support is an important factor in the choice of breastfeeding and its success. The more affirmation a mother receives from members of her social network the better she copes with breastfeeding (Arlotti et al, 1998; Humphreys, Thompson, Miner, 1998, Tarkka, Paunonen, Laippala, 1999).

- Give praise for positive mother-infant interactions related to breastfeeding.

  Maternal confidence is an important factor in the continuation of breastfeeding (Dennis, Faux, 1999). "Strategies that promote not only the initiation, but also the successful con-

- = **Independent;** ▲ = **Collaborative**

tinuation of breastfeeding, are particularly important in helping the mother achieve competence and mastery in this important aspect of mothering" (Brandt, Andrews, Kvale, 1998).

- Do not provide samples of formula at discharge.
  Commercial discharge packs are associated with poor lactation success, especially in vulnerable subgroups such as first-time mothers and low-income women (Chezem, Friesen, 1998; Zimmerman 1999; Donnelly et al, 2000).
- Provide a nurse-initiated contact within two days of discharge from hospital.
  Outreach of this type is associated with breastfeeding success (American Academy of Pediatrics, 1997; Kuan et al, 1999; Locklin, Jansson, 1999).

Multicultural

- Assess for the influence of cultural beliefs, norms, and values on current breastfeeding practices.
  The client's knowledge of breastfeeding may be based on cultural perceptions, as well as influences from the larger social context (Leininger, 1996).
- Assess for when the mother wishes to begin breastfeeding.
  Usual hospital practice is to begin breastfeeding immediately, but some cultures don't regard colostrum as appropriate for newborns and may prefer to wait until milk is present at about 3 days of age (Pillitteri, 1999).
- Validate the client's concerns about the amount of milk taken. Some cultures may add semisolid food within the first month of life as a result of concerns that the infant is not getting enough to eat and the perception that "big is healthy" (Stuart, Laraia, 2001; Higgins, 2000; Bentley et al, 1999; Giger, Davidhizar, 1995).

Client/Family Teaching

- Include the father and other family members in education about breastfeeding.
  Allaying the misconceptions and the social embarrassment associated with breastfeeding can encourage fathers to be more supportive (Shepherd, Power, Carter, 2000).
- Teach client the importance of maternal nutrition.
  Dieting during lactation can have a negative impact on milk production (Gonzalez-Cossio et al, 1998).
- Teach client to be aware of infant's subtle hunger cues (e.g., quiet-alert state, rooting, sucking, hand-to-mouth activity) and to nurse whenever signs are apparent.
  Feedings are initiated more easily when the infant is hungry and in the quiet-alert state (Brandt, Andrews, Kvale, 1998). The infant brings certain characteristics to the breastfeeding experience, which contribute to breastfeeding success (Milligan et al, 2000).
- Review guidelines for frequency of feedings (every 2 to 3 hours, or at least 8 feedings per 24 hours).
  In the first few days, frequent and regular stimulation of the breasts is important to establish an adequate milk supply (Janken et al, 1999).
- Review guidelines for duration of feeding (e.g., until suckling and swallowing slow down).
  The mother should be taught to use infant cues of satiety rather than arbitrary time limits (Powers, Slusser, 1997).
- Provide anticipatory guidance about common breastfeeding problems.
  Lack of knowledge about detection, prevention, and treatment of these problems can lead to premature termination of breastfeeding (Cox, Turnbull, 1998).

• = Independent; ▲ = Collaborative

- Provide anticipatory guidance about common infant behaviors.
  Lack of knowledge about infant growth spurts, temperament, sleep/wake cycles, and intro-duction of other foods can create parental anxiety and lead to premature termination of breastfeeding (Carey, 1998; Milligan et al, 2000).
- Provide information about additional breastfeeding resources.
  Breastfeeding classes, books, materials, and breastfeeding support groups, which provide current and accurate information, can enhance maternal success and satisfaction with the breastfeeding process (Cox, Turnbull, 1998, Zimmerman, 1999).

WEB SITES FOR EDUCATION

MERLIN See the MERLIN web site for World Wide Web resources for client education.

REFERENCES   American Academy of Pediatrics Work Group on Breastfeeding: Breastfeeding and the use of human milk, *Pediatrics* 100:1035, 1997.

Arlotti JP et al: Breastfeeding among low-income women with and without peer support, *J Community Health Nurs* 15:163, 1998.

Bentley M et al: Infant feeding practices of low-income, African-American, adolescent mothers: an ecologi-cal, multigenerational perspective, *Soc Sci Med* 49(8):1085-1100, 1999.

Brandt KA, Andrews CM, Kvale J: Mother-infant interaction and breast-feeding outcome 6 weeks after birth, *J Obstet Gynecol Neonatal Nurs* 27:169, 1998.

Carey WB: Teaching parents about infant temperament, *Pediatrics* 102(5 suppl E):1311-1316, 1998.

Chezem J, Friesen C: Lactation duration: influences of human milk replacements and formula samples on women planning postpartum employment, *J Obstet Gynecol Neonatal Nurs* 27:646, 1998.

Cox SG, Turnbull CJ: Developing effective interactions to improve breast-feeding outcomes, *Breastfeed Rev* 6(2):11-22, 1998.

Dennis CL, Faux S: Development and psychometric testing of the Breastfeeding Self-Efficacy Scale, *Res Nurs Health* 22(5):399-409, 1999.

Donnelly A et al: Commercial hospital discharge packs for breastfeeding women, *Cochrane Database Syst Rev* (2):CD002075, 2000.

Duffy EP, Percival P, Kershaw E: Positive effects of an antenatal group teaching session on postnatal nipple pain, nipple trauma and breast feeding rates, *Midwifery* 13(4):189-196, 1997.

Giger JN, Davidhizar RE: *Transcultural nursing,* ed 2, St Louis, 1995, Mosby.

Gonzalez-Cossio T et al: Impact of food supplementation during lactation on infant breast-milk intake and on the proportion of infants exclusively breast-fed, *J Nutr* 128:1692, 1998.

Higgins B: Puerto Rican cultural beliefs: influence on infant feeding practices in western New York, *J Trans-cultural Nurs* 11(1), 2000.

Humphreys AS, Thompson NJ, Miner KR: Intention to breastfeed in low-income pregnant women: the role of social support and previous experience, *Birth* 25(3):169-174, 1998.

Janken JK et al: Changing nursing practice through research utilization: consistent support for breastfeeding mothers, *Appl Nurs Res* 12:22, 1999.

Kuan LW et al: Health system factors contributing to breastfeeding success, *Pediatrics* 104(3):e28, 1999.

Lavergne NA: Does application of tea bags to sore nipples while breastfeeding provide effective relief? *J Obstet Gynecol Neonatal Nurs* 26:53-58, 1997.

Leininger MM: *Transcultural nursing: theories, research and practices,* ed 2, Hilliard, Ohio, 1996, McGraw-Hill.

Locklin MP, Jansson MJ: Home visits: strategies to protect the breastfeeding newborn at risk, *J Obstet Gynecol Neonatal Nurs* 28:33, 1999.

Milligan RA et al: Breastfeeding duration among low income women, *J Midwifery Womens Health* 45(3):246-252, 2000.

Neifert, MR: The optimization of breast-feeding in the perinatal period, *Clin Perinatol* 25(2):303-326. 1998.

• = **Independent;** ▲ = **Collaborative**

Pillitteri A: Nutritional needs of the newborn. In Pillitteri A, editor: *Maternal & child health nursing: care of the childbearing & childrearing family,* Philadelphia, 1999, JB Lippincott.

Powers NG, Slusser W: Breastfeeding update 2: clinical lactation management, *Pediatr Rev* 18:147-161, 1997.

Pugh LC, Milligan RA: Nursing intervention to increase the duration of breastfeeding, *Appl Nurs Res* 11:190, 1998.

Righard L: Are breastfeeding problems related to incorrect breastfeeding technique and the use of pacifiers and bottles? *Birth* 25:40, 1998.

Scott KD, Klaus PH, Klaus MH: The obstetrical and postpartum benefits of continuous support during childbirth, *J Womens Health Gend Based Med* 8(10):1257-1264, 1999.

Shepherd CK, Power KG, Carter H: Examining the correspondence of breastfeeding and bottle-feeding couples' infant feeding attitudes, *J Adv Nurs* 31(3):651-660, 2000.

Stuart GW, Laraia MT: Therapeutic nurse-patient relationship. In Stuart GW, Laraia MT, editors: *Principles and practice of psychiatric nursing,* St Louis, 2001, Mosby, p 30.

Susin LR et al: Does parental breastfeeding knowledge increase breastfeeding rates? *Birth* 26(3):149-156, 1999.

Tarkka MT, Paunonen M, Laippala P: Factors related to successful breastfeeding by first-time mothers when the child is 3 months old, *J Adv Nurs* 29(1):113-118, 1999.

Trado MG, Hughes RB: A phenomenological study of breastfeeding WIC recipients in South Carolina, *Adv Pract Nurs* Q 2:31, 1996.

Wilson-Clay B: Clinical use of silicone nipple shields, *J Hum Lact* 12(4):279-285, 1996.

Zimmerman DR: You can make a difference: increasing breastfeeding rates in an inner-city clinic, *J Hum Lact* 15(3):217-220, 1999.

Ineffective Breastfeeding

Vicki E. McClurg and Virginia R. Wall

NANDA   **Definition** Dissatisfaction or difficulty a mother, infant, or child experiences with the breastfeeding process

Defining Characteristics

Unsatisfactory breastfeeding process; nonsustained suckling at the breast; resisting latching on; unresponsive to comfort measures; persistence of sore nipples beyond first week of breastfeeding; observable signs of inadequate infant intake; insufficient emptying of each breast per feeding; infant inability to latch on to maternal breast correctly; infant arching and crying at the breast; infant exhibiting fussiness and crying within the first hour after breastfeeding; actual or perceived inadequate milk supply; no observable signs of oxytocin release; insufficient opportunity for suckling at the breast

Related Factors (r/t)

Nonsupportive partner/family; previous breast surgery; infant receiving supplemental feedings with artificial nipple; prematurity; previous history of breastfeeding failure; poor infant sucking reflex; maternal breast anomaly; maternal anxiety or ambivalence; interruption in breastfeeding; infant anomaly; knowledge deficit

NOC   **Outcomes (Nursing Outcomes Classification)**

Suggested NOC Labels

Breastfeeding Establishment: Infant; Breastfeeding Establishment: Maternal; Breastfeeding Maintenance; Breastfeeding Weaning; Knowledge: Breastfeeding

 • = Independent; ▲ = Collaborative

Example NOC Outcome
Accomplishes **Breastfeeding Establishment: Infant** as evidenced by the following indicators: Proper alignment and latch on/Proper areolar grasp/Proper areolar compression/Correct suck and tongue placement/Swallowing a minimum of 5 to 10 minutes per breast/Minimum eight feedings per day/Six or more urinations per day/ Age appropriate weight gain (Rate each indicator of **Breastfeeding Establishment: Infant:** 1 = not adequate, 2 = slightly adequate, 3 = moderately adequate, 4 = substantially adequate, 5 = totally adequate [see Section I])

Client Outcomes

- Achieves effective breastfeeding
- Verbalizes/demonstrates techniques to manage breastfeeding problems
- Infant manifests signs of adequate intake at the breast
- Mother manifests positive self-esteem in relation to the infant feeding process
- Mother explains a safe alternative method of infant feeding if unable to continue exclusive breastfeeding

NIC Interventions (Nursing Interventions Classification)

Suggested NIC Labels
Breastfeeding Assistance

Example NIC Interventions—Breastfeeding Assistance
- Discuss with parents an estimate of effort and length of time they would like to put toward breastfeeding
- Provide early mother/infant contact opportunity to breastfeed within 2 hours after birth

Nursing Interventions and Rationales

Refer to care plan for **Effective Breastfeeding**

- Assess for presence/absence of related factors or conditions that would preclude breastfeeding.
  Some conditions (e.g., certain maternal drugs, maternal HIV-positive status, infant galactosemia) may preclude breastfeeding, in which case the infant needs to be started on a safe alternative method of feeding (Riordan, Auerbach, 2000; Lawrence, 2000).
- Assess breast and nipple structure.
  Normal nipple and breast structure or early detection and treatment of abnormalities with continuing support are important for successful breastfeeding (Vogel, Hutchison, Mitchell, 1999).
- Evaluate and record the mother's ability to position, give cues, and help the infant latch on.
  Correct positioning and getting the infant to latch on is critical for getting breastfeeding off to a good start and contributes to breastfeeding success (Duffy, Percival, Kershaw, 1997; Brandt, Andrews, Kvale, 1998).
- Evaluate and record the infant's ability to properly grasp and compress the areola with lips, tongue, and jaw.
  The infant must have a "competent suck" in order to achieve successful breastfeeding. The jaws must compress the milk sinuses beneath the areola. To do this the jaws must be well back on the areola with the tongue over the lower gum, forming a trough around the

• = Independent; ▲ = Collaborative

breast, and the lips must be flanged and sealed around the breast (Palmer, VandenBerg, 1998; Lau, Hurst, 1999; Hill, Kurkowski, Garcia, 2000).

- Evaluate and record the infant's suckling and swallowing pattern at the breast.
  When the infant sucks adequately, there is muscular movement visible above the ears. When breast milk is actively flowing, infants suck at a rate of once per second, and swallowing increases as milk supply increases (Palmer, VandenBerg, 1998; Lau, Hurst, 1999; Hill, Kurkowski, Garcia, 2000).
- Evaluate and record signs of oxytocin release.
  The let-down reflex (tingling sensation in the breasts, milk dripping from the breasts, and uterine cramping) is indication of oxytocin release and is necessary for transfer of milk to the infant (Uvnas-Moberg, Eriksson, 1996; Nissen et al, 1998; Neville, 1999).
- Evaluate and record infant's state at the time of feeding.
  Infants breastfeed best when in the quiet-alert state. Difficulties arise when trying to breastfeed a sleepy infant or a ravenously hungry and crying infant (Brandt, Andrews, Kvale, 1998).
- Assess knowledge regarding psychophysiology of lactation and specific treatment measures for underlying problems.
  Support and teaching must be individualized to the client's level of understanding. The mother must acquire knowledge and become cognitively and emotionally ready (Cox, Turnbull, 1998).
- Assess psychosocial factors that may contribute to ineffective breastfeeding (e.g., anxiety, goals and values/lifestyle that contribute to ambivalence about breastfeeding).
  The attitude of the mother toward breastfeeding is critical in achieving successful lactation, influencing milk production, and facilitating the art of breastfeeding (Brandt, Andrews, Kvale, 1998).
- Assess support person network.
  Social support is an important factor in successful breastfeeding (Trado, Hughes, 1996; Arlotti et al, 1998).
- Promote comfort and relaxation to reduce pain and anxiety.
  Discomfort associated with breastfeeding can cause some women to discontinue breastfeeding prematurely. Promoting comfort and relaxation can lead to more successful breastfeeding (Lavergne, 1997).
- Provide support by actively helping the mother to correctly position the baby to attain a good latch on the nipple and encouraging her to continue trying.
  Many problems that can lead to discontinuing breastfeeding can be prevented by giving a high level of practical and emotional support to the mother (Janken et al, 1999).
- Bring infant to a quiet-alert state through alerting techniques (e.g., provide variety in auditory, visual, and kinesthetic stimuli by unwrapping the infant, placing the infant upright, or talking to the infant) or consoling techniques as needed.
  A variety of stimuli can bring the infant to a quiet-alert state. Repetition can soothe a crying baby, thus making it easier to initiate breastfeeding (Brandt, Andrews, Kvale, 1998).
- Enhance the flow of milk. Teach the mother to massage breast or burp infant and switch to other breast when infant's swallowing slows down.
  The perception of inadequate milk supply can lead to early weaning. Infants should breastfeed from both breasts at each feeding. Breast massage can enhance the flow of milk and stimulate production (Riordan, Auerbach, 2000).

• = **Independent**; ▲ = **Collaborative**

- Evaluate adequacy of infant intake.
  Infant intake can be measured by objective criteria such as number and quality of feedings, infant elimination and weight gain appropriate for age, as well as test-weights when necessary (Meier et al, 2000).
- Discourage supplemental bottle feedings and encourage exclusive, effective breastfeeding.
  Supplemental feedings can interfere with the infant's desire to breastfeed, increase the risk of allergies, and convey the subtle message that the mother's breast milk is not adequate (American Academy of Pediatrics, 1997; Chezem et al, 1998).
- Acknowledge mother's feelings and support her decision to continue or choose an alternate plan.
  Mastering infant feeding is an important first step in mothering, and the mother needs to be empowered so that she feels competent and capable of making intelligent decisions (Brandt, Andrews, Kvale, 1998; Mozingo et al, 2000).
- ▲ Make appropriate referrals and ensure close follow-up.
  Collaborative practice with neonatal nutritionists, physical or occupational therapist, home visiting nurses, or lactation specialists will help ensure feeding and parenting success (American Academy of Pediatrics, 1997; Pugh, Milligan, 1998; Locklin, Jansson, 1999).
- If unsuccessful in achieving effective breastfeeding, help client accept and learn an alternate method of infant feeding.
  Once the decision has been made to provide an alternate method of infant feeding, the mother needs support and education (Brandt, Andrews, Kvale, 1998; Mozingo et al, 2000).

Multicultural

- Assess for the influence of cultural beliefs, norms, and values on breastfeeding attitudes.
  The client's knowledge of breastfeeding may be based on cultural perceptions, as well as influences from the larger social context (Leininger, 1996).
- Assess whether the client's concerns about the amount of milk taken during breastfeeding is contributing to dissatisfaction with the breastfeeding process.
  Some cultures may add semisolid food within the first month of life as a result of concerns that the infant is not getting enough to eat and the perception that "big is healthy" (Higgins, 2000; Bentley et al, 1999).
- Assess the influence of family support on the decision to continue or discontinue breastfeeding.
  Women are the keepers and transmitters of culture in families. Female family members can play a dominant role in how infants are fed (Pillitteri, 1999).
- Validate the client's feelings regarding the difficulty or dissatisfaction with breastfeeding.
  Validation lets the client know that the nurse has heard and understands what was said and promotes the nurse-client relationship (Stuart, Laraia, 2001; Giger, Davidhizar, 1995).

Client/Family Teaching

- Provide instruction in correct positioning.
  "Correct positioning is perhaps the most critical single measure for getting breastfeeding off to a good start. Many problems can be attributed to carelessness or inattention to this simple aspect of breastfeeding" (Righard, 1998).
- Reinforce and add to knowledge base regarding underlying problems and specific treatment measures.

• = **Independent**; ▲ = **Collaborative**

If mother understands rationale for recommended treatment, she may be more likely to comply with recommendations and less likely to perceive the problem as insurmountable (Cox, Turnbull, 1998; Susin et al, 1999).

- Provide education to support persons as needed.

Informational support providers help the mother achieve a more positive outcome (Trado, Hughes, 1996; Tarkka, Paunonen, Laippala, 1999; Zimmerman 1999).

WEB SITES FOR EDUCATION

See the MERLIN web site for World Wide Web resources for client education.

REFERENCES American Academy of Pediatrics Work Group on Breastfeeding: Breastfeeding and the use of human milk, *Pediatrics* 100:1035, 1997.

Arlotti JP et al: Breastfeeding among low-income women with and without peer support, *J Community Health Nurs* 15:163, 1998.

Bentley M et al: Infant feeding practices of low-income, African-American, adolescent mothers: an ecological, multigenerational perspective, *Soc Sci Med* 49(8):1085-1100, 1999.

Brandt KA, Andrews CM, Kvale J: Mother-infant interaction and breastfeeding outcome 6 weeks after birth, *J Obstet Gynecol Neonatal Nurs* 27:169, 1998.

Chezem J et al: Lactation duration: influences of human milk replacements and formula samples on women planning postpartum employment, *J Obstet Gynecol Neonatal Nurs* 27:646, 1998.

Cox SG, Turnbull CJ: Developing effective interactions to improve breastfeeding outcomes, *Breastfeeding Rev* 6(2):11-22, 1998.

Duffy EP, Percival P, Kershaw E: Positive effects of an antenatal group teaching session on postnatal nipple pain, nipple trauma and breastfeeding rates, *Midwifery* 13(4):189-196, 1997.

Giger JN, Davidhizar RE: *Transcultural nursing,* ed 2, St Louis, 1995, Mosby.

Higgins, B: Puerto Rican cultural beliefs: influence on infant feeding practices in western New York, *J Transcultural Nurs* 11(1), 2000.

Hill AS, Kurkowski TB, Garcia J: Oral support measures used in feeding the preterm infant, *Nurs Res* 49(1):2-10, 2000.

Janken JK et al: Changing nursing practice through research utilization: consistent support for breastfeeding mothers, *Appl Nurs Res* 12:22, 1999.

Lavergne NA: Does application of tea bags to sore nipples while breastfeeding provide effective relief? *J Obstet Gynecol Neonatal Nurs* 26:53-58, 1997.

Lau C, Hurst N: Oral feeding in infants, *Curr Probl Pediatr* 29(4):105-124, 1999.

Lawrence RA: Breastfeeding: benefits, risks and alternatives, *Curr Opin Obstet Gynecol* 12(6):519-524, 2000.

Leininger MM: *Transcultural nursing: theories, research and practices,* ed 2, Hilliard, Ohio, 1996, McGraw-Hill.

Locklin MP, Jansson MJ: Home visits: strategies to protect the breastfeeding newborn at risk, *J Obstet Gynecol Neonatal Nurs* 28:33, 1999.

Meier PP et al: Nipple shields for preterm infants: effect on milk transfer and duration of breastfeeding, *J Hum Lact* 16(2):106-114, quiz 129-131, 2000.

Mozingo JN et al: "It wasn't working": women's experiences with short-term breastfeeding, *MCN Am J Matern Child Nurs* 25(3):120-126, 2000.

Neville MC: Physiology of lactation, *Clin Perinatol* 26(2):251-279, 1999.

Nissen E et al: Oxytocin, prolactin, milk production and their relationship with personality traits in women after vaginal delivery or Cesarean section, *J Psychosom Obstet Gynaecol* 19:49, 1998.

North American Nursing Diagnosis Association: *Taxonomy 1,* St Louis, 1990 (revised), NANDA.

Palmer MM, VandenBerg KA: A closer look at neonatal sucking, *Neonatal Netw* 17(2):77-79, 1998.

Pillitteri A: Nutritional needs of the newborn. In Pillitteri A, editor: *Maternal & child health nursing: care of the childbearing & childrearing family,* Philadelphia, 1999, JB Lippincott.

Pugh LC, Milligan RA: Nursing intervention to increase the duration of breastfeeding, *Appl Nurs Res* 11:190, 1998.

• = Independent; ▲ = Collaborative

Righard L: Are breastfeeding problems related to incorrect breastfeeding technique and the use of pacifiers and bottles? *Birth* 25:40, 1998.

Riordan J, Auerbach KG: *Breastfeeding and human lactation,* ed 2, Boston, 2000, Jones and Bartlett.

Stuart GW, Laraia MT: Therapeutic nurse-patient relationship. In Stuart GW, Laraia MT, editors: *Principles and practice of psychiatric nursing,* St Louis, 2001, Mosby, p 30.

Susin LR et al: Does parental breastfeeding knowledge increase breastfeeding rates? *Birth* 26(3):149-156, 1999.

Tarkka MT, Paunonen M, Laippala P: Factors related to successful breastfeeding by first-time mothers when the child is 3 months old, *J Adv Nurs* 29(1):113-118, 1999.

Trado MG, Hughes RB: A phenomenological study of breastfeeding WIC recipients in South Carolina, *Adv Pract Nurs Q* 2:31, 1996.

Uvnas-Moberg K, Eriksson M: Breastfeeding: physiological, endocrine and behavioural adaptations caused by oxytocin and local neurogenic activity in the nipple and mammary gland, *Acta Paediatr* 85(5):525-530, 1996.

Vogel A, Hutchison BL, Mitchell EA: Factors associated with the duration of breastfeeding, *Acta Paediatr* 88(12):1320-1326, 1999.

Zimmerman DR: You can make a difference: increasing breastfeeding rates in an inner-city clinic, *J Hum Lact* 15(3):217-220, 1999.

Interrupted Breastfeeding

Vicki E. McClurg and Virginia R. Wall

NANDA   **Definition** Break in the continuity of the breastfeeding process as a result of inability or inadvisability to put baby to breast for feeding

Defining Characteristics

Infant does not receive nourishment at the breast for some or all feedings; maternal desire to maintain lactation and provide (or eventually provide) her breast milk for her infant's nutritional needs; separation of mother and infant; lack of knowledge regarding expression and storage of breast milk

Related Factors (r/t)

Maternal or infant illness; prematurity; maternal employment; contraindications to breastfeeding (e.g., drugs, true breast milk jaundice); need to abruptly wean infant (with intent to resume at later date)

NOC   ## Outcomes (Nursing Outcomes Classification)

Suggested NOC Labels

Breastfeeding Establishment: Infant; Breastfeeding Establishment: Maternal; Breastfeeding Maintenance; Knowledge: Breastfeeding; Parent-Infant Attachment

> **Example NOC Outcome**
> Accomplishes **Breastfeeding Establishment: Infant** as evidenced by the following indicators: Proper alignment and latch on/Proper areolar grasp/Proper areolar compression/Correct suck and tongue placement/Swallowing a minimum of 5 to 10 minutes per breast/Minimum eight feedings per day/Six or more urinations per day/ Age appropriate weight gain (Rate each indicator of **Breastfeeding Establishment: Infant:** 1 = not adequate, 2 = slightly adequate, 3 = moderately adequate, 4 = substantially adequate, 5 = totally adequate [see Section I])

• = Independent; ▲ = Collaborative

Client Outcomes

Infant

- Receives mother's breast milk if not contraindicated by maternal conditions (e.g. certain drugs, infections) or infant conditions (e.g. true breast milk jaundice)

Maternal

- Initiates or maintains lactation
- Achieves effective breastfeeding or satisfaction with the breastfeeding experience
- Demonstrates effective methods of breast milk collection and storage

NIC Interventions (Nursing Interventions Classification)

Suggested NIC Labels

Bottle Feeding; Emotional Support; Lactation Counseling

> **Example NIC Interventions—Lactation Counseling**
> - Instruct parents on how to differentiate between perceived and actual insufficient milk supply
> - Provide formula information for temporary low supply problems

Nursing Interventions and Rationales

- Evaluate and record mother's desire to begin or continue breastfeeding.
  Maternal commitment to breastfeed is associated with breastfeeding success (Brandt, Andrews, Kvale, 1998; Hill, 2000; Mozingo et al, 2000).
- Evaluate advisability of initiating or reinstituting breastfeeding.
  Some conditions (e.g., certain maternal drugs; HIV-positive status; active, untreated tuberculosis; infant galactosemia) may be contraindications to breastfeeding. Some conditions (e.g., infant cleft palate or maternal breast surgery) may make it difficult to exclusively breastfeed (Lawrence, Howard, 1999; Riordan, Auerbach, 1999; Davis, Okuboye, Ferguson, 2000; Lawrence, 2000).
- Evaluate infant's ability to breastfeed and interest in breastfeeding.
  The infant must be able to demonstrate the ability to breastfeed and interest in breastfeeding in order for the mother to reinstitute breastfeeding. The interplay between mother and baby is an important factor in breastfeeding success (Williams, 1997; Meyer, Anderson, 1999; Thoyre, 2000).
- Evaluate whether the mother is being supported in her decision to continue breastfeeding.
  Relactating after an interruption is often stressful; the mother will benefit from social support of her efforts (Trado, Hughes, 1996; Mozingo et al, 2000).
- Assess the mother's emotional response to events that caused interruption.
  Feelings of grief, guilt, anxiety, and failure are common and may need to be addressed for breastfeeding to be successful (Kavanaugh et al, 1997; Seideman et al, 1997; Brandt, Andrews, Kvale, 1998; Mozingo et al, 2000).
- Develop a satisfactory feeding plan with the mother to allow for continued breastfeeding. This may include Kangaroo Care for part of each day.
  Involvement of the mother in planning helps her to feel as though she is able to participate in caretaking (Baker, Rasmussen, 1997; Kavanaugh et al, 1997; Meyer, Anderson, 1999; Griffin et al, 2000; Thoyre, 2000).

• = Independent; ▲ = Collaborative

- Assess and record mother's knowledge of breast milk expression techniques.
  During interruption, the mother needs to maintain lactation by expressing milk via either hand expression or via manual or electric breast pumping (Hill, Aldag, Chatterton, 1996, 1999; Baker, Rasmussen, 1997).
- Assess and record mother's knowledge of how to handle (store, transport) breast milk safely.
  If expressed breast milk is to be fed to infant, mother must demonstrate storage and handling techniques which ensure that milk remains fresh and uncontaminated (Baker, Rasmussen, 1997; Gromada, Spangler, 1998; Riordan, Auerbach, 2001; Guttman, Zimmerman, 2000).
- Assess equipment needs.
  The health care professional needs to base pumping recommendations on each mother's situation and needs (Biancuzzo, 1999; Hill, Aldag, Chatterton, 1999; Riordan, Auerbach, 2001; Guttmann, Zimmerman, 2000).
- Provide resource information (support groups, equipment and supply rental or sales).
  The mother needs to have this information to enable her to follow through on plan of care and receive support as needed (Trado, Hughes, 1996; Biancuzzo, 1999).
- ▲ Help mother identify and obtain social support.
  Support is important to mothers of high-risk infants, and they may need assistance with identifying individuals in their social network who could help provide that support (Logsdon, Davis, 1998).
- ▲ Make appropriate referrals and ensure close follow-up.
  Collaborative practice with neonatal nutritionists, physical or occupational therapist, home visiting nurses, or lactation specialists will help ensure feeding and parenting success (American Academy of Pediatrics, 1997; Elliott, Reimer, 1998; Pugh, Milligan, 1998; Locklin, Jansson, 1999).
- Promote emotional resolution through encouragement to verbalize feelings.
  Mother should be encouraged that breastfeeding can be a rewarding experience (Kavanaugh et al, 1997; Brandt, Andrews, Kvale, 1998; Mozingo et al, 2000).

Multicultural

- Assess for the influence of cultural beliefs, norms, and values on current decision to stop breastfeeding.
  The client's decision to halt breastfeeding may be based on cultural perceptions, as well as influences from the larger social context (Leininger, 1996).
- Assess the influence of family support on the decision to continue or discontinue breastfeeding.
  Women are the keepers and transmitters of culture in families. Female family members can play a dominant role in how infants are fed (Pillitteri, 1999).
- Assess whether the client's concerns about the amount of milk taken during breastfeeding is contributing to decision to stop breastfeeding.
  Some cultures may add semisolid food within the first month of life as a result of concerns that the infant is not getting enough to eat and the perception that "big is healthy" (Higgins, 2000; Bentley et al, 1999).
- Validate the client's feelings with regard to the difficulty of or her dissatisfaction with breastfeeding.
  Validation lets the client know that the nurse has heard and understands what was said and promotes the nurse-client relationship (Stuart, Laraia, 2001; Giger, Davidhizar, 1995).

• = **Independent**; ▲ = **Collaborative**

Client/Family Teaching

- Teach mother effective methods to express breast milk.

  The mother needs to be taught how to continue lactation during the interruption of breastfeeding (Furman, Minich, Hack, 1998; Biancuzzo, 1999).

- Teach mother safe breast milk handling techniques.

  The mother needs to be taught how to handle breast milk so that she can provide a safe product for her infant (Baker, Rasmussen, 1997; Gromada, Spangler, 1998; Guttman, Zimmerman, 2000).

- Provide anticipatory guidance for common problems associated with interrupted breastfeeding (e.g., incomplete emptying of milk glands, diminishing milk supply, infant difficulty with resuming breastfeeding, or infant refusal of alternative feeding method).

  Knowing what to expect will help the mother cope with any difficulties that may arise (Chezem et al, 1998; Furman, Minich, Hack, 1998; Kliethermes et al, 1999; Thoyre, 2000).

- Provide education to support persons as needed.

  Informational support providers help the mother achieve a more positive outcome (Trado, Hughes, 1996; Logsdon, Davis, 1998; Guttman, Zimmerman, 2000; Hill, 2000).

WEB SITES FOR EDUCATION

MERLIN   See the MERLIN web site for World Wide Web resources for client education.

REFERENCES   American Academy of Pediatrics Work Group on Breastfeeding: Breastfeeding and the use of human milk, *Pediatrics* 100:1035, 1997.

Baker BJ, Rasmussen TW: Organizing and documenting lactation support of NICU families, *J Obstet Gynecol Neonatal Nurs* 26:515, 1997.

Bentley M et al: Infant feeding practices of low-income, African-American, adolescent mothers: an ecological, multigenerational perspective, *Soc Sci Med* 49(8):1085-1100, 1999.

Biancuzzo M: Selecting pumps for breastfeeding mothers, *J Obstet Gynecol Neonatal Nurs* 28:417-426, 1999.

Brandt KA, Andrews CM, Kvale J: Mother-infant interaction and breastfeeding outcome 6 weeks after birth, *J Obstet Gynecol Neonatal Nurs* 27:169, 1998.

Chezem J, Friesen C: Lactation duration: influences of human milk replacements and formula samples on women planning postpartum employment, *J Obstet Gynecol Neonatal Nurs* 27:646-651, 1998.

Davis LJ, Okuboye S, Ferguson SL: Healthy people 2010: examining a decade of maternal & infant health, *AWHONN Lifelines* 4(3):26-33, 2000.

Elliott S, Reimer C: Postdischarge telephone follow-up program for breastfeeding preterm infants dischaged from a special care nursery, *Neonatal Netw* 17(6):41-45, 1998.

Furman L, Minich NM, Hack M: Breastfeeding of very low birth weight infants, *J Hum Lact* 14(1):29-34, 1998.

Giger JN, Davidhizar RE: *Transcultural nursing*, ed 2, St Louis, 1995, Mosby.

Griffin TL et al: Mothers' performing creamatocrit measures in the NICU: accuracy, reactions, and cost, *J Obstet Gynecol Neonatal Nurs* 29:249-257, 2000.

Gromada KK, Spangler AK: Breastfeeding twins and higher-order multiples, *J Obstet Gynecol Neonatal Nurs* 27:441-449, 1998.

Guttman N, Zimmerman DR: Low-income mothers' views on breastfeeding, *Soc Sci Med* 50:1457-1473, 2000.

Higgins B: Puerto Rican cultural beliefs: influence on infant feeding practices in western New York, *J Transcultural Nurs* 11(1), 2000.

Hill PD: Update on breastfeeding: healthy people 2010 objectives, *MCN* 25:248-251, 2000.

Hill PD, Aldag JC, Chatterton RT: The effect of sequential and simultaneous breast pumping on milk volume and prolactin levels: a pilot study, *J Hum Lact* 12:193, 1996.

• = Independent; ▲ = Collaborative

Hill PD, Aldag JC, Chatterton RT: Effects of pumping style on milk production in mothers of non-nursing preterm infants, *J Hum Lact* 15:209-216, 1999.

Kavanaugh K et al: The rewards outweigh the efforts: breastfeeding outcomes for mothers of preterm infants, *J Hum Lact* 13:15, 1997.

Kliethermes PA et al: Transitioning preterm infants with nasogastric tube supplementation: increased likelihood of breastfeeding, *J Obstet Gynecol Neonatal Nurs* 28:264-273, 1999.

Lawrence RA: Breastfeeding: benefits, risks and alternatives, *Curr Opin Obstet Gynecol* 12(6):519-524, 2000.

Lawrence RA, Howard CR: Given the benefits of breastfeeding, are there any contraindications? *Clin Perinatol* 26:479-490, 1999.

Leininger MM: *Transcultural nursing: theories, research and practices,* ed 2, Hilliard, Ohio, 1996, McGraw-Hill.

Locklin MP, Jansson MJ: Home visits: strategies to protect the breastfeeding newborn at risk, *J Obstet Gynecol Neonatal Nurs* 28:33, 1999.

Logsdon MC, Davis DW: Guiding mothers of high-risk infants in obtaining social support, *MCN* 23:195-199, 1998.

Meyer K, Anderson GC: Using kangaroo care in a clinical setting with fullterm infants having breastfeeding difficulties, *MCN* 24:190-192, 1999.

Mozingo JN et al: "It wasn't working": women's experiences with short-term breastfeeding, *MCN Am J Matern Child Nurs* 25(3):120-126, 2000.

Pillitteri A: Nutritional needs of the newborn. In Pillitteri A, editor: *Maternal & child health nursing: care of the childbearing & childrearing family,* Philadelphia, 1999, JB Lippincott.

Pugh LC, Milligan RA: Nursing intervention to increase the duration of breastfeeding, *Appl Nurs Res* 11:190, 1998.

Riordan J, Auerbach KG: *Breastfeeding and human lactation,* ed 2, Boston, 2001, Jones and Bartlett.

Seideman RY et al: Parent stress and coping in NICU and PICU, *J Pediatr Nurs* 12:169-177, 1997.

Stuart GW, Laraia MT: Therapeutic nurse-patient relationship. In Stuart GW, Laraia MT, editors: *Principles and practice of psychiatric nursing,* St Louis, 2001, Mosby, p 30.

Thoyre SM: Mothers' ideas about their role in feeding their high-risk infants, *J Obstet Gynecol Neonatal Nurs* 29:613-624, 2000.

Trado MG, Hughes RB: A phenomenological study of breastfeeding WIC recipients in South Carolina, *Adv Pract Nurs Q* 2:31, 1996.

Williams N: Maternal psychological issues in the experience of breastfeeding, *J Hum Lact* 13:57-60, 1997.

Ineffective Breathing pattern

Betty J. Ackley

NANDA   **Definition** Inspiration and/or expiration that does not provide adequate ventilation

Defining Characteristics

Decreased inspiratory/expiratory pressure; decreased minute ventilation; use of accessory muscles to breathe; nasal flaring; dyspnea; altered chest excursion; shortness of breath; assumption of a three-point position; pursed-lip breathing; prolonged expiration phases; increased anteroposterior diameter; respiratory rate (adults <11 or >24; infants <25 or >60; ages 1 to 4 <20 or >30; ages 5 to 14 <14 or >25); depth of breathing (adults V_T 500 ml at rest; infants 6 to 8 ml/kg); timing ratio; decreased vital capacity

Related Factors (r/t)

Hyperventilation; hypoventilation syndrome; bony deformity; pain; chest wall deformity; anxiety; decreased energy/fatigue; neuromuscular dysfunction; musculoskeletal impairment; perception/cognitive impairment; obesity; spinal cord injury; body position; neurological immaturity; respiratory muscle fatigue

• = **Independent**; ▲ = **Collaborative**

NOC **Outcomes (Nursing Outcomes Classification)**

Suggested NOC Labels

Respiratory Status: Ventilation; Vital Signs Status; Respiratory Status: Airway Patency

Example NOC Outcome

Achieves appropriate **Respiratory Status: Ventilation** as evidenced by the following indicators: Respiratory rate IER*/Respiratory rhythm IER/Depth of inspiration/Chest expansion symmetrical/Ease of breathing/Accessory muscle use not present/Chest retraction not present/Ausculated breath sounds IER/Tidal volume IER/Vital capacity IER (Rate each indicator of **Respiratory Status: Ventilation:** 1 = extremely compromised, 2 = substantially compromised, 3 = moderately compromised, 4 = mildly compromised, 5 = not compromised [see Section I])

*In Expected Range

Client Outcomes

- Demonstrates a breathing pattern that supports blood gas results within the client's normal parameters
- Reports ability to breathe comfortably
- Demonstrates ability to perform pursed-lip breathing and controlled breathing and use relaxation techniques effectively
- Identifies and avoids specific factors that exacerbate episodes of ineffective breathing patterns

NIC **Interventions (Nursing Interventions Classification)**

Suggested NIC Labels

Airway Management; Respiratory Monitoring

Example NIC Interventions—Airway Management
- Encourage slow, deep breathing; turning; and coughing
- Monitor respiratory and oxygenation status as appropriate

Nursing Interventions and Rationales

- Monitor respiratory rate, depth, and ease of respiration.
  Normal respiratory rate is 12 to 16 breaths/min in the adult. When the respiratory rate exceeds 24 breaths/min, there is often significant respiratory or cardiovascular disease. See Defining Characteristics for guidelines for children.
- Note pattern of respiration. If client is dyspneic, note what seems to cause the dyspnea, the way in which the client deals with the condition, and how the dyspnea resolves or gets worse.
  A normal respiratory pattern is regular in a healthy adult. To assess dyspnea, it is important to consider all of its dimensions, including antecedents, mediators, reactions, and outcomes (McCord, Cronin-Stubbs, 1992; Meek, 1999).
- ▲ Attempt to determine if client's dyspnea is physiological or psychogenic in cause.
  There are two distinct categories of antecedents to dyspnea: physiological and psychogenic. Psychogenic dyspnea includes dyspnea caused by anxiety, fear, or anger (McCord, Cronin-Stubbs, 1992). Psychogenic dyspnea is commonly known as hyperventilation.

• = **Independent;** ▲ = **Collaborative**

Psychogenic dyspnea–hyperventilation

- Assess cause of hyperventilation by asking client about current emotions and psychological state.
  Hyperventilation can be caused by factors including anxiety, fear, pain, and anger (McCord, Cronin-Stubbs, 1992).
- Ask client to breathe with you to slow down respiratory rate. Maintain eye contact and give reassurance.
  By making the client aware of respirations and giving support, the client may gain control of the breathing rate.
- ▲ Consider having client use a paper bag to breathe into and rebreathe expired air or help to do diaphragmatic breathing.
  Rebreathing air with increased levels of carbon dioxide helps raise the carbon dioxide level in the body and combats the respiratory alkalosis that follows hyperventilation (Forrest, Ricketts, 1995).
- ▲ If pain is the cause of hyperventilation, provide medication routinely as ordered to prevent severe pain. Use distraction techniques to help client deal with pain. See interventions for **Acute Pain.**
  An increased respiratory rate is one sign of pain. Providing pain relief will cause the respiratory rate to return to normal.
- ▲ If client has chronic problems with hyperventilation, numbness and tingling in extremities, dizziness, and other signs of panic attacks, refer for counseling.
  Cognitive behavioral therapy for hyperventilation and panic attacks has been shown to be beneficial (Forrest, Ricketts, 1995).

Physiological dyspnea

- ▲ Ensure that client in acute dyspneic state has received medications, oxygen, and any other treatment needed.
  Pharmacological treatment of dyspnea exists but may not suffice to relieve dyspnea (Bruera et al, 2000; Janssens, 2000).
- Determine severity of dyspnea using a rating scale such as the modified Borg scale, rating dyspnea 0 (best) to 10 (worst) in severity. An alternative scale is the the Visual Analogue Scale (VAS) with dyspnea rated as 0 (best) to 100 (worst).
  In a study in an emergency room, the modified Borg scale correlated well with clinical measurements of respiratory function and was found helpful by both clients and nurses (Kendrick, Baxi, and Smith, 2000). Another study comparing the Borg and the VAS scales found that they measured symptoms reproducibly during steady-state exercise and can detect the effect of a drug intervention (Grant et al, 1999).
- Using touch on the shoulder, coach the client to slow respiratory rate, demonstrating slower respirations; making eye contact with the client; and communicating in a calm, supportive fashion.
  Anxiety can exacerbate dyspnea, causing the client to enter into a dyspneic panic state (Gift, Moore, Soeken, 1992; Bruera et al, 2000). The nurse's presence, reassurance, and help in controlling the client's breathing can be very beneficial (Truesdell, 2000).
- Demonstrate and encourage the client to use pursed-lip breathing.
  Pursed-lip breathing results in increased use of intercostal muscles, decreased respiratory rate, increased tidal volume, and improved oxygen saturation levels (Breslin, 1992). Pursed-lip breathing can result in increased exercise performance (Casciari et al, 1981), and it empowers the client to self manage dyspnic incidences (Truesdell, 2000).

- **= Independent; ▲ = Collaborative**

- Note abdominal breathing, use of accessory muscles, nasal flaring, retractions, irritability, confusion, or lethargy.
  These symptoms signal increasing respiratory difficulty and increasing hypoxia.
- Observe color of tongue, oral mucosa, and skin.
  Cyanosis of the tongue and oral mucosa is central cyanosis and generally represents a medical emergency. Peripheral cyanosis of nail beds or lips may or may not be serious (Carpenter, 1993).
- Auscultate breath sounds, noting decreased or absent sounds, crackles, or wheezes.
  These abnormal lung sounds can indicate a respiratory pathology associated with an altered breathing pattern.
- ▲ Monitor client's oxygen saturation and blood gases.
  An oxygen saturation of less than 90% (normal being 95% to 100%) or a Po_2 of less than 80 mm Hg (normal being 80 to 100 mm Hg) indicates significant oxygenation problems that may result in altered breathing patterns.
- ▲ Monitor for presence of pain and provide pain medication for comfort as needed.
  Pain causes the client to hyperventilate and take shallow breaths that predispose the client to atelectasis.
- Position client in an upright or semi-Fowler's position.
  *An upright position facilitates lung expansion. See nursing interventions for **Impaired Gas exchange** for further information on positioning.*
- ▲ Administer oxygen as ordered.
  Oxygen therapy helps decrease dyspnea through reduction in the central drive mediated via peripheral chemoreceptors in the carotid body (Meek, 1999).
- ▲ Increase client's activity to walking 3 times per day as tolerated. Assist client to use oxygen during activity as needed.
  *See nursing interventions for **Activity intolerance.** Supervised exercise has been shown to decrease dyspnea and increase tolerance to activity (Meek, 1999).*
- Schedule rest periods before and after activity.
  Respiratory clients with dyspnea are easily exhausted and need additional rest.
- ▲ Evaluate client's nutritional status. Refer to a dietitian if needed. Use nutritional supplements to increase nutritional level if need indicated.
  Improved nutrition may help increase inspiratory muscle function and decrease dyspnea (Meek, 1999).
- Provide small, frequent feedings.
  Small feedings are given to avoid compromising ventilatory effort and to conserve energy. Clients with dyspnea often do not eat sufficient amounts of food because their priority is breathing.
- Offer a fan to move the air in the environment.
  The movement of cool air on the face may help relieve dyspnea in pulmonary clients (Meek, 1999).
- Encourage client to take deep breaths at prescribed intervals and do controlled coughing.
- Help the client with chronic respiratory disease to evaluate dypnea experience to determine if similar to previous incidences of dyspnea and to recognize that he or she made it through those incidences.
  The focus of attention on sensations of breathlessness has an impact on judgment used to determine the intensity of the sensation (Meek, 2000).

• = Independent; ▲ = Collaborative

- See **Ineffective Airway clearance** if client has a problem with increased respiratory secretions.
- ▲ If chronic pulmonary disease is interfering with quality of life, refer client for pulmonary rehabilitation. Pulmonary rehabilitation programs that include desensitization to dyspnea and guided mastery with monitored exercise are preferable.
  Pulmonary rehabilitation has been shown to improve exercise capacity, ability to walk, and sense of well-being (Fishman, 1994; American Thoracic Society, 1999; Janssens, 2000). The processes of desensitization and guided mastery for control of dyspnea have helped clients learn to be in control of their condition and have increased the amount of activity they can tolerate (Carrieri-Kohlman et al, 1993).

Geriatric

- Encourage ambulation as tolerated.
  Immobility is often harmful to the elderly because it decreases ventilation and increases stasis of secretions (Foyt, 1992; Tempkin, Tempkin, Goodman, 1997).
- Encourage elderly clients to sit upright or stand and to avoid lying down for prolonged periods during the day.
  Thoracic aging results in decreased lung expansion; an erect position fosters maximal lung expansion.

Home Care Interventions

- Assist client and family with identifying other factors that precipitate or exacerbate episodes of ineffective breathing patterns (i.e., stress, allergens, stairs, activities that have high energy requirements).
  Awareness of precipitating factors helps clients avoid them and decreases risk of episodes.
- Assess client knowledge of and compliance with medication regimen.
- ▲ Teach client and family the importance of maintaining regimen and having prn drugs easily accessible at all times.
  Appropriate and timely use of medications can decrease the risk of exacerbating ineffective breathing.
- Assess coping skills and refer client for counseling if necessary.
  Many clients with chronic respiratory disease develop depression.
- ▲ Identify an emergency plan including when to call the physician or 911.
  Having a ready emergency plan reassures the client and promotes client safety.
- ▲ Refer client to outpatient pulmonary rehabilitation program or a home-based training program for COPD.
  Outpatient rehabilitation programs can achieve worthwhile benefits including decreased perception of dyspnea, increased walking distance, and less fatigue, with benefits persisting for as long as 2 years (Glell et al, 2000). A simple home-based program of exercise training can help COPD patients achieve improvement in exercise tolerance, dyspnea, and quality of life (Hernandez et al, 2000).
- ▲ Refer to occupational therapy for evaluation and teaching of energy conservation techniques.
- ▲ Refer for home health aide services as needed to support energy conservation.
  Energy conservation decreases the risk of exacerbating ineffective breathing.
- Provide family with support for care of client with chronic or terminal illness.
  Severe compromise to respiratory function creates fear in clients and caregivers. Excessive fear inhibits effective coping.

- = **Independent;** ▲ = **Collaborative**

Client/Family Teaching

- Teach pursed-lip and controlled breathing techniques.
  Pursed-lip breathing results in increased use of intercostal muscles, decreased respiratory rate, increased tidal volume, and improved oxygen saturation levels (Breslin, 1992).
- Using a prerecorded tape, teach client progressive muscle relaxation techniques.
  Relaxation therapy can help reduce dyspnea and anxiety (Gift, Moore, Soeken, 1992).
- Teach about dosage, actions, and side effects of medications.
  Inhaled steroids and bronchodilators can have undesirable side effects, especially when taken in inappropriate doses.
- Teach client to identify and avoid specific factors that exacerbate ineffective breathing patterns, such as exposure to other sources of air pollution (especially smoking).

WEB SITES FOR EDUCATION

$\mathcal{Merlin}$ See the MERLIN web site for World Wide Web resources for client education.

REFERENCES American Thoracic Society: Pulmonary rehabilitation—1999, *Am J Respir Crit Care Med* 159(5 Pt 1):1666-1682, 1999.

Breslin EH: The pattern of respiratory muscle recruitment during pursed-lip breathing, *Chest* 101(1):75-78, 1992.

Bruera E et al: The frequency and correlates of dyspnea in patients with advanced cancer, *J Pain Symptom Manage* 19(5):357-362, 2000.

Carpenter KD: A comprehensive review of cyanosis, *Crit Care Nurse* 13:66, 1993.

Carrieri-Kohlman V et al: Desensitization and guided mastery: treatment approaches for the management of dyspnea, *Heart Lung* 22(3):226-232, 1993.

Casciari RJ et al: Effects of breathing retraining in patients with chronic obstructive pulmonary disease, *Chest* 79(4):393-398, 1981.

Fishman AP: Pulmonary rehabilitation research, *Respir Crit Care Med* 149:825-833, 1994.

Forrest J, Ricketts T: A cognitive approach to panic disorder, *Nurs Times* 91(45):27-30, 1995.

Foyt MM: Impaired gas exchange in the elderly, *Geriatr Nurs* 13:262, 1992.

Gift A, Moore T, Soeken K: Relaxation to reduce dyspnea and anxiety in COPD patients, *Nurs Res* 41(4):242, 1992.

Glell R et al: Long-term effects of outpatient rehabilitation of COPD: a randomized trial, *Chest* 117(4), 2000.

Grant S et al: A comparison of the reproducibility and the sensitivity to change of visual analogue scales, Borg scales, and Likert scales in normal subjects during submaximal exercise, *Chest* 116(5), 1999.

Hernandez MTE et al: Results of a home-based training program for patients with COPD, *Chest* 188(1), 2000.

Janssens JP, Muralt BD, Titelion V: Management of dyspnea in severe chronic obstructive pulmonary disease, *J Pain Symptom Manage* 19(5):378-392, 2000.

Kendrick KR, Baxi SC, Smith RM: Usefulness of the modified 1-10 Borg scale in assessing the degree of dyspnea in patients with COPD and asthma, *J Emerg Nurs* 26(3):216-222, 2000.

McCord M, Cronin-Stubbs D: Operationalizing dyspnea: focus on measurement, *Heart Lung* 21(2):167-179, 1992.

Meek PM: Influence of attention and judgment on perception of breathlessness in healthy individuals and patients with chronic obstructive pulmonary disease, *Nurs Res* 49(1):11-19, 2000.

Meek PM et al: Dyspnea: mechanisms, assessment, and management: a consensus statement, *Am J Respir Crit Care Med* 159:321-340, 1999.

Tempkin T, Tempkin A, Goodman H: Geriatric rehabilitation, *Nurse Pract Forum* 8(2):59-63, 1997.

Truesdell S: Helping patients with COPD manage episodes of acute shortness of breath, *MedSurg Nurs* 9(4):178-182, 2000.

• = Independent; ▲ = Collaborative

Decreased Cardiac output

Linda L. Straight and Betty J. Ackley

NANDA   **Definition** Inadequate blood pumped by the heart to meet metabolic demands of the body

Defining Characteristics

Altered heart rate/rhythm: dysrhythmias (tachycardia, bradycardia); palpitations; EKG changes; altered preload: jugular vein distention; fatigue; edema; murmurs; increased/decreased central venous pressure (CVP); increased/decreased pulmonary artery wedge pressure (PAWP); weight gain; altered afterload: cold/clammy skin; shortness of breath/dyspnea; oliguria; prolonged capillary refill; decreased peripheral pulses; variations in blood pressure readings; increased/decreased systemic vascular resistance (SVR); increased/decreased pulmonary vascular resistance (PVR); skin color changes; altered contractility: crackles; cough; orthopnea/paroxysmal nocturnal dyspnea; cardiac output <4 L/min; cardiac index <2.5 L/min; decreased ejection fraction, stroke volume index (SVI), left ventricular stroke work index (LVSWI); S_3 or S_4 sounds; behavioral/emotional: anxiety; restlessness

Related Factors (r/t)

Myocardial infarction or ischemia, valvular disease, cardiomyopathy, serious dysrhythmia, ventricular damage, altered preload or afterload, pericarditis, sepsis, congenital heart defects, vagal stimulation, stress, anaphylaxis, cardiac tamponade

NOC   **Outcomes (Nursing Outcomes Classification)**

Suggested NOC Labels

Cardiac Pump Effectiveness; Circulatory Status; Tissue Perfusion: Abdominal Organs; Tissue Perfusion: Peripheral; Vital Signs Status

> **Example NOC Outcome**
> Accomplishes **Cardiac Pump Effectiveness** as evidenced by the following indicators: BP IER*/Heart rate IER/Cardiac index IER/Ejection fraction IER/Activity tolerance IER/Peripheral pulses strong/NVD not present/Dysrhythmias not present/Abnormal heart sounds not present/Angina not present/Peripheral edema not present/Pulmonary edema not present (Rate each indicator of **Cardiac Pump Effectiveness:** 1 = extremely compromised, 2 = substantially compromised, 3 = moderately compromised, 4 = mildly compromised, 5 = not compromised [see Section I])

*In Expected Range

Client Outcomes

- Demonstrates adequate cardiac output as evidenced by BP and pulse rate and rhythm within normal parameters for client; strong peripheral pulses; and an ability to tolerate activity without symptoms of dyspnea, syncope, or chest pain
- Remains free of side effects from the medications used to achieve adequate cardiac output
- Explains actions and precautions to take for cardiac disease

NIC   **Interventions (Nursing Interventions Classification)**

Suggested NIC Labels

Cardiac Care; Cardiac Care: Acute; Circulatory Care

• = **Independent;** ▲ = **Collaborative**

Example NIC Interventions—Cardiac Care
- Evaluate chest pain (e.g., intensity, location, radiation, duration, and precipitating and alleviating factors)
- Document cardiac dysrhythmias

Nursing Interventions and Rationales

- Monitor for symptoms of heart failure and decreased cardiac output, including diminished quality of peripheral pulses, cool skin and extremities, increased respiratory rate, presence of paroxysmal nocturnal dyspnea or orthopnea, increased heart rate, neck vein distention, decreased level of consciousness, and presence of edema.
  As these symptoms of heart failure progress, cardiac output declines (Murphy, Bennett, 1992; Ahrens, 1995).
- Listen to heart sounds; note rate, rhythm, presence of S_3, S_4, and lung sounds (noting presence of crackles).
  The new onset of a gallop rhythm, tachycardia, and fine crackles in lung bases can indicate onset of heart failure (Janowski, 1996). If client develops pulmonary edema, there will be coarse crackles on inspiration and severe dyspnea.
- Observe for confusion, restlessness, agitation, dizziness.
  Central nervous system disturbances may be noted with decreased cardiac output (Alspach, 1998).
- Observe for chest pain or discomfort; note location, radiation, severity, quality, duration, associated manifestations such as nausea, and precipitating and relieving factors.
  Chest pain/discomfort is generally indicative of an inadequate blood supply to the heart, which can compromise cardiac output. Clients with heart failure can continue to have chest pain with angina or can reinfarct.
- ▲ If chest pain is present, have client lie down, monitor cardiac rhythm, give oxygen, run a strip, medicate for pain, and notify the physician.
  These actions can increase oxygen delivery to the coronary arteries and improve client prognosis.
- ▲ Place on cardiac monitor; monitor for dysrhythmias, especially atrial fibrillation.
  Atrial fibrillation is common in heart failure (Janowski, 1996).
- ▲ Monitor hemodynamic parameters for an increase in pulmonary wedge pressure, an increase in systemic vascular resistance, or a decrease in cardiac output and index.
  Hemodynamic parameters give a good indication of cardiac function.
- ▲ Titrate inotropic and vasoactive medications within defined parameters to maintain contractility, preload, and afterload per physician's order.
  By following parameters, the nurse ensures maintenance of a delicate balance of medications that stimulate the heart to increase contractility, maintaining adequate perfusion of the body.
- Monitor intake and output. If client is acutely ill, measure hourly urine output and note decreases in output.
  Decreased cardiac output results in decreased perfusion of the kidneys, with a resulting decrease in urine output.
- ▲ Note results of EKG and chest x-ray.
  EKG can reveal previous MI, or evidence of left ventricular hypertrophy, indicating aortic stenosis or chronic systemic hypertension. x-ray may provide information on pulmonary

• = Independent; ▲ = Collaborative

edema, pleural effusions, or enlarged cardiac silhouette found in dilated cardiomyopathy or large pericardial effusion (Fuster et al, 2000).

▲ Note results of diagnostic imaging studies such as echocardiogram, radionuclide imaging or dobutamine stress echocardiography.
The echocardiogram is the most important imaging tool for evaluating patients with symptoms of heart failure because overall systolic function and chamber size can be evaluated quickly. In addition, global versus regional left ventricular function, valvular abnormalities, and diastolic function can be defined, assisting in differential diagnosis. (Fuster et al, 2000). An ejection fraction in a healthy heart is approximately 50%. Most patients experiencing heart failure have an ejection fraction of <40% (Janowski, 1996).

▲ Watch laboratory data closely, especially arterial blood gases and electrolytes, including potassium.
Client may be receiving cardiac glycosides and the potential for toxicity is greater with hypokalemia; hypokalemia is common in heart clients because of diuretic use (Lessig, Lessig, 1998).

▲ Monitor lab work such as complete blood count, sodium level, and serum creatinine.
Routine blood work can provide insight into the etiology of heart failure and extent of decompensation. A low serum sodium level often is observed with advanced heart failure and can be a poor prognostic sign (Fuster et al, 2000). Serum creatinine levels will elevate in clients with severe heart failure because of decreased perfusion to the kidneys. Creatinine may also elevate because of ACE inhibitors (Ahrens, 1995).

▲ Administer oxygen as needed per physician's order.
Supplemental oxygen increases oxygen availability to the myocardium (Prizant-Weston, Castiglia, 1992).

• Place client in semi-Fowler's position or position of comfort.
Elevating the head of the bed may decrease the work of breathing, and also decrease venous return and preload.

▲ Check blood pressure, pulse, and condition before administering cardiac medications such as angiotensin converting enzyme (ACE) inhibitors, digoxin, and beta-blockers such as carvedilol. Notify physician if heart rate or blood pressure is low before holding medications.
It is important that the nurse evaluate how well the client is tolerating current medications before administering cardiac medications; do not hold medications without physician input. The physician may decide to have medications administered even though the blood pressure or pulse rate has lowered.

• During acute events, ensure client remains on bed rest or maintains activity level that does not compromise cardiac output.
In severe heart failure, restriction of activity often facilitates temporary recompensation (Massie, Amidon, 1998).

▲ Gradually increase activity when client's condition is stabilized by encouraging slower paced activities or shorter periods of activity with frequent rest periods following exercise prescription; observe for symptoms of intolerance. Take blood pressure and pulse before and after activity and note changes.
*Activity of the cardiac client should be closely monitored. See **Activity intolerance**.*

▲ Serve small sodium-restricted, low-cholesterol meals. Give only small amounts of caffeine-containing beverages (1 or 2 cups per 24 hours) if no resulting dysrhythmia.
Sodium-restricted diets help decrease fluid volume excess. Low-cholesterol diets help decrease atherosclerosis, which causes coronary artery disease. Clients with cardiac disease tolerate

• = **Independent;** ▲ = **Collaborative**

smaller meals better because they require less cardiac output to digest. One cup of caffein-ated coffee has generally not been found to have any significant effect (Schneider, 1987; Powell, 1993).

▲ Monitor bowel function. Provide stool softeners as ordered. Caution client not to strain when defecating.
Decreased activity can cause constipation. Straining when defecating that results in the Valsalva maneuver can lead to dysrhythmia, decreased cardiac function, and sometimes death.

• Have clients use a commode or urinal for toileting and avoid use of a bedpan.
Getting out of bed to use a commode or urinal does not stress the heart any more than staying in bed to toilet. In addition, getting the client out of bed minimizes complications of immobility and is often preferred by the client (Winslow, 1992).

• Provide a restful environment by minimizing controllable stressors and unnecessary disturbances. Schedule rest periods after meals and activities.
Rest periods decrease oxygen consumption (Prizant-Weston, Castiglia, 1992).

• Weigh client at same time daily (after voiding).
An accurate daily weight is a good indicator of fluid balance. Increased weight and sever-ity of symptoms can signal decreased cardiac function with retention of fluids.

• Assess for presence of anxiety; see interventions for **Anxiety** to facilitate reduction of anxiety in clients and family.

• Consider using music to decrease anxiety and improve cardiac function.
Music has been shown to reduce heart rate, blood pressure, anxiety, and cardiac complica-tions (Guzzetta, 1994).

▲ Closely monitor fluid intake including IV lines. Maintain fluid restriction if ordered.
In clients with decreased cardiac output, poorly functioning ventricles may not tolerate increased fluid volumes.

▲ Refer to heart failure program or cardiac rehabilitation program for education, evalu-ation, and guided support to increase activity and rebuild life.
Exercise can help many patients with heart failure. Whereas rest was commonly recom-mended a few years ago, it has become clear that inactivity can worsen the skeletal muscle myopathy in these patients. A carefully monitored exercise program can improve both func-tional capacity (Bellardinelli et al, 1999) and left ventricular function (Giannuzzi et al, 1997). Exercise-based cardiac rehabilitation programs appear to be effective in reducing cardiac deaths, but the evidence base is weakened by poor quality trials (Jolliffe et al, 2000).

Geriatric

• Observe for atypical pain; the elderly often have jaw pain instead of chest pain or may have silent myocardial infarctions with symptoms of dyspnea or fatigue.
The elderly have altered pain pathways and often do not experience the usual chest pain of cardiac patients (Carnevali, Patrick, 1993).

• Observe for syncope, dizziness, palpitations, or feelings of weakness associated with a irregular heart rhythm.
Dysrhythmias are common in the elderly (Carnevali, Patrick, 1993).

▲ Observe for side effects from cardiac medications.
The elderly have difficulty with metabolism and excretion of medications due to decreased function of the liver and kidneys; therefore toxic side effects are more common.

• = **Independent**; ▲ = **Collaborative**

Home Care Interventions

▲ Begin discharge planning as soon as possible with case manager or social worker to assess home support systems and the need for community or home health services. Support services may be needed to assist with home care, meal preparations, housekeeping, personal care, transportation to doctor visits, or emotional support.

Clients often need help upon discharge. The existing social support network needs to be assessed and assistance provided as needed to meet client needs and to keep the support persons from being overwhelmed (Campbell, 1998). Being discharged to home without adequate support has been shown to be related to readmission of elderly patients (Jaarsma, 1996).

▲ Assess or refer to case manager or social worker to evaluate client ability to pay for prescriptions.

The cost of drugs may be a factor to fill prescriptions and adhere to a treatment plan (Campbell, 1998).

▲ Continue to monitor client for exacerbation of heart failure when discharged home.

Transition to home can create increased stress and physiological instability related to diagnosis.

• Assess client for understanding and compliance with medical regimen, including medications, activity level, and diet.

• Instruct family and client about the disease process, complications of disease process, information on medications, need for weighing daily, and when it is appropriate to call doctor.

Early recognition of symptoms facilitates early problem solving and prompt treatment (Janowski, 1996). Clients with heart failure need intensive guideline gased education about these topics to help prevent readmission to the hospital (Moser, 2000).

▲ Identify emergency plan, including use of CPR.

Decreased cardiac output can be life threatening.

• Help family adapt daily living patterns to establish life changes that will maintain improved cardiac functioning in the client.

Transition to the home setting can cause risk factors such as inappropriate diet to reemerge.

▲ Refer to physical therapy for strengthening exercises if client is not involved in cardiac rehabilitation.

▲ Refer to medical social services as necessary for counseling about the impact of severe or chronic cardiac disease.

Social workers can assist the client and family with acceptance of life changes.

Client/Family Teaching

• Teach symptoms of heart failure and appropriate actions to take if client becomes symptomatic.

• Teach importance of smoking cessation and avoidance of alcohol intake.

Clients who continue to smoke increase their chance of dying by at least 50%, and alcohol depresses heart contractility (Janowski, 1996). Smoking cessation advice and counsel given by nurses can be effective, and should be available to clients to help stop smoking (Rice, Stead, 2000).

• Teach stress reduction (e.g., imagery, controlled breathing, muscle relaxation techniques).

• Explain necessary restrictions, including consumption of a sodium-restricted diet, guidelines on fluid intake, and the avoidance of Valsalva's maneuver. Teach the

• = Independent; ▲ = Collaborative

importance of pacing activities, work simplification techniques, and the need to rest between activities to prevent becoming overly fatigued.

Sodium retention leading to fluid overload is a common cause of hospital readmission (Bennett et al, 2000).

▲ Assist client in understanding the need for and how to incorporate lifestyle changes. Refer to cardiac rehabilitation for assistance with coping and adjustment.

Psychoeducational programs including information on stress management and health education have been shown to reduce long term mortality and recurrence of myocardial infarction in heart patients (Benson, 2000).

• Teach client actions, side effects, and importance of consistently taking cardiovascular medications.

Medications can prolong the lives of heart failure clients but often are not taken, resulting in hospital readmissions (Agency for Health Care Policy and Research, 1994).

• Provide client/family with advance directive information to consider.

Allow client to give advance directions about medical care or designates who should make medical decisions if he or she should lose decision-making capacity (Alspach, 1998).

▲ Instruct client on importance of getting a pneumonia shot (usually one per lifetime) and yearly flu shots as prescribed by physician.

Clients with decreased cardiac output are considered higher risk for complications or death if they do not get immunization injections.

• Instruct client/family on the need to weigh daily and keep a weight log. Ask if client has a scale at home; if not, assist in getting one. Instruct on establishing baseline weight on own scale when gets home.

Daily weighing is an essential aspect of self-management. A scale is necessary (Campbell, 1998). Scales vary; the client needs to establish a baseline weight on his or her home scale.

• Provide specific written materials and self-care plan for client/caregivers to use for reference.

Consult dietitian or assist client in understanding the need for a sodium-restricted diet. Provide alternatives for salt such as spices, herbs, lemon juice, or vinegar. Although the initial elimination of salt from the diet is very difficult for a person use to its taste, the taste of salt can be unlearned. The above can enhance the taste appeal of food while the preference for salt is changing (Peckenpaugh, Poleman, 1999).

• Instruct family regarding cardiopulmonary resuscitation.

WEB SITES FOR EDUCATION

MERLIN See the MERLIN web site for World Wide Web resources for client education.

REFERENCES Agency for Health Care Policy and Research (AHCPR): *Guidelines for patients with heart failure,* AHCPR Publication No 94-0612, Rockville, Md, 1994, U.S. Department of Health and Human Services.

Ahrens SG: Managing heart failure: a blueprint for success, *Nursing* 25:26, 1995.

Alspach JG, editor: *Core curriculum for critical care nursing,* ed 5, Philadelphia, 1998, WB Saunders.

Bellardinelli R et al: A randomized, controlled trial of long-term moderate exercise training in chronic heart failure: effects on functional capacity, quality of life, and clinical outcome, *Circulation* 99(9):1173-1182, 1999.

Bennett SJ et al: Self-care strategies for symptom management in patients with chronic heart failure, *Nurs Res* 49(3):139-145, 2000.

Benson G: Review: psychoeducational programmes reduce long term mortality and recurrence of myocardial infarction in cardiac patients, *Evidence-Based Nurs* 3(3):80, 2000.

• = Independent; ▲ = Collaborative

Campbell R et al: Discharge planning and home follow-up of the elderly patient with heart failure, *Geriatr Nurs* 33(3):497-509, 1998.

Carnevali DL, Patrick M: *Nursing management for the elderly,* ed 3, Philadelphia, 1993, JB Lippincott.

Fuster V et al: *Hurst's the heart,* ed 10, New York, 2000, McGraw-Hill.

Giannuzzi P et al: Attenuation of unfavorable modeling by exercise training in postinfarction patients with left ventricular dysfunction: results of the Exercise in Left Ventricular Dysfunction (ELVD) Trial, *Circulation* 96(6):1790-1797, 1997.

Guzzetta CE: Soothing the ischemic heart, *Am J Nurs* 94:24, 1994.

Jaarsma T et al: Readmission of older heart failure patients, *Prog Cardiovasc Nurs* 11(1):15-20, 1996.

Janowski MJ: Managing heart failure, *RN* 59:34, 1996.

Jolliffe JA et al: Exercise-based rehabilitation for coronary heart disease (Cochrane Review). In: *The Cochrane Library,* 4:CD001800, 2000.

Lessig ML, Lessig PM: The cardiovascular system. In Alspach JG, editor: *Core curriculum for critical care nursing,* ed 5, Philadelphia, 1998, WB Saunders.

Massie B, Amidon TM: Heart. In Tierney L, McPhee S, Papadakis M, editors: *Current medical diagnosis and treatment,* ed 37, 1998, Stamford, Conn, Appleton & Lange.

Moser DK: Heart failure management: optimal health care delivery programs, *Annu Rev Nurs Res* 18:91-126, 2000.

Murphy T, Bennett EJ: Low-tech, high-touch perfusion assessment, *Am J Nurs* 92:36, 1992.

Peckenpaugh NJ, Poleman C: *Nutrition essentials and diet therapy,* ed 8, Philadelphia, 1999, WB Saunders.

Powell AH: What's that brewing in the CCU? Working smart, *Am J Nurs* 93:16, 1993.

Prizant-Weston M, Castiglia K: Hemodynamic regulation. In Bulechek GM, McCloskey JC, editors: *Nursing interventions: essential nursing treatments,* Philadelphia, 1992, WB Saunders.

Rice VH, Stead LF: Nursing interventions for smoking cessation (Cochrane Review) In: *The Cochrane Library,* (2):CD001188, 2000.

Schneider JR: Effects of caffeine ingestion on heart rate, blood pressure, myocardial oxygen consumption, and cardiac rhythm in acute myocardial infarction patients, *Heart Lung* 16:167, 1987.

Winslow EH: Panning bedpans, *Am J Nurs* 92:16G, 1992.

Caregiver role strain

Betty J. Ackley

NANDA   **Definition** Difficulty in performing caregiver role

Defining Characteristics
Caregiving activities

Apprehension about possible institutionalization of care receiver; apprehension about the future regarding care receiver's health and the caregiver's ability to provide care; difficulty performing/completing required tasks; apprehension about care receiver's care if caregiver becomes ill or dies; preoccupation with care routine

Caregiver health status—physical

GI upset; weight change; rash; hypertension; cardiovascular disease; diabetes; fatigue; headaches

Caregiver health status—emotional

Impaired individual coping; feeling depressed; disturbed sleep; anger; stress; somatization; increased nervousness; increased emotional lability; impatience; lack of time to meet personal needs; frustration

Caregiver health status—socioeconomic

Withdraws from social life; changes in leisure activities; low work productivity; refuses career advancement

• = Independent; ▲ = Collaborative

Caregiver-care receiver relationship

Grief/uncertainty regarding changed relationship with care receiver; difficulty watching care receiver go through the illness

Family processes

Family conflict; concerns about family members

Related Factors (r/t)

Care receiver health status

Illness severity; illness chronicity; increasing care needs/dependency; unpredictability of illness course; instability of care receiver's health; problem behaviors; psychological or cognitive problems; addiction or codependency

Caregiving activities

Amount of activities; complexity of activities; 24-hour care responsibilities; ongoing changes in activities; discharge of family members to home with significant care needs; years of caregiving; unpredictability of care situation

Caregiver health status

Physical problems; psychological or cognitive problems; addiction or codependency; marginal coping patterns; unrealistic expectations of self; inability to fulfill one's own or others' expectations

Socioeconomic

Isolation from others; competing role commitments; alienation from family, friends, and co-workers; insufficient recreation resources

Caregiver-care receiver relationship

History of poor relationship; presence of abuse or violence; unrealistic expectations of caregiver by care receiver; mental status of elder inhibiting conversation

Family processes

History of marginal family coping; history of family dysfunction

Resources   Inadequate physical environment for providing care; inadequate equipment for providing care; inadequate transportation; inadequate community resources; insufficient finances; lack of support; caregiver is not developmentally ready for caregiver role; inexperience with caregiving; insufficient time; lack of knowledge of or difficulty with accessing community resources; lack of caregiver privacy, emotional strength, physical energy, assistance, and support

NOC   Outcomes (Nursing Outcomes Classification)

Suggested NOC Labels

Caregiver Emotional Health; Caregiver Endurance Potential; Caregiver Lifestyle Disruption; Caregiver Performance: Direct Care; Caregiver Performance: Indirect Care; Caregiver Physical Health; Caregiver Stressors; Caregiver Well-Being; Role Performance

> **Example NOC Outcome**
> Demonstrates increased **Caregiver Emotional Health** with plans for a positive future as evidenced by the following indicators: Satisfaction with life/Sense of control/Self-esteem/Free of Anger/Free of guilt/Free of depression/Perceived social connectedness/Perceived spiritual well-being (Rate each indicator of **Caregiver Emotional Health:** 1 = extremely compromised, 2 = substantially compromised, 3 = moderately compromised, 4 = mildly compromised, 5 = not compromised [see Section I])

• = Independent; ▲ = Collaborative

Client Outcomes

- Caregiver maintains physical and psychological health
- Caregiver identifies resources available to help in giving care
- Care receiver obtains appropriate care

NIC   Interventions (Nursing Interventions Classification)

Suggested NIC Labels

Caregiver Support

> **Example NIC Interventions—Caregiver Support**
> - Determine caregiver's acceptance of role; accept expressions of negative emotion

Nursing Interventions and Rationales

- Monitor quality of care for adequacy and need for improvement.
- Determine physical and psychological health of caregiver. Use an evaluation tool to determine caregiver coping (Moos, 1992), caregiver burden (Zarit et al, 1980), or the Bakas Caregiver Outcomes Scale (Bakas, Champion, 1999).
- Watch for signs of depression in the caregiver, especially if poor marital relationship. Intervene to help the caregiver cope.

    One study done on caregivers of stroke clients demonstrated that caregiver problems are similar at 1, 3, and 6 months. Intervening early to help the caregiver can result in improved care for the stroke client and, it is hoped, improved health for the caregiver (Teel, Duncan, Lai, 2001). Refer to the care plan for **Hopelessness.** *Caregiving may weaken the immune system and predispose the caregiver to illness in some situations; the incidence of depression in family caregivers is estimated to be 40% to 50% (Stevens, Walsh, Baldwin, 1993; Knop, Bergman-Evans, McCabe, 1998). Psychiatric nurses can play an important role in the assessment and treatment of caregiver depression (Buckwalter, 1999).*

- Observe for signs of addiction or codependency in caregiver or care receiver.
- Arrange for a home health nurse to provide nursing care and case management following discharge.

    Home health nurses can decrease the burden of caregiving and depression in elderly caregivers (Mignor, 2000).

- Arrange for intervals of respite care for caregiver; encourage use if available.

    Respite care is beneficial to caregivers, if they can be convinced to use it (Sayles-Cross, DeLorme, 1995; Hayes, 1999).

- Help caregiver to identify supports and be assertive in using them.

    Caregivers sometimes feel abandoned (Given et al, 1990) and need assistance to activate their support system (Kleffel, 1998).

- Encourage caregiver to grieve over loss of care receiver's function. Give caregiver permission to share angry feelings in a safe environment. Refer to nursing interventions for **Grieving.**

    Caregivers grieve the loss of function of their loved one, especially when dementia is involved (Liken, Collins, 1993; Narayan et al, 2001).

- Identify with caregiver the factors that can and cannot be controlled.
- Help caregiver find personal time to meet own needs and learn stress management techniques.

• = Independent; ▲ = Collaborative

Self-care is important for the caregiver. Practicing personal wellness measures can increase stamina, energy, and self-esteem and enhance the quality of care given (Ruppert, 1996).

- Support the female caregiver in setting boundaries, determining legitimate caregiving role, trusting own judgment, and attending to one's own voice—being true to self as well as to the care receiver.

  Women in caregiving roles can develop "fraying connections" and lose sense of self when own needs are not met (Wuest, 1998).

- Encourage caregiver to use humor to cope when appropriate, including use of cartoons, stories, and jokes.

  Humor is a healthy distancing technique, helping the caregiver to feel liberated from oppressive stimuli. It can help relieve pain, loss, grief, or unpleasantness (Buffum, Brod, 1998).

- Encourage caregiver to talk about feelings, concerns, and fears. Acknowledge frustration associated with caregiver responsibilities.

  Professionals need to listen to caregiving spouses and note expressions of positive and negative responses to caregiving (Narayan et al, 2001).

- Observe for any evidence of caregiver or care receiver violence; if evidence is present, speak with caregiver and care receiver separately.

  Caregiver violence is possible, especially if the care receiver was violent to the caregiver in the past (Brandle, Raymond, 1997).

- Involve the family in discharge planning.

  Caregivers who reported involvement in discharge planning reported better acceptance of the caregiving role and better health (Bull, Hansen, Gross, 2000).

- ▲ Arrange for follow-up care after discharge, including the services of a case management team, to provide medical and social services to caregiver and client.

  A program after discharge that supports the caregiver has been shown to delay nursing home placements, possibly delay some deaths, and save money (Oktay, Volland, 1990). Providing care to a seriously ill family member is a severe financial strain and often depletes most or all of the family savings (Covinsky, 1994).

- Give caregiver permission to arrange custodial care in an extended care facility if necessary; support both caregiver and care receiver during this difficult transition.

  Placing a loved one in an extended care facility can relieve the burden of care but does not relieve the stress resulting from financial concerns, guilt, loss of control, or lack of support (Stevens, Walsh, Baldwin, 1993).

Geriatric

- Monitor caregiver for psychological distress and signs of depression, especially if caring for a mentally impaired elder or if there was an unsatisfactory marital relationship before caregiving.

  Those caring for mentally impaired elders for an extended time with minimal social support are at high risk for psychological distress or depression (Baille, Norbeck, Barnes, 1988). A difficult marriage before caregiving predisposes the caregiver to depression (Knop, Bergman-Evans, McCabe, 1998).

- Assess the health of the caregiver at intervals, especially if he or she has chronic illness in addition to caregiving role.

  The elderly can be overly self-sufficient, especially if they live in rural areas, and elderly caregivers can develop poor health as a result (Silveira, Winstead-Fry, 1997).

- Recognize that it is hard for the elderly to accept any change in caregivers or in environment.

• = Independent; ▲ = Collaborative

- Help caregiver identify ways to equitably distribute workload among family or significant others.

Multicultural

- Assess for the influence of cultural beliefs, norms, values, and expectations on the family's experience of caregiving.
  How the family views caregiving may be based on cultural perceptions (Leininger, 1996).
- Assess for conflicts between the caregiver's cultural obligations to provide care and competing factors like employment.
  Conflicts between cultural expectations and competing factors can increase caregiving stress (Jones, 1996).
- Negotiate with the client regarding the aspects of caregiving that can be modified and still honor cultural beliefs.
  Give and take with the client will lead to culturally congruent care (Leininger, 1996).
- ▲ Refer family to social services or other supportive services to assist with the impact of caregiving.
  Black caregivers of dementia clients evidence less desire than others to institutionalize their family members and are more likely to report unmet service needs (Hinrichsen, Ramirez, 1992). Black and white families of dementia clients report restricted social activity (Haley et al, 1995).
- ▲ Encourage family to use support groups or other service programs.
  Studies indicate that minority families of clients with dementia use few support programs even though these programs could have a positive impact on caregiver well-being (Cox, 1999).
- Validate the family's feelings regarding the impact of caregiving on family and personal lifestyle.
  Validation lets the client know that the nurse has heard and understands what was said (Stuart, Laraia, 2001).

Home Care Interventions

- Assess client and caregiver at every visit for quality of care provided and signs of caregiver stress. Document all observations objectively.
  The changing level of support from institutional care to home care and the length of time that care is needed may precipitate cumulative caregiver burden (Silveira, Winstead-Fry, 1997).
- Form a trusting and supportive relationship with caregiver. Allow caregiver to verbalize frustrations.
  Providing attention to the caregiver can decrease caregiver stress and reduce the risk of caregiver violence.
- Provide caregiver with necessary information and education regarding client's disease, medications, and what to expect.
  This can help the client and caregiver establish routines more quickly and get the situation under control (Bull, Jervis, 1997).
- Assist caregiver and client with arranging care so that it is compatible with other household patterns.
  With the right tools, the caregiver is better able to plan and have confidence in the caregiver role, thus decreasing potential frustration (Hogstel, 1990; Humphrey, 1994).
- ▲ Refer client to home health aide services for activities of daily living (ADLs) assistance and light housekeeping. Allow caregiver to gain confidence in respite provider.

- **= Independent;** ▲ **= Collaborative**

Home health aide services can provide physical relief and respite for the caregiver (Boland, Sims, 1996).

▲ Refer to a caregivers support group if available or recommend an online support group—see suggested web sites listed on the MERLIN web site.
Caregiver support groups can help caregivers cope with stress, increase their own self-care, and find hope (Kleffel, 1998). Because members read and send messages 24 hours a day every day of the week, online support groups offer the advantage of immediate communication with others offering support. When nurses assist with online support groups, the groups can help caregivers learn, give them a sense of community, and encourage a sense of empowerment (White, Dorman, 2000).

▲ Refer to case managers as necessary for community resource assistance, financial planning, and supportive counseling for both client and caregiver.
Individualized counseling in problem solving by nurses was shown to be effective for reducing the number of admissions to nursing homes (Roberts et al, 1999).

NOTE: Families of terminally ill clients are especially vulnerable to caregiver role strain because timing of the impending death is unpredictable, and caregiver effort and resources are disproportionately spent early in the caregiving process.

Client/Family Teaching

- Teach caregiver methods for managing behavioral symptoms if care receiver has dementia. Refer to care plan for **Chronic Confusion.**
  Caregivers can be taught to understand and manage problem behavior (Mastrian, Ritter, Diemling, 1996).
- Teach caregiver how to provide physical care needed.
▲ Refer to counseling or support groups to assist in adjusting to caregiver role.

WEB SITES FOR EDUCATION

See the MERLIN web site for World Wide Web resources for client education.

REFERENCES Baille V, Norbeck JS, Barnes LE: Stress, social support, and psychological distress of family caregivers of the elderly, *Nurs Res* 37(4):217-222, 1988.

Bakas T, Champion V: Development and psychometric testing of the Bakas caregiving outcomes scale, *Nurs Res* 48(5):250-258, 1999.

Boland D, Sims S: Family caregiving at home as a solitary journey, *Image J Nurs Sch* 28:55, 1996.

Brandle B, Raymond J: Unrecognized elder abuse victims: older abused women, *J Case Manage* 6(2):62-68, 1997.

Buckwalter KC et al: A nursing intervention to decrease depression in family caregivers of person with dementia, *Arch Psychiatr Nurs* 13(2):80-88, 1999.

Buffum MD, Brod M: Humor and well-being in spouse caregivers of patients with Alzheimer's disease, *Appl Nurs Res* 11(1):12-17, 1998.

Bull MJ, Hansen HE, Gross CR: Differences in family caregiver outcomes by their level of involvement in discharge planning, *Appl Nurs Res* 13(2):76-81, 2000.

Bull MJ, Jervis LL: Strategies used by chronically ill older women and their caregiving daughters in managing posthospital care, *J Adv Nurs* 25:541-547, 1997.

Covinsky KE: The impact of serious illness on patient's families, *JAMA* 272:1839, 1994.

Cox C: Race and caregiving: patterns of service use by African-American and white caregivers of persons with Alzheimer's, *J Gerontol Soc Work* 32(2):5-19, 1999.

Given B et al: Responses of elder spouse caregivers, *Res Nurs Health* 13:77-85, 1990.

Haley WE et al: Psychological, social, and health impact of caregiving: a comparison of black and white dementia family caregivers and noncaregivers, *Psychol Aging* 10(4):540-552, 1995.

• = **Independent;** ▲ = **Collaborative**

Hayes JM: Respite for caregivers: a community-based model in a rural setting, *J Gerontol Nurs* pp 22-25, Jan 1999.

Hinrichsen GA, Ramirez M: Black and white dementia caregivers: a comparison of their adaptation, *Gerontologist* 32(3):375-381, 1992.

Hogstel M: *Geropsychiatric nursing,* St Louis, 1990, Mosby.

Humphrey CJ: *Home care nursing handbook,* ed 2, Gaithersburg, Md, 1994, Aspen.

Jones PS: Asian American women caring for elderly parents, *J Family Nurs* 2(1):56-75, 1996.

Kleffel D: Lives on hold: evaluation of a caregivers' support program, *Home Health Nurse* 16(7):465-472, 1998.

Knop DS, Bergman-Evans B, McCabe BW: In sickness and in health: an exploration of the perceived quality of the marital relationship, coping, and depression in caregivers of spouses with Alzheimer's disease, *J Psychosoc Nurs Ment Health Serv* 36(1):16-21, 1998.

Leininger MM: *Transcultural nursing: theories, research and practices,* ed 2, Hilliard, Ohio, 1996, McGraw-Hill.

Liken MA, Collins CE: Grieving: facilitating the process for dementia caregivers, *J Psychosoc Nurs Ment Health Serv* 31(1):21-26, 1993.

Mastrian KG, Ritter C, Diemling GT: Predictors of caregiver health strain, *Home Health Nurse* 14(3):209-217, 1996.

Mignor D: Effectivenss of use of home health nurses to decrease burden and depression of elderly caregivers, *J Psychosoc Nurs* 38(7):34-43, 2000.

Moos RH: *Coping responses inventory adult form manual,* Palo Alto, Calif, 1992, Center for Health Care Evaluation, Stanford University and Department of Veterans Affairs Medical Center.

Narayan S et al: Subjective responses to caregiving for a spouse with dementia, *J Gerontol Nurs* 27(3):19-28, 2001.

Oktay JS, Volland PT: Post-hospital program for the frail elderly and their caregivers: a quasi-experimental evaluation, *Am J Public Health* 80(1):39-46, 1990.

Roberts J et al: Problem-solving counseling for caregivers of the cognitively impaired: effective for whom? *Nurs Res* 48(3):162-172, 1999.

Ruppert RA: Caring for the lay caregiver, *Am J Nurs* 96(3):40-46, 1996.

Sayles-Cross S, DeLorme J: Worried, worn out, and angry: providing relief for caregivers, *ABNF J* 6:74-77, 1995.

Silveira JM, Winstead-Fry P: The needs of patients with cancer and their caregivers in rural areas, *Oncol Nurs Forum* 24(1):71-76, 1997.

Stevens GL, Walsh RA, Baldwin BA: Family caregivers of institutionalized and noninstitutionalized elderly individuals, *Nurs Clin North Am* 28(2):349-362, 1993.

Stuart GW, Laraia MT: Therapeutic nurse-patient relationship. In Stuart GW, Lauria MT, editors: *Principles and practice of psychiatric nursing,* St Louis, 2001, Mosby, p 30.

Teel CS, Duncan P, Lai SM: Caregiving experiences after stroke, *Nurs Res* 50(1):53-60, 2001.

White MH, Dorman SM: Online support for caregivers: analysis of an internet Alzheimer mailgroup, *Comput Nurs* 18(4):168-175, 2000.

Wuest J: Setting boundaries: a strategy for precarious ordering of women's caring demands, *Res Nurs Health* 21(1):39-49, 1998.

Zarit SH et al: Relatives of the impaired elderly: correlates of feelings of burden, *Gerontologist* 20(6):649-655, 1980.

Risk for Caregiver role strain

NANDA   **Definition**   Caregiver is vulnerable for felt difficulty in performing the family caregiver role

Risk Factors

Caregiver is not developmentally ready for caregiver role (e.g., a young adult needing to provide care for middle-aged); inadequate physical environment for providing care (e.g., housing, transportation, community services, equipment); unpredictable illness course or instability in care receiver's health; psychological or cognitive problems in care receiver;

• = **Independent;** ▲ = **Collaborative**

presence of situational stressors that normally affect families (e.g., significant loss, disaster, or crisis; economic vulnerability; major life events); presence of abuse or violence; premature birth/congenital defect; past history of poor relationship between caregiver and care receiver; marginal family adaptation or dysfunction before the caregiving situation; marginal caregiver's coping patterns; lack of respite and recreation for caregiver; inexperience with caregiving; caregiver is female; addiction or codependency; care receiver exhibits deviant, bizarre behavior; caregiver's competing role commitments; caregiver health impairment; illness severity of care receiver; caregiver is spouse; complexity/amount of caregiving tasks; developmental delay or retardation of care receiver or caregiver; discharge of family member with significant home care needs; duration of caregiving required; family/caregiver isolation

NOC Outcomes (Nursing Outcomes Classification)

Suggested NOC Labels

Caregiver Emotional Health; Caregiver Endurance Potential; Caregiver Lifestyle Disruption; Caregiver Performance: Direct Care; Caregiver Performance: Indirect Care; Caregiver Physical Health; Caregiver Stressors; Caregiver Well-Being; Role Performance

Example NOC Outcome

Maintain **Caregiver Emotional Health** with plans for a positive future as evidenced by the following indicators: Satisfaction with life/Sense of control/Self-esteem/Free of Anger/Free of guilt/Free of depression/Perceived social connectedness/Perceived spiritual well-being (Rate each indicator of **Caregiver Emotional Health:** 1 = extremely compromised, 2 = substantially compromised, 3 = moderately compromised, 4 = mildly compromised, 5 = not compromised [see Section I])

Client Outcomes

- Caregiver maintains physical and psychological health
- Caregiver identifies resources available to help in giving care
- Care receiver obtains appropriate care

NIC Interventions (Nursing Interventions Classification)

Suggested NIC Labels

Caregiver Support; Family Support; Home Maintenance Assistance; Normalization Promotion; Respite Care; Support Group

Example NIC Interventions—Caregiver Support

- Determine caregiver's acceptance of role
- Accept expressions of negative emotion

Nursing Interventions and Rationales, Home Care Interventions, Client/Family Teaching

See care plan for **Caregiver role strain**.

WEB SITES FOR EDUCATION

MERLIN See the MERLIN web site for World Wide Web resources for client education.

• = Independent; ▲ = Collaborative

Impaired Comfort–pruritis

Betty J. Ackley

Definition   State in which an individual experiences an uncomfortable sensation in response to a noxious stimulus (Carpenito, 1993)

Defining Characteristics
Verbalization or demonstration of discomfort, itching, reddened irritated skin

Related Factors (r/t)
Chemical irritants, dry skin

NOC   **Outcomes (Nursing Outcomes Classification)**
Suggested NOC Labels
Comfort Level

> **Example NOC Outcome**
> Reports **Comfort Level** as evidenced by the following indicators: Reported physical well-being/Reported satisfaction with symptom control (Rate each indicator of **Comfort Level:** 1 = none, 2 = limited, 3 = moderate, 4 = substantial, 5 = extensive [see Section I])

Client Outcomes
- States he or she is comfortable, itching relieved
- Explains methods to decrease itching

NIC   **Interventions (Nursing Interventions Classification)**
Suggested NIC Labels
Pruritis Management

> **Example NIC Interventions—Pruritis Management**
> - Apply medicated creams and lotions as appropriate
> - Instruct client to limit bathing to once or twice a week as appropriate

Nursing Interventions and Rationales
- Determine cause of pruritus (e.g., dry skin, contact with irritating substance, medication side effect, insect bite, infection, symptom of systemic disease).
  The etiology of pruritus helps direct treatment. Pruritus may be caused by serious illnesses such as renal failure, liver failure, malignancy, or diabetes (Eaglestein, McKay, Pariser, 1994), as well as by dry skin and various skin conditions.
- Apply soaks with washcloths wrung out in cool water or ice water as needed.
  The application of cool or cold washcloths can depress the itching sensation.
- Keep client's fingernails short; have client wear mitts if necessary.
  Scratching with fingernails can excoriate the area and increase skin damage.
- Leave pruritic area open to the air if possible.
  Covering the area with a nonventilated dressing can increase itching sensation and warmth in the area.
- Use nonallergenic mild soap and use it sparingly.
  Many soaps can be irritating to the skin and increase the itching sensation.

• = Independent; ▲ = Collaborative

- Keep skin well lubricated. After bathing while the skin is still moist, apply nonallergenic moisturizers such as Medilan that are alcohol free and available in cream or ointment form. Apply moisturizers daily.

  These agents lubricate the skin surface and make the skin feel smoother and less dry (Hardy, 1996). Medilan is a hypoallergenic lanolin that has soothing and hydrating properties. It can be helpful for the treatment of eczema and other dry skin conditions (Stone, 2000). Creams and ointments are more effective than lotions because they contain less water (Frantz, Gardner, 1994). Daily application of moisturizers can have the persistent clinical effect of relieving dry skin (Tabata et al, 2000).

- Provide distraction techniques such as music, television, or massage.

  These activities help to temporarily distract the client from the itching sensation. Massage has been helpful for some people with atopic dermatitis (Koblenzer, 1999).

- Consult with physician for medication to relieve itching.

  Medications such as topical steroids or antihistamines can be helpful (Koblenzer, 1999).

Geriatric

- Limit number of complete baths to one every other day. Use a tepid water temperature of 90° to 105° F for bathing.

  Excessive bathing, especially in hot water, depletes aging skin of moisture and increases dryness.

- Use a superfatted soap such as Dove, Tone, Basis, or Caress.

  Superfatted soaps help retain moisture in dry, elderly skin (Hardy, 1996).

- Increase fluid intake within cardiac or renal limits to a minimum of 1500 ml/day.

  Dry skin is caused by loss of fluid through the skin; increasing fluid intake rehydrates the skin. Adequate hydration helps decrease itching (Koblenzer, 1999).

- Use a humidifier or a container of water on heat source to increase humidity in the environment, especially during winter.

  Increasing moisture in the air helps to keep moisture in the skin (Hardy, 1996). During times of cold weather and low humidity, dermatitis of the hands is common (Uter, Gefeller, Schwanitz, 1998).

Multicultural

- Assess for the influence of cultural beliefs, norms, and values on the client's perceptions of skin and/or hair status and practices.

  What the client considers normal and abnormal skin and hair condition may be based on cultural perceptions (Leininger, 1996).

- Identify and clarify cultural language used to describe skin and hair.
- Assess skin for ashy appearance.

  Black skin and the skin of other people of color will appear ashy as a result of the flaking off of the top layer of the epidermis (Smith, Burns, 1999; Jackson, 1998).

- Encourage use of lanolin-based lotions for black clients with dry skin.

  Vaseline may clog the pores and cause cellulitis or other skin problems (Jackson, 1998).

- Offer hair oil and lanolin-based lotion for dry scalp and skin.

  Black skin seems to produce less oil than lighter colored skin; therefore blacks may use more lubricants as a normal part of skin hygiene (Smith, Burns, 1999).

- Use soap sparingly if the skin is dry.

  Black skin tends to be dry, and soap will exacerbate this condition (Jackson, 1998).

• = **Independent;** ▲ = **Collaborative**

Home Care Interventions

- Assist client and family with identifying and avoiding irritants that exacerbate pruritus (e.g., wool).
  Avoiding irritants decreases discomfort of pruritus (Koblenzer, 1999).
- Teach family to use mild, nonscented, and nonbleach laundry products.
  Chemical irritants increase discomfort of pruritus.
- Keep temperature of home moderated. Use a humidifier.
  Overheated home environments increase sweating, which adds salts to the skin and increases irritation. Increasing moisture in the air helps to keep moisture in the skin (Hardy, 1996).

Client/Family Teaching

- Teach techniques to use when client is uncomfortable, including relaxation techniques, guided imagery, hypnosis, and music therapy.
  Interventions such as progressive muscle relaxation training, guided imagery, hypnosis, and music therapy can effectively decrease the itching sensation.
- Teach client with pruritus to substitute rubbing, pressure, or vibration for scratching when itching is severe and irrepressible.
- Teach client to see primary care practitioner if itching persists and no cause is found.
  Itching can be a symptom of other conditions (Eaglestein, McKay, Pariser, 1994; Koblenzer, 1999).

WEB SITES FOR EDUCATION

MERLIN See the MERLIN web site for World Wide Web resources for client education.

REFERENCES Carpenito JL: *Nursing diagnosis: application to clinical practice,* ed 5, Philadelphia, 1993, JB Lippincott.

Eaglestein WH, McKay M, Pariser DM: The problems that plague aging skin, *Patient Care* 28:89-120, 1994.

Frantz RA, Gardner S: Clinical concerns: management of dry skin, *J Gerontol Nurs* 9:15-18, 1994.

Hardy MA: What can you do about your patient's dry skin? *J Gerontol Nurs* 5:11, 1996.

Jackson F: The ABC's of black hair and skin care, *ABNF J* 9(5):100-104, 1998.

Koblenzer CS: Itching and atopic skin, *J Allergy Clin Immunol* 104:S109-S112, 1999.

Leininger MM: *Transcultural nursing: theories, research and practices,* ed 2, Hilliard, Ohio, 1996, McGraw-Hill.

Smith W, Burns C: Managing the hair and skin of African-American pediatric clients, *J Pediatr Health Care* 13:72-78, 1999.

Stone L: Product focus: Medilan—a hypoallergenic lanolin for emollient therapy, *Br J Nurs* 9(1)54-57, 2000.

Tabata N et al: Biophysical assessment of persistent effects of moisturizers after their daily applications: evaluation of corneotherapy, *Dermatology* 200(4):308-313, 2000.

Uter W, Gefeller O, Schwanitz HJ: An epidemiological study of the influence of season on the occurrence of irritant skin changes of the hands, *Br J Dermatol* 138(2):266-272, 1998.

Impaired verbal Communication

Gail B. Ladwig

NANDA **Definition** Decreased, delayed, or absent ability to receive, process, transmit, and use a system of symbols

- • = **Independent;** ▲ = **Collaborative**

Defining Characteristics

Willful refusal to speak; disorientation in the three spheres of time, space, person; inability to speak dominant language; does not or cannot speak; speaks or verbalizes with difficulty; inappropriate verbalizations; difficulty forming words or sentences (e.g., aphonia, dyslalia, dysarthria); difficulty expressing thoughts verbally (e.g., aphasia, dysphasia, apraxia, dyslexia); stuttering; slurring; dyspnea; absence of eye contact or difficulty in selective attending; difficulty in comprehending and maintaining the usual communication pattern; partial or total visual deficit; inability or difficulty in use of facial or body expressions

Related Factors (r/t)

Decrease in circulation to brain; brain tumor; physical barrier (e.g., tracheostomy, intubation); anatomical defect; cleft palate; alteration of the neuromuscular visual system; auditory system; phonatory apparatus; psychological barriers (e.g., psychosis, lack of stimuli); cultural difference; differences related to developmental age; side effects of medication; environmental barriers; absence of significant others; altered perceptions; lack of information; stress; alteration of self-esteem or self-concept; physiological conditions; alteration of central nervous system; weakening of musculoskeletal system; emotional conditions

NOC Outcomes (Nursing Outcomes Classification)

Suggested NOC Labels

Communication Ability; Communication: Expressive Ability; Communication: Receptive Ability

> ### Example NOC Outcome
> Demonstrates **Communication Ability** as evidenced by the following indicators: Use of spoken language/Use of written language/Acknowledgment of messages received/Exchanges messages with others (Rate each indicator of **Communication Ability:** 1 = extremely compromised, 2 = substantially compromised, 3 = moderately compromised, 4 = mildly compromised, 5 = not compromised [see Section I])

Client Outcomes

- Uses effective communication techniques
- Uses alternative methods of communication effectively
- Demonstrates congruency of verbal and nonverbal behavior
- Demonstrates understanding even if not able to speak
- Expresses desire for social interactions

NIC Interventions (Nursing Interventions Classification)

Suggested NIC Labels

Active Listening; Communication Enhancement: Hearing Deficit; Communication Enhancement: Speech Deficit

> ### Example NIC Interventions—Communication Enhancement
> - Listen attentively
> - Validate understanding of messages by asking client to repeat what was said

Nursing Interventions and Rationales

▲ When client is having difficulty communicating, assess and refer for consultation for hearing problems. Hearing loss might be suspected when a person does not always

• = Independent; ▲ = Collaborative

hear sounds such as ringing telephone or doorbell, turns his or her ear toward the source of sound, frequently asks the speaker to repeat, turns the television or radio up too loud, or shows obvious signs of confusion or misunderstanding of speech. *People with hearing disorders do not hear sounds clearly. Such disorders may range from hearing speech sounds faintly or in a distorted way to profound deafness (American Speech-Language-Hearing Association, 2001).*

- Involve a familiar person when attempting to communicate with a person who has difficulty with communication. Ask about deviations in behaviors.
  The involvement of a familiar person may be reassuring and assist in interpretation of communications, whether behavior is typical or new. Sometimes deviations from normal behavior indicate a change in health status or a need (Hahn, 1999).
- ▲ Determine language spoken; obtain language dictionary or interpreter if possible and accepted by the client.
  For clear understanding, the nurse and client must speak the same language or have a means of understanding each others' language. The lack of fluency in the English language of many patients and the lack of bilingual or multilingual nurses are major sources of miscommunication, even with the use of interpreters and translated health information. Many immigrant women find the use of interpreters unacceptable, and nurses are concerned with legal issues (Maltby, 1999).
- Listen carefully. Validate verbal and nonverbal expressions.
  Client satisfaction studies have repeatedly shown that what clients want most from their nurses is common courtesy—someone who really listens to their fears and concerns and treats them like a real person, not a disease (Long, Greeneich, 1994). Listening carefully to patients gives nurses valuable tools for intervening in the lives of their patients (Walden-McBride, McBride, 2000).
- Anticipate client's needs until effective communication is possible.
  Anticipation of client's needs increases client satisfaction (Long, Greeneich, 1994).
- Use simple communication, speak in a well-modulated voice, smile, and show concern for the client.
  Such techniques have been described by clients as demonstrating caring (Clark, 1993).
- Involve clients with mental retardation in communication when possible by asking open-ended questions to elicit answers.
  Sometimes people with mental retardation answer "yes" to both yes and no questions. If you ask many yes and no questions, validate the answers by asking pertinent open-ended questions (Hahn, 1999).
- Observe behavioral cues for pain (e.g., hair pulling, face slapping, facial grimacing).
  Accurately reading cues may help to identify pain (Hahn, 1999).
- Observe behavioral communication cues in infants.
  In one study, greater pain was strongly associated with tears, stiff posture, guarding, and fisting in infants up to 12 months of age (Fuller et al, 1996).
- Maintain eye contact at client's level, reading client's eyes as able.
  Sitting down is an effective way of listening and helps to build trust (Robinson, 1993).
- When working with the hearing impaired, remove masks and reduce background noise whenever possible.
  One study of hearing impaired children receiving dental care indicated that removing masks while talking, reducing background noise, and learning to use simple signs may improve communication with hearing-impaired children (Champion, Holt, 2000).

- **= Independent; ▲ = Collaborative**

- Assess whether a person is averse to touch (tactile defensiveness), which is common among children or adults with pervasive developmental delays or autism.
  The use of touch may not work if someone experiences tactile defensiveness (Hahn, 1999).
- Use touch as appropriate. Holding a client's hand or stroking the arm is a simple, nonintrusive way of showing empathy and concern.
  Touch that conveys caring is an appropriate way of communicating, unless the person touched shows discomfort (Wells, 1996).
- Use presence. Spend time with client, allow time for responses, and make call light readily available.
  Nursing presence, one-to-one interaction, connecting with the client's experience, going beyond the scientific data, and knowing what will work and when to act all support the nurse-client relationship and affirm their respective selves. As a result, the client grows in awareness of his own being (Doona, Chase, Haggerty, 1999).
- Explain all health care procedures.
  The nurse cannot assume that a person does not understand, even if that person is non-verbal. A person's receptive language skills may be better than expressive language skills (Hahn, 1999).
- Obtain communication equipment such as electronic devices, letterboards, picture boards, and magic slates.
  Alternative methods of communication are necessary when the client is unable to use verbal communication.
- Establish an alternative method of communication such as writing or pointing to letters, word phrases, picture cards, or simple drawings of basic needs.
  Alternative methods of communication are necessary when the client is unable to use verbal communication. A booklet of drawings (visual language) representing the most common needs was used with a group of 34 patients affected by severe dysarthria or motor aphasia causing severe language disorders. Most of these patients used this booklet to express their basic needs, which resulted in a lower degree of anxiety in these patients (Marquez-Rebollo, Tornel-Costa, 1997).
- Provide pencil and paper for letter writing to facilitate expression of feelings.
  Letter writing has been used with patients who have had amputations to help them to successfully express feelings (Hatipoglu, Temiz, 1995).
- ▲ It may be helpful to consult with a speech therapist. Supplement the work of speech therapist with appropriate exercises.
  Consultation and collaboration with a specialist may be necessary to provide the best approach to improving communication. The main conclusion of this review is that speech and language therapy treatment for people with aphasia after a stroke has not been shown either to be clearly effective or clearly ineffective within a randomized controlled trial (Greener, Enderby, Whurr, 2000).
- Give praise for progress noted. Ignore mistakes and watch for frustration or fatigue.
  Positive reinforcement increases confidence, which can increase communication (Boss, 1991).
- Encourage family to bring in familiar pictures or calendars.
- Establish an understanding of client's symbolic speech (especially with schizophrenic clients). Ask client to clarify particular statements.
  Clarification is a necessary communication skill. Psychoeducation covers the practical problems of living with schizophrenia. Families learn when to ignore problem behaviors and when to intervene (Huddleston, 1992).

• = Independent; ▲ = Collaborative

- If there is a comprehension deficit, keep environment quiet when communicating and get client's attention before attempting to communicate (e.g., touch client's shoulder, call client's name).
  When the client is confused, a distracting environment interferes with communication. It is necessary to get the client's full attention before any communication can take place (Boss, 1991).
- Use "affection therapy" when the client cannot express thoughts or ideas. Provide frequent and regular reminders that client is wanted and cared about (e.g., physical signs of affection such as a hug or a friendly comment before and after every interaction regardless of client's performance).
  When clients are unable to communicate their thoughts and feelings adequately, they may whistle, swear, and make other noises incessantly. "Affection therapy" works when behavior modification techniques do not (Armstrong, 1991).
- Do not raise your voice or shout at the client.
  A loud voice can be frightening and decrease communication.

Geriatric

- ▲ Carefully assess client for hearing difficulty using an audio scope.
  The prevalence of hearing impairment in hospitalized elderly patients was found to be very high during screening with an audio scope (Lim, Yap, 2000).
- ▲ Encourage client to wear prescribed eyeglasses and hearing aids.
  Auditory and visual disorders are prevalent among older people. About 40% of adults aged 65 and older have a hearing loss sufficient to interfere with daily conversation (Erber, 1994). About 20% in the same age range experience low vision and reduced visual fields, which can prevent clear perception of a communication partner at a conversational distance (Erber, 1994).
- When communicating with client, face toward his or her unaffected side or better ear.
  Correct positioning increases the client's awareness of the interaction and enhances the client's ability to interact.
- Provide sufficient light and remove distractions such as glare and background noise.
  Background noise further impairs the elderly client's hearing.
- Use low voice tones and recognize that perception of the sounds "f," "s," "th," "ch," "sh," "b," "t," "p," "k," and "d" is impaired with hearing loss that results from aging.
  Presbycusis decreases the ability to hear high-pitched sounds and the consonant sounds listed in the preceding paragraph. Perception of consonants is important to understanding language.
- Allow time for thought comprehension when communicating with client.
  Older clients do not like to be rushed. They fare much better in a calm, consistent environment that functions at a moderately slow pace (Bailey, Bailey, 1993).
- Schedule time to listen to client's life story.
  This is a means of finding out what is important to client. The practice of nursing comes alive by listening to individual stories. Each person's story is created out of personal life experiences (Running, 1996).

Multicultural

- Assess for the influence of cultural beliefs, norms, and values on the client's communication process.
  What the client considers normal and abnormal communication may be based on cultural perceptions (Leininger, 1996).
- Assess the use of personal space needs, communication styles, acceptable body language, eye contact, perception of touch, and use of paraverbals when communicating with the client.

• = **Independent**; ▲ = **Collaborative**

Nurses need to consider these when interpreting verbal and nonverbal messages (Siantz, 1991). Native Americans may consider avoidance of direct eye contact as a sign of respect and asking questions to be rude and intrusive (Seiderman et al, 1996).

- Use extreme care when using touch.
  Touch is believed by some cultures to be a source of illness. Touching a baby's head requires parental permission in some Southeast Asian cultures. Many Latinos believe that excessive admiration of a child without touching will result in physical illness to the child (mal de ojo—evil eye). In some Islamic and Latino cultures, physical touch between a nurse and client is acceptable only if the individuals are the same sex (Kelley, 1998).
- Modify communication approach to the client's particular culture.
  Modification of communication will convey respect to the client (Siantz, 1991).
- Use an interpreter if the client speaks a different language.
  An experienced interpreter will allow for accurate translation.
- Use therapeutic communication techniques that emphasize acceptance, offer the self, validate the client's concerns, and convey respect.
  Validation lets the client know that the nurse has heard and understands what was said, and it promotes the nurse-client relationship (Stuart, Laraia, 2001; Giger, Davidhizar, 1995). Studies show that even when language is not a barrier, some ethnic clients may be reluctant to discuss their beliefs and practices because of fear of criticism or ridicule (Evans, Cunningham, 1996).

Home Care Interventions

- ▲ Continue with speech therapy services per physician order. Support speech therapy plan of care.
  With appropriate support, clients can continue to make significant progress toward resuming normal or improved communication function.
- Assess family for possible role changes resulting from communication impairment of family member.
  An impairment that prevents a family member from fulfilling the usual role can change the family constellation.
- When possible, encourage family to include client in family activities using enhanced communication techniques with sensitivity.
  Involving the client in family activities promotes earlier return to normal life patterns, but doing so in an awkward or embarrassing way can diminish interest.
- ▲ Refer to medical social services as necessary for help in obtaining funds for communication devices and counseling for dealing with long-term impact of communication changes in family.

Client/Family Teaching

- Teach client and family techniques to increase communication.
  Alternative methods of communication are necessary when the client is unable to use verbal communication.
- Teach basic signs to indicate needs, such as "eat," "drink," "toilet," "more," "finished."
  Sometime clients with mental retardation are taught basic signs for communication (Hahn, 1999).
- Encourage significant others to use touch, such as holding client's hand or stroking the arm.
  Incorporating relatives into this aspect of care provides continuity with the client's real life and fulfills the relatives' need to demonstrate care (MacGinley, 1993).

• = **Independent;** ▲ = **Collaborative**

▲ Teach client how to use communication devices.

▲ Refer client to a speech-language pathologist or audiologist.

A thorough evaluation by a speech-language pathologist or audiologist is needed to determine a person's communication strengths and weaknesses. After this evaluation, the speech-language pathologist or audiologist will be able to provide a plan for meeting individual needs (American Speech-Language-Hearing Association, 2001).

WEB SITES FOR EDUCATION

ᶴₘₑᵣₗᵢₙ See the MERLIN web site for World Wide Web resources for client education.

REFERENCES   American Speech-Language-Hearing Association: *Stroke,* retrieved from the World Wide Web on May 29, 2001. Web site: www.asha.org/speech/disabilities/Stroke.cfm.

Armstrong C: Emotional changes following brain injury: psychological and neurological components of depression, denial and anxiety, *J Rehab* 57:15, 1991.

Bailey DS, Bailey DR: *Therapeutic approaches to the care of the mentally ill,* ed 3, Philadelphia, 1993, FA Davis.

Boss BJ: Managing communication disorders in stroke, *Nurs Clin North Am* 26:985, 1991.

Champion J, Holt R: Dental care for children and young people who have a hearing impairment, *Br Dent J* 189(3):155-159, 2000.

Clark S: Challenges in critical care nursing: helping patients and families cope, *Crit Care Nurs* S2:2, 1993.

Doona M, Chase S, Haggerty L: Nursing presence, *J Holistic Nurs* 17(1):54-69, 1999.

Erber N: Conversation as therapy for older adults in residential care: the case for intervention, *Eur J Disord Commun* 29:269, 1994.

Evans CA, Cunningham BA: Caring for the ethnic elder, *Geriatr Nurs: Am J Care Aging* 17(3):105-110, 1996.

Fuller B et al: Relationship of cues to assessed infant pain level, *Clin Nurs Res* 5(1):43-66, 1996.

Giger JN, Davidhizar RE: *Transcultural nursing,* ed 2, St Louis, 1995, Mosby.

Greener J, Enderby P, Whurr R: Speech and language therapy for aphasia following stroke, *Cochrane Database Syst Rev* 2:CD000425, 2000.

Hahn J: Cueing in to patient language, *Reflections* 25(1):8-11, 1999.

Hatipoglu S, Temiz Z: Amputee's diary, *Image J Nurs Sch* 27:248, 1995.

Huddleston J: Family and group psychoeducational approaches in the management of schizophrenia, *Clin Nurs Spec* 6:118, 1992.

Kelley J: Cultural and ethnic considerations. In Frisch NC, Frisch LE, editors: *Psychiatric mental health nursing,* Albany, NY, 1998, Delmar, pp 106-117.

Leininger MM: *Transcultural nursing: theories, research and practices,* ed 2, Hilliard, Ohio, 1996, McGraw-Hill.

Lim JK, Yap KB: Screening for hearing impairment in hospitalised elderly, *Ann Acad Med Singapore* 29(2):237-241, 2000.

Long C, Greeneich D: Four strategies for keeping patients satisfied, *Am J Nurs* 94:27, 1994.

MacGinley K: Nursing care of the patient with altered body image, *Brit J Nurs* 2:1098, 1993.

Maltby HJ: Interpreters: a double-edged sword in nursing practice, *J Transcult Nurs* 10(3):248-254, 1999.

Marquez-Rebollo MC, Tornel-Costa MC: Design of a non-verbal method of communication using cartoons, *Rev Neurol* 25(148):2045-2047, 1997.

Robinson K: Denial: an adaptive response, *Dimens Crit Care Nurs* 12:102, 1993.

Running A: "The measure of my day" critiqued by the oldest old, *Image J Nurs Sch* 28:71, 1996.

Seiderman RY et al: Assessing American Indian families, *MCN Am J Matern Child Nurs* 21(6):274-279, 1996.

Siantz ML: How can we be more aware of culturally specific body language and use this awareness therapeutically? *J Psychosoc Nurs* 29(11):38-39, 1991.

Stuart GW, Laraia MT: Therapeutic nurse-patient relationship. In Stuart GW, Lauria MT, editors: *Principles and practice of psychiatric nursing,* St Louis, 2001, Mosby, p 30.

Walden-McBride DL, McBride JL: Listening for the patient's story: the psychosocial story of a patient with end-stage heart disease, *J Psychosoc Nurs Ment Health Serv* 38(11):26-31, 2000.

Wells E: Assisting parents when a child dies in the ICU, *Crit Care Nurs* 16:58, 1996.

• = **Independent;** ▲ = **Collaborative**

Decisional Conflict

Gail B. Ladwig

 Definition Uncertainty about course of action to be taken when choice among competing actions involves risk, loss, or challenge to personal life values

Defining Characteristics

Verbalizes uncertainty about choices; verbalizes undesired consequences of alternative actions being considered; vacillation between alternative choices; delayed decision making; verbalizes feelings of distress while attempting to make a decision; self-focusing; physical signs of distress or tension (e.g., increased heart rate, increased muscle tension, restlessness); questioning of personal values and beliefs while attempting to make a decision

Related Factors (r/t)

Support system deficit; perceived threat to value system; lack of experience or interference with decision making; multiple or divergent sources of information; lack of relevant information; unclear personal values/beliefs

NOC ## Outcomes (Nursing Outcomes Classification)

Suggested NOC Labels
Decision Making; Information Processing; Participation: Health Care Decisions

> ### Example NOC Outcome
> Demonstrates **Decision Making** as evidenced by the following indicators: Identifies relevant information/Identifies alternatives/Identifies potential consequences of each alternative/Identifies resources necessary to support each alternative (Rate each indicator of **Decision Making:** 1 = never demonstrated, 2 = rarely demonstrated, 3 = sometimes demonstrated, 4 = often demonstrated, 5 = consistently demonstrated [see Section I])

Client Outcomes

- States the advantages and disadvantages of choices
- Shares fears and concerns regarding choices and responses of others
- Makes an informed choice

NIC ## Interventions (Nursing Interventions Classification)

Suggested NIC Labels
Decision-Making Support

> ### Example NIC Interventions—Decision-Making Support
> - Inform client of alternative views or solutions
> - Facilitate client's articulation of goals for care

Nursing Interventions and Rationales

- Observe for factors causing or contributing to conflict (e.g., value conflicts, fear of outcome, poor problem-solving skills).
  Baseline data are important in directing interventions; no single set of values is appropriate for all individuals. Values clarification emphasizes the client's capacity for intelligent, self-directed behavior (Dossey et al, 1988).

- = Independent; ▲ = Collaborative

- Work with and allow clients to make decisions in a way that is comfortable for them, such as deferring (allowing others to decide), delaying (choosing an alternative that meets basic requirements), or deliberating (looking at all alternatives).
  Individual clients confronting health care choices have unique decision-making styles (Pierce, 1993). Involving clients in health care decisions makes a potentially significant and enduring difference to health care outcomes (Elwyn et al, 2000).
- Give client time and permission to express feelings associated with decision making.
  Decisions become more difficult when feelings are repressed. Once client relieves some of the stress talking through problems and releasing pent-up emotions, the decision process often becomes easier (Burnard, 1992).
- Explore client's perception of the future with regard to different decisions.
  Perceiving the future helps the client focus on what is important. Accurate time orientation (the ability to view the future on the basis of present and past experience) indicates that the client will have better coping skills (Haber et al, 1992).
- Demonstrate reassurance with unconditional respect for and acceptance of client's values, spiritual beliefs, and cultural norms.
  Good communication with and reassurance of client are nursing skills that promote trust and orientation and reduce anxiety (Harvey, 1996).
- Encourage client to list the advantages and disadvantages of each alternative.
  Listing alternatives helps clients learn how to problem solve. Clients might not believe they have alternatives and may need assistance exploring options (Chez, 1994).
- ▲ Initiate health teaching and referrals when needed.
  All interventions need to be individualized, and sometimes referrals are necessary.
- Facilitate communication between client and family members regarding the final decision; offer support to person actually making the decision.
  Studies suggest that clients' decisions are rarely the same as those of their friends and family members; therefore, when possible, clients are best suited to determine their own life support treatment (Beland, Froman, 1995).
- Provide detailed benefits and risks using functional terms and probabilities tailored to clinical risk plus steps for considering the issues and means for making a decision, including values clarification and decision aides when clients are faced with difficult treatment choices.
  It is concluded that tailored decision aids prepare women for decision making better than do general pamphlets (O'Connor et al, 1998). Decision aids improve knowledge, reduce decisional conflict, and stimulate patients to be more active in decision making without increasing their anxiety (O'Connor et al, 1999).

Geriatric

- Work with clients in setting goals for their plans of care.
  Goal-centered advance medical planning can be initiated in nursing homes by asking residents or their surrogates to prioritize their goals of care. These prioritizations can form the foundation for specific patterns of care (Gillick, Berkman, Cullen, 1999).
- Discuss with client and family the importance of discussing and recording end-of-life decisions.
  These decisions are of extreme importance to an aging client. Discussing these issues gives the client both a sense of control and the opportunity to prepare for the inevitable (Dossey et al, 1988).

  • = **Independent;** ▲ = **Collaborative**

- If end-of-life discussions are being avoided, describe the possible consequences.
  Participants in this study thought that a Do Not Resuscitate decision should be discussed with patients and also with relatives if appropriate. However, there was ambivalence about whether individuals would like to be involved personally in such a decision because of the anxiety this would produce (Phillips, Woodward, 1999).
- Discuss the purpose of a living will and advance directives.
  Elderly clients and their significant others need to know how to legally make end-of-life decisions. (NOTE: Laws differ in each state.) Research has demonstrated that the presence of an advance directive can be very helpful for decreasing family stress when end-of-life decisions need to be made (Tilden et al, 2001).
- ▲ Discuss choices or changes to be made (e.g., moving in with children, into a nursing home, or into an adult foster care home).
  Exploring options gives the client and family a sense of control. For a change to be effective, it must be accepted and owned by the client (Fleury, 1991).
- Teach family members how to be supportive of final decision or how to refrain from being destructive if unable to be supportive.
  It is important to support the decisions that the client makes.

Multicultural

- Assess for the influence of cultural beliefs, norms, and values on the client's decision-making conflict.
  Cultural influences may interfere with the client's decision-making process (Wright, Cohen, Caroselli, 1997; Leininger, 1996).
- Identify who will be involved in the decision-making process.
  In a group of frail elderly, ethnic variations were found with regard to the family member identified as the decision maker (Hornug et al, 1998). Contrary to expectations, Latinas will often make decisions related to prenatal care and services (Browner, Preloran, Cox, 1999). Korean-American clients and other Asian clients may consider some decisions to be a family affair (D'Avanzo et al, 2001; Blackhall et al, 1999).
- ▲ Use cross-cultural decision aids whenever possible.
  Consumer-based cross-cultural decision aids inform patients of potential risks and benefits so that they can make value- and evidence-integrated decisions (Lawrence et al, 2000). In one study, Latinas' assessment of risk and uncertainty with procedures was associated with decisions to refuse certain procedures (Browner, Preloran, Cox, 1999).
- Validate the client's feelings regarding the decisional conflict.
  Validation lets the client know that the nurse has heard and understands what was said, and it promotes the nurse-client relationship (Stuart, Laraia, 2001; Giger, Davidhizar, 1995).

Home Care Interventions

- ▲ Before providing any home care, assess client plan for advance directives (living will and power of attorney). If plan exists, place copy in client file. If no plan exists, offer information on advance directives according to agency policy. Refer for assistance in completing advance directives as necessary. Do not witness living will.
  This is a legal requirement of COBRA legislation.
- Determine relevance of conflict to plan of care.
- Assess client and family for consensus (or lack of) regarding issue in conflict.
- ▲ If decision is relevant to plan of care, primary nurse or medical social services may evaluate the need for and call a family conference. If consensus cannot be reached,

• = **Independent**; ▲ = **Collaborative**

continue efforts to resolve the conflict. Clients, unless medically incompetent (by legal guidelines) or under authorized power of attorney, may make their own decisions. *Guided family conferences allow all persons affected by the decision to be heard and the value system of the client to be validated. The nurse or social worker serves as the facilitator and client advocate.*

▲ If not relevant to the plan of care, refer to community support appropriate to type of decision and client need.

Client/Family Teaching

• Instruct the client and family members to provide advance directives in the following areas:
  ▪ Person to contact in an emergency
  ▪ Preference (if any) to die at home or in the hospital
  ▪ Desire to sign a living will
  ▪ Desire to donate an organ
  ▪ Funeral arrangements (i.e., burial, cremation)
  While clients are still out in the community, complete advance directives through their family physicians or through area agencies on aging. Make these decisions before the crisis occurs (Maloney, 2001).

• Inform family of treatment options; encourage and defend self-determination.
  The Patient Self-Determination Act, effective since December 1991, has changed the importance of introducing life support options to patients (Beland, Froman, 1995).

• Identify reasons for family decisions regarding care. Explore ways in which family decisions can be respected.
  Family issues need to be identified to provide optimal care (e.g., establish whether the family understands the prognosis, has unresolved issues with the client, is waiting for someone to come from out of town, and whether other issues must be resolved before final decisions can be made [Campbell, 1994]).

▲ Recognize and allow client to discuss the choice of complementary therapies available, such as spiritual, relaxation, imagery, exercise, lifestyle, diet (e.g., macrobiotic, vegetarian), and nutritional supplementation.
  Discussing these health practices in a nonjudgmental manner increases client's coping skills and ability to make decisions about his or her health care. A study of cancer patients found that the patients unanimously believed that complementary therapies helped to improve their quality of life by helping them to cope more effectively with stress, decreasing the discomforts of treatment and illness, and giving them a sense of control (Sparber et al, 2000).

• Include families in patient care conferences. As a client's condition changes, it may be necessary to rethink the goal of treatment. It may change from restoration and cure to stabilization of functioning or preparation for comfortable and dignified death.
  Families who are consistently apprised of changes in a client's condition and assisted with exploring what these changes mean are more likely than others to trust the recommendation of the care team to withdraw or withhold further aggressive treatment (Taylor, 1995).

WEB SITES FOR EDUCATION

MERLIN See the MERLIN web site for World Wide Web resources for client education.

• = **Independent;** ▲ = **Collaborative**

REFERENCES   Beland K, Froman R: Preliminary validation of a measure of life support preferences, *Image J Nurs Sch* 27:307, 1995.

Blackhall LJ et al: Ethnicity and attitudes towards life sustaining technology, *Soc Sci Med* 48(12):1779-1789, 1999.

Browner CH, Preloran HM, Cox SJ: Ethnicity, bioethics, and prenatal diagnosis: the amniocentesis decisions of Mexican-origin women and their partners, *Am J Public Health* 89(11):1658-1666, 1999.

Burnard PL: *Counseling: a guide to practice in nursing,* Oxford, England, 1992, Butterworth-Heinemann.

Campbell M: Making an end-of-life difference, *Crit Care Nurse* 14:111, 1994.

Chez N: Helping the victim of domestic violence, *Am J Nurs* 94:33, 1994.

D'Avanzo CE et al: Developing culturally informed strategies for substance-related interventions. In Naegle MA, D'Avanzo CE, editors: *Addictions and substance abuse: strategies for advanced practice nursing,* St Louis, 2001, Mosby, pp 59-104.

Dossey B et al: *Holistic nursing: a handbook for practice,* Gaithersburg, Md, 1988, Aspen.

Elwyn G et al: Shared decision making and the concept of equipoise: the competences of involving patients in healthcare choices, *Br J Gen Pract* 50(460):892-899, 2000.

Fleury J: Empowering potential: a theory of wellness motivation, *Nurs Res* 40:268, 1991.

Giger JN, Davidhizar RE: *Transcultural nursing,* ed 2, St Louis, 1995, Mosby.

Gillick M, Berkman S, Cullen L: A patient-centered approach to advance medical planning in the nursing home, *J Am Geriatr Soc* 47(2):227-230, 1999.

Haber J et al: *Comprehensive psychiatric nursing,* ed 4, St Louis, 1992, Mosby.

Harvey M: Managing agitation in critically ill patients, *Am J Crit Care* 5:7, 1996.

Hornug CA et al: Ethnicity and decision makers in a group of frail elderly, *J Am Geriatr Soc* 46(3):280-286, 1998.

Lawrence VA et al: A cross-cultural consumer based decision aid for screening mammography, *Prev Med* 30(3):200-208, 2000.

Leininger MM: *Transcultural nursing: theories, research and practices,* ed 2, Hilliard, Ohio, 1996, McGraw-Hill.

Maloney J: A time for deciding: the reality of the patient self-determination act, *Health & Hum Dev Online,* retrieved from the World Wide Web on May 29, 2001. Web site: www.hhdev.psu.edu/research/Deciding/htm.

O'Connor A et al: Randomized trial of a portable, self-administered decision aid for postmenopausal women considering long-term preventive hormone therapy, *Med Decis Making* 18(3):295-303, 1998.

O'Connor AM et al: Decision aids for patients facing health treatment or screening decisions: systematic review, *BMJ* 319(7212):731-734, 1999.

Phillips K, Woodward V: The decision to resuscitate: older people's views, *J Clin Nurs* 8(6):753-761, 1999.

Pierce P: Deciding on breast cancer treatment: a description of decision behavior, *Nurs Res* 42:1, 1993.

Sparber A et al: Use of complementary medicine by adult patients participating in cancer clinical trials, *Oncol Nurs Forum* 27(4):623-630, 2000.

Stuart GW, Laraia MT: Therapeutic nurse-patient relationship. In Stuart GW, Lauria MT, editors: *Principles and practice of psychiatric nursing* St Louis, 2001, Mosby, p 30.

Taylor C: Medical futility and nursing, *Image J Nurs Sch* 27:301, 1995.

Tilden VP et al: Family decision making to withdraw life-sustaining treatments from hospitalized patients, *Nurs Res* 50(2):105-115, 2001.

Wright F, Cohen S, Caroselli C: Diverse decisions: how culture affects ethical decision-making, *Crit Care Nurs Clin North Am* 9(1):63-74, 1997.

Parental role Conflict

Peggy A. Wetsch and Mary Markle

NANDA   **Definition**   Parent experience of role confusion and conflict in response to crisis

Defining Characteristics

Expresses concerns about changes in parental role, family functioning, family communication, family health; expresses concerns/feelings of inadequacy with regard to providing for child's physical and emotional needs during hospitalization or at home; reluctant to participate in usual caregiving activities, even with encouragement and

• = Independent; ▲ = Collaborative

support; demonstrates disruption in care and caregiving routines; expresses concern about perceived loss of control regarding decisions relating to child; verbalizes or demonstrates feelings of guilt, anger, fear, anxiety, and frustration concerning the effect of the child's illness on family processes

Related Factors (r/t)

Change in marital status; home care of child with special needs (e.g., apnea monitoring, postural drainage, hyperalimentation); interruptions of family life as a result of home care regimens (e.g., treatments, caregivers, lack of respite, specialized care center policies); separation from child as a result of chronic illness; intimidation by invasive or restrictive modalities (e.g., isolation, intubation)

NOC   Outcomes (Nursing Outcomes Classification)

Suggested NOC Labels

Caregiver Adaptation to Child Institutionalization; Caregiver Home Care Readiness; Coping; Parenting; Psychosocial Adjustment: Life Change; Role Performance

> **Example NOC Outcome**
> Achieves **Caregiver Adaptation to Child Institutionalization** as evidenced by: Participation in care as desired/Trust in nonfamily caregivers/Caregivers' resolution of guilt (Rate each indicator of **Caregiver Adaptation to Child Institutionalization:** 1 = no adaptation, 2 = limited adaptation, 3 = moderate adaptation 4 = substantial adaptation, 5 = extensive adaptation [see Section I])

Client Outcomes

- Expresses feelings and perceptions regarding impacts of illness, disability, and/or hospitalization on parental role
- Participates in hospital/home care of as much as able to given the availability of resources and support systems
- Exhibits assertiveness and responsibility in active family decision making regarding care of the child
- Describes and selects available resources to support parental management of child/ family needs

NIC   Interventions (Nursing Interventions Classification)

Suggested NIC Labels

Crisis Intervention; Parenting Promotion; Role Enhancement

> **Example NIC Interventions—Parenting Promotion**
> - Assist parents with role transition and expectations of parenthood
> - Assist family members to use existing support mechanisms

Nursing Interventions and Rationales

- Assess parents' previous coping behaviors.
  Having previous success with coping gives parents a feeling of competence. Identifying ineffective or absent coping behaviors allows development of interventions. Research indicates that parents who cope successfully are better able to promote the adjustment and recovery of the child (Ladebauche, 1992).
- Explore parent/family sources of stress, usual methods of coping, and perceptions of illness/condition. Capitalize on strengths identified. Involve both parents in assessment.

• = **Independent;** ▲ = **Collaborative**

Identification of parents' perceptions of the magnitude of circumstances, perceived degree of adequacy, and usual coping methods can support strategies that promote active constructive coping or help nurse to develop approaches to build/strengthen coping ability. Maintaining an optimistic outlook is important for parents who are caring for a chronically ill child at home (Ray, Ritchie, 1993; Bond, Phillips, Rollins, 1994; Heaman, 1995; Melnyk, 1995).

- Consider use of family theory as a framework to help guide interventions (e.g., family stress theory, role theory, social exchange theory).
  Theory helps to identify the focus, means, and goals of nursing practice. It enhances communication and increases autonomy and accountability to care (Gillis et al, 1989; Meleis, 1991).
- Sustain parental involvement in shared decision making with regard to care by using the following steps:
  Incorporate parents' information concerning child's typical routines, behaviors, fears, likes, and dislikes.
  - Provide clear and direct firsthand information concerning child's condition and progress.
  - Normalize the home/hospital environment as much as possible.
  - Collaborate in care by providing choices when possible.
  Involving parents in a child's caregiving and in decision making helps increase parental feelings of control and decrease feelings of stress. Noting parents' questions and nonverbal cues to determine need for improved communication is important (Sims et al, 1992; Shellabarger, Thompson, 1993; Bond, Phillips, Rollins, 1994).
- Seek and support parental participation in care.
  As parents of disabled children gain knowledge and become more involved in caregiving activities, their caregiver identity emerges. Parents eventually emerge as the central persons in their children's lives. Parental participation has been demonstrated to have a positive effect on a child's reactions to procedures, resulting in improved cooperation and decreases in upset behaviors and child's level of disturbed activity (Moynihan, Nalcerio, Kiley, 1995; Perkins, 1993; Jones, Maestri, McCoy, 1994).
- Provide support for each parent's primary coping strategies.
  Mothers tend to focus more on strategies related to social support, whereas fathers are inclined to analyze situations (Heaman, 1995).
- ▲ Offer respite care to assist parents in maintaining sufficient energy and personal resources to continue caregiving responsibilities.
  Medically fragile or technology-dependent children, and children with chronic health problems and resultant disabilities, receive most of their care at home by family members, frequently at severe economic and psychological costs (Coffman, Folden, 1992; Folden, Coffman, 1993).
- ▲ Determine older-than-average mother's support systems and self-expectations for motherhood. Pay particular attention to relationships with spouse or partner, family, and friends.
  Social support has a positive influence on early parenting for primiparas >35 years of age. Older primiparas with high self-expectations, low satisfaction with parenting, or inadequate social support systems may be at risk (Ferris, Reece, 1994).
- Be available to discuss concerns, and be a good listener.
  The parent is more likely to verbalize concerns when the nurse is not hurried. Open communication is essential for the identification of potential coping problems (Ladebauche, 1992).

• = **Independent**; ▲ = **Collaborative**

▲ Encourage parent to meet own needs of rest, nutrition, and hygiene. Provide facilities so that parent may stay with sick child (e.g., cot, reclining chair).
A parent is unable to meet the child's needs when the basic self-needs are unmet.

• Demonstrate safe places where parent may touch or stroke child. Encourage parent to talk or sing to child. Adjust equipment so that parent is able to hold child, and provide a comfortable chair, preferably a rocking chair. Provide opportunities and offer praise for successful caregiving.
Involvement in child's care will give parents a sense of control in the hospital environment.

▲ Refer parents to available telephone counseling services.
Telephone counseling services can provide confidential advice to families who might otherwise have no access to help for dealing with a child's problems (Jones, Maestri, McCoy, 1994).

Multicultural

• Acknowledge racial/ethnic differences at the onset of care.
Acknowledgement of race/ethnicity issues will enhance communication, establish rapport, and promote treatment outcomes (D'Avanzo et al, 2001).

• Assess for the influence of cultural beliefs, norms, and values on the client's perceptions of parent role.
What the client considers normal or abnormal parental role may be based on cultural perceptions (Leininger, 1996). Some Mexican-American families may engage in an intergenerational family ritual called "La Cuarentena," which lasts for 40 days after birth and involves prescriptions for maternal food, clothing, and paternal role (Niska, Snyder, Lia-Hoagberg, 1998).

• Acknowledge that value conflicts from acculturation stresses may contribute to increased anxiety and significant conflict with parental role.
Challenges to traditional beliefs and values are anxiety provoking (Charron, 1998). Less acculturated parents may experience conflict with their more acculturated children as the children demand greater independence and freedom (True, 1995).

• Validate the client's feelings with regard to parental role confusion and conflict.
Validation lets the client know that the nurse has heard and understands what was said, and it promotes the nurse-client relationship (Stuart, Laraia, 2001; Giger, Davidhizar, 1995).

Client/Family Teaching

• Furnish clear explanations about condition, disease or disability, associated treatments, and prognosis. Describe circumstances involving emotional and physical reactions of the child and types of family member reactions that might be anticipated in response to condition or crisis. Provide ample time for skill practice.
Providing information to families decreases confusion and anxiety, increases understanding, and allows a feeling of competence and control. Providing information about the disease and treatment process helps build parents' feelings of confidence (Baker, 1994).

• For parents of children with chronic disabilities, tailor educational opportunities based on the experiential phase (protection, survival, or development of the parent as central person) of the parents as they develop an identity as the central caregiver for their child.
As parents of physically and/or cognitively disabled children gain knowledge and become more involved in caregiving activities, their caregiver identity emerges (Perkins, 1993).

▲ Involve parents in formal and/or informal social support situations, including parent-to-parent groups, community agencies, and counseling resources.
Parents of children with special health care needs are uniquely equipped to help each other learn day-to-day coping skills. Use of available social supports in the community can help parents to achieve successful outcomes (Coffman, Folden, 1992; Hartman, Radin, McConnell, 1992).

• = **Independent;** ▲ = **Collaborative**

REFERENCES   Baker NA: Avoid collisions with challenging families, *Matern Child Nurs* 19:97, 1994.

Bond N, Phillips P, Rollins JA: Family centered care at home for families with children who are technology dependent, *Pediatr Nurs* 20:123, 1994.

Charron HS: Anxiety disorders. In Varcarolis EM, editor: *Foundations of psychiatric mental health nursing,* ed 3, Philadelphia, 1998, WB Saunders, pp 447-448.

Coffman S, Folden SL: Respite care for medically fragile children, *J Home Health Care Pract* 5:16, 1992.

D'Avanzo et al: Developing culturally informed strategies for substance-related interventions. In Naegle MA, D'Avanzo CE, editors: *Addictions and substance abuse: strategies for advanced practice nursing,* St Louis, 2001, Mosby, pp 59-104.

Ferris A, Reece C: Nutritional consequences of chronic maternal conditions during pregnancy and lactation: lupus and diabetes, *J Clin Nutr* 59:4658, 1994.

Folden SL, Coffman S: Respite care for families of children with disabilities, *J Pediatr Health Care* 7:103, 1993.

Giger JN, Davidhizar RE: *Transcultural nursing,* ed 2, St Louis, 1995, Mosby.

Gillis C et al: *Toward a science of family nursing,* Menlo Park, Calif, 1989, Addison-Wesley.

Hartman AF, Radin MB, McConnell B: Parent-to-parent support: a critical component of health care services for families, *Issues Compr Pediatr Nurs* 15(1):55, 1992.

Heaman DJ: Perceived stressors and coping strategies of parents who have children with developmental disabilities: a comparison of mothers with fathers, *J Pediatr Nurs* 10:311, 1995.

Jones LC, Maestri BO, McCoy K: Why parents use the warm line, *Matern Child Nurs* 18:258, 1994.

Ladebauche P: Unit-based family support groups: a reminder, *Matern Child Nurs* 17:18, 1992.

Leininger MM: *Transcultural nursing: theories, research and practices,* ed 2, Hilliard, Ohio, 1996, McGraw-Hill.

Meleis A: *Theoretical nursing,* Philadelphia, 1991, JB Lippincott.

Melnyk BM: Parental coping with childhood hospitalization: a theoretical framework to guide research and clinical interventions, *Matern Child Nurs* 23:123, 1995.

Moynihan P, Nalcerio L, Kiley K: Parent participation, *Nurs Clin North Am* 30:231, 1995.

Niska K, Snyder M, Lia-Hoagberg B: Family ritual facilitates adaptation to parenthood, *Public Health Nurs* 15(5):329-337, 1998.

Perkins MT: Parent-nurse collaboration: using the caregiver identity emergence phases to assist parents of hospitalized children with disabilities, *J Pediatr Nurs* 8:2, 1993.

Ray LD, Ritchie JA: Caring for chronically ill children at home: factors that influence parents' coping, *J Pediatr Nurs* 8:217, 1993.

Shellabarger SG, Thompson TL: The critical times: meeting parental communication needs throughout the NICU experience, *Neonatal Netw* 12:39, 1993.

Sims SL et al: Decision making in home health care, *West J Nurs Res* 14:186, 1992.

Stuart GW, Laraia MT: Therapeutic nurse-patient relationship. In Stuart GW, Lauria MT, editors: *Principles and practice of psychiatric nursing,* St Louis, 2001, Mosby, p 30.

True RH: Mental health issues of Asian/Pacific island women. In Adams DL, editor: *Health issues for women of color: a cultural diversity perspective,* Thousand Oaks, Calif, 1995, Sage, pp 102-105.

Acute Confusion

Kimberly Hickey and Gail B. Ladwig

NANDA   **Definition**   Abrupt onset of a cluster of global, transient changes and disturbances in attention, cognition, psychomotor activity, level of consciousness, or the sleep/wake cycle

• = Independent; ▲ = Collaborative

Defining Characteristics

Lack of motivation to initiate and/or follow through with goal-directed or purposeful behavior; fluctuation in psychomotor activity; misperceptions; fluctuation in cognition; increased agitation or restlessness; fluctuation in level of consciousness; fluctuation in sleep-wake cycle; hallucinations

Related Factors (r/t)

>60 years of age; dementia; alcohol abuse; abuse; delirium; uncontrolled pain; multiple morbidities and medications

NOC   **Outcomes (Nursing Outcomes Classification)**

Suggested NOC Labels

Cognitive Ability; Distorted Thought Control; Information Processing; Memory; Neurological Status: Consciousness; Safety Behavior: Personal; Sleep

> **Example NOC Outcome**
> Demonstrates **Cognitive Ability** as evidenced by the following indicators: Communicates clearly and appropriately for age and ability/Attentiveness/Orientation (Rate each indicator of **Cognitive Ability:** 1 = extremely compromised, 2 = substantially compromised, 3 = moderately compromised, 4 = mildly compromised, 5 = not compromised [see Section I])

Client Outcomes

- Cognitive status restored to baseline
- Obtains adequate amount of sleep
- Demonstrates appropriate motor behavior
- Maintains functional capacity

NIC   **Interventions (Nursing Interventions Classification)**

Suggested NIC Labels

Delirium Management; Delusion Management

> **Example NIC Interventions—Delirium Management**
> - Orient to time, place, and person
> - Present information in small, concrete portions

Nursing Interventions and Rationales

- Assess client's behavior and cognition systematically and continually throughout the day and night as appropriate.
  Rapid onset and fluctuating course are hallmarks of delirium (Murphy, 2000). The Confusion Assessment Method is sensitive, specific, reliable, and easy to use (Inouye et al, 1990). Nurses play a vital role in assessing acute confusion because they provide 24-hours-a-day care and see the client in a variety of circumstances (Marr, 1992). Delirium always involves acute change in mental status; therefore knowledge of the client's baseline mental status is key in assessing delirium (Flacker, Marcantonio, 1998).
- Perform an accurate mental status exam that includes the following:
  - Overall appearance, manner, and attitude
  - Behavior observations and level of psychomotor behavior
  - Mood and affect (presence of suicidal or homicidal ideation as observed by others and reported by client)

- = Independent; ▲ = Collaborative

- Insight and judgment
- Cognition as evidenced by level of consciousness, orientation (to time, place, and person), thought process and content (perceptual disturbances such as illusions and hallucinations, paranoia, delusions, abstract thinking)
- Attention

Abnormal attention is an important diagnostic feature of delirium (Flacker, Marcantonio, 1998). Delirium is a state of mind, while agitation is a behavioral manifestation. Some clients may be delirious without agitation and may actually have withdrawn behavior (a hypoactive form of delirium). Others may have a mixed hypoactive/hyperactive type of delirium (O'Keefe, Lavan, 1999). Missing a diagnosis of delirium can have serious consequences. Delirium in adults should be considered a medical emergency (Rosen, 1994).

▲ Assess and report possible physiological alterations (e.g., sepsis, hypoglycemia, hypotension, infection, changes in temperature, fluid and electrolyte imbalances, medications with known cognitive and psychotropic side effects).

Such alterations may be contributing to confusion and must be corrected (Matthiesen et al, 1994). Medications are considered the most common cause of delirium in the ICU (Harvey, 1996).

▲ Treat underlying causes of delirium in collaboration with the health care team: Establish/maintain normal fluid and electrolyte balance; establish/maintain normal nutrition, body temperature, oxygenation (if patients experience low oxygen saturation treat with supplemental oxygen), blood glucose levels, blood pressure.

▲ Communicate client status, cognition, and behavioral manifestations to all necessary providers. Monitor for any trending of these.

Recognize that client's fluctuating cognition and behavior is a hallmark for delirium and is not to be construed as client preference for caregivers (Inouye et al, 1990). Careful monitoring may allow for various symptoms to be related to various causes and interventions (Rapp, Iowa Veterans Affairs Nursing Research Consortium, 1997).

▲ Lab results should be closely monitored and physiological support provided as appropriate.

Once acute confusion has been identified, it is vital to recognize and treat the associated underlying causes (Rapp, Iowa Veterans Affairs Nursing Research Consortium, 1997).

- Establish or maintain elimination patterns.

Disruption of elimination may be a cause for confusion (Rapp, Iowa Veterans Affairs Nursing Research Consortium, 1997). Changes in elimination patterns may also be a symptom of acute confusion. Prompt response to requests for assistance with elimination in addition to timed voids may assist in maintaining regular elimination, orientation, and patient safety (Rosen, 1994).

- Plan care that allows for appropriate sleep-wake cycle.

Disruptions in usual sleep and activity patterns should be minimized as those clients with nocturnal exacerbations endure more complications from delirium.

▲ Review medication.

Medication is one of the most important modifiable factors that can cause delirium, especially use of anticholinergics, antipsychotics, and hypnosedatives (Flacker, Marcantonio, 1998).

- Decrease caffeine intake.

Decreasing caffeine intake helps to reduce agitation and restlessness (Rapp, Iowa Veterans Affairs Nursing Research Consortium, 1997).

• = Independent; ▲ = Collaborative

- Modulate sensory exposure and establish a calm environment.
  Extraneous lights and noise can give rise to agitation, especially if misperceived. Sensory overload or sensory deprivation can result in increased confusion (Rosen, 1994). Clients with a hyperactive form of delirium often have increased irritability and startle responses and may be acutely sensitive to light and sound (Casey et al, 1996).
- Manipulate the environment to make it as familiar to the patient as possible. Use a large clock and calendar. Encourage visits by family and friends. Place familiar objects in sight.
  An environment that is familiar provides orienting clues, maintains an appropriate balance of sensory stimulation, and secures safety (Rosen, 1994).
- Identify self by name at each contact; call patient by his or her preferred name.
  Appropriate communication techniques for clients at risk for confusion (Rapp, Iowa Veterans Affairs Nursing Research Consortium, 1997).
- Use orientation techniques. However, if client becomes distressed or argumentative about what is real, do not argue with the client. Rather, explore the emotion behind the client's non–reality-based statements (Rosen, 1994).
- Offer reassurance to the client and use therapeutic communication at frequent intervals.
  Client reassurance and communication are nursing skills that promote trust and orientation and reduce anxiety (Harvey, 1996).
- Provide supportive nursing care.
  Delirious patients are unable to care for themselves as a result of their confusion. Their care and safety needs must be anticipated by the nurse (Foreman, 1999).
- Identify, evaluate, and treat pain quickly (see care plan for **Acute Pain**).
  Untreated pain is a potential cause for delirium.

Geriatric

- Mobilize client as soon as possible; provide active and passive range of motion.
  Older clients who had a low level of physical activity before injury are at a particular risk for acute confusion (Matthiesen et al, 1994).
- ▲ Provide sufficient medication to relieve pain.
  Older clients may give inaccurate pain histories; underreport symptoms; not want to bother the nurse; and exhibit restlessness, agitation, or increased confusion (Matthiesen et al, 1994).
- Because anxiety and sensory impairment decrease the older client's ability to integrate new information, explain hospital routines and procedures slowly and in simple terms, repeating information as necessary (Matthiesen et al, 1994).
- Provide continuity of care when possible (e.g., provide the same caregivers, avoid room changes).
  Continuity of care helps decrease the disorienting effects of hospitalization (Matthiesen et al, 1994).
- If clients know that they are not thinking clearly, acknowledge the concern.
  Confusion is very frightening (Matthiesen et al, 1994).
- Do not use the intercom to answer a call light.
  The intercom may be frightening to an older confused client (Matthiesen et al, 1994).
- Keep client's sleep-wake cycle as normal as possible (e.g., avoid letting client take daytime naps, avoid waking clients at night, give sedatives but not diuretics at bedtime, provide pain relief and backrubs).
  Acute confusion is accompanied by disruption of the sleep-wake cycle (Matthiesen et al, 1994).

• = Independent; ▲ = Collaborative

- Maintain normal sleep/wake patterns (treat with bright light for 2 hours in the early evening).
  This facilitates normal sleep/wake patterns (Rapp, Iowa Veterans Affairs Nursing Research Consortium, 1997).

Home Care Interventions

- Monitor for acute changes in cognition and behavior.
  An acute change in cognition and behavior is the classic presentation of delirium. It should be considered a medical emergency.

Client/Family Teaching

▲ Teach family to recognize signs of early confusion and seek medical help.
  Early intervention prevents long-term complications (Rapp, Iowa Veterans Affairs Nursing Research Consortium, 1997).

WEB SITES FOR EDUCATION

 See the MERLIN web site for World Wide Web resources for client education.

REFERENCES Casey DA et al: Delirium: quick recognition, careful evaluation, and appropriate treatment, *Postgrad Med* 100(1):121-124, 128, 133-134, 1996 (symposium: fourth of four articles on psychiatric disorders).

Flacker JM, Marcantonio ER: Delirium in the elderly: optimal management, *Drugs Aging* 13(2):119-130, 1998.

Foreman MD et al: Standard of practice protocol: acute confusion/delirium, *Geriatr Nurs* 20:147-152, 1999.

Harvey M: Managing agitation in critically ill patients, *Am J Crit Care* 5:7, 1996.

Inouye SK et al: Clarifying confusion: the Confusion Assessment Method—a new method for detection of delirium, *Ann Intern Med* 113(12):941-948, 1990.

Marr J: Acute confusion, *Nurs Times* 88:16-18, 1992.

Matthiesen V et al: Acute confusion: nursing intervention in older patients, *Orthop Nurs* 13:25, 1994.

Murphy BA: Delirium, *Emerg Med Clin North Am* 18:243-252, 2000.

O'Keefe ST, Lavan JN: Clinical significance of delirium subtypes in older people, *Age Aging* 28(2):115-119, 1999.

Rapp C, Iowa Veterans Affairs Nursing Research Consortium: *Acute confusion/delirium*, Iowa City, 1997, University of Iowa. Web site: www.guidelines.gov/FRAMESETS/guideline_fs.asp?guideline=000536

Rosen SL: Managing delirious older adults in the hospital, *Med Surg Nurs* 3(3):181-189, 1994.

Chronic Confusion

Kimberly Hickey, Betty J. Ackley, and Nancy English

NANDA **Definition** Irreversible, long-standing, and/or progressive deterioration of intellect and personality characterized by a decreased ability to interpret environmental stimuli and a decreased capacity for intellectual thought processes, which manifest as disturbances of memory, orientation, and behavior

Defining Characteristics

Altered interpretation/response to stimuli; clinical evidence of organic impairment; altered personality; impaired memory (short and long term); impaired socialization; no change in level of consciousness

• = Independent; ▲ = Collaborative

Related Factors (r/t)

Multi-infarct dementia; Korsakoff's psychosis; head injury; Alzheimer's disease; cerebrovascular accident

NOC **Outcomes (Nursing Outcomes Classification)**

Suggested NOC Labels

Cognitive Orientation; Information Processing; Memory; Neurological Status: Consciousness

Client Outcomes

- Remains content and free from harm
- Functions at maximal cognitive level
- Participates in activities of daily living at the maximum of functional ability

NIC **Interventions (Nursing Interventions Classification)**

Suggested NIC Labels

Dementia Management; Environmental Management; Reality Orientation; Surveillance: Safety

> **Example NIC Interventions—Dementia Management**
> - Use distraction rather than confrontation to manage behavior
> - Give one simple direction at a time

Nursing Interventions and Rationales

- Determine client's cognitive level using a screening tool such as the Mini Mental State Exam (MMSE).
  Using a standard evaluation tool such as the MMSE can help determine the client's abilities and assist with planning appropriate nursing interventions (Agostinelli et al, 1994; Espino et al, 1998).
- ▲ Gather information about client pre-dementia functioning, including social situation, physical condition, and psychological functioning.
  Knowing the client's background can help the nurse identify agenda behavior and use validation therapy, which will provide guidance for reminiscence. Background information may help the nurse to understand client's behavior if client becomes delusional and hallucinates.
- Assess the client for signs of depression: insomnia, poor appetite, flat affect, and withdrawn behavior.
  As many as 50% of clients with dementia have depressive symptoms (Cleeland, 1997).
- Ensure that client is in a safe environment by removing potential hazards such as sharp objects and harmful liquids.
  Clients with dementia lose the ability to make good judgments and can easily harm self or others.
- Place an identification bracelet on client.
  Clients with dementia wander and can become lost; identification bracelets increase client safety.
- Avoid exposing client to unfamiliar situations and people as much as possible. Maintain continuity of caregivers. Maintain routines of care through established mealtimes, bathing, and sleeping schedules. Send familiar person with client when client goes for diagnostic testing or into unfamiliar environments.

• = Independent; ▲ = Collaborative

Situational anxiety associated with environmental, interpersonal, or structural change can escalate into agitated behavior (Gerdner, Buckwalter, 1994).

- Keep environment quiet and nonstimulating; avoid using buzzers and alarms if possible. Minimize sights and sounds that have a high potential for misinterpretation such as buzzers, alarms, and overhead paging systems.
Sensory overload can result in agitated behavior in a client with dementia. Misinterpretation of the environment can also contribute to agitation.

- Begin each interaction with client by identifying self and calling client by name. Approach client with a caring, loving, and accepting attitude and speak calmly and slowly.
Dementia clients can sense feelings of compassion. A calm, slow manner projects a feeling of comfort to the client (Stolley, 1994).

- Touch client gently, stroking hand or arm in a soothing fashion if acceptable in client's culture.

- Give one simple direction at a time and repeat as necessary. Use verbal and physical prompts, and model the desired action if needed and possible.
People with dementia need time to assimilate and interpret your directions. If you rephrase your question, you give them something new to process, increasing their confusion (Stolley, 1994).

- Break down self-care tasks into simple steps (e.g., instead of saying, "Take a shower," say to client, "Please follow me. Sit down on the bed. Take off your shoes. Now take off your socks. . . .").
Dementia clients are unable to follow complex commands; breaking down an activity into simple steps makes completing the activity more feasible (Agostinelli et al, 1994).

- Keep questions simple; yes or no questions are often preferable to open-ended questions. Use positive statements and actions and avoid negative communication.
Negative feedback leads to increased confusion and agitation. It is more effective to go along with the client and then redirect as necessary.

- If eating in the dining room causes increased agitation, let client leave and eat in a quieter environment with a smaller number of people.
The noise and confusion in a large dining room can be overwhelming for a dementia client and can result in agitated behavior. It is preferable to have dementia clients eat in small groups (Sloane, 1998).

- Provide finger food if patient has difficulty using eating utensils or if unable to sit to eat.
Feeding oneself is a complex task and may prove challenging for someone with significant dementia (Finley, 1997).

- Provide boundaries by placing red or yellow tape on the floor or by using a stop sign.
Boundaries help the client identify safe areas; older clients can more easily see red and yellow than other colors.

- Assess the etiology of wandering before or rather than attempting to control the wandering.
Wandering indicates a problem and need for intervention; therefore the reason for the wandering behavior needs to be determined (Algase, 1999).

- Write client's name in large block letters in the room and on client's clothing and possessions. Use symbols rather than words to identify areas such as the bathroom or kitchen.

• = **Independent**; ▲ = **Collaborative**

- Limit visitors to two and provide them with guidelines on appropriate topics to discuss and how to best communicate with client. (See Client/Family Teaching for how to converse with a memory-impaired person.)
- Set up scheduled quiet periods in a recliner or room. Use blankets and other environmental cues to define rest periods.
  Quiet times allow the client's anxiety and building tension levels to decrease (Hall et al, 1995). Fatigue has been associated with the onset of increased confusion and agitation (Stolley, 1994).
- Provide quiet activities, such as listening to classical or religious music, or other cues that promote relaxation in the afternoon or early evening.
  An increase in confusion and agitation, referred to as sundowning syndrome, may occur in the late afternoon and early evening. Quiet activities can provide a calming environment.
- Provide simple activities for the client, such as folding washcloths and sorting or stacking activities. Avoid misleading and frightening stimuli, which may include television, mirrors, and pictures of people or animals.
  Repetitive activities give the client with dementia a positive outlet for behavior (Burgener et al, 1998). Dementia clients see, hear, and perceive a different world than other people. They may not recognize themselves in the mirror and be afraid of the stranger they see so close to them.
- Consider using doll therapy. Ask family members to bring a large, safe doll or stuffed animal such as a teddy bear.
  Doll therapy can be soothing to some dementia clients (Bailey, 1992; Paulanka, Griffin, 1993).
- If client becomes increasingly confused and agitated, perform the following steps:
  - ▲ Monitor client for physiological causes, including acute hypoxia, pain, medication effects, malnutrition, infections such as urinary tract infection, fatigue, electrolyte disturbances, and constipation. An acute change in behavior is a medical emergency and should be evaluated.
    Many physiological factors can result in increased agitation of clients with dementia (Gerdner, Buckwalter, 1994; Alexopoulos et al, 1998).
  - ▪ Monitor for psychological causes, including changes in environment, caregiver, and routine; demands to perform beyond capacity; and multiple competing stimuli (including discomfort).
    It is important for the nurse to recognize precipitating events and subsequent behavior to prevent further incidents of agitation (Bair et al, 1999).
  - ▪ Avoid confrontations with the client; allow client to dissipate energy by performing repetitive tasks or by pacing.
- If client is delusional or hallucinating, do not confront him or her with reality. Use validation therapy to verbally reflect back the emotions that the client appears to be experiencing. Use statements such as, "It must be frightening to see a fire at the end of your bed," "I can see that you are afraid," "I will stay with you," or "Can you tell me more about what is going on right now?"
  Orienting the client to reality can increase agitation; validation therapy conveys empathy and understanding and can help determine the internal stimulus that is creating the change in behavior (Feil, 1993). In one study, training in validation therapy for staff resulted in decreased doses of psychotherapeutic medications and incidences of behavior problems (Fine, Rouse-Bane, 1995).

• = Independent; ▲ = Collaborative

- Decrease stimuli in the environment (e.g., turn off television, take client to a quiet place). Institute activities associated with pleasant emotions, such as playing soft music the client likes, looking through a photo album, providing favorite food, or using simulated presence therapy.
  Decreasing stimuli can decrease agitation. Reassuring activities, such as simulated presence therapy wherein client listens to a tape of a loved one's phone conversation, can help bring about pleasant emotions that soothe the client (Woods, Ashley, 1995).
- Avoid using restraints if at all possible.
  Restraints are not benign interventions and should be used sparingly and judiciously only when alternatives to manage the behaviors have been tried and been unsuccessful. Side effects include falls, increased confusion, deconditioning, and incontinence (Tinetti, Liu, Ginter, 1992).
- ▲ Use prn or low dose regular dosing of psychotropic or antianxiety drugs only as a last resort. They are effective in managing symptoms of psychosis and aggressive behavior. Start with the lowest possible dose.
  Psychotropic drugs such as haloperidol (Haldol) and resperidone (Risperdol) may decrease client function and have side effects that need to be monitored (Katz et al, 1999).
- ▲ Avoid use of anticholinergic medications such as Benadryl.
  Anticholinergic medications have a high side effect profile that includes disorientation, urinary retention, and excessive drowsiness (Nurses Drug Alert, 1995). The anticholinergic side effects outweigh the antihistaminic effects.
- For predictable difficult times, such as during bathing and grooming, try the following:
  - ▪ Massage the client's hands lovingly or use therapeutic touch to relax the client.
    Hand massage and therapeutic touch have been shown to induce relaxation that may allow care activities to take place without difficulty (Snyder, Egan, Burns, 1995).
  - ▪ Use positive behavioral reinforcement for each of the small steps involved in bathing, such as praising client for walking toward the shower, sitting in the shower chair, and removing items of clothing.
    Positive behavioral reinforcement for desired behavior is effective for clients with dementia (Boehm et al, 1995). Consider a towel bath if shower or tub bathing is too stressful for client (Hall, Buckwalter, 1999).
  - ▪ Treat the client with the utmost respect and give individualized care.
    Treating confused clients with respect and individualizing care can decrease aggression and increase nursing staff satisfaction (Maxfield, Lewis, Cannon, 1996).
- For early dementia clients with primarily symptoms of memory loss, see care plan for **Impaired Memory.** For clients with self-care deficits, see appropriate care plan **(Feeding Self-care deficit, Dressing/grooming Self-care deficit, Toileting Self-care deficit).**

Geriatric

NOTE: Most of the preceding interventions apply to the geriatric client.
- Use reminiscence and life review therapeutic interventions; ask questions about client's work, child rearing, or time spent in the service. Ask questions such as "What was really important to you as you look back?"
  Reminiscence and life review can help an older person reframe and accept life events (Burnside, Haight, 1994).

Multicultural

- Assess for the influence of cultural beliefs, norms, and values on the family or caregiver understanding of chronic confusion or dementia.

• = **Independent;** ▲ = **Collaborative**

What the family considers normal and abnormal health behavior may be based on cultural perceptions (Leininger, 1996).

- Inform client family or caregiver of the meaning of and reasons for common behavior observed in clients with dementia.
  An understanding of dementia behavior will enable the client family/caregiver to provide the client with a safe environment.
- ▲ Refer family to social services or other supportive services to assist with meeting the demands of caregiving for the client with dementia.
  Black caregivers of dementia clients may evidence less desire than others to institutionalize their family members and are more likely to report unmet service needs (Hinrichsen, Ramirez, 1992). Families of dementia clients may report restricted social activity (Haley et al, 1995).
- ▲ Encourage family to make use of support groups or other service programs.
  Studies indicate that some minority families of clients with dementia may use few support programs even though these programs could have a positive impact on caregiver well-being (Cox, 1999).
- Validate the family members' feelings with regard to the impact of client behavior on family lifestyle.
  Validation lets the client know that the nurse has heard and understands what was said, and it promotes the nurse-client relationship (Stuart, Laraia, 2001; Giger, Davidhizar, 1995).

Home Care Interventions

NOTE: Keeping the client as independent as possible is important. However, because community-based care is usually less structured than institutional care, in the home setting, the goal of maintaining safety for the client takes on primary importance.

- Provide support to family of client with chronic and disabling condition.
- ▲ If client will require extensive supervision on an ongoing basis, evaluate client for day care programs. Refer family to medical social services to assist with this process if necessary.
  Day care programs provide safe, structured care for the client and respite for the family. Respite care for caregivers is an essential part of successful long-term care for a confused client.
- Encourage family to include client in family activities when possible. Reinforce use of therapeutic communication guidelines (see Client/Family Teaching) and sensitivity to the number of people present.
  These steps help the client maintain dignity and lead to familiar socialization of the client.
- Assess family caregivers for caregiver burden.
  Caring for a loved one with a dementing process is highly stressful. Respite care is a necessary component to the overall care plan.

Client/Family Teaching

- Recommend that the family develop a memory aid wallet or booklet for client that contains pictures and text that chronicle the client's life.
  Using memory aids such as wallets or booklets helps dementia clients make more factual statements and stay on topic, and it decreases the number of confused, erroneous, and repetitive statements (Bouregois, 1992).

• = Independent; ▲ = Collaborative

- Teach family how to converse with a memory-impaired person. Guidelines include the following:
  - Ask client to have a conversation with you.
  - Guide conversation to specific, nonthreatening topics and redirect the conversation back on topic when client begins to ramble.
  - Reassure and help out when the client gets stuck or cannot find the right words.
  - Smile and act interested in what client is saying even if unsure what it means.
  - Thank client for talking.
  - Avoid quizzing client or asking a lot of specific questions.
  - Avoid correcting or contradicting something that was stated even if it is wrong.

  These guidelines can help family interact more effectively with client and decrease frustration levels (Bouregois, 1992).
- Teach family how to set up environment and use care techniques/interventions listed so that client will experience a progressively lowered stress threshold.

  Alzheimer's clients are unable to deal with stress; decreasing stress can decrease confusion and changes in behavior (Hall, 1991; Stolley, 1994).
- Discuss with the family what to expect as the dementia progresses.
- Counsel the family about resources available with regard to end-of-life decisions and legal concerns.
- ▲ Inform family that as dementia progresses, hospice care may be available in the terminal stages in the home to help the caregiver.

  Hospice services in the late stages of dementia can help support the family with nursing services and visitation by primary care provider, home health aides, social services, volunteer visitors, and a spiritual counselor if desired as the client is dying (Boyd, Vernon, 1998).

  NOTE: The nursing diagnoses **Impaired Environmental interpretation syndrome** and **Chronic Confusion** are very similar in definition and interventions. **Impaired Environmental interpretation syndrome** must be interpreted as a syndrome where other nursing diagnoses would also apply. **Chronic Confusion** may be interpreted as the human response to a situation or situations that require a level of cognition no longer available to the individual. Further research is underway to make this distinction clear to the practicing nurse.

WEB SITES FOR EDUCATION

MERLIN See the MERLIN web site for World Wide Web resources for client education.

REFERENCES
Agostinelli B et al: Targeted interventions: use of the Mini-Mental State Exam, *J Gerontol Nurs* 20(8):15-23, 1994.

Alexopoulos GS et al: Treatment of agitation in older persons with dementia, *Postgrad Med* 103(4 suppl): 1-22, 1998.

Algase D: Wandering: a dementia-compromised behavior, *J Gerontol Nurs* 25(9):10-16, 46-51, 1999.

Author unknown: Delirium with single dose of diphenhydramine, *Nurses Drug Alert* 19(1):4-5, 1995.

Bailey J: To find a soul, *Nursing 92* 7:63, 1992.

Bair B et al: Interventions for disruptive behaviors, *J Gerontol Nurs* 25(1):13-21, 1999.

Boehm S et al: Behavioral analysis and nursing interventions for reducing disruptive behaviors of patients with dementia, *Appl Nurs Res* 8(3):118-122, 1995.

Bouregois MS: *Conversing with memory impaired individuals using memory aids: a memory aid workbook,* Gaylord, Mich, 1992, Northern Speech Services.

Boyd CO, Vernon GM: Primary care of the older adult with end-stage Alzheimer's disease, *Nurse Pract* 23(4):63-76, 1998.

• = **Independent;** ▲ = **Collaborative**

Burgener SC et al: Effective caregiving approaches for patients with Alzheimer's disease, *Geriatr Nurs* 19(3):121-125, 1998.

Burnside I, Haight B: Reminiscence and life review: therapeutic interventions for older people, *Nurse Pract* 19(4):55-61, 1994.

Cleeland EA: Depression in people with dementia, *Home Healthcare Nurse* 15:781, 1997.

Cox C: Race and caregiving: patterns of service use by African-American and white caregivers of persons with Alzheimer's, *J Gerontol Soc Work* 32(2):5-19, 1999.

Espino DV et al: Diagnostic approach to the confused elderly patient, *Am Fam Physician* 57(6):1358-1366, 1998.

Feil N: *The validation breakthrough: simple techniques for communicating with people with Alzheimer's-type dementia,* Baltimore, 1993, Health Professions.

Fine J, Rouse-Bane S: Using validation techniques to improve communication with cognitively impaired older adults, *J Gerontol Nurs* 21(6):39-45, 1995.

Finley B: Nutritional needs of the person with Alzheimer's disease: practical approaches to quality care, *J Am Diet Assoc* 97(10 suppl), 1997.

Gerdner LA, Buckwalter KC: A nursing challenge: assessment and management of agitation in Alzheimer's patients, *J Gerontol Nurs* 20(4):11-20, 1994.

Giger JN, Davidhizar RE: *Transcultural nursing,* ed 2, St Louis, 1995, Mosby.

Haley WE et al: Psychological, social, and health impact of caregiving: a comparison of black and white dementia family caregivers and noncaregivers, *Psychol Aging* 10(4):540-552, 1995.

Hall GR: This hospital patient has Alzheimer's, *Am J Nurs* 91(10):45-52, 1991.

Hall GR et al: Standardized care plan: managing Alzheimer's patients at home, *J Gerontol Nurs* 21(1):37-47, 1995.

Hall GR, Buckwalter KC: *Bathing persons with dementia,* Iowa City, 1999, University of Iowa Gerontological Nursing Interventions Research Center.

Hinrichsen GA, Ramirez M: Black and white dementia caregivers: a comparison of their adaptation, *Gerontologist,* 32(3):375-381, 1992.

Katz IR et al: Comparison of Risperidone and placebo for psychosis and behavioral disturbances with dementia: a randomized, double-blind trial: *J Clin Psychiatry* 60(2):107-115, 1999.

Leininger MM: *Transcultural nursing: theories, research and practices,* ed 2, Hilliard, Ohio, 1996, McGraw-Hill.

Maxfield MC, Lewis RE, Cannon S: Training staff to prevent aggressive behavior of cognitively impaired elderly patients during bathing and grooming, *J Gerontol Nurs* 22(1):37-43, 1996.

Paulanka BJ, Griffin LS: Behavioral responses of memory impaired clients to selected nursing interventions, *Phys Occup Ther Geriatr* 12:65, 1993.

Sloane PD: Advances in the treatment of Alzheimer's disease, *Am Fam Physician* 58(7):1577-1588, 1998.

Snyder M, Egan EC, Burns KR: Interventions for decreasing agitation behaviors in persons with dementia, *J Gerontol Nurs* 21(7):34-40, 1995.

Stolley JM: When your patient has Alzheimer's disease, *Am J Nurs* 94(8):34-40, 1994.

Stuart GW, Laraia MT: Therapeutic nurse-patient relationship. In Stuart GW, Laraia MT, editors: *Principles and practice of psychiatric nursing,* St Louis, 2001, Mosby, p 30.

Tinetti ME, Liu WL, Ginter SF: Mechanical restraint use and fall-related injuries among residents of skilled nursing facilities, *Ann Intern Med* 116:369, 1992.

Woods P, Ashley J: Simulated presence therapy: using selected memories to manage problem behaviors in Alzheimer's disease patients, *Geriatr Nurs* 16(1):9-14, 1995.

Constipation

Betty J. Ackley and Kathie D. Hesnan

NANDA   **Definition** A decrease in a person's normal frequency of defecation, accompanied by difficult or incomplete passage of stool and/or passage of excessively hard, dry stool

• = Independent; ▲ = Collaborative

Defining Characteristics

Change in bowel pattern; bright red blood with stool; presence of soft paste-like stool in rectum; distended abdomen; dark, black, or tarry stool; increased abdominal pressure; percussed abdominal dullness; pain with defecation; decreased volume of stool; straining with defecation; decreased frequency; dry, hard, formed stool; palpable rectal mass; feeling of rectal fullness or pressure; abdominal pain; unable to pass stool; anorexia; headache; change in abdominal growing (borborygmi); indigestion; atypical presentation in older adults (e.g., change in mental status, urinary incontinence, unexplained falls, elevated body temperature); severe flatus; generalized fatigue; hypoactive or hyperactive bowel sounds; palpable abdominal mass; abdominal tenderness with or without palpable muscle resistance; nausea and/or vomiting; oozing liquid stool

Related Factors (r/t)

Functional   Recent environmental changes; habitual denial/ignoring of urge to defecate; insufficient physical activity; irregular defecation habits; inadequate toileting (e.g., timeliness, positioning for defecation, privacy); abdominal muscle weakness

Psychological   Depression; emotional stress; mental confusion

Pharmacological

Antilipemic agents; laxative overdose; calcium carbonate; aluminum-containing antacids; nonsteroidal antiinflammatory agents; opiates; anticholinergics; diuretics; iron salts; phenothiazines; sedatives; sympathomimetics; bismuth salts; antidepressants; calcium channel blockers

Mechanical   Rectal abscess or ulcer; pregnancy; rectal anal fissures; tumors; megacolon (Hirschsprung's disease); electrolyte imbalance; rectal prolapse; prostate enlargement; neurological impairment; rectal anal stricture; rectocele; postsurgical obstruction; hemorrhoids; obesity

Physiological   Poor eating habits; decreased motility of gastrointestinal tract; inadequate dentition or oral hygiene; insufficient fiber intake; insufficient fluid intake; change in usual foods and eating patterns; dehydration

NOC   **Outcomes (Nursing Outcomes Classification)**

Suggested NOC Labels

Bowel Elimination; Hydration

> **Example NOC Outcome**
> Constipation relieved as evidenced by **Bowel Elimination** and the following indicators: Elimination pattern in expected range/Stool soft and formed/Passes stool without aids/Ease of stool passage (Rate each indicator of **Bowel Elimination:** 1 = extremely compromised, 2 = substantially compromised, 3 = moderately compromised, 4 = mildly compromised, 5 = not compromised [see Section I])

Client Outcomes

- Maintains passage of soft, formed stool every 1 to 3 days without straining
- States relief from discomfort of constipation
- Identifies measures that prevent or treat constipation

NIC   **Interventions (Nursing Interventions Classification)**

Suggested NIC Labels

Constipation/Impaction Management

• = Independent; ▲ = Collaborative

Nursing Interventions and Rationales

- Observe usual pattern of defecation including time of day, amount and frequency of stool, consistency of stool, history of bowel habits or laxative use; diet including fluid intake; exercise patterns; personal remedies for constipation; obstetrical/gynecological history; surgeries; alterations in perianal sensation; present bowel regimen.

  There often are multiple reasons for constipation; the first step is assessment of usual patterns of bowel elimination.

- Have the client or family keep a diary of bowel habits including time of day; usual stimulus; consistency, amount, and frequency of stool; fluid consumption; and use of any aids to defecation.

  A diary of bowel habits is valuable in treatment of constipation (Wong, Kadakia, 1999).

▲ Review client's current medications.

  Many medications affect normal bowel function, including opiates, antidepressants, antihypertensives, anticholinergics, diuretics, anticonvulsants, antacids containing aluminum, iron supplements, and muscle relaxants (Wong, Kadakia, 1999).

- Palpate for abdominal distention, percuss for dullness, and auscultate bowel sounds.

  In clients with constipation the abdomen is often distended with a palpable colon (Held, 1995).

▲ Check for impaction; perform digital removal per physician's order.

  If impaction is present, use cleansing regimen until you obtain a very soft stool. If using an enema, the client must be able to bodily retain the fluid. If the client has poor sphincter tone, use a cone tip–irrigating bag to assist the client in retaining the fluids. This also decreases the amount of fluid necessary for cleansing.

- Provide privacy for defecation. Assist the client to the bathroom and close the door if possible.

  Bowel elimination is a very private act, and a lack of privacy can contribute to constipation (Weeks, Hubbartt, Michaels, 2000).

- Encourage fiber intake of 25 g/day for adults. Emphasize foods such as fresh fruits, beans, vegetables, and bran cereals. Add fiber to diet gradually.

  Fiber helps prevent constipation by giving stool bulk. Add fiber to diet gradually because a sudden increase can cause bloating, gas, and diarrhea (Doughty, 1996). A daily fiber intake of 25 g can increase frequency of stools in clients with constipation (Anti, 1998). Dietary supplements of fiber in the form of bran or wheat fiber are helpful for women experiencing constipation with pregnancy (Jewell, Young, 2000).

- Encourage a fluid intake of 1.5 to 2 L/day (6 to 8 glasses of liquids per day). If oral intake is low, gradually increase fluid intake. Fluid intake must be within the cardiac and renal reserve.

  Adequate fluid intake is necessary to prevent hard, dry stools. Increasing fluid intake to 1.5 to 2 L/day along with fiber intake of 25 g can significantly increase frequency of stools in clients with constipation (Anti, 1998; Weeks, Hubbartt, Michaels, 2000).

- Encourage client to be out of bed as soon as possible, and to own activities of daily living (ADLs) as able. Encourage exercises such as turning and changing positions in bed, lifting their hips off the bed, doing range of motion exercises, alternating lifting

- = **Independent;** ▲ = **Collaborative**

each knee to the chest, doing wheelchair lifts, doing waist twists, stretching arms away from body, and pulling in the abdomen while taking deep breaths.

Activity, even minimal, increases peristalsis, which is necessary to prevent constipation (Yakabowich, 1990; Weeks, Hubbartt, Michaels, 2000).

- At each meal, sprinkle bran over client's food as allowed by client and prescribed diet. Ensure that client receives adequate fluid (1500 ml/day) along with bran.

  The number of bowel movements is increased and the use of laxatives is decreased in a client who eats wheat bran (Schmelzer, 1990; Wong, Kadakia, 1999). A study done on institutionalized elderly male clients with chronic constipation demonstrated that with bran use, clients were able to discontinue use of oral laxatives (Howard, West, Ossip-Klein, 2000).

- If sprinkling bran over the food is not effective, try this mixture: 1 cup Kellogg's All Bran cereal, 1 cup applesauce, 1 cup prune juice. Mix together, and give 2 tablespoons per day. Keep refrigerated. Always check with the primary care practitioner before initiating this intervention. It is important that the client also have sufficient fluids.

  This mixture has been shown to be effective even with short-term use in elderly clients recovering from acute conditions. NOTE: Giving fiber without sufficient fluid has resulted in impaction/bowel obstruction (Gibson et al, 1995). A number of bran mixtures have been shown to effectively decrease constipation (Beverley, Travis, 1992; Gibson et al, 1995), including a mixture called power pudding (Neal, 1995).

- Initiate a regular schedule for defecation, using the client's normal evacuation time whenever possible. Offer hot coffee, hot lemon water, or prune juice before breakfast, or while sitting on the toilet if necessary. An optimal time for many individuals is 30 minutes after breakfast because of the gastrocolic reflex.

  A schedule gives the client a sense of control, but more importantly it promotes evacuation before drying of stool and constipation occur (Doughty, 1992). Hot liquids can stimulate peristasis and result in defecation (Weeks, Hubbartt, Michaels, 2000).

- Emphasize to the client the necessary ingredients for a normal bowel regimen (e.g., fluid, fiber, activity, and regular schedule for defecation).

  Help client onto bedside commode or toilet with client's hips flexed and feet flat. Have client deep breathe through mouth to encourage relaxation of the pelvic floor muscle and use the abdominal muscles to help evacuation.

▲ Provide laxatives, suppositories, and enemas as needed and as ordered only; establish a client goal of eliminating their use. Avoid soapsuds enemas, or use a low concentration of castile soap only.

  Use of laxatives should be avoided (Schaefer, Cheskin, 1998). Soapsuds enemas can cause damage to the colonic mucosa (Schmelzer, Wright, 1993). The use of a soapsuds enema was shown to increase stool output as compared with tap water enemas in preoperative liver transplant patients; amount of mucosal irritation was unknown (Schmelzer et al, 2000).

▲ For the stable neurological client, consider use of a bowel routine of Therevac enema or suppositories every other day, or performing digital stimulation with physician's permission. For persistent constipation, refer to physician for evaluation.

  Use of the Therevac SB mini-enema was found to cut time needed for bowel care by as much as one hour or more as compared with use of suppositories (Dunn, Galka, 1994).

• = Independent; ▲ = Collaborative

Geriatric

- Explain the importance of fiber intake, fluid intake, and activity for soft, formed stool.
  Fiber intake, fluid intake, and activity are often decreased in elderly clients. Increasing fiber and fluids can effectively prevent constipation in the elderly (Rodrigues-Fisher, Bourguignon, Good, 1993).
- Determine client's perception of normal bowel elimination; promote adherence to a regular schedule.
  Misconceptions regarding the frequency of bowel movements can lead to anxiety and overuse of laxatives.
- Explain Valsalva's maneuver and the reason it should be avoided.
  Valsalva's maneuver can cause bradycardia and even death in cardiac patients.
- Respond quickly to client's call for help with toileting.
- Avoid regular use of enemas in the elderly.
  Enemas can cause fluid and electrolyte imbalances (Yakabowich, 1990) and damage to the colonic mucosa (Schmelzer, Wright, 1993).
- ▲ Use opioids cautiously. If ordered, use stool softeners and bran mixtures to prevent constipation.
  Use of opioids can cause constipation (Schaefer, Cheskin, 1998).
- Position client on toilet or commode and place a small footstool under the feet.
  Placing a small footstool under the feet increases intraabdominal pressure and makes defecation easier for an elderly client with weak abdominal muscles.

Home Care Interventions

- Put client in bathroom to toilet when possible.
  Bowel elimination is a very private act, and a lack of privacy can contribute to constipation (Weeks, Hubbartt, Michaels, 2000).
- ▲ Carefully monitor bowel patterns of clients under pain management with opioids. Introduce a bowel management program at first sign of constipation.
  Constipation is a major problem for terminally ill or hospice clients who may need very high doses of opioids for pain management.
- When using a bowel program, establish a pattern that is very regular and allows client to be part of family unit.
  Regularity of program promotes psychological and/or physiological "readiness" to evacuate. Families of home care clients often cannot proceed with normal daily activities until bowel programs are complete.

Client/Family Teaching

- Instruct client on normal bowel function and the necessity of fluid, fiber, and activity in a bowel program.
- Encourage client to heed defecation warning signs and develop a regular schedule of defecation by using a stimulus such as a warm drink or prune juice.
  Most cases of constipation are mechanical and result from habitual neglect of impulses that signal appropriate time for defecation. This results in accumulation of a large, dry fecal mass (Wright, Thomas, 1995).
- Encourage client to avoid long-term use of laxatives and enemas and to gradually withdraw from their use if used regularly.
- If not contraindicated, teach client how to do bent-leg sit-ups to increase abdominal tone; also encourage client to contract abdominal muscles frequently throughout the day. Help client develop a daily exercise program to increase peristalsis.

• = **Independent**; ▲ = **Collaborative**

WEB SITES FOR EDUCATION

 See the MERLIN web site for World Wide Web resources for client education.

REFERENCES   Anti M: Water supplementation enhances the effect of high-fiber diet on stool frequency and laxative consumption in adult patients with functional constipation, *Hepatogastroenterology* 45(21):727-732, 1998.

Beverley L, Travis I: Constipation: proposed natural laxative mixtures, *J Gerontol Nurs* 18(10):5-12, 1992.

Doughty D: A step-by-step approach to bowel training, *Progressions* 4:12, 1992.

Doughty D: A physiologic approach to bowel training, *J Wound Ostomy Continence Nurs* 23(1):46-56, 1996.

Dunn KL, Galka ML: A comparison of the effectiveness of There-vac SB and bisacodyl suppositories in SCI patients' bowel programs, *Rehabil Nurs* 19:334-338, 1994.

Gibson CJ et al: Effectiveness of bran supplement on the bowel management of elderly rehabilitation patients, *J Gerontol Nurs* 21(10):21-25, 1995.

Held JL: Preventing and treating constipation, *Nursing* 3:26, 1995.

Howard LV, West D, Ossip-Klein DJ: Chronic constipation management for institutionalized older adults, *Geriatr Nurs* 21(2):78-82, 2000.

Jewell DJ, Young G: Interventions for treating constipation in pregnancy, *Cochrane Database Syst Rev* CD001142, DJ9, 2000.

Neal LJ: "Power pudding": natural laxative therapy for the elderly who are homebound, *Home Healthcare Nurse* 13(3):66-71, 1995.

Rodrigues-Fisher L, Bourguignon C, Good BV: Dietary fiber nursing intervention: prevention of constipation in older adults, *Clin Nurs Res* 2:464, 1993.

Schaefer DC, Cheskin LJ: Constipation in the elderly, *Am Fam Physician* 58(4):907-914, 1998.

Schmelzer M: Effectiveness of wheat bran in prevention of constipation in hospitalized orthopaedic surgery patients, *Orthop Nurs* 15:10, 1990.

Schmelzer M et al: Colonic cleansing, fluid absorption, and discomfort following tap water and soapsuds enemas, *Applied Nurs Res* 13(2):83-91, 2000.

Schmelzer M, Wright K: Working smart, *Am J Nurs* 93:55, 1993.

Weeks SK, Hubbartt E, Michaels TK: Keys to bowel success, *Rehabil Nurs* 25(2):66-69, 2000.

Wong PN, Kadakia S: How to deal with chronic constipation, *Postgrad Med* 106(6):199-210, 1999.

Wright PS, Thomas SL: Constipation and diarrhea: the neglected symptoms, *Semin Oncol Nurs* 11(4):289-297, 1995.

Yakabowich M: Prescribe with care: the role of laxatives in the treatment of constipation, *J Gerontol Nurs* 16:4, 1990.

Perceived Constipation

Betty J. Ackley and Kathie D. Hesnan

NANDA   **Definition**   The state in which an individual makes a self-diagnosis of constipation and ensures a daily bowel movement through the abuse of laxatives, enemas, and suppositories

Defining Characteristics

Expectation of a daily bowel movement that results in an overuse of laxatives, enemas, and suppositories; expectation of a bowel movement at the same time every day

Related Factors (r/t)

Cultural or family beliefs; faulty appraisals; impaired thought processes

• = Independent; ▲ = Collaborative

NOC Outcomes (Nursing Outcomes Classification)
Suggested NOC Labels
Bowel Elimination; Health Beliefs; Health Beliefs: Perceived Threat

> **Example NOC Outcome**
> Demonstrates appropriate **Bowel Elimination** as shown by the following indicators:
> Elimination pattern in expected range/Stool soft and formed/Passes stool without
> aids/Ease of stool passage (Rate each indicator of **Bowel Elimination:** 1 = ex-
> tremely compromised, 2 = substantially compromised, 3 = moderately compro-
> mised, 4 = mildly compromised, 5 = not compromised [see Section I])

Client Outcomes

- Regularly defecates soft, formed stool without using any aids
- Explains the need to decrease or eliminate the use of laxatives, suppositories, and
  enemas
- Identifies alternatives to laxatives, enemas, and suppositories for ensuring
  defecation
- Explains that defecation does not have to occur every day

NIC Interventions (Nursing Interventions Classification)
Suggested NIC Labels
Bowel Management; Medication Management

> **Example NIC Interventions—Bowel Management**
> - Note preexistent bowel problems, bowel routine, and use of laxatives

Nursing Interventions and Rationales

- Observe pattern of food intake and also usual pattern of defecation (e.g., timing,
  consistency, amount, and frequency of stool passage; diet; fluid intake).
  *A bowel record provides both the client and the health care provider a way to assess the
  present bowel program, identify areas of concern, and develop an individualized bowel
  program (Wong, Kadakia, 1999).*
- Determine client's perception of an appropriate defecation pattern.
  *The client may need to be taught that one bowel movement every 1 to 3 days is normal
  (Wong, Kadakia, 1999).*
- ▲ Monitor use of laxatives, suppositories, or enemas and suggest use of increased fiber
  intake along with increased fluids to 2 L/day.
  *Chronic use of laxatives may alter colonic myenteric plexus function and should be
  avoided. (Wright, Thomas, 1995; Schaefer, Cheskin, 1998). Increasing fiber intake to 25
  g/day along with increasing fluid intake can help patients with chronic constipation (Anti
  et al, 1998; Wong, Kadakia, 1999).*
- Encourage client to promptly respond to the defecation reflex.
  *Not responding to the urge to defecate can be a contributing factor to constipation (Battle,
  Hanna, 1989; Basta, Anderson, 1998).*
- ▲ Obtain a dietary referral for analysis and input on how to improve diet to receive
  adequate fiber and nutrition.

• = Independent; ▲ = Collaborative

▲ Assess for signs of depression, a sedentary lifestyle, and obesity, all of which can contribute to constipation. Refer for counseling and encourage activity (walking for at least 30 minutes at least 5 days a week).
Increased activity increases bowel motility, which decreases constipation (Wright, Thomas, 1995; Wong, Kadakia, 1999).

• Provide privacy for defecation and encourage client to avoid using a bedpan if possible.
Many individuals need privacy to defecate. Using a bedpan makes it more difficult to use the abdominal muscles to help evacuate the rectum, and the client may have a feeling of incomplete emptying (Weeks, Hubbartt, Michaels, 2000).

▲ Observe for potential disturbed body image or the use of laxatives to control or decrease weight; refer for counseling if needed.

Home Care Interventions

• Obtain family and client histories of bowel or other patterned behavior problems.
History may reveal psychological etiology to constipation (e.g., withholding).

• Observe family cultural patterns related to eating and bowel habits.
Cultural patterns may control bowel habits.

• Contract with the client and/or a responsible family member regarding use of laxatives. Have client maintain a bowel pattern diary. Observe for diarrhea or frequent evacuation.
Intermittent care does not allow for 24-hour supervision. Contracting allows guided control of care by client in partnership with the nurse, and the diary promotes more accurate reporting.

▲ Teach family to carry out bowel program per physician orders.
Refer for home health aide services to assist with personal care, including bowel program if appropriate.

• Identify contingency plan for bowel care if client is dependent on outside persons for such care.

Client/Family Teaching

• Explain normal bowel function and the necessary ingredients for a regular bowel regimen (e.g., fluid, fiber, activity, and regular schedule for defecation).

• Work with client and family to develop a diet that fits lifestyle and includes increased fiber.

• Teach client that it is not necessary to have daily bowel movements and that the passage of anywhere from three stools each day to three stools each week is considered normal.

• Explain to client the harmful effects of the continual use of defecation aids.

• Encourage client to gradually decrease use of usual laxatives and enemas and to set a date to have eliminated all defecation aids.

• Determine a method of increasing client's fluid intake and fit this practice into client's lifestyle.

• Explain Valsalva's maneuver and why it should be avoided.

• Work with client and family to design a bowel training routine that is based on previous patterns (before laxative or enema abuse) and incorporates warm fluids, increased fiber, increased fluids, privacy, and a predictable routine.

Additional Nursing Interventions and Rationales, Client/Family Teaching

See care plan for **Constipation.**

• = Independent; ▲ = Collaborative

REFERENCES Anti M et al: Water supplementation enhances the effect of high-fiber diet on stool frequency and laxative consumption in adult patients with functional constipation, *Hepatogastroenterology* 45(21):727-732, 1998.

Battle E, Hanna C: Evaluation of a dietary regimen for chronic constipation, *J Gerontol Nurs* 6:527, 1989.

Basta S, Anderson DL: Mechanisms and management of constipation in the cancer patient, *J Pharm Care Pain Symptom Control* 6(3):21-41, 1998.

Schaefer DC, Cheskin LJ: Constipation in the elderly, *Am Fam Physician* 58(4):907-914, 1998.

Weeks SK, Hubbartt E, Michaels TK: Keys to bowel success, *Rehabil Nurs* 25(2):66-69, 2000.

Wong PW, Kadakia S: How to deal with chronic constipation: a stepwise method of establishing and treating the source of the problem, *Postgrad Med* 106(6):199-200, 203-204, 207-210, 1999.

Wright PS, Thomas SL: Constipation and diarrhea: the neglected symptoms, *Semin Oncol Nurs* 11(4):289-294, 1995.

Risk for Constipation

Betty J. Ackley

NANDA **Definition** At risk for a decrease in a person's normal frequency of defecation accompanied by difficult or incomplete passage of stool and/or passage of excessively hard, dry stool

Related Factors (r/t)

Functional Recent environmental changes; habitual denial/ignoring of urge to defecate; insufficient physical activity; irregular defecation habits; inadequate toileting (e.g., timeliness, positioning for defecation, privacy); abdominal muscle weakness

Psychological Emotional stress; mental confusion; depression

Physiological Poor eating habits; decreased motility of gastrointestinal tract; inadequate dentition or oral hygiene; insufficient fiber intake; insufficient fluid intake; change in usual foods and eating patterns; dehydration

Pharmacological

Phenothiazides; antilipemic agents; laxative overuse; calcium carbonate; aluminum-containing antacids; nonsteroidal antiinflammatory agents; opiates; anticholinergics; iron salts; sedatives; sympathomimetics; bismuth salts; antidepressants; calcium channel blockers; anticonvulsants

Mechanical Rectal abscess or ulcer; pregnancy; postsurgical obstruction; rectal anal fissures; tumors; megacolon (Hirschsprung's disease); electrolyte imbalance; rectal prolapse; prostate enlargement; neurological impairment; rectal anal stricture; rectocele; tumors; hemorrhoids; obesity

NOC **Outcomes (Nursing Outcomes Classification)**
Suggested NOC Labels
Bowel Elimination

• = Independent; ▲ = Collaborative

> **Example NOC Outcome**
> Constipation relieved as evidenced by **Bowel Elimination** and the following indicators: Elimination pattern in expected range/Stool soft and formed/Passes stool without aids/Ease of stool passage (Rate each indicator of **Bowel Elimination:** 1 = extremely compromised, 2 = substantially compromised, 3 = moderately compromised, 4 = mildly compromised, 5 = not compromised [see Section I])

Client Outcomes

- Maintains passage of soft, formed stool every 1 to 3 days without straining
- Identifies measures that prevent constipation

NIC   Interventions (Nursing Interventions Classification)

Suggested NIC Labels

Constipation/Impaction Management

> **Example NIC Interventions—Constipation Management**
> - Identify factors (e.g., medications, bed rest, and diet) that may cause or contribute to constipation
> - Monitor for signs and symptoms of constipation

Nursing Interventions and Rationales

- Observe usual pattern or have patient keep diary of defecation, including time of day; usual stimulus; consistency, amount, and frequency of stool; type, amount, and time of food consumed; fluid intake; history of bowel habits or laxative use; diet; exercise patterns; personal remedies for constipation; obstetrical/gynecological history; medications; surgeries; alterations in perianal sensation; present bowel regimen.
  A bowel record provides both the client and the health care provider a way to assess the present bowel program, identify areas of concern, and develop an individualized bowel program (Wong, Kadakia, 1999).
- ▲ Review client's current medications.
  Many medications affect normal bowel function, including opiates, antidepressants, antihypertensives, anticholinergics, diuretics, anticonvulsants, antacids containing aluminum, iron supplements, and muscle relaxants (Wong, Kadakia, 1999).
- Palpate for abdominal distention, percuss for dullness, and auscultate bowel sounds.
  In clients with constipation the abdomen is often distended with a palpable colon (Held, 1995).
- Assess for anxiety or embarrassment regarding defecation.
- Encourage adequate fiber intake of 25 g/day for adults; emphasize foods such as fresh fruits, vegetables, and bran cereals. Add fiber to diet gradually.
  Fiber helps prevent constipation by giving stool bulk. Add fiber gradually because a sudden increase can cause bloating, gas, and diarrhea (Doughty, 1992). A daily fiber intake of 25 g can increase frequency of stools in clients with constipation (Anti et al, 1998; Wong, Kadakia, 1999).
- Encourage a fluid intake of 1.5 to 2 L/day; if oral intake is low, gradually increase fluid intake. Fluid intake must be within the cardiac and renal reserve.
  Adequate fluid intake is necessary to prevent hard, dry stools. Increasing fluid intake to 1.5 to 2 L/day, along with fiber intake of 25 g/day, can significantly increase frequency of stools in clients with constipation (Anti et al, 1998; Weeks, Hubbartt, Michaels, 2000).

• = **Independent;** ▲ = **Collaborative**

- Encourage ambulation and/or a daily exercise program.
  Activity, even minimal activity such as waist twists, increases peristalsis, which is necessary for the prevention of constipation (Yakabowich, 1990; Weeks, Hubbartt, Michaels, 2000).
- At each meal, sprinkle bran over client's food as allowed by client and prescribed diet.
  The number of bowel movements is increased and the use of laxatives is decreased in a client who eats wheat bran (Schmelzer, 1990; Wong, Kadakia, 1999). A study done on institutionalized elderly male clients with chronic constipation demonstrated that with bran use, clients were able to discontinue use of oral laxatives (Howard, West, Ossip-Klein, 2000).
- Initiate a regular schedule for defecation, using the client's normal evacuation time whenever possible. An optimal time for many individuals is 30 minutes after breakfast because of the gastrocolic reflex.
  A defecation schedule gives the client a sense of control, but more important it promotes evacuation before drying of stool and constipation occur (Doughty, 1992; Weeks, Hubbartt, Michaels, 2000).
- Help client onto bedside commode or toilet with client's hips flexed and feet flat. Have client deep breathe through mouth to encourage relaxation of the pelvic floor muscle and use the abdominal muscles to help evacuation.

Geriatric

- Explain the importance of fiber intake, fluid intake, and activity for soft, formed stool.
  Activity, fiber, and fluid intake are often decreased in elderly clients. Increasing fiber and fluids can be effective in preventing constipation in the elderly (Rodrigues-Fisher, Bourguignon, Good, 1993).
- Determine client's perception of normal bowel elimination; promote adherence to a regular schedule.
  Misconceptions regarding the frequency of bowel movements can lead to anxiety and overuse of laxatives.
- Explain Valsalva's maneuver and the reason it should be avoided.
  Valsalva's maneuver can cause bradycardia and even death in cardiac patients.
- Respond quickly to client's call for help with toileting.
- Avoid regular use of enemas in the elderly.
  Enemas can cause fluid and electrolyte imbalances (Yakabowich, 1990) and damage to the colonic mucosa (Schmelzer, Wright, 1993).
- ▲ Use opioids cautiously. If ordered, use stool softeners and bran mixtures to prevent constipation.
  Opioids can cause constipation (Schaefer, Cheskin, 1998).
- Position client on toilet or commode and place a small footstool under the feet.
  Placing a small footstool under the feet increases intraabdominal pressure and makes defecation easier for an elderly client with weak abdominal muscles.

Home Care Interventions

- Put client in bathroom to toilet when possible.
  Use of purpose-specific surroundings increases psychological stimulus to evacuate and privacy is more easily protected (Weeks, Hubbartt, Michaels, 2000).
- ▲ Carefully monitor bowel patterns of clients under pain management with opioids. Introduce a bowel management program at first sign of constipation.
  Constipation is a major problem for terminally ill or hospice clients who may need very high doses of opioids for pain management.

• = **Independent;** ▲ = **Collaborative**

- When using a bowel program, establish a pattern that is very regular and allows client to be part of family unit.
  Regularity of program promotes psychological and/or physiological "readiness" to evacuate. Families of home care clients often cannot proceed with normal daily activities until bowel programs are complete.

Client/Family Teaching

- Instruct client on normal bowel function and the necessity of fluid, fiber, and activity in a bowel program.
- Encourage client to heed defecation warning signs and develop a regular schedule of defecation by using a stimulus such as a warm drink or prune juice.
  Many cases of constipation are mechanical and result from habitual neglect of impulses that signal the need for defecation. This results in accumulation of a large, dry fecal mass (Wright, Thomas, 1995; Basta, Anderson, 1998).
- If not contraindicated, teach client how to do bent-leg sit-ups to increase abdominal tone; also encourage client to contract abdominal muscles frequently throughout the day. Help client develop a daily exercise program to increase peristalsis.

WEB SITES FOR EDUCATION

⟡MERLIN See the MERLIN web site for World Wide Web resources for client education.

REFERENCES   Anti M et al: Water supplementation enhances the effect of high-fiber diet on stool frequency and laxative consumption in adult patients with functional constipation, *Hepatogastroenterology* 45(21):727-732, 1998.

Basta S, Anderson DL: Mechanisms and management of constipation in the cancer patient, *J Pharm Care Pain Symptom Control* 6(3): 21-41, 1998.

Doughty D: A step-by-step approach to bowel training, *Progressions* 4:12, 1992.

Held JL: Preventing and treating constipation, *Nursing* 3:26, 1995.

Howard LV, West D, Ossip-Klein DJ: Chronic constipation manangement for older institutionalized adults, *Geriatr Nurs* 21(2):78-82, 2000.

Rodrigues-Fisher L, Bourguignon C, Good BV: Dietary fiber nursing intervention: prevention of constipation in older adults, *Clin Nurs Res* 2:464, 1993.

Schaefer DC, Cheskin LJ: Constipation in the elderly, *Am Fam Physician* 58(4):907-914, 1998.

Schmelzer M: Effectiveness of wheat bran in prevention of constipation in hospitalized orthopaedic surgery patients, *Orthop Nurs* 15:10, 1990.

Schmelzer M, Wright K: Working smart, *Am J Nurs* 93:55, 1993.

Weeks SK, Hubbartt E, Michaels TK: Keys to bowel success, *Rehabil Nurs* 25(2):66-69, 2000.

Wong PN, Kadakia S: How to deal with chronic constipation, *Postgrad Med* 106(6):199-210, 1999.

Wright PS, Thomas SL: Constipation and diarrhea: the neglected symptoms, *Semin Oncol Nurs* 11(4):289-294, 1995.

Yakabowich M: Prescribe with care: the role of laxatives in the treatment of constipation, *J Gerontol Nurs* 16:4, 1990.

Ineffective Coping

Gail B. Ladwig and Jill M. Barnes

NANDA   **Definition** Inability to form a valid appraisal of stressors, inadequate choices of practiced responses, and/or inability to use available resources

• = Independent; ▲ = Collaborative

Defining Characteristics

Lack of goal-directed behavior/resolution of problem, including inability to attend, difficulty with organized information, sleep disturbance, abuse of chemical agents; decreased use of social support; use of forms of coping that impede adaptive behavior; poor concentration; fatigue; inadequate problem solving; verbalized inability to cope or ask for help; inability to meet basic needs; destructive behavior toward self or others; inability to meet role expectations; high illness rate; change in usual communication patterns; risk taking

Related Factors (r/t)

Gender differences in coping strategies; inadequate level of confidence in ability to cope; uncertainty; inadequate social support created by characteristics of relationships; inadequate level of perception of control; inadequate resources available; high degree of threat; situational crises; maturational crises; disturbance in pattern of tension release; inadequate opportunity to prepare for stressor; inability to conserve adaptive energies; disturbance in pattern of appraisal of threat

NOC   Outcomes (Nursing Outcomes Classification)

Suggested NOC Labels

Coping; Decision Making; Impulse Control; Information Processing

> **Example NOC Outcome**
> Demonstrates **Coping** as evidenced by: Identifies effective and ineffective coping patterns and modifies lifestyle as needed (Rate each indicator of **Coping**: 1 = never demonstrated, 2 = rarely demonstrated, 3 = sometimes demonstrated, 4 = often demonstrated, 5 = consistently demonstrated [see Section I])

Client Outcomes/Goals

- Verbalizes ability to cope and asks for help when needed
- Demonstrates ability to solve problems and participates at usual level in society
- Remains free of destructive behavior toward self or others
- Communicates needs and negotiates with others to meet needs
- Discusses how recent life stressors have overwhelmed normal coping strategies
- Has illness and accident rates not excessive for age and developmental level

NIC   Interventions (Nursing Interventions Classification)

Suggested NIC Labels

Coping Enhancement; Decision-Making Support

> **Example NIC Interventions—Coping Enhancement**
> - Assist the client in developing an objective appraisal of the event
> - Explore with the client previous methods of dealing with problems

Nursing Interventions and Rationales

- Observe for causes of ineffective coping such as poor self-concept, grief, lack of problem-solving skills, lack of support, or recent change in life situation.
  Situational factors must be identified to gain an understanding of the client's current situation and to aid client with coping effectively (Norris, 1992).

• = Independent; ▲ = Collaborative

- Observe for strengths such as the ability to relate the facts and to recognize the source of stressors.

  Clients and family members who are coping with critical injuries often feel defeated, hopeless, and like a failure; therefore it is imperative to verbally commend them for their strengths and use those strengths to aid functioning (Leske, 1998).

- Monitor risk of harming self or others and intervene appropriately. See care plan for **Risk for Suicide.**

  Situational factors can lead to depression or risk for suicide. Identification of such factors leads to appropriate referral or help (Norris, 1992). A client with hopelessness and an inability to problem solve often runs the risk of suicide (Buchanan, 1991). In these cases immediate referral for mental health care is essential (Norris, 1992).

- Help client set realistic goals and identify personal skills and knowledge.

  Involving clients in decision making helps them move toward independence (Connelly et al, 1993).

- Use empathetic communication, and encourage client/family to verbalize fears, express emotions, and set goals.

  Acknowledging and empathizing creates a supportive environment that enhances coping (Feeley, Gottlieb, 1998). Clients report increased satisfaction and empowerment, greater compliance with mutually agreed-upon goals, and less anxiety and depression when communication is empathic (Wells-Federman et al, 1995). Acknowledgment of feelings communicates support and conveys that clients are understood (Leske, 1998).

- Encourage client to make choices and participate in planning of care and scheduled activities.

  Participation gives a feeling of control and increases self-esteem.

- Provide mental and physical activities within the client's ability (e.g., reading, television, radio, crafts, outings, movies, dinners out, social gatherings, exercise, sports, games).

  Interventions that enhance body awareness such as exercise, proper nutrition, and muscular relaxation may be effective for treating anxiety and depression (Wells-Federman et al, 1995).

- If the client is physically able, encourage moderate aerobic exercise.

  Aerobic exercise increases one's ability to cope with acute stress (Anshel, 1996).

- Use touch with permission. Give client a back massage using slow, rhythmic stroking with hands. Use a rate of 60 strokes a minute for 3 minutes on 2-inch wide areas on both sides of the spinous process from the crown to the sacral area.

  A gentle touch can display acceptance and empathy (Hopkins, 1994). Slow stroke back massage decreased heart rate, decreased systolic and diastolic blood pressure, and increased skin temperature at significant levels. The conclusion is that relaxation is induced by slow stroke back massage (Meek, 1993).

- Provide information regarding care before care is given.

  In traumatic situations, families have a need for information and explanations (Hopkins, 1994). Providing information prepares the family for understanding the situation and possible outcomes (Leske, 1998). Adequate information and training before and after treatment reduces anxiety and fear (Herranz, Gavilan, 1999).

- Discuss changes with client before making them.

  Communication with the medical staff provides patients and families with understanding of the medical condition (Grootenhuis, Last, 1997).

• = Independent; ▲ = Collaborative

- Discuss client's/family's power to change a situation or the need to accept a situation.
  Such a discussion helps the client maintain self-esteem and look at the situation realistically with the aid of a trusted individual (Norris, 1992). In threatening situations, people search for reasons for the event(s). This search is an effort to make sense of the event, gain control, and cope (Grootenhuis, Last, 1997).
- Use active listening and acceptance to help client express emotions such as crying, guilt, and anger (within appropriate limits).
  Active listening provides the client and/or family a nonjudgmental person to listen to them and relieve their guilt feelings (Hopkins, 1994). Acknowledgment of feelings communicates support and conveys that they are understood (Leske, 1998).
- Avoid false reassurance; give honest answers and provide only the information requested.
  Identification of previously used effective coping mechanisms allow the nurse to focus attention on necessary education and referral (Norris, 1992).
- Encourage client to describe previous stressors and the coping mechanisms used.
  Describing previous experiences strengthens effective coping and helps eliminate ineffective coping mechanisms.
- Be supportive of coping behaviors; allow client time to relax.
  A supportive presence creates a supportive environment to enhance coping (Feeley, Gottlieb, 1998).
- Help clients to define what meaning their symptoms might have for them.
  In one study, the importance of helping clients find meaning in their suffering experiences was identified as a strategy perceived as helpful with a group of patients who had the diagnosis of multiple sclerosis (Pollock, Sands, 1997).
- Encourage use of cognitive behavioral relaxation (e.g., music therapy, guided imagery).
  Relaxation techniques, desensitization, and guided imagery can help clients cope, increase their sense of control, and allay anxiety (Narsavage, 1997). Relaxation with guided imagery is a technique used with increasing frequency to help individuals improve their performance and control their responses to stressful situations (Rees, 1993). Music is not a cure, but it can lift the human spirit, comfort the heart, and inspire the soul. Imagery is useful for relaxation and distraction (Fontaine, 1994). The provision of information and general mastery may play a role in decreasing helplessness and dysfunctional coping (Nicassio et al, 1997).
- Use distraction techniques during procedures that cause client to be fearful.
  Distraction is used to direct attention toward a pleasurable experience and block the attention of the feared procedure (DuHamel, Redd, Johnson-Vickberg, 1999).
- Use systematic desensitization when introducing new people, places, or procedures that may cause fear and altered coping.
  Fear of new things diminishes with repeated exposure (DuHamel, Redd, Johnson-Vickberg, 1999).
- Provide the client/family with a video of any feared procedure to view before the procedure. Ensure that the video shows a patient of similar age and background.
  Videos provide the client/family with the information necessary to eliminate fear of the unknown (DuHamel, Redd, Johnson-Vickberg, 1999).
- ▲ Refer for counseling as needed.
  Arranging for referral assists the client in working with the system, and resource use helps to develop problem-solving and coping skills (Feeley, Gottlieb, 1998).

• = **Independent;** ▲ = **Collaborative**

Geriatric

- Engage client in reminiscence.
  Reminiscence can activate past sources of self-esteem and aid in coping (Nugent, 1995).
- Be aware of client's fear of illness. Identify and reinforce patterns the elderly client has previously used to respond to stress. Allow client time to reminisce about past successes. The elderly client has had a lifetime of experience dealing with stressful events.
  A standard reminiscence interview and one that focused on successfully met challenges reduced state anxiety and enhanced coping self-efficacy when measured against both attention-placebo and no-intervention control groups (Rybarczyk, Auerbach, 1990).
- Assess and report possible physiological alterations (e.g., sepsis, hypoglycemia, hypotension, infection, changes in temperature, fluid and electrolyte imbalances, medications with known cognitive and psychotropic side effects).
  Such alterations may be contributing to confusion and must be corrected (Matthiesen et al, 1994). Medications are considered the most common cause of delirium in the ICU (Harvey, 1996).
- Determine if the individual is displaying a change in personality as a manifestation of difficulty with coping. An older individual's responses to age-related stress will depend on the balance of personality strengths and weaknesses.
  Severe or multiple stresses in late life may overwhelm an individual's coping skills and lead to personality change (Agronin, 1998).
- ▲ Increase and mobilize support available to the elderly client. Encourage interaction with family and friends.
  Friends and relatives have shared many of the older person's life experiences. Such mutual interests and overlapping memories can serve to stimulate and focus conversation and contribute effectively to the client's self-esteem (Erber, 1994). Support from family, friends, and the medical community aids coping ability (Grootenhuis, Last, 1997).
- Maintain continuity of care by keeping the number of caregivers to a minimum.
  Consistency in caregivers helps decrease anxiety and fosters trust by providing the client and family with familiar faces (Hopkins, 1994).

Multicultural

- Assess for the influence of cultural beliefs, norms, and values on the client's perceptions of effective coping.
  The client's coping behavior may be based on cultural perceptions of normal and abnormal coping behavior (Leininger, 1996; D'Avanzo et al, 2001).
- Assess for intergenerational family problems that can overwhelm coping abilities.
  Intergenerational family problems put families at risk of dysfunction (Seiderman et al, 1996; Evans, Cunningham, 1996).
- Encourage spirituality as a source of support for coping.
  Many African-Americans and Latinos identify spirituality, religiousness, prayer, and church-based approaches as coping resources (Samuel-Hodge et al, 2000; Bourjolly, 1998; Mapp, Hudson, 1997).
- Negotiate with the client with regard to the aspects of coping behavior that will need to be modified.
  Give and take with the client will lead to culturally congruent care (Leininger, 1996).
- Identify which family members the client can rely on for support.
  Many Latinos, Native Americans, and African-Americans rely on family members to cope with stress (Abraido-Lanza, Guier, Revenson, 1996; Seiderman et al, 1996).

• = Independent; ▲ = Collaborative

- Assess the influence of fatalism on the client's coping behavior.
  Fatalistic perspectives, which involve the belief that you cannot control your own fate, may influence health behaviors in some African-American and Latino populations (Phillips, Cohen, Moses, 1999; Harmon, Castro, Coe, 1996).

Home Care Interventions

- Observe family for coping behavior patterns. Obtain family and client history as able.
  Obtaining a family assessment provides a wealth of information regarding current family functions and can guide interventions (Leske, 1998).
- ▲ Assess for suicidal tendencies. Refer for mental health care immediately if indicated. Identify an emergency plan should the client become suicidal.
  A suicidal client is not safe in the home environment unless supported by professional help.
- ▲ Refer to medical social services for evaluation and counseling, which will promote adequate coping as part of the medical plan of care. If no primary medical diagnosis has been made, request medical social services to assist with community support contacts.
- ▲ If the client is involved with the mental health system, actively participate in mental health team planning.
  Based on knowledge of the home and family, home care nurses can often advocate for clients. These nurses are often requested to monitor medications and therefore need to know the plan of care.
- ▲ Refer patient/family to support groups.
  Support groups foster the sharing of common experiences and help to build mutual support. They are particularly helpful when others within the family are unable to provide support because of their own grieving or coping needs (Leske, 1998).
- ▲ If monitoring medications, contract with client or solicit assistance from a responsible caregiver. Pre-pouring of medications may be helpful with some clients.
  Successful contracting provides the client with control of care and promotes self-esteem while establishing responsibility for desired actions.
  NOTE: All of the previously mentioned interventions may be applied in the home setting. Home care may offer psychiatric nursing or the services of a licensed clinical social worker under special programs. Traditionally, insurance does not reimburse for counseling that is not related to a medical plan of care unless it falls under one of the programs just described. Public health agencies generally do not have the clinical support needed to offer psychiatric nursing services to clients. Clients are usually treated in the ambulatory mental health system.

Client/Family Teaching

- Teach clients to problem solve. Have them define the problem and cause and list the advantages and disadvantages of their options.
- Provide seriously ill clients and their families with needed information regarding their condition and treatment.
  Information is an important need of families of critically ill patients (Henneman, Cardin, 1992). In one study, information structured to meet individual needs reduced anxiety and increased satisfaction with the information provided (McGaughey, Harrisson, 1994).
- Teach relaxation techniques.
  Problem-solving skills promote the client's sense of control. Relaxation decreases stress and enhances coping (Fontaine, 1994).

• = **Independent;** ▲ = **Collaborative**

- Suggest listening to music.
  Listening to music has been found to decrease total mood disturbances scores (profile of mood states [POMS] scores). A decrease in POMS scores is indicative of decreased distress and a mood improvement (McNair, Lorr, Droppleman, 1992).
- Teach process imagery (purposely evoking a mental image of a desired effect).
  Using process imagery, a person can look at an old problem in a totally different way, making new connections and freeing the problem from the original memory. Imagery engenders a feeling of control and gives the client an effective tool for self-care (Stephens, 1993).
- Work closely with the client to develop appropriate educational tools that address individualized coping strategies.
  Collaboration between client and staff in the production of client information can improve client understanding and empower the client and family to take an active part in treatment (Willock, Grogan, 1998).
- ▲ Teach client about available community resources (e.g., therapists, ministers, counselors, self-help groups).
  Resource use helps to develop problem-solving and coping skills (Feeley, Gottlieb, 1998). Client and family teaching that promotes the ability to understand and carry out any necessary medical, rehabilitative, or daily living activities contributes to a sense of mastery, competency, and control and is vital to discharge planning and community-based assessments (Norris, 1992). Praying and religion are frequently used effective coping strategies (Grootenhuis, Last, 1997).

WEB SITES FOR EDUCATION

Merlin See the MERLIN web site for World Wide Web resources for client education.

REFERENCES   Abraido-Lanza AF, Guier C, Revenson TA: Coping and social support resources among Latinas with arthritis, *Arthritis Care Res* 9(6):501-508, 1996.

Agronin ME: Personality and psychopathology in late life, *Geriatrics* 53(suppl 1):S35-40, 1998.

Anshel MH: Effect of chronic aerobic exercise and progressive relaxation on motor performance and affect following acute stress, *Behav Med* 21(4):186-196, 1996.

Bourjolly JN: Differences in religiousness among black and white women with breast cancer, *Social Work in Health Care* 28(1):21-39, 1998.

Buchanan D: Suicide: a conceptual model for an avoidable death, *Arch Psychiatr Nurs* 5:341, 1991.

Connelly L et al: A place to be yourself: empowerment from the client's perspective, *Image J Nurs Sch* 25:297, 1993.

D'Avanzo CE et al: Developing culturally informed strategies for substance-related interventions. In Naegle MA, D'Avanzo CE, editors: *Addictions and substance abuse: strategies for advanced practice nursing*, St Louis, Mosby, pp 59-104.

DuHamel KN, Redd WH, Johnson-Vickberg SM: Behavioral interventions in the diagnosis, treatment and rehabilitation of children with cancer, *Acta Oncol* 38(6):719-734, 1999.

Erber NP: Conversation as therapy for older adults in residential care: the case for intervention, *Eur J Disord Commun* 29:269, 1994.

Evans CA, Cunningham BA: Caring for the ethnic elder, *Geriatr Nurs: Am J Care Aging* 17(3):105-110, 1996.

Feeley N, Gottlieb LN: Classification systems for health concerns, nursing strategies, and client outcomes: nursing practice with families who have a child with chronic illness, *Can J Nurs Res* 30(1):45-59, 1998.

Fontaine D: Recognition, assessment, and treatment of anxiety in the critical care setting, *Crit Care Nurse* 3(suppl):7, 1994.

• = Independent; ▲ = Collaborative

Grootenhuis MA, Last BF: Adjustment and coping by parents of children with cancer: a review of the literature, *Support Care Cancer* 5(6):466-484, 1997.

Harmon MP, Castro FG, Coe K: Acculturation and cervical cancer: knowledge, beliefs, and behaviors of Hispanic women, *Women and Health* 24(3):37-57, 1996.

Harvey M: Managing agitation in critically ill patients, *Am J Crit Care* 5(1):7-18, 1996.

Henneman EA, Cardin S: Need for information: interventions for practice, *Crit Care Nurs Clin North Am* 4(4):615-621, 1992.

Herranz J, Gavilan J: Psychosocial adjustment after laryngeal cancer surgery, *Ann Otol Rhinol Laryngol* 108(10):990-997, 1999.

Hopkins AG: The trauma nurse's role with families in crisis, *Crit Care Nurs* 14(2):35-43, 1994.

Leininger MM: *Transcultural nursing: theories, research and practices,* ed 2, Hilliard, Ohio, 1996, McGraw-Hill.

Leske JS: Treatment for family members in crisis after critical injury, *AACN Clin Issues* 9(1):129-139, 1998.

Mapp I, Hudson R: Stress and coping among African-American and Hispanic parents of deaf children, *American Annals of the Deaf* 142(1):48-56, 1997.

Matthiesen V et al: Acute confusion: nursing intervention in older patients, *Orthop Nurs* 13:25, 1994.

McGaughey J, Harrisson S: Understanding the pre-operative information needs of patients and their relatives in intensive care units, *Intens Crit Care Nurs* 3:186-194, 1994.

McNair D, Lorr M, Droppleman L: *Manual for the profile of mood states (POMS),* San Diego, 1992, Educational Testing Service.

Meek S: Effects of slow stroke back massage on relaxation in hospice clients, *Image J Nurs Sch* 25:17, 1993.

Narsavage GL: Promoting functions in clients with chronic lung disease by increasing their perceptions of control, *Holistic Nurs Pract* 12(1):17-26, 1997.

Nicassio PM et al: A comparison of behavioral and educational interventions for fibromyalgia, *J Rheumatol* 24(10):2000-2007, 1997.

Norris J: Nursing interventions for self-esteem disturbances, *Nurs Diag* 3:48, 1992.

Nugent E: Reminiscence as a nursing intervention, *J Psychosoc Nurs* 33(11):7-11, 44-45, 1995.

Phillips JM, Cohen MZ, Moses G: Breast cancer screening and African-American women: fear, fatalism, and silence, *Oncol Nurs Forum* 26(3):561-571, 1999.

Pollock SE, Sands D: Adaptation to suffering: meaning and implications for nursing, *Clin Nurs Res* 6(2):171-185, 1997.

Rees BL: An exploratory study of the effectiveness of a relaxation with guided imagery protocol, *J Holistic Nurs* 11(3):271-276, 1993.

Rybarczyk BD, Auerbach SM: Reminiscence interviews as stress management interventions for older patients undergoing surgery, *Gerontologist* 4:522-528, 1990.

Samuel-Hodge CD et al: Influences on day-to-day self-management of type 2 diabetes among African-American women: spirituality, the multi-caregiver role, and other social context factors, *Diabetes Care* 23(7):928-933, 2000.

Seiderman RY et al: Assessing American Indian families, *MCN Am J Matern Child Nurs* 21(6):274-279, 1996.

Stephens R: Imagery: a strategic intervention to empower clients—review of research literature, *Clin Nurse Spec* 7:170, 1993.

Wells-Federman C et al: The mind-body connection: the psychophysiology of many traditional nursing interventions, *Clin Nurse Spec* 9:59, 1995.

Willock J, Grogan S: Involving families in the production of patient information literature, *Prof Nurse* 13(6):351-354, 1998.

Ineffective community Coping

Margaret Lunney

NANDA   **Definition** Pattern of community activities (for adaptation and problem solving) that is unsatisfactory for meeting the demands or needs of the community

• = Independent; ▲ = Collaborative

Defining Characteristics

Expressed community powerlessness; community not meeting its own expectations; deficits of community participation; deficits in communication methods; excessive community conflicts; expressed difficulty in meeting demands for change; expressed vulnerability; high illness rates; stressors perceived as excessive; increased social problems (e.g., homicides, vandalism, arson, terrorism, robbery, infanticide, abuse, divorce, unemployment, poverty, militancy, mental illness)

Related Factors (r/t)

Natural or manmade disasters; ineffective or nonexistent community systems (e.g., lack of emergency medical, transportation, or disaster planning systems); deficits in community social support services and resources; inadequate resources for problem solving

NOC   Outcomes (Nursing Outcomes Classification)

Suggested NOC Labels

Community Competence; Community Health Status

> **Example NOC Outcome**
> Demonstrates **Community Competence** as evidenced by the following indicators:
> Prevalence of health promotion programs/Health status of infants, children, adolescents, adults, elders/Attendance at programs for healthy states (Rate each indicator of **Community Competence:** 1 = poor demonstration, 2 = fair demonstration, 3 = average demonstration, 4 = good demonstration, 5 = excellent demonstration [see Section I])

Community Outcomes

- Participate in community actions to improve power resources
- Develop improved communication with each other
- Participate in problem solving
- Demonstrate cohesiveness in problem solving
- Develop new strategies for problem solving
- Express power to deal with change and manage problems

NIC   Interventions (Nursing Interventions Classification)

Suggested NIC Labels

Environmental Management: Community; Health Policy Monitoring

NIC Interventions developed for use with individuals can be adapted for use with communities: Coping Enhancement; Culture Brokerage; Mutual Goal Setting; Support System Enhancement

> **Example NIC Interventions—Coping Enhancement**
> - Explore with the client previous methods of dealing with life problems
> - Assist the client to solve problems in a constructive manner

Nursing Interventions and Rationales

NOTE: The diagnosis of **Ineffective Coping** does not apply and should not be used when stress is being imposed by external sources or circumstance. If the community is a victim of circumstances, using the nursing diagnosis **Ineffective Coping** is equivalent to blaming the victim. See care plans for **Ineffective community Therapeutic regimen management** and **Readiness for enhanced community Coping**.

- = Independent; ▲ = Collaborative

- Establish a collaborative/partnership relationship with the community (see care plan for **Ineffective community Therapeutic regimen management** for references).
  Maximum involvement of people in their own health care is an essential component of primary health care, the internationally accepted health care model. Conflict is best managed by community members.
- Participate with community members in the identification of stressors and assessment of distress.
  It may be possible to reduce or eliminate some of the stressors. Not all stressors produce distress. Distress is negatively associated with perceived health and perceived health is predictive of health decline (morbidity, disability, and mortality) (Farmer, Ferraro, 1997).
- Determine the extent of stress proliferation (i.e., primary stressors associated with contextual circumstances such as poverty) and secondary stressors related to the primary stressors (e.g., poor nutrition and housing conditions).
  Stress proliferation may lead to ineffective coping (Pearlin, Aneshensel, Leblanc, 1997). Nurses can help communities to prevent primary stressors from leading to secondary stressors.
- Work with community members to increase awareness of ineffective coping behaviors (e.g., conflicts that prevent community members from working together, anger and hate that paralyzes the community).
  Problem solving is essential for effective coping. Behaviors that interfere with problem solving can be modified by community members in partnership with nurses and other health providers (Anderson, McFarlane, 2000; Chinn, 2001; Wallerstein, 2000).
- Provide support to the community and help community members to identify and mobilize additional supports.
  Social support is associated with positive coping strategies (Pender, 1996). Adequate social support may help to prevent primary stressors from leading to secondary stressors (Pearlin, Aneshensel, Leblanc, 1997).
- Advocate for the community in multiple arenas (e.g., television, newspapers, governmental agencies).
  Advocacy is a specific form of caring that enhances power resources for community coping. Power resources include knowledge, motivation, belief system (hope), physical strength and reserve, psychological stamina and support network, positive self-concept, and energy (Miller, 1999).
- Write grant proposals to help community members obtain funds for programs that reduce stress or improve coping. (See Coley, Scheinberg, 2000, for program proposal writing methods).
  The programs that are necessary may be expensive and funds may not be available without the support of public or privately funded grants.
- Work with members of the community to identify and develop coping strategies that promote a sense of power (e.g., obtaining sources for funding, collaborating with other communities).
  Power is an essential aspect of coping. According to Barrett's nursing theory of power, "power is being aware of what one is choosing to do, feeling free to do it, and doing it intentionally" (Caroselli, Barrett, 1998). A first step in power enhancement is for the community to identify and develop its own coping strategies (Chinn, 2001).
- Obtain police support for community partnerships toward healthy coping.
  In some communities, police programs have led to innovative programs that contribute to community health (Frommer, Papouchado, 2000).

• = Independent; ▲ = Collaborative

Multicultural

- Acknowledge the stresses unique to racial/ethnic communities.
  Targeted alcohol and tobacco marketing, high levels of unemployment, lack of health insurance, and racism are stressors unique to culturally diverse communities (D'Avanzo et al, 2001).
- Identify the health services and information that are currently available in the community.
  This will assist with focusing efforts and promote wise use of valuable resources (National Institutes of Health, 1998).
- Work with members of the community to prioritize and target health goals specific to the community.
  This will increase feelings of control over and a sense of ownership of programs (Anderson, McFarlane, 2000; Chinn, 2001; National Institutes of Health, 1998).
- Approach community leaders and members of color with respect, warmth, and professional courtesy.
  Instances of disrespect and lack of caring have special significance for individuals of color (D'Avanzo et al, 2001).
- Establish and sustain partnerships with key individuals within communities when developing and implementing programs.
  Local leaders are excellent sources of information and will enhance the credibility of programs (National Institutes of Health, 1998).
- Use community church settings as a forum for advocacy, teaching, and program implementation.
  Church based interventions have been very successful. (Havas et al, 1994).
- Request political leaders to become part of the partnership process.
  The Carnegie Commission on Preventing Deadly Conflict established the importance of political leaders working to prevent community conflicts and violence (Hamburg, George, Ballentine, 1999).
- Protect children from exposure to community conflicts.
  In a 15-month study of 97 urban 6- to 10-year-old boys who had witnessed community violence and antisocial behavior, reports of witnessing community conflicts were associated with child antisocial behavior, including children from families with low family conflict (Miller et al, 1999).

Community teaching

- Teach strategies for stress management.
  Explain the relationship of enhancing power resources and coping.

WEB SITES FOR EDUCATION

　See the MERLIN web site for World Wide Web resources for client education.

REFERENCES   Anderson ET, McFarlane J: *Community as partner: theory and practice in nursing*, ed 3, Philadelphia, 2000, Lippincott, Williams & Wilkins.
Caroselli C, Barrett EAM: A review of the power as knowing participation in change literature, *Nurs Sci Q* 11(1):9-16, 1998.
Chinn PL: *Peace and power: building communities for the future*, ed 5, Boston, 2001, Jones & Bartlett.
Coley SM, Scheinberg CA: *Proposal writing*, ed 2, Thousand Oaks, Calif, 2000, Sage.

• = Independent; ▲ = Collaborative

D'Avanzo CE et al: Developing culturally informed strategies for substance-related interventions. In Naegle MA, D'Avanzo CE, editors: *Addictions and substance abuse: strategies for advanced practice nursing,* St Louis, 2001, Mosby, pp 59-104.

Farmer MM, Ferraro KF: Distress and perceived health: mechanisms of health decline, *J Health Soc Behav* 39:298-311, 1997.

Frommer P, Papouchado K: Police as contributors to healthy communities, *Aiken, South Carolina, Public Health Rep* 115(2-3):249-252, 2000.

Havas S et al: 5 a day for better health: a new research initiative, *J Am Diet Assoc* 94(1):32-36, 1994.

Hamburg DA, George A, Ballentine K: Preventing deadly conflict: the critical role of leadership, *Arch Gen Psychiatry* 56(11):971-976, 1999.

Miller JF: *Coping with chronic illness: overcoming powerlessness,* ed 3, Philadelphia, 1999, FA Davis.

Miller LS et al: Witnessed community violence and anti-social behavior in high risk, urban boys, *J Clin Child Psychol* 28(1):2-11, 1999.

National Institutes of Health: *Sauld para su corazon: bringing heart health to Latinos—a guide for building community programs,* DHHS Publication No. 98-3796, Washington, DC, 1998, U.S. Government Printing Office.

Pearlin L, Aneshensel CS, Leblanc AJ: The forms and mechanisms of stress proliferation: the case of AIDS caregivers, *J Health Soc Behav* 38:223-236, 1997.

Pender NJ: *Health promotion in nursing practice,* ed 3, Stamford, Conn, 1996, Appleton & Lange.

Wallerstein N: A participatory evaluation model for healthier communities: developing indicators for New Mexico, *Public Health Rep* 115(2-3):199-204, 2000.

Readiness for enhanced community Coping

Margaret Lunney

NANDA **Definition** Pattern of community activities for adaptation and problem solving that is satisfactory for meeting the demands or needs of the community but that can also be improved for management of current and future problems and stressors

Defining Characteristics

One or more of the following characteristics that indicate effective coping: positive communication between community/aggregates and larger community; programs available for recreation and relaxation; resources sufficient for managing stressors; agreement that community is responsible for stress management; active planning by community for predicted stressors; active problem solving by community when faced with issues; positive communication among community members

NOC **Outcomes (Nursing Outcomes Classification)**
Suggested NOC Labels
Community Competence; Community Health Status

Example NOC Outcome
Demonstrates **Community Competence** as evidenced by the following indicators: Prevalence of health promotion programs/Health status of infants, children, adolescents, adults, elders/Attendance at programs for healthy states (Rate each indicator of **Community Competence:** 1 = poor demonstration, 2 = fair demonstration, 3 = average demonstration, 4 = good demonstration, 5 = excellent demonstration [see Section I])

• = Independent; ▲ = Collaborative

Community Outcomes

- Develops enhanced coping strategies
- Maintains effective coping strategies for management of stress

NIC ## Interventions (Nursing Interventions Classification)

Suggested NIC Labels

Environmental Management: Community; Health Policy Monitoring

NIC Interventions developed for use with individuals can be adapted for use with communities: Coping Enhancement; Culture Brokerage; Mutual Goal Setting; Support System Enhancement

> **Example NIC Interventions—Coping Enhancement**
> - Explore with the client previous methods of dealing with life problems
> - Assist the client to solve problems in a constructive manner

Nursing Interventions and Rationales

NOTE: Interventions depend on the specific aspects of community coping that can be enhanced (e.g., planning for stress management, communication, development of community power, community perceptions of stress, community coping strategies).

- Establish a collaborative partnership with the community (see care plan for **Ineffective community Therapeutic regimen management** for references).
- Describe the role of community/public health nurse in working with healthy communities (Stanhope, Lancaster, 1999).
  Members of society are not familiar with nurses' roles in public health.
- Help the community to obtain funds for additional programs. (See Coley, Scheinberg, 2000, for proposal writing methods.)
  Healthy communities may need additional funding sources to strengthen community resources.
- Encourage positive attitudes toward the community through the media and other sources.
  Negative attitudes or stigmas create additional stress and deficits in social support (Lubkin, 1998).
- Help community members to collaborate with one another for power enhancement and coping skills.
  Community members may not have sufficient skills to collaborate for enhanced coping. Effective collaboration skills can be promoted by health care providers (Courtney et al, 1996; Chinn, 2001).
- Encourage critical thinking.
  Critical thinking supports problem-solving ability.
- Demonstrate optimum use of the power resources of knowledge, motivation, belief system (hope), physical strength and reserve, psychological stamina and support network, positive self-concept, and energy.
  Optimum use of power resources supports coping (Miller, 1999). Community members benefit from observations of nurse's use of resources.
- Collaborate with community members to improve educational levels within the community.
  In a study of 18 randomly selected communities and 900 elders living in those communities, higher educational levels were associated with less stress pertaining to health, and fewer help-

• = Independent; ▲ = Collaborative

ers were needed by educated elderly (Preston, Bucher, 1996). Higher educational levels are associated with lower levels of emotional and physical distress (Ross, Van Willigen, 1997).

Multicultural

- Acknowledge the stresses unique to racial/ethnic communities.
  Targeted alcohol and tobacco marketing, high levels of unemployment, lack of health insurance, and racism are stressors unique to culturally diverse communities (D'Avanzo et al, 2001).
- Identify what health services and information are currently available in the community.
  This will assist with focusing efforts and promote wise use of valuable resources (National Institutes of Health, 1998).
- Work with members of the community to prioritize and target health goals specific to the community.
  This will increase feelings of control over and sense of ownership of programs (National Institutes of Health, 1998).
- Approach community leaders and members of color with respect, warmth, and professional courtesy.
  Instances of disrespect and lack of caring have special significance for individuals of color (D'Avanzo et al, 2001).
- Establish and sustain partnerships with key individuals within communities when developing and implementing programs.
  Local leaders are excellent sources of information and will enhance the credibility of programs (National Institutes of Health, 1998).
- Use community church settings as a forum for advocacy, teaching, and program implementation.
  Church-based interventions have been very successful in communities of color (Havas et al, 1994).

Community teaching

- Review coping skills, power for coping, and the use of power resources.

WEB SITES FOR EDUCATION

MERLIN   See the MERLIN web site for World Wide Web resources for client education.

REFERENCES   Chinn PL: *Peace and power: building communities for the future,* ed 5, Boston, 2001, Jones & Bartlett.

Coley SM, Scheinberg CA: *Proposal writing,* ed 2, Thousand Oaks, Calif, 2000, Sage.

Courtney R et al: The partnership model: working with individuals, families, and communities toward a new vision of health, *Public Health Nurs* 13:177-186, 1996.

D'Avanzo CE et al: Developing culturally informed strategies for substance-related interventions. In Naegle MA, D'Avanzo CE, editors: *Addictions and substance abuse: strategies for advanced practice nursing,* St Louis, 2001, Mosby, pp 59-104.

Havas S et al: 5 a day for better health: a new research initiative, *J Am Dietetic Assoc* 94(1):32-36, 1994.

Lubkin IM: *Chronic illness: impact and interventions,* ed 4, Boston, 1998, Jones & Bartlett.

Miller JF: *Coping with chronic illness: overcoming powerlessness,* ed 3, Philadelphia, 1999, FA Davis.

National Institutes of Health: *Sauld para su corazon: bringing heart health to Latinos—a guide for building community programs,* DHHS Publication No. 98-3796, Washington, DC, 1998, U.S. Government Printing Office.

Preston DB, Bucher JA: The effects of community differences on health status, health stress, and helping networks in a sample of 900 elderly, *Public Health Nurs* 13:72-79, 1996.

Ross CE, Van Willigen M: Education and subjective quality of life, *J Health Soc Behav* 38:275-297, 1997.

Stanhope M, Lancaster J: *Community health & public health nursing,* ed 5, St Louis, 1999, Mosby.

• = Independent; ▲ = Collaborative

Defensive Coping

Gail B. Ladwig and Jill M. Barnes

 Definition Repeated projection of falsely positive self-evaluations based on a self-protective pattern that defends against underlying perceived threats to positive self-regard

Defining Characteristics

Grandiosity; rationalization of failures; hypersensitivity to slight/criticism; denial of obvious problems/weaknesses; projection of blame/responsibility; lack of follow-through or participation in treatment or therapy; superior attitude toward others; hostile laughter or ridicule of others; difficulty in perception of reality, reality/testing; difficulty establishing/maintaining relationships

Related Factors (r/t)

Situational crises; psychological impairment; substance abuse

NOC Outcomes (Nursing Outcomes Classification)

Suggested NOC Labels

Coping; Decision Making; Impulse Control; Information Processing

> **Example NOC Outcome**
> Demonstrates **Coping** as evidenced by the following indicators: Identifies effective and ineffective coping patterns/Modifies lifestyle as needed (Rate each indicator of **Coping:** 1 = never demonstrated, 2 = rarely demonstrated, 3 = sometimes demonstrated, 4 = often demonstrated, 5 = consistently demonstrated [see Section I])

Client Outcomes

- Accepts responsibility for actions
- Accepts constructive criticism without feeling personally rejected
- Interacts with others
- Participates in therapy and establishes realistic goals

NIC Interventions (Nursing Interventions Classification)

Suggested NIC Labels

Self-Awareness Enhancement

> **Example NIC Interventions—Self-Awareness Enhancement**
> - Encourage client to recognize and discuss thoughts and feelings
> - Assist client to identify behaviors that are self-destructive

Nursing Interventions and Rationales

- Assess for the presence of denial as a coping mechanism.
  Denial is a defensive avoidance of emotion. It can be beneficial as a coping mechanism, but total denial can be detrimental (Robinson, 1999).
- Determine whether the patient has a positive or negative overall appraisal of the event.
  A negative appraisal of the event can lead to anxiety, depression, and other symptomatology (Mazur et al, 1999).
- Develop a trusting, therapeutic relationship with the client/family.
  A genuine connection can ease defensiveness or uneasiness (Robinson, 1999).

• = Independent; ▲ = Collaborative

- Ask appropriate questions to assess whether denial is being used in association with alcoholism.
  A short, sensitive tool is the CAGE questionnaire. (The most widely used tool is the Michigan Alcoholism Screening Test [MAST]. Although it is a very reliable and valid tool, it is not practical for use by a bedside nurse for purposes of assessment.)
- An affirmative answer to two or more of the following questions is considered a basis for suspicion of alcohol abuse:

  C   Have you ever felt you ought to cut down on drinking?
  A   Have people annoyed you by criticizing your drinking?
  G   Have you ever felt bad or guilty about your drinking?
  E   Have you ever had a drink first thing in the morning to steady your nerves or get rid of a hangover (eye opener)?

  There are several screening instruments that have been extensively used and found to be superior to the use of biochemical markers or laboratory tests for the early detection of alcohol or other drug abuse. The CAGE questionnaire is a quick and easy tool for bedside nurses (Burns, 1993). Because alcoholics often employ denial, they are unlikely to produce an accurate response when asked directly how much they drink. Questions must be asked differently to obtain more accurate data. The CAGE questionnaire is a practical tool for a bedside nurse (Kovach, Weiss, 1991).
- Determine client's perception of the problem, and then provide reality-based examples of the true situation (i.e., witnesses to an accident, blood alcohol levels, problems caused by alcohol).
  Reframing and awareness-raising are techniques used to restructure cognitions to aid in coping (Feeley, Gottlieb, 1998). Ascribing meaning, altering one's self-perception, and relating the critical event to alcohol is necessary for the alcoholic to transcend denial (Wing, 1995).
- Help client to identify the situations or people that trigger feelings of defensiveness; acknowledge that these are triggers, and emphasize that the client is ultimately responsible for personal behavior.
  Refocusing on the real cause of anger can help the client to reduce his or her anger and enhance coping (Hopkins, 1994). Identifying exact situations and feelings helps direct interventions. An emphasis on helping the individual attain a sense of control may facilitate change, ensuring the use constructive rather than obstructive denial (Russell, 1993).
- ▲ Encourage client self-worth by using group or individual therapy, role-playing, one-to-one interactions, and role modeling.
  Role-playing can help the client to identify coping and problem-solving skills (Feeley, Gottlieb, 1998).
- Support strengths and normal observations with "I note that. . ." or "I want you to notice. . . ." Tell clients when they do something well.
  Listening and providing feedback creates a supportive environment for the client (Feeley, Gottlieb, 1998). By promoting the client's strengths the nurse will be assisting the client to become more secure in the surroundings. As the client's security level increases, the need to use denial decreases (Robinson, 1993).
- Teach client to use positive thinking by blocking negative thoughts with the word "Stop!" and inserting positive thoughts (e.g., "I'm a good [person, friend, student]").
  Once clients learn to recognize negative and distorted thoughts, they can learn to interrupt or stop this self-defeating behavior and replace it with realistic and positive appraisals (Norris, 1992).

• = Independent; ▲ = Collaborative

▲ Provide feedback regarding others' perceptions of the client's behavior through group or milieu therapy or one-to-one interactions.

Listening and providing feedback creates a supportive environment for the client (Feeley, Gottlieb, 1998). Motivation, sharing of experiences, camaraderie with and support from peers, and knowledge of not being alone have been identified as advantages of group learning (Payne, 1993).

• Encourage client to use "I" statements and to accept responsibility for and consequences of actions.

"I" statements encourage personal responsibility and help the client to overcome defensiveness. All clients have the capacity for change (Murray, Bair, 1993).

• Encourage emotional expression after a traumatic event.

If emotions are bottled up, the person cannot fully overcome the trauma until they are expressed (Johal, Bennett, 1999).

Geriatric

• Assess client for anger and identify previous outlets for anger.

Anger is a normal reaction to loss. Allowing clients to vent and refocus their anger on its real cause can enhance coping (Hopkins, 1994). Use of appropriate familiar outlets for anger can help a client dissipate emotions.

• Explore new outlets for anger, including physical activities within client's capabilities (e.g., hitting a pillow, woodworking, sanding, scrubbing floors).

Physical activities help the client direct anger outward instead of holding it inside.

• Assess client for dementia or depression.

Dementia and depression need to be identified if the nurse is to intervene appropriately (Norris, 1992). Symptoms of dementia or depression may be masked by inappropriate coping techniques. Depression may be overlooked because there is a focus on the physiological problems of aging (Abraham, Neudorfer, Currie, 1992).

Multicultural

• Assess for the influence of cultural beliefs, norms, and values on the client's feelings of defensiveness.

The client's defensive behavior may be based on cultural perceptions of treatment (Leininger, 1996).

• Acknowledge racial/ethnic differences at the onset of care.

Acknowledgement of race/ethnicity issues will enhance communication, establish rapport, and promote treatment outcomes (D'Avanzo et al, 2001).

• Use therapeutic communication techniques that emphasize acceptance, offer the self, validate the client's concerns, and convey respect.

Studies show that even when language is not a barrier, some ethnic clients may be reluctant to discuss their beliefs and practices because of fear of criticism or ridicule (Evans, Cunningham, 1996).

• Give a rationale when assessing ethnically diverse clients about alcohol use/misuse or other sensitive topics.

Blacks and other people of color may expect white caregivers to hold negative and preconceived ideas about people of color. Giving a rationale for questions asked will help alleviate this perception (D'Avanzo et al, 2001).

Home Care Interventions

• Include in initial assessment client and family histories of mental health problems.
• Observe family dynamics for dysfunctional and supportive communication.

• = Independent; ▲ = Collaborative

In the context of some family patterns of communication, defensive coping may be a learned behavior.

▲ Refer to a mental health professional for possible psychodrama therapy, especially if difficulty coping with a traumatic event.
Psychodrama has been shown to help people begin to reframe their feelings of victimization as feelings of survival and begin to see the future as hopeful (Carbonell, Parteleno-Barehmi, 1999).

▲ In the absence of primary medical diagnoses, refer to medical social services for assistance with contacting appropriate community services.

▲ If medical diagnoses coexist with defensive coping, confirm and validate client's mental health plan and progress. Medical social services may or may not be necessary depending on community support.

▲ Contract with client for administration of medications. Observe for abuse.
Successful contracting provides control and improved self-esteem, as well as a vehicle for reinforcing clients' responsibility for their actions.

▲ Refer to therapist for debriefing if a traumatic or critical event has occurred.
Critical incident debriefing has decreased the number of psychological problems caused by traumatic events (Johal, Bennett, 1999).

Client/Family Teaching

▲ Teach client the actions and side effects of medications and the importance of taking them as prescribed, even when the client is feeling good.
Carrying out the medical regimen is critical, and an assessment of the family's ability to do so should be made before discharge (Norris, 1992). The client needs to know that feeling good may result from the medications and that it is important to continue taking them.

▲ Refer client to appropriate therapist for grandiose and possibly harmful symptoms such as promiscuity, insomnia, euphoria, overspending, and alcohol or drug abuse.
Arranging for referrals helps clients work the system and, in turn, therapy helps clients develop problem-solving and coping skills (Feeley, Gottlieb, 1998). Harmful behaviors need appropriate intervention from a qualified professional. Resource personnel should be consulted to assist with identifying and altering patterns of alcohol abuse and addressing the problems that alcoholism creates (Kovach, Weiss, 1991).

▲ Work with client's support group to identify harmful behaviors and to seek help for client if unable to control behavior.
To ensure safety and compliance, the client's support group needs to be involved in the treatment plan.

• When a traumatic event has occurred, encourage the use of written disclosure. Instruct the person to write about the event over a period of days.
Written disclosure has been found to decrease the number of office visits and complaints of physical and psychological symptoms following the event (Johal, Bennett, 1999).

WEB SITES FOR EDUCATION

🖳 MERLIN See the MERLIN web site for World Wide Web resources for client education.

REFERENCES   Abraham I, Neudorfer M, Currie L: Effects of group interventions on cognition and depression in nursing home residents, *Nurs Res* 41:196, 1992.
Burns CM: Assessment and screening for drug abuse: guidelines for the primary care nurse practitioner, *Nurse Pract Forum* 4(4):199-206, 1993.

• = Independent; ▲ = Collaborative

Carbonell DM, Pareleno-Barehmi C: Psychodrama groups for girls coping with trauma, *Int J Group Psycho-ther* 49(3):285-306, 1999.

D'Avanzo CE et al: Developing culturally informed strategies for substance-related interventions. In Naegle MA, D'Avanzo CE, editors: *Addictions and substance abuse: strategies for advanced practice nursing*, St Louis, 2001, Mosby, pp 59-104.

Evans CA, Cunningham BA: Caring for the ethnic elder, *Geriatr Nurs: Am J Care Aging* 17(3):105-110, 1996.

Feeley N, Gottlieb LN: Classification systems for health concerns, nursing strategies, and client outcomes: nursing practice with families who have a child with chronic illness, *Can J Nurs Res* 30(1):45-59, 1998.

Hopkins AG: The trauma nurse's role with families in crisis, *Crit Care Nurs* 14(2):35-43, 1994.

Johal SS, Bennett P: Written disclosure: a way of coping with traumatic stress, *Nurs Stand* 13(37):43-44, 1999.

Kovach G, Weiss K: Denying alcoholism, *Focus Crit Care AACN* 18:469, 1991.

Leininger MM: *Transcultural nursing: theories, research and practices*, ed 2, Hilliard, Ohio, 1996, McGraw-Hill.

Mazur E et al: Cognitive moderators of children's adjustment to stressful divorce events: the role of negative cognitive errors and positive illusions, *Child Dev* 70(1):231-245, 1999.

Murray RB, Bair M: Use of therapeutic milieu in a community setting, *J Psychosoc Nurs Ment Health Serv* 31:11, 1993.

Norris J: Nursing intervention for self-esteem disturbances, *Nurs Diag* 3:48, 1992.

Payne J: The contribution of group learning to the rehabilitation of spinal cord injured adults, *Rehabil Nurs* 18:375, 1993.

Robinson AW: Getting to the heart of denial, *Am J Nurs* 99(5):38-42, 1999.

Robinson K: Denial: an adaptive response, *Dimens Crit Care Nurs* 12:102, 1993.

Russell G: The role of denial in clinical practice, *J Adv Nurs* 18:938, 1993.

Wing D: Transcending alcoholic denial, *Image J Nurs Sch* 27:121, 1995.

Compromised family Coping

Beverly Pickett, Gail B. Ladwig, and Mary Markle

NANDA   **Definition** Usually supportive primary person (family member or close friend) provides insufficient, ineffective, or compromised support, comfort, assistance, or encouragement that may be needed by the client to manage or master adaptive tasks related to a health challenge

Defining Characteristics

Objective   Significant person attempts assistive or supportive behaviors with less than satisfactory results; significant person displays protective behavior disproportionate (too little or too much) to client's abilities or need for autonomy; significant person withdraws or enters into limited or temporary personal communication with client at the time of need

Subjective   Client expresses or confirms a concern or complaint about significant other's response to his or her health problem; significant person describes or confirms an inadequate understanding or knowledge base, which interferes with effective assistance or support-ive behaviors; significant person describes preoccupation with personal reaction (e.g., fear, anticipatory grief, guilt, or anxiety) to client's illness, disability, other situational or developmental crises)

Related Factors (r/t)

Temporary preoccupation of a significant person who tries to manage emotional con-flicts and personal suffering and is unable to perceive or act effectively with regard to client's needs; temporary family disorganization and role changes; prolonged disease or disability progression that exhausts supportive capacity of significant person; other situ-

• = Independent; ▲ = Collaborative

ational or developmental crises or problems the significant person may be facing; inadequate or incorrect information or understanding by a primary person; lack of support given by client to the significant person

NOC **Outcomes (Nursing Outcomes Classification)**

Suggested NOC Labels

Family Coping; Family Normalization; Family Participation in Professional Care

> **Example NOC Outcome**
> Demonstrates **Family Coping** as evidenced by the following indicators: Manages problems/Involves family members in decision making/Believes he or she can manage problems (Rate each indicator of **Family Coping:** 1 = never demonstrated, 2 = rarely demonstrated, 3 = sometimes demonstrated, 4 = often demonstrated, 5 = consistently demonstrated [see Section I])

Client Outcomes

- Verbalizes internal resources to help deal with the situation (family or significant person)
- Verbalizes knowledge and understanding of illness, disability, or disease (family or significant person)
- Provides support and assistance as needed (family or significant person)
- Identifies need for and seeks outside support (family or significant person)

NIC **Interventions (Nursing Interventions Classification)**

Suggested NIC Labels

Family Involvement; Family Mobilization; Family Support

> **Example NIC Interventions—Family Support**
> - Facilitate communication of concerns/feelings between client and family or between family members
> - Provide assistance in meeting basic needs for family such as shelter, food, and clothing

Nursing Interventions and Rationales

- Assess the strengths and deficiencies of the family system.
  Assessments allow for anticipatory care and guidance to help members acquire and maintain supports and coping strategies (Ducharmes, Rowat, 1992; Thomas, 2000).
- Consider use of family theory as a framework to help guide interventions (e.g., family stress theory, social exchange theory).
  Theory helps to identify the focus, means, and goals of nursing practice. It enhances communication and increases autonomy and accountability to care (Gillis et al, 1989; Meleis, 1991).
- Observe for cause of family problems.
  Ongoing assessment provides clues about underlying feelings (Barry, 1989).
- Assist significant person with expanding repertoire of coping skills.
  Coping skills can decrease the family's vulnerability to stress and can strengthen and maintain family resources that protect the family.
- Help family members recognize the need for help and teach them how to ask for it.
  Recognizing the need for help and knowing how to ask for it enables family members to maintain control (Szabo, Strang, 1999).

• = Independent; ▲ = Collaborative

- Assess how family members interact with each other; observe verbal and nonverbal communication and individual and group responses to stress.
  Understanding how families cope with stress is important. One person's problems affect the entire family (Mears, 1990).
- Help family members identify strengths and make a list that each member can refer to for positive reinforcement.
  Positive feedback from one family member reinforces a particular action or behavior of another member.
- Encourage family members to verbalize feelings. Spend time with them, sit down and make eye contact, and offer coffee and other nourishment.
  The expression of feelings helps family caregivers to regain and maintain control (Szabo, Strang, 1999). Acceptance of nourishment indicates a beginning acceptance of the situation.
- Talk with family about the importance of sharing feelings and ways to do so (e.g., role-playing, writing a letter to significant other).
  Sharing feelings allows the family an opportunity to communicate in an effective yet non-threatening manner.
- Involve client and family in the planning of care as much as possible.
  Involving the client and family in the care plan or treatment regimen encourages compliance with treatment and enhances the client's feeling of control (Barry, 1989).
- Provide privacy during family visits. If possible, maintain flexible visiting hours to accommodate more frequent family visits.
- If possible, arrange staff assignments so the same staff members have contact with the family. Familiarize other staff members with the situation in the absence of the usual staff member.
  Providing privacy, maintaining flexible hours, and arranging consistent staff assignments will reduce stress, enhance communication, and facilitate the building of trust.
- Determine whether family is suffering from additional stressors (e.g., childcare issues, financial problems).
- ▲ Refer family to appropriate resources for assistance as indicated (e.g., counseling, psychotherapy, financial or spiritual support).
  If family members do not know who to contact, many useful services may be underused (Mears, 1990).
- Encourage family-centered care of clients during and after discharge.
  Family-centered care supports families by building on their strengths and respecting their different coping methods (Ahmann, 1994).

Geriatric

- Assess physical, emotional, and spiritual needs of significant person and meet needs while visiting (e.g., ensure that a person with diabetes eats meals).
  Meeting the needs of the significant person will optimize individual health and well-being, thus enhancing the health and well-being of the family.
- Assist in finding transportation to enable family members to visit.
- If family member is homebound and unable to visit, encourage alternative contact (e.g., telephone, cards and letters, e-mail) to provide ongoing scheduled progress reports.
  Reducing loneliness and isolation has many positive psychosocial and physical health benefits (Bulechek, McCloskey, 1992).

• = Independent; ▲ = Collaborative

Home Care Interventions

- During time of compromised coping, increase visits to ensure safety of client, support of family, and assistance with coping strategies.
  Increased time for expressions of support, active listening, and empathy can nurture the client and family and move them toward more effective coping.

▲ Assess the needs of the caregiver in the home. Intervene to meet needs as appropriate to total case management and explore all available resources that may be used to provide adequate home care (e.g., parish nursing as an effective adjunct, home health aide services to relieve caregiver's fatigue). Encourage caregivers not to neglect their own physical, mental and spiritual health, and give more specific information about client needs and ways to meet them.
  Meeting the needs of caregivers supports their ability to meet the needs of the client.

▲ Refer family to medical social services for evaluation and supportive counseling.
  Dedicating time for nurturing the caregivers and reassuring the client allows them to express feelings and feel hope.

▲ Serve as an advocate, mentor, and role model for caregiving. Write down or contract for the care needed by the client.
  Therapeutic use of self by the nurse and concrete task definition and assignment reinforce positive coping strategies and allow caregivers to feel less guilty when tasks are delegated to multiple caregivers.

▲ When a terminal illness is the precipitating factor for ineffective coping, offer hospice services and support groups as possible resources.
  Nonjudgmental support from helpers with no agenda allows verbalization of feelings. The hospice paradigm addresses the physical, emotional, and spiritual needs of the dying and their loved ones.

- Support positive individual and family coping efforts.
  Positive feedback reinforces desired behaviors and supports the family unit.

Client/Family Teaching

- Provide truthful information for family and significant people regarding client's specific illness or condition, including anticipatory guidance for expected outcomes.
  Research on families' needs identified as most important by all family members pointed to the need to receive information (Daly et al, 1994).

- Promote individual and family relaxation and stress reduction strategies.
  The immune system weakens in response to stress; relaxation elicits the opposite, healthful response (Bulechek, McCloskey, 1992).

- Involve client and family in planning of care as often as possible; mutual goal setting is often an effective strategy.
  Family members of any trauma client admitted to the level I trauma center of one hospital are invited by the trauma staff to attend weekly multidisciplinary meetings. By the use of these meetings, family concerns can become a positive care factor, and the tasks of nurses, doctors, and social workers are made easier (Boettcher, Schiller, 1990).

Multicultural

- Acknowledge racial/ethnic differences at the onset of care.
  Acknowledgement of race/ethnicity issues will enhance communication, establish rapport, and promote treatment outcomes (D'Avanzo et al, 2001).

• = **Independent;** ▲ = **Collaborative**

- Approach families of color with respect, warmth, and professional courtesy.
  Instances of disrespect and lack of caring have special significance for families of color (D'Avanzo et al, 2001).
- Assess for the influence of cultural beliefs, norms, and values on the family's perceptions of coping.
  What the family considers normal and abnormal coping behavior may be based on cultural perceptions (Leininger, 1996).
- Give rationale when assessing families with regard to sensitive issues.
  Blacks and other people of color may expect white caregivers to hold negative and preconceived ideas about them. Giving a rationale for questions asked will help alleviate this perception (D'Avanzo et al, 2001).
- Use a family-centered approach when working with Latino, Asian, African-American, and Native American clients.
  Latinos may perceive family as a source of support, solver of problems, and source of pride. Asian Americans may regard the family as the primary decision-maker and influence on individual family members (D'Avanzo et al, 2001). Native American families may be extended structures that exert powerful influences over functioning (Seiderman et al, 1996).
- Facilitate modeling and role-playing for family regarding healthy ways to communicate and interact.
  It is helpful for families and the client to practice communication skills in a safe environment before trying them in a real-life situation (Rivera-Andino, Lopez, 2000).
- Validate the family's feelings regarding the impact of client illness on family lifestyle.
  Validation lets the client know that the nurse has heard and understands what was said, and it promotes the nurse-client relationship (Stuart, Laraia, 2001; Giger, Davidhizar, 1995).
- Work to provide caregivers who understand the importance of cultural beliefs and values the family may hold.
  There are differences in some cultures regarding health beliefs, practices, and values (Andrews, 1992; Camphinha-Bacote, Narayan, 2000).

WEB SITES FOR EDUCATION

MERLIN See the MERLIN web site for World Wide Web resources for client education.

REFERENCES Ahmann E: Family centered care: the time has come, *Pediatr Nurs* 20(6), 1994.
Andrews M: Cultural perspectives of nursing in the 21st century, *J Prof Nurse* 8(1):7-15, 1992.
Barry P: Psychosocial nursing assessment and intervention, Philadelphia, 1989, JB Lippincott.
Boettcher M, Schiller W: The use of a multidisciplinary group meeting for families of critically ill trauma patients, *Intens Care Nurs* 6(3):129, 1990.
Bulechek G, McCloskey J: *Advanced nursing interventions*, Philadelphia, 1992, WB Saunders.
Camphinha-Bacote J, Narayan M: Culturally competent health care at home, *Home Care Prov* 5(6):213-219, 2000.
Daly K et al: The effect of two nursing interventions on families of ICU patients, *Clin Nurs Res* 3(4):414, 1994.
D'Avanzo CE et al: Developing culturally informed strategies for substance-related interventions. In Naegle MA, D'Avanzo CE, editors: *Addictions and substance abuse: strategies for advanced practice nursing*, St Louis, 2001, Mosby, pp 59-104.
Ducharmes F, Rowat K: Conjugal support, family coping behaviors and the well-being of elderly couples, *Can J Nurs Res* 24:5, 1992.
Giger JN, Davidhizar RE: *Transcultural nursing*, ed 2, St Louis, 1995, Mosby.
Gillis C et al: *Toward a science of family nursing*, Menlo Park, Calif, 1989, Addison-Wesley.

• **= Independent;** ▲ **= Collaborative**

Leininger MM: *Transcultural nursing: theories, research and practices,* ed 2, Hilliard, Ohio, 1996, McGraw-Hill.

Mears D: Enhancing family coping skills, *Nurs Homes* 39:32, 1990.

Meleis A: *Theoretical nursing,* Philadelphia, 1991, JB Lippincott.

Rivera-Andino J, Lopez L: When culture complicates care, *RN* 63(7):47-49, 2000.

Seiderman RY et al: Assessing American Indian families, *Am J Maternal/Child Nurs* 21(6):274-279, 1996.

Szabo V, Strang V: Experiencing control in caregiving, *Image J Nurs Sch* 31(1):71, 1999.

Stuart GW, Laraia MT: Therapeutic nurse-patient relationship. In Stuart GW, Laraia MT, editors: *Principles and practice of psychiatric nursing,* St Louis, 2001, Mosby, p 30.

Thomas D et al: Parish nursing assessment—what should you know? *Home Health Nurs Manage* 4(5):11-13, 2000.

Disabled family Coping

Beverly Pickett, Gail B. Ladwig, and Mary Markle

 Definition Behavior of a significant person (family member or other primary person) that disables his or her capacity and client's capacity to effectively address tasks essential to either persons' adaptation to the health challenge

Defining Characteristics

Intolerance; agitation; depression; aggression; hostility; taking on illness signs of client; rejection; psychosomaticism; neglectful relationships with other family members; neglectful care of the client with regard to basic human needs and/or illness treatment; distortion of reality regarding client's health problem, including extreme denial about its existence or severity; impaired restructuring of a meaningful life for self; impaired individualization; prolonged over-concern for client; desertion; decisions and actions that are detrimental to economic or social well-being; carrying on usual routines, disregarding client's needs; abandonment; client's development of helpless, inactive dependence; disregarding needs

Related Factors (r/t)

Significant person with chronically unexpressed feelings of guilt, anxiety, hostility, despair, etc.; arbitrary handling of family's resistance to treatment, which tends to solidify defensiveness by dealing inadequately with underlying anxiety; dissonant or discrepant coping styles for dealing with adaptive tasks by the significant person and client or among significant people; highly ambivalent family relationships

NOC   **Outcomes (Nursing Outcomes Classification)**

Suggested NOC Labels

Family Coping; Caregiver Well-Being; Family Normalization; Neglect Recovery

Example NOC Outcome

Demonstrates **Family Coping** as evidenced by the following indicators: Manages problems/Involves family members in decision making (Rate each indicator of **Family Coping:** 1 = never demonstrated, 2 = rarely demonstrated, 3 = sometimes demonstrated, 4 = often demonstrated, 5 = consistently demonstrated [see Section I])

• = Independent; ▲ = Collaborative

Client Outcomes

- Expresses realistic understanding and expectations of the client (family or significant person)
- Participates positively in client's care within the limits of his or her abilities (family)
- Identifies responses that are harmful (family or significant person)
- Acknowledges and accepts the need for assistance with circumstances (significant person)
- Expresses feelings openly, honestly, and appropriately (significant person)

NIC Interventions (Nursing Interventions Classification)

Suggested NIC Labels

Family Involvement; Family Mobilization; Family Support

> **Example NIC Interventions—Family Support**
> - Facilitate communication of concerns/feelings between client and family or between family members
> - Provide assistance in meeting basic needs for family such as shelter, food, and clothing

Nursing Interventions and Rationales

- Observe for causative and contributing factors.
  Ongoing assessments provide clues about underlying feelings (Barry, 1989).
- Review the client's background.
  The client's background is largely responsible for reactions (Lipkin, Cohen, 1992).
- Identify patterns of family behaviors and interactions before the illness occurred.
  Most family members have certain roles that are disrupted by illnesses and hospitalizations; this disruption results in shifts in family functioning.
- Consider use of family theory as a framework to help guide interventions (e.g., family stress theory, social exchange theory).
  Theory helps to identify the focus, means, and goals of nursing practice. It enhances communication and increases autonomy and accountability to care (Gillis et al, 1989; Meleis, 1991).
- Identify current behaviors of family members, such as withdrawal (e.g., not visiting, briefly visiting, ignoring client when visiting), anger and hostility toward client and others, or expression of guilt.
  Many of these behaviors are defense mechanisms used by the ego to protect itself until it can fully accept the implications of the illness.
- Note other stressors in family (e.g., financial, job-related).
  This information allows the nurse to develop an appropriate plan of care.
- Encourage family members to verbalize feelings by discussing ways to solve problems associated with client's condition.
  Many families find it difficult to maintain open and empathic communication during times of acute stress. Interventions that help mobilize family strengths, such as problem-solving communication, may effectively promote the adaptation of families of critically injured patients (Leske, Jiricka, 1998).
- Serve as a role model for interpersonal skills that will help the family members improve their verbal interactions.
  Interpersonal skills such as active listening, warmth, employing friendliness, empathy, consideration, and competence are essential for promoting a therapeutic relationship.

• = Independent; ▲ = Collaborative

- Provide consistent structure for family interactions (e.g., length of visits, number of visitors, content of interactions).
  Consistency and structure provide stability during times of stress and crisis.
- Help family identify its personal strengths.
  Individual coping skills assist in adjusting to life crises.
- ▲ Encourage family members to participate in appropriate support programs (e.g., chronic obstructive pulmonary disease [COPD], arthritis I Can Cope, Alzheimer's support groups).
  Support group participation develops coping skills, enhances communication skills, and facilitates exchange of useful information (Northouse, Peters-Golden, 1993).
- ▲ Provide continuity of care by maintaining effective communication between staff members. Initiate regular multidisciplinary client-care conferences that involve the client and family in problem solving.
  Continuity of care enhances health status. Involvement of client and family in case conferences is proactive and empowering.
- ▲ Serve as case manager to explore and use all available resources appropriate for situation (e.g., community mental health services, reimbursement options).
  Resources will provide the family with information and assistance if necessary and appropriate.
- Observe for any symptoms of elder or child abuse or neglect.
  Abuse can take several forms, such as physical assaults that may or may not result in injury, verbal attacks, isolation, and social and emotional neglect.
- ▲ Prompt reporting of abuse according to local and state law is necessary.
  In most states, reporting abuse is mandated by law.

Geriatric

- ▲ Refer family to appropriate senior community resources (e.g., senior centers, Medicare assistance, meal programs, parish nursing, charitable organizations).
  Many federal, state, and local community-based resources for seniors are underused.
- ▲ If actual or potential abuse or neglect is an issue, report it to the appropriate agency.
  The purpose of protective services is to preserve the family.
- ▲ Encourage family member to participate in appropriate support groups (e.g., COPD, Arthritis I Can Cope, Alzheimer's support groups).
  Support groups provide people with a setting in which they can discuss their illness-related problems with other people who have the same illness.
- Work with family to manage common challenges related to normal aging.
  Having knowledge of normative developmental challenges of aging can reduce the stress such challenges place on families.

Multicultural

- Work to provide caregivers who understand the importance of cultural beliefs and values the family may hold.
  Cultures can differ with regard to health beliefs, practices, and values (Andrews, 1992; Camphinha-Bacote, Narayan, 2000).
- Acknowledge racial/ethnic differences at the onset of care.
  Acknowledgement of race/ethnicity issues will enhance communication, establish rapport, and promote treatment outcomes (D'Avanzo et al, 2001).
- Approach families of color with respect, warmth, and professional courtesy.
  Instances of disrespect and lack of caring have special significance for families of color (D'Avanzo et al, 2001).

• = Independent; ▲ = Collaborative

- Assess for the influence of cultural beliefs, norms, and values on the family's perceptions of coping.
  What the family considers normal and abnormal coping behavior may be based on cultural perceptions (Leininger, 1996).
- Give rationale when assessing families with regard to sensitive issues.
  Blacks and other people of color may expect white caregivers to hold negative and preconceived ideas about blacks. Giving a rationale for questions asked will help alleviate this perception (D'Avanzo et al, 2001).
- Use a family-centered approach when working with Latino, Asian, African-American, and Native American clients.
  Latinos may perceive family as a source of support, solver of problems, and source of pride. Asian Americans may regard the family as the primary decision-maker and influence on individual family members (D'Avanzo et al, 2001). Native American families may be extended structures that exert powerful influences over functioning (Seiderman et al, 1996).
- Facilitate modeling and role-playing for family regarding healthy ways to communicate and interact.
  It is helpful for family members and the client to practice communication skills in a safe environment before trying them in a real-life situation (Rivera-Andino, Lopez, 2000).
- Validate the feelings of family members or significant caregivers regarding the impact of client illness on family lifestyle.
  Validation lets the client know that the nurse has heard and understands what was said, and it promotes the nurse-client relationship (Stuart, Laraia, 2001; Giger, Davidhizar, 1995).

Home Care Interventions

NOTE: This diagnosis presents the complex and difficult problem of securing an appropriate response by the family to a client's illness and caregiving needs. The same problem in the home setting creates an unusually high risk for abuse of the client. The nurse is cautioned that the margin of time for planning and effectively supporting the family unit to avoid abuse may be minimal or even negligible.

- If the client has been in an institution, establish empathetic contact with the client and family before discharge.
  Contact with the family in a nonthreatening manner helps establish a trusting relationship, easing the transition to home.
- During time of compromised coping, increase visits to assess safety of client and family, provide assistance with coping strategies, identify dysfunctional coping mechanisms, and intervene as necessary.
  Increased opportunity for interaction and appropriate intervention will enhance safety and health status of client and family. Frequent assessment of the client's health status promotes early detection and treatment of problems. Changes in the client's health status (especially any deterioration in status) can precipitate more problems with the family or caregiver and place the client at greater risk.
- ▲ Identify any changes in skills needed for client care and support caregiving efforts. Assess the needs of the caregiver in the home. Intervene to meet needs as appropriate to total case management and explore all available resources that may be used to provide adequate home care (e.g., add home health aide services, coordinate services

• = **Independent;** ▲ = **Collaborative**

with mental health agencies, encourage caregivers not to neglect their own physical, mental, and spiritual health, and give more specific information about client needs and ways to meet them).

Support from the nurse by teaching and positive feedback helps caregivers to have a realistic perception of client expectations and shows them they are valued for efforts made; meeting the needs of caregivers supports their ability to meet the needs of the client; home health aides may be used as role models for caregiving and can observe the status of the client and family. Caution the home health aide to document objectively.

▲ Serve as an advocate, mentor, and role model for appropriate behavior. Write down or contract for the care needed by the client.

Therapeutic use of self by the nurse and concrete task definition and assignment reinforce positive coping strategies.

▲ When a terminal illness is the precipitating factor for ineffective coping, offer hospice services and support groups as possible resources.

Nonjudgmental support from helpers with no agenda allows verbalization of feelings. The hospice paradigm addresses the physical, emotional, and spiritual needs of the dying and their loved ones.

• Support positive individual and family coping efforts.

Positive feedback reinforces desired behaviors and supports the family unit.

Client/Family Teaching

• Encourage family members to ask for a break in caregiving and to spend time away from client.

Caregivers who were able to maintain control recognized when they were losing control and needed a break from caregiving (Szabo, Strang, 1999).

• Provide truthful information regarding illness of client to family; use anticipatory guidance to prepare for expected outcomes.

Information is an important need of families of critically ill patients. Meeting this need requires a multidisciplinary approach and an environment that values the delivery of humanistic care (Henneman, Cardin, 1992). Families need a framework that can serve as a measure against which they can monitor progress (Northouse, Peters-Golden, 1993).

• Involve client and family in planning of care as often as possible; mutual goal setting is often an effective strategy.

Family members of any trauma client admitted to the level I trauma center are invited by the trauma staff to attend weekly multidisciplinary meetings. In this way family concerns can become a positive care factor, and the tasks of nurses, doctors, and social workers are made easier (Boettcher, Schiller, 1990).

• Discuss with family appropriate ways to demonstrate feelings.

Learning basic components of therapeutic communication helps family members to express feelings appropriately.

• Help family identify the health care needs of the client and family; teach skills needed to address health care needs.

Once needs are identified, skill mastery by family will optimize health status. Skill mastery is an empowering and positive coping mechanism.

• Promote individual and family relaxation and stress reduction strategies.

The immune system weakens in response to stress; relaxation elicits the opposite, healthful response (Bulechek, McCloskey, 1992).

• = **Independent;** ▲ = **Collaborative**

REFERENCES   Andrews M: Cultural perspectives of nursing in the 21st century, *J Prof Nurs* 8(1):7-15, 1992.

Barry P: Psychosocial nursing assessment and intervention, Philadelphia, 1989, JB Lippincott.

Boettcher M, Schiller W: The use of a multidisciplinary group meeting for families of critically ill trauma patients, *Intens Care Nurs* 6(3):129, 1990.

Bulechek G, McCloskey J: *Advanced nursing interventions,* Philadelphia, 1992, WB Saunders.

Camphinha-Bacote J, Narayan M: Culturally competent health care at home, *Home Care Prov* 5(6):213-219, 2000.

D'Avanzo CE et al: Developing culturally informed strategies for substance-related interventions. In Naegle MA, D'Avanzo CE, editors: *Addictions and substance abuse: strategies for advanced practice nursing,* St Louis, 2001, Mosby, pp 59-104.

Giger JN, Davidhizar RE: *Transcultural Nursing,* ed 2, St Louis, 1995, Mosby.

Gillis C et al: *Toward a science of family nursing,* Menlo Park, Calif, 1989, Addison-Wesley.

Henneman EA, Cardin S: Need for information: interventions for practice, *Crit Care Nurs Clin North Am* 4(4):615, 1992.

Leininger MM: *Transcultural nursing: theories, research and practices,* ed 2, Hilliard, Ohio, 1996, McGraw-Hill.

Leske J, Jiricka M: Impact of family demands and family strengths and capabilities on family well-being and adaptation after critical injury, *Am J Crit Care* 7(5):383, 1998.

Lipkin G, Cohen R: *Effective approaches to patient's behavior,* New York, 1992, Springer.

Meleis A: *Theoretical nursing,* Philadelphia, 1991, JB Lippincott.

Northouse L, Peters-Golden H: Cancer and the family: strategies to assist spouses, *Semin Oncol Nurs* 9:74, 1993.

Rivera-Andino J, Lopez L: When culture complicates care, *RN* 63(7):47-49, 2000.

Seiderman RY et al: Assessing American Indian families, *MJN Am J Matern Child Nurs* 21(6):274-279, 1996.

Stuart GW, Laraia MT: Therapeutic nurse-patient relationship. In Stuart GW, Laraia MT, editors: *Principles and practice of psychiatric nursing,* St Louis, 2001, Mosby, p 30.

Szabo V, Strang V: Experiencing control in caregiving, *Image J Nurs Sch* 31(1):71, 1999.

Readiness for enhanced family Coping

Beverly Pickett, Gail B. Ladwig, and Mary Markle

NANDA   **Definition** Effective management of adaptive tasks by family member involved with the client's health challenge who now exhibits desire and readiness for enhanced health and growth with regard to self and in relation to client

Defining Characteristics

Expresses interest in making contact on a one-to-one basis or on a mutual-aid group basis with another person who has experienced a similar situation; attempts to describe growth impact of crisis on his or her own values, priorities, goals, or relationships; moves in direction of health promotion and health-enriching lifestyle that supports and monitors maturational processes; audits and negotiates treatment programs and generally chooses experiences that optimize wellness

Related Factors (r/t)

Needs sufficiently gratified and adaptive tasks effectively addressed to enable goals of self-actualization to surface

• = **Independent**; ▲ = **Collaborative**

Outcomes (Nursing Outcomes Classification)

Suggested NOC Labels

Family Coping; Family Normalization; Family Participation in Professional Care

> **Example NOC Outcome**
> Demonstrates **Family Coping** as evidenced by the following indicators: Manages problems/Involves family members in decision making/Uses stress reduction techniques (Rate each indicator of **Family Coping:** 1 = never demonstrated, 2 = rarely demonstrated, 3 = sometimes demonstrated, 4 = often demonstrated, 5 = consistently demonstrated [see Section I])

Client Outcomes

- States a plan for growth (family)
- Performs tasks needed for change (family)
- States positive effects of changes made (family)

NIC **Interventions (Nursing Interventions Classification)**

Suggested NIC Labels

Family Involvement; Family Mobilization; Family Support

> **Example NIC Interventions—Family Support**
> - Facilitate communication of concerns/feelings between client and family or between family members
> - Identify and respect family's coping mechanisms

Nursing Interventions and Rationales

- Observe traits family possesses that will help initiate change, such as having a positive attitude or stating that change is possible.
  The nurse can then identify the strengths on which the family may rely and build upon, and weaknesses from which the family needs protection.
- Consider use of family theory as a framework to help guide interventions (e.g., family stress theory, social exchange theory).
  Theory helps to identify the focus, means, and goals of nursing practice. It enhances communication and increases autonomy and accountability to care (Gillis et al, 1989; Meleis, 1991).
- Allow family members time to verbalize their concerns; provide one-to-one interaction with the family.
  Interactions allow family to gather and impart information, decrease anxiety, and provide input for plan of care.
- Provide truthful information and constructive advice about the client's illness and treatment.
  Having knowledge about the illness helps family members to develop their coping strategies (Van Hammond, Deans, 1995).
- When a family member is having surgery, give the family a 5- to 10-minute progress report about halfway through a surgical procedure.
  Family members in this experimental group reported lower state-anxiety scores (p < 0.001) and had significantly lower MAP levels (p < 0.001) and heart rates (p < 0.01) compared with the control and attention groups. Progress reports appear to be a beneficial independent

• = **Independent;** ▲ = **Collaborative**

nursing intervention for reducing anxiety in family members during the intraoperative waiting period (Leske, 1995).

- Allow family to attend invasive procedures and resuscitation efforts.
  This facilitates effective coping of family members during the crisis of critical illness (Twibell, 1998).
- Have family members share responsibility for change and encourage all to have input.
  It is important to view the entire family as a system as well as individual stakeholders when trying to promote positive change.
- Encourage family members to write down their goals.
  The more involved the family is in goal development, the greater the probability that their goals will be achieved.
- Explore with the family members ways to attain their goals (e.g., adult education classes; enrichment courses; family activities such as sports, cooking, or reading; sharing time together).
- Educate client and family regarding illness and take time to answer questions.
  Empowerment of family members through education increases the family's knowledge and understanding and ability to deal with the illness (Van Hammond, Deans, 1995).
- Encourage leisure time free of obligatory tasks to enjoy each other's company; because everyone is busy, family members might need to set up a schedule for leisure time.
- Help family members communicate with each other using techniques they are comfortable with, such as role-playing, letter writing, or tape recording messages.
  These techniques give the family an opportunity to communicate in an effective yet non-threatening manner.
- ▲ Identify groups that discuss similar problems and concerns (e.g., Al-Anon, Arthritis I Can Cope).
  Such groups allow family members to discuss issues and concerns with others who share the same lived experience.

Geriatric

- Encourage family members to reminisce with the older family member.
- Start and maintain a log of anecdotal stories about the older family member.
- Encourage children in family to spend time with and share activities with the older family member.
  These activities allow for knowledge of and respect for one another; they support the normative developmental tasks of aging.
- ▲ Refer family to parenting classes and classes for coping with older parents.
  Such groups allow family members to discuss the challenges of aging parents with others who share the same lived experience.

Multicultural

- Acknowledge racial/ethnic differences at the onset of care.
  Acknowledgement of race/ethnicity issues will enhance communication, establish rapport, and promote treatment outcomes (D'Avanzo et al, 2001).
- Approach families of color with respect, warmth, and professional courtesy.
  Instances of disrespect and lack of caring have special significance for families of color (D'Avanzo et al, 2001).
- Assess for the influence of cultural beliefs, norms, and values on the family's perceptions of coping.

• = **Independent**; ▲ = **Collaborative**

What the family considers normal and abnormal coping behavior may be based on cultural perceptions (Leininger, 1996).

- Use a family-centered approach when working with Latino, Asian, African-American, and Native American clients.
  Latinos may perceive family as a source of support, solver of problems, and source of pride. Asian Americans may regard the family as the primary decision-maker and influence on individual family members (D'Avanzo et al, 2001). Native American families may be extended structures that exert powerful influences over functioning (Seiderman et al, 1996).
- Facilitate modeling and role-playing for family with regard to healthy ways to communicate and interact.
  It is helpful for family members and the client to practice communication skills in a safe environment before trying them in a real-life situation (Rivera-Andino, Lopez, 2000).
- Validate family members' feelings regarding the impact of client illness on family lifestyle.
  Validation lets the client know that the nurse has heard and understands what was said, and it promotes the nurse-client relationship (Stuart, Laraia, 2001; Giger, Davidhizar, 1995).

Home Care Interventions

The nursing interventions described previously in the care plan for **Compromised family Coping** should be used in the home environment with adaptations as necessary.

Client/Family Teaching

- Teach that it is normal for changes in family relationships to occur. Work with family to manage common challenges related to family dynamics.
  Having knowledge of normative family dynamics promotes growth and self-actualization and supports effective coping.
- Promote individual and family relaxation and stress reduction strategies.
  The immune system weakens in response to stress; relaxation elicits the opposite, healthful response (Bulechek, McCloskey, 1992).

WEB SITES FOR EDUCATION

MERLIN See the MERLIN web site for World Wide Web resources for client education.

REFERENCES Bulechek G, McCloskey J: *Advanced nursing interventions,* Philadelphia, 1992, WB Saunders.
D'Avanzo CE et al: Developing culturally informed strategies for substance-related interventions. In Naegle MA, D'Avanzo CE, editors: *Addictions and substance abuse: strategies for advanced practice nursing,* St Louis, 2001, Mosby, pp 59-104.
Giger JN, Davidhizar RE: *Transcultural nursing,* ed 2, St Louis, 1995, Mosby.
Gillis C et al: *Toward a science of family nursing,* Menlo Park, Calif, 1989, Addison-Wesley.
Leininger MM: *Transcultural nursing: theories, research and practices,* ed 2, Hilliard, Ohio, 1996, McGraw-Hill.
Leske JS: Effects of intraoperative progress reports on anxiety levels of surgical patients' family members, *Appl Nurs Res* 8(4):169, 1995.
Meleis A: *Theoretical nursing,* Philadelphia, 1991, JB Lippincott.
Rivera-Andino J, Lopez L: When culture complicates care, *RN* 63(7):47-49, 2000.
Seiderman RY et al: Assessing American Indian families, *MCN Am J Matern Child Nurs* 21(6):274-279, 1996.
Stuart GW, Laraia MT: Therapeutic nurse-patient relationship. In Stuart GW, Laraia MT, editors: *Principles and practice of psychiatric nursing,* St Louis, 2001, Mosby, p 30.
Twibell RS: Family coping during critical illness, *Dimens Crit Care Nurs* 17(2):100, 1998.
Van Hammond T, Deans C: A phenomenological study of families and psychoeducation support groups, *J Psychosoc Nurs* 33(10):7-12, 1995.

• = **Independent;** ▲ = **Collaborative**

Ineffective Denial

Gail B. Ladwig and Jill M. Barnes

 Definition The conscious or unconscious attempt to reduce anxiety or fear by disavowing the knowledge or meaning of an event, leading to the detriment of health

Defining Characteristics

Delays seeking or refuses health care attention to the detriment of health; does not perceive personal relevance of symptoms or danger; displaces source of symptoms to other organs; displays inappropriate affect; does not admit fear of death or invalidism; makes dismissive gestures or comments when speaking of distressing events; minimizes symptoms; unable to admit impact of disease on life pattern; uses home remedies (self-treatment) to relieve symptoms; displaces fear of impact of condition

Related Factors (r/t)

Fear of consequences; chronic or terminal illness; actual or perceived fear of possible losses (e.g., job, significant other); refusal to acknowledge substance abuse problem; fear of the social stigma associated with disease

NOC Outcomes (Nursing Outcomes Classification)

Suggested NOC Labels

Acceptance: Health Status; Anxiety Control; Health Beliefs: Perceived Threat; Symptom Control Behavior

> **Example NOC Outcome**
>
> Demonstrates **Anxiety Control** as evidenced by the following indicators: Eliminates precursors of anxiety/Reports absence of physical manifestations of anxiety/Controls anxiety response (Rate each indicator of **Anxiety Control:** 1 = never demonstrated, 2 = rarely demonstrated, 3 = sometimes demonstrated, 4 = often demonstrated, 5 = consistently demonstrated [see Section I])

Client Outcomes/Goals

- Seeks out health care attention when needed
- Uses home remedies only when appropriate
- Displays appropriate affect and verbalizes fears
- Acknowledges substance abuse problem and seeks help

NIC Interventions (Nursing Interventions Classification)

Suggested NIC Labels

Anxiety Reduction

> **Example NIC Interventions—Anxiety Reduction**
> - Use a calm reassuring approach
> - Stay with the patient to promote safety and reduce fear

Nursing Interventions and Rationales

- Assess client's understanding of symptoms and illness.
  The use of denial can cause practical problems and hinder realistic planning for the future if the patient chooses to deny his or her illness and/or its potential outcomes (Morley, 1997).

• = **Independent;** ▲ = **Collaborative**

- Spend time with client, allow time for responses.
  Nursing presence, one-to-one interaction, connecting with the client's experience, going beyond the scientific data, and knowing what will work and when to act all support the nurse-client relationship and affirm their respective selves. As a result, the client grows in awareness of his own being (Doona, Chase, Haggerty, 1999).
- Assess whether the use of denial is helping or hindering the patient's care.
  Denial can allow coping in the face of stress; however, total denial can be life-threatening (Robinson, 1999).
- Allow client to express and use denial as a coping mechanism.
  This may be the only psychologically safe way of coping with the unimaginable (Davidhizar, Newman-Giger, 1998). Denial can allow a person to cope with reality while relieving stress; however, total denial can be destructive (Morley, 1997). At certain stages of an illness, denial may be appropriate. Denial is common and sometimes necessary immediately following the diagnosis of cancer; denial controls the overwhelming information until other coping mechanisms can be mobilized (Weisman, 1992).
- Assess for subtle signs of denial (e.g., urealistic display of optimism, downplaying of symptoms, inability to admit one's own fear).
  Not all signs of denial are obvious (Robinson, 1999).
- Avoid confrontation.
  Challenging a patient's denial may cause an increase in anxiety (Robinson, 1999). Challenging denial when the patient finds it intolerable to consider reality can cause overwhelming distress (Morley, 1997).
- Develop a trusting, therapeutic relationship with the client/family.
  A genuine connection can ease defensiveness or uneasiness (Robinson, 1999).
- Ask appropriate questions to assess whether denial is being used in association with alcoholism. A short, sensitive tool is the CAGE questionnaire. (The most widely used tool is the Michigan Alcoholism Screening Test [MAST]. Although it is a very reliable and valid tool, it is not practical for use by a bedside nurse for purposes of assessment.)
- An affirmative answer to two or more of the following questions is considered a basis for suspicion of alcohol abuse:

C	Have you ever felt you ought to cut down on drinking?
A	Have people annoyed you by criticizing your drinking?
G	Have you ever felt bad or guilty about your drinking?
E	Have you ever had a drink first thing in the morning to steady your nerves or get rid of a hangover (eye opener)?

  There are several screening instruments that have been extensively used and found to be superior to the use of biomechanical markers or laboratory tests for the early detection of alcohol or other drug abuse. The CAGE questionnaire is a quick and easy tool for bedside nurses (Burns, 1993). Because alcoholics often employ denial, they are unlikely to produce an accurate response when asked directly how much they drink. Nurses must ask questions differently to obtain more accurate data. The CAGE questionnaire is a practical tool for the bedside nurse (Kovach, Weiss, 1991).
- Sit at eye level.
  Eye-level communication promotes emotional comfort (Ringsven, Bond, 1991).
- Use touch if appropriate and with permission. Touch client's hand or arm.
  Touch conveys empathy. Human beings are often hungry for touch (Karnes, Gyulay, 1993).

• = Independent; ▲ = Collaborative

- Explain signs and symptoms of illness; as necessary, reinforce use of prescribed treatment plan.

  Because of the fluctuation of denial in relation to the current threats, information may need to be repeated over time (Morley, 1997).

- Have the client make choices regarding treatment and actively involve him or her in the decision-making process.

  Making their own decisions empowers clients, regardless of the severity of the crisis they are dealing with (Burgess, 1994). An emphasis on helping the individual attain a sense of control may facilitate change, ensuring the use of constructive rather than obstructive denial (Russell, 1993).

- Help the client recognize existing and additional sources of support; allow time for adjustment.

  The resilience and strengths of the family are what should be noted first (Burgess, 1994).

▲ If appropriate, refer family to a skilled mental health counselor for help in planning an intervention to observe whether denial has been or is being used as a coping mechanism in other areas of life.

  Clients who are ill use denial in a number of ways and situations, and in varying degrees (Davidhizar, Newman-Giger, 1998). Denial can be an adaptive response that helps the client cope (Robinson, 1993).

Geriatric

- Identify recent losses of client, because grieving may prolong denial. Encourage client to take one day at a time.

  Unresolved grief may be compounded when a grieving individual encounters a crisis (Davidhizar, Newman-Giger, 1998). An elderly client may have experienced multiple losses and need supportive care and extra time to adapt (Ringsven, Bond, 1991).

- Encourage client to verbalize feelings.

  Verbalization allows the client to release emotions and develop a sense of control.

- Encourage communication among family members.

  Once communication has begun, it helps with accepting the unacceptable (Davidhizar, Newman-Giger, 1998).

- Recognize denial.

  Some nurses may be able to recognize denial during an interview or assessment (Davidhizar, Newman-Giger, 1998).

- Use reality-focusing techniques.

  When patient talks about unrealistic goals or hopes, do not reply or foster them (Robinson, 1993).

Multicultural

- Assess for the influence of cultural beliefs, norms, and values on the client's understanding of and ability to acknowledge health status.

  Willingness to acknowledge health status may be based on cultural perceptions (Leininger, 1996).

- Discuss with the client those aspects of his or her health behavior/lifestyle that will remain unchanged by health status.

  Aspects of the client's life that are meaningful and valuable to him or her should be understood and preserved without change (Leininger, 1996).

• = Independent; ▲ = Collaborative

- Negotiate with the client regarding the aspects of health behavior that will need to be modified as a result of health status.
  Give and take with the client will lead to culturally congruent care (Leininger, 1996).
- Assess the role of fatalism on the client's ability to acknowledge health status.
  Fatalistic perspectives, which involve the belief that you cannot control your own fate, may influence health behaviors in some African-American and Latino populations (Phillips, Cohen, Moses, 1999; Harmon, Castro, Coe, 1996).
- Validate the client's feelings of anxiety and fear related to health status.
  Validation lets the client know that the nurse has heard and understands what was said, and it promotes the nurse-client relationship (Stuart, Laraia, 2001; Giger, Davidhizar, 1995).

Home Care Interventions

- Observe family interaction and roles. Assess whether denial is being used to meet the needs of another family member.
  The home setting can provide a wealth of information to health care providers (Burgess, 1994). In dysfunctional families, inappropriate or ineffective coping methods may be employed to meet the social needs of the dysfunctional unit.
- ▲ Refer client and family to medical social services for evaluation and treatment as indicated per physician order.
  It may be necessary to involve the entire family to effectively treat the client.
- ▲ Refer client/family for follow-up if prolonged denial is a risk.
  Prolonged denial almost always interferes with successful treatment. Only when denial subsides does the patient regain control (Robinson, 1999).
- ▲ Identify an emergency plan, including how to contact hotlines and receive emergency services.
  Denial may be abandoned when the need for emergency care is perceived by the client or the family.
- Encourage communication between family members, particularly when dealing with the loss of a significant person.
  Once they start talking about the deceased, what they remember about him or her, and how they feel about death, they begin to accept the unacceptable (Davidhizar, Newman-Giger, 1998).

Client/Family Teaching

- ▲ Teach signs and symptoms of illness and appropriate responses (e.g., taking medication, going to the emergency room, calling the physician).
  Discharge information may seem threatening to a client in denial; however, it is important that the patient receive the information. Linking therapy to an increase in control may assist in getting the information across (Cook, 1994). Lack of knowledge about the condition or illness may result in unrealistic goals and hopes. Education is necessary (Robinson, 1993).
- Teach family members that denial may continue throughout the adjustment to home and not to be confrontational.
  Denial is normal especially during phases of adjustment and reprimanding can lead to increased frustration and further denial (Robinson, 1999).
- ▲ If problem is substance abuse, refer to an appropriate community agency (e.g., Alcoholics Anonymous).
  Groups of peer role models confront denial and reinforce that alcohol is a problem (Wing, 1995).

- = **Independent;** ▲ = **Collaborative**

- Teach families of clients with brain injuries that denial has been associated with damage to the right hemisphere. The client may exhibit inappropriate affect and anxiety.

  Denial may have an underlying physical cause and may be a necessary coping mechanism to maintain emotional stability and motivation (Armstrong, 1991).

WEB SITES FOR EDUCATION

 See the MERLIN web site for World Wide Web resources for client education.

REFERENCES Armstrong C: Emotional changes following brain injury: psychological and neurological components of depression, denial and anxiety, *J Rehab* 57:15, 1991.

Burgess D: Denial and terminal illness, *Am J Hospice Palliative Care* 11(2):46-48, 1994.

Burns CM: Assessment and screening for substance abuse: guidelines for the primary care nurse practitioner, *Nurse Pract Forum* 4(4):199-206, 1993.

Cook EA: Understanding your patient's denial, *Nursing* 24(4):66-67, 1994.

Davidhizar R, Newman-Giger J: Patients' use of denial: coping with the unacceptable, *Nurs Standard* 12(43):44-46, 1998.

Doona M, Chase S, Haggerty L: Nursing presence, *J Holistic Nurs* 17(1):54-69, 1999.

Giger JN, Davidhizar RE: *Transcultural nursing*, ed 2, St Louis, 1995, Mosby.

Harmon MP, Castro FG, Coe K: Acculturation and cervical cancer: knowledge, beliefs, and behaviors of Hispanic women, *Women and Health* 24(3):37-57, 1996.

Karnes B, Gyulay J: Healing the dying person—theoretical and practical approaches to emotional, mental, and spiritual dimensions, *Am J Hosp Care* 1(4):28. In Meek S: Effects of slow stroke back massage on relaxation in hospice clients, *Image J Nurs Sch* 25:7, 1993.

Kovach G, Weiss K: Denying alcoholism, *Focus Crit Care AACN* 18:469, 1991.

Leininger MM: *Transcultural nursing: theories, research and practices*, ed 2, Hilliard, Ohio, 1996, McGraw-Hill.

Morley C: The use of denial by patients with cancer, *Prof Nurse* 12(5):380-381, 1997.

Phillips JM, Cohen MZ, Moses G: Breast cancer screening and African-American women: fear, fatalism, and silence, *Oncol Nurs Forum* 26(3):561-571, 1999.

Ringsven M, Bond D: *Gerontology and leadership skills for nurses*, Albany, NY, 1991, Delmar.

Robinson AW: Getting to the heart of denial, *Am J Nurs* 99(5):38-42, 1999.

Robinson K: Denial: an adaptive response, *Dimens Crit Care Nurs* 12:102, 1993.

Russell GC: The role of denial in clinical practice, *J Adv Nurs* 18:938, 1993.

Stuart GW, Laraia MT: Therapeutic nurse-patient relationship. In Stuart GW, Laraia MT, editors: *Principles and practice of psychiatric nursing*, St Louis, 2001, Mosby, p 30.

Weisman A: Coping with cancer, *Image J Nurs Sch* 24:19, 1992.

Wing D: Transcending alcoholic denial, *Image J Nurs Sch* 27:121, 1995.

Impaired Dentition

Gail B. Ladwig and Betty J. Ackley

NANDA **Definition** Disruption in tooth development/eruption patterns or structural integrity of individual teeth

Defining Characteristics

Excessive plaque; crown or root caries; halitosis; tooth enamel discoloration; toothache; loose teeth; excessive calculus; incomplete eruption for age (may be primary or perma-

• = **Independent;** ▲ = **Collaborative**

nent teeth); malocclusion or tooth misalignment; premature loss of primary teeth; worn down or abraded teeth; tooth fracture(s); missing teeth or complete absence; erosion of enamel; asymmetrical facial expression

Related Factors (r/t)

Ineffective oral hygiene; sensitivity to heat or cold; barriers to self-care; nutritional deficits; dietary habits; genetic predisposition; selected prescription medications; premature loss of primary teeth; excessive intake of fluorides; chronic vomiting; chronic use of tobacco, coffee, tea, red wine; lack of knowledge regarding dental health; excessive use of abrasive cleaning agents; bruxism

NOC Outcomes (Nursing Outcomes Classification)

Suggested NOC Labels

Oral Health; Self-Care: Oral Health

> **Example NOC Outcome**
>
> Accomplishes **Oral Health** as evidenced by the following indicators: Cleanliness of teeth/Cleanliness of gums/Cleanliness of dentures/Tooth integrity/Gum integrity (Rate each indicator of **Oral Health:** 1 = extremely compromised, 2 = substantially compromised, 3 = moderately compromised, 4 = mildly compromised, 5 = not compromised [see Section I])

Client Outcomes

- Teeth clean, gums healthy pink color, mouth has pleasant odor
- Able to masticate foods without difficulty
- Free of pain originating from teeth
- Demonstrates measures can take to improve dental hygiene

NIC Interventions (Nursing Interventions Classification)

Suggested NIC Labels

Oral Health Maintenance; Oral Health Promotion: Oral Health Restoration

> **Example NIC Interventions—Oral Health Maintenance**
> - Establish a mouth care routine
> - Arrange for dental check-ups as needed

Nursing Interventions and Rationales

▲ Inspect oral cavity/teeth at least once daily and note any discoloration, presence of debris, amount of plaque buildup, presence of lesions, edema, or bleeding, intactness of teeth. Refer to a dentist or periodontist as appropriate.
  Systematic inspection can identify impending problems (Bhaskar, Lilly, Pratt, 1990).

- Monitor client's nutritional and fluid status to determine if adequate.
  Malnutrition predisposes clients to dental disease.

- Assess client for underlying medical condition that may be causing halitosis.
  Halitosis may indicate a serious underlying medical condition necessitating medical referral (Ayers, Colquhoun, 1998).

- Determine client's mental status and manual dexterity; if client is unable to care for self, dental hygiene must be provided by nursing personnel. The nursing diagnosis **Bathing/hygiene Self-care deficit** is then also applicable.

• = **Independent;** ▲ = **Collaborative**

- Determine client's usual method of oral care.
  Whenever possible, build on client's existing knowledge base and current practices to develop an individualized plan of care.
- If client is unable to brush own teeth, follow this procedure:
  1. Use a soft bristle baby toothbrush
  2. Use tapwater or saline as a solution
  3. Brush teeth in an up and down manner
  4. Suction as needed
  Avoid using foam sticks to clean teeth; use only to swab out the oral cavity.
  Use of this nursing protocol results in improved oral hygiene in a vulnerable population (Stiefel et al, 2000). Foam sticks are not effective for removing plaque (Roberts, 2000).
- If client is free of bleeding disorders and is able to swallow, encourage client to brush teeth with a soft toothbrush using a fluoride-containing toothpaste after every meal and to floss teeth daily.
  The toothbrush is the most important tool for oral care; toothbrushing is the most effective method of reducing plaque and controlling periodontal disease (Armstrong, 1994).
- Direct the toothbrush vertically toward the tooth surfaces.
  One study demonstrated that brushing with the toothbrush bristles perpendicular to the surface of the teeth has a high efficacy of plaque removal and maintains good gingival condition (Sasahara, Kawamura, 2000).
- The tongue must also be cleaned when performing oral hygiene maintenance. Brush tongue with soft toothbrush and follow with a mouth rinse. Use tap water or saline only for a mouth rinse. Avoid the use of hydrogen peroxide, lemon glycerin swabs, or alcohol-based mouthwashes.
  Tongue cleaning and optional use of an efficacious mouth rinse will lead to breath improvement (Rosenberg, 1996). Hydrogen peroxide can damage oral mucosa and is extremely foul tasting (Tombes, Gallucci, 1993; Winslow, 1994). Lemon and glycerine swabs are drying to the oral mucous membranes (Roberts, 2000).
- If platelet numbers are decreased, or if client is edentulous, use moistened toothettes for oral care.
  A toothbrush can cause soft tissue injury and bleeding in clients with low numbers of platelets (Armstrong, 1994).
- Provide scrupulous dental care to critically ill clients.
  Cultures of the teeth of critically ill clients have yielded significant bacterial colonization, which can cause nosocomial pneumonia (Scannapieco, Stewart, Mylotte, 1992).
- If teeth are nonfunctional for chewing, modification of oral intake (e.g., edentulous diet, soft diet) may be necessary. The nursing diagnosis **Imbalanced Nutrition: less than body requirements** may apply.
- If client is unable to swallow, keep suction nearby when providing oral care.
- See care plan for **Impaired Oral mucous membrane.**

Geriatric

- Consider recommending use of an ultrasonic toothbrush if any impairment of manual dexterity exists.
  Use of an ultrasonic toothbrush was shown to reduce plaque and bleeding in a study of 12 patients >65 years of age (Whitmyer et al, 1998).
- Carefully observe oral cavity and lips for abnormal lesions when providing dental care.

• = Independent; ▲ = Collaborative

Malignant lesions in the mouth are common in the elderly, especially if there is a history of smoking or alcohol use. The elderly are least likely to see a dentist, and often lesions are painless until they invade other structures (Aubertin, 1997).

• Ensure that dentures are removed and cleaned regularly, preferably after every meal and before bedtime.
Dentures left in the mouth at night impede circulation to the palate and predispose the client to oral lesions.

• Recognize that halitosis in older adults is a common condition that may have oral or non-oral sources.
Bad breath may reflect serious local or systemic conditions, including gingivitis, periodontal disease, diabetic acidosis, hepatic failure, or respiratory infection. Non-oral sources require treatment of the underlying cause, whereas suspected oral sources require referral for a dental evaluation (Durham, Malloy, Hodges, 1993).

Infants/children

• Expectant mothers should eat a healthy, balanced diet that is rich in calcium.
A set of teeth is in place when the baby is born. The teeth usually start to form in the gums during the second trimester of pregnancy. To encourage the development of good, strong teeth, expectant mothers should eat a healthy, balanced diet that is rich in calcium (Koop, 2001).

Infant oral hygiene

• Gently wipe baby's gums with a washcloth or sterile gauze at least once a day.
Wiping gums prevents bacterial buildup in the mouth (Koop, 2001). Infants of breastfeeding mothers need early and consistent mouth care when the teeth erupt. This study was not able to determine a definite time when breast fed infants should be weaned after eruption of teeth to prevent caries; therefore early and consistent mouth care is imperative (Valaitis et al, 2000).

• Never allow child to fall asleep with a bottle containing milk, formula, fruit juice, or sweetened liquids. If child needs a comforter between regular feedings, at night, or during naps, fill a bottle with cool water or give the child a clean pacifier recommended by your dentist or physician. Never give child a pacifier dipped in any sweet liquid. Avoid filling child's bottle with liquids such as sugar water and soft drinks.
Decay in infants and children is referred to as baby bottle tooth decay. It can destroy the teeth and most often occurs in the upper front teeth, but other teeth may also be affected. Decay occurs when sweetened liquids are given and are left clinging to an infant's teeth for long periods. Many sweet liquids cause problems, including milk, formula, and fruit juice. Bacteria in the mouth use these sugars as food. They then produce acids that attack the teeth. Each time your child drinks these liquids, acids attack for 20 minutes or longer. After many attacks, the teeth can decay. It's not just what is put in the child's bottle that causes decay, but how often—and for how long (American Dental Association, 2001).

• When multiple teeth appear, brush with small toothbrush with small (pea-sized) amount of flouride toothpaste.

Older children

▲ Talk with your dentist about dental sealants. They can help prevent cavities in permanent teeth.
Sealants should be available to all children regardless of socioeconomic status. In this study, children of low socioeconomic status in this study had a higher rate of caries in primary and permanent teeth than children of higher socioeconomic status (Gillcrist, Brumley, Blackford, 2001).

• = Independent; ▲ = Collaborative

- Use dental floss to help prevent gum disease. Talk with your dentist about when to start. Do not permit your child to smoke or chew tobacco. Set a good example—don't use tobacco products yourself. If a permanent tooth is knocked out, rinse it gently and put it back into the socket or in a glass of cold milk or water. See a dentist immediately (Consumer Information, 2001).
- Drink fluoridated water when possible.
  Drinking water fluoridation is associated with an increase in the percentage of 5-year-old children with no experience of tooth decay (Gray, Davies-Slowik, 2001).

Multicultural

- Assess for the influence of cultural beliefs, norms, and values on the client's understanding of dental care.
  What the client considers normal and abnormal dental care may be based on cultural perceptions (Leininger, 1996).
- Assess for access to dental care insurance.
  Poverty and lack of dental care insurance may prevent the obtainment of dental care (Woolfolk et al, 1999).
- Assess for dental anxiety.
  Anxiety is a major reason for infrequent dental check-ups (Woolfolk et al, 1999).
- Validate the client's feelings with regard to dental health and access to dental care.
  Validation lets the client know that the nurse has heard and understands what was said, and it promotes the nurse-client relationship (Stuart, Laraia, 2001; Giger, Davidhizar, 1995).

Home Care Interventions

- Assess client patterns for daily and professional dental care and related patterns (e.g., smoking, nail biting). Assess for environmental influences on dental status (e.g., fluoride).
  Many dental problems are preventable with good dental hygiene and care. Behaviors to preserve oral health in old age are essential (Barmes, 2000).
- Assess client facilities and financial resources for providing dental care.
  Lack of appropriate facilities or financial resources is a barrier to positive dental care patterns. Provision for dental care may be missing from health care plans or unavailable to the uninsured.
- Request dietary log from client, adding column for type of food (i.e., soft, pureed, regular).
- Observe typical meal to assess first-hand the impact of impaired dentition on nutrition.
  Clients, especially the elderly, are often hesitant to admit nutritional changes that may be embarrassing.
- Identify mechanical needs for food preparation and ease of ingestion/digestion to meet client dental/nutritional needs.
  Assist client with accessing financial or other resources to support optimum dental and nutritional status.

Client/Family Teaching

- Teach how to inspect the oral cavity and monitor for problems with the teeth and gums.
- Teach how to implement a personal plan of dental hygiene, including a schedule of care.

- **= Independent; ▲ = Collaborative**

Encouragement and reinforcement of dental care are important to oral outcomes (Armstrong, 1994).

- Teach clients of all ages the need to decrease intake of sugary foods and brush teeth regularly.

  One study demonstrated that intake of foods such as caramel toffees and sugar lumps increased the number of organisms on the teeth significantly. Just one day of withdrawl of normal oral hygiene resulted in an approximately ten-fold increase in the number of microorganisms on the teeth (Beighton et al, 1999).

- Inform individuals who are considering tongue piercing of the potential complications such as chipping and cracking of teeth and possible trauma to the gingiva.

  These are examples of possible complications that individuals should be informed about (De Moor, De Witte, De Bruyne, 2000).

WEB SITES FOR EDUCATION

MERLIN See the MERLIN web site for World Wide Web resources for client education.

REFERENCES American Dental Association: *Preventing baby bottle tooth decay,* retrieved from the World Wide Web on May 26, 2001, Web site:www.ada.org/public/topics/bottle.html.

Armstrong TS: Stomatitis in the bone marrow transplant patient, *Cancer Nurs* 17:403, 1994.

Aubertin MA: Oral cancer screening in the elderly: the home healthcare nurse's role, *Home Healthcare Nurse* 15(9):595, 1997.

Ayers KM, Colquhoun AN: Halitosis: causes, diagnosis, and treatment, *NZ Dent J* 94(418):156-160, 1998.

Beighton D et al: The influence of specific foods and oral hygiene on the microflora of fissures and smooth surfaces of molar teeth: a 5-day study, *Caries Res* 33(5):349-356, 1999.

Barmes DE: Public policy on oral health and old age: a global view, *J Public Health Dent* 60(4):335-337, 2000.

Bhaskar SN, Lilly GE, Pratt LW: A practical, high-yield mouth exam, *Patient Care* 24:53-74, 1990.

Consumer information: *Child health guide: put prevention into practice,* Rockville, Md, Agency for Health Care Policy and Research, retrieved from the World Wide Web on May 26, 2001. Web site: www.ahcpr.gov/ppip/ppchild.htm#dental.

De Moor RJ, De Witte AM, De Bruyne MA: Tongue piercing and associated oral and dental complications, *Endod Dent Traumatol* 16(5):232-237, 2000.

Durham TM, Malloy T, Hodges ED: Halitosis: knowing when "bad breath" signals systemic disease, *Geriatrics* 48(8):55-59, 1993.

Giger JN, Davidhizar RE: *Transcultural nursing,* ed 2, St Louis, 1995, Mosby.

Gillcrist JA, Brumley DE, Blackford JU: Community socioeconomic status and children's dental health, *J Am Dent Assoc* 132(2):216-222, 2001.

Gray MM, Davies-Slowik J: Changes in the percentage of 5-year-old children with no experience of decay in Dudley towns since the implementation of fluoridation schemes in 1987, *Br Dent J* 190(1):30-32, 2001.

Koop CE: *Kids' dental health,* retrieved from the World Wide Web on Feb 20, 2001. Web site: drkoop.com/wellness/prevcenter/care/child-dental.asp.

Leininger MM: *Transcultural nursing: theories, research and practices,* ed 2, Hilliard, Ohio, 1996, McGraw-Hill.

Roberts J: Developing an oral assessment and intervention tool for older people, *Br J Nurs* 9(18):2033-2040, 2000.

Rosenberg M: Clinical assessment of bad breath: current concepts, *J Am Dental Assoc* 127(4):475-482, 1996. (Published erratum appears in *J Am Dental Assoc* 127[5]:570, 1996.)

Sasahara H, Kawamura M: Behavioral dental science: the relationship between tooth-brushing angle and plaque removal at the lingual surfaces of the posterior teeth in the mandible, *J Oral Sci* 42(2):79-82, 2000.

Scannapieco FA, Stewart EM, Mylotte JM: Colonization of dental plaque by respiratory pathogens in medical intensive care patients, *Crit Care Med* 20:740, 1992.

Stiefel KA et al: Improving oral hygiene for the seriously ill patient: implementing research-based practice, *Medsurg Nurs* 9(1):40-43, 46, 2000.

Stuart GW, Laraia MT: Therapeutic nurse-patient relationship. In Stuart GW, Laraia MT, editors: *Principles and practice of psychiatric nursing,* St Louis, 2001, Mosby, p 30.

• = **Independent;** ▲ = **Collaborative**

Tombes MB, Gallucci B: The effects of hydrogen peroxide rinses on the normal oral mucosa, *Nurs Res* 42:332, 1993.

Valaitis R et al: A systematic review of the relationship between breastfeeding and early childhood caries, *Can J Public Health* 91(6):411-417, 2000.

Whitmyer CC et al: Clinical evaluation of the efficacy and safety of an ultrasonic toothbrush system in an elderly patient population, *Geriatr Nurs* 19:1, 1998.

Winslow EH: Research for practice: don't use H_2O_2 for oral care, *Am J Nurs* 94(3):19, 1994.

Woolfolk MW et al: Determining dental checkup frequency, *J Am Dental Assoc* 130(5):715-723, 1999.

Risk for delayed Development

Gail B. Ladwig and Mary Markle

NANDA **Definition** At risk for delay of 25% or more in one or more of the areas of social or self-regulatory behavior or cognitive, language, gross, or fine motor skills.

Risk Factors

Prenatal Maternal age <15 or >35 years; substance abuse; infections; genetic or endocrine disorders; unplanned or unwanted pregnancy; lack of, late, or poor prenatal care; inadequate nutrition; illiteracy; poverty; depression or other mental disorders; lack of knowledge; domestic abuse

Individual Prematurity; seizures; congenital or genetic disorders; positive drug screening test; brain damage (e.g., hemorrhage in postnatal period, shaken baby, abuse, accident); vision impairment; hearing impairment or frequent otitis media; chronic illness; technology dependence; failure to thrive; inadequate nutrition; foster or adopted child; lead poisoning; chemotherapy; radiation therapy; natural disaster; behavior disorders; substance abuse

Environmental Poverty; violence

Caregiver Abuse; mental illness; mental retardation or severe learning disability

NOC **Outcomes (Nursing Outcomes Classification)**

Suggested NOC Labels

Child Development: 2 Months; 4 Months; 6 Months; 12 Months; 2 Years; 3 Years; 4 Years; 5 Years; Middle Childhood (5-11 Years); Adolescence (12-17 Years)

> **Example NOC Outcome**
> Demonstrates **Child Development** as evidenced by the following indicators: Appropriate milestones of physical, cognitive, and psychosocial age appropriate progression (Rate each indicator of **Child Development:** 1 = extreme delay from expected range, 2 = substantial delay from expected range, 3 = moderate delay from expected range, 4 = mild delay from expected range, 5 = no delay from expected range [see Section I])

Client Outcomes

- Describe realistic, age-appropriate patterns of development (parents/primary caregiver)

• = Independent; ▲ = Collaborative

- Promote activities and interactions that support age-related developmental tasks (parents/primary caregiver)

NIC   Interventions (Nursing Interventions Classification)

Suggested NIC Labels

Developmental Enhancement

> **Example NIC Interventions—Developmental Enhancement**
> - Teach caregivers about normal developmental milestones and associated behaviors
> - Enhance parental effectiveness

Nursing Interventions and Rationales

Refer to care plan for **Delayed Growth and development.**

NOTE: Determination of the etiology for delayed development is critical because it will direct the selection of interventions for treating the diagnosis. Parenting skill deficits, lack of consistency between caregivers, and hospitalization versus a chronic medical condition/developmental disability will necessitate different strategies. A hospitalization experience with regressive behaviors can be a transient occurrence as opposed to a chronic situation, which may have more severe and longer delays requiring more in-depth intervention. Parenting skills and consistent expectations between multiple caregivers can be addressed by more intensive education efforts (Stutts, 1994; Seideman, Kleine, 1995).

Multicultural

- Acknowledge racial/ethnic differences at the onset of care.
  Acknowledgement of race/ethnicity issues will enhance communication, establish rapport, and promote treatment outcomes (D'Avanzo et al, 2001).
- Assess for the influence of cultural beliefs, norms, and values on the client's perceptions of child development.
  What the client considers normal and abnormal child development may be based on cultural perceptions (Leininger, 1996).
- Use a neutral, indirect style when addressing areas in which improvement is needed (such as a need for verbal stimulation) when working with clients.
  Using indirect statements such as "Other mothers have tried. . ." or "I had a client who tried 'X' and it seemed to work very well" will assist in avoiding resentment from the parent (Seiderman et al, 1996).
- Assess whether exposure to community violence is contributing to developmental problems.
  Exposure to community violence has been associated with increases in aggressive behavior and depression (Gorman-Smith, Tolan, 1998).
- Validate the client's feelings and concerns related to child's development.
  Validation lets the client know that the nurse has heard and understands what was said, and it promotes the nurse-client relationship (Stuart, Laraia, 2001; Giger, Davidhizar, 1995).

Client/Family Teaching

- Encourage mothers to abstain from alcohol and cocaine use during pregnancy; refer to treatment programs for substance abuse.

• = Independent; ▲ = Collaborative

Findings indicate that deficiencies in motor development remain detectable at 2 years of age in children exposed to drugs prenatally. Although other environmental variables may influence motor development, children exposed to cocaine and to alcohol in utero may encounter developmental challenges that impede later achievement (Arendt et al, 1999).

- Encourage adequate antepartum and postpartum care for both mother and child.
  Access to prenatal and postnatal health care promotes optimal growth and development (Bland, 2000; Starfield, 1992).
- Counsel parents, siblings, and caregivers about the importance of smoking cessation and the necessity of eliminating all secondhand smoke exposure.
  Cigarette smoke is a well-known carcinogen that also contributes to chronic respiratory infections in children (Gergen et al, 1998).
- Teach caregivers of children appropriate developmental interactions; use anticipatory guidance to facilitate preparation for developmental milestones.
  Children with IQ scores ≥90 had more developmentally appropriate interaction by caregivers (P = 0.043) and higher scores on six of eight subscales and Total HOME (P = 0.05) than the group of children with IQ scores <90. Conclusions: Two postnatal factors, home environment and caregiver-child interaction, were associated with full-scale IQ scores ≥90, whereas prenatal and natal factors were not. These potentially malleable postnatal factors can be targeted for change to improve cognitive outcome of inner-city children (Hurt et al, 1998).

WEB SITES FOR EDUCATION

᛭ᴹᴱᴿᴸᴵᴺ See the MERLIN web site for World Wide Web resources for client education.

REFERENCES Arendt R et al: Motor development of cocaine-exposed children at age two years, *Pediatrics* 103(1):86-92, 1999.

Bland M et al: Late third trimester treatment of rectovaginal group B streptococci with benzathine penicillin G, *Am J Obstet Gynecol* 183(2):372-376, 2000.

D'Avanzo CE et al: Developing culturally informed strategies for substance-related interventions. In Naegle MA, D'Avanzo CE, editors: *Addictions and substance abuse: strategies for advanced practice nursing,* St Louis, 2001, Mosby, pp 59-104.

Gergen PJ et al: The burden of environmental tobacco smoke exposure on the respiratory health of children 2 months through 5 years of age in the United States, *Pediatrics* 101(2):E8, 1998.

Giger JN, Davidhizar RE: *Transcultural nursing,* ed 2, St Louis, 1995, Mosby.

Gorman-Smith D, Tolan P: The role of exposure to community violence and developmental problems among inner city youth, *Dev Psychopathol* 10(1):101-116, 1998.

Hurt H et al: Inner-city achievers: who are they? *Arch Pediatr Adolesc Med* 152(10):993-997, 1998.

Leininger MM: *Transcultural nursing: theories, research and practices,* ed 2, Hilliard, Ohio, 1996, McGraw-Hill.

Seideman RJ, Kleine PF: A theory of transformed parenting: parenting a child with developmental delay/mental retardation, *Nurs Res* 44:38, 1995.

Seiderman RY et al: Assessing American Indian families, *MCN Am J Matern Child Nurs* 21(6):274-279, 1996.

Starfield B: Primary care, New York, 1992, Oxford University Press.

Stuart GW, Laraia MT: Therapeutic nurse-patient relationship. In Stuart GW, Laraia MT, editors: *Principles and practice of psychiatric nursing,* St Louis, 2001, Mosby, p 30.

Stutts AL: Selected outcomes of technology dependent children receiving home care and prescribed child care services, *Pediatr Nurs* 20:501, 1994.

• = Independent; ▲ = Collaborative

Diarrhea

Betty J. Ackley

NANDA   **Definition**   Passage of loose, unformed stools

Defining Characteristics

Hyperactive bowel sounds; at least three loose liquid stools per day; urgency; abdominal pain; cramping

Related Factors (r/t)

Psychological   High stress levels and anxiety

Situational   Alcohol abuse; toxins; laxative abuse; radiation; tube feedings; adverse effects of medications; contaminants; travel

Physiological   Inflammation; malabsorption; infectious processes; irritation; parasites

NOC   **Outcomes (Nursing Outcomes Classification)**

Suggested NOC Labels

Bowel Elimination; Electrolyte and Acid-Base Balance; Fluid Balance; Hydration; Treatment Behavior: Illness or Injury

> **Example NOC Outcome**
> Demonstrates appropriate **Bowel Elimination** as shown by the following indicators: Elimination pattern in expected range/Stool soft and formed/Diarrhea not present/ Control of bowel movements/Comfort of stool passage/Painful cramps not present (Rate each indicator of **Bowel Elimination:** 1 = extremely compromised, 2 = substantially compromised, 3 = moderately compromised, 4 = mildly compromised, 5 = not compromised [see Section I])

Client Outcomes

- Defecates formed, soft stool every day to every third day
- Maintains a rectal area free of irritation
- States relief from cramping and less or no diarrhea
- Explains cause of diarrhea and rationale for treatment
- Maintains good skin turgor and weight at usual level
- Contains stool appropriately (if previously incontinent)

NIC   **Interventions (Nursing Interventions Classification)**

Suggested NIC Labels

Diarrhea Management

> **Example NIC Interventions—Diarrhea Management**
> - Evaluate medication profile for gastrointestinal side effects
> - Suggest trial elimination of foods containing lactose

Nursing Interventions and Rationales

- Assess pattern of defecation or have client keep a diary that includes the following: time of day defecation occurs; usual stimulus for defecation; consistency, amount, and frequency of stool; type of, amount of, and time food consumed; fluid intake; history of bowel habits and laxative use; diet; exercise patterns; obstetrical/gynecological,

• = Independent; ▲ = Collaborative

medical, and surgical histories; medications; alterations in perianal sensations; and present bowel regimen.

Assessment of defecation pattern will help direct treatment (Mertz et al, 1995; Hogan, 1998).

▲ Identify cause of diarrhea if possible (e.g., viral, rotavirus, human immunodeficiency virus [HIV]); food; medication effect; radiation therapy; protein malnutrition; laxative abuse; stress). See Related Factors (r/t).

Identification of the underlying cause is imperative because the treatment and expected outcome depend on it. If the onset of diarrhea is sudden with no obvious cause, a colonoscopy is recommended to rule out colon cancer. When reviewing medication, assess for medications that increase peristalsis, such as metoclopramide (Reglan). HIV infection is also commonly associated with diarrhea (Anastasi, 1993).

▲ If client has watery diarrhea, a low-grade fever, abdominal cramps, and a history of antibiotic therapy, consider possibility of *Clostridium difficile* infection.

C. difficile *infection and pseudomembranous colitis have become increasingly common because of the frequent use of broad-spectrum antibiotics (Vogel, 1995; Gantz, Gerding, Johnson, 1998).*

• Use Standard Precautions when caring for clients with diarrhea to prevent spread of infectious diarrhea; use gloves and handwashing.

C. difficile *has been shown to be contagious and at times epidemic. One study of medical patients demonstrated that more than 30% developed nosocomial diarrhea after admission to a nursing unit, and the majority of cases were caused by* C. difficile *(McFarland, 1995).* C. difficile *is spread by direct or indirect contact, placing other clients at risk for infection (Miller, Walton, Tordecilla, 1998).*

▲ Obtain stool specimens as ordered to either rule out or diagnose an infectious process (e.g., ova and parasites, *C. difficile* infection, bacterial cultures).

▲ If client has infectious diarrhea, avoid using medications that slow peristalsis.

If an infectious process is occurring, such as C. difficile *infection or food poisoning, medication to slow down peristalsis should generally not be given (Bliss et al, 2000). The increase in gut motility helps eliminate the causative factor, and use of antidiarrheal medication could result in a toxic megacolon (Gantz, Gerding, Johnson, 1998).*

• Observe and record number and consistency of stools per day; if desired, use a fecal incontinence collector for accurate measurement of output.

Documentation of output provides a baseline and helps direct replacement fluid therapy.

• Inspect, palpate, percuss, and auscultate abdomen; note whether bowel sounds are frequent.

• Assess for dehydration by observing skin turgor over sternum and inspecting for longitudinal furrows of the tongue. Watch for excessive thirst, fever, dizziness, lightheadedness, palpitations, excessive cramping, bloody stools, hypotension, and symptoms of shock.

Severe diarrhea can cause deficient fluid volume with extreme weakness (Hogan, 1998) and cause death in the very young, the chronically ill, and the elderly.

▲ Observe for symptoms of sodium and potassium loss (e.g., weakness, abdominal or leg cramping, dysrhythmia). Note results of electrolyte laboratory studies.

Stool contains electrolytes; excessive diarrhea causes electrolyte abnormalities that can be especially harmful to clients with existing medical conditions.

▲ Monitor and record intake and output; note oliguria and dark, concentrated urine. Measure specific gravity of urine if possible.

• = **Independent;** ▲ = **Collaborative**

Dark, concentrated urine, along with a high specific gravity of urine, is an indication of deficient fluid volume.

- Weigh client daily and note decreased weight.
  An accurate daily weight is an important indicator of fluid balance in the body (Metheny, 2000).
- Give clear fluids as tolerated (e.g., clear soda, Jell-O), serving at lukewarm temperature.
- ▲ For children with diarrhea, give oral rehydration therapy liquids (Pedialyte) as directed by physician.
  Oral rehydration therapy is effective for treating mild to moderate dehydration in children with diarrhea and may help prevent the need for hospitalization with administration of IVs (Larson, 2000).
- ▲ If diarrhea is associated with cancer or cancer treatment, once infectious cause of diarrhea is ruled out, provide medications as ordered to stop diarrhea.
  The loss of proteins, electroytes, and water from diarrhea in a cancer client can lead to rapid deterioration and possibly fatal dehydration (Kornblau et al, 2000).
- ▲ If diarrhea is chronic and there is evidence of malnutrition, consult with primary care practitioner for a dietary consult and possible use of a hydrolyzed formula to maintain nutrition while the gastrointestinal system heals.
  A hydrolyzed formula contains protein that is partially broken down to small peptides or amino acids for people who cannot digest nutrients (Cataldo, DeBruyne, Whitney, 1999).
- Encourage client to eat small, frequent meals and to consume foods that normally cause constipation and are easy to digest (e.g., bananas, crackers, pretzels, rice, potatoes, applesauce). Encourage client to avoid milk products, foods high in fiber, and caffeine (dark sodas, tea, coffee, chocolate).
  Bland, starchy foods are initially recommended when starting to eat solid food again (Rice, 1994).
- Provide a readily available bedpan, commode, or bathroom.
- ▲ Maintain perirectal skin integrity. Cleanse with a mild cleansing agent (perineal skin cleanser). Apply protective ointment prn (Haisfield-Wolfe, Rund, 2000). If skin is still excoriated and desquamated, apply a wound hydrogel. Avoid the use of rectal Foley catheters.
  Moisture-barrier ointments protect the skin from excoriation. Rectal Foley catheters can cause rectal necrosis, sphincter damage, or rupture, and the nursing staff may not have the time to properly follow the necessary and very time-consuming steps of their care (Bosley, 1994; Fiers, 1996).
- ▲ If client is receiving a tube feeding, do not assume it is the cause of diarrhea. Perform a complete assessment to rule out other causes such as medication effects, sorbitol in medications, or an infection.
  Research has shown that tube feedings do not usually cause diarrhea (Campbell, 1994). However, sorbitol in medication has been linked to diarrhea (Drug Watch, 1994).
- ▲ If client is receiving a tube feeding, suggest formulas that contain a bulking agent such as Jevity. Note rate of infusion, and prevent contamination of feeding by rinsing container every 8 hours and replacing it every 24 hours.
  Rapid administration of tube feeding and contaminated feedings have been associated with diarrhea. Bulking agents are useful in tube feedings to prevent diarrhea (Doughty, 1991; Bockus, 1993).

• = Independent; ▲ = Collaborative

Geriatric

▲ Evaluate medications client is taking. Recognize that many medications can result in diarrhea, including digitalis, propranolol, ACE inhibitors, Hx-receptor antagonists, NSAIDS, anticholinergic agents, oral hypoglycemia agents, antibiotics, and others.

A drug-associated cause should always be considered when treating diarrhea in the older person; many drugs can result in diarrhea (Ratnaike, 2000).

▲ Monitor client closely to detect whether an impaction is causing diarrhea; remove impaction as ordered.

Impactions are more common in the elderly than in younger clients. It is very important that the client be checked for impaction before being given any antidiarrheal medication (Carnaveli, Patrick, 1993).

▲ Seek medical attention if diarrhea is severe or persists for more than 24 hours, or if client has symptoms of dehydration or electrolyte disturbances such as lassitude, weakness, or prostration.

Elderly clients can dehydrate rapidly. The greatest concern for elderly clients with severe diarrhea is hypokalemia. Hypokalemia is treatable but when missed can be fatal (Carnaveli, Patrick, 1993).

• Provide emotional support for clients who are having trouble controlling unpredictable episodes of diarrhea.

Diarrhea can be a great source of embarrassment to the elderly and can lead to social isolation and a feeling of powerlessness (Carnaveli, Patrick, 1993).

Home Care Interventions

• Assess the home for general sanitation and methods of food preparation. Reinforce principles of sanitation for food handling.

• Assess for methods of handling soiled laundry if client is bedbound or has been incontinent. Instruct or reinforce Standard Precautions with family and bloodborne pathogen precautions with agency caregivers.

The Bloodborne Pathogen Regulations of the Occupational Safety and Health Administration (OSHA) identify legal guidelines for caregivers.

• When assessing medication history, include over-the-counter drugs, both general and those currently being used to treat the diarrhea. Instruct clients not to mix over-the-counter medications when self-treating.

Mixing over-the-counter medications can further irritate the gastrointestinal system, intensifying the diarrhea or causing nausea and vomiting.

Client/Family Teaching

• Encourage avoidance of coffee, spices, milk products, and foods that irritate or stimulate the gastrointestinal tract.

▲ Teach appropriate method of taking ordered antidiarrheal medications; explain side effects.

• Explain how to prevent the spread of infectious diarrhea (e.g., careful handwashing, appropriate handling and storage of food).

• Help client to determine stressors and set up an appropriate stress reduction plan.

• Teach signs and symptoms of dehydration and electrolyte imbalance.

• Teach perirectal skin care.

• = Independent; ▲ = Collaborative

REFERENCES Anastasi J: Diarrhea in acquired immune deficiency syndrome (AIDS), *Ostomy Wound Manage* 39:14-23, 1993.

Bliss DZ et al: Fecal incontinence in hospitalized patients who are acutely ill, *Nurs Res* 49(2):101-107, 2000.

Bockus S: When your patient needs tube feeding: making the right decision, *Nursing* 93:34-42, 1993.

Bosley C: Three methods of stool management for patients with diarrhea, *Ostomy Wound Manage* 40:52, 1994.

Campbell C: Research for practice: diarrhea not always linked to tube feedings, *Am J Nurs* 94(4):59, 1994.

Carnaveli DL, Patrick M: Nursing management for the elderly, ed 3, Philadelphia, 1993, JB Lippincott.

Cataldo CB, DeBruyne LK, Whitney EN: Nutrition and diet therapy, Belmont, Calif, 1999, Wadsworth.

Doughty D: Maintaining normal bowel function in the patient with cancer, *J ET Nurs* 18:90, 1991.

Drug Watch: Sorbitol: missing link to diarrhea, *Am J Nurs* 10:50, 1994.

Fiers S: Breaking the cycle: the etiology of incontinence dermatitis and evaluating and using skin care products, *Ostomy Wound Manage* 42:32, 1996.

Gantz NM, Gerding DN, Johnson PC: Managing and containing *Clostridium difficile* disease, *Patient Care* pp 171-182, April 15, 1998.

Haisfield-Wolfe ME, Rund C: A nursing protocol for the management of perineal-rectal skin alterations, *Clin J Oncol Nurs* 4(1):15-33, 2000.

Hogan CM: The nurse's role in diarrhea management, *Oncol Nurs Forum* 25(5):879-885, 1998.

Kornblau S et al: Management of cancer treatment-related diarrhea: issues and therapeutic strategies, *J Pain Symptom Manage* 19(2):118-128, 2000.

Larson CE: Evidence-based practice: safety and efficacy of oral rehydration therapy for the treatmet of diarrhea and gastroenteritis in pediatrics, *Pediatr Nurs* 26(2):177-179, 2000.

McFarland LV: Epidemiology of infectious and iatrogenic nosocomial diarrhea in a cohort of general medicine patients, *Am J Infect Control* 23:295, 1995.

Mertz HR et al: Validation of a new measure of diarrhea, *Digest Dis Sci* 40:1873, 1995.

Metheny N: Fluid and electrolyte balance: nursing considerations, ed 4, Philadelphia, 2000, JB Lippincott.

Miller JM, Walton JC, Tordecilla LL: Recognizing and managing *Clostridium difficile*-associated diarrhea, *Medsurg Nurs* 7(6):348-356, 1998.

Ratnaike RN: Drug-induced diarrhea in older persons, *Clin Geriatr* 8(1):67-76, 2000.

Rice KH: Oral rehydration therapy: a simple, effective solution, *J Pediatr Nurs* 9:349-356, 1994.

Vogel LC: Antibiotic-induced diarrhea, *Orthop Nurs* 14:38-41, 1995.

Risk for Disuse syndrome

Betty J. Ackley

NANDA   **Definition** A state in which an individual is at risk for a deterioration of body systems as the result of prescribed or unavoidable musculoskeletal inactivity

Risk Factors

Paralysis; altered level of consciousness; mechanical immobilization; prescribed immobilization; severe pain (NOTE: complications from immobility can include pressure ulcer, constipation, stasis of pulmonary secretions, thrombosis, urinary tract infection and/or retention, decreased strength or endurance, orthostatic hypotension, decreased range of joint motion, disorientation, disturbed body image, and powerlessness)

Related Factors (r/t)

See Risk Factors

• = **Independent;** ▲ = **Collaborative**

NOC   **Outcomes (Nursing Outcomes Classification)**

Suggested NOC Labels

Immobility Consequences: Physiological; Mobility Level; Neurological Status: Consciousness; Pain Level: Endurance

> **Example NOC Outcome**
> Develops minimal **Immobility Consequences: Physiological** as evidenced by the presence of the following indicators: Pressure ulcers/Constipation/Decreased nutrition status/Urinary calculi/Decreased muscle strength (Rate each indicator of **Immobility Consequences: Physiological:** 1 = severe, 2 = substantial, 3 = moderate, 4 = slight, 5 = none [see Section I])

Client Outcomes

- Maintains full range of motion in joints
- Maintains intact skin, good peripheral blood flow, and normal pulmonary function
- Maintains normal bowel and bladder function
- Expresses feelings about imposed immobility
- Explains methods to prevent complications of immobility

NIC   **Interventions (Nursing Interventions Classification)**

Suggested NIC Labels

Energy Management; Exercise Therapy: Joint Mobility; Exercise Therapy: Muscle Control

> **Example NIC Interventions—Energy Management**
> - Determine client's physical limitations
> - Determine client's significant other's perception of causes of fatigue

Nursing Interventions and Rationales

- Have client do exercises in bed if not contraindicated (e.g., flexing and extending feet and quadriceps, performing gluteal and abdominal sitting exercises, lifting small weights to maintain muscle strength).
  Unused muscles lose about one eighth of their strength for each week of bed rest; the muscles atrophy, change shape, and shorten, and muscle fatigue occurs more readily (Harper, Lyles, 1988; Corcoran, 1991). In-bed exercises help maintain muscle strength and tone (Metzlar, Harr, 1996). Strength improvement in response to resisted exercise is possible even in the very elderly, extremely sedentary client with multiple chronic diseases and functional disabilities. Increased strength can help prevent falls (Connelly, 2000).
- ▲ If not contraindicated by client's condition, obtain referral to physical therapy for use of tilt table to provide weight bearing on long bones.
  The upright position helps maintain bone strength, increase circulation, and prevent postural hypotension. The best way to prevent osteoporosis is to begin weight-bearing exercises as soon as possible (Jiricka, 1994).
- Perform range of motion exercises for all possible joints at least twice daily; perform passive or active range of motion exercises as appropriate.
  If not used, muscles weaken and shorten and are predisposed to contractures; if nonuse continues, the contracture eventually involves the tendons, ligaments, and joint capsules and limits the range of motion (Jiricka, 1994).

• = Independent; ▲ = Collaborative

▲ Use high-top sneakers or specialized boots from the occupational therapy department to prevent footdrop; remove shoes twice daily to provide foot care.
Sneakers or boots help keep the foot in normal anatomical alignment; footdrop can make it difficult or impossible to walk after bed rest.

• Position client so that joints are in normal anatomical alignment at all times.
Improper positioning can damage peripheral nerves and blood vessels, as well as cause joint deformities (Metzlar, Harr, 1996).

▲ Get client up in chair as soon as appropriate; use a stretcher-chair if necessary. Assist client to walk as soon as medically possible.
Almost all clients can get out of bed now with use of the stretcher-chair, which converts from a stretcher to a chair. Bed rest is almost always harmful to clients; early mobilization is better than bed rest for most health conditions (Allen, Glasziou, Del Mar, 1999).

▲ Consider use of a continuous lateral rotation therapy bed.
Continuous lateral rotation therapy has been shown to be effective for the prevention of pneumonia in transplant clients (Whiteman et al, 1995) and deep vein thrombosis in spinal cord injury clients (Von Rueden, Harris, 1995).

▲ If at all possible, help the client begin a walking program, using a physical therapist as needed.
Early mobilization has been shown to improve the outcome for clients after treatment of medical conditions and procedures (Allen, Glasziou, Del Mar, 1999).

• Be very careful when helping client into a chair and when transferring. Be sure to lock beds and wheelchairs. Recognize that there is a high probability for falls.
Nonambulatory clients have a substantially greater number of serious falls than their ambulatory peers. 87% of falls with injuries involved equipment misuse such as not locking beds and wheelchairs; 82% occurred while seated or transferring; 54% occurred at chair or bed height only (Thapa et al, 1996).

• Minimize cardiovascular deconditioning by positioning clients as close to the upright position as possible several times daily.
The hazards of bed rest in the elderly are multiple, serious, quick to develop, and slow to reverse. Decondition of the cardiovascular system occurs within days and involves fluid shifts, fluid loss, decreased cardiac output, decreased peak oxygen uptake, and increased resting heart rate (Resnick, 1998a).

• When getting client up after bed rest, do so slowly and watch for signs of postural hypotension, tachycardia, nausea, diaphoresis, or syncope. Take the blood pressure lying, sitting, and standing, waiting 2 minutes between each reading.
Sitting or standing after 3 or 4 days of bed rest results in postural hypotension because of cardiovascular reflex dysfunction (Jiricka, 1994; Metzlar, Harr, 1996).

▲ Obtain assistive devices to help client reach and maintain as much mobility as possible.

• Turn client at least every 2 hours and carefully observe skin condition, especially bony prominences. Turning clients is of paramount importance to prevent all of the complications of bed rest (Metzlar, Harr, 1996). Routine turning has been demonstrated to reduce the length of stay of critical care patients (Von Reuden, Harris, 1995). Systematic inspection can identify impending problems early (Bryant, 1993).

• Provide client with a pressure-relieving horizontal support surface.
Support surfaces can help to relieve pressure. If foam is used, it must be 4 inches thick, or use a static air mattress or low–air-loss surface as appropriate (Maklebust, Sieggreen,

• = **Independent**; ▲ = **Collaborative**

1996). More research is needed to set definitive guidelines with regard to which pressure-relieving horizontal support surfaces are most effective (Maklebust, 1999).

▲ To prevent DVT, use antiembolism stockings or a sequential compression system for legs as ordered. Recognize that may also need to consult with physician for order of anticoagulant.
These stockings can be helpful for preventing DVT. If DVT risk is high, consult with physician regarding need for intermittent pneumatic compression of the calves or subcutaneous administration of heparin (Brock, 1994; Ecklund, 1995). A combination of an anticoagulant and mechanical methods to prevent DVT has been shown to be most effective in postoperative clients (Hyers, 1999).

• Monitor peripheral circulation and especially note color, pulse, and calf or thigh swelling; check Homans' sign, but recognize that it is an unreliable sign of DVT.
Because of venous stasis, pressure of mattress against veins, and hypercoagulability of blood, bed rest predisposes the client to deep vein thrombosis (Harper, Lyles, 1988). Deep vein thrombosis may result in pulmonary embolism in an immobilized client (Metzlar, Harr, 1996).

• Have client cough and deep breathe or use incentive spirometry every 2 hours while awake.
Bed rest compromises breathing because of decreased chest expansion and decreased size of thoracic compartment; deep breathing helps prevent complications (Jiricka, 1994).

• Monitor respiratory functions, noting breath sounds and respiratory rate. Percuss for new onset of dullness in lungs.
Immobility results in hypoventilation, which predisposes the client to atelectasis, the pooling of respiratory secretions, and thus pneumonia (Corcoran, 1991; Tempkin, Tempkin, Goodman, 1997).

• Note bowel function daily. Provide increased fluids, fiber, and natural laxatives such as prune juice as needed.
Constipation is common in immobilized clients because of decreased activity and food intake.

• Increase fluid intake to 2000 ml/day within the client's cardiac and renal reserve.
Adequate fluids help prevent kidney stones and constipation and help counteract dehydration associated with bed rest (Rubin, 1988).

• Encourage intake of a balanced diet with adequate amounts of fiber and protein.
Reduced muscular activity and lowered metabolism generally reduce the appetite of a client on bed rest (Rubin, 1988).

Geriatric

• Recognize the importance of keeping elderly clients active if possible.
In the elderly, 10% to 15% of muscle strength can be lost for every week that muscles are resting completely (Mobily, Kelley, 1991).

▲ Refer to physical therapy for an individualized strength training program.

• Monitor for signs of depression: flat affect, poor appetite, insomnia, many somatic complaints.
Depression can commonly accompany decreased mobility and function in the elderly (Resnick, 1998b).

• Keep careful track of bowel function in the elderly; do not allow client to become constipated.
The elderly can easily develop impactions as a result of immobility.

• = Independent; ▲ = Collaborative

Home Care Interventions

NOTE: Care for all body systems for the immobilized or otherwise at risk client must continue in the home as stated in the previously mentioned interventions. The primary nurse monitors and adjusts the plan of care accordingly per physician orders.

- Become oriented to all programs of care for client before discharge from institutional care. Confirm the immediate availability of all necessary assistive devices for home. *Continuity in management of care promotes success in meeting client-centered goals.*
- Perform complete physical assessment and recent history at initial visit. *A complete assessment validates status of client upon discharge and defines client problems needing immediate intervention.*
- ▲ Refer to physical and occupational therapies for immediate evaluations of client's potential for independence and functioning in the home setting and for follow-up care. *Early identification of client needs allows for early intervention.*
- Allow client to have as much input and control of the plan of care as possible. *Client perception of control increases self-esteem and motivation to follow medical plan of care.*
- Assess knowledge of all care with caregivers. Review as necessary. *Having the necessary knowledge and skills to perform care decreases caregiver role strain and supports safety of the client.*
- ▲ Support family of client in assumption of caregiver activities. Refer for home health aide services for assistance and respite as appropriate. Refer to medical social services as appropriate.

Client/Family Teaching

- Teach how to perform range-of-motion exercises in bed if not contraindicated.
- Teach family how to turn and position client.

NOTE: Nursing diagnoses that are commonly relevant when the client is on bed rest include **Constipation, Risk for impaired Skin integrity, Disturbed Sensory perception; Disturbed Sleep pattern, Adult Failure to thrive,** and **Powerlessness.**

WEB SITES FOR EDUCATION

MERLIN See the MERLIN web site for World Wide Web resources for client education.

REFERENCES   Allen C, Glasziou P, Del Mar C: Bed rest: a potentially harmful treatment needing more careful attention, *Lancet* 354(9186):1229-1233, 1999.

Bryant R, editor: *Acute and chronic wounds,* St Louis, 1993, Mosby.

Brock JD: Compression stockings: do they prevent DVT? *Am J Nurs* 94:25, 1994.

Connelly DM: Resisted exercise training of institutionalized older adults for improved strength and functional mobility: a review, *Topics Geriatr Rehabil* 15(3):6-28, 2000.

Corcoran PJ: Use it or lose it: the hazards of bed rest and inactivity, *West J Med* 154:536-538, 1991.

Ecklund MM: Optimizing the flow of care for prevention and treatment of deep vein thrombosis and pulmonary embolism. *AACN Clin Issues* 6(4)588-601, 1995.

Harper CM, Lyles YM: Physiology and complications of bed rest, *J Am Geriatr Soc* 36:1047, 1988.

Hyers TM: Venous thromboembolism. *Am J Respir Crit Care Med* 159:1-14, 1999.

Jiricka MK: Alterations in activity intolerance. In Porth CM, editor: Pathophysiology: concepts of altered health states, Philadelphia, 1994, JB Lippincott.

Maklebust JA: An update on horizontal patient support surfaces, *Ostomy Wound Manage* 45(1A):70S, 1999.

Maklebust JA, Sieggreen M: *Pressure ulcers: guidelines for prevention and nursing management,* ed 2, 1996, Springhouse.

Metzlar DJ, Harr J: Positioning your patient properly, *Am J Nurs* 96:33-37, 1996.

Mobily PR, Kelley LS: Iatrogenesis in the elderly: factors of immobility, *J Gerontol Nurs* 17:5-11, 1991.

• = **Independent;** ▲ = **Collaborative**

Resnick B: Predictors of functional ability in geriatric rehabilitation patients, *Rehabil Nurs* 23(1):21, 1998a.

Resnick N: *Geriatric medicine in current medical diagnosis and treatment,* ed 37, Stamford, Conn, 1998b, Appleton & Lange.

Rubin M: The physiology of bed rest, *Am J Nurs* 88:50-55, 1988.

Tempkin T, Tempkin A, Goodman H: Geriatric rehabilitation, *Nurs Pract Forum* 8(2):59, 1997.

Thapa P et al: Injurious falls in nonambulatory nursing home residents: a comparative study of circumstances, incidence, and risk factors, *J Am Geriatr Soc* 44:273, 1996.

Von Rueden KT, Harris JR: Pulmonary dysfunction related to immobility in the trauma patient, *AACN Clin Issues* 6:212-226, 1995.

Whiteman K et al: Effects of continuous lateral rotation therapy on pulmonary complications in liver transplant patients, *Am J Crit Care* 4:133-139, 1995.

Deficient Diversional activity

Betty J. Ackley

 Definition The state in which an individual experiences decreased stimulation from or interest or engagement in recreational or leisure activities

Defining Characteristics

Usual hobbies cannot be undertaken in hospital; patient's statements regarding boredom and the wish for something to do, to read, etc.

Related Factors (r/t)

Environmental lack of diversional activity as a result of long-term hospitalization or frequent or lengthy treatments

NOC Outcomes (Nursing Outcomes Classification)

Suggested NOC Labels

Leisure Participation; Play Participation; Social Involvement

> **Example NOC Outcome**
> Enjoys **Leisure Participation** as evidenced by the following indicators: Expression of satisfaction with leisure activities/Reports of relaxation from leisure activities/ Reports of restfulness of leisure activities (Rate each indicator of **Leisure Participation:** 1 = not adequate, 2 = slightly adequate, 3 = moderately adequate, 4 = substantially adequate, 5 = totally adequate [see Section I])

Client Outcome/Goal

▪ Engages in personally satisfying diversional activities

NIC Interventions (Nursing Interventions Classification)

Suggested NIC Labels

Recreation Therapy; Self-Responsibility Facilitation

> **Example NIC Interventions—Recreation Therapy**
> ▪ Assist client to identify meaningful recreational activities
> ▪ Provide safe recreational equipment

• = Independent; ▲ = Collaborative

Nursing Interventions and Rationales

- Observe for symptoms of deficient diversional activity: yawning, restlessness, flat facial expression, and statements of boredom (Radziewicz, 1992).
- Observe ability to engage in activities that require good vision and use of hands. *Diversional activities must be tailored to the client's capabilities.*
- Discuss activities with client that are interesting and feasible in the present environment.
- Encourage client to share feelings about situation of inactivity away from usual life activities.
  Work and hobbies provide structure and continuity to life; the client can feel a sense of loss when unable to engage in usual activities.
- Encourage a mix of physical and mental activities (e.g., crafts, videotapes). Provide activities that are entertaining, such as videotapes, joke books, or a "humor room." *Humor can help clients reduce anxiety and survive in a high technology environment (Radziewicz, 1992).*
- Use "bread therapy" —have clients bake bread with a breadmaker two times per day or prn.
  Assembling the ingredients is a group activity can be therapeutic. The smell of bread baking gives a homelike, loving atmosphere to a health care environment.
- Encourage client to schedule visitors so that they are not all present at once or at inconvenient times.
  A schedule prevents the client from becoming exhausted from frequent company.
- Provide reading material, television, radio, and books on tape.
- Provide virtual reality experiences for children, which can be used as distraction techniques during chemotherapy treatments. Recommend programs such as Magic Carpet, Sherlock Holmes Mystery, and Seventh Guest.
  Virtual reality experiences as a distraction technique can be effective and result in positive clinical outcomes (Schneider, Workman, 2000).
- If clients are able to write, have them keep journals; if clients are unable to write, have them record thoughts on tape.
  Keeping a journal is diversional and can also help the client deal with the many feelings that result from hospitalization or confinement. A journal can also help the client gain perspective on the situation.
- ▲ Request recreational or art therapist to assist with providing diversional activities. *Recreational therapists specialize in helping people have fun. Art therapy can be effective for helping people express emotions, as well as provide diversion (Shaw, Wilkinson, 1996).*
- ▲ Request an order for a child life specialist or, if not available, a play therapist for children. Encourage activities such as video projects, use of computer-based support groups for children, such as Starbright World, a computer network where children interact virtually, sharing their experiences and escaping hospital routines.
  Therapeutic play is extremely important for children, especially children isolated after bone marrow transplantation (Kuntz et al, 1996). A child life specialist can provide psychosocial assessment and care and therapeutic activities to help children progress developmentally when hospitalized or isolated (Rode et al, 1998).
- Provide a change in scenery; get client out of room as much as possible.
  A lack of sensory stimulation and diversity have significantly adverse effects on clients (Hamilton, 1992).

• = Independent; ▲ = Collaborative

- Structure the environment as needed to promote optimal comfort and sensory diversity (e.g., have family bring in posters, banners, or a sound system; change lighting; change direction bed faces).
  Modification of the environment is sometimes necessary for the well-being of the client (Williams, 1988).
- Recommend activities in which the client can watch movement of animals and develop involvement (e.g., bird-watching, keeping a fish tank).
- Work with family to provide music that is enjoyable to the client.
  Music can help catalyze the client's own self-healing capacity (Guzzetta, 1987) and can help clients find a means to express themselves in a musical activity (Paul, Ramsey, 2000).
- Structure client's schedule around personal wishes for time of care, relaxation, and participation in fun activities.
  Increased client control fosters increased client self-esteem.
- Spend time with the client when possible or arrange for a friendly visitor.
  Simply being available for the client as a fellow human being is important and helpful (Gardner, 1992).

Geriatric

- If client is able, arrange for him or her to attend a group senior citizen exercise session for progressive strength training, even if exercise can only be done while seated.
  Strength training can help seniors improve balance, coordination, range of motion, flexibility, and spatial awareness while receiving social support and having fun (Brill, 1999).
- Encourage involvement in senior citizen activities (e.g., AARP, YMCA, church groups, Gray Panthers). Arrange transportation to activities as needed.
- Encourage clients to use their ability to help others by volunteering.
  Assisting others can help the client grow as a generative human being.
- Provide an environment that promotes activity (e.g., one that has adequate lighting for crafts, large-print books); allow periods of solitude and privacy.
  - Periods of solitude are important for emotional well-being in the elderly.
- Use reminiscence and pet therapy either individually or in groups.
  Reminiscence therapy can increase social interaction, self-esteem, and self-care activities (Hamilton, 1992; Puentes, 1998). Elderly individuals who have or can interact with pets are healthier and live longer than those who do not.

Multicultural

- Assess for the influence of cultural beliefs, norms, and values on the client's leisure activity interests.
  Leisure interests or hobbies may be based on cultural preferences (Leininger, 1996).
- Validate the client's feelings and concerns related to their lack of stimulation or interest in leisure activities.
  Validation lets the client know that the nurse has heard and understands what was said and promotes the nurse-client relationship (Stuart, Laraia, 2001; Giger, Davidhizar, 1995).

Home Care Interventions

NOTE: Many of the previously listed interventions should be administered in the home setting (e.g., modifying the environment to stimulate the client, scheduling visitors to allow for rest and activity). Some adaptations will be necessary.

• = Independent; ▲ = Collaborative

- Assess the family's ability to respond to client's psychosocial needs for stimulation. Assist as able.
  Individuals and caregivers provide care through the context of their own cultural experiences.
- ▲ Refer to occupational therapy to assist the client and family with identifying diversional activities within the capability of the client and family.
  Some services require the consultation of specialty prepared professionals.
- Introduce (or continue) friendly volunteer visitors if the client is willing and able to have the company.
  Simply being available for the client as a fellow human being is important and helpful (Gardner, 1992).

Client/Family Teaching

- Work with client and family on learning diversional activities that client is interested in (e.g., knitting, hooking rugs, writing memoirs).
- If client is in isolation, give the client complete information on why isolation needed, how it should be done, and especially guidelines for visitors.
  In one study, 21 clients who were in isolation identified their greatest needs, which were for more information about the isolation regulations and the need for guidelines for visitors so that visitors would be comfortable and continue to visit (Ward, 2000).

WEB SITES FOR EDUCATION

ᶮMERLIN See the MERLIN web site for World Wide Web resources for client education.

REFERENCES   Brill PA: Effective approach toward prevention and rehabilitation in geriatrics, *Activities Adaptation Aging* 23(4):21, 1999.

Gardner DL: Presence. In Bulechek GM, McCloskey JC, editors: Nursing interventions: essential nursing treatments, Philadelphia, 1992, WB Saunders.

Giger JN, Davidhizar RE: *Transcultural nursing*, ed 2, St Louis, 1995, Mosby.

Guzzetta CE: *Effects of relaxation and music therapy on coronary care patients admitted with presumptive acute myocardial infarction*, Grant NU-00824, Rockville, Md, 1987, Department of Health and Human Services Division of Nursing.

Hamilton DB: Reminiscence therapy. In Bulechek GM, McCloskey JC, editors: *Nursing interventions: essential nursing treatments*, Philadelphia, 1992, WB Saunders.

Kuntz N et al: Therapeutic play and bone marrow transplantation, *J Pediatr Nurs* 11(6):359, 1996.

Leininger MM: *Transcultural nursing: theories, research and practices*, ed 2, Hilliard, Ohio, 1996, McGraw-Hill.

Paul S, Ramsey D: Music therapy in physical medicine and rehabilitation, *Australian Occup Ther J* 47(3):111-118, 2000.

Puentes WJ: Incorporating simple reminiscence techniques into acute care nursing practice, *J Gerontol Nurs* 2:15, 1998.

Radziewicz RM: Using diversional activities to enhance coping, *Cancer Nurs* 15(4):293, 1992.

Rode D et al: The therapeutic use of technology, *Am J Nurs* 12:32, 1998.

Schneider SM, Workman, ML: Virtual reality as a distraction intervention for older children receiving chemotherapy, *Pediatr Nurs* 26(6):593-597, 2000.

Shaw R, Wilkinson W: Therapy and rehabilitation: building the pyramids—palliative care patients' perceptions of making art, *Int J Palliat Nurs* 2(4):217, 1996.

Stuart GW, Laraia MT: Therapeutic nurse-patient relationship. In Stuart GW, Laraia MT, editors: *Principles and practice of psychiatric nursing*, St Louis, 2001, Mosby, p 30.

Ward D: Infection control: reducing the psychological effects of isolation, *Br J Nurs* 9(3):162-170, 2000.

Williams MA: The physical environment and patient care, *Am Rev Nurs Res* 6:61, 1988.

• = Independent; ▲ = Collaborative

Disturbed Energy field

Helen Kelley and Gail B. Ladwig

 Definition A disruption of the flow of energy surrounding a person's being, which results in a disharmony of mind and spirit

Defining Characteristics

Temperature change (warmth/coolness); visual changes (image/color); disruption of the field (vacant/hold/spike/bulge), movement (wave/spike/tingling/dense/flowing), sounds (tone/words)

NOC Outcomes (Nursing Outcomes Classification)

Suggested NOC Labels

Spiritual Well-Being; Well-Being

> **Example NOC Outcome**
> Demonstrates **Well-Being** as evidenced by the following indicators: Satisfaction with physiological functioning/Satisfaction with psychological functioning/Satisfaction with ability to relax (Rate each indicator of **Well-Being:** 1 = extremely compromised, 2 = substantially compromised, 3 = moderately compromised, 4 = mildly compromised, 5 = not compromised [see Section I])

Client Outcomes

- States sense of well-being
- States feeling of relaxation
- States decreased pain
- States decreased tension
- Demonstrates evidence of physical relaxation (e.g., decreased blood pressure, pulse, respiration rate, muscle tension)

NIC Interventions (Nursing Interventions Classification)

Suggested NIC Labels

Therapeutic Touch

> **Example NIC Interventions—Therapeutic Touch**
> - Focuses awareness on inner self
> - Focuses awareness on the intention to facilitate wholeness and healing at all levels of consciousness

Nursing Interventions and Rationales

Refer to care plans for **Anxiety, Acute Pain,** and **Chronic Pain**

- Administer therapeutic touch as described in following discussion (may also include healing touch and Reiki practice).
  Therapeutic touch is the knowledgeable and purposeful patterning of the patient environmental energy field process (Meehan, 1992). Therapeutic touch relieves discomfort and distress and facilitates healing. For some patients, therapeutic touch may serve as a beneficial adjuvant nursing intervention (Meehan, 1998). Therapeutic touch has been shown to induce relaxation, decrease anxiety, and speed healing (Dalglish, 1999).

• = Independent; ▲ = Collaborative

Guidelines for Therapeutic Touch

There are two general guidelines to follow when in training for the use of therapeutic touch. Krieger (1979) recommends that nurses who use therapeutic touch should have had at least 6 months of experience in an acute care setting. Learning should be guided by a nurse who has at least 2 years of experience with therapeutic touch; preferably a Master's degree in nursing; and conforms to the practice guidelines requiring 30 hours of instruction in theory, 30 hours of supervised practice with relatively healthy individuals, and successful completion of written and practice evaluations (Kunz, Krieger, 1975-1990). The Nurse Healers Professional Associates recommend that practitioners complete a beginning workshop addressing the cognitive and therapeutic aspects of therapeutic touch. A minimum of 12 hours of instruction with a certificate of training is recommended. Family members can be instructed on basic soothing and comforting measures in less time.

Administer therapeutic touch by performing the following steps:

1. Centering in the present moment: Shift awareness from the physical environment to an inner focus on the center within self, a center of calm and balance through which nurses perceive themselves and the client as a unitary whole.
   The nurse's attitude becomes clear, and the gentle, compassionate attention and focused intent help the client. Although there is awareness of the physical environment, it is not the primary focus (Meehan, 1992). This study suggests that therapeutic touch (TT), when provided by the nurse in the clinical setting, can promote feelings of comfort, peace, calm, and security among patients (Hayes, Cox, 1999).

2. Assessment: Pass palmar surface of hands 2 to 4 inches over the client's body from head to toe.
   This qualitative analysis of findings indicates that the experiences of giving and receiving TT can be classified within two categories: the cognitive (knowing in the widest sense); and conative (instinct and feeling). The key constructs that emerged in this study are associated with feelings such as tingling, warmth, coolness, comfort, peace, calm, and security. Formulation of the two main categories, cognitive and conative, emphasize the relationship associated with what is known by the mind and instinctively felt by the body (Hayes, Cox, 1999). Validation study cues include heat, decreased or disrupted energy flow, cold, tingling, pulsating, congestion, heaviness, unbalance, decreased flow, and field symmetry (Mornhinweg, 1996).

3. Treatment (unruffling): Use hands to brush or smooth out the energy flow. Sweep the hands downward and out of the field from head to toe, and concentrate on the areas of disturbance that were identified during the assessment.
   Areas of static congestion in the energy flow are relieved, and the field is prepared for the reception of healing energy. Clients mobilize their own resources for self-healing, and pain, anxiety, and discomfort are diminished (Jurgens, Meehan, Wilson, 1987).

4. Direction and modulation of energy: Rest hands on or near the body area where a block of congestion is detected or in other areas of energy imbalance. Facilitate transfer of energy to these areas.
   This step corrects energy imbalances (Krieger, 1979).

5. Stop: Stop procedure when there are no longer any clues or when client indicates it is time to stop. Place hands over the solar plexus (just above the waist) and focus specifically on facilitating the flow of healing energy to the client.
   This final phase allows for rest and evaluation (Jurgens, Meehan, Wilson, 1987).

• = **Independent;** ▲ = **Collaborative**

Multicultural

- Assess for the influence of cultural beliefs, norms, and values on the client's sense of disharmony of mind and spirit.
  The client's sense of disharmony may have cultural roots (Leininger, 1996).
- Assess for the presence of specific culture-bound syndromes that may manifest as disturbances in energy or spirit.
  Voodoo death, evil eye, and trance dissociation are some of the culture-bound syndromes that have symptoms of disharmony of mind and spirit (Arnault, 1998).
- Validate the client's feelings and concerns related to sense of disharmony or energy disturbance.
  Validation lets the client know that the nurse has heard and understands what was said, and it promotes the nurse-client relationship (Stuart, Laraia, 2001; Giger, Davidhizar, 1995).

Home Care Interventions

See Guidelines for Therapeutic Touch.

- Help the client and family accept therapeutic touch as a healing intervention.
  Consultation and collaboration with a specialist may be the best approach to nursing care. Numerous studies have reported positive outcomes of Healing Touch as a noninvasive complementary therapy (Umbreit, 2000).
- Assist the family with providing an appropriate space in which therapeutic touch can be administered.

Client/Family Teaching

- Teach the TT process to family members.
  Family members can use this skill to assist with care and comfort of the client. It helps people move to a higher level of self-care by putting them back in control of their own health and well-being. This health maintenance technique can be used anytime, anywhere, for self and others (Gottesman, 1992). TT enables caregivers to embrace their compassion and to touch people with effect (Dalglish, 1999).
- Teach that when working with the very young, old, or ill, or in the head area, TT should be gentle and used only for short periods.
  Under these circumstances the client is particularly sensitive to TT (Boguslawski, 1980; Borelli, Heidt, 1981). Exercise caution when using TT with patients who may exhibit an extreme sensitivity to the process (e.g., premature infants, frail elderly, psychotic clients) (Sayer-Adams, 1994).
- Teach client how to use guided imagery.
  The nurse can facilitate healing by helping the client recontact and reclaim parts of the self (resolve energy disturbance) through guided imagery (Rancour, 1994).
- Teach client to to use deep breating to relax. Ask client to have the disease, affected organ, or symptom assume an image. After the image has been identified, ask client to speak with the image to address an unresolved issue.
  By describing a previously unacknowledged part of the self, liberated energy can transform resistance, defenses, and disease into self-acceptance, peace, and wholeness (Remen, 1994).

WEB SITES FOR EDUCATION

MERLIN   See the MERLIN web site for World Wide Web resources for client education.

• = **Independent;** ▲ = **Collaborative**

REFERENCES   Arnault DS: Framework for culturally relevant psychiatric nursing. In Varcarolis EM, editor: *Foundations of psychiatric mental health nursing* ed 3, Philadelphia, 1998, WB Saunders, pp 133-140.

Boguslawski M: Therapeutic touch: a facilitator of pain relief, *Top Clin Nurs* 2:27, 1980.

Borelli M, Heidt P: *Therapeutic touch: a book of readings,* New York, 1981, Springer.

Dalglish S: Therapeutic touch in an acute care community hospital, *Can Nurse* 95(3):57-58, 1999.

Giger JN, Davidhizar RE: *Transcultural nursing,* ed 2, St Louis, 1995, Mosby.

Gottesman C: Energy balancing through touch for health, *J Holistic Nurs* 10(4):306, 1992.

Hayes J, Cox C: The experience of therapeutic touch from a nursing perspective, *Br J Nurs* 8(18):1249, 1999.

Jurgens A, Meehan T, Wilson H: Therapeutic touch as a nursing intervention, *Holistic Nurse Pract* 2:1, 1987.

Krieger D: *The therapeutic touch: how to use your hands to heal,* Englewood Cliffs, NJ, 1979, Prentice Hall.

Kunz D, Krieger D: Annual invitational workshops on therapeutic touch, Graysville, NY, 1975-1990, Pumpkin Hollow Foundation.

Leininger MM: *Transcultural nursing: theories, research and practices,* ed 2, Hilliard, Ohio, 1996, McGraw-Hill.

Meehan T: Therapeutic touch. In Bulechek G, McCloskey J: *Nursing interventions: essential nursing treatments,* Philadelphia, 1992, JB Lippincott.

Meehan T: Therapeutic touch as a nursing intervention, *J Adv Nurs* 28(1):117, 1998.

Mornhinweg G: Energy field disturbance validation study, *Healing Touch Newsletter* 6:11, 1996.

Rancour P: Interactive guided imagery with oncology patients, *J Holistic Nurs* 12:149, 1994.

Remen N: Psychosynthesis and healing, *J Holistic Nurs* 12:150, 1994.

Sayer-Adams J: Complementary therapies: therapeutic touch nursing function, *Nurs Standard* 8:25, 1994.

Stuart GW, Laraia MT: Therapeutic nurse-patient relationship. In Stuart GW, Laraia MT, editors: *Principles and practice of psychiatric nursing,* St Louis, 2001, Mosby, p 30.

Umbreit AW: Healing touch: applications in the acute care setting, *AACN Clin Issues* 11(1):105-119, 2000.

Impaired Environmental interpretation syndrome

Betty J. Ackley and Nancy English

NANDA   **Definition**   Consistent lack of orientation to person, place, time, or circumstances for more than 3 to 6 months, necessitating a protective environment

Defining Characteristics

Chronic confusional states; consistent disorientation in known and unknown environments; loss of occupation or social functioning resulting from memory decline; slow to respond to questions; inability to follow simple directions/instructions, concentrate, or reason

Related Factors (r/t)

Depression; dementia (e.g., Alzheimer's, multi-infarct, Pick's disease, AIDS, Parkinson's disease, alcoholism)

NOC   **Outcomes (Nursing Outcomes Classification)**

Suggested NOC Labels

Cognitive Orientation; Concentration; Information Processing; Memory; Neurological Status: Consciousness

> **Example NOC Outcome**
> Improves **Concentration** as evidenced by the following indicators: Maintains focus without being distracted/Responds appropriately to visual cues/Responds appropriately to language cues/Draws a circle (on command)/Drawns a pentagon (on command) (Rate each indicator of **Concentration:** 1 = never demonstrated, 2 = rarely demonstrated, 3 = sometimes demonstrated, 4 = often demonstrated, 5 = consistently demonstrated [see Section I])

• = Independent; ▲ = Collaborative

Client Outcomes

- Remains content and free from harm
- Functions at maximal cognitive level
- Independently participates in activities of daily living (ADLs) at the maximum of functional ability

 Interventions (Nursing Interventions Classification)

Suggested NIC Labels

Dementia Management; Environmental Management; Reality Orientation; Surveillance: Safety

> **Example NIC Interventions—Dementia Management**
> - Encourage client to verbalize memories of loss, both past and current
> - Help client to identify personal coping strategies

Nursing Interventions and Rationales, Home Care Interventions, Client/Family Teaching, Web Sites For Education

See care plan for **Chronic Confusion**.

Adult Failure to thrive

Gail B. Ladwig

NANDA **Definition** Progressive functional deterioration of a physical and cognitive nature with remarkably diminished ability to live with multisystem diseases, cope with ensuing problems, and manage care

Defining Characteristics

Anorexia—does not eat meals when offered; states does not have an appetite, is not hungry, or "I don't want to eat"; inadequate nutritional intake—eating less than body requirements; consumption of minimal to no food at most meals (i.e., consumes less than 75% of normal requirements); weight loss (from baseline weight)—5% unintentional weight loss in 1 month or 10% unintentional weight loss in 6 months; physical decline (decline in bodily function)—evidence of fatigue, dehydration, incontinence of bowel and bladder; frequent exacerbations of chronic health problems (e.g., pneumonia, urinary tract infections); cognitive decline (decline in mental processing) as evidenced by problems with responding appropriately to environmental stimuli, demonstrated difficulty in reasoning, decision making, judgment, memory, and concentration; decreased perception; decreased social skills; social withdrawal—noticeable decrease from usual past behavior in attempts to form or participate in cooperative and interdependent relationships (e.g., decreased verbal communication with staff, family, friends); decreased participation in ADLs that the older person once enjoyed; self-care deficit—no longer looks after or takes charge of physical cleanliness or appearance; difficulty performing simple self-care tasks; neglect of home environment and/or financial responsibilities; apathy as evidenced by lack of observable feeling or emotion in terms of normal ADLs

• = Independent; ▲ = Collaborative

and environment; altered mood state—expresses feelings of sadness, being low in spirit; expresses loss of interest in pleasurable outlets such as food, sex, work, friends, family, hobbies, or entertainment; verbalizes desire for death

Related Factors (r/t)

Depression; apathy; fatigue

NOC **Outcomes (Nursing Outcomes Classification)**

Suggested NOC Labels

Physical Aging Status; Psychosocial Adjustment: Life Change; Will to Live

> **Example NOC Outcome**
> Demonstrates **Will to Live** as evidenced by the following indicators: Expression of determination to live/Expression of hope/Use of strategies to compensate for problems associated with disease (Rate each indicator of **Will to Live:** 1 = extremely compromised, 2 = substantially compromised, 3 = moderately compromised, 4 = mildly compromised, 5 = not compromised [see Section I])

Client Outcomes

- Resumes highest level of functioning possible
- Consumes adequate dietary intake for weight and height
- Maintains usual weight
- Has adequate fluid intake with no signs of dehydration
- Participates in ADLs
- Participates in social interactions
- Maintains clean personal and home environment
- Expresses feelings associated with losses

NIC **Interventions (Nursing Interventions Classification)**

Suggested NIC Labels

Hope Instillation; Mood Management; Self-Care Assistance

> **Example NIC Interventions—Hope Installation**
> - Help client/family to identify areas of hope in life
> - Involve the client actively in own care

Nursing Interventions and Rationales

▲ Elderly clients who have failure to thrive (FTT) should be evaluated by review of the patient's ADLs, cognitive function, and mood; a targeted history and physical examination; and selected laboratory studies.
Early recognition and management of FTT can reduce the risk of further functional deterioration, hospitalization, or nursing home placement (Palmer, Foley, 1990).

▲ Assess possible causes for adult FTT and treat any underlying problems such as depression, malnutrition, and illnesses that are caused by physical and cognitive changes.
The characteristics of FTT in the elderly are malnutrition (undernutrition), loss of physical and cognitive function, and depression (Groom, 1993). Malnutrition is a frequent condition, both widely represented in the geriatric population and underestimated in diagnostic and therapeutic work-up, and is known to affect health status and life expectancy of elderly people (Vetta et al, 1999). An initial clinical assessment that combines multiple

• = Independent; ▲ = Collaborative

and varied sources of information is recommended to evaluate patients with suspected dementia (U.S. Department of Health and Human Services, 1996).

▲ Assess for signs of fatigue and sensory changes that may indicate an infection is present that may be related to undetected diabetes mellitus.
Older adults may never exhibit the classic signs of polyuria, polydipsia, polyphagia, and weight loss; instead they may develop an infection and complain of fatigue and sensory changes (Faherty, 1994).

▲ Assess for all etiologies including depression using a geriatric depression scale. Be alert for depression in clients newly admitted to nursing homes.
The geriatric depressions scale is recommended to determine the presence of depression (Jamison, 1997). Depression in newly admitted nursing home residents is a frequently overlooked area of nursing concern (Ryden et al, 1998). New depression may be the first sign of impending cognitive dysfunction (Sarkisian, Lachs, 1996).

• Note if the client is irritable and is blaming others.
Recent findings in nursing research support the presence of these behaviors as symptomatic of depression (Proffitt, Augspurger, Byrne, 1996).

▲ Provide cognitive therapy for clients who are identified as depressed. Reinforce their value as a person and provide reality as to "who they really are."
Clients who are depressed can be helped by examining "who they are" as compared to "who they believe they are" (Drake, Price, Drake, 1996).

• Instill hope and encourage the expression of positive thoughts.
The findings from this study of 1002 older disabled women suggest that positive emotions can protect older persons against adverse health outcomes. Of the women studied, 351 were described as emotionally vital, and among the women without a specific disability at baseline, emotional vitality was associated with a significantly decreased risk for incident disability performing ADLs (RR = 0.81, 95% CI = 0.66-0.99), for incident disability walking ¼ mile (RR = 0.73, 95% CI = 0.59-0.92), and for incident disability lifting/carrying 10 pounds (RR = 0.77, 95% CI = 0.63-0.95). Emotional vitality was also associated with a lower risk of dying (RR = 0.56, 95% CI = 0.39-0.80). These results were not simply caused by the absence of depression because protective health effects remained when emotionally vital women were compared with 334 women who were not emotionally vital and not depressed (Penninx et al, 2000).

• Monitor elderly client's weight and note any unexplained weight loss.
The FTT of an elderly client is usually accompanied by weight loss that occurs without immediate explanation (Palmer, Foley, 1990).

• Play soothing music during mealtimes to increase the amount of food eaten.
One study suggested that dinner music, particularly soothing music, can reduce irritability, fear, panic, and depressed mood and can stimulate the appetite of demented patients in a nursing home. In this study the patients were less irritable, anxious, and depressed during the periods when music was playing (Ragneskog et al, 1996).

• Note changes in the elderly client's appetite and assess for depression.
Depression can lead to FTT by two routes: a direct path of decreased appetite as a symptom of depression and an indirect path of increasing disability as an effect of depression (Katz, DiFilippo, 1997).

• Offer comfort foods and happy hour: foods associated with bygone years, intended to trigger recollections of pleasant childhood experiences and feelings of caring and healing, and a "happy hour" beverage, presented in a social milieu.

• = Independent; ▲ = Collaborative

These are two approaches that have demonstrated effectiveness in stimulating oral intake in the FTT client (Wood, Vogen, 1998).

- Provide appropriate nutrition for the client whose obesity may be affecting physical performance and thus has limited ability to perform ADLs, which leads to functional dependence.
  Malnutrition includes obesity (overnutrition); obesity among older persons is defined as being ≥30% above ideal body weight. Obesity may contribute to the previously mentioned problems (Still, Apovian, Jensen, 1997).

- Encourage clients to reminiscence about past experiences.
  Reminiscing helps to foster social relatedness (Jamison, 1997). A standard reminiscence interview and one that focused on successfully met challenges reduced state anxiety and enhanced coping self-efficacy (Rybarczyk, Auerbach, 1990).

- Encourage clients to pray if they wish.
  Various studies have discovered that various groups of people have used prayer for managing their symptoms of aging or illness (Meraviglia, 1999).

- Encourage elderly clients to interact with others on a regular basis. Have them participate in activities for seniors in their community.
  FTT of an elderly client is usually accompanied by social withdrawal (Palmer, Foley, 1990).

- Help clients to participate in activities by assessing motivation and helping them to identify reasons to participate such as better mobility, more independence, feelings of well-being.
  Motivation has been identified as an important factor in the older adult's ability to perform functional activities (Resnick, 1998).

- Provide physical touch for clients. Touch their hand or arm when speaking with them; offer hugs with permission.
  Touch helps with integration and fosters social relatedness. Tactile stimulation benefits the older adult's psychological well-being (Jamison, 1997).

- Administer therapeutic touch (TT).
  Results of this study of (n = 16) patients in the advanced stages of dementia of the Alzheimer's type (DAT), showed that discomfort levels decreased significantly after five therapeutic touch sessions, becoming significantly lower than levels in the control group (n = 10) (Giasson et al, 1999).

- Refer to care plans for **Imbalanced Nutrition: less than body requirements, Hopelessness,** and **Disturbed Energy field.**

Multicultural

- Assess for the influence of cultural beliefs, norms, and values on the family's or caregiver's understanding of FTT.
  What the family considers normal and abnormal health behavior may be based on cultural perceptions (Leininger, 1996).

- Validate the family's feelings and concerns related to the FTT symptoms.
  Validation lets the family know that the nurse has heard and understands what was said, and it promotes the nurse-client relationship (Stuart, Laraia, 2001; Giger, Davidhizar, 1995).

Home Care Interventions

- Assess and track areas of decreased functioning resulting from failure to thrive. Ensure that all symptomatology is considered for necessary action.
  Clients may change response to stressors/needs with changes in environment or interventions.

- = **Independent;** ▲ = **Collaborative**

- Give permission for role activity changes. Negotiate and clarify role expectations and reevaluate as necessary.
  Failure to thrive may require an extended period of recovery. Chronic illness often requires role changes to preserve a functional unit. Comfort level with role activities supports continued recovery.
- Provide support for family/caregivers.
  Support for caregivers decreases caregiver burden.
- ▲ Refer to medical social services or mental health counseling and/or community support groups. If necessary, contract with client to attend sessions.
  Counseling support can increase coping ability; group participation provides support and offers new problem-solving strategies to the client.
- ▲ Refer to home health aide services for assistance with ADLs throughout the duration of decreased participation.
  Maintaining ADLs and the integrity of the environment prevents further decline in status of those areas and decreases frustration as the client recovers and resumes responsibility for them.

Client/Family Teaching

- If adult FTT is related to dementia, help the caregiver to understand the diagnosis and help to identify needs that the caregiver will have to assist client with, such as nutrition, maintenance of adequate fluid intake, toileting, self-care, and safety.
  When the etiology of adult FTT is dementia, the caregiver needs to be educated on how to handle (Jamison, 1997).
- Instruct the family on the use of verbal cues to encourage eating, such as "Pick up your spoon; use the spoon to scoop up the pudding; now put the spoon with the pudding in your mouth."
  Verbal cueing is effective for improving nutritional status (Jamison, 1997).
- ▲ Discuss the possibility with the physician of a drug holiday when the etiology is delirium.
  Delirium may resolve with a drug holiday (Jamison, 1997).
- ▲ Provide referral for evaluation of hearing and appropriate hearing aids.
  This study of 60 subjects >65 years of age (mean age 79 years) living in nursing homes demonstrated that hearing loss affects the communication, sociability, and psychological aspects of quality of life (Tsuruoka et al, 2001).
- ▲ Refer for psychotherapy and possible medication if the etiology is depression.
  Treatment of the etiology is necessary; the previously mentioned are treatments that may be used for depression (Jamison, 1997).

WEB SITES FOR EDUCATION

$MERLIN See the MERLIN web site for World Wide Web resources for client education.

REFERENCES Drake RE, Price JL, Drake RE: Helping depressed clients discover personal power, *Perspect Psychiatr Care* 32(4):30, 1996.
Faherty B: Myths and facts about older adults, *Nursing 1994* 24(4):75, 1994.
Giger JN, Davidhizar RE: *Transcultural nursing*, ed 2, St Louis, 1995, Mosby.
Giasson M et al: Therapeutic touch, *Infirm Que* 6(6):38-47, 1999.
Groom DD: Elder care: a diagnostic model for failure to thrive, *J Gerontol Nurs* 19:6, 1993.
Jamison M: Failure to thrive in older adults, *J Gerontol Nurs* 23(2):13, 1997.

• = Independent; ▲ = Collaborative

Katz IR, DiFilippo S: Neuropsychiatric aspects of failure to thrive in late life, *Clin Geriatr Med* 13:4, 1997.

Leininger MM: *Transcultural nursing: theories, research and practices,* ed 2, Hilliard, Ohio, 1996, McGraw-Hill.

Meraviglia M: Critical analysis of spirituality and its empirical indicators, prayer and meaning in life, *J Holistic Nurs* 17(1):18, 1999.

Palmer RM, Foley JM: Failure to thrive in the elderly: diagnosis and management, *Geriatrics* 45:9, 1990.

Penninx BW et al: The protective effect of emotional vitality on adverse health outcomes in disabled older women, *J Am Geriatr Soc* 48(11):1359-1366, 2000.

Proffitt C, Augspurger P, Byrne M: Geriatric depression: a survey of nurses' knowledge and assessment practices, *Issues Ment Health Nurs* 17(2):123, 1996.

Ragneskog H et al: Influence of dinner music on food intake and symptoms common in dementia, *Scand J Caring Sci* 10(1):11, 1996.

Resnick B: Functional performance of older adults in a long-term care setting, *Clin Nurs Res* 7(3):230, 1998.

Rybarczyk BD, Auerbach SM: Reminiscence interviews as stress management interventions for older patients undergoing surgery, *Gerontologist* 30(4):522, 1990.

Ryden MB et al: Assessment of depression in a population at risk newly admitted nursing home residents, *J Gerontol Nurs* 24(2):21, 1998.

Sarkisian C, Lachs M: "Failute to thrive" in older adults, *Ann Intern Med* 124(12):1072, 1996.

Still C, Apovian C, Jensen G: Failure to thrive in older adults, *Ann Intern Med* 126(8):668, 1997.

Stuart GW, Laraia MT: Therapeutic nurse-patient relationship. In Stuart GW, Laraia MT, editors: *Principles and practice of psychiatric nursing,* St Louis, 2001, Mosby, p 30.

Tsuruoka H et al: Hearing impairment and quality of life for the elderly in nursing homes, *Auris Nasus Larynx* 28(1):45-54, 2001.

U.S. Department of Health and Human Services: Recognition and initial assessment of Alzheimer's disease and related dementia, Clinical practice guideline No. 19 [302], Rockville, Md, 1996, Public Health Service, AHCPR.

Vetta F et al: The impact of malnutrition on the quality of life in the elderly, *Clin Nutr* 18(5):259, 1999.

Wood P, Vogen BD: Feeding the anorectic client: comfort foods and happy hour, *Geriatr Nurs* 19(4):192-194, 1998.

Risk for Falls

Betty J. Ackley and Teepa Snow

NANDA   **Definition** Increased susceptibility to falling that may cause physical harm

Risk Factors

Adults History of falls; wheelchair use; ≥65 years of age; female (if elderly); lives alone; lower limb prosthesis; use of assistive devices (e.g., walker, cane)

Physiological Presence of acute illness; postoperative conditions; visual difficulties; hearing difficulties; arthritis; orthostatic hypotension; sleeplessness; faintness when turning or extending neck; anemias; vascular disease; neoplasms (i.e., fatigue/limited mobility, urgency and/or incontinence, diarrhea, decreased lower extremity strength, posprandial blood sugar changes, foot problems, impaired physical mobility, impaired balance, difficulty with gait, unilateral neglect, proprioceptive deficits, neuropathy)

Cognitive Diminished mental status (e.g., confusion, delerium, dementia, impaired reality testing)

Medication Antihypertensive agents; ACE-inhibitors; diuretics; tricyclic antidepressants; alcohol use; antianxiety agents; opiates; hypnotics or tranquilizers

Environment Restraints; weather conditions (e.g., wet floors/ice); throw/scatter rugs; cluttered environment; unfamiliar, dimly lit room; no antislip material in bath and/or shower

• = Independent; ▲ = Collaborative

Children (<2 years of age)

Male gender when <1 year of age; lack of auto restraints; lack of gate on stairs; lack of window guard; bed located near window; unattended infant on bed/changing table/sofa; lack of parental supervision

Related Factors (r/t)

See Risk Factors.

NOC **Outcomes (Nursing Outcomes Classification)**

Suggested NOC Labels

Safety Behavior: Fall Prevention; Knowledge: Child Safety

> **Example NOC Outcome**
>
> Accomplishes **Safety Behavior: Fall Prevention** as evidenced by the following indicators: Correct use of assistive devices/Elimination of clutter, spills, glare from floors/Use of safe transfer procedures (Rate each indicator of **Safety Behavior: Fall Prevention:** 1 = not adequate, 2 = slightly adequate, 3 = moderately adequate, 4 = substantially adequate, 5 = totally adequate [see Section I])

Client Outcomes

- Remains free of falls
- Changes environment to minimize the incidence of falls
- Explains methods to prevent injury

NIC **Interventions (Nursing Interventions Classification)**

Suggested NIC Labels

Fall Prevention; Dementia Management; Surveillance: Safety

> **Example NIC Interventions—Fall Prevention**
> - Assist unsteady individual with ambulation.
> - Monitor gait, balance, and fatigue level with ambulation

Nursing Interventions and Rationales

- Determine risk of falling by using an evaluation tool such as the Fall Risk Assessment (Farmer, 2000), The Conley Scale (Conley, Schultz, Selvin, 1999), or the FRAINT Tool for fall risk assessment (Parker, 2000).
  Risk factors for falling include recent history of falls, confusion, depression, altered elimination patterns, cardiovascular/respiratory disease impairing perfusion or oxygenation, postural hypotension, dizziness or vertigo, primary cancer diagnosis, and altered mobility (Hendrich et al, 1995; Wilson, 1998; Farmer, 2000). Predictors of fall risk in the community included atrial fibrillation, neurological problems, living alone, and not adhering to a regular exercise program (Resnick, 1999).
- Screen all clients for stability and mobility skills (supine to sit, sitting supported and unsupported, sit to stand, standing, walking and turning around, transferring, stooping to floor and recovering, and sitting down). Use tools such as the Balance Scale by Tinetti or the Get Up and Go Scale by Mathais.
  It is helpful to determine the client's functional abilities and then plan for ways to improve problem areas or determine methods to ensure safety (Lewis et al, 1994; Macknight, Rockwood, 1996).
- Recognize that when people attend to another task while walking, such as carrying a

• = Independent; ▲ = Collaborative

cup of water, clothing, or supplies, they are more likely to fall.
Those who slow down when given a carrying task are at a higher risk for subsequent falls (Lundin-Olsson, Nysberg, Gustafson, 1998).

- Be careful when getting a mostly immobile client up. Be sure to lock the bed and wheelchair and have sufficient personnel to protect client from falls.
The most important preventative measure to reduce the risk of injurious falls for nonambulatory residents involves increasing safety measures while transferring, including careful locking of equipment such as wheelchairs and beds before moves (Thapa et al, 1996). These immobile clients commonly sustain the most serious injuries when they fall.

- Identify clients likely to fall by placing a "Fall Precautions" sign on the doorway and by keying the Kardex and chart. Use a "high-risk fall" arm band and room marker to alert staff for increased vigilance and mobility assistance.
These steps alert the nursing staff of the increased risk of falls (Cohen, Guin, 1991).

- If necesssary to place the client in a wrist or vest restraint, use increased vigilance and watch for falls.
The risk of falling is highest soon after a client has been placed in a mechanical restraint (Arbesman, Wright, 1999).

▲ Evaluate client's medications to determine whether medications increase the risk of falling; consult with physician regarding client's need for medication if appropriate.
Polypharmacy, or taking more than four medications, has been associated with increased falls. Medications increasing the risk of falls include diuretics, hypnotics, sedatives, opiates, antidepressants, and psychotropic and antihypertension agents (Wilson, 1998). Medications such as benzodiazapines and antipsychotic and antidepressant medications given to promote sleep actually increase the rate of falls (Capezuti, 1999b). Use of selective serotonin reuptake inhibitors and tricyclic antidepressants resulted in increased incidences of falls in a nursing home setting (Thapa et al, 1998; Liu et al, 1998).

- Thoroughly orient client to environment. Place call light within reach and show how to call for assistance; answer call light promptly.

- Use $1/4$- to $1/2$-length side rails only, and maintain bed in a low position. Ensure that wheels are locked on bed and commode. Keep dim light in room at night.
Use of full side rails can result in the client climbing over the rails, leading with the head, and sustaining a head injury. Siderails with widely spaced vetical bars and siderails not situated flush with the mattress have been associated with asphxiation deaths because of rail and in-bed entrapment and should not be used (Todd, Ruhl, Gross, 1997; Hanger, Ball, Wood, 1999; Capezuti, 1999a).

- Routinely assist client with toileting on his or her own schedule. Always take client to bathroom on awakening, before bedtime, and before administering sedatives (Wilson, 1998). Keep the path to the bathroom clear, label the bathroom, and leave the door open.
The majority of falls are related to toileting. It is more acceptable to fall than to "wet yourself." Studies have indicated that falls are often linked to the need to eliminate in a hurry (Cohen, Guin, 1991; Wilson, 1998).

▲ Avoid use of restraints; obtain a physician's order if restraints are necessary.
Restrained elderly clients often experience an increased number of falls, possibly as a result of muscle deconditioning or loss of coordination (Tinetti, Liu, Ginter, 1992; Wilson, 1998). If elderly clients are restrained and fall, they can sustain severe injuries, including strangulation, asphyxiation, or head injury from leading with their heads to get out of the bed (DiMaio, Dana, Bix, 1986; Evans, Strumpf, 1990). Restraint-free extended care

• = **Independent;** ▲ = **Collaborative**

facilities were shown to have fewer residents with activities of daily living (ADLs) deficiencies and fewer residents with bowel or bladder incontinence than facilities that use restraints (Castle, Fogel, 1998). Restraint use can lead to depression, anger, infection, pressure ulcers, deconditioning, and sometimes death (Rogers, Bocchino, 1999). The risk of falling is highest soon after a client is placed in a mechanical restraint (Arbesman, Wright, 1999). No differences in nighttime fall rates was shown between a group that was restrained versus a similar group that was not restrained (Capezuti et al, 1999b).

- In place of restraints, use the following:
  - Alarm systems with ankle, above the knee, or wrist sensors
  - Bed or wheelchair alarms
  - Increased observation of client
  - Locked doors to unit
  - Low or very low height beds
  - Border-defining pillow/mattress to remind the client to stay in bed

  These alternatives to restraints can be helpful to prevent falls (Commodore, 1995; Wilson, 1998; Capezuti et al, 1999a).
- If client is extremely agitated, consider using a special safety bed that surrounds client. If client has a traumatic brain injury, use the Emory cubicle bed.

  Special beds can be an effective alternative to restraints and can help keep the client safe during periods of agitation (Williams, Morton, Patrick, 1990).
- If client has a new onset of confusion (delirium), provide reality orientation when interacting. Have family bring in familiar items, clocks, and watches from home to maintain orientation.

  *Reality orientation can help prevent or decrease the confusion that increases risk of falling for clients with delirium. See interventions for **Acute Confusion.***
- If client has chronic confusion with dementia, use validation therapy that reinforces feelings but does not confront reality.

  *Validation therapy is for clients with dementia (Fine, Rouse-Bane, 1995). See Interventions for **Chronic Confusion.***
- Ask family to stay with client to prevent client from accidentally falling or pulling out tubes.
- If client is unsteady on feet, use a walking belt or two nursing staff members when ambulating the client.

  The client can walk independently with a walking belt, but the nurse can rapidly ensure safety if the knees buckle.
- Place a fall-prone client in a room that is near the nurses' station.

  Such placement allows more frequent observation of the client.
- Help clients sit in a stable chair with arm rests. Avoid use of wheelchairs and geri-chairs except for transportation as needed.

  Clients are likely to fall when left in a wheelchair or geri-chair because they may stand up without locking the wheels or removing the footrests. Wheelchairs do not increase mobility; people just sit in them the majority of the time (Lipson, Braun, 1993; Simmons et al, 1995).
- Ensure that the chair or wheelchair fits the build, abilities, and needs of the client to ensure propulsion with legs or arms and ability to reach the floor, eliminating footrests and minimizing problems with shearing.

  The seating system should fit the needs of the client so that the client can move the wheels, stand up from the chair without falling, and not be harmed by the chair. Footrests can

• = Independent; ▲ = Collaborative

cause skin tears and bruising, as well as postural alignment and sitting posture problems (Lipson, Braun, 1993; Rader, Jones, Miller, 2000).

- Avoid use of wheelchairs as much as possible because they can serve as a restraint device. Most people in wheelchairs do not move.
  Wheelchairs unfortunately serve as a restraint device. A study has shown that only 4% of residents in wheelchairs were observed to propel them independently and only 45% could propel them, even with cues and prompts. Another study showed that no residents could unlock wheelchairs without help, the wheelchairs were not fitted to residents, and residents were not trained in propulsion (Simmons et al, 1995).
- ▲ Refer to physical therapy for strengthening exercises and gait training to increase mobility.
  Gait training in physical therapy has been shown to be effective for preventing falls (Galinda-Ciocon, Ciocon, Galinda, 1995; Wilson, 1998).

Geriatric

- Encourage client to wear glasses and use walking aids when ambulating.
- Help the client obtain and wear a specially designed hip protector when ambulating. Hip protectors are worn in a specially designed stretchy undergarment containing a pocket on each side for placement of the protector.
  The risk of a hip fracture in the elderly can be reduced by use of an anatomically designed external hip protector when ambulating (Kannus et al, 2000).
- Consider use of a "Merri-walker" adult walker that surrounds body if client is mobile but unsafe because of wobbling.
- If client experiences dizziness because of orthostatic hypotension when getting up, teach methods to decrease dizziness, such as rising slowly, remaining seated several minutes before standing, flexing feet upward several times while sitting, sitting down immediately if feeling dizzy, and trying to have someone present when standing.
  The elderly develop decreased baroreceptor sensitivity and decreased ability of compensatory mechanisms to maintain blood pressure when standing up, resulting in postural hypotension (Aaronson, Carlon-Wolfe, Schoener, 1991; Matteson, McConnell, Linton, 1997).
- ▲ If client is experiencing syncope, determine symptoms that occur before syncope, and note medications that client is taking. Refer for medical care.
  The circumstances surrounding syncope often suggest the cause. Use of many medications, including diuretics, antihypertensives, digoxin, beta-blockers, and calcium channel blockers can cause syncope. Use of the tilt table can be diagnostic in incidences of syncope (Cox, 2000).
- ▲ Refer to physical therapy for strength training, using free weights or machines.
  Strength improvement in response to resisted exercise is possible even in the very elderly, extremely sedentary client, with multiple chronic diseases and functional disabilities. Increased strength can help prevent falls (Connelly, 2000).

Home Care Interventions

- If client was identified as a fall risk in the hospital, recognize that there is a high incidence of falls after discharge, and use all measures possible to reduce the incidence of falls.
  The rate of falls is substantially increased in the geriatric client who has been recently hospitalized, especially during the first month after discharge (Mahoney et al, 2000).
- Assess home environment for threats to safety: clutter, slippery floors, scatter rugs, unsafe stairs and stairwells, blocked entries, dim lighting, extension cords (across pathway), high beds, pets, and pet excrement. Use antiskid acrylic floor wax, nonskid rugs, and skid-proof strips near the bed to prevent slippage.

• = **Independent**; ▲ = **Collaborative**

Clients suffering from impaired mobility, impaired visual acuity, and neurological dysfunction, including dementia and other cognitive functional deficits, are all at risk for injury from common hazards.

▲ Instruct client and family or caregivers on how to correct identified hazards. Refer to occupational therapy services for assistance if needed. Notify landlord or code enforcement office of structural building hazards as necessary.

• If client is at risk for falls, use gait belt and additional persons when ambulating. *Gait belts decrease the risk of falls during ambulation.*

• Install motion sensitive lighting that turns on automatically when the client gets out of bed to go to the bathroom.

• Have client wear supportive low heeled shoes with good traction when ambulating. *Supportive shoes provide the client with better balance and protect the client from instability on uneven surfaces.*

▲ Refer to physical therapy services for client and family education of safe transfers and ambulation and for strengthening exercises (for client) for ambulation and transfers.

• Provide a signaling device for clients who wander or are at risk for falls. If client lives alone, provide a Lifeline or similar call device. *Orienting a vulnerable client to a safety net relieves anxiety of the client and caregiver and allows for rapid response to a crisis situation.*

• Provide medical identification bracelet for clients at risk for injury from dementia, seizures, or other medical disorders.

Client/Family Teaching

• Teach client how to safely ambulate at home, including using safety measures such as hand rails in bathroom.

• Teach client the importance of maintaining a regular exercise program such as walking. *Lack of a consistent exercise program was one of the variables associated with a higher incidence of falls (Resnick, 1999).*

WEB SITES FOR EDUCATION

MERLIN See the MERLIN web site for World Wide Web resources for client education.

REFERENCES Aaronson L, Carlon-Wolfe W, Schoener S: Pressures that fall on rising, *Geriatr Nurs* 12:67, 1991.

Arbesman MD, Wright C: Mechanical restraints, rehabilitation therapies, and staffing adequacy as risk factors for falls in an elderly hospitalized population, *Rehabil Nurs* 24(3):122-128, 1999.

Capezuti E et al: Individualized interventions to prevent bed-related falls and reduce siderail use, *J Gerontol Nurs* 25(11):26-34, 1999a.

Capezuti E et al: Outcomes of nighttime physical restraint removal for severely impaired nursing home residents, *Am J Alzheimers Dis* 14(3):157-164, 1999b.

Castle NG, Fogel B: Characteristics of nursing homes that are restraint free, *Gerontologist* 38(2):181-188, 1998.

Cohen L, Guin P: Implementation of a patient fall prevention program, *J Neurosci Nurs* 23:315, 1991.

Commodore DI: Falls in the elderly population: a look at incidence, risks, healthcare costs, and preventive strategies, *Rehabil Nurs* 20:84, 1995.

Conley D, Schultz AA, Selvin R: The challenge of predicting patients at risk for falling: development of the Conley Scale, *MedSurg Nurs* 8(6):348-355, 1999.

Connelly DM: Resisted exercise training of institutionalized older adults for improved strength and functional mobility: a review, *Topics Geriatr Rehabil* 15(3):6-28, 2000.

Cox MM: Uncovering the cause of syncope, *Patient Care* 30:39-60, 2000.

DiMaio V, Dana S, Bix R: Death caused by restraint vests, *JAMA* 255:905, 1986.

• = Independent; ▲ = Collaborative

Evans L, Strumpf N: Myths about elder restraint, *Image J Nurs Sch* 22:124, 1990.

Farmer BC: Try this: fall risk assessment, *J Gerontol Nurs* 26(7):6-7, 2000.

Fine JI, Rouse-Bane S: Using validating techniques to improve communication with cognitively impaired older adults, *J Gerontol Nurs* 21:39, 1995.

Galinda-Ciocon DJ, Ciocon JO, Galinda DJ: Gait training and falls in the elderly, *J Gerontol Nurs* 21:11, 1995.

Hanger HC, Ball MC, Wood LA: An analysis of falls in the hospital: can we do without bedrails? *J Am Geriatr Soc* 47(5):529-531, 1999.

Hendrich A et al: Hospital falls: development of a predictive model for clinical practice, *Appl Nurs Res* 8:129, 1995.

Kannus P et al: Prevention of hip fracture in elderly people with use of a hip protector, *New Engl J Med* 343(21):1506-1513, 2000.

Lewis BJ et al: *The functional tool book,* Washington, DC, 1994, Learn.

Lipson J, Braun S: *Toward a restraint-free environment: reducing the use of physical and chemical restraint in long-term care and acute settings,* Baltimore, 1993, Health Professions Press.

Liu et al: Use of selective serotonin-reuptake inhibitors of tricyclic antidepressants and risk for hip fractures in elderly people, *Lancet* 351, 1998.

Lundin-Olsson L, Nysberg L, Gustafson Y: Attention, frailty, and falls: the effect of a manual task on basic mobility, *J Am Geriatr Soc* 46:758-761, 1998.

MacKnight C, Rockwood K: Mobility and balance in the elderly: a guide to bedside assessment, *Postgrad Med* 99(3):269-271, 275-276, 1996.

Mahoney JE et al: Temporal association between hospitalization and rate of falls after discharge, *Arch Intern Med* 160(18):2788-2795, 2000.

Matteson MA, McConnell ES, Linton AD: *Gerontological nursing,* ed 2, Philadelphia, 1997, WB Saunders.

Parker R: Assessing the risk of falls among older inpatients, *Professional Nurse* 15(8):511-514, 2000.

Rader J, Jones D, Miller L: The importance of individualized wheelchair seating for frail older adults, *J Gerontol Nurs* 26(11):24-47, 2000.

Resnick B: Falls in a community of older adults, *Clin Nurs Res* 8(3):251-265, 1999.

Rogers PD, Bocchino NL: Restraint free care—is it possible? *Am J Nurs* 99(10):27-33, 1999.

Simmons S et al: Wheelchairs as mobility restraints: predictors of wheelchair activity in nonambulatory nursing home residents, *J Am Geriatr Soc* 43:384, 1995.

Thapa P et al: Injurious falls in nonambulatory nursing home residents: a comparative study of circumstances, incidence, and risk factors, *J Am Geriatr Soc* 44:273-278, 1996.

Thapa et al: Antidepressants and the risk of falls among nursing home residents, *N Engl J Med* 339, 1998.

Tinetti ME, Liu WL, Ginter SF: Mechanical restraint use and fall-related injuries among residents of skilled nursing facilities, *Ann Intern Med* 116:369-374, 1992.

Todd JF, Ruhl CE, Gross TP: Injury and death associated with hospital bed side-rails: reports of the US Food and Drug Administration from 1985 to 1995, *Am J Public Health* 87(10):1675-1677, 1997.

Williams LM, Morton GA, Patrick CH: The Emory cubicle bed: an alternative to restraints for agitated traumatically brain injured clients, *Rehabil Nurs* 15:30, 1990.

Wilson EB: Preventing patient falls, *AACN Clin Issues* 9(1):100-108, 1998.

Dysfunctional Family processes: alcoholism

Jane Maria Curtis and Gail Ladwig

 Definition The state in which the psychosocial, spiritual, and physiological functions of the family unit are chronically disorganized, leading to conflict, denial of problems, resistance to change, ineffective problem solving, and a series of self-perpetuating crises

Defining Characteristics
Roles and Relationships

Inconsistent parenting/low perception of parental support; ineffective spouse communication/marital problems; intimacy dysfunction; deterioration in family

• = Independent; ▲ = Collaborative

relationships/disturbed family dynamics; altered role function/disruption of family roles; closed communication systems; chronic family problems; family denial; lack of cohesiveness; neglected obligations; lack of skills necessary for relationships; reduced ability of family members to relate to each other for mutual growth and maturation; family unable to meet security needs of its members; disrupted family rituals; economic problems; family does not demonstrate respect for individuality and autonomy of its members; triangulating family relationships; pattern of rejection

Behavioral   Refusal to get help/inability to accept and receive help appropriately; inadequate understanding or knowledge of alcoholism; ineffective problem-solving skills; loss of control of drinking; manipulation; rationalization/denial of problems; blaming; inability to meet emotional needs of its members; alcohol abuse; broken promises; criticizing; dependency; impaired communication; difficulty with intimate relationships; enabling to maintain drinking; expression of anger inappropriately; isolation; inability to meet spiritual needs of its members; inability to express or accept wide ranges of feelings; inability to deal with traumatic experiences constructively; inability to adapt to change; immaturity; harsh self-judgment; lying; lack of dealing with conflict; lack of reliability; nicotine addiction; orientation toward tension relief rather than achievement of goals; seeking approval and affirmation; difficulty having fun; agitation; chaos; contradictory, paradoxical communication; diminished physical contact; disturbances in academic performance in children; disturbances in concentration; escalating conflict; failure to accomplish current or past developmental tasks/difficulty with life cycle transitions; family special occasions are alcohol centered; controlling communication/power struggles; self-blaming; stress-related physical illnesses; substance abuse other than alcohol; unresolved grief; verbal abuse of spouse or parent

Feelings   Insecurity; lingering resentment; mistrust; vulnerability; rejection; repressed emotions; responsibility for alcoholic's behavior; shame/embarrassment; unhappiness; powerlessness; anger/suppressed rage; anxiety, tension, or distress; emotional isolation/loneliness; frustration; guilt; hopelessness; hurt; decreased self-esteem/worthlessness; hostility; lack of identity; fear; loss; emotional control by others; misunderstood; moodiness; abandonment; being different from other people; being unloved; confused love and pity; confusion; failure; depression; dissatisfaction

Related Factors (r/t)

Abuse of alcohol; genetic predisposition; lack of problem-solving skills; family history of alcoholism; resistance to treatment; biochemical influences; addictive personality

NOC   ## Outcomes (Nursing Outcomes Classification)

Suggested NOC Labels

Family Coping; Family Functioning; Family Health Status; Substance Addiction Consequences

> **Example NOC Outcome**
> Demonstrates **Family Coping** as evidenced by the following indicators: Confronts problems/Regulates behavior of members/Absence of substance abuse (Rate each indicator of **Family Coping:** 1 = never demonstrated, 2 = rarely demonstrated, 3 = sometimes demonstrated, 4 = often demonstrated, 5 = consistently demonstrated [see Section I])

• = Independent; ▲ = Collaborative

Client Outcomes
Family

- Develops relationship with nurse that demonstrates at least minimal level of trust
- Demonstrates an understanding of alcoholism as a family illness and the severity of the threat to emotional and physical health of family members
- Develops belief in feasibility and effectiveness of efforts to address alcoholism
- Begins to change dysfunctional patterns by moving from inappropriate to appropriate role relationships, improving cohesion among family members, decreasing conflict and social isolation, and improving coping behaviors
- Maintains improvements

NIC   Interventions (Nursing Interventions Classification)
Suggested NIC Labels
Family Process Maintenance; Substance Use Treatment

> **Example NIC Interventions—Family Process Maintenance**
> - Identify effects of role changes on family processes
> - Assist family members to use existing support measures
> - Encourage client to take control over own behavior
> - Help family members recognize that chemical dependency is a family disease
> - Identify support groups in the community for long-time substance abuse treatment

Nursing Interventions and Rationales

- Demonstrate high levels of empathy and expectancy of positive outcomes in interactions with family members.

  Empathy as evidenced by respect, warmth, sympathetic understanding, supportiveness, caring, concern, commitment, and interest has been found to be the most important caregiver trait that affects motivation for treatment among alcoholic clients. The client's perception that the caregiver wants to help and that a positive outcome can be achieved increases commitment and willingness to be influenced (Miller, 1985). A Swiss campaign used a short intervention approach that focused on an empathic and open discussion of drinking habits. This approach is efficient; takes little time; and, for nondependent patients, can considerably reduce the quantity of alcohol consumed (Stoll, Wick, 2000).

- When completing a family assessment, include demographic data, physical and emotional health of individuals, current family structure and roles, communication patterns, relationships among members, current stressors and conflicts, family cohesion, coping behaviors, shared interests and activities, resources and supports, knowledge of the problem, and expectations for recovery.

  Assessment factors are included under interventions because it has been noted that assessment questions initiate a family process of self-examination and family problem solving and also provide assessment data (Craft, Willadsen, 1992). Most families are not aware of their adjustment to the addictive behavior, and family structure and function may be altered (e.g., a child assumes a parent's role in absence of parent appropriateness). In addition, individual family members or the family unit itself may be experiencing biological, cognitive, or spiritual responses that require separate interventions (American Nurses Association, 1987; Captain, 1989). The range of possible nursing interventions required for family members is extremely broad; the nurse is advised to consult the Standards of Addictions Nursing for assistance (American Nurses Association, 1987).

• = Independent; ▲ = Collaborative

- Screen clients for at-risk drinking during routine primary care visits. At-risk drinking is defined as consuming an average of two or more drinks per day (chronic drinking), or two or more occasions of consuming five or more drinks in the past month (binge drinking), or, in the past month, one or more occasion of driving after consuming three or more drinks (drinking and driving).

  At least one in ten patients making routine primary care visits have drinking practices that place them at risk for negative consequences from drinking. In this study, 3439 patients with advance appointments in 23 primary care practices completed a health survey before their visit (Curry et al, 2000).

- Educate family members about alcoholism, being careful not to label or stigmatize them.

  Children of alcoholics frequently build up defenses, shame, guilt, and loneliness. They need to be reassured that they did not cause the alcoholism and are not responsible for solving the problem. Labeling them may tend to draw attention away from cultural differences, customs, values, and beliefs that make the family and its members unique (SAMHSA's National Clearinghouse for Alcohol and Drug Information).

- Educate family members about available educational and support programs.

  A program aimed at early intervention and problem behaviors in preschool children in alcoholic families indicates that prevention programming is more appropriately family based rather than aimed at individuals (Nye, Zucker, Fitzgerald, 1999).

- Stress individual self-focus as a first step in problem resolution.

  Health Beliefs Model Research confirms that client understanding of the severity of the threat to personal and family health and a belief in the feasibility and effectiveness of treatment are important motivating factors in changing health-related behavior (Damrosch, 1991; Giuffra, 1993). Family members can benefit themselves, the family as a whole, and the client through self-focus and participation in education and support activities (Captain, 1989; Williams, 1989). The perception of choice enhances motivation and improves compliance and outcome (Miller, 1985).

- Help family to restructure family patterns of interaction and function to support the development of consistency, a predictable environment, emotional nurturance, and positive modeling.

  Studies indicate that consistency, a predictable environment, emotional nurturance, and positive social modeling may act as ameliorating factors in the dysfunctional environment (Roberts, 1992; Sielhamer, Jacob, Dunn, 1993). Clinical reports and research also indicate that recovery is partially contingent on the restructuring of family interaction patterns. In assisting the family, the generalist nurse becomes a role model, counselor, educator, and promoter of effective interactions, self-care, and referral sources by using principles of nursing care derived from medical, surgical, psychiatric, and community health nursing. The nurse specialist, who has had specialty training and advanced education, may serve as family therapist (American Nurses Association, 1987).

- Assist with stabilization and maintenance of positive change in the family. Instruct the alcoholic's family members before client's discharge to give verbal messages that convey concern about the alcoholic's problem drinking, their observations of the alcoholic's past episodes of drinking, and wishes and support for abstinence.

  This intervention method can help the alcoholic face the reality of his or her drinking problem and alcohol dependence and thus remain longer in long-range rehabilitation programs, which is a prerequisite for successful recovery from alcohol dependence. Patients'

• = Independent; ▲ = Collaborative

maintenance of abstinence was significantly better only when both they and their family members attended hospital outpatient follow-up sessions and/or self-help group meetings (Ino, Hayasida, 2000).

- Focus on the continued use of resources, which may become apparent as family dynamics change.
- To form a basis for realistic and objective evaluation of family changes, continue to provide education pertinent to the appropriate stage of family improvement.
- Support increasing social contacts and family recreational activities, and use contracting or homework assignment techniques to encourage positive behaviors.
- Monitor family closely for return to old patterns of behavior.

  The improvement of family interaction is an important condition for maintaining change. Family cohesion is fostered through the sharing of positive and fun experiences and is a critical factor in lasting recovery (Captain, 1989). A return to previous behavior patterns, termed relapse, occurs most frequently within the first 3 months. Factors that have been useful in relapse prevention are education, social support, skills training, reinforcement, recreational activities, and the practice of new behaviors (Jones, 1990). Continuation and compliance are behaviors that are influenced by maintaining contact with an empathetic caregiver (Miller, 1985). There is evidence that success is achieved only after several relapses, and the effort to succeed is enhanced by knowledge skills training, support and self-help groups, and other techniques (Damrosch, 1991).

- Provide activities that are physical in nature, such as adventure therapy and therapeutic camping, as part of a substance abuse treatment program.

  This study shows that the 10-month follow-up relapse rate was 31% for the experimental group and 58% for the comparison group. There were significant improvements in autonomic arousal, frequency of negative thoughts, and alcohol craving. These results add to the limited body of research supporting outdoor adventure and therapeutic camping experiences integrated with traditional relapse prevention activities as an adjunct to substance abuse treatment (Bennett, Cardone, Jarczyk, 1998).

- ▲ Refer for possible use of medications such as Disulfiram, Naltrexone, and Acamprosate to control problem drinking.

  Controlled clinical trials of Disulfiram reveal mixed findings. There is little evidence that Disulfiram enhances abstinence, but there is evidence that it reduces the number of drinking days. When measured, compliance is a strong predictor of outcome. Trials of Naltrexone in the treatment of alcoholism are recent and of generally good quality. There is good evidence that Naltrexone reduces relapse and number of drinking days in alcohol-dependent subjects. There is some evidence that Naltrexone reduces craving and enhances abstinence in alcohol-dependent subjects. There is good evidence that Naltrexone has a favorable harms profile. Trials of Acamprosate in alcohol dependence are large but limited to European populations. There is good evidence that Acamprosate enhances abstinence and reduces drinking days in alcohol-dependent subjects. There is minimal evidence for the effects of Acamprosate on craving or rates of severe relapse in alcohol-dependent subjects. There is good evidence that Acamprosate is reasonably well tolerated and without serious harm (Agency for Healthcare Research and Quality).

Geriatric

- Include assessment of possible alcohol abuse when assessing elderly family members.

  Alcohol abuse and alcoholism are common but under recognized problems among older adults. One third of older alcoholic persons develop a problem with alcohol in later life,

• = Independent; ▲ = Collaborative

while the other two thirds grow older with the medical and psychosocial sequelae of early-onset alcoholism (Rigler, 2000).

Multicultural

- Acknowledge racial/ethnic differences at the onset of care.
  Acknowledgement of race/ethnicity issues will enhance communication, establish rapport, and promote treatment outcomes (D'Avanzo et al, 2001).
- Approach families of color with respect, warmth, and professional courtesy.
  Instances of disrespect and lack of caring have special significance for families of color (D'Avanzo, 2001).
- Give rationale when assessing black families about alcohol use and misuse.
  Many blacks may expect white caregivers to hold negative and preconceived ideas. Giving a rationale for questions asked will help alleviate this perception (D'Avanzo et al, 2001).
- Use a family-centered approach when working with Latino, Asian, African-American, and Native American clients.
  Latinos may perceive family as a source of support, solver of problems, and source of pride. Asian Americans may regard the family as the primary decision-maker and influence on individual family members (D'Avanzo et al, 2001). Native American families may be extended structures that could exert powerful influences over functioning (Seiderman et al, 1996).
- When working with Asian clients, provide opportunities for the family to save face.
  This will allow the family to not have to own the shame of the alcohol problem. Asian families may avoid situations that bring shame on the family unit (D'Avanzo et al, 2001).

Home Care Interventions

NOTE: In the community setting, alcoholism as an etiology for dyfunctional family processes must be considered in two categories. The first is when the client suffers personally from the illness; the second is when a significant other suffers from the illness, that is, the client is not the active alcoholic but may be dependent on the alcoholic for caregiving. The listed considerations apply to both situations with appropriate adaptation for the circumstances.

- Identify client and family expectations of the home care nurse and nurse expectations of the client and family by use of a well-defined contract. Be specific and realistic. Adjust the contract only with clear consent and understanding of the client/family.
  A well-defined contract supports success in meeting goals and encourages positive family dynamics. A contract defines conditions under which care can be safely provided and under which care cannot continue. Safety of the staff should never be jeopardized.
- Establish well-defined contingency and emergency plans for the care of client.
  Clinical safety of the client between visits is a primary goal of the home care nurse (Stanhope, Lancaster, 1996).
- Request concrete, measurable tasks of client and family for caregiving.
- ▲ Refer for medical social work services at outset of care.
  The social worker can help identify, set the structure for, and guide appropriate client/family and client/family/nurse interactions that will promote the plan of care throughout the length of the stay.
- Acknowledge without judging when resolution of alcoholism is not a goal of care.
  It is usually not appropriate for terminally ill or hospice clients or their families to change family life patterns. Recognizing this fact nonjudgmentally helps the client or family use remaining energy to complete other end-of-life work.

• = **Independent;** ▲ = **Collaborative**

REFERENCES   Agency for Healthcare Research and Quality (AHRQ): *Evidence Report/Technology Assessment Number 3: Pharmacotherapy for Alcohol Dependence,* AHCPR Publication No. 99-E004, retrieved from the World Wide Web Jan 16, 2000. (AHCPR Pub No. 99-E003 current as of January 1999.) Web site: www.ahcpr.gov/clinic/index.html#evidence

American Nurses Association: Task Force on Substance Abuse Nursing Practice: *The care of clients with addictions: dimensions of nursing practice,* Kansas City, Mo, 1987, The Association.

Bennett LW, Cardone S, Jarczyk J: Effects of a therapeutic camping program on addiction recovery, *J Subst Abuse Treat* 15(5):469-474, 1998.

Captain C: Family recovery from alcoholism: mediating family factors, *Nurs Clin North Am* 24:55, 1989.

Craft MJ, Willadsen JA: Interventions related to family, *Nurs Clin North Am* 27:517, 1992.

Curry SJ et al: At-risk drinking among patients making routine primary care visits, *Prev Med* 31(5):595-602, 2000.

D'Avanzo CE et al: Developing culturally informed strategies for substance-related interventions. In Naegle MA, D'Avanzo CE, editors: *Addictions and substance abuse: strategies for advanced practice nursing,* St Louis, 2001, Mosby, pp 59-104.

Damrosch S: General strategies for motivating people to change their behavior, *Nurs Clin North Am* 26:833, 1991.

Giuffra MJ: Nursing strategies with alcohol and drug problems in the family. In Naegle MA, editor: *Substance abuse in education in nursing, vol III,* Pub No 15-2464, New York, 1993, National League for Nursing Press.

Ino A, Hayasida M: Before-discharge intervention method in the treatment of alcohol dependence, *Alcohol Clin Exp Res* 24(3):373-376, 2000.

Jones J: A proposed model of relapse prevention for adolescents who abuse alcohol, *J Child Adol Psychiatr Ment Health Nurs* 3:139, 1990.

Miller WR: Motivation for treatment: a review with special emphasis on alcoholism, *Psychol Bull* 198:84, 1985.

Nye CL, Zucker RA, Fitzgerald HE: Early family-based intervention in the path to alcohol problems: rationale and relationship between treatment process characteristics and child and parenting outcomes, *J Stud Alcohol Suppl* 13:10-21, 1999.

Rigler SK: Alcoholism in the elderly, *Am Fam Physician* 61(6):1710-1716, 1883-1884, 1887-1888, 2000.

Roberts BJ: Adult children of alcoholics, *J Am Acad Nurse Pract* 4:22, 1992.

SAMHSA's National Clearinghouse for Alcohol and Drug Information—a service of the Substance Abuse and Mental Health Services Administration. Web site: www.samhsa.gov/

Seiderman RY et al: Assessing American Indian families, *MCN Am J Matern Child Nurs* 21(6):274-279, 1996.

Sielhamer RA, Jacob T, Dunn NJ: The impact of alcohol consumption on parent-child relationships in families of alcoholics, *J Stud Alcohol* 54:189, 1993.

Stanhope M, Lancaster J, editors: *Community health nursing: promoting health of aggregates, families, and individuals,* ed 4, St Louis, 1996, Mosby.

Stoll B, Wick HD: Short intervention approach: one way of reducing excessive alcohol consumption, *Abhangigkeiten* Feb 2000.

Williams E: Strategies for intervention, *Nurs Clin North Am* 24:95, 1989.

Interrupted Family processes

Beverly Pickett, Gail B. Ladwig, and Mary Markle

NANDA   **Definition** Change in family relationships and/or functioning

Defining Characteristics

Changes in: power alliances; assigned tasks; effectiveness in completing assigned tasks; mutual support; availability for affective responsiveness and intimacy; patterns and rituals,

• = **Independent;** ▲ = **Collaborative**

participation in problem solving; participation in decision making; communication patterns; availability for emotional support; satisfaction with family; stress-reduction behaviors; expressions of conflict with and/or isolation from community resources; somatic complaints; expressions of conflict within family

Related Factors (r/t)

Power shift of family members; family roles shift; shift in health status of a family member; developmental transition and/or crisis; situational transition and/or crisis; informal or formal interaction with community; modification in family social status; modification in family finances

NOC   Outcomes (Nursing Outcomes Classification)

Suggested NOC Labels

Family Coping; Family Environment: Internal; Family Functioning; Family Normalization; Parenting; Psychosocial Adjustment: Life Changes; Role Performance

> **Example NOC Outcome**
> Demonstrates **Family Coping** as evidenced by the following indicators: Confronts problems/Manages problems/Involves family members in decision making (Rate each indicator of **Family Coping:** 1 = never demonstrated, 2 = rarely demonstrated, 3 = sometimes demonstrated, 4 = often demonstrated, 5 = consistently demonstrated [see Section I])

Client Outcomes

- Expresses feelings (family)
- Identifies ways to cope effectively and use appropriate support systems (family)
- Treats impaired family member as normally as possible to avoid overdependence (family)
- Meets physical, psychosocial, and spiritual needs of members or seeks appropriate assistance (family)
- Demonstrates knowledge of illness or injury, treatment modalities, and prognosis (family)
- Participates in the development of the plan of care to the best of ability (significant person)

NIC   Interventions (Nursing Interventions Classification)

Suggested NIC Labels

Family Integrity Promotion; Family Process Maintenance; Normalization Promotion

> **Example NIC Interventions—Family Process Maintenance**
> - Identify effects of role changes on family processes
> - Assist family members to use existing support measures

Nursing Interventions and Rationales

- Observe for cause of change in family's normal pattern of functioning.
  Ongoing assessment of family members can provide important clues about a possible family disruption. Assessment factors are included under interventions because it has been noted that assessment questions initiate a family process of self-examination and family problem solving and also provide assessment data (Craft, Willadsen, 1992).

• = Independent; ▲ = Collaborative

- Assess the strengths and deficiencies of the family system.
  The nurse can then help client and family with acquiring and maintaining support and coping strategies (Ducharme, Rowat, 1992).
- Consider use of family theory as a framework to help guide interventions (e.g., family stress theory, social exchange theory).
  Theory helps to identify the focus, means, and goals of nursing practice. It enhances communication and increases autonomy and accountability to care (Gillis et al, 1989; Meleis, 1991).
- Discuss with the family members how they have handled previous crises.
  Such a discussion gives the nurse clues and information that can help in plan of care. Families that have a broad and diverse array of coping behaviors are more likely than others to meet needs and have a good outcome (Coleman, Taylor, 1995).
- Spend time with family members; allow them to verbalize their feelings.
  Interactions help the client and family feel relieved and allow anxiety levels to decrease. Critical care nurses can provide support for families after the death of a loved one (Coolican, Politoski, 1994).
- Acknowledge the stages of grief when there is a change of health status in a family member; counsel family members that it is normal to be angry, afraid, etc.
  It is important to understand the wide range of feelings experienced during normal grief and to reassure those experiencing such feelings.
- Encourage family members to list their personal strengths.
  A list of strengths provides information that family members can refer to for positive feedback.
- Involve family members in the care and information/patient teaching sessions with the client.
  Family-focused activities can help families cope better with the hospital experience (Worthington, 1995).
- Encourage family to visit client; adjust visiting hours to accommodate family's schedule (e.g., schedule around work, school, babysitting needs).
- Assist with sleeping arrangements if family is spending the night; provide a place to lie down, pillows, and blankets.
- Allow and encourage family to assist in the client's care. Allow family presence during invasive procedures and resuscitation.
  Assisting with client's care helps maintain family's connectedness. Strategies to facilitate effective coping of family members during the crisis of critical illness include family attendance during invasive procedures and resuscitation efforts (Twibell, 1998).
- Have family members participate in client conferences that involve all members of the health care team.
  Conferences allow for distribution of information, input by all members at one time, and a decrease in anxiety levels of family members.
- ▲ Serve as case manager to explore and use all available resources appropriate for situation (e.g., counseling, social services, self-help groups, pastoral care).
  Family members are often unaware of the wide array of services available in many communities.

Geriatric

- Teach family members about impact of developmental events (e.g., retirement, death, change in health status, and household composition).

• = Independent; ▲ = Collaborative

Knowledge regarding normative developmental challenges of aging can reduce the stress such challenges place on families.

- Support group problem solving among family members and include the older member.
  Problem solving is an effective method to manage stressors for family members of all ages.
- ▲ Refer family for counseling with a psychotherapist who is knowledgeable about gerontology.
- Refer to care plan for **Readiness for enhanced family Coping.**

Multicultural

- Assess for the influence of cultural beliefs, norms, and values on the family's perceptions of normal functioning.
  What the family considers normal and abnormal family functioning may be based on cultural perceptions (Leininger, 1996).
- With the client's consent, facilitate a group meeting for family members to discuss how the family is functioning.
  A family meeting opens communication and lets each family member know it is okay to talk about what is happening (Rivera-Andino, Lopez, 2000).
- Facilitate modeling and role-playing for client and family regarding healthy ways to start a discussion about the client's prognosis.
  It is helpful for families and the client to practice communication skills in a safe environment before trying them in a real-life situation (Rivera-Andino, Lopez, 2000).
- Identify and acknowledge the stresses unique to racial/ethnic families.
  Financial difficulties and maintaining cultural values are two of the most common family stressors cited by women of color (Majumdar, Ladak, 1998).
- Offer frequent gestures of support to family members.
  Black mothers of seriously ill children identified support from the health care team as their highest source of satisfaction (Miles, Wilson, Docherty, 1999).
- Encourage the family members to demonstrate and offer caring and support to each other.
  The familial characteristics of care and support are associated with fostering resiliency in black families. Resilience is the ability to experience adverse conditions and successfully overcome them (Calvert, 1997).
- Validate the family's feelings regarding concerns about current crisis and family functioning.
  Validation lets the client know that the nurse has heard and understands what was said, and it promotes the nurse-client relationship (Stuart, Laraia, 2001; Giger, Davidhizar, 1995).

Home Care Interventions

The nursing interventions described previously for **Compromised family Coping** should be used in the home environment with adaptations as necessary.

Client/Family Teaching

Refer to Client/Family Teaching for **Compromised family Coping** and **Readiness for enhanced family Coping** for suggestions that may be used with minor adaptations.

WEB SITES FOR EDUCATION

MERLIN See the MERLIN web site for World Wide Web resources for client education.

• = Independent; ▲ = Collaborative

REFERENCES   Calvert WJ: Protective factors within the family, and their role in fostering resiliency in African American adolescents, *J Cult Divers* 4(4):110-117, 1997.

Coleman W, Taylor E: Family-focused pediatrics: issues, challenges, and clinical methods, *Pediatr Clin North Am* 42(1):119-129, 1995.

Coolican MB, Politoski G: Donor family programs, *Crit Care Nurs Clin North Am* 6(3):613-623, 1994.

Craft MJ, Willadsen JA: Interventions related to family, *Nurs Clin North Am* 27:517, 1992.

Ducharme F, Rowat K: Conjugal support, family coping behaviors and the well being of elderly couples, *Can J Nurs Res* 24:5, 1992.

Giger JN, Davidhizar RE: *Transcultural nursing,* ed 2, St Louis, 1995, Mosby.

Gillis C et al: *Toward a science of family nursing,* Menlo Park, Calif, 1989, Addison-Wesley.

Leininger MM: *Transcultural nursing: theories, research and practices,* ed 2, Hilliard, Ohio, 1996, McGraw-Hill.

Majumdar B, Ladak S: Management of family and workplace stress experienced by women of color from various cultural backgrounds, *Can J Public Health* 89(1):48-52, 1998.

Meleis A: *Theoretical nursing,* Philadelphia, 1991, JB Lippincott.

Miles MS, Wilson SM, Docherty SL: African American mothers' responses to hospitalization of an infant with serious health problems, *Neonatal Netw* 18(8):17-25, 1999.

Rivera-Andino J, Lopez L: When culture complicates care, *RN* 63(7):47-49, 2000.

Stuart GW, Laraia MT: Therapeutic nurse-patient relationship. In Stuart GW, Laraia MT, editors: *Principles and practice of psychiatric nursing,* St Louis, 2001, Mosby, p 30.

Twibell RS: Family coping during critical illness, *Dimens Crit Care Nurs* 17(2):100-112, 1998.

Worthington R: Effective transitions for families: life beyond the hospital, *Pediatr Nurs* 21:8, 1995.

Fatigue

Betty J. Ackley

NANDA   **Definition** An overwhelming, sustained sense of exhaustion and decreased capacity for physical and mental work at usual level

Defining Characteristics

Inability to restore energy even after sleep; lack of energy or inability to maintain usual level of physical activity; increase in rest requirements; tired; inability to maintain usual routines; verbalization of an unremitting and overwhelming lack of energy; lethargic or listless; perceived need for additional energy to accomplish routine tasks; increase in physical complaints; compromised concentration; disinterest in surroundings, introspection; decreased performance; compromised libido; drowsy; feelings of guilt for not keeping up with responsibilities

Related Factors (r/t)

Psychological Boring lifestyle; stress; anxiety; depression

Environmental Humidity; lights; noise; temperature

Situational Negative life events; occupation

Physiological Sleep deprivation; pregnancy; poor physical condition; disease states (cancer, HIV, multiple sclerosis); increased physical exertion; malnutrition; anemia

NOC   **Outcomes (Nursing Outcomes Classification)**

Suggested NOC Labels

Endurance; Concentration; Energy Conservation; Nutritional Status: Energy

• = Independent; ▲ = Collaborative

> **Example NOC Outcome**
> Demonstrates **Endurance** as evidenced by the following indicators: Performance of usual routine/Activity/Rested appearance/Blood oxygen level within normal limits/Expresses feelings about loss/Verbalizes acceptance of loss/Describes meaning of the loss or death/Reports decreased preoccupation with loss/Expresses positive expectations about the future (Rate each indicator of **Endurance:** 1 = extremely compromised, 2 = substantially compromised, 3 = moderately compromised, 4 = mildly compromised, 5 = not compromised [see Section I])

Client Outcomes

- Verbalizes increased energy and improved well-being
- Explains energy conservation plan to offset fatigue

NIC Interventions (Nursing Interventions Classification)

Suggested NIC Labels

Energy Management

> **Example NIC Interventions—Energy Management**
> - Determine patient's physical limitations
> - Determine patient's significant other's perception of causes of fatigue

Nursing Interventions and Rationales

- Assess severity of fatigue on a scale of 0 to 10; assess frequency of fatigue, activities associated with increased fatigue, ability to perform activities of daily living (ADLs), times of increased energy, ability to concentrate, mood, and usual pattern of activity. If client has cancer, consider use of an instrument such as the Profile of Mood State short form fatigue subscale, the Multidimensional Assessment of Fatigue, the Lee Fatigue Scale, or the Multidimensional Fatigue Inventory.
  These assessments have all shown to have good internal reliability. The Profile of Mood State Short Form Fatigue Scale was the strongest performer in one study (Meek et al, 2000).
- Evaluate adequacy of nutrition and sleep. Encourage the client to get adequate rest. Refer to **Imbalanced Nutrition: less than body requirements** or **Disturbed Sleep pattern** if appropriate. NOTE: Sometimes clients with chronic fatigue syndrome can sleep excessively and need support to limit sleeping.
  The most commonly suggested treatment for fatigue is rest (Nail, Winningham, 1995). Inadequate nutrition or poor sleep can contribute to fatigue.
- ▲ Determine with help from the primary care practitioner whether there is a physiological or psychological cause of fatigue that could be treated, such as anemia, electrolyte imbalance, hypothyroidism, depression, or medication effect.
  The presence of fatigue is associated with biological, psychological, social, and personal factors (Belza et al, 1993). Fatigue should not be tolerated if it can be readily reversed with treatment.
- ▲ Work with the physician to determine if the client has chronic fatigue syndrome. The Centers for Disease Control and Prevention defines chronic fatigue syndrome as:

  Clinically evaluated, unexplained, persistent, or relapsing chronic fatigue (over six months duration) that is of new or definite onset (has not been lifelong); is not the result of ongoing exertion; is not alleviated by rest; and results in substantial reduction in previous levels of occupational,

• = Independent; ▲ = Collaborative

educational, social, or personal activities. In addition, four or more the following symptoms must concurrently be present for over six months: impaired memory or concentration, sore throat, tender cervical or axial lymph nodes, muscle pain, multijoint pain, new headaches, unrefreshing sleep, and postexertion malaise lasting more than 24 hours (Walker, 1999).

- Encourage client to express feelings about fatigue; use active listening techniques and help identify sources of hope.
  Fatigue has been associated with depression, anxiety, anger, and mood disturbances (Potempa, 1993; Fisher, 1997).
- Encourage client to keep a journal of activities, symptoms of fatigue, and feelings.
  The journal helps the client monitor progress toward resolving or coping with fatigue and express feelings, which helps with adjustment (Jones, 1992).
- Assist client with ADLs as necessary; encourage independence without causing exhaustion.
- Help client set small, easily achieved short-term goals such as writing two sentences in a journal daily or walking to the end of the hallway twice daily.
- ▲ With physician's approval, refer to physical therapy for carefully monitored aerobic exercise program.
  Aerobic exercise and physical therapy can reduce fatigue in some oncology clients (MacVicar, 1989; Mock et al, 1994; Schwartz, 1998, 2000). An exercise program for patients receiving radiation treatments for cancer of the breast also helped improve emotional health and increased sleep (Mock et al, 1997) A customized exercise program can be helpful to the client with chronic fatigue syndrome (Jain, DeLisa, 1998).
- ▲ Refer client to diagnosis-appropriate support groups such as National Chronic Fatigue Syndrome Association or Multiple Sclerosis Association.
  Support groups can help clients deal with body changes and cope with the frequent depression that accompanies fatigue (Jones, 1992; Jain, DeLisa, 1998).
- Help client identify essential and nonessential tasks and determine what can be delegated.
- Give client permission to limit social and role demands if needed (e.g., switch to part-time employment, hire cleaning service).
  The nurse can help the client look at life realistically to balance available energy and energy demands.
- ▲ For cardiac client, recognize that fatigue is common following a myocardial infarction (Lee et al, 2000). Refer to cardiac rehabilitation for carefully prescribed and monitored exercise program.
  Carefully monitored exercise is thought to decrease symptoms of fatigue in heart patients (Friedman, King, 1995).
- For fatigue with multiple sclerosis, encourage energy conservation, "recharging efforts," excellent self-care, and keeping the temperature cool (Stuifbergen, Rogers, 1997).
- For attentional fatigue, suggest restorative activities such as sitting outside, bird-watching, and gardening (Erickson, 1996).
  Being outside and enjoying nature can help people recover their strength and think more clearly.
- ▲ If not coping well, refer for cognitive therapy to help deal with symptoms of fatigue and help change negative thought patterns.
  Cognitive therapy can be effective for clients with chronic fatigue syndrome (Fisher, 1997; Walker, 1999), also for clients with HIV (Rose et al, 1998).

• = **Independent;** ▲ = **Collaborative**

▲ If fatigue is associated with chemotherapy, be sure to treat nausea, vomiting, and pain effectively and prevent mouth sores if possible.
Increased fatigue was seen in breast cancer clients receiving chemotherapy if they were also experiencing unrelieved pain, had nausea with vomiting, or developed mouth sores (Jacobsen et al, 1999).

▲ Refer client to occupational therapy to learn new energy-conserving ways to perform tasks.
Occupational therapy can help clients learn energy conserving techniques so that clients can perform ADLs without exhaustion.

▲ If client is very weak, refer to physical therapy for prescription and use of a mobility aid such as a walker.

Geriatric

• Identify recent losses; monitor for depression as a possible contributing factor to fatigue.
Depression and fatigue are closely correlated; the elderly are more prone to depression because they frequently experience significant losses as they age.

▲ Review medications for side effects.
Certain medications (e.g., beta-blockers, antihistamines, pain medications) may cause fatigue in the elderly.

Home Care Interventions

• Assess client's history and current patterns of fatigue as they relate to the home environment.
Fatigue may be more pronounced in specific settings for physical or psychological reasons (e.g., rooms associated with loss of loved ones).

• Assess home for environmental and behavioral triggers of increased fatigue (e.g., stairs required to reach bathroom, patterns of movement around home, cleaning activities that require high energy).

▲ When assisting client with adapting to home and daily patterns, avoid activities of high energy output. Refer to occupational therapy to accomplish this if necessary.

• Assist client with identifying or creating a safe, restful place within the home that can be used routinely (e.g., a room with familiar, nonthreatening, or nonfrightening belongings).

▲ Refer cancer clients to a community-based pain and fatigue management program, such as the I Feel Better program, if available.
A program such as I Feel Better was received with enthusiasm and rapid enrollment by cancer clients (Grant et al, 2000).

Client/Family Teaching

• Share information about fatigue and how to live with it, including need for positive self-talk.
Client education legitimizes fatigue and enhances client's control through self-care and positive self talk (Fisher, 1997).

• Teach strategies for energy conservation (e.g., sitting instead of standing during showering, storing items at waist level).

• Teach client to carry a pocket calendar, make lists of required activities, and post reminders around the house.
Chronic fatigue is often associated with memory loss and sometimes difficulty thinking (Jain, DeLisa, 1998).

• Teach the importance of following a healthy lifestyle with adequate nutrition and rest, pain relief, and appropriate exercise to decrease fatigue.

• = Independent; ▲ = Collaborative

• Teach stress-reduction techniques such as controlled breathing, imagery, and use of music. See **Anxiety** care plan if appropriate; anxiety is correlated with increased fatigue.

WEB SITES FOR EDUCATION

Merlin See the MERLIN web site for World Wide Web resources for client education.

REFERENCES Belza BL et al: Correlates of fatigue in older adults with rheumatoid arthritis, *Nurs Res* 42(2):93-99, 1993.

Erickson JM: Anemia, *Semin Oncol Nurs* 12(1):2, 1996.

Fisher L: Chronic fatigue syndrome, *Prof Nurse* 12(8):578-581, 1997.

Friedman MM, King KK: Correlates of fatigue in older women with heart failure, *Heart Lung* 24(6):512-518, 1995.

Grant M et al: Developing a community program on cancer pain and fatigue, *Cancer Pract* 8(4):187-194, 2000.

Jacobsen PB et al: Fatigue in women receiving adjuvant chemotherapy for breast cancer: characteristics, course, and correlates, *J Pain Symptom Manage* 18(4):233-242, 1999.

Jain SS, DeLisa JA: Chronic fatigue syndrome: a literature review from a physiatric perspective, *Am J Phys Med Rehabil* 77(2):160-166, 1998.

Jones CA: These patients truly need our help, *RN* 55:46-53, 1992.

Lee H et al: Fatigue, mood, and hemodynamic patterns after myocardial infarction, *Applied Nurs Res* 13(2):60-69, 2000.

MacVicar M: Effects of aerobic interval training on cancer patients' functional capacity, *Nurs Res* 38:348, 1989.

Meek PM et al: Psychometric testing of fatigue instruments for use with cancer patients, *Nurs Res* 49(4):181-190, 2000.

Mock et al: A nursing rehabilitation program for women with breast cancer receiving adjuvant chemotherapy, *Oncol Nurs Forum* 21:899-907, 1994.

Mock et al: Effects of exercise on fatigue, physical functioning, and emotional distress during radiation therapy for breast cancer, *Oncol Nurs Forum* 24(6):991-1000, 1997.

Nail LM, Winningham ML: Fatigue and weakness in cancer patients: the symptom experience, *Semin Oncol Nurs* 11(4):272, 1995.

Potempa KM: Chronic fatigue, *Annu Rev Nurs Res* 11:57-72, 1993.

Rose L et al: The fatigue experience: persons with HIV infection, *J Adv Nurs* 28(2):295-304, 1998.

Schwartz AL: Patterns of exercise and fatigue in physically active cancer survivors, *Oncol Nurs Forum* 25(3):485-491, 1998.

Schwartz AL: Daily fatigue patterns and effect of exercise in women with breast cancer, *Cancer Pract* 8(1):16-24, 2000.

Stuifbergen AK, Rogers S: The experience of fatigue and strategies of self-care among persons with multiple sclerosis, *Appl Nurs Res* 10(1):2-10, 1997.

Walker TL: Chronic fatigue syndrome, *Am J Nurs* 99(3):70-75, 1999.

Fear

Pam B. Schweitzer and Gail B. Ladwig

NANDA   **Definition** Response to perceived threat that is consciously recognized as a danger

Defining Characteristics

Report of: apprehension; increased tension; decreased self-assurance; excitement; being scared; jitteriness; dread; alarm; terror; panic

• = **Independent**; ▲ = **Collaborative**

Cognitive	Identifies object of fear; stimulus believed to be a threat; diminished productivity, learning ability, problem-solving ability
Behaviors	Increased alertness; avoidance or attack behaviors; impulsiveness; narrowed focus on "it" (i.e., the focus of the fear)
Physiological	Increased pulse; anorexia; nausea; vomiting; diarrhea; muscle tightness; fatigue; increased respiratory rate and shortness of breath; pallor; increased perspiration; increased systolic blood pressure; pupil dilation; dry mouth

Related Factors (r/t)

Natural/innate origin (e.g., sudden noise, height, pain, loss of physical support); learned response (e.g., conditioning, modeling from or identification with others); separation from support system in potentially stressful situation (e.g., hospitalization, hospital procedures); unfamiliarity with environmental experience(s); language barrier; sensory impairment; innate releasers (neurotransmitters); phobic stimulus

NOC Outcomes (Nursing Outcomes Classification)

Suggested NOC Labels

Fear Control

> **Example NOC Outcome**
> Demonstrates **Fear Control** as evidenced by the following indicators: Eliminates precursors of fear/Seeks information to reduce fear/Plans coping strategies for fearful situations (Rate each indicator of **Fear Control:** 1 = never demonstrated, 2 = rarely demonstrated, 3 = sometimes demonstrated, 4 = often demonstrated, 5 = consistently demonstrated [see Section I])

Client Outcomes

- Verbalizes known fears
- States accurate information about the situation
- Identifies, verbalizes, and demonstrates those coping behaviors that reduce own fear
- Reports and demonstrates reduced fear

NIC Interventions (Nursing Interventions Classification)

Suggested NIC Labels

Anxiety Reduction; Coping Enhancement; Security Enhancement

> **Example NIC Interventions—Anxiety Reduction**
> - Use a calm reassuring approach
> - Stay with the patient to promote safety and reduce fear

Nursing Interventions and Rationales

- Assess source of fear with client.
  Fear is a normal response to actual or perceived danger and helps mobilize protective defenses.
- Have the client draw the object of their fear. This is a reliable assessment tool for children.
  Because human figure drawings are reliable tools for assessing anxiety and fears in children, practitioners should incorporate these drawings as part of their routine assessments of fearful children (Carroll, Ryan-Wenger, 1999).
- Discuss situation with client and help distinguish between real and imagined threats to well-being.

- = Independent; ▲ = Collaborative

The first step in helping the client deal with fear is to collect information about the situation and its effect on the client and significant others (Bailey, Bailey, 1993).

- If irrational fears based on incorrect information are present, provide accurate information.
  Correcting mistaken beliefs reduces anxiety (Beck, Emery, 1985).
- If client's fear is a reasonable response, empathize with client. Avoid false reassurances and be truthful.
  Reassure clients that seeking help is both a sign of strength and a step toward resolution of the problem (Bailey, Bailey, 1993).
- If possible, remove the source of the client's fear with accurate and appropriate amounts of information.
  Clients' uncertainty regarding the outcomes can lead to feelings of distress. In one study, the major strategy used to reduce distress was information management, in which the amount and type of incoming information was controlled (Shaw, Wilson, O'Brien, 1994). Fear is a normal response to actual or perceived danger; if the threat is removed, the response will stop.
- If possible, help the client confront the fear.
  Self-discovery enhances feelings of control.
- Stay with clients when they express fear; provide verbal and nonverbal (touch and hug with permission) reassurances of safety if safety is within control.
  The nurse's presence and touch demonstrate caring and diminish the intensity of feelings such as fear (Olson, Sneed, 1995). Of 376 patients surveyed in 20 family practices throughout Ontario, Canada, 66% believe touch is comforting and healing and view distal touches (on the hand and shoulder) as comforting (Osmun et al, 2000).
- Explain all activities, procedures (in advance when possible), and issues that involve the client; use nonmedical terms; calm, slow speech; and verify client's understanding.
  Deficient knowledge or unfamiliarity is one factor associated with fear (Johnson, 1972; Garvin, Huston, Baker, 1992; Whitney, 1992).
- Explore coping skills used previously by client to deal with fear; reinforce these skills and explore other outlets.
  Methods of coping with anxiety that have previously been successful are likely to be helpful again (Clunn, Payne, 1982).
- Provide backrubs for clients to decrease anxiety.
  The dependent variable, anxiety, was measured before back massage, immediately following, and 10 minutes later on four consecutive evenings. There was a statistically significant difference in the mean anxiety (STAI) score between the back massage group and the no-intervention group (Fraser, Kerr, 1993).
- Provide massage before procedures to decrease anxiety.
  Massage was done by parents before venous puncture of hospitalized preschoolers and school-age children. The results obtained indicated that massage had significant effect on nonverbal reactions, especially those related to muscular relaxation. (Garcia, Horta, Farias, 1997).
- Use therapeutic touch (TT) and healing touch techniques.
  Various techniques that involve intention to heal, laying on of hands, clearing the energy field surrounding the body, and transfer of healing energy from the environment through the healer to the subject can reduce anxiety (Fishel, 1998). Anxiety was reduced significantly in a TT group but was unchanged in a TT placebo group. Healing touch may be one of the most useful nursing interventions available to reduce anxiety (Fishel, 1998).

• = **Independent;** ▲ = **Collaborative**

▲ Refer for cognitive behavioral group therapy.
In this study of 253 persons with neck or back pain, the experimental group who received the standardized six-session cognitive behavioral group sessions had significantly better results with regard to fear avoidance beliefs than the comparison group (Linton, Ryberg, 2001).

• Animal-assisted therapy (AAT) can be incorporated into the care of perioperative patients.
In a study done on perioperative clients, interacting with animals was shown to reduce blood pressure and cholesterol, decrease anxiety, and improve a person's sense of well-being (Miller, Ingram, 2000).

• Refer to care plans for **Anxiety** and **Death Anxiety**

Geriatric

• Establish a trusting relationship so that all fears can be identified.
An elderly client's response to a real fear may be immobilizing.

• Monitor for dementia and use appropriate interventions.
Fear may be an early indicator of disorientation or impaired reality testing in elderly clients.

• Note if the client is irritable and is blaming others.
Recent findings in nursing research support the presence of these other behaviors as symptoms of depression (Proffitt, Augspurger, Byrne, 1996).

• Provide a protective and safe environment, use consistent caregivers, and maintain the accustomed environmental structure.
Elderly clients tend to have more perceptual impairments and adapt to changes with more difficulty than younger clients, especially during an illness.

• Observe for untoward changes if antianxiety drugs are taken.
Advancing age renders clients more sensitive to both the clinical and toxic effects of many agents.

Multicultural

• Assess for the presence of culture-bound anxiety/fear states.
The context in which anxiety/fear is experienced, its meaning, and responses to it are culturally mediated (Kavanagh, 1999; Charron, 1998).

• Assess for the influence of cultural beliefs, norms, and values on the client's perspective of a stressful situation.
What the client considers stressful may be based on cultural perceptions (Leininger, 1996).

• Identify what triggers fear response.
Arab Muslim clients may express a high correlation between fear and pain (Sheets, El-Azhary, 1998).

• Identify how the client expresses fear.
Research indicates that the expression of fear may be culturally mediated (Shore, Rapport, 1998).

• Validate the client's feelings regarding fear.
Validation lets the client know that the nurse has heard and understands what was said, and it promotes the nurse-client relationship (Stuart, Laraia, 2001; Giger, Davidhizar, 1995).

Home Care Interventions

• During initial assessment, determine whether current or previous episodes of fear relate to the home environment (e.g., perception of danger in home or neighborhood or of relationships that have a history in the home).

• = **Independent;** ▲ = **Collaborative**

Investigating the source of the fear allows the client to verbalize feelings and the nurse to determine appropriate interventions.

- Identify with client what steps may be taken to make the home a "safe" place to be. *Identifying a given area as a safe place reduces fear and anxiety when the client is in that area.*
- ▲ Encourage the client to seek or continue appropriate counseling to reduce fear associated with stress or to resolve alterations in thought processes. *Correcting mistaken beliefs reduces anxiety.*
- ▲ Encourage the client to have a trusted companion, family member, or caregiver present in the home for periods when fear is most prominent. Pending other medical diagnoses, a referral to homemaker/home health aide services may meet this need. *Creating periods when fear and anxiety can be reduced allows the client periods of rest and supports positive coping.*
- Offer to sit with a terminally ill client quietly as needed by the client or family, or provide hospice volunteers to do the same. *Terminally ill clients and their families often fear the dying process. The presence of a nurse or volunteer lets clients know they are not alone. Fears are reduced, and the dying process becomes more easily tolerated.*

Client/Family Teaching

- Teach client the difference between warranted and excessive fear. *Different interventions are indicted for rational and irrational fears.*
- Teach stress management interventions to clients who experience emotions of fear. *Acute stress caused by strong emotions such as fear can sometimes cause sudden death in people with underlying coronary artery disease (Pashkow, 1999).*
- Teach families to share personal stories about an illness using the computer-based psychoeducational application experience journal. *The educational journal was reported to be useful for increasing understanding of familial feelings for families facing pediatric illness (DeMaso et al, 2000).*
- Teach client to visualize or fantasize absence of the fear or threat and successful resolution of the conflict or outcome of the procedure.
- Teach client to identify and use distraction or diversion tactics when possible. *Early interruption of the anxious response prevents escalation (Pope, 1995).*
- Teach clients to use guided imagery when they are fearful: have them use all senses to visualize a place that is "comfortable and safe" for them. *Results from this study showed that the psychological intervention of guided imagery significantly improved subjects' perceived quality of life and decreased fears (Moody, Fraser, Yarandi, 1993).*
- Teach client to allow fearful thoughts and feelings to be present until they dissipate. *Purposefully and repetitively allowing and even devoting time and energy to a thought reduces associated anxiety (Beck, Emery, 1985).*
- ▲ Teach use of appropriate community resources in emergency situations (e.g., hotlines, emergency rooms, law enforcement, judicial systems). *Serious emergencies need immediate assistance to ensure the client's safety.*
- ▲ Encourage use of appropriate community resources in nonemergency situations (e.g., family, friends, neighbors, self-help and support groups, volunteer agencies, churches, recreation clubs and centers, seniors, youths, others with similar interests).
- Teach client appropriate use of ordered medications.

• = Independent; ▲ = Collaborative

WEB SITES FOR EDUCATION

ᶫᵉᴿᴸᴵᴺ See the MERLIN web site for World Wide Web resources for client education.

REFERENCES Bailey DS, Bailey DR: *Therapeutic approaches to the care of the mentally ill,* ed 3, Philadelphia, 1993, FA Davis.

Beck AT, Emery G: *Anxiety disorder and phobias: a cognitive perspective,* New York, 1985, Basic Books.

Carroll M, Ryan-Wenger N: School-age children's fears, anxiety, and human figure drawings, *J Pediatr Health Care* 13(1):24, 1999.

Charron HS: Anxiety disorders. In Varcarolis EM, editor: *Foundations of psychiatric mental health nursing,* ed 3, Philadelphia, 1998, WB Saunders, pp 447-448.

Clunn PA, Payne DB: *Psychiatric mental health nursing,* Garden City, NJ, 1982, Medical Examination.

DeMaso DR et al: The experience journal: a computer-based intervention for families facing congenital heart disease, *Am Acad Child Adolesc Psychiatr* 39(6):727-734, 2000.

Fishel A: Nursing management of anxiety and panic, *Nurs Clin North Am* 33(1):135, 1998.

Fraser J, Kerr JR: Psychophysiological effects of back massage on elderly institutionalized patients, *J Adv Nurs* 18(2):238, 1993.

Garcia RM, Horta AL, Farias F: The effect of massage before venipuncture on the reaction of pre-school and school children, *Rev Esc Enferm USP* 31(1):119, 1997.

Garvin BJ, Huston GP, Baker CF: Information used by nurses to prepare patients for a stressful event, *Appl Nurs Res* 5:158, 1992.

Giger JN, Davidhizar RE: *Transcultural nursing,* ed 2, St Louis, 1995, Mosby.

Johnson J: Effects of structuring patient's expectations on their reactions to threatening events, *Nurs Res* 21:499, 1972.

Kavanagh KH: The role of cultural diversity in mental health nursing. In Fontaine KL, Fletcher JS, editors: *Mental health nursing* ed 4, Menlo Park, Calif, 1999, Addison-Wesley, pp 57-59.

Leininger MM: *Transcultural nursing: theories, research and practices,* ed 2, Hilliard, Ohio, 1996, McGraw-Hill.

Linton SJ, Ryberg M: A cognitive-behavioral group intervention as prevention for persistent neck and back pain in a non-patient population: a randomized controlled trial, *Pain* 90(1-2):83-90, 2001.

Miller J, Ingram L: Perioperative nursing and animal-assisted therapy, *AORN J* 72(3):477-483, 2000.

Moody L, Fraser M, Yarandi H: Effects of guided imagery in patients with chronic bronchitis and emphysema, *Clin Nurs Res* 2(4):478, 1993.

Olson M, Sneed N: Anxiety and therapeutic touch, *Issues Ment Health Nurs* 16(2):97, 1995.

Osmun WE et al: Patients' attitudes to comforting touch in family practice, *Can Fam Physician* 46(12):2411-2416, 2000.

Pashkow F: Is stress linked to heart disease? the evidence grows stronger, *Cleveland Clin J Med* 66(2):75, 1999.

Pope DS: Music noise and the human voice in the nurse-patient environment, *Image J Nurs Sch* 27:291, 1995.

Proffitt C, Augspurger P, Byrne M: Geriatric depression: a survey of nurses' knowledge and assessment practices, *Issues Ment Health Nurs* 17(2):123, 1996.

Shaw C, Wilson S, O'Brien M: Information needs prior to breast biopsy, *Clin Nurs Res* 3(2):119, 1994.

Sheets DL, El-Azhary RA: The Arab Muslim client: implications for anesthesia, *AANA J* 66(3):304-312, 1998.

Shore GN, Rapport MD: The fear survey schedule for children-revised (FSSC-HI): ethnocultural variations in children's fearfulness, *J Anxiety Disord* 12(5):437-461, 1998.

Stuart GW, Laraia MT: Therapeutic nurse-patient relationship. In Stuart GW, Laraia MT, editors: *Principles and practice of psychiatric nursing,* St Louis, 2001, Mosby, p 30.

Whitney G: Concept analysis of fear, *Nurs Diag* 3:159, 1992.

Deficient Fluid volume

Betty J. Ackley

NANDA **Definition** Decreased intravascular, interstitial, and/or intracellular fluid (refers to dehydration, water loss alone without change in sodium level)

• = Independent; ▲ = Collaborative

Defining Characteristics

Decreased urine output; increased urine concentration; weakness; sudden weight loss (except in third-spacing); decreased venous filling; increased body temperature; decreased pulse volume/pressure; change in mental state; elevated hematocrit; decreased skin/tongue turgor; dry skin/mucous membranes; thirst; increased pulse rate; decreased blood pressure

Related Factors (r/t)

Active fluid volume loss; failure of regulatory mechanisms

NOC   Outcomes (Nursing Outcomes Classification)

Suggested NOC Labels

Electrolyte and Acid-Base Balance; Fluid Balance; Hydration; Nutritional Status: Food and Fluid Intake

> **Example NOC Outcome**
>
> Maintains **Fluid Balance** as evidenced by the following indicators: Skin hydration/ Moist mucous membranes/Orthostatic hypotension not present/24-hour intake and output balanced/Urine specific gravity WNL* (Rate each indicator of **Fluid Balance:** 1 = extremely compromised, 2 = substantially compromised, 3 = moderately compromised, 4 = mildly compromised, 5 = not compromised [see Section I])

*WNL = Within Normal Limits

Client Outcomes

- Maintains urine output >1300 ml/day (or at least 30 ml/hr)
- Maintains normal blood pressure, pulse, and body temperature
- Maintains elastic skin turgor; moist tongue and mucous membranes; and orientation to person, place, time
- Explains measures that can be taken to treat or prevent fluid volume loss
- Describes symptoms that indicate the need to consult with health care provider

NIC   Interventions (Nursing Interventions Classification)

Suggested NIC Labels

Fluid Management; Hypovolemia Management; Shock Management: Volume

> **Example NIC Interventions—Fluid Management**
> Monitor hydration status (e.g., moist mucous membranes, adequacy of pulses, and orthostatic blood pressure) as appropriate

Nursing Interventions and Rationales

▲ Monitor for the existence of factors causing deficient fluid volume (e.g., gastrointestinal losses, difficulty maintaining oral intake, fever, uncontrolled type II diabetes, diuretic therapy).
Early identification of risk factors and early intervention can decrease the occurrence and severity of complications from deficient fluid volume. The gastrointestinal system is a common site of abnormal fluid loss (Metheny, 2000).

▲ Watch for early signs of hypovolemia, including weakness, muscle cramps, and postural hypotension.
Late signs include oliguria; abdominal or chest pain; cyanosis; cold, clammy skin; and confusion (Fauci et al, 1998).

• = Independent; ▲ = Collaborative

- Monitor total fluid intake and output every 8 hours (or every hour for the unstable client).
  A urine output of <30 ml/hr is insufficient for normal renal function and indicates hypovolemia or onset of renal damage (Metheny, 2000).
- Watch trends in output for 3 days; include all routes of intake and output and note color and specific gravity of urine.
  Monitoring for trends for 2 to 3 days gives a more valid picture of the client's hydration status than monitoring for a shorter period (Metheny, 2000). Dark-colored urine with increasing specific gravity reflects increased urine concentration.
- Monitor daily weight for sudden decreases, especially in the presence of decreasing urine output or active fluid loss. Weigh client on same scale with same type of clothing at same time of day, preferably before breakfast.
  Body weight changes reflect changes in body fluid volume. A 1-pound weight loss reflects a fluid loss of about 500 ml (Metheny, 2000).
- Monitor vital signs of clients with deficient fluid volume every 15 minutes to 1 hour for the unstable client (every 4 hours for the stable client). Observe for decreased pulse pressure first, then hypotension, tachycardia, decreased pulse volume, and increased or decreased body temperature.
  A decreased pulse pressure is an earlier indicator of shock than is the systolic blood pressure (Mikhail, 1999). Decreased intravascular volume results in hypotension and decreased tissue oxygenation. The temperature will be decreased as a result of decreased metabolism, or it may be increased if there is infection or hypernatremia present (Metheny, 2000).
- Check orthostatic blood pressures with client lying, sitting, and standing.
  A 15 mm Hg drop when upright or an increase of 15 beats/minute in the pulse rate are seen with deficient fluid volume (Metheny, 2000).
- Monitor for inelastic skin turgor, thirst, dry tongue and mucous membranes, longitudinal tongue furrows, speech difficulty, dry skin, sunken eyeballs, weakness (especially of upper body), and confusion.
  Tongue dryness, longitudinal tongue furrows, dryness of the mucous membranes of the mouth, upper body muscle weakness, thirst, confusion, speech difficulty, and sunkenness of eyes are symptoms of deficient fluid volume (Metheny 2000).
- Provide frequent oral hygiene, at least twice a day (if mouth is dry and painful, provide hourly while awake).
  Oral hygiene decreases unpleasant tastes in the mouth and allows the client to respond to the sensation of thirst.
- Provide fresh water and oral fluids preferred by client (distribute over 24 hours [e.g., 1200 ml on days, 800 ml on evenings, and 200 ml on nights]); provide prescribed diet; offer snacks (e.g., frequent drinks, fresh fruits, fruit juice); instruct significant other to assist client with feedings as appropriate.
  The oral route is preferred for maintaining fluid balance (Metheny, 2000). Distributing the intake over the entire 24 hour period and providing snacks and preferred beverages increases the likelihood that the client will maintain the prescribed oral intake.
- Provide free water with tube feedings as appropriate (50 to 100 ml every 4 hours).
  This provides water for replacement of intravascular or intracellular volume as necessary. Tube feeding has been found to increase the risk for dehydration (Lavizzo-Mourey, Johnson, Stolley, 1988; Sheehy, Perry, Cromwell, 1999).

• = Independent; ▲ = Collaborative

▲ Institute measures to rest the bowel when client is vomiting or has diarrhea (e.g., restrict food or fluid intake when appropriate, decrease intake of milk products). Hydrate client with ordered IV solutions if prescribed.
The most common cause of deficient fluid volume is gastrointestinal loss of fluid. At times it is preferable to allow the gastrointestinal system to rest before resuming oral intake. Hydration should be maintained. (See care plan for **Diarrhea** *or* **Nausea.***)*

▲ Provide oral replacement therapy as ordered with a glucose-electrolyte solution when client has acute diarrhea or nausea/vomiting. Provide small, frequent quantities of slightly chilled solutions.
Maintenance of oral intake stabilizes the ability of the intestines to digest and absorb nutrients; glucose-electrolyte solutions increase net fluid absorption while correcting deficient fluid volume (Cohen et al, 1995).

▲ Administer antidiarrheals and antiemetics as appropriate.
The gastrointestinal tract is a common site for fluid loss. The goal is to stop the loss that results from vomiting or diarrhea.

▲ If client requires IV fluid replacement, maintain patent IV access, set an appropriate IV infusion flow rate, and administer at a constant flow rate as ordered.
Isotonic IV fluids such as 0.9% N/S or lactated ringers allow replacement of intravascular volume (Metheny, 2000).

• Assist with ambulation if client has postural hypotension.
Postural hypotension can cause dizziness, which places the client at higher risk for injury.

• Promote skin integrity (e.g., monitor areas for breakdown, ensure frequent weight shifts, prevent shearing, promote adequate nutrition).
Deficient fluid volume decreases tissue oxygenation, which makes the skin more vulnerable to breakdown.

Critically ill

▲ Monitor central venous pressure, right atrial pressure, and pulmonary wedge pressure for decreases.
Hemodynamic parameters are sensitive indicators of intravascular fluid volume, and hemodynamic measurements are especially needed in the client with cardiac or renal problems (Metheny, 2000).

▲ Monitor serum and urine osmolality, serum sodium, blood urea nitrogen (BUN)/creatinine ratio, and hematocrit for elevations.
These are all measures of concentration and will be elevated with decreased intravascular volume (Fauci et al, 1998).

▲ When ordered, initiate a fluid challenge of crystalloids for replacement of intravascular volume; monitor client's response to prescribed fluid therapy and fluid challenge, especially noting vital signs, urine output, and lung sounds.
A fluid challenge can help the client with deficient fluid volume regain intravascular volume quickly, but the client must be carefully observed to ensure that he or she does not go into fluid volume overload. In trauma clients, if there is no clinical improvement after 2 L of crystalloids, then generally a blood transfusion should be initiated (Jordan, 2000).

• Position client flat with legs elevated when hypotensive, if not contraindicated.
This position enhances venous return, thus contributing to the maintenance of cardiac output.

▲ If trauma client, monitor lactic acid levels as ordered, along with watching for signs of fluid deficit and shock.

• **= Independent;** ▲ **= Collaborative**

Increased lactic acid levels can help identify occult hypoperfusion, which results in decreased survival and increased incidence of respiratory complications and multiple organ failure in trauma clients (Mikhail, 1999; Blow et al, 1999).

▲ Consult physician if signs and symptoms of deficient fluid volume persist or worsen. *Prolonged deficient fluid volume increases the risk for development of complications, including shock, multiple organ failure, and death.*

Geriatric

▲ Monitor elderly clients for deficient fluid volume carefully, noting new onset of weakness, dizziness, or dry mouth with longitudinal furrows.
The elderly are predisposed to deficient fluid volume because of decreased fluid in body, decreased thirst sensation, and decreased ability to concentrate urine (Bennett, 2000; Sheehy, Perry, Cromwell, 1999).

• Check skin turgor of elderly client on the forehead or sternum; also look for the presence of longitudinal furrows on the tongue and dry mucous membranes.
Elderly people commonly have decreased skin turgor from normal age-related loss of elasticity; therefore checking skin turgor on the arm is not reflective of fluid volume (Bennett, 2000). The presence of longitudinal furrows or dry mucous membranes is a good indication of dehydration in the elderly (Bennett, 2000; Sheehy, Perry, Cromwell, 1999).

• Encourage fluid intake by offering fluids regularly to cognitively impaired clients.
The elderly have a decreased thirst sensation (Metheny, 2000), and short-term memory loss may impede the client's memory of fluid intake.

• Incorporate regular hydration into daily routines (e.g., extra glass of fluid with medication or social activities).
Integration of hydration into regular routines increases the chance that the client will meet the daily fluid requirements.

▲ Monitor elderly clients for excess fluid volume during the treatment of deficient fluid volume: listen to lung sounds, watch for edema, and note vital signs.
The elderly client has a decreased ability to adapt to rapid increases in intravascular volume and can quickly develop heart failure.

Home Care Interventions

▲ Determine if it is appropriate to intervene for defecient fluid volume or allow the client to die comfortably without fluids as desired.
Deficient fluid volume may be a symptom of impending death in terminally ill clients. The deficit may result in a mild euphoria, and a more comfortable death (Bennett, 2000).

• Teach family members how to monitor output in the home (e.g., use of commode "hat" in the toilet, urinal, or bedpan, or use of catheter and closed drainage). Instruct them to monitor both intake and output.
An accurate measure of fluid intake and output is an important indicator of client fluid status (Metheny, 2000).

• When weighing client, use same scale each day. Be sure scale is on a flat (not cushioned) surface. Do not weigh client with scale placed on any kind of rug. Use bed or chair scales for clients who are unable to stand.
An accurate daily weight is an excellent reflection of fluid balance (Metheny, 2000).

▲ Teach family about complications of deficient fluid volume and when to call physician.

▲ If the client is receiving IV fluids, there must be a responsible caregiver in the home. Teach caregiver about administration of fluids, complications of IV administration (e.g., fluid volume overload, speed of medication reactions), and when to call for as-

• = Independent; ▲ = Collaborative

sistance. Assist caregiver with administration for as long as necessary to maintain client safety.

Administration of IV fluids in the home is a high-technology procedure and requires sufficient professional support to ensure safety of the client.

▲ Identify an emergency plan, including when to call 911.

Some complications of deficient fluid volume cannot be reversed in the home and are life-threatening. Clients progressing toward hypovolemic shock will need emergency care.

Client/Family Teaching

- Instruct client to avoid rapid position changes, especially from supine to sitting or standing.
- Teach client and family about appropriate diet and fluid intake.
- Teach client and family how to measure and record intake and output accurately.
- Teach client and family about measures instituted to treat hypovolemia and to prevent or treat fluid volume loss.
▲ Instruct client and family about signs of deficient fluid volume that indicate they should contact health care provider.

WEB SITES FOR EDUCATION

MERLIN   See the MERLIN web site for World Wide Web resources for client education.

REFERENCES   Bennett JA: Dehydration: hazards and benefits, *Geriatr Nurs* 21(2):84-88, 2000.

Blow O et al: The golden hours and the silver day: detection and correction of occult hypoperfusion within 24 hours improves outcome from major trauma, *J Trauma* 47(5):964-969, 1999.

Cohen M et al: Use of a single solution for oral rehydration and maintenance therapy of infants with diarrhea and mild to moderate dehydration, *Pediatr* 95:639, 1995.

Fauci AS et al, editors: *Harrison's principles of internal medicine,* ed 14, New York, 1998, McGraw-Hill.

Jordan KS: Fluid resuscitation in acutely injured patients, *J Intravenous Nurs* 23(2):81-87, 2000.

Lavizzo-Mourey RM, Johnson J, Stolley P: Risk factors for dehydration among elderly nursing home residents, *J Am Geriatr Soc* 36(3):213-218, 1988.

Metheny N: *Fluid and electrolyte balance: nursing considerations,* ed 4 Philadelphia, 2000, JB Lippincott.

Mikhail J: Resuscitation endpoints in trauma, *AACN Clin Issues* 10(1):10-21, 1999.

Sheehy CM, Perry PA, Cromwell SL: Dehydration: biological considerations, age-related changes, and risk factors in older adults, *Biol Res Nurs* 1(1):30-37, 1999.

Excess Fluid volume

Betty J. Ackley and Martha A. Spies

NANDA   **Definition** Increased isotonic fluid retention

Defining Characteristics

Jugular vein distention; decreased hemoglobin and hematocrit; weight gain over short period; changes in respiratory pattern, dyspnea or shortness of breath; orthopnea; abnormal breath sounds (rales or crackles); pulmonary congestion; pleural effusion; intake exceeds output; S_3 heart sound; change in mental status; restlessness; anxiety; blood pressure changes; pulmonary artery pressure changes; increased central venous pressure;

• = **Independent;** ▲ = **Collaborative**

oliguria; azotemia; specific gravity changes; altered electrolytes; edema, may progress to anascara; positive hepatojugular reflex

Related Factors (r/t)

Compromised regulatory mechanism; excess fluid intake; excess sodium intake

NOC Outcomes (Nursing Outcomes Classification)

Suggested NOC Labels

Electrolyte and Acid-Base Balance; Fluid Balance; Hydration

> **Example NOC Outcome**
> Maintains **Fluid Balance** as evidenced by the following indicators: Peripheral edema not present/Neck vein distention not present/Body weight stable/24-hour intake and output balanced/Urine specific gravity WNL*/Adventitious breath sounds not present (Rate each indicator of **Fluid Balance:** 1 = extremely compromised, 2 = substantially compromised, 3 = moderately compromised, 4 = mildly compromised, 5 = not compromised [see Section I])

*Within Normal Limits

Client Outcomes

- Remains free of edema, effusion, anascara; weight appropriate for client
- Maintains clear lung sounds; no evidence of dyspnea or orthopnea
- Remains free of jugular vein distention, positive hepatojugular reflex, and gallop heart rhythm
- Maintains normal central venous pressure, pulmonary capillary wedge pressure, cardiac output, and vital signs
- Maintains urine output within 500 ml of intake and normal urine osmolality and specific gravity
- Remains free of restlessness, anxiety, or confusion
- Explains measures that can be taken to treat or prevent excess fluid volume, especially fluid and dietary restrictions and medications
- Describes symptoms that indicate the need to consult with health care provider

NIC Interventions (Nursing Interventions Classification)

Suggested NIC Labels

Fluid Management; Fluid Monitoring

> **Example NIC Interventions—Fluid Monitoring**
> - Weigh daily and monitor trends
> - Maintain accurate intake and output record

Nursing Interventions and Rationales

- Monitor location and extent of edema; use a millimeter tape in the same area at the same time each day to measure edema in extremities.
  Heart failure and renal failure are usually associated with dependent edema because of increased hydrostatic pressure; dependent edema will cause swelling in the legs and feet of ambulatory clients and the presacral region of clients on bed rest. Dependent edema was found to demonstrate the greatest sensitivity as a defining characteristic for excess fluid volume (Rios et al, 1991). Generalized edema (e.g., in the upper extremities and eyelids)

• = Independent; ▲ = Collaborative

is associated with decreased oncotic pressure as a result of nephrotic syndrome. Measuring the extremity with a millimeter tape is more accurate than using the 1 to 4 scale (Metheny, 2000).

• Monitor daily weight for sudden increases; use same scale and type of clothing at same time each day, preferably before breakfast.
Body weight changes reflect changes in body fluid volume. Clinically it is extremely important to get an accurate body weight of a client with fluid imbalance (Metheny, 2000).

• Monitor lung sounds for crackles, monitor respirations for effort, and determine the presence and severity of orthopnea.
Pulmonary edema results from excessive shifting of fluid from the vascular space into the pulmonary interstitial space and alveoli. Pulmonary edema can interfere with the oxygen–carbon dioxide exchange at the alveolar-capillary membrane (Metheny, 2000), resulting in dyspnea and orthopnea.

▲ With head of bed elevated 30 to 45 degrees, monitor jugular veins for distention in the upright position; assess for positive hepatojugular reflex.
Increased intravascular volume results in jugular vein distention, even in a client in the upright position, and also a positive hepatojugular reflex.

▲ Monitor central venous pressure, mean arterial pressure, pulmonary artery pressure, pulmonary capillary wedge pressure, and cardiac output; note and report trends indicating increasing pressures over time.
Increased vascular volume with decreased cardiac contractility increases intravascular pressures, which are reflected in hemodynamic parameters. Over time, this increased pressure can result in uncompensated heart failure.

▲ Monitor vital signs; note decreasing blood pressure, tachycardia, and tachypnea. Monitor for gallop rhythms. If signs of heart failure are present, see nursing care plan for **Decreased Cardiac output.**
Heart failure results in decreased cardiac output and decreased blood pressure. Tissue hypoxia stimulates increased heart and respiratory rates.

▲ Monitor serum osmolality, serum sodium, blood urea nitrogen (BUN)/creatinine ratio, and hematocrit for decreases.
These are all measures of concentration and will decrease (except in the presence of renal failure) with increased intravascular volume. In clients with renal failure the BUN will increase because of decreased renal excretion.

• Monitor intake and output; note trends reflecting decreasing urine output in relation to fluid intake.
Accurately measuring intake and output is very important for the client with fluid volume overload.

• Monitor client's behavior for restlessness, anxiety, or confusion; use safety precautions if symptoms are present.
When excess fluid volume compromises cardiac output, the client will experience tissue hypoxia. Cerebral tissue is extremely sensitive to hypoxia, and the client may demonstrate restlessness and anxiety before any physiological alterations occur. When the excess fluid volume results in hyponatremia, the cerebral function will also be altered because of cerebral edema (Fauci et al, 1998).

▲ Monitor for the development of conditions that increase the client's risk for excess fluid volume.

• = **Independent**; ▲ = **Collaborative**

Common causes are heart failure, renal failure, and liver failure, all of which result in decreased glomerular filtration rate and fluid retention. Other causes are increased intake of oral or IV fluids in excess of the client's cardiac and renal reserve levels, increased levels of antidiuretic hormone, or movement of fluid from the interstitial space to the intravascular space (Fauci et al, 1998). Early detection allows the institution of specific treatment measures before the client develops pulmonary edema.

▲ Provide a restricted-sodium diet as appropriate if ordered.
Restricting the sodium in the diet will favor the renal excretion of excess fluid. Take care to avoid hyponatremia. Decreasing sodium can be more important that restricting fluid intake (Fauci et al, 1998).

▲ Monitor serum albumin level and provide protein intake as appropriate.
Serum albumin is the main contributor to serum oncotic pressure, which favors the movement of fluid from the interstitial space into the intravascular space. When serum albumin is low, peripheral edema may be severe.

▲ Administer prescribed loop, thiazide, and/or potassium-sparing diuretics as appropriate; these may be given intravenously or orally.
Therapeutic responses to diuretic therapy include natriuresis, diuresis, elimination of edema, vasodilation, reduction of cardiac filling pressures, decreased renal vasculature resistance, and increased renal blood flow (Cody, Kubo, Pickworth, 1994; DePriest, 1997).

▲ Monitor for side effects of diuretic therapy: orthostatic hypotension (especially if client is also receiving angiotensin-converting enzyme [ACE] inhibitors) and electrolyte and metabolic imbalances (hyponatremia, hypocalcemia, hypomagnesemia, hyperuricemia, and metabolic alkalosis). In clients receiving loop or thiazide diuretics, observe for hypokalemia. Observe for hyperkalemia in clients receiving a potassium-sparing diuretic, especially with the concurrent administration of an ACE inhibitor.
The blood pressure reduction in response to ACE inhibitors is greater in the presence of sodium depletion and diuretic therapy. The incidence of electrolyte and metabolic imbalances ranges from 14% to 60%; the most common is hypokalemia (Cody, Kubo, Pickworth, 1994).

▲ Implement fluid restriction as ordered, especially when serum sodium is low; include all routes of intake. Schedule fluids around the clock, and include the type of fluids preferred by the client.
Fluid restriction may decrease intravascular volume and myocardial workload. Overzealous fluid restriction should not be used because hypovolemia can worsen heart failure. In one study, instituting fluid restriction, distributing fluids over a 24-hour period, and using a fluid restriction when the client had hyponatremia all had high intervention content validity scores for the fluid management intervention label (Cullen, 1992). Client involvement in planning will enhance participation in the necessary fluid restriction.

▲ Maintain the rate of all IV infusions carefully.
This is done to prevent inadvertant exacerbation of excess fluid volume.

• Turn clients with dependent edema frequently (i.e., at least every 2 hours).
Edematous tissue is vulnerable to ischemia and pressure ulcers (Cullen, 1992).

• Provide for scheduled rest periods.
Bed rest can induce diuresis related to diminished peripheral venous pooling, resulting in increased intravascular volume and glomerular filtration rate (Metheny, 2000).

• Promote a positive body image and good self-esteem.
*Visible edema may alter the client's body image (Cullen, 1992). See the care plan for **Disturbed Body image**.*

• = **Independent**; ▲ = **Collaborative**

▲ Consult with physician if signs and symptoms of excess fluid volume persist or worsen.
Because excess fluid volume can result in pulmonary edema, it must be treated promptly and aggressively (Fauci et al, 1998).

Geriatric

• Recognize that the presence of risk factors for excess fluid volume is particularly serious in the elderly.
Decreased cardiac output and stroke volume are normal aging changes that increase the risk for excess fluid volume (Metheny, 2000).

Home Care Interventions

• Assess client and family knowledge of disease process causing excess fluid volume. Teach about disease process and complications of excess fluid volume, including when to contact physician.
Knowledge of disease and complications promotes early detection of and intervention for pending problems.

• Assess client and family knowledge and compliance with medical regimen, including medications, diet, rest, and exercise. Assist family with integrating restrictions into daily living.
Knowledge promotes compliance. Assistance with integration of cultural values, especially those related to foods, with medical regimen promotes compliance and decreased risk of complications.

• If client is confined to bed rest or has difficulty reclining, follow previously mentioned positioning recommendations.

▲ Teach and reinforce knowledge of medications. Instruct client not to use over-the-counter medications (e.g., diet medications) without first consulting the physician. Instruct client to make primary physician aware of medications ordered by other physicians.
There is potential for undesirable interaction among multiple medications, especially when use of over-the-counter and other prescribed medications is not monitored.

▲ Identify emergency plan for rapidly developing or critical levels of excess fluid volume when diuresing is not safe at home.
When out of control, excess fluid volume can be life threatening.

▲ Teach about signs and symptoms of both excess and deficient fluid volume and when to call physician.
Fluid volume balance can change rapidly with aggressive treatment.

Client/Family Teaching

▲ Describe signs and symptoms of excess fluid volume and actions to take if they occur.
Teach the importance of fluid and sodium restrictions. Help client and family to devise a schedule for intake of fluids throughout entire day. Refer to dietitian concerning implementation of low-sodium diet.

▲ Teach how to take diuretics correctly: take one dose in the morning and second dose (if taken) no later than 4 PM. Adjust potassium intake as appropriate for potassium-losing or potassium-sparing diuretics. Note the appearance of side effects such as weakness, dizziness, muscle cramps, numbness and tingling, confusion, hearing impairment, palpitations or irregular heartbeat, and postural hypotension.
Emphasise the need to consult with health care provider before taking over-the-counter medications (Byers, Goshorn, 1995; Dunbar, Jacobson, Deaton, 1998).

• = **Independent;** ▲ = **Collaborative**

REFERENCES   Byers J, Goshorn J: How to manage diuretic therapy, *Am J Nurs* 95(2):38-44, 1995.
Cody R, Kubo S, Pickworth K: Diuretic treatment for the sodium retention of congestive heart failure, *Arch Int Med* 154:1905-1914, 1994.
Cullen L: Interventions related to fluid and electrolyte imbalance, *Nurs Clin North Am* 27:569-597, 1992.
DePriest J: Reversing oliguria in critically ill patients, *Postgrad Med* 102(3):245-258, 1997.
Dunbar SB, Jacobson LH, Deaton C: Heart failure: strategies to enhance patient self-management, *AACN Clin Issues* 9(2):244-256, 1998.
Fauci AS et al, editors: *Harrison's principles of internal medicine,* ed 14, New York, 1998, McGraw-Hill, pp 268-269, 1292-1293.
Metheny N: *Fluid and electrolyte balance: nursing considerations,* ed 4, Philadelphia, 2000, JB Lippincott.
Rios H et al: Validation of defining characteristics of four nursing diagnoses using a computerized data base, *J Prof Nurs* 7:293-299, 1991.

Risk for deficient Fluid volume

Betty J. Ackley

    Definition At risk for experiencing vascular, cellular, or intracellular dehydration

Risk Factors

Factors influencing fluid needs (e.g., hypermetabolic state); extremes of age; extremes of weight; excessive losses of fluid through normal routes (e.g., diarrhea); loss of fluids through abnormal routes (e.g., indwelling tubes); deviations affecting access, intake, or absorption of fluids (e.g., physical immobility); knowledge deficiency regarding fluid volume; medication (e.g., diuretics)

Related Factors (r/t)

See Risk Factors

NOC **Outcomes (Nursing Outcomes Classification)**

Suggested NOC Labels

Fluid Balance; Hydration; Knowledge: Treatment Regimen

> **Example NOC Outcome**
> Maintains **Fluid Balance** as evidenced by the following indicators: Skin hydration/ Moist mucous membranes/Orthostatic hypotension not present/24-hour intake and output balanced/Urine specific gravity WNL* (Rate each indicator of **Fluid Balance:** 1 = extremely compromised, 2 = substantially compromised, 3 = moderately compromised, 4 = mildly compromised, 5 = not compromised [see Section I])

*Within Normal Limits

Client Outcomes

- Maintains urine output >1300 ml/day (or at least 30 ml/hr)
- Maintains normal blood pressure, pulse, and body temperature

• = Independent; ▲ = Collaborative

- Maintains elastic skin turgor; moist tongue and mucous membranes; and orientation to person, place, time
- Explains measures that can be taken to treat or prevent fluid volume loss
- Describes symptoms that indicate the need to consult with health care provider

NIC **Interventions (Nursing Interventions Classification)**

Suggested NIC Labels

Fluid Management; Fluid Monitoring, Hypovolemia Management

> **Example NIC Interventions—Fluid Management**
> Monitor hydration status (e.g., moist mucous membranes, adequacy of pulses, and orthostatic blood pressure) as appropriate

Nursing Interventions and Rationales, Home Care Interventions, Client/Family Teaching

See care plan for **Deficient Fluid volume.**

Geriatric

- ▲ Aim for 1500 ml of oral liquids per day unless contraindicated by a medical condition such as congestive heart failure.
- Allow adequate time for eating and drinking at meals.
  Meals can provide two thirds of daily fluids if clients are encouraged to consume liquids and have sufficient time to do so (Bennett, 2000).
- Provide water that is freely available on the bedside or beside the chair.
- Offer fluids regularly throughout the day.
  Elderly clients may not think to serve themselves liquids but may consume them when offered (Bennett, 2000).
- Encourage consumption of fluids with medications.
  In one study it was shown that liquids consumed with medication made the difference between adequate and inadequate fluid intake for some clients (Lavizzo-Mourey, Johnson, Stolley, 1988).
- Ensure that clients who are immobile or restrained get adequate fluids.
  These are methods to increase fluid intake in the elderly and prevent defecient fluid volume (Bennett, 2000).

WEB SITES FOR EDUCATION

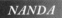 See the MERLIN web site for World Wide Web resources for client education.

REFERENCES   Bennett JA: Dehydration: hazards and benefits, *Geriatr Nurs* 21(2):84-88, 2000.
Lavizzo-Mourey RJ, Johnson J, Stolley P: Risk factors for dehydration among elderly nursing home residents, *J Am Geriatr Society* 36(3):213-218, 1988.

Risk for imbalanced Fluid volume

Terri Foster and Betty J. Ackley

NANDA   **Definition** At risk for a decrease, increase, or rapid shift from one to the other of intravascular, interstitial, and/or intracellular fluid (refers to body fluid loss, gain, or both)

- **= Independent; ▲ = Collaborative**

Risk Factors

Major invasive procedures

NOC   **Outcomes (Nursing Outcomes Classification)**
Suggested NOC Labels

Fluid Balance; Electrolyte and Acid-Base Balance; Hydration

> **Example NOC Outcome**
> Maintains **Fluid Balance** as evidenced by the following indicators: BP IER*/
> Peripheral pulses palpable/Skin hydration/Moist mucous membranes/Serum electro-
> lytes WNL†/Hematocrit WNL/Peripheral edema not present/Neck vein distention
> not present/Body weight stable/24-hour intake and output balanced/Urine specific
> gravity WNL/Adventitious breath sounds not present (Rate each indicator of **Fluid
> Balance:** 1 = extremely compromised, 2 = substantially compromised, 3 = moder-
> ately compromised, 4 = mildly compromised, 5 = not compromised [see Section I])

*In Expected Range
†Within Normal Limits

Client Outcomes

- Lung sounds clear, respiratory rate 12 to 20, and free of dyspnea postoperatively
- Maintains urine output of at least 30 to 50 ml/hour, 1300 ml/24 hours
- Blood pressure, pulse rate, and pulse oximetry within preoperative limits
- Laboratory values within expected range
- Nonedematous extremities and dependent areas
- Mental orientation unchanged from preoperative status

NIC   **Interventions (Nursing Interventions Classification)**
Suggested NIC Labels

Autotransfusion; Electrolyte Management; Fluid Management; Fluid Monitoring; Hypovolemia Management; Intravenous Therapy; Shock Management: Volume

> **Example NIC Interventions—Fluid Management**
> - Maintain accurate intake and output record
> - Monitor vital signs

Nursing Interventions and Rationales

- Carefully assess the client's preoperative status.
  *A history of aspirin, nonsteroidal antiinflammatory usage, or anticoagulant therapy can
  affect bleeding, as can a history of hemophilia, von Willebrand's disease, or disseminated
  intravascular coagulation. Use of laxatives, preoperative dehydration, infection, abnormal
  drainage, or hemorrhage can lead to hypotension during anesthesia induction if not corrected preoperatively. Preoperative vomiting, fever, sweating, or third-spacing resulting
  from a bowel obstruction, ascites, pleural effusion, or pulmonary edema can also lead to
  fluid and electrolyte imbalances if undetected. If the caregiver is unaware of preexisting
  excess fluid volume as in heart or liver disease, renal failure, hormonal disturbances, or
  from iatrogenic causes, fluid overload could occur (Rothrock, 1996).*
- Monitor vital signs, noting especially pulse rate and blood pressure. If systolic blood
  pressure is <100, notify anesthesiologist.

• = **Independent;** ▲ = **Collaborative**

The blood pressure and pulse rate are an indication of fluid volume. Low pressures and increased pulse rate are seen in hypovolemia, which can be dangerous in the surgical client. A blood pressure <90 mm Hg for more than 1 hour can result in acute renal failure post-operatively in the cardiac surgery client (Suen et al, 1998).

- In the critically ill surgical client with a pulmonary artery catheter, monitor pressures, especially wedge pressure.

  Pulmonary artery pressures are helpful for determining fluid balance, including preload and afterload, and they can help to guide fluid administration and administration of vasoactive IV drips such as dopamine.

▲ If hypotension develops, administer fluid challenge as ordered, giving a specified amount of IV fluid, such as 0.9% normal saline rapidly IV, and watching response in vital signs, lung sounds, and urine output.

  A fluid challenge can help reverse deficient fluid volume rapidly.

- Keep all IV fluids on a volumetric pump.

  This is done to ensure that IVs do not "run in" and fluid-overload the client and so that client receives sufficient fluids.

- Carefully keep track of input and output of fluids during surgery.

  The intake and output chart provides a means of evaluating fluid balance (Clancy, McVicar, 1997).

▲ Measure urine output hourly. If urine output is <30 ml/hr or 0.5 ml/kg/hr, notify anesthesiologist.

  Urine output is an indicator of fluid balance in the body. If output falls below 30 ml/hr, it may indicate deficient fluid volume, which can result in systemic hypoperfusion, decreased oxygen delivery, and organ system failure (Rothrock, 1996; Weissman, 1994). Assessment, accurate documentation of intake and output, and management of fluid and electrolyte imbalances is crucial to prevent serious problems (Kumar, 2001).

- If large amounts of fluid or tissues are being removed during surgery, be especially vigilant in watching for signs of hypovolemia and hypokalemia.

  When large amounts of fluids are removed from the body, the possibility of hypovolemia exists (Trott et al, 1998). Removing large amounts of fluids during surgery increases renal flow (Meeker, Rothrock, 1999).

▲ If large amounts of hypotonic irrigation solutions (e.g., glycine) are used during surgery, carefully keep track of fluid inflow and outflow. If there is a deficit of 1000 ml or more in outflow, request an order for a serum sodium (Kriplani et al, 1998) and also a serum osmolality (Metheny, 2000).

  TURP syndrome: Watch for symptoms of headache, visual changes, agitation, lethargy, vomiting, muscle twitching, bradycardia, diminished pupillary reflexes, hypertension and respiratory distress (Metheny, 2000).

- Endometrial ablation: If client is undergoing general anesthesia, watch for symptoms of decreased body temperature, decreased oxygen saturation, dilated pupils, and tremulousness (Metheny, 2000).

  Serious fluid overload and dilutional hyponatremia can develop in surgeries such as trans-urethral resections of the prostate, transcervical resection of the endometrium, or a hysteroscopy as a result of the absorption of large amounts of irrigation solution into the vascular system, which can cause permanent morbidity or death (Indman et al, 1998; Kriplani et al, 1998; Meeker, Rothrock, 1999). Saline cannot be used for irrigation in these procedures because it conducts electrical current and electrosurgical cautery is used during the procedure (Meeker, Rothrock, 1999).

- Observe the surgical client for signs of hyperkalemia: cardiac dysrhythmias, heart block, asystole, abdominal distention, and weakness.

Massive blood transfusions, tissue breakdown from surgery, crush injuries, or burns can lead to hyperkalemia (Meeker, Rothrock, 1999). Clients who have undergone bilateral thyroid surgery should be observed for hypocalcemia (Kumar, 2001).

- Observe closely for signs of hypokalemia in clients who have been under prolonged stress or who have lost GI fluids. Hypokalemia commonly causes dysrhythmias.

Stress and/or GI fluid loss in surgical clients make them susceptible to hypokalemia.

- Recognize that the surgical client may develop hyponatremia related to inappropriate antidiuretic hormone (ADH) secretion, which can be caused by trauma, thrombosis, abscesses, hemorrhages, or hematomas (Leite, 2001).

ADH, which acts on the kidneys to control water loss/retention, is an important factor in surgical clients under stress (Kumar, 2001).

- Accurately measure blood loss intraoperatively.

Weighing sponges is a reliable means of estimating blood loss and gauging replacement needs (Meeker, Rothrock, 1999).

Geriatric

- Be especially vigilant when monitoring vital signs and fluids in elderly surgical clients.

The elderly have depressed homeostatic mechanisms to regulate fluid balance during surgery, and many have renal insufficiency or heart failure, which can result in increased morbidity and sometimes mortality postoperatively (Metheny, 2000).

Pediatric

- Monitor pediatric surgical clients closely for signs of fluid loss.

Small losses can be life-threatening to these clients (Kumar, 2001).

WEB SITES FOR EDUCATION

MERLIN See the MERLIN web site for World Wide Web resources for client education.

REFERENCES   Clancy J, McVicar A: Homeostasis: the key concept to physiological control, *Br J Theatre Nurs* 7(8):27-32, 1997.

Indman PD et al: Complications of fluid overload from resectoscopic surgery, *J Am Assoc Gynecol Laparosc* 5(1):63-67, 1998.

Kriplani A et al: Biochemical, hemodynamic and hematological changes during transcervical resection of the endometrium using a 1.5% glycine as the irrigation solution, *Eur J Obstet Gynecol Reprod Biol* 80(1):99-104, 1998.

Kumar N: *Monitoring fluids and electrolytes in the surgical patient,* web site: www.advancefornurses.com/ls1.html?issue=22 (accessed March 5, 2001).

Leite W: *Fluid and electrolyte disorders—part I: disorders of sodium balance,* web site: www.medstudents.com.br/cirur/cirur1.htm (accessed March 5, 2001).

Meeker MH, Rothrock JC: *Alexander's care of the patient in surgery,* ed 11, St Louis 1999, Mosby.

Metheny NM: *Fluid and electrolyte balance: nursing considerations,* ed 4, Philadelphia, 2000, JB Lippincott.

Rothrock JC: *Perioperative nursing care plans,* ed 2, St Louis, 1996, Mosby.

Suen WS et al: Risk factors for development of acute renal failure requiring dialysis in patients undergoing cardiac surgery, *Angiology* 49(10):789-800, 1998.

Trott WA et al: Safety considerations and fluid resuscitation in liposuction: an analysis of 53 consecutive patients, *Plast Reconstr Surg* 102(6):220-229, 1998.

Weissman C: Ensuring perioperative fluid homeostasis in critically ill patients, *J Crit Illness* 9(12):183-190, 1994.

• = **Independent**; ▲ = **Collaborative**

Impaired Gas exchange

Betty J. Ackley

NANDA   **Definition**   Excess or deficit in oxygenation and/or carbon dioxide elimination at the alveolar-capillary membrane

Defining Characteristics

Visual disturbances; decreased carbon dioxide; dyspnea; abnormal arterial blood gases; hypoxia; irritability; somnolence; restlessness; hypercapnia; tachycardia; cyanosis (in neonates only); abnormal skin color (pale, dusky); hypoxemia; hypercarbia; headache on awakening; abnormal rate, rhythm, depth of breathing; diaphoresis; abnormal arterial pH; nasal flaring

NOC   Outcomes (Nursing Outcomes Classification)

Suggested NOC Labels

Respiratory Status: Gas Exchange; Respiratory Status: Ventilation; Tissue Perfusion: Pulmonary; Vital Signs Status; Electrolyte and Acid-Base Balance

> **Example NOC Outcome**
> Achieves appropriate **Respiratory Status: Gas Exchange** as evidenced by the following indicators: Mental status IER*/Restlessness not present/Cyanosis not present/Somnolence not present/PaO_2 WNL†/$PaCO_2$ WNL/Arterial pH WNL/O_2 saturation WNL/End tidal CO_2 IER (Rate each indicator of **Respiratory Status:** 1 = extremely compromised, 2 = substantially compromised, 3 = moderately compromised, 4 = mildly compromised, 5 = not compromised [see Section I])

*In Expected Range
†Within Normal Limits

Client Outcomes

- Demonstrates improved ventilation and adequate oxygenation as evidenced by blood gases within client's normal parameters
- Maintains clear lung fields and remains free of signs of respiratory distress
- Verbalizes understanding of oxygen and other therapeutic interventions

NIC   Interventions (Nursing Interventions Classification)

Suggested NIC Labels

Airway Management; Oxygen Therapy; Respiratory Monitoring; Acid-Base Management

> **Example NIC Interventions—Acid-Base Management**
> - Monitor for symptoms of respiratory failure (e.g., low PaO_2 and elevated $PaCO_2$ levels and respiratory muscle fatigue)
> - Monitor determinants of tissue oxygen delivery (e.g., PaO_2 SaO_2 and hemoglobin levels and cardiac output) if available

Nursing Interventions and Rationales

- Monitor respiratory rate, depth, and effort, including use of accessory muscles, nasal flaring, and abnormal breathing patterns.

• = Independent; ▲ = Collaborative

Increased respiratory rate, use of accessory muscles, nasal flaring, abdominal breathing, and a look of panic in the client's eyes may be seen with hypoxia.

- Auscultate breath sounds q ___ h(rs).
  Presence of crackles and wheezes may alert the nurse to an airway obstruction, which may lead to or exacerbate existing hypoxia.
- Monitor client's behavior and mental status for onset of restlessness, agitation, confusion, and (in the late stages) extreme lethargy.
  Changes in behavior and mental status can be early signs of impaired gas exchange (Misasi, Keyes, 1994). In late stages the client becomes lethargic, somnolent, and then comatose (Pierson, 2000).
- ▲ Monitor oxygen saturation continuously, using pulse oximeter. Note blood gas results as available.
  An oxygen saturation of <90% (normal: 95% to 100%) or a partial pressure of oxygen of <80 (normal: 80 to 100) indicates significant oxygenation problems.
- Observe for cyanosis in skin; especially note color of tongue and oral mucous membranes.
  Central cyanosis of tongue and oral mucosa is indicative of serious hypoxia and is a medical emergency. Peripheral cyanosis in extremities may or may not be serious (Carpenter, 1993).
- If client is acutely dyspneic, coach the client to slow respiratory rate using touch on the shoulder, demonstrating slower respirations while making eye contact with the client, and communicating in a calm, supportive fashion.
  Anxiety can exacerbate dyspnea, causing the client to enter into a dyspneic panic state (Gift, Moore, Soeken, 1992; Bruera et al, 2000). The nurse's presence, reassurance, and help in controlling the client's breathing can be very beneficial (Truesdell, 2000).
- Demonstrate and encourage the client to use pursed-lip breathing.
  Pursed-lip breathing results in increased use of intercostal muscles, decreased respiratory rate, increased tidal volume, and improved oxygen saturation levels (Breslin, 1992). Pursed-lip breathing can result in increased exercise performance (Casciarai et al, 1981), and it empowers the client to self-manage dyspneic incidences (Truesdell, 2000).
- Position client with head of bed elevated, in a semi-Fowler's position as tolerated.
  Semi-Fowler's position allows increased lung expansion because the abdominal contents are not crowding the lungs.
- If client has unilateral lung disease, alternate semi-Fowler's position with lateral position (with a 10- to 15-degree elevation and "good lung down" for 60 to 90 minutes). This method is contraindicated for clients with a pulmonary abscess or hemorrhage or interstitial emphysema.
  Gravity and hydrostatic pressure cause the dependent lung to become better ventilated and perfused, which increases oxygenation (Lasater-Erhard, 1995; Yeaw, 1992).
- If client has a bilateral lung disease, position in either a semi-Fowler's or side-lying position, which increases oxygenation as indicated by pulse oximetry (or if client has pulmonary catheter, venous oxygen saturation). Turn client every 2 hours. Monitor mixed venous oxygen saturation closely after turning. If it drops below 10% or fails to return to baseline promptly, turn the client back into a supine position and evaluate oxygen status.
  Turning is important to prevent complications of immobility, but in critically ill clients with low hemoglobin levels or decreased cardiac output, turning on either side can result

• = **Independent;** ▲ = **Collaborative**

in desaturation (Winslow, 1992). Critically ill clients should be turned carefully and watched closely (Gawlinski, Dracup, 1998).

- If client is obese or has ascites, consider positioning client in reverse Trendelenburg position at 45 degrees for periods as tolerated.
  A study demonstrated that use of the reverse Trendelenburg position at 45 degrees resulted in increased tidal volumes and decreased respiratory rates in a group of intubated clients with obesity, abdominal distention, and ascites (Burns et al, 1994; Winslow, 1996).
- Consider positioning the client prone with upper thorax and pelvis supported, allowing the abdomen to protrude. Monitor oxygen saturation, and turn back if desaturation occurs. Do not put in prone position if client has multisystem trauma.
  Partial pressure of arterial oxygen has been shown to increase in the prone position, possibly because of greater contraction of the diaphragm and increased function of ventral lung regions (Douglas et al, 1977; Lasater-Erhard, 1995; Curley, 1999). Prone positioning improves hypoxemia significantly (Dupont et al, 2000). In one study clients with multisystem trauma had serious iatrogenic injuries with prone positioning, including wound dehiscence, chest wall pressure necrosis, and a cardiac arrest (Offner et al, 2000).
- If client is acutely dyspneic, consider having client lean forward over a bedside table, if tolerated.
  Leaning forward can help decrease dyspnea, possibly because gastric pressure allows better contraction of the diaphragm (Celli, 1998). The tripod position can be helpful during times of dyspnea (Dunn, 2001).
- Help client deep breathe and perform controlled coughing. Have client inhale deeply, hold breath for several seconds, and cough two to three times with mouth open while tightening the upper abdominal muscles as tolerated.
  This technique can help increase sputum clearance and decrease cough spasms (Celli, 1998). Controlled coughing uses the diaphragmatic muscles, making the cough more forceful and effective.
  NOTE: If client has excessive fluid in respiratory system, see interventions for **Ineffective Airway clearance.**
- ▲ Monitor the effects of sedation and analgesics on client's respiratory pattern; use judiciously.
  Both analgesics and medications that cause sedation can depress respiration at times. However, these medications can be very helpful for decreasing the sympathetic nervous system discharge that accompanies hypoxia.
- Schedule nursing care to provide rest and minimize fatigue.
  The hypoxic client has limited reserves; inappropriate activity can increase hypoxia.
- ▲ Administer humidified oxygen through appropriate device (e.g., nasal cannula or face mask per physician's order); watch for onset of hypoventilation as evidenced by increased somnolence after initiating or increasing oxygen therapy.
  A client with chronic lung disease may need a hypoxic drive to breathe and may hypoventilate during oxygen therapy.
- Provide adequate fluids to liquefy secretions within the client's cardiac and renal reserve.
  If client is severely debilitated from chronic respiratory disease, consider use of a wheeled walker to help in ambulation.
- Use of a wheeled walker has been shown to result in significant decrease in disability, hypoxemia, and breathlessness during a 6-minute walk test (Honeyman, Barr, Stubbing, 1996).

• = Independent; ▲ = Collaborative

▲ Monitor nutritional status. Refer client for a dietary consult if needed.
Many clients with emphysema are malnourished. Improved nutrition can help improve inspiratory muscle function (Meeks et al, 1999).

▲ If chronic pulmonary disease is interfering with quality of life, refer client for pulmonary rehabilitation. Pulmonary rehabilitation programs that include desensitization to dyspnea and guided mastery with monitored exercise are preferable.
Pulmonary rehabilitation has been shown to improve exercise capacity, ability to walk, and sense of well-being (Fishman, 1994; American Thoracic Society, 1999; Janssens, de-Muralt, Titelion, 2000). The processes of desensitization and guided mastery for control of dyspnea have helped clients learn to be in control of their condition and have increased the amount of activity they can tolerate (Carrieri-Kohlman et al, 1993).

▲ Refer client to pulmonary rehabilitation team if client has chronic respiratory disease.
This team is multidisciplinary, and working together can help increase exercise capacity, decrease dyspnea, improve quality of life, and decrease admissions to the hospital (Celli, 1998).

NOTE: If client becomes ventilator-dependent, see care plan for **Impaired spontaneous Ventilation.**

Geriatric

▲ Use central nervous system depressants carefully to avoid decreasing respiration rate.
An elderly client is prone to respiratory depression.

▲ Maintain low-flow oxygen therapy.
An elderly client is susceptible to oxygen-induced respiratory depression.

• Encourage client to stop smoking.
There are substantial health benefits for elderly clients who stop smoking (Foyt, 1992).

Home Care Interventions

• Assess the home environment for irritants that impair gas exchange. Help the client to adjust home environment as necessary (e.g., installing air filter to decrease presence of dust).

▲ Refer client to occupational therapy as necessary to assist with adapting to home environment and energy conservation.

• Assist client with identifying and avoiding situations that exacerbate impairment of gas exchange (e.g., stress-related situations, proximity to noxious gas fumes such as chlorine bleach).
Irritants in the environment decrease the client's effectiveness in accessing oxygen during breathing.

• Instruct client to limit exposure to persons with respiratory infections.

▲ Instruct family in complications of disease and importance of maintaining medical regimen, including when to call physician.

• Assess nutritional status. Instruct client to eat several small meals daily and to use dietary supplements as necessary.
Clients with decreased oxygenation have little energy to use for eating and will avoid meals. Malnutrition significantly affects the aerobic capacity of muscle and exercise tolerance in clients with chronic obstructive pulmonary disease (COPD) (Palange et al, 1995). When nutritional status is clearly improved, it is accompanied by improvements in strength of the respiratory muscles and, in some studies, increased distance of walking (Larson, Leidy, 1998).

• = Independent; ▲ = Collaborative

▲ Refer client for home health aide services as necessary to assist with activities of daily living (ADLs).
Clients with decreased oxygenation have decreased energy to carry out personal and role activities.

▲ Assess family role changes and coping ability. Refer client to medical social services as appropriate for assistance in adjusting to chronic illness.
Inability to maintain pre-illness level of social involvement leads to frustration and anger in the client and may create a threat to the family unit. In one study, clients with chronic lung problems were described as negative, helpless, confused, and socially obstreperous by their family members (Leidy, Traver, 1996).

▲ Refer to outpatient pulmonary rehabilitation program, or a home-based training program for COPD.
Outpatient rehabilitation programs can achieve worthwhile benefits, including decreased perception of dyspnea, increased walking distance, and less fatigue, with benefits that persist for a period of 2 years (Glell et al, 2000). A simple home-based program of exercise training can achieve improvement in exercise tolerance, dyspnea, and quality of life for COPD patients (Hernandez et al, 2000). In mild COPD, a weight-training program was shown to result in increased strength and increased exercise tolerance (Clark et al, 2000).

• Support family of client with chronic illness.
Severely compromised respiratory functioning causes fear and anxiety in clients and their families. Reassurance from the nurse can be helpful.

Client/Family Teaching

• Teach client these techniques to use during acute dyspneic episodes:
  ▪ Pursed-lip breathing and controlled diaphragmatic breathing: Have client watch pulse oximetry to note improvement in oxygenation with breathing techniques.
    Controlled breathing techniques can help control anxiety and decrease panic and dyspnea (Celli, 1998; Dunn, 2001).
  ▪ Progressive muscle relaxation with or without guided imagery.
    Progressive relaxation eases the workload of muscles that are not being used to breathe, reducing the body's oxygen requirement (Dunn, 2001).
  ▪ Assistive breathing technique: Fold arms just below ribcage and push into belly while exhaling, then release during inhalation; repeat process until breathing becomes more controlled.
    This technique can help push the diaphragm up and force out the trapped air that was causing the feeling of pressure (Dunn, 2001).

• Instruct client to keep home temperature above 68° F and to avoid cold weather.
Cold air temperatures cause constriction of the blood vessels and increased moisture, impairing the client's ability to absorb oxygen.

• Teach clients to keep humidity levels in their homes between 40% and 50%, using a humidifier or dehumidifier as needed.
Both high humidity and low humidity can affect the ability of the COPD client to breathe comfortably (Dunn, 2001).

• Teach client energy conservation techniques and the importance of alternating rest periods with activity. See nursing interventions for **Fatigue.**

▲ Teach the importance of not smoking. Be aggressive in approach, and ask client to set a date for smoking cessation. Recommend nicotine replacement therapy (nicotine

• = Independent; ▲ = Collaborative

patch or gum). Refer client to smoking cessation programs. Encourage clients who relapse to keep trying to quit.

All health care clinicians should be aggressive in helping smokers quit (Agency for Health Care Policy Research, 1996).

▲ Instruct family regarding home oxygen therapy if ordered (e.g., delivery system, liter flow, safety precautions). If need for oxygen is chronic, encourage use of a portable system. Explain advantages of transtracheal oxygen delivery systems. Encourage client to use oxygen as ordered.

Clients with portable oxygen therapy spent more time outside and walked futher than people with fixed delivery systems (Vergeret, Brambilla, Mounier, 1989). Clients with transtracheal oxygen delivery systems were more independent than those with fixed delivery systems and had increased morale (Bloom et al, 1989; Larson, Leidy, 1998). Clients who used oxygen for longer periods had decreased mortality (Pierson, 2000).

• Teach client relaxation therapy techniques to help reduce stress responses and panic attacks resulting from dyspnea.

Relaxation therapy includes progressive muscle relaxation, autogenic techniques, visualization, and diaphragmatic breathing. This therapy can help to modify the symptoms of dyspnea and help the client deal with feelings associated with the chronic disease (Jerman, Haggerty, 1993).

WEB SITES FOR EDUCATION

Merlin See the MERLIN web site for World Wide Web resources for client education.

REFERENCES   Agency for Health Care Policy Research: *Smoking cessation: Clinical Practice Guideline No. 18,* U.S. Government Printing Office No. 017-026-00159-0, 1996, The Agency.

American Thoracic Society: Dyspnea mechanisms, assessment, and management: a consensus statement, *Am J Respir Crit Care Med* 159:321-340, 1999.

Bloom et al: Transtracheal oxygen delivery and patients with chronic obstructive pulmonary disease, *Respir Med* 4:281-288, 1989.

Breslin EH: The pattern of respiratory muscle recruitment during pursed lip breathing *Chest* 101(1):75-78, 1992.

Bruera E et al: The frequency and correlates of dyspnea in patients with advanced cancer, *J Pain Symptom Manage* 19(5):357-363, 2000.

Burns SM et al: Effect of body position on spontaneous respiratory rate and tidal volume in patients with obesity, abdominal distention and ascites, *Am J Crit Care* 3:102-107, 1994.

Carpenter KD: A comprehensive review of cyanosis, *Crit Care Nurse* 13:66-72, 1993.

Carrieri-Kohlman V et al: Desensitization and guided mastery: treatment approaches for the management of dyspnea, *Heart Lung* 22(3):226-233, 1993.

Casciari RJ et al: Effects of breathing retraining in patients with chronic obstructive pulmonary disease, *Chest* 79(4):393-398, 1981.

Celli BR: Pulmonary rehabilitation for COPD, *Postgrad Med* 103(4):159-175, 1998.

Clark CJ et al: Skeletal muscle strength and endurance in patients with mild COPD and the effects of weight training, *Eur Respir J* 15(1):92-97, 2000.

Curley MA: Prone positioning of patients with acute respiratory distress syndrome: a systematic review, *Am J Crit Care* 8(6):397-405, 1999.

Douglas W et al: Improved oxygenation in patients with acute respiratory failure: the prone position, *Am Rev Respir Dis* 115:559, 1977.

Dunn N: Keeping COPD patients out of the ER, *RN* 64(2):33-37, 2001.

Dupont H et al: Short-term effect of inhaled nitric oxide and prone positioning on gas exchange in patients with severe acute respiratory distress syndrome, *Crit Care Med* 28(2):304-308, 2000.

• = Independent; ▲ = Collaborative

Foyt MM: Impaired gas exchange in the elderly, *Geriatr Nurs* 13:262, 1992.

Gawlinski A, Dracup K: Effect of positioning on SvO2 in the critically ill patient with a low ejection fraction, *Nurs Res* 47(5):293-298, 1998.

Gift AG, Moore T, Soeken K: Relaxation to reduce dyspnea and anxiety in COPD patients, *Nurs Res* 41(4):242, 1992.

Glell R et al: Long-term effects of outpatient rehabilitation of COPD: a randomized trial, *Chest* 117(4):976-983, 2000.

Hernandez MTE et al: Results of a home-based training program for patients with COPD, *Chest* 118(1):106-114, 2000.

Honeyman P, Barr P, Stubbing DG: Effect of a walking aid on disability, oxygenation, and breathlessness in patients with chronic airflow limitation, *J Cardiopulm Rehab* 16:63-67, 1996.

Janssens JP, deMuralt B, Titelion V: Management of dyspnea in severe chronic obstructive pulmonary disease, *J Pain Symptom Manage* 19(5):378-392, 2000.

Jerman A, Haggerty MC: Relaxation and biofeedback: coping skills training. In Casaburi R, Petty L, editors: *Principles and practice of pulmonary rehabilitation,* Philadelphia, 1993, WB Saunders.

Larson JL, Leidy NK: Chronic obstructive pulmonary disease: strategies to improve functional status, *Annu Rev Nurs Res* 16:253-286, 1998.

Lasater-Erhard M: The effect of patient position on arterial oxygen saturation, *Crit Care Nurse* 15(5):31-36, 1995.

Leidy NK, Traver GA: Adjustment and social behavior in older adults with chronic obstructive pulmonary disease: the family's perspective, *J Adv Nurs* 23:252-259, 1996.

Meeks PM et al: Dyspnea: mechanisms, assessment, and management—a consensus statement, *Am J Respir Crit Care Med* 159:321-340, 1999.

Misasi RS, Keyes JL: The pathophysiology of hypoxia, *Crit Care Nurse* 14:55-64, 1994.

Offner PJ et al: Complications of prone ventilation in patients with multisystem trauma with fulminant acute respiratory distress syndrome. *J Trauma Injury Infect Crit Care* 48(2):224-228, 2000.

Palange P et al: Nutritional state and exercise tolerance in patients with COPD, *Chest* 107:1206-1212, 1995.

Pierson DJ: Pathophysiology and clinical effects of chronic hypoxia: state-of-the-art conference on long-term oxygen therapy, part 1, *Resp Care* 45(1):39-51, 2000.

Truesdell S: Helping patients with COPD manage episodes of acute shortness of breath, *Medsurg Nurs* 9(4):178-182, 2000.

Vergeret J, Brambilla C, Mounier L: Portable oxygen therapy: use and benefit in hypoxaemic COPD patients on long-term oxygen therapy, *Eur Resp J* 2:20-25, 1989.

Winslow EH: Turn for the worse, *Am J Nurs* 92:16C, 1992.

Winslow EH: High Fowler's won't always ease breathing, *Am J Nurs* 96:59, 1996.

Yeaw P: Good lung down, *Am J Nurs* 92:27, 1992.

Grieving

Betty J. Ackley

Definition   A state in which an individual or group of individuals reacts to an actual or perceived loss, which may be a person, object, function, status, relationship, or body part

NOTE: Grieving is not an official NANDA nursing diagnosis, but it is included because the authors believe that grieving is part of the normal human response to loss and that nurses can use interventions to help the client grieve. Grieving is a wellness-oriented nursing diagnosis (Arnold, 1996).

Defining Characteristics

Verbal expression of distress at loss; anger; sadness; crying; difficulty in expressing loss; alterations in eating habits, sleep patterns, dream patterns, activity levels, or libido;

• = Independent; ▲ = Collaborative

reliving of past experiences; interference with life function; alterations in concentration or pursuit of tasks

Related Factors (r/t)

Actual or perceived object loss, which may include people, possessions, job, status, home, ideals, or parts and processes of the body

NOC Outcomes (Nursing Outcomes Classification)

Suggested NOC Labels

Grief Resolution; Hope; Mood Equilibrium; Psychosocial Adjustment: Life Change

> **Example NOC Outcome**
>
> Accomplishes **Grief Resolution** with plans for a positive future as evidenced by the following indicators: Expresses feelings about loss/Verbalizes acceptance of loss/Describes meaning of the loss or death/Reports decreased preoccupation with loss/Expresses positive expectations about the future (Rate each indicator of **Grief Resolution:** 1 = not at all, 2 = to a slight extent, 3 = to a moderate extent, 4 = to a great extent, 5 = to a very great extent [see Section I])

Client Outcomes

- Expresses feelings of guilt, fear, anger, or sadness
- Identifies problems associated with grief (e.g., changes in appetite, insomnia, loss of libido, decreased energy, alteration in activity level)
- Plans for future one day at a time
- Functions at normal developmental level and performs activities of daily living (ADLs)

NIC Interventions (Nursing Interventions Classification)

Suggested NIC Labels

Grief Work Facilitation; Grief Work Facilitation: Perinatal Death

> **Example NIC Interventions—Grief Work Facilitation**
> - Encourage the client to verbalize memories of the loss, both past and current
> - Assist client to identify personal coping strategies

Nursing Interventions and Rationales

- Allow family members to participate in care of the body if desired. Help survivors say goodbye in the most loving and caring way possible.
  These experiences can help facilitate positive outcomes from grieving.
- Allow family "holding" behaviors, including taking photographs of the deceased or clipping a piece of hair.
  Holding behaviors can help the family preserve the fact and meaning of the loved one's existence (Carter, 1989).
- Help bereaved client survive during times of acute grief. Ensure that client maintains sufficient nutrition, and help client determine a routine to make it through each day.
  A newly bereaved person can be stunned and helpless (Gifford, Cleary, 1990). It is common for a newly bereaved person to eat minimally for several days (Rodebaugh, Schwindt, Valentine, 1999), but after that it is important that they eat to maintain health.
- Encourage client to share memories of the person or loss by saying, "Tell me about your wife [or husband, parent]." Do an in-depth personal interview to learn about client and loved one or loss.

• = Independent; ▲ = Collaborative

A personal history can help a nurse understand the unique loss that the person has experienced, the meaning of the loss to the individual, and the strengths the person brings to the situation (Solari-Twadell et al, 1995). Bereaved clients need someone to listen to them while they sort out the complex emotional reactions to the new reality.

- Actively listen to the client's expression of grief; do not interrupt, do not tell own story, and do not offer meaningless platitudes such as, "It will be better this way." *These behaviors do not help and can often hurt (Gifford, Cleary, 1990; Hoffman, 1997).*
- Encourage client to "cry out" his or her grief and express feelings, including sadness and anger. *Grief is work and is best treated as an active process in which the grieving client expresses and feels the grief (Grainger, 1990).*
- If client or family members are expressing anger, try not to react in anger. Instead, allow feelings to be expressed, listen to the expressions of anger, and accept their right to those feelings. Try lowering the voice and slowing the rate of speech as you respond back to the client/family. *It is not therapeutic to respond to anger with anger. Instead, strive to be therapeutic, helping the client/family express the anger and gain control of themselves by modeling calm behavior (Rueth, Hall, 1999).*
- Help client identify previous successful personal coping strategies. *Coping strategies used previously are helpful in dealing with loss.*
- ▲ Refer client for spiritual counseling if desired. *Spiritual counseling can help the client gain perspective about the loss and give comfort.*
- Provide information about the grief process, including the stages of grieving: denial, anger, bargaining, and acceptance (Kubler-Ross, 1969) or reeling, feeling, dealing, and healing (Rodebaugh, Schwindt, Valentine, 1999). Help client realize that spasms of grief can come at any time, that most people don't go through the stages in a predictable fashion, and that the grieving process takes time and is painful. *This information helps normalize the grief experience and provides clients with hope that they can survive (Gifford, Cleary, 1990; Rodebaugh, Schwindt, Valentine, 1999).*
- Help client determine the best way and where to find social support. Encourage client to continue to use supports for 1 to 2 years. *Social support has been identified as an important predictor of positive bereavement (Cooley, 1992; Steen, 1998).*
- ▲ Assess for causes of dysfunctional grieving (e.g., sudden death, highly dependent or ambivalent relationship with deceased, lack of coping skills, lack of social support, previous physical or mental health problems, death of child, death of wife, death by suicide). Refer for counseling, starting 2 to 8 weeks after loss and for up to 3 months following bereavement (Steen, 1998). Refer to care plan for **Dysfunctional Grieving.** *Life circumstances can interfere with normal grieving (Steen, 1998).*
- Assess for signs of depression: feelings of worthlessness, inability to eat or sleep, sleeping all the time. *Depression can occur in nearly half of all grieving people, and 10% of people who are grieving suffer major depression (Steen, 1998).*
- Encourage family members to set aside time to talk with one another about the loss without criticizing or belittling one another's feelings.

• = **Independent;** ▲ = **Collaborative**

Once these feelings are shared, family members can begin to accept the unacceptable (Gifford, Cleary, 1990). Help families to grieve as a system, not just as individual mourners (Steen, 1998).

▲ Identify available community resources, including bereavement groups from local hospitals and hospice. Volunteers who provide bereavement support can also be effective.
Support groups can have positive effects on bereavement outcomes (Heiney, Dunaway, Webster, 1995; Hoffman, 1997; Stewart, 1995).

▲ Recognize times when you as a nurse are affected by loss and need grief resolution. Attend a grief resolution group, ask for help from pastoral care, speak with a kind friend who is supportive, or seek counseling.
Nursing staff can experience unresolved grief from the death of a client or may suffer other losses that require grief resolution so that they can function effectively and be able to give to others (Hittle, 1995).

Geriatric

• Use reminiscence therapy in conjunction with the expression of emotions.
Reminiscence therapy can help the client look back at past experiences and use coping techniques that were effective in the past (Puentes, 1998).

• Identify previous losses, and assess client for depression.
Losses and changes associated with aging often occur in rapid succession without adequate recovery time (Hegge, Fischer, 2000). Having more than two concurrent losses increases the incidence of unresolved grief (Herth, 1990). The grieving elderly widow may develop depression resulting in poor nutrition, noncompliance with medications, decreasing cognition, and multiple health problems (Fischer, Hegge, 2000).

• Evaluate the social support system of the elderly client. If support system is minimal, help client determine how to increase available support.
The elderly who have poor grieving outcomes often do not live with family members and have a minimal support system. The support of family (especially children) and friends is a common way for elderly widows to cope with a loss (Hegge, Fischer, 2000).

Multicultural

• Assess for the influence of cultural beliefs, norms, and values on the client's grief and mourning practices.
Grieving practices may be based on cultural perceptions (Leininger, 1996). Great emphasis may be placed on attendance at funerals for some blacks; many Native American tribes may hold long somber wakes during which food and memorial gifts are distributed; Chinese and Japanese families may have specific funeral rituals that must be followed precisely to ensure safe passage of their loved one; Latinos may hold wakes, utilize prayer during a novena, and light candles in honor of the dead; in West Indian/Caribbean cultures death arrangements may be made by a kinsman of the deceased (McQuay, 1995).

• Assess for the influence of cultural beliefs, norms, and values on the client's expressions of grief.
Blacks may be expected to act "strong" and go about the business of life after a death; Native Americans may not talk about the death because of beliefs that such talk will detract from spirituality and bring bad luck; Latinos may wear black and act subdued during their luto/mourning period; Southeast Asian families may wear white when mourning (McQuay, 1995).

• Identify whether the client had been notified of health status and was able to be present at deathbed.

• = **Independent;** ▲ = **Collaborative**

Not being present during terminal illness and death can disrupt grief process (McQuay, 1995).
- Validate the client's feelings regarding the loss.
  Validation lets the client know that the nurse has heard and understands what was said, and it promotes the nurse-client relationship (Stuart, Laraia, 2001; Giger, Davidhizar, 1995).

Home Care Interventions
- If the agency has served the deceased as a client, allow primary caregivers to attend services.
  Families experiencing the loss of a loved one perceive staff attendance at services as a significant statement of caring and support.
- Plan first home visit within 10 days following loss by client, guided by type of loss and schedule of family following loss.
  Support is a contributing factor to completion of grief work. The nurse can provide support and guidance.
- If the loss is of a loved one, allow client to express feelings about the loss through interaction with the home environment (e.g., looking at pictures, keeping special chairs or clothing).
  Symbols of the lost loved one can be comforting and allow the bereaved to accept the loss in stages.
- ▲ Refer the bereaved to hospice bereavement programs.
  Support can be provided by groups of people sharing similar pain. Bereavement programs can support the bereaved through the first full year following the loss using personal contact, telephone calls, and cards.
- ▲ Refer the client to medical social services as necessary for losses not related to deaths.
  Support is helpful to grief work for all types of losses. Social workers can assist the client with planning for financial changes as a result of job losses and help with community referrals as appropriate.
- ▲ Refer the bereaved spouse to an Internet self-help group if desired.
  An Internet-based self-help group can help the bereaved spouse cope, receive support, develop a sense of family, share information, and help others (Bacon, Condon, Fernsler, 2000).

WEB SITES FOR EDUCATION

$\overset{\$}{\text{MERLIN}}$ See the MERLIN web site for World Wide Web resources for client education.

REFERENCES   Arnold J: Rethinking grief: nursing implications for health promotion, *Home Health Nurse* 14(10):777-785, 1996.
Bacon ES, Condon EH, Fernsler JI: Young widows' experience with an internet self-help group, *J Psychosoc Nurs* 38(7):24-33, 2000.
Carter SL: Themes of grief, *Nurs Res* 38(6):354-358, 1989.
Cooley ME: Bereavement care: a role for nurse, *Cancer Nurs* 15(2):125-129, 1992.
Fischer C, Hegge M: The eldery woman at risk, *AJN* 100(6):54-57, 2000.
Gifford BJ, Cleary BB: Supporting the bereaved, *Am J Nurs* 90(2):49-53, 1990.
Giger JN, Davidhizar RE: *Transcultural nursing*, ed 2, St Louis, 1995, Mosby.
Grainger RD: Successful grieving, *Am J Nurs* 90(9):12, 1990.
Hegge M, Fischer C: Grief responses of senior and elderly widows: practice implications, *J Gerontol Nurs* 26(2):35-43, 2000.
Heiney SP, Dunaway C, Webster J: Good grieving: an intervention program for grieving children, *Oncol Nurs Forum* 22:649-655, 1995.
Herth K: Relationship of hope, coping styles, concurrent losses, and setting to grief resolution in the elderly widow(er), *Res Nurs Health* 13:109-117, 1990.
Hittle JM: Grieving together, *Am J Nurs* 95(7):55-57, 1995.

- **= Independent;** ▲ **= Collaborative**

Hoffman C: Volunteers providing bereavement support, *Caring* 16(11):48-50, 1997.

Kubler-Ross E: *On death and dying,* New York, 1969, Macmillan.

Leininger MM: *Transcultural nursing: theories, research and practices,* ed 2, Hilliard, Ohio, 1996, McGraw-Hill.

McQuay JE: Cross-cultural customs and beliefs related to health crises, death, and organ donation/transplantation: a guide to assist health care professionals understand different responses and provide cross-cultural assistance, *Crit Care Nurs Clin North Am* 7(3):581-594, 1995.

Puentes WJ: Incorporating simple reminiscence techniques into acute care nursing practice, *J Gerontol Nurs* 24(2):15-20, 1998.

Rodebaugh LS, Schwindt RG, Valentine FM: How to handle grief, *Nursing* 99(10):52-53, 1999.

Rueth TW, Hall SE: Dealing with the anger and hostility of those who grieve, *Am J Hosp Palliat Care* 16(6):743-746, 1999.

Solari-Twadell PA et al: The pinwheel model of bereavement, *Image* 27(4):323-326, 1995.

Steen KF: A comprehensive approach to bereavement, *Nurse Pract* 23(3):54-64, 1998.

Stewart ES: Family-centered care for the bereaved, *Pediatr Nurs* 21(2):181-184, 1995.

Stuart GW, Laraia MT: Therapeutic nurse-patient relationship. In Stuart GW, Laraia MT, editors: *Principles and practice of psychiatric nursing,* St Louis, 2001, Mosby, p 30.

Anticipatory Grieving

Betty J. Ackley

NANDA   **Definition**   Intellectual and emotional responses and behaviors by which individuals, families, and communities work through the process of modifying self-concept based on the perception of potential loss

Defining Characteristics

Expression of distress at potential loss; sorrow; guilt; denial of potential loss; anger; altered communication patterns; potential loss of significant object (e.g., people, possessions, job, status, home, ideals, parts and processes of the body); denial of the significance of the loss; bargaining; alteration in eating habits, sleep patterns, dream patterns, activity level, libido; difficulty taking on new or different roles; resolution of grief before the reality of loss

Related Factors (r/t)

Perceived or actual impending loss of people, objects, possessions, job, status, home, ideals, or parts and processes of body (Carpenito, 1993)

NOC   **Outcomes (Nursing Outcomes Classification)**

Suggested NOC Labels

Grief Resolution; Coping; Family Coping; Family Environment: Internal; Psychosocial Adjustment: Life Change

> **Example NOC Outcome**
>
> Accomplishes **Grief Resolution** with plans for a positive future as evidenced by the following indicators: Expresses feelings about loss/Verbalizes acceptance of loss/Describes meaning of the loss or death/Reports decreased preoccupation with loss/Expresses positive expectations about the future (Rate each indicator of **Grief Resolution:** 1 = not at all, 2 = to a slight extent, 3 = to a moderate extent, 4 = to a great extent, 5 = to a very great extent [see Section I])

• = **Independent;** ▲ = **Collaborative**

Client Outcomes

- Expresses feelings of guilt, anger, or sorrow
- Identifies problems associated with anticipatory grief (e.g., changes in activity, eating, or libido)
- Seeks help in dealing with anticipated problems
- Plans for the future one day at a time

NIC Interventions (Nursing Interventions Classification)

Suggested NIC Labels

Grief Work Facilitation; Grief Work Facilitation: Perinatal Death

> **Example NIC Interventions—Grief Work Facilitation**
> - Encourage the client to verbalize memories of the loss, both past and current
> - Assist client to identify personal coping strategies

Nursing Interventions and Rationales

- If grief results from impending death of a loved one, allow family members to stay with loved one during the dying process if desired, and help them determine appropriate times to take breaks.
  Families often feel disorganized and helpless; they need support from nurses to be with the dying person (Walters, 1995).
- Encourage family members to touch dying client if they are comfortable with doing so.
  Sharing personal space with touch can help establish connectedness and help with grieving (Walters, 1995).
- Encourage family members to listen carefully to messages given by the dying loved one; they may hear symbolic or obscure language referring to the dying process.
  As people approach death, they develop an understanding of how their death will unfold, and they communicate this awareness in symbolic language (Callanan, 1994).
- If dying client is denying seriousness of his or her condition, do not negate the denial.
  Denial protects clients from hopelessness and may be their coping mechanism to deal with reality. Not everyone needs to go through the stages of dying (McClement, Degner, 1995).
- Help dying client to maintain hope by focusing on the moment, reviewing his or her assets, and maintaining important relationships.
  Hope is not a cure for the dying; hope maintains a connection to the world (McClement, Degner, 1995).
- Help family members to let the loved one go if appropriate; give the loved one permission to die.
  Sometimes dying people wait until they know their family members are strong enough to accept the loss before they allow themselves to die (Callanan, 1994).
- Use therapeutic communication with open-ended questions such as: "What are your thoughts and fears?"
  Nurses need to give a grieving client permission and opportunity to talk about the anticipated loss.
- Actively listen to client's/family's expression of grief; do not interrupt, do not tell own story, and do not offer meaningless platitudes such as: "It will be better this way."
  Just being with the client/family and listening can be the most helpful thing the nurse does (Furman, 2000). Behaviors such as telling own story and meaningless platitudes do not help and can often hurt (Gifford, Cleary, 1990).

• = Independent; ▲ = Collaborative

- Encourage client to "cry out" grief and express feelings, including sadness or anger.
  Grief is work and is best treated as an active process in which the grieving client expresses and feels the grief.
- Encourage client to take care of any unfinished business if appropriate. Client can talk to dying person or use simulated conversations to resolve issues.
  Unfinished business must be resolved before the grieving client can heal and move on (Grainger, 1990).
- Help client build memories. This can be done a number of ways, including:
  - Love letters—letters to be opened on family birthdays or other special days after death
  - Audiotaped or videotaped recordings—to share memories and say goodbye
  - Journaling—an autobiography that can be read by children and loved ones
  - Planning own funeral
  - Writing own obituary
  - Leaving a legacy—designating money for favorite causes
  These are creative ways to nurture family relationships by leaving mementos for loved ones (Brant, 1998).
- ▲ Assess for spiritual distress, and refer client for spiritual counseling if desired and appropriate.
  Spiritual support can help clients; the nurse should approach the client with a nonjudgmental, listening ear and refer to the appropriate spiritual leader (Brant, 1998).
- Help client/family determine how to best obtain social support.
  Social support has been identified as an important predictor of positive bereavement (Cooley, 1992; Costello, 1999).
- Identify problems with eating or sleeping, and intervene with suggestions as appropriate.
  A grieving client can feel stunned and helpless and be unable to consume food for a period (Gifford, Cleary, 1990).
- Encourage caregiver of a dying person to live one day at a time and recognize that mourning is occurring while caring for the loved one. Help caregiver express feelings of loss, and encourage caregiver to practice self-care. Refer to care plan for **Caregiver role strain** if appropriate.
  Caregivers grieve as they give care to the dying person. They can develop an increased intimacy and involvement in the relationship, which can help them obtain a positive bereavement outcome (Brown, Powell-Cope, 1993; Costello, 1999).

Multicultural

- Assess for the influence of cultural beliefs, norms, and values on the client's grief and mourning practices.
  Grieving practices may be based on cultural perceptions (Leininger, 1996). Great emphasis may be placed on attendance at funerals for some blacks; many Native American tribes may hold long somber wakes during which food and memorial gifts are distributed; Chinese and Japanese families may have specific funeral rituals that must be followed precisely to ensure safe passage of their loved one; Latinos may hold wakes, utilize prayer during a novena, and light candles in honor of the dead; in West Indian/Caribbean cultures death arrangements may be made by a kinsman of the deceased (McQuay, 1995).
- Assess for the influence of cultural beliefs, norms, and values on the client's expressions of grief.
  Blacks may be expected to act "strong" and go about the business of life after a death; Native Americans may not talk about the death because of beliefs that such talk will

• = Independent; ▲ = Collaborative

detract from spirituality and bring bad luck; Latinos may wear black and act subdued during their luto/mourning period; Southeast Asian families may wear white when mourning (McQuay, 1995).

- Identify whether significant family members have been notified of health status and are able to be present.
  Not being present during terminal illness and death can disrupt grief process (McQuay, 1995).
- Validate the client's feelings regarding the impending loss.
  Validation lets the client know that the nurse has heard and understands what was said, and it promotes the nurse-client relationship (Stuart, Laraia, 2001; Giger, Davidhizar, 1995).

Home Care Interventions

NOTE: Hospice care encourages individuals and families to experience final days in the setting of choice. All of the previously mentioned interventions can and should be applied in the home setting when that is the setting of choice.

- ▲ When potential loss is of a loved one, refer grieving client to hospice volunteer services for support.
  Social support has been identified as the most important predictor of positive bereavement (Cooley, 1992). Hospice volunteers are available to the grieving person, and support is their only agenda.

Client/Family Teaching

- Teach caregivers that they are doing anticipatory grieving as they care for their loved one, which is part of the reason care can be so difficult. The grief can become more acute as death approaches.
  Anticipatory grief allows adaptation to the loss to begin before the loved one's death (Costello, 1999).

WEB SITES FOR EDUCATION

MERLIN See the MERLIN web site for World Wide Web resources for client education.

REFERENCES Brant JM: The art of palliative care: living with hope, dying with dignity, *Oncol Nurs Forum* 25(6):995-1003, 1998.
Brown MA, Powell-Cope G: Themes of loss and dying in caring for a family member with AIDS, *Res Nurs Health* 16:179-191, 1993.
Callanan M: Farewell messages: dealing with death, *Am J Nurs* 94(5):19-20, 1994.
Carpenito JL: *Nursing diagnosis: applications to clinical practice,* ed 5, Philadelphia, 1993, JB Lippincott.
Cooley ME: Bereavement care: a role for nurses, *Cancer Nurs* 15:125, 1992.
Costello J: Anticipatory grief: coping with the impending death of a partner, *Int J Palliat Nurs* 5(5):223-231, 1999.
Furman J: Taking a holistic approach to the dying time, *Nursing* 30(6):46-49, 2000.
Gifford BJ, Cleary BB: Supporting the bereaved, *Am J Nurs* 90:49, 1990.
Giger JN, Davidhizar RE: *Transcultural nursing,* ed 2, St Louis, 1995, Mosby.
Grainger RD: Successful grieving, *Am J Nurs* 90:12, 1990.
Leininger MM: *Transcultural nursing: theories, research and practices,* ed 2, Hilliard, Ohio, 1996, McGraw-Hill.
McClement SE, Degner LF: Expert nursing behaviors in care of the dying adult in the intensive care unit, *Heart Lung* 24(5):408-419, 1995.
McQuay JE: Cross-cultural customs and beliefs related to health crises, death, and organ donation/transplantation: a guide to assist health care professionals understand different responses and provide cross-cultural assistance, *Crit Care Nurs Clin North Am* 7(3):581-594, 1995.
Stuart GW, Laraia MT: Therapeutic nurse-patient relationship. In Stuart GW, Laraia MT, editors: *Principles and practice of psychiatric nursing,* St Louis, 2001, Mosby, p 30.
Walters AJ: A hermeneutic study of the experiences of relatives of critically ill patients, *J Adv Nurs* 22:998-1005, 1995.

• = **Independent;** ▲ = **Collaborative**

Dysfunctional Grieving

Betty J. Ackley

NANDA **Definition** Extended unsuccessful use of intellectual and emotional responses by which individuals, families, and communities attempt to work through the process of modifying self-concept based on the perception of loss

NOTE: It is now recognized that sometimes what was previously diagnosed as **Dysfunctional Grieving** might instead be **Chronic Sorrow,** in which grief lingers and is reactivated at intervals (Eakes, Burke, Hainsworth, 1998). Refer to the nursing diagnosis **Chronic Sorrow** if appropriate.

Defining Characteristics

Repetitive use of ineffectual behaviors associated with attempts to reinvest in relationships; crying; sadness; reliving of past experiences with little or no reduction (diminishment) of intensity of the grief; labile affect; expression of unresolved issues; interference with life functioning; verbal expression of distress at loss; idealization of lost object (e.g., people, possessions, job, status, home, ideals, parts and processes of the body); difficulty in expressing loss; denial of loss; anger; alterations in eating habits, sleep patterns, dream patterns, activity level, libido, concentration and/or pursuit of tasks; developmental regression; expression of guilt; prolonged interference with life functioning; onset or exacerbation of somatic or psychosomatic responses

Related Factors (r/t)

Actual or perceived object loss (e.g., people, possessions, job, status, home, ideals, parts and processes of the body)

NOC **Outcomes (Nursing Outcomes Classification)**

Suggested NOC Labels

Grief Resolution; Family Coping; Coping; Psychosocial Adjustment: Life Change

> **Example NOC Outcome**
> Accomplishes **Grief Resolution** with plans for a positive future as evidenced by the following indicators: Expresses feelings about loss/Verbalizes acceptance of loss/ Describes meaning of the loss or death/Reports decreased preoccupation with loss/ Expresses positive expectations about the future (Rate each indicator of **Grief Resolution:** 1 = not at all, 2 = to a slight extent, 3 = to a moderate extent, 4 = to a great extent, 5 = to a very great extent [see Section I])

Client Outcomes

- Expresses appropriate feelings of guilt, fear, anger, or sadness
- Identifies problems associated with grief (e.g., changes in appetite, insomnia, nightmares, loss of libido, decreased energy, alteration in activity levels)
- Seeks help in dealing with grief-associated problems
- Plans for future one day at a time
- Identifies personal strengths
- Functions at a normal developmental level and performs activities of daily living (ADLs) after an appropriate length of time

• = Independent; ▲ = Collaborative

NIC **Interventions (Nursing Interventions Classification)**
Suggested NIC Labels
Grief Work Facilitation; Grief Work Facilitation: Perinatal Death; Guilt Work Facilitation

> **Example NIC Interventions—Grief Work Facilitation**
> - Encourage the client to verbalize memories of the loss, both past and current
> - Assist client to identify personal coping strategies

Nursing Interventions and Rationales

- Assess client's state of grieving. Utilize a tool such as the Hogan Grief Reaction Checklist, or the Grief Experience Inventory.
  These are commonly used measures of grief that have shown to effectively measure grief (Hogan, Greenfield, Schmidt, 1988; Gamino, Sewell, Easterling, 2000).
- Assess for causes of dysfunctional grieving (e.g., sudden bereavement [less than 2 weeks to prepare for the oncoming loss], highly dependent or ambivalent relationship with the deceased, inadequate coping skills, lack of social support, previous physical or mental health problems, death of a child, loss of spouse).
  Life circumstances can interfere with normal grieving and be risk factors for dysfunctional grieving (Steele, 1992; Stewart, 1995; Gamino, Sewell, Easterling, 2000).
- Observe for the following reactions to loss, which predispose a client to dysfunctional grieving:
  - Delayed grieving: the bereaved exhibits little emotion and continues with a busy life
  - Inhibited grieving: the bereaved exhibits various physical conditions and does not feel grief
  - Chronic grieving: the behaviors of the normal grief period continue beyond a reasonable time
  These maladaptive grief reactions indicate that the client needs help with grief work (Gifford, Cleary, 1990).
- Identify problems of eating and sleeping; ensure that basic human needs are being met.
  Losses often interrupt appetite and sleep (Bateman et al, 1992; Gifford, Cleary, 1990).
- Develop a trusting relationship with client by using therapeutic communication techniques.
  An accepting, trusting relationship facilitates communication and serves as a foundation for healing.
- Establish a defined time to meet and discuss feelings about the loss and to perform grief work.
- Encourage client to "cry out" grief and to talk about feelings of anger, sadness, and guilt.
  Grief is work and is best treated as an active process in which the bereaved expresses and feels the grief. Expression of guilt or anger is necessary for progressing through the grieving process and feeling better (Bateman et al, 1992).
- ▲ Assess for spiritual distress, and refer client to appropriate spiritual leader.
  Intrinsic spirituality can help the client grieve (Gamino, Sewell, Easterling, 2000); the nurse should approach the client with a nonjudgmental, listening ear and refer client to the appropriate spiritual leader (Brant, 1998).
- Help client recognize that although sadness will occur at intervals for the rest of his or her life, it will become bearable.

• = **Independent;** ▲ = **Collaborative**

The sadness associated with chronic sorrow is permanent, but as the grief resolves, there can be times of satisfaction and even happiness (Grainger, 1990; Teel, 1991). Grief has a lasting nature; it changes and softens but never ends (Carter, 1989).

- Help client complete the following "guilt work" exercises:
  - Identifying "if onlys" and putting them into perspective
  - Dealing with "I didn't do" by looking at what was accomplished
  - Forgiving self; say to client, "You are being awfully hard on yourself; try not to hurt yourself over something you could not have controlled"

The client may need to resolve guilt before successfully grieving and moving on with life.

- Help client review past experiences, role changes, and coping skills.
- Encourage client to keep a journal and write about their bereavement experience.

Writing projects can be helpful for clients who are grieving, especially for those experiencing the unique bereavement of suicidal death (Range, Kovac, Marion, 2000).

- Help client to identify own strengths for use in dealing with loss; reinforce these strengths.
- If client or family members are expressing anger, try not to react in anger. Instead, allow feelings to be expressed, listen to the expressions of anger, and accept their right to those feelings. Try lowering the voice and slowing the rate of speech as you respond back to the client/family.

It is not therapeutic to respond to anger with anger. Instead, strive to be therapeutic, helping the client/family express the anger and gain control of themselves by modeling calm behavior (Rueth, Hall, 1999).

- Expect client to meet responsibilities; give positive reinforcement.
- Help client to identify areas of hope in life and to determine their purposes if possible.

A significant positive relationship has been found between the level of grief resolution and the level of hope (Herth, 1990). Grieving people who have little purpose in life often experience more anger than individuals with more purpose.

- ▲ Encourage client to make time to talk to family members about the loss with the help of professional support as needed and without criticizing or belittling one another's feelings about the loss.

Once these feelings are shared, family members can begin to accept the unacceptable (Gifford, Cleary, 1990).

- ▲ Identify available community resources, including bereavement groups from local hospitals and hospice.

Support groups can have positive effects on bereavement for both children and adults (Cooley, 1992; Heiney, Dunaway, Webster, 1995; Stewart, 1995).

- ▲ Identify whether client is experiencing depression, suicidal tendencies, or other emotional disorders. Refer client for counseling as appropriate.

Counseling, including use of relaxation therapy, desensitization, and biofeedback in addition to traditional psychotherapy, has been shown to be helpful (Arnette, 1996). Depression syndromes occur in almost one half of all grieving people, and 10% suffer major depression (Steen, 1998). Cognitive behavior therapy can be helpful for traumatic grief (Jacobs, Prigerson, 2000).

Geriatric

- Use reminiscence therapy in conjunction with the expression of emotions (Puentes, 1998).
- Identify previous losses and assess client for depression. Signs of depression are often masked by somatic complaints.

• = Independent; ▲ = Collaborative

Losses and changes associated with older age often occur in rapid succession without adequate recovery time. Having more than two concurrent losses increases the incidence of unresolved grief (Herth, 1990). The elderly often express grief in the form of somatic complaints (Steen, 1998).

- Evaluate the social support system of the elderly client. If support system is minimal, help client determine how to increase available support.
  The elderly who have poor grieving outcomes often do not live with family members and have a minimal support system.

Multicultural

- Assess for the influence of cultural beliefs, norms, and values on the client's grief and mourning practices.
  Grieving practices may be based on cultural perceptions (Leininger, 1996). Great emphasis may be placed on attendance at funerals for some blacks; many Native American tribes may hold long somber wakes during which food and memorial gifts are distributed; Chinese and Japanese families may have specific funeral rituals that must be followed precisely to ensure safe passage of their loved one; Latinos may hold wakes, utilize prayer during a novena, and light candles in honor of the dead; in West Indian/Caribbean cultures death arrangements might be made by a kinsman of the deceased (McQuay, 1995).
- Assess for the influence of cultural beliefs, norms, and values on the client's expressions of grief.
  Blacks may be expected to act "strong" and go about the business of life after a death; Native Americans may not talk about the death because of beliefs that such talk will detract from spirituality and bring bad luck; Latinos may wear black and act subdued during their luto/mourning period; Southeast Asian families may wear white when mourning (McQuay, 1995).
- Identify whether the client had been notified of health status and was able to be present during death and illness.
  Not being present during terminal illness and death can disrupt grief process (McQuay, 1995).
- Validate the client's feelings regarding the loss.
  Validation lets the client know that the nurse has heard and understands what was said, and it promotes the nurse-client relationship (Stuart, Laraia, 2001; Giger, Davidhizar, 1995).

Home Care Interventions

- Encourage client to make choices about daily living and the home environment that acknowledge the loss.
  Helping with grief work allows client to accept reality of loss and realize that grieving is a healthy response.
- Evaluate the long-term support system of the bereaved client. Encourage client to interact with the support system at defined intervals.
  Regular contact with support systems allows for regular expression of feelings and grief resolution.
- ▲ Refer client to or encourage continued interaction with hospice volunteers and bereavement programs as continuing forms of support.
- ▲ Refer client to medical social services, especially the hospice program social worker, for assistance with grief work.
  Consulting with or referring to specialty services is sometimes the best way to provide care.

• = **Independent;** ▲ = **Collaborative**

REFERENCES Arnette JD: Physiological effects of chronic grief: a biofeedback treatment approach, *Death Stud* 20:59-72, 1996.

Bateman A et al: Dysfunctional grieving, *J Psychosoc Nurs* 30(12):5-9, 1992.

Brant JM: The art of palliative care: living with hope, dying with dignity, *Oncol Nurs Forum* 25(6):995, 1998.

Carter SL: Themes of grief, *Nurs Res* 38(6):354-358, 1989.

Cooley ME: Bereavement care: a role for nurses, *Cancer Nurs* 15:125, 1992.

Eakes GG, Burke ML, Hainsworth MA: Theory: middle-range theory of chronic sorrow, *Image J Nurs Sch* 30:179, 1998.

Gamino LA, Sewell KW, Easterling LW: Scott and White Grief Study—phase 2: toward an adaptive model of grief, *Death Stud* 24:633-660, 2000.

Gifford BJ, Cleary B: Supporting the bereaved, *Am J Nurs* 90:49, 1990.

Giger JN, Davidhizar RE: *Transcultural nursing,* ed 2, St Louis, 1995, Mosby.

Grainger RD: Successful grieving, *Am J Nurs* 90:12, 1990.

Heiney SP, Dunaway NC, Webster J: Good grieving: an intervention program for grieving children, *Oncol Nurs Forum* 22(4):649-655, 1995.

Herth K: Relationship of hope, coping styles, concurrent losses, and setting to grief resolution in the elderly widow(er), *Res Nurs Health* 13:109, 1990.

Hogan NS, Greenfield DB, Schmidt LA: Validation of the Hogan Grief Reaction Checklist, *Death Stud* 25(1):1-32, 2001.

Jacobs S, Prigerson H: Psychotherapy of traumatic grief: a review of evidence for psychotherapeutic treatments, *Death Stud* 24:479-495, 2000.

Leininger MM: *Transcultural nursing: theories, research and practices,* ed 2, Hilliard, Ohio, 1996, McGraw-Hill.

McQuay JE: Cross-cultural customs and beliefs related to health crises, death, and organ donation/transplantation: a guide to assist health care professionals understand different responses and provide cross-cultural assistance, *Crit Care Nurs Clin North Am* 7(3):581-594, 1995.

Puentes WJ: Incorporating simple reminiscence techniques into acute care nursing practice, *J Gerontol Nurs* 24(2):15-20, 1998.

Range LM, Kovac SH, Marion MS: Does writing about the bereavement lessen grief following sudden, unintentional death? *Death Stud* 24:115-134, 2000.

Rueth TW, Hall SE: Dealing with the anger and hostility of those who grieve, *Am J Hosp Palliat Care* 16(6):743-746, 1999.

Steele L: Risk factor profile for bereaved spouses, *Death Stud* 16:387, 1992.

Steen KF: A comprehensive approach to bereavement, *Nurse Pract* 23(3):54-64, 1998.

Stewart ES: Family-centered care for the bereaved, *Pediatr Nurs* 21:181, 1995.

Stuart GW, Laraia MT: Therapeutic nurse-patient relationship. In Stuart GW, Laraia MT, editors: *Principles and practice of psychiatric nursing,* St Louis, 2001, Mosby, p 30.

Teel CS: Chronic sorrow: analysis of the concept, *J Adv Nurs* 16:1311, 1991.

Delayed Growth and development

Peggy A. Wetsch and Mary Markle

NANDA **Definition** Deviations from age group norms

Defining Characteristics

Altered physical growth; delay or difficulty in performing skills (motor, social, expressive) typical of age group; inability to perform self-care or self-control activities appropriate for age; flat affect; listlessness; decreased responses

• = Independent; ▲ = Collaborative

Related Factors (r/t)

Prescribed dependence; indifference; separation from significant others; environmental and stimulation deficiencies; effects of physical disability; inadequate caretaking; inconsistent responsiveness; multiple caretakers

NOC **Outcomes (Nursing Outcomes Classification)**

Suggested NOC Labels

Child Development: 2 Months, 4 Months, 6 Months, 12 Months, 2 Years, 3 Years, 4 Years, 5 Years, Middle Childhood (5-11 Years), Adolescence (12-17 Years); Growth; Physical Maturation: Female; Physical Maturation: Male

> **Example NOC Outcome**
> Demonstrates **Growth** as evidenced by indicators of normal increase in body size and weight (Rate indicator of **Growth:** 1 = extreme deviation from expected range, 2 = substantial deviation from expected range, 3 = moderate deviation from expected range, 4 = mild deviation from expected range, 5 = no deviation from expected range [see Section I])

Client Outcomes

- Describes realistic, age-appropriate patterns of growth and development (parents/primary caregiver)
- Promotes activities and interactions that support age-related developmental tasks (parents/primary caregiver)
- Displays consistent, sustained achievement of age-appropriate behaviors (social, interpersonal, and/or cognitive) and/or motor skills (child/adolescent)
- Achieves realistic developmental and/or growth milestones based on existing abilities, extent of disability, and functional age (mentally and/or physically challenged)
- Exhibits limited temporary behavioral regression that reverses shortly after episode of illness/hospitalization (child/adolescent)
- Attains steady gains in growth patterns (child/adolescent)

NIC **Interventions (Nursing Interventions Classification)**

Suggested NIC Labels

Developmental Care and Enhancement; Nutritional Therapy

> **Example NIC Interventions—Developmental Enhancement**
> - Teach caregivers about normal developmental milestones and associated behaviors
> - Enhance parental effectiveness

Nursing Interventions and Rationales

NOTE: Determination of the etiologic basis for delayed growth and development is critical because it will direct the selection of interventions for treating the client. Parenting skill deficits, lack of consistency between caregivers, and hospitalization versus a chronic medical condition/developmental disability will necessitate different strategies. A hospitalization experience with regressive behaviors can be a transient occurrence, as opposed to a chronic situation, which may have more severe and longer delays requiring more in-depth intervention. Parenting skills and consistent expectations between multiple caregivers can be addressed by more intensive education efforts (Seideman, Kleine, 1995; Stutts, 1994).

• = **Independent;** ▲ = **Collaborative**

- Identify child at risk for or with actual developmental delays using standard developmental screening surveillance tests.

  Developmental surveillance is a flexible, ongoing process that involves the use of both skilled observation of the child and concerns of parents, health professionals, teachers, and others to identify children at risk for variation in normal growth and development (Curry, Duby, 1994).

- Interview parents to determine risk for or actual deviations in normal development. Note and emphasize positive attributes of parents/family.

  Early intervention into developmental issues is beneficial to both parents and children and leads to improved outcomes (Curry, Duby, 1994). Accepting the family's value system with respect will support and encourage parents/family to increase their involvement (Reis, 1993).

- Compare height and weight measurements regularly for child or adolescent to established age-appropriate norms and previous measurements over time.

  This process identifies delayed growth patterns and deviations from the norm (U.S. Public Health Service, 1995).

▲ Initiate referrals for a more comprehensive growth and/or development evaluation if indicated.

  Presence of a risk factor alone does not always obviate the need for referrals. The number and weight of risk factors and normal differences of each child must be considered (Curry, Duby, 1994).

▲ Identify coexisting health or medical conditions that may be contributing to the alteration in growth and/or development, and refer client to appropriate health care discipline for management.

  Treatment of underlying or coexisting conditions, such as metabolic disorders, obstructive sleep apnea, parasitic infestations, or brain injury, may facilitate return to previous developmental levels or growth patterns (Spahis, 1994).

- Examine parental/caregiver expectations of future learning, ability, and developmental achievements of children with developmental disabilities.

  Initiation of measures to support or enhance family/child motivation and ability increases achievement (Edwards-Beckett, 1994).

- Assist family with discerning child's regressive responses to illness, hospitalization, or chronic health conditions. Explain manifestations of regression, magical thinking, separation anxiety, and fears.

  A child may regress to earlier developmental levels. Children's responses differ from those of adults depending on the child's stage of cognitive development and previous encounters. When parents are able to attribute their child's usual reactions to stress and illness, they are better able to support the child (Ziegler, Prior, 1994).

- Provide meaningful stimulation for hospitalized infants and children.

  Stimulation is essential to the development of gross- and fine-motor adaptive skills, language, and personal-social functioning in infants and children. Disruption of this process for infants, even those without preexisting developmental delays, can occur without intervention. Hospitalized infants are often subjected to understimulation or an overabundance of meaningless stimulation (Slusher, McClure, 1995).

▲ Engage child in appropriate play activities. Refer child to play/recreational therapist (if available) for supplemental strategies.

  Play is the work of childhood. It supports the development of expanding gross- and fine-motor skills and social and interactional behaviors (LeVieux-Anglin, Sawyer, 1993).

• = Independent; ▲ = Collaborative

- Enlist and encourage parents and/or family involvement as participants in care, particularly for hospitalized infants, toddlers, preschoolers, or school-age children, whenever possible without exceeding the parent's/family's emotional and physical limits.
  Frequent and consistent parent/family contact and care diminish normal separation anxiety. Most infants and toddlers find this presence comforting and as a result are better able to cope with the situation and stress (Craft, Willadsen, 1992).
- Model age and cognitively appropriate caregiver skills by doing the following:
  - Communicating with child at an appropriate cognitive level of development
  - Giving the child tasks and responsibilities appropriate to age or functional age level
  - Instituting safety devices such as assistive equipment
  - Encouraging child to perform activities of daily living (ADLs) as appropriate
  These actions illustrate parenting and child-rearing skills and behaviors for parents and family members (McCloskey, Bulechek, 1992).
- Furnish an environment that promotes additional sleep and rest opportunities.
  A balance of sleep, rest, and activity is essential for sustained progression of growth and development (White et al, 1990).

Multicultural

- Acknowledge racial/ethnic differences at the onset of care.
  Acknowledgement of race/ethnicity issues will enhance communication, establish rapport, and promote treatment outcomes (D'Avanzo et al, 2001).
- Assess for the influence of cultural beliefs, norms, and values on the client's perceptions of child development.
  What the client considers normal and abnormal child development may be based on cultural perceptions (Leininger, 1996).
- Use a neutral, indirect style when addressing areas where improvement is needed (such as a need for verbal stimulation) when working with Native American clients.
  Using indirect statements such as "Other mothers have tried. . ." or "I had a client who tried 'X' and it seemed to work very well" will assist in avoiding resentment from the parent (Seiderman et al, 1996).
- Assess whether exposure to community violence is contributing to developmental problems.
  Exposure to community violence has been associated with increases in aggressive behavior and depression in children (Gorman-Smith, Tolan, 1998).
- Validate the client's feelings and concerns related to child's development.
  Validation lets the client know that the nurse has heard and understands what was said, and it promotes the nurse-client relationship (Stuart, Laraia, 2001; Giger, Davidhizar, 1995).

Client/Family Teaching

- Provide anticipatory guidance for parents/caregivers regarding expectations for realistic attainment of growth and development milestones. Clarify expectations and correct misconceptions.
  Parents/caregivers who understand both what is normal and realistic for their child are better equipped to provide a nurturing, supportive environment (Denehy, 1990).
- Have parents/caregivers rehearse coping strategies with approaching developmental milestones and acknowledge positive actions/behaviors.

• = Independent; ▲ = Collaborative

As children progress to another developmental stage, such as adolescence, families are challenged to master developmental tasks that seem enigmatic. Anticipating and preparing can strengthen their ability to mediate situations and enhance achievement (Reisch, Forsyth, 1992).

• Teach methods of providing meaningful stimulation for infants and children.
Stimulation is essential to the development of gross-motor and fine-motor adaptive skills, language, and personal-social functioning in infants and children (Slusher, McClure, 1995).

• Advise client with regard to age-appropriate activities and play, nutrition, discipline, and safety, and support growth and development.
Parents are then better equipped to promote the growth and development of the child (McCloskey, Bulechek, 1992).

▲ Elicit involvement of parents/caregivers in social support groups and parenting classes. Furnish information about community resources.
Support groups and other opportunities to obtain guidance serve to empower parents and clarify and reinforce knowledge and parenting skills (Kinney, Mannetter, Carpenter, 1992; McCloskey, Bulechek, 1992).

WEB SITES FOR EDUCATION

MERLIN   See the MERLIN web site for World Wide Web resources for client education.

REFERENCES   Craft MJ, Willadsen JA: Interventions related to family. In Bulechek GM, McCloskey JC, editors: Symposium on nursing interventions, *Nurs Clin North Am* 27:517-540, 1992.

Curry DM, Duby JC: Developmental surveillance by pediatric nurses, *Pediatr Nurs* 20:40-44, 1994.

D'Avanzo CE et al: Developing culturally informed strategies for substance-related interventions. In Naegle MA, D'Avanzo CE, editors: *Addictions and substance abuse: strategies for advanced practice nursing,* St Louis, 2001, Mosby, pp 59-104.

Denehy JA: Anticipatory guidance. In Craft MJ, Denehy JA, editors: *Nursing interventions for infants and children,* Philadelphia, 1990, WB Saunders.

Edwards-Beckett J: Caregivers' expectations of future learning of dependents with a developmental disability, *J Pediatr Nurs* 9:27, 1994.

Giger JN, Davidhizar RE: *Transcultural nursing,* ed 2, St Louis, 1995, Mosby.

Gorman-Smith D, Tolan P: The role of exposure to community violence and developmental problems among inner city youth, *Dev Psychopathol* 10(1):101-116, 1998.

Kinney CK, Mannetter R, Carpenter MA: Support groups. In Bulechek GM, McCloskey JC, editors: *Nursing interventions: essential nursing treatment,* Philadelphia, 1992, WB Saunders.

Leininger MM: *Transcultural nursing: theories, research and practices,* ed 2, Hilliard, Ohio, 1996, McGraw-Hill.

LeVieux-Anglin L, Sawyer EH: Incorporating play interventions into nursing care, *Pediatr Nurs* 19:459, 1993.

McCloskey JC, Bulechek GM, editors: *Nursing interventions classification (NIC),* St Louis, 1992, Mosby.

Reis M: The neglected preschooler, *Can Nurse* 89:42, 1993.

Reisch SK, Forsyth DM: Preparing to parent the adolescent: a theoretical overview, *J Child Adolesc Psychiatr Ment Health Nurs* 5:31, 1992.

Seideman RJ, Kleine PF: A theory of transformed parenting: parenting a child with developmental delay/mental retardation, *Nurs Res* 44:38, 1995.

Seiderman RY et al: Assessing American Indian families, *MCN Am J Matern Child Nurs* 21(6):274-279, 1996.

Slusher IL, McClure MJ: Infant stimulation during hospitalization, *J Pediatr Nurs* 7:276, 1995.

Spahis J: Sleepless nights: obstructive sleep apnea in pediatric patient, *J Pediatr Nurs* 20:469, 1994.

Stuart GW, Laraia MT: Therapeutic nurse-patient relationship. In Stuart GW, Laraia MT, editors: *Principles and practice of psychiatric nursing,* St Louis, 2001, Mosby, p 30.

• = Independent; ▲ = Collaborative

Stutts AL: Selected outcomes of technology-dependent children receiving home care and prescribed child care services, *J Pediatr Nurs* 20:501, 1994.

U.S. Public Health Service: Body measurement, *J Am Acad Nurs Pediatr* 7:339, 1995.

White MA et al: Sleep onset latency and distress in hospitalized children, *Nurs Res* 39:134, 1990.

Ziegler DB, Prior MM: Preparation for surgery and adjustment to hospitalization, *Nurs Clin North Am* 29:655, 1994.

Risk for disproportionate Growth

Gail B. Ladwig and Mary Markle

NANDA   **Definition** At risk for growth above the 97th percentile or below the 3rd percentile for age, crossing two percentile channels; disproportionate growth

Risk Factors

Prenatal Congenital/genetic disorders; maternal malnutrition; multiple gestation; teratogen exposure; substance use/abuse

Individual Infection; prematurity; malnutrition; organic and inorganic factors; caregiver and/or individual maladaptive feeding behaviors; anorexia; insatiable appetite; infection; chronic illness; substance abuse

Environmental Deprivation; teratogen; lead poisoning; poverty; violence; natural disasters

Caregiver Abuse; mental illness; mental retardation or severe learning disability

NOC   **Outcomes (Nursing Outcomes Classification)**

Suggested NOC Labels

Child Development: 2 Months, 4 Months, 6 Months, 12 Months, 2 Years, 3 Years, 4 Years, 5 Years, Middle Childhood (5-11 Years), Adolescence (12-17 Years); Growth; Physical Maturation: Female; Physical Maturation: Male

Example NOC Outcome

Demonstrates **Growth** as evidenced by indicators of normal increase in body size and weight (Rate each indicator of **Growth:** 1 = extreme deviation from expected range, 2 = substantial deviation from expected range, 3 = moderate deviation from expected range, 4 = mild deviation from expected range, 5 = no deviation from expected range [see Section I])

Client Outcomes

- States information related to possible teratogenic agents
- States information related to adequate nutrition
- Seeks help from appropriate professionals for nutritional needs

NIC   **Interventions (Nursing Interventions Classification)**

Suggested NIC Labels

Nutritional Monitoring; Teaching: Infant Nutrition; Toddler Nutrition; Nutritional Monitoring

Example NIC Interventions—Nutritional Monitoring

Teaching: Infant Nutrition; Toddler Nutrition; Nutritional Monitoring

• = **Independent;** ▲ = **Collaborative**

Nursing Interventions and Rationales

NOTE: Management of a risk diagnosis necessitates approaches using primary and secondary prevention. Primary prevention interventions, which include such activities as nutrition counseling, focus on thwarting the development of disease or condition. Secondary prevention is achieved through screening, monitoring, and surveillance (Shortridge, Valanis, 1992).

▲ Look for exposure to toxic agents during pregnancy:
- Prenatal: give mother information on known teratogenic agents
- Infectious agents: rubella, cytomegalovirus (CMV), other viral conditions (e.g., AIDS virus), syphilis, toxoplasmosis
- Therapeutics: thalidomide, aminopterin/amethopterin, warfarin (anticoagulant), phenytoin (anticonvulsant), trimethadione/paramethadione, valproate, iodides (thyroid medication), tetracycline (antibiotic), vitamin A (isotretinoin), diethylstilbesterol (DES; also causes cancer), x-rays
- Maternal conditions: AIDS, phenylketonuria, diabetes mellitus
- Illicit drugs: alcohol, crack, LSD, PCP, mescaline

Exposure during pregnancy to these agents has proven to be responsible for causing harmful effects in the unborn child (Blatt, 1999).

• Provide for adequate nutrition and nutrition monitoring in clients with developmental disorders.

When nutrition therapy is given in the early stages of diagnosis and treatment of cerebral palsy, growth delays may be prevented or remediated (Sanders et al, 1990). Nutrient needs may be altered as a result of long-term medication therapy for conditions such as epilepsy, recurrent urinary or respiratory infections, chronic constipation, and behavioral problems (American Dietetic Association, 1999).

▲ Provide for adequate nutrition for clients with active intestinal inflammation.

Nutrition is clearly disturbed by active intestinal inflammation. Appetite is reduced, yet energy substrates are diverted into the inflammatory process, thus weight loss is characteristic. The nutritional disturbance represents part of a profound defect of somatic function. Linear growth and pubertal development in children are notably retarded, body composition is altered, and there may be significant psychosocial disturbance. Increasing evidence shows that an aggressive nutritional program may in itself be sufficient to reduce the mucosal inflammatory response. Recent evidence suggests that enteral nutrition alone may reduce many proinflammatory cytokines to normal levels and allow mucosal healing (Murch, Walker-Smith, 1998).

▲ Provide for adequate nutrition for pediatric/adolescent clients on chronic oral glucocorticoid therapy (e.g., those treated for chronic severe asthma).

Growth may be inhibited by chronic use of these agents; however, recent studies suggest inhaled use of such agents does not affect long-term growth (Prescriber's Letter, 2000).

▲ Provide tube feedings per physician's order when appropriate for clients with neuromuscular impairment.

Feeding problems that arise from neuromuscular dysfunction, obstructive lesions, and/or psychological factors often reduce food intake, inhibit optimal growth and development, result in poor weight maintenance in adults, and increase the risk of malnutrition. Persons with cerebral palsy frequently have hyperactive gag reflex, tongue thrust, poor lip closure, gastroesophageal reflux, and inability to chew. Recurrent aspiration pneumonia is not uncommon. Tube feedings should be considered as a means to promote increased growth, but

• = **Independent**; ▲ = **Collaborative**

use requires ongoing nutrition monitoring and may present other medical and developmental concerns.
Refer to care plan for **Delayed Growth and development.**

Multicultural

- Assess for the influence of cultural beliefs, norms, values, and expectations on the parent's perception of normal growth and development.
  How the parent views normal growth and development may be based on cultural perceptions (Leininger, 1996).
- Negotiate with the client regarding which aspects of healthy nutrition can be modified and still honor cultural beliefs.
  Give and take with the client will lead to culturally congruent care (Leininger, 1996).
- Assess whether the parent has concerns about the amount of food eaten.
  Some cultures may add semisolid food within the first month of life because of concerns that the infant is not getting enough to eat and the perception that "big is healthy" (Higgins, 2000; Bentley et al, 1999).
- Assess the influence of family support on patterns of nutritional intake.
  Women are the keepers and transmitters of culture in families. Female family members can play a dominant role in how children and infants are fed (Pillitteri, 1999).

Client/Family Teaching

- Provide anticipatory guidance for parents/caregivers regarding expectations for normative patterns of growth. Clarify expectations and correct misconceptions.
  Parents/caregivers with this knowledge will be able to recognize and report early deviations in normal growth, allowing for more timely intervention.
- ▲ Refer client to a registered dietitian for nutritional counseling.
  Help from qualified professionals is often needed to meet the nutritional needs of clients with deviations in normal growth.
- Teach families the importance of taking measures to prevent lead poisoning: Wash before preparing the child's food. Wash the child's hands before serving food. Wash bottle nipples and pacifiers frequently, especially if they fall on the floor. Wash the child's toys frequently. Stomp your feet before coming in the house to clean your shoes of outside soil that may carry lead from exterior house paint. Damp mop frequently along baseboards, around door frames, under windowsills, and around iron radiators. Wash windowsills and window wells frequently. The window well is the depression behind the windowsill where the window fits when it is closed. Move the crib away from window wells. Always damp mop before sweeping or vacuuming. Home vacuum cleaners do not trap lead dust; they blow it into the air.
  Child's exposure to ingested lead can be lowered by following these instructions (Stapleton, 1998).

WEB SITES FOR EDUCATION

᛭MERLIN See the MERLIN web site for World Wide Web resources for client education.

REFERENCES   American Dietetic Association: *Nutrition in comprehensive program planning for persons with developmental disabilities (1996-1999),* retrieved from the World Wide Web March 29, 1999. Web site: www.eatright.org/adap0297b.html
Bentley M et al: Infant feeding practices of low-income, African-American, adolescent mothers: an ecological, multigenerational perspective, *Soc Sci Med* 49(8):1085-1100, 1999.

• = Independent; ▲ = Collaborative

Blatt R: What is a teratogen? *The Gene Letter* 1:3, 1996, retrieved from the World Wide Web March 29, 1999. Web site: www.geneletter.org/1196/teratogen.htm

Higgins B: Puerto Rican cultural beliefs: influence on infant feeding practices in western New York, *J Transcult Nurs* 11(1):19-30, 2000.

Leininger MM: *Transcultural nursing: theories, research and practices,* ed 2, Hilliard, Ohio, 1996, McGraw-Hill.

Murch SH, Walker-Smith JA: Nutrition in inflammatory bowel disease, *Baillieres Clin Gastroenterol* 12(4):719-738, 1998.

Pillitteri A: Nutritional needs of the newborn. In Pillitteri A, editor: *Maternal & child health nursing: care of the childbearing & childrearing family,* Philadelphia, 1999, Lippincott, Williams & Wilkins, pp 654-666.

Prescriber's Letter, National Institutes of Health: Childhood Asthma Management Program (CAMP), *New Engl J Med* 7(11):62, 2000.

Sanders K et al: Growth response to enteral feeding by children with cerebral palsy, *JPEN J* 14:23-26, 1990.

Shortridge L, Valanis B: The epidemiological model applied in community health nursing. In Stanhope M, Lancaster J, editors: *Community health nursing: process and practice for promoting health,* ed 3, St Louis, 1992, Mosby.

Stapleton R: *Help prevent childhood lead poisoning: a resource for parents,* 1998. Web site: nolead.home.mindspring.com/whatcani.htm#what can i do

Ineffective Health maintenance

Suzanne Skowronski and Gail B. Ladwig

NANDA **Definition** The inability to identify, manage, or seek out help to maintain health

Defining Characteristics

History of lack of health-seeking behavior; reported or observed lack of equipment, financial, and/or other resources; reported or observed impairment of personal support systems; expressed interest in improving health behaviors; demonstrated lack of knowledge regarding basic health practices; demonstrated lack of adaptive behaviors to internal and external environmental changes; reported or observed inability to take responsibility for meeting basic health practices in any or all functional pattern areas

Related Factors (r/t)

Disabled family coping, perceptual-cognitive impairment (complete or partial lack of gross or fine motor skills); lack of or significant alteration in communication skills (written, verbal, or gestural); unachieved developmental tasks; lack of material resources; dysfunctional grieving; disabling spiritual distress; inability to make deliberate and thoughtful judgments; ineffective coping

NOC **Outcomes (Nursing Outcomes Classification)**

Suggested NOC Labels

Health Beliefs: Perceived Resources; Health-Promoting Behavior, Health-Seeking Behavior

> **Example NOC Outcome**
> Demonstrates **Health-Seeking Behavior** as evidenced by the following indicators: Completes health-related tasks/Performs self-screening when indicated/Contacts health professionals when indicated (Rate each indicator of **Health-Seeking Behavior:** 1 = never demonstrated, 2 = rarely demonstrated, 3 = sometimes demonstrated, 4 = often demonstrated, 5 = consistently demonstrated [see Section I])

• = Independent; ▲ = Collaborative

Client Outcomes

- Discusses fear of or blocks to implementing a health regimen
- Follows mutually agreed upon health care maintenance plan
- Meets goals for health care maintenance

NIC **Interventions (Nursing Interventions Classification)**

Suggested NIC Labels

Health System Guidance; Support System Enhancement; Health Education

> **Example NIC Interventions—Health Education**
> - Prioritize identified learner needs based on client preference, skills of nurse, resources available, and likelihood of successful goal attainment
> - Emphasize immediate or short-term positive health benefits to be received from positive lifestyle behaviors rather than long-term benefits or negative effects of noncompliance

Nursing Interventions and Rationales

- Assess client's feelings, values, and reasons for not following prescribed plan of care. See Related Factors.
  A factor to assess when examining client responsibility is the level of dissatisfaction with current lifestyle and readiness for change (Clark, 1996).
- Assess for family patterns, economic issues, and cultural patterns that influence compliance with a given medical regimen.
  Responsiveness to clients enables the nurse to gain an understanding of clients' lives and to cultivate their connections to a responsive community, encouraging clients to not get into "receiving" behaviors (Smith-Battle, 1997).
- Help client determine how to arrange a daily schedule that incorporates the new health care regimen (e.g., taking pills before meals).
- ▲ Refer client to social services for financial assistance if needed.
  Information-seeking behavior is a strategy that many people use as a means of coping with and reducing stress when coping with an illness such as cancer (van der Molen, 1999).
- ▲ Identify support groups related to the disease process (e.g., Reach to Recovery for a woman who has had a mastectomy).
- Help client to choose healthy lifestyle and to have appropriate diagnostic screening tests.
  This study identified that women who adopt a healthy lifestyle and practice preventive healthy behaviors can reduce the risks of some cancers and other diseases such as heart disease and sexually transmitted infections (Furniss, 2000).
- ▲ Identify complementary healing modalities such as herbal remedies, acupuncture, healing touch, yoga, or cultural shamans that the client uses in addition to or instead of the prescribed allopathic regimen.
  Expenditures for alternative medicine professional services increased 45% from 1990 to 1997. Total visits to alternative medical practitioners exceeded total visits to all U.S. primary care practitioners (Eisenberg et al, 1998). A widening recognition of the mind-body-spirit connection in western medicine has resulted in a growing interest in ancient health practices such as yoga (Herrick, Ainsworth, 2000).
- ▲ Refer client to community agencies for appropriate follow-up care (e.g., day treatment or adult day health program).

- **= Independent; ▲ = Collaborative**

Increased social support has been related to a reduction in mortality rates and incidences of physical and mental illness (Callaghan, Morrissey, 1993). This study showed a positive response when using a community youth setting, such as the girl scouts, to prevent disordered eating behaviors (Neumark-Sztainer et al, 2000).

- Obtain or design educational material that is appropriate for the client; use pictures if possible.
  Verbal reinforcement of personalized written instructions appears to be the best intervention. In one study, the use of computer-generated, personalized instructions improved adherence when compared with the use of handwritten instructions (Hayes, 1998).
- Ensure that follow-up appointments are scheduled before the client is discharged; discuss a way to ensure that appointments are kept.
  The client brings to the learning situation a unique personality, established social interaction patterns, cultural norms and values, and environmental influences (Bohny, 1997).

Geriatric

- Assess sensory deficits and psychomotor skills in terms of client's ability to comply with a health program.
  Barriers to health promotion in people with chronic illness were fatigue, time, safety, and lack of accessible facilities (Stuifbergen, 1997).
- Discuss "symptoms of daily living" in addition to the major illness.
  Older adults are unlikely to report day-to-day symptoms such as headaches because they do not view them as illness. However, these day-to-day complaints may foretell more serious problems (Musil et al, 1988).
- Recognize resistance to change in lifelong patterns of personal health care.
  The client brings to the learning situation a unique personality, established social interaction patterns, cultural norms and values, and environmental influences (Bohny, 1997).
- Discuss with client realistic goals for changes in health maintenance.
  The focus of a chronic illness may be care rather than cure. In this study of 86 people, the oldest old may have increased optimism but decreased satisfaction. They have a sense of realism about the tasks of aging and have a present-focused orientation (Lennings, 2000).
- Consider the age of the client when suggesting screening for disease.
  Even assuming that the mortality reduction with screening persists in the elderly, 80% of the benefit is achieved before 80 years of age for colon cancer, before 75 years of age for breast cancer, and before 65 years of age for cervical cancer. The small benefit of screening in the elderly may be outweighed by the harms: anxiety, additional testing, and unnecessary treatment (Rich, Black, 2000).

Multicultural

- Assess for the influence of cultural beliefs, norms, and values on the client's ability to modify health behavior.
  What the client considers normal and abnormal health behavior may be based on cultural perceptions (Leininger, 1996).
- Discuss with the client those aspects of their health behavior/lifestyle that will remain unchanged by their health status.
  Aspects of the client's life that are meaningful and valuable to him or her should be understood and preserved without change (Leininger, 1996).
- Negotiate with the client regarding the aspects of health behavior that will need to be modified.
  Give and take with the client will lead to culturally congruent care (Leininger, 1996).

• = Independent; ▲ = Collaborative

- Assess the role of fatalism on the client's ability to modify health behavior.
  Fatalistic perspectives, which involve the belief that you cannot control your own fate, may influence health behaviors in some African-American and Latino populations (Phillips, Cohen, Moses, 1999; Harmon, Castro, Coe, 1996).
- Validate the client's feelings regarding the impact of health status on current lifestyle.
  Validation lets the client know that the nurse has heard and understands what was said, and it promotes the nurse-client relationship (Stuart, Laraia, 2001; Giger, Davidhizar, 1995).

Home Care Interventions

- Provide aids to assist with compliance (e.g., prepare medication schedules and put a week's medication in daily containers).
- Provide sufficient outside supports (e.g., written notices, calendars, planned ride shares) to assist with follow-through of the agreed-upon actions.
  Cues play a significant role in stimulating completion of desired health actions.
- Establish a written contract with client to follow the agreed-upon health care regimen.
  Written agreements reinforce the verbal agreement and serve as a reference.
- Meet with client following the proposed actions to review the contract and determine the next course of action. Do this until the client is able to initiate and follow through independently.
  Successful completion of contracts promotes improved self-esteem and positive coping.

Client/Family Teaching

- Provide family with lists of addresses for information to be obtained from the Internet. (Most libraries have Internet access with printing capabilities.)
  Internet-based technologies have emerged as potentially powerful tools to enable meaningful communication and proactive partnership in care for various medical conditions (Patel, 2001). A study of 469 Internet postings of patients with implantable defibrillators showed that they used the Internet for practical information seeking and support in coping (Dickerson, Flaig, Kennedy, 2000).
- Have client and family demonstrate at least twice any procedures to be done at home.
  Practice of a procedure exposes problems, enhances skill levels, and promotes confidence in new behaviors.
- Explain nonthreatening material before introducing more anxiety-producing possible side effects of the disease or medical regimen.
  An individual's perception of barriers and benefits has consistently been most predictive of subsequent behavior (Fenn, 1998).

WEB SITES FOR EDUCATION

MERLIN See the MERLIN web site for World Wide Web resources for client education.

REFERENCES Bohny B: A time for self-care: role of the home healthcare nurse, *Home Healthc Nurse* 15(4):281-286, 1997.
Callaghan P, Morrissey G: Social support and health: a review, *J Adv Nurs* 203:18, 1993.
Clark C: *Wellness practitioner: concepts, research and strategies,* New York, 1996, Springer.
Dickerson SS, Flaig DM, Kennedy MC: Therapeutic connection: help seeking on the Internet for persons with implantable cardioverter defibrillators, *Heart Lung* 29(4):248-255, 2000.

• = Independent; ▲ = Collaborative

Eisenberg M et al: Trends in alternative medicine use in the United States 1990-1997, *JAMA* 280(18):1569-1575, 1998.

Fenn M: Health promotion: theoretical perspectives and clinical applications, *Holist Nurs Pract* 12(2):1-7, 1998.

Furniss K: Tomatoes, Pap smears, and tea? adopting behaviors that may prevent reproductive cancers and improve health, *J Obstet Gynecol Neonatal Nurs,* 29(6):641-652, 2000.

Giger JN, Davidhizar RE: *Transcultural nursing,* ed 2, St Louis, 1995, Mosby.

Harmon MP, Castro FG, Coe K: Acculturation and cervical cancer: knowledge, beliefs, and behaviors of Hispanic women, *Women Health* 24(3):37-57, 1996.

Hayes K: Randomized trial of geragogy-based medication instruction in the emergency department, *Nurs Res* 47(4):211-218, 1998.

Herrick CM, Ainsworth AD: Invest in yourself: yoga as a self-care strategy, *Nurs Forum* 35(2):32-36, 2000.

Leininger MM: *Transcultural nursing: theories, research and practices,* ed 2, Hilliard, Ohio, 1996, McGraw-Hill.

Lennings CJ: Optimism, satisfaction and time perspective in the elderly, *Int J Aging Hum Dev* 51(3):167-181, 2000.

Musil CM et al: Health problems and health actions among community-dwelling older adults: results of a health diary study, *Appl Nurs Res* 11(3):138-147, 1988.

Neumark-Sztainer D et al: Primary prevention of disordered eating among preadolescent girls: feasibility and short-term effect of a community-based intervention, *J Am Diet Assoc* 100(12):1466-1473, 2000.

Patel AM: Using the Internet in the management of asthma, *Curr Opin Pulm Med* 7(1):39-42, 2001.

Phillips JM, Cohen MZ, Moses G: Breast cancer screening and African American women: fear, fatalism, and silence, *Oncol Nurs Forum* 26(3):561-571, 1999.

Rich JS, Black WC: When should we stop screening? *Eff Clin Pract* 3(2):78-84, 2000.

Smith-Battle L: The responsive use of self in community health nursing practice, *Adv Nurs Sci* 10(2):75-88, 1997.

Stuart GW, Laraia MT: Therapeutic nurse-patient relationship. In Stuart GW, Laraia MT, editors: *Principles and practice of psychiatric nursing,* St Louis, 2001, Mosby, p 30.

Stuifbergen A: Health promotion: an essential component of rehabilitation for persons with chronic disabling conditions, *Adv Nurs Sci* 19(4):138-147, 1997.

van der Molen B: Relating information needs to the cancer experience, 1: information as a key coping strategy, *Eur J Cancer Care (Engl)* 8(4):238-244, 1999.

Health-seeking behaviors

Suzanne Skowronski and Gail B. Ladwig

 Definition Active seeking (by a person in stable health) of ways to alter personal health habits and/or the environment in order to move toward a higher level of health

NOTE: Stable health is defined as achievement of age-appropriate illness-prevention measures; report of good or excellent health from client; and control of signs and symptoms of disease, if present.

Defining Characteristics

Expressed or observed desire to seek a higher level of wellness for self or family; demonstrated or observed lack of knowledge of health-promoting behaviors; stated or observed unfamiliarity with wellness community resources; expressed concern about the effect of current environmental conditions on health status; expressed or observed desire for increased control of health practice

Related Factors (r/t)

Role change; change in developmental level (e.g., marriage, parenthood, empty-nest syndrome, retirement); lack of knowledge regarding need for preventive health behaviors,

• = Independent; ▲ = Collaborative

appropriate health screenings, optimal nutrition, weight control, regular exercise program, stress management, supportive social network, and responsible role participation

NOC ## Outcomes (Nursing Outcomes Classification)

Suggested NOC Labels

Health-Promoting Behavior, Health-Seeking Behavior; Adherence Behavior; Health Beliefs; Health Orientation

> **Example NOC Outcome**
>
> Demonstrates **Health-Seeking Behavior** as evidenced by the following indicators: Completes health related tasks/Performs self-screening when indicated/Contacts health professionals when indicated (Rate each indicator of **Health-Seeking Behavior:** 1 = never demonstrated, 2 = rarely demonstrated, 3 = sometimes demonstrated, 4 = often demonstrated, 5 = consistently demonstrated [see Section I])

Client Outcomes

- Maintains ideal weight and is knowledgeable about nutritious diet
- Explains ways to fit newly prescribed change in health habits into lifestyle
- Lists community resources available for assistance with achieving wellness
- Explains ways to include wellness behaviors in current lifestyle

NIC ## Interventions (Nursing Interventions Classification)

Suggested NIC Labels

Health System Guidance; Support System Enhancement; Health Education

> **Example NIC Interventions—Health Education**
> - Prioritize identified learner needs based on client preference, skills of nurse, resources available, and likelihood of successful goal attainment
> - Emphasize immediate or short-term positive health benefits to be received by positive lifestyle behaviors rather than long-term benefits or negative effects of noncompliance

Nursing Interventions and Rationales

- Discuss client's beliefs about health and his or her ability to maintain health.
  An individual's belief in his or her ability to accomplish a desired action is predictive of performance (Fenn, 1998).
- Identify barriers and benefits to being healthy.
  An individual's perception of barriers and benefits has consistently been most predictive of behavior changes (Fenn, 1998).
- Identify environmental and social factors that the client perceives as health promoting.
  Exposure to a health-promoting environment had statistically significant direct and indirect effects (Conrad et al, 1996).

Nutrition

- Determine client's height and weight. Compare results with standard weight for age and height.
- Encourage client to eat a diet that contains fresh foods, is low in saturated (visible) fat, and contains no added salt.
  Saturated fats and cholesterol are strongly associated with cardiovascular disease, obesity, diabetes, and hypertension (Clark, 1996).

• = Independent; ▲ = Collaborative

- Assess the role that stress plays in overeating and weight cycling.
  Women who weight cycle are triggered to overeat by unpleasant feelings or tension stress, while normal weight subjects tend to overeat in social situations (Smith-Battle, 1997).

Exercise

▲ Advise client to consult with physician for testing to determine ability to tolerate a specific regimen.
  Previous bone injuries or inflammatory disease may rule out jogging and aerobic exercises.
- Explore weightlifting options with client to increase muscle strength and stamina.
- Help client focus on enjoyment of exercise. Set up a support and reward system.
  An individual's perception of barriers and benefits has consistently been most predictive of subsequent behavior (Fenn, 1998).
- Encourage aerobic exercises that increase heart rate within the prescribed limit. Encourage client to exercise at least 3 times per week for 20 or more minutes using exercises that the client prefers (e.g., walking, jogging, aerobics, swimming, bicycling, yoga, Tai Chi).
  Brisk walking is superior to jogging or running because walking causes fewer injuries and has shown to be more effective for weight loss (Clark, 1996, p 175). Yoga and Tai Chi are stretching exercises that promote energy and muscle balance. A widening recognition of the mind-body-spirit connection in Western medicine has resulted in a growing interest in ancient health practices such as yoga (Herrick, Anisworth, 2000).

Stress management

- Ask client to define stress in terms of lifestyle events and assign events a value on a scale from 1 to 5.
  This exercise helps to distinguish between anxiety as a personality trait and anxiety as a coping response to threatening events.
- Determine ways in which the client relieves stress and evaluate their effectiveness.
  Stress management techniques are of two types, those that focus on body systems and those that focus on handling stress differently through behavior responses (Clark, 1996, p 69).
- Determine client's social support network.
  Exposure to a health-promoting environment had statistically significant direct and indirect effects (Conrad et al, 1996).
- Teach stress-relieving techniques (e.g., deep and slow breathing, progressive muscle relaxation, meditation, imagery, problem solving).
  Stress management addresses the sources of tension in physical performance, emotional expression, transcendent spiritual experiences, social relationships, and the surrounding environment.

Smoking, drinking, self-medication

- Discuss risk-taking behaviors of smoking, drinking, and self-medication.
- Discuss frequency of risk-taking habits.
  People move through a series of behaviors—precontemplation, preparation, action, and maintenance—in their effort to change or adopt a new behavior (Fenn, 1998, p 5).
▲ Refer clients who smoke to Smoke Enders or a similar community-based program. Discuss ways in which client can deal with change in behavior.
  Although complete cessation of smoking is preferred, sustained reduction is likely to reduce the risk of disease and is a valuable public health outcome (Wakefield et al, 1992).
▲ Refer clients who drink alcohol excessively to Alcoholics Anonymous. Identify a support person to help client into the organization.

• = Independent; ▲ = Collaborative

Posttreatment from alcohol use is a major life transition that requires extensive coping efforts, social support, and environmental control (Murphy, 1993).

- Identify patterns of self-medication with over-the-counter medications, herbal remedies, and excessive use of prescribed medications.
  Medications and herbal preparations are most effective when taken as intended. Combining remedies predisposes client to unwanted side effects.

Health-seeking behaviors

- Teach stress-relieving techniques (e.g., deep and slow breathing, progressive muscle relaxation, exercise, medication, power strategies, problem solving, imagery, verbalization of feelings, spiritual practice [prayer]).
  Stress management addresses the sources of tension in physical performance, emotional expression, transcendent spiritual experiences, social relationships, and the surrounding environment.

Health screening, appropriate health care

- Assess frequency of illness-preventing practices, such as yearly physical examinations, dental examinations, flu shots, monthly breast self-examinations (and mammograms as recommended) for women, testicular self-examinations and prostate examinations for men, screening for familial diseases such as glaucoma and elevated cholesterol. See care plan for **Ineffective Health maintenance.**
  The CDC recommends yearly flu vaccination for adults with chronic disease, those >65 years of age, and children ≥2 years of age with chronic illness (Morbidity and Mortality Weekly Report, 1984). Reducing uncertainty about Self-Breast Examination (SBE) is seen as a key to promote SBE (Babrow, Kline, 2000).

Geriatric

- Assess client's awareness of deficits that may result from normal aging (e.g., changes in sleep patterns or frequency of urination, loss of visual acuity in night driving, loss of hearing, dietary changes, memory changes, loss of significant others).
  If symptoms of health problems are not viewed as an illness, older adults are unlikely to report them to the health care provider. Annual checkups focusing on disease symptoms may fail to uncover day-to-day complaints that foretell more serious problems (Musil, 1998).
- Identify coping mechanisms that promote wellness and place control of life choices back with the client. Discuss ways to prepare for retirement security.
  An active sense of accountability for one's own well-being provides the necessary motivation to pursue a health-enhancing lifestyle (Walker, 1993).
- Find suitable housing that provides support, safety, protection, meals, and social events.
  Only 5% of older adults live in an institution at any one time. The risk of institutionalization increases with age (Walker, 1993).
- ▲ Give client information about community resources for the elderly (e.g., transportation to appointments, Meals-on-Wheels, home visitors, pets, American Association of Retired Persons, Elder Hostel, Internet addresses).
  The aging process occurs throughout the lifespan. The elderly client hopes to be independent and useful as long as possible without being a burden on others. The web site www.healthfinder.org/justforyou/seniors.htm offers health information for seniors on a variety of topics.
- ▲ Assess the environment for signs of elder abuse and report as appropriate.
  Activities categorized as mistreatment include force-feeding; overmedication/ undermedication; withholding care or needed therapies; and failure to provide health devices such as dentures, glasses, or ambulatory support devices (Rosenblatt, 1997).

- = **Independent;** ▲ = **Collaborative**

- Teach health-protecting behaviors to the elderly.
  The Surgeon General recommends receiving flu vaccines yearly and pneumonia vaccines once in a lifetime, wearing seat belts, installing smoke detectors, preventing falls, not smoking, decreasing alcohol consumption, and using medications safely (U.S. Department of Health and Human Services, 1991).
- ▲ Consider the age of the client when suggesting screening for disease.
  Even assuming that the mortality reduction with screening persists in the elderly, 80% of the benefit is achieved before 80 years of age for colon cancer, before 75 years of age for breast cancer, and before 65 years of age for cervical cancer. The small benefit of screening in the elderly may be outweighed by the harms: anxiety, additional testing, and unnecessary treatment (Rich, Black, 2000).

Multicultural

- Assess for the influence of cultural beliefs, norms, and values on the client's beliefs about health behavior.
  What the client considers normal and abnormal health behavior may be based on cultural perceptions (Leininger, 1996).
- Acknowledge and praise those aspects of behavior/lifestyle that are health-promoting.
  Aspects of the client's life that are meaningful and valuable to him or her should be understood and preserved without change (Leininger, 1996).
- Negotiate with client the aspects of health behavior that will require further modification.
  Give and take with the client will lead to culturally congruent care (Leininger, 1996).
- Validate the client's feelings regarding the impact of health behavior on current lifestyle.
  Validation lets the client know that the nurse has heard and understands what was said, and it promotes the nurse-client relationship (Stuart, Laraia, 2001; Giger, Davidhizar, 1995).

Home Care Interventions

NOTE: All the previously listed nursing interventions are applicable to the home care setting. For more information, see Home Care Interventions for **Ineffective Health maintenance.**

Client/Family Teaching

- Discuss the role of environmental and social factors in supporting a healthy family life.
  The people are the community. Reciprocal relationships to build community education with a view to prevention is key to enhancing health (Davis, 1998).
- Provide and review pamphlets about health-seeking opportunities and wellness and provide family with lists of addresses for information to be obtained on the Internet. (Most libraries have Internet access with printing capabilities.)
  Internet-based technologies have emerged as potentially powerful tools to enable meaningful communication and proactive partnership in care for various medical conditions (Patel, 2001). A study of 469 Internet postings of patients with implantable defibrillators showed that they used the Internet for practical information seeking and support in coping (Dickerson, Flaig, Kennedy, 2000).
- Identify physical and emotional threats to family security (e.g., domestic violence, child abuse, school violence).
  According to Maslow's hierarchy of needs, wellness and health-promoting behaviors can be met only when personal and social safety and security issues are resolved.

• = Independent; ▲ = Collaborative

REFERENCES   Babrow AS, Kline KN: From "reducing" to "coping with" uncertainty: reconceptualizing the central challenge in breast self-exams, *Soc Sci Med* 51(12):1805-1816, 2000.

Clark C: *Wellness practitioner: concepts, research and strategies,* New York, 1996, Springer.

Conrad KM et al: The work site environment as a cue to smoking reduction, *Res Nurs Health* 19(1):21-31, 1996.

Davis R: Community caring: an ethnographic study within an organizational culture, *Public Health Nurs* 14(2):92-100, 1998.

Dickerson SS, Flaig DM, Kennedy MC: Therapeutic connection: help seeking on the Internet for persons with implantable cardioverter defibrillators, *Heart Lung* 29(4):248-255, 2000.

Fenn M: Health promotion: theoretical perspectives and clinical applications, *Holist Nurs Pract* 12(2):1-7, 1998.

Giger JN, Davidhizar RE: *Transcultural nursing,* ed 2, St Louis, 1995, Mosby.

Herrick CM, Ainsworth AD: Invest in yourself: yoga as a self-care strategy, *Nurs Forum* 35(2):32-36, 2000.

Leininger MM: *Transcultural nursing: theories, research and practices,* ed 2, Hilliard, Ohio, 1996, McGraw-Hill.

Morbidity and Mortality Weekly Report, *New Engl J Med* 33:275, 1984.

Murphy S: Coping strategies of abstainers from alcohol up to 3 years post treatment, *Image J Nurs Sch* 25:32, 1993.

Musil C: Health problems and health actions among community dwelling older adults: results of a health diary study, *Appl Nurs Res* 11(3):138-147, 1998.

Patel AM: Using the Internet in the management of asthma, *Curr Opin Pulm Med* 7(1):39-42, 2001.

Rich JS, Black WC: When should we stop screening? *Eff Clin Pract* 3(2):78-84, 2000.

Rosenblatt D: Elder mistreatment, *Crit Care Nurs Clin North Am* 9(2):183-192, 1997.

Smith-Battle L: The responsive use of self in community health nursing practice, *Adv Nurs Sci* 10(2):75-88, 1997.

Stuart GW, Laraia MT: Therapeutic nurse-patient relationship. In Stuart GW, Laraia MT, editors: *Principles and practice of psychiatric nursing,* St Louis, 2001, Mosby, p 30.

U.S. Department of Health and Human Services: *Healthy People 2000 national health promotion and disease prevention objectives,* DHHS No (PHS) 91-50212, Washington, DC, 1991, U.S. Government Printing Office.

Wakefield M et al: Workplace smoking restrictions, occupational status and reduced cigarette consumption, *J Occup Med* 34:693-697, 1992.

Walker S: Wellness for elders, *Holist Nurs Pract* 38:7, 1993.

Impaired Home maintenance

Suzanne Skowronski and Gail B. Ladwig

NANDA   **Definition** The inability to independently maintain a safe and growth-promoting immediate environment

Defining Characteristics
Subjective   Household members express difficulty with maintaining their home in a comfortable fashion; household members describe outstanding debts or financial crises; household requests assistance with home maintenance

Objective   Disorderly surroundings; unwashed or unavailable cooking equipment, clothes, or linen; accumulation of dirt, food wastes, or hygienic wastes; offensive odors; inappropriate household temperature; overtaxed family members (e.g., exhausted, anxious); lack of necessary equipment or aids; presence of vermin or rodents; repeated hygienic disorders, infestations, or infections

• = Independent; ▲ = Collaborative

Related Factors (r/t)

Individual/family member with disease or injury; unfamiliarity with neighborhood resources; lack of role modeling; lack of knowledge; insufficient family organization or planning; inadequate support systems; impaired cognitive or emotional functioning; insufficient finances

`NOC` Outcomes (Nursing Outcomes Classification)

Suggested NOC Labels

Parenting; Parenting: Social Safety; Role Performance; Self-Care: Instrumental Activities of Daily Living (IADLs)

> **Example NOC Outcome**
> Demonstrates **Family Functioning** as evidenced by the following indicators: Regulates behavior of members/Obtains adequate resources to meet needs of family members (Rate each indicator of **Family Functioning:** 1 = never demonstrated, 2 = rarely demonstrated, 3 = sometimes demonstrated, 4 = often demonstrated, 5 = consistently demonstrated [see Section I])

Client Outcomes

- Wears clean clothing, eats nutritious meals, and has a sanitary and safe home
- Has the resources to cope physically and emotionally with the chronic illness process
- Uses community resources to assist with treatment needs

`NIC` Interventions (Nursing Interventions Classification)

Suggested NIC Labels

Home Maintenance Assistance

> **Example NIC Interventions—Home Maintenance Assistance**
> - Provide information on how to make home safe and clean
> - Help family use social support network

Nursing Interventions and Rationales

- Establish a plan of care with client and family based on the client's needs and the caregiver's capabilities.
  Broad categories of health promotion identified by a study of persons with chronic illness were physical activity, nutritional strategies, life adjustment, maintenance of a positive attitude, and interpersonal support (Stuifbergen, 1997).
- Assess family members' concerns, especially those of the primary caregiver, about long-term home care issues.
  The stress of caregiving may be so intense that the burden of caring is not automatically reduced when the elder is institutionalized (Sayles-Cross, 1993).
- Set up a system of relief for the main caregiver in the home and plan for sharing household duties.
  The caregiving career does not have a specific endpoint: it lasts as long as the chronically ill person is cared for at home (Lindgren, 1993).
- Encourage social relationships with family and friends, even if by phone.
  Social distance and high cost of caring were associated with tension and potential for conflict between caregivers and family members (Sayles-Cross, 1993).

• = Independent; ▲ = Collaborative

- Assess the characteristics of the current caregiving stage.
  The encounter stage calls for rapid adjustment, the enduring stage is the heavy duty caring phase, the exit stage requires the caregiver to relinquish most duties (Lindgren, 1993).
- ▲ Initiate referral to community agencies as needed, including housekeeping aides, Meals-on-Wheels, wheelchair-compatible transportation, and oxygen therapy.
  Barriers to health promotion in people with chronic illness are fatigue, time, safety, and lack of accessible facilities (Stuifbergen, 1997, p 14).
- ▲ Obtain adaptive equipment and telemedical equipment, as appropriate, to help family members continue to maintain the home environment.
  Telemedicines available in the home are the infusion pump, pulse oximeter, 12-lead EKG, and telestethoscope" (McNeal, 1998).
- ▲ Refer client to social services to help with debt consolidation or financial concerns.
  Financial help ranges from Medicaid and private insurance to specific foundations such as Shriners Burn Center for Children. Hospital discharge planners are an important resource for coordinating agencies.
- Ask family to identify support people who can help with home maintenance.
  Church, nursing home health agencies, and hospice organizations are sources for reliable in-home support.
- ▲ Community health agencies can evaluate whether the home is safe enough for providing health care to a chronically ill person, can provide direct care, and can assist with resource coordination.

Geriatric

- ▲ Explore community resources to assist with home care (e.g., senior centers, Department of Aging, hospital discharge planners, the Internet, church parish nurse, or Stephen's program).
  Promoting health of populations has always required an organic relationship to the community and knowledge of specific populations (Smith-Battle, 1997). An Internet resource is geriatrician Dr. Stall's web site: www.acsu.buffalo.edu~drstall/nutrition.html.
- Visit client's home to assess safety features (e.g., no throw rugs, safety bars in the bathroom, stair borders that distinguish each step, adequate nonglare light).
  The eye retina changes with age, making it easier to perceive red and yellow colors. With age, some glare occurs in bright light and contrast and shadows blur.
- ▲ Encourage regular eye examinations.
  Early detection of eye changes is imperative to prevent irreversible damage (Age Net).
- The following interventions should be considered for those with low or failing sight:
  Reduce Glare
  - Use nonglare light bulbs
  - Remove wax from floors to reduce glare
  - Encourage client to wear sunglasses
  - Use sheer curtains or blinds
  Proper Lighting
  - Use night-lights in the bedroom, bathroom, and hallways
  - Use dimmer switches and three-way bulbs to control light
  - Put bright lights at the top and bottom of staircase
  - Use consistent lighting to minimize shadows

- **= Independent; ▲ = Collaborative**

Color Contrast
- Use colored tape to define steps
- Paint walls and staircase to contrast with floor
- Put glow-in-the-dark tape on light switches and door knobs
- Use colored dishes

Low Vision Aids

Encourage client to:
- Use magnifiers to improve near vision
- Hang magnifiers around the neck for convenience when sewing, doing crafts, or reading
- Request large print medication labels, books, and phones
- Use handrails on stairs
- Keep flashlights in a convenient location

Vision loss can cause less hardship if adaptive strategies and aides are used. Use of aides increases safety and promotes a sense of independence (Age Net).

▲ During the home visit, be alert for signs of elder abuse. Report any findings.
Activities categorized as mistreatment include force-feeding; overmedication/ undermedication; withholding care or needed therapies; failure to provide safety precautions; failure to provide health devices such as dentures, glasses, or ambulatory devices (Rosenblatt, 1997).

• See care plan for **Risk for Injury.**

Multicultural

• Acknowledge the stresses unique to racial/ethnic communities.
Targeted alcohol and tobacco marketing, high levels of unemployment, lack of health insurance, and racism are stresses unique to culturally diverse communities and often accompany poor housing (D'Avanzo et al, 2001; Zambrana, Dorrington, Hayes-Bautista, 1995). One in 10 Latino children live in a "severely distressed neighborhood," compared with 1 in 63 non-Hispanic white children (The Annie E. Casey Foundation, 1994).

• Identify what services and information are currently available in the community to assist with housing needs.
This will assist with focusing efforts and promote the wise use of valuable resources (National Heart, Lung, and Blood Institute of the National Institutes of Health, 1998).

• Approach families of color with respect, warmth, and professional courtesy.
Instances of disrespect and lack of caring have special significance for individuals of color (D'Avanzo et al, 2001).

Home Care Interventions

NOTE: By definition this nursing diagnosis consists of primarily community-based interventions. Home care and public health nursing are two community resources that can assist the family to restore or improve home management. The previous interventions incorporate these resources.

Client/Family Teaching

• Teach caregiver the need to set aside some personal time every day to meet own needs.
Constant vigilance was found to be one of the primary caregiver burdens for parents of technologically dependent (e.g., gastrostomy, tracheostomy, peritoneal dialysis) children at home (Burke et al, 1991).

• Encourage family members to perform home maintenance activities (e.g., cooking, cleaning, fire prevention).

• = Independent; ▲ = Collaborative

When one family member becomes ill and requires home care, the roles of other family members may change.

- Identify support groups within the community to assist families in the caregiver career.

  New caregivers could benefit from support groups that address adjustments at this stage. Support groups may not be the answer if caregivers are "veterans" and they discuss extensive caregiving frustrations (Lindgren, 1993).

▲ Provide written instructions for medication management and side effects, written instructions for equipment brought to the home, and resource phone numbers for emergency needs.

  Verbal reinforcement of personalized written instructions appears to be the best intervention. In one study, the use of computer-generated, personalized instructions improved adherence when compared with the use of handwritten instructions (Hayes, 1998).

WEB SITES FOR EDUCATION

See the MERLIN web site for World Wide Web resources for client education.

REFERENCES   Age Net: *Visual changes,* retrieved from the World Wide Web March 7, 2001. Web site: www.agenet.com/Visual_Changes.html

Burke S et al: Hazardous secrets and reluctantly taking charge; parenting a child with repeated hospitalizations, *Image* 23:39, 1991.

The Annie E. Casey Foundation: *Kids count data book: state profiles of child well-being,* ed 5, Baltimore, 1994, The Foundation.

D'Avanzo CE et al: Developing culturally informed strategies for substance-related interventions. Naegle MA, D'Avanzo CE, editors: *Addictions and substance abuse: strategies for advanced practice nursing,* St Louis, 2001, Mosby, pp 59-104.

Hayes K: Randomized trial of geragogy-based medication instruction in the emergency department, *Nurs Res* 47(4):211-218, 1998.

Lindgren C: The caregiver career, *Image* 25:214, 1993.

McNeal G: Telecommunication techniques in high-tech home care, *Adv Pract Nurse* 10(3):279-286, 1998.

National Heart, Lung, and Blood Institute of the National Institutes of Health: *Salud para su corazon: bringing heart health to Latinos—a guide for building community programs,* NIH Publication No. 98-3796, Washington, DC, November 1998, U.S. Department of Health and Human Services.

Rosenblatt D: Elder mistreatment, *Crit Care Nurs Clin North Am* 9(2):183-192, 1997.

Sayles-Cross S: Perceptions of familial caregivers of elder adults, *Image* 25:88, 1993.

Smith-Battle L: The responsive use of self in community health nursing practice, *Adv Nurs Sci* 10(2):75-88, 1997.

Stuifbergen A: Health promotion: an essential component of rehabilitation for persons with chronic disabling conditions, *Adv Nurs Sci* 19(4):1-20, 1997.

Zambrana RE, Dorrington C, Hayes-Bautista D: Family and child health: a neglected vision. In Zambrana RE, editor: *Understanding Latino families,* Thousand Oaks, Calif, 1995, Sage, pp 157-176.

Hopelessness

Gail B. Ladwig and Jill M. Barnes

NANDA   **Definition** A subjective state in which an individual sees limited or unavailable alternatives or personal choices and is unable to mobilize energy on own behalf

• = Independent; ▲ = Collaborative

Defining Characteristics

Passivity; decreased verbalization; decreased affect; verbal cues (e.g., saying "I can't," sighing); closing eyes; decreased appetite; decreased response to stimuli; increased/decreased sleep; lack of initiative; lack of involvement in care; passively allowing care; shrugging in response to speaker; turning away from speaker

Related Factors (r/t)

Abandonment; prolonged activity restriction creating isolation; lost beliefs in transcendent values/God; long-term stress; failing or deteriorating physiological condition

NOC   Outcomes (Nursing Outcomes Classification)

Suggested NOC Labels

Decision Making; Hope; Mood Equilibrium; Nutritional States: Food and Fluid Intake; Quality of Life; Sleep

> **Example NOC Outcome**
> Has a presence of **Hope** as evidenced by the expression of a positive orientation, faith, and will to live (Rate indicator of **Hope:** 1 = no expression, 2 = limited expression, 3 = moderate expression, 4 = substantial expression, 5 = extensive expression [see Section I])

Client Outcomes

- Verbalizes feelings, participates in care
- Makes positive statements (e.g., "I can" or "I will try")
- Makes eye contact, focuses on speaker
- Maintains appropriate appetite for age and physical health
- Sleeps appropriate amount of time for age and physical health

NIC   Interventions (Nursing Interventions Classification)

Suggested NIC Labels

Hope Instillation

> **Example NIC Interventions—Hope Instillation**
> - Assist client/family to identify areas of hope in life
> - Demonstrate hope by recognizing the client's intrinsic worth and viewing the client's illness as only one facet of the individual
> - Expand the client's repertoire of coping mechanisms

Nursing Interventions and Rationales

▲ Monitor and document potential for suicide. (Refer client for appropriate treatment if potential for suicide is identified.) See care plan for **Risk for self-directed Violence** for specific interventions.
Hopelessness is directly associated with suicidal behavior and also with a variety of other dysfunctional personal characteristics (Fritsch et al, 2000). Previous suicide attempts and hopelessness are the most powerful clinical predictors of future completed suicide (Malone et al, 2000).

• Assess the client for and point out reasons for living.
Interventions that increase the awareness of reasons for living may decrease hopelessness and decrease risk for suicide (Malone et al, 2000).

• Assess for impaired problem-solving ability and dysfunctional attitude.

• = Independent; ▲ = Collaborative

Impaired problem-solving ability and dysfunctional attitude have been shown to correlate with hopelessness (Cannon et al, 1999).

- Evaluate client by realistically assessing the predicament or threat.
  Understanding the etiologic basis of the client's hopelessness is important in order to intervene (Wake, Miller, 1992). Unless there is a threat that is acknowledged and assessed, hope does not exist (Morse, Doberneck, 1995).

- Determine appropriate approaches based on the underlying condition or situation that is contributing to feelings of hopelessness. Either encourage a positive mental attitude (discourage negative thoughts) or brace client for negative outcomes (i.e., client may need to accept some long-term limitations).
  Truthful information is generally preferred by families; surprise information regarding a change in status may cause the family to worry that information is being withheld from them (Johnson, Roberts, 1996). A person awaiting a transplant may need to express only hope or optimism, whereas a person with an injury with long-term effects, such as a spinal-cord injury, may need to prepare for possible negative outcomes and slow progress (Morse, Doberneck, 1995).

- Assist client with looking at alternatives and setting goals that are important to him or her.
  Mutual goal setting ensures that goals are attainable and helps to restore a cognitive-temporal sense of hope (Johnson, Dahlen, Roberts, 1997). Clients who do not know what to hope for are without hope. Thus an integral part of developing hope is determining and setting goals. The significance of the goal to the individual is complex and critical to sustaining hope (Morse, Doberneck, 1995).

- In dealing with possible long-term deficits, work with the client to set small, attainable goals.
  Mutual goal setting ensures that goals are attainable and helps to restore a cognitive-temporal sense of hope (Johnson, Dahlen, Roberts, 1997). Clients with spinal cord injury focused hope only on small gains, one step at a time. "Every little step I took was more important to me than what I had in the end" (Morse, Doberneck, 1995).

- Spend one-on-one time with client. Use empathy; try to understand what a client is saying, and communicate this understanding to the client.
  Experiencing warmth, empathy, genuineness, and unconditional positive regard can inspire hope (Cutcliffe, 1998). Empathy allows the nurse to communicate understanding without expressing feelings of judgment (Johnson, Roberts, 1996).

- Encourage expression of feelings, and acknowledge acceptance of them.
  Active listening is a tool used by nurses to enable them to listen to all ideas and feelings without judgment. Active listening may help clients to express themselves (Johnson, Roberts, 1996). A client's ability to express a negative emotion can be a very healthy sign; strong emotions are potentially dangerous if not expressed (Barry, 1994).

- Give client time to initiate interactions. After an appropriate amount of time is allowed, approach client in an accepting and nonjudgmental manner.
  Clients who have feelings of hopelessness need extra time to initiate relationships and sometimes are not able to. Approaching the client in an unhurried, nonjudgmental manner allows the client to feel secure and provides an atmosphere conducive to venting fears and asking questions (Anderson, 1992).

- Encourage client to participate in group activities.
  Group activities provide social support and help the client to identify alternative ways to problem-solve.

- **= Independent;** ▲ **= Collaborative**

- Encourage exercise of the mind to alleviate boredom. Watching or listening to the news, listening to music, and writing letters help to relieve the monotony of hospitalization.
  Focusing attention outside the self can decrease thoughts of hopelessness (Wake, Miller, 1992). Boredom may become a serious problem, leading to apathy, loss of hope, and depression (Anderson, 1992).
- Review client's strengths with client. Have client list own strengths on a note card and carry this list for future reference.
  Having individual worth affirmed inspires hope (Cutcliffe, 1998). Listing strengths provides reinforcement of positive self-regard.
- Use humor as appropriate.
  Humor is an effective intervention for hopelessness (Hunt, 1993).
- Involve family and significant others in plan of care.
  The importance of the need for hope has been emphasized by families during the critical illness of a family member (Johnson, Roberts, 1996). Frequent meetings between the staff and family can create a safe, positive atmosphere for the discussion of feelings (Anderson, 1992).
- Encourage family and significant others to express care, hope, and love for client.
  Helping the family to provide client reinforcement, to understand the client's feelings, and to be physically present and involved in care are strategies that enable the family to alter the client's hope state (Wake, Miller, 1992). Clients awaiting transplants had only one alternative, and that was hoping to receive a transplant. These clients solicited mutually supportive relationships. They sought social and emotional support from staff, family, clergy, and friends, and it was the intensity of these social relationships that enabled them to survive the precarious nature of their physical conditions (Morse, Doberneck, 1995).
- Use touch, if appropriate and with permission, to demonstrate caring, and encourage the family to do the same.
  Human touch and human presence may in some way directly and/or indirectly restore the human-centered dignity and affirmation of being that is necessary for the emergence of hope (Cutcliffe, 1998).
- For additional interventions, see care plans for **Spiritual distress, Readiness for enhanced Spiritual well-being,** and **Disturbed Sleep pattern.**

Geriatric

- Assess for clinical signs and symptoms of depression; differentiate depression from functional or organic dementia.
  Hopelessness and suicidal wishes in older adults are present with high levels of depressive symptoms suggestive of treatable pathology (Uncapher et al, 1998). It can be difficult to distinguish depression from dementia in people >65 years of age because some symptoms (e.g., disorientation, memory loss, and distractibility) may suggest dementia. Concurrent medical illnesses, prescription medications, and concealed alcohol or substance abuse can also appear to be dementia (Agency for Health Care Policy and Research, 1993).
- ▲ If depression is suspected, confer with primary physician regarding referral for mental health.
  In older adults, hopelessness and suicidal wishes are present with high levels of depressive symptoms suggestive of treatable pathology (Uncapher et al, 1998).
- Take threats of self-harm or suicide seriously.
  The elderly have the highest rate of completed suicide of all age groups (Uncapher et al, 1998). Hopelessness is often linked to depression and suicidal ideation in the elderly.

• = Independent; ▲ = Collaborative

Elderly people who are depressed or have experienced recent losses and live alone are at the highest risk (Uncapher et al, 1998).

- Identify significant losses that might be leading to feelings of hopelessness.
- Discuss stages of emotional responses to multiple losses.
- Use reminiscence and life-review therapies to identify past coping skills.
  Help clients acknowledge positive accomplishments and review survival of past illnesses to promote hope for dealing with current illness (Johnson, Dahlen, Roberts, 1997). Reminiscence can activate past sources of self-esteem and aid coping (Nugent, 1995). Memories and reminiscence have been used successfully with elderly persons to evoke pleasure and achieve therapeutic goals (Woods, Ashley, 1995).
- Express hope to client, and give positive feedback whenever appropriate.
  Sharing hope with a client who is experiencing hopelessness was identified as helpful for redirecting thoughts (Wake, Miller, 1992).
- Identify client's past and current sources of spirituality. Help client explore life and identify those experiences that are noteworthy. Clients may want to read the Bible or have it read to them.
  Spirituality is often identified by clients as a bridge between hopelessness and a sense of meaning (Fryback, Reinert, 1999).
- Use simulated presence therapy (SPT). SPT is a personalized audiotape composed of a family member's or caregiver's portion of a telephone conversation and soundless spaces that correspond to the client's side of the conversation. On the SPT audiotape, a caregiver "converses" about cherished memories, loved ones, family antidotes, and other valued experiences of the client's life. The SPT audiotape is played by using headphones and a lightweight automatic-reverse cassette player that is inserted into a hip pack. (SPT is a patented product of SIM-PRES Inc., Boston, Massachusetts.)
  Recorded messages can be used for proximity enhancement. Proximity enhancement helps to remove the threat of distant loved ones at a time of trauma (Johnson, Roberts, 1996). SPT builds on strengths of cognitively impaired elderly people because it relies on their remote memory, which is more likely to be retained than their recent memory. SPT produces a positive environment for cognitively impaired elderly people; the selected memories of SPT seem to provide enough stimulation to evoke the elder's interest, involvement, and pleasure (Woods, Ashley, 1995).
- Encourage visits from children.
  Children stimulate a sense of hope in many older adults (Gaskins, Forte, 1995).
- Position clients by window, take them outside, or encourage activities such as gardening (if ability allows).
  Any change in environment breaks the monotony that can lead to hopelessness (Wake, Miller, 1992). Enjoyment of nature fosters hope (Gaskins, Forte, 1995).

Multicultural

- Assess for the influence of cultural beliefs, norms, and values on the client's feelings of hopelessness.
  The client's expressions of hopelessness may be based on cultural perceptions (Leininger, 1996).
- Assess the role of fatalism on the client's expression of hopelessness.
  Fatalistic perspectives, which involve the belief that you cannot control your own fate, may influence health behaviors in some African-American and Latino populations, (Phillips, Cohen, Moses, 1999; Harmon, Castro, Coe, 1996).

• = **Independent;** ▲ = **Collaborative**

- Encourage spirituality as a source of support for hopelessness.
  Blacks and Latinos may identify spirituality, religiousness, prayer, and church-based approaches as coping resources (Samuel-Hodge et al, 2000; Bourjolly, 1998; Mapp, Hudson, 1997).
- Validate the client's feelings regarding the impact of health status on current lifestyle.
  Validation lets the client know that the nurse has heard and understands what was said, and it promotes the nurse-client relationship (Stuart, Laraia, 2001; Giger, Davidhizar, 1995).

Home Care Interventions

- Assess for isolation within the family unit. Encourage client to participate in family activities. If client cannot participate, encourage him or her to be in the same area and watch family activities. If possible, move client's bed or primary sitting place to active household area.
  Participation in events increases energy and promotes a sense of belonging.
- ▲ If depression is suspected, confer with primary physician regarding referral for mental health.
  In older adults, hopelessness and suicidal wishes are present with high levels of depressive symptoms suggestive of treatable pathology (Uncapher et al, 1998).
- Reminisce with client about his or her life.
  Help clients acknowledge positive accomplishments and review survival of past illnesses to promote hope for dealing with current illness (Johnson, Dahlen, Roberts, 1997). Reminiscence can activate past sources of self-esteem and aid coping (Nugent, 1995).
- Identify areas in which client can have control. Allow client to set achievable goals in these areas.
  Restoring control over the illness can increase the physiological sense of hope (Johnson, Dahlen, Roberts, 1997).
- If illness precipitated the hopelessness, discuss knowledge of and previous experience with the disease. Help client to identify own strengths.
  Uncertainty is a danger when it results in pessimism. Knowledge of and previous experience with the disease decrease uncertainty.
- Provide plant or pet therapy if possible.
  Caring for pets or plants helps to redefine the client's identity and makes him or her feel needed and loved.
- ▲ Provide a safe environment so client cannot harm self. (See also no-suicide contract in following section). Provide one-to-one contact when necessary. Refer client for immediate mental health treatment if needed.
  Hopelessness is an accurate indicator of suicidal risk. A safe environment reassures the client.

Client/Family Teaching

- Provide information regarding client's condition, treatment plan, and progress.
  Honest information regarding these issues in terms that the family can understand can give the family a sense of control and may allay some anxiety (Johnson, Roberts, 1996).
- Teach use of stress reduction techniques, relaxation, and imagery. Many cassette tapes on relaxation and meditation are available. Assist the client with relaxation based on the client's preference from the initial assessment.
  These techniques reduce physical stressors, which in turn increases the physiological sense of hope (Johnson, Dahlen, Roberts, 1997). Relaxation techniques, desensitization, and guided imagery can help clients cope, increase their control, and allay anxiety (Narsavage, 1997).

• = **Independent;** ▲ = **Collaborative**

- Encourage families to express love, concern, and encouragement, and allow client to vent feelings.

  Helping the family to provide positive client reinforcement, to understand the client's feelings, and to be physically present and involved in care are strategies that enable the family to alter the client's hope state (Wake, Miller, 1992). One study showed that hope is partially sustained through relationships with the social network—families. The availability of significant sources of support can perpetuate hopefulness with cardiac transplant recipients (Hirth, Stewart, 1994).

- ▲ Refer client to self-help groups such as I Can Cope and Make Today Count.

  These groups allow the client to recognize the love and care of others, and they promote a sense of belonging (Bulechek, McCloskey, 1992).

- ▲ Supply a crisis phone number, and secure a no-suicide contract from the client stating that the crisis number will be used if thoughts of self-harm occur.

  A no-suicide contract is one type of intervention used with clients who have suicidal thoughts (Valente, 1989).

WEB SITES FOR EDUCATION

MERLIN See the MERLIN web site for World Wide Web resources for client education.

REFERENCES   Agency for Health Care Policy and Research: *Clinical practice guideline: depression in primary care,* Publ 93-0550, vol 1, *Detection and diagnosis,* Rockville, Md, 1993, U.S. Department of Health and Human Services.

Anderson SB: Guillain-Barré syndrome: giving the patient control, *J Neurosci Nurs* 24:158, 1992.

Barry P: *Mental health and mental illness,* ed 5, Philadelphia, 1994, JB Lippincott.

Bourjolly JN: Differences in religiousness among black and white women with breast cancer, *Soc Work Health Care* 28(1):21-39, 1998.

Bulechek G, McCloskey J: Nursing interventions: essential nursing treatments, ed 2, Philadelphia, 1992, JB Lippincott.

Cannon B et al: Dysfunctional attitudes and poor problem solving skills predict hopelessness in major depression, *J Affect Disord* 55(1):45-49, 1999.

Cutcliffe JR: Hope, counseling and complicated bereavement reactions, *J Adv Nurs* 28(4):754-761, 1998.

Fritsch S et al: Personality characteristics of adolescent suicide attempters, *Child Psychiatry Hum Dev* 30(4):219-235, 2000.

Fryback PB, Reinert BR: Spirituality and people with potentially fatal diagnoses, *Nurs Forum* 34(1):13-22, 1999.

Gaskins S, Forte L: The meaning of hope: implications for nursing practice and research, *J Gerontol Nurs* 21:17, 1995.

Giger JN, Davidhizar RE: *Transcultural nursing,* ed 2, St Louis, 1995, Mosby.

Harmon MP, Castro FG, Coe K: Acculturation and cervical cancer: knowledge, beliefs, and behaviors of Hispanic women, *Women Health* 24(3):37-57, 1996.

Hirth A, Stewart M: Hope and social support as coping resources for adults waiting for cardiac transplantation, *Can J Nurs Res* 26:31, 1994.

Hunt AH: Humor as a nursing intervention, *Cancer Nurs* 16:34, 1993.

Johnson LH, Dahlen R, Roberts SL: Supporting hope in congestive heart failure patients, *Dimens Crit Care Nurs* 16(2):65-78, 1997.

Johnson LH, Roberts SL: Hope facilitating strategies for the family of the head injury patient, *J Neurosci Nurs* 28(4):259-265, 1996.

Leininger MM: *Transcultural nursing: theories, research and practices,* ed 2, Hilliard, Ohio, 1996, McGraw-Hill.

Malone KM et al: Protective factors against suicidal acts in major depression: reasons for living, *Am J Psychiatry* 157(7):1084-1088, 2000.

• = Independent; ▲ = Collaborative

Mapp I, Hudson R: Stress and coping among African American and Hispanic parents of deaf children, *Am Ann Deaf* 142(1):48-56, 1997.

Morse J, Doberneck B: Delineating the concept of hope, *Image* 27:277, 1995.

Narsavage GL: Promoting function in clients with chronic lung disease by increasing their perception of control, *Holist Nurs Pract* 12(1):17-26, 1997.

Nugent E: Reminiscence as a nursing intervention, *J Psychosoc Nurs* 33(11):7-11, 44-45, 1995.

Phillips JM, Cohen MZ, Moses G: Breast cancer screening and African American women: fear, fatalism, and silence, *Oncol Nurs Forum* 26(3):561-571, 1999.

Samuel-Hodge CD et al: Influences on day-to-day self-management of type 2 diabetes among African-American women: spirituality, the multi-caregiver role, and other social context factors, *Diabetes Care* 23(7):928-933, 2000.

Stuart GW, Laraia MT: Therapeutic nurse-patient relationship. In Stuart GW, Laraia MT, editors: *Principles and practice of psychiatric nursing*, St Louis, 2001, Mosby, p 30.

Uncapher H et al: Hopelessness and suicidal ideation in older adults, *Gerontologist* 38(1):62-71, 1998.

Valente SM: Adolescent suicide: assessment and intervention, *J Child Adolesc Psychiatr Ment Health Nurs* 2:34, 1989.

Wake MM, Miller JF: Treating hopelessness: nursing strategies from six countries, *Clin Nurs Res* 1(4):347-365, 1992.

Woods P, Ashley J: Simulated presence therapy: using selected memories to manage problem behaviors in Alzheimer's disease patients, *Geriatr Nurs* 16(1):9-14, 1995.

Hyperthermia

Marcia LaHaie and Terry VandenBosch

 Definition Body temperature elevated above normal range

NOTE: Elevated body temperature can be either fever or hyperthermia. Fever is a normal response in which the core body temperature elevates at least 1.5 to 2 degrees above an individual's normal temperature ($>100.5°$ F). This elevation is in response to a chemical signal (endogenous pyrogen) released as a part of an inflammatory response, such as in infection or tissue injury. Because there is a proportional enhancement of the immune system for each degree of temperature elevation, fever is believed to be adaptive to $104°$ F (Kluger, 1991; Kluger et al, 1996). Hyperthermia is an abnormal increase in core body temperature, usually above $104°$ F, that occurs as a result of disorders of temperature control. Causes include brain trauma, heat stroke, or malignant hyperthermia of anesthesia. Hyperthermia is not adaptive (Holtzclaw, 1992) and should be treated as a medical emergency.

Defining Characteristics

Fever: core body temperature elevated at least 1.5 to 2 degrees above an individual's normal temperature ($>100.5°$ F)

Hyperthermia: Body temperature $>104°$ F with flushed or hot skin, increased respiratory rate, tachycardia

Related Factors (r/t)

Fever: Infection, tissue injury, illness or trauma, dehydration, blood transfusion, medication, increased metabolic rate

Hyperthermia: Exposure to hot environment, vigorous activity, inappropriate clothing, inability or decreased ability to perspire, brain injury, medications or anesthesia, severe illness or trauma

• = **Independent;** ▲ = **Collaborative**

Outcomes (Nursing Outcomes Classification)

Suggested NOC Labels

Thermoregulation; Thermoregulation: Neonate

> **Example NOC Outcome**
>
> Accomplishes **Thermoregulation** as evidenced by the following indicators: Body temperature WNL*/Skin temperature IER†/Skin color changes not present/ Hydration adequate/Reported thermal comfort (Rate each indicator of **Thermoregulation:** 1 = extremely compromised, 2 = substantially compromised, 3 = moderately compromised, 4 = mildly compromised, 5 = not compromised [see Section I])

*Within Normal Limits
†In Expected Range

Client Outcomes

- Maintains oral temperature within adaptive levels (below 104° F), or lower depending on the presence of cardiopulmonary illness, or depending on patient comfort
- Remains free of dehydration

Interventions (Nursing Interventions Classification)

Suggested NIC Labels

Fever Treatment; Malignant Hyperthermia Precautions; Temperature Regulation

> **Example NIC Interventions—Fever Treatment**
> - Institute a continuous core temperature monitoring device as appropriate
> - Monitor for decreasing levels of consciousness

Nursing Interventions and Rationales

- Take afebrile hospitalized client's temperature at least once a day, between 5 PM and 7 PM, or according to institutional standards.
  Temperature screening for afebrile patients can be based on daily circadian rhythm patterns (Beaudry, VandenBosch, Anderson, 1995).
- Take and record febrile client's temperature every 4 to 6 hours while awake.
  Recognizing the pattern of a fever can help determine the source (Holtzclaw, 1992; Cunha, 1996).
- Take a temperature reading anytime a client experiences other signs/symptoms of a possible infectious process, and if the client has chills.
  Shivering indicates a rising body temperature.
- ▲ Notify physician of temperature according to institutional standards or written orders, or when temperature reaches 100.5° F.
- ▲ Administer antipyretic medication for patient comfort, per physician orders, or for infection-induced fever of 104° F. Acetaminophen may be the preferred antipyretic to aspirin.
  Elimination of fever will interfere with its enhancement of the immune response (Klein, Cunha, 1996). Acetaminophen was better than aspirin for reducing fever in endotoxemia and did not affect the humoral response of the subjects (Pernerstorfer et al, 1999).
- ▲ Assess client for a history of febrile seizures; antipyretics should be used more aggressively only for clients with a positive history.

• = **Independent;** ▲ = **Collaborative**

In adults, there is very little evidence that fever, seizures, and neurological damage are associated (Powers, Scheld, 1996). Children who have a high fever (>104° F) at the time of an initial febrile seizure are less likely to have a recurrence than children who have a more moderate fever (El-Radhi et al, 1986).

▲ Assess fluid loss and facilitate oral intake or administer intravenous fluids to accomplish fluid replacement.
Increased metabolic rate and diaphoresis associated with fever cause loss of body fluids.

• When diaphoresis is present, assist the client with bathing and changing into dry clothing.
Bathing and clothing changes increase comfort and decrease the possibility of continued shivering caused by water evaporation from the skin.

▲ Notify physician of changes in the client's mental status.
A change in mental status may indicate the onset of septic shock.

▲ Do not use external cooling measures such as ice packs, tepid water baths, or removal of blankets and clothing for fever management unless fever is >104° F; these measures cause shivering and are ineffective.
If the client's temperature drops as a result of external cooling measures, the hypothalamus resets the body temperature at a higher level, which results in more shivering (Klien, Cunha, 1996). Shivering results in significantly increased oxygen consumption (Holtzclaw, 1993).

▲ Use a cooling blanket if client's fever is >105° F or if a high body temperature is related to a disorder of temperature regulation.
Cooling blankets are used when the client's oral temperature exceeds 105°F and cannot be controlled by antipyretics (Styrt, Sugarman, 1990), or when the fever is caused by a heat-related illness or is neurologically related (Morgan, 1990).

Geriatric

• A temperature of 1.5° to 2° above baseline should be considered a fever in the elderly.
The elderly may have a low baseline body temperature. They do not manifest fever in the same manner as younger adults. The temperature response is often blunted in the elderly because of changes in physiology resulting from aging (Norman, Yoshikawa, 1996).

• Assess for other signs/symptoms of infection in addition to or in the absence of fever.
Because fever may not be present, other signs/symptoms may be the only indication of an infectious process.

▲ Assist the client to seek medical attention immediately if fever is present. To diagnose the fever source, assess for possible precipitating factors, including changes in medication, environmental changes, and recent medical interventions or infectious exposures.
Fever in the elderly, especially the very old, is much more likely than in younger persons to be an indication of a serious bacterial infection (Norman, Yoshikawa, 1996). Hyperthermia can be precipitated by many medications prescribed for the elderly (Harchelroad, 1993).

• In hot weather, encourage clients to drink 8 to 10 glasses of fluid per day (within the cardiac and renal reserve) regardless of whether they are thirsty. Assess for the need/presence of fans or air conditioning.
The elderly (and children) are more susceptible to heat than are younger adults because of a decreased sensitivity to heat, decreased sweat gland function, and decreased thirst (Brody,

• = **Independent;** ▲ = **Collaborative**

1994). The number of geriatric deaths rises as environmental temperatures increase in the hot summer months (Bull, Morton, 1978; Worfolk, 2000).

▲ In hot weather, watch elderly clients for signs of heat exhaustion: temperature 100° to 102° F, orthostatic BP signs, weakness, restlessness, faintness, thirst, nausea, and vomiting. If signs are present, move to a cool place, have client lie down, give sips of water, check orthostatic BPs, sponge with tepid water, and notify the physician.
The elderly are predisposed to heat exhaustion and should be watched carefully for its occurrence; if present, it should be treated promptly (Worfolk, 2000).

▲ In hot weather monitor client for onset of heat stroke: core temperature >105° F; skin hot and dry; tachycardia; tachypnea; and changes in mentation with confusion, delirium, hallucinations, seizures, or coma. If present, have the client lie down; call 911 because it is a medical emergency; and institute cooling measures such as application of ice bags at the neck, axillae, and groin until help arrives. Do not give water because client may aspirate.
Heat stroke is always a medical emergency and can be deadly (Worfolk, 2000).

Home Care Interventions

• Assess whether the client or family has a thermometer. Instruct as needed in type of thermometer (non–mercury-containing preferred; sublingual or tympanic rather than skin patches) and how to use/read accurately.
An accurate temperature is one indicator of the client's condition.

▲ Teach client and family to use acetaminophen rather than aspirin or ibuprofen for fever reduction at home to prevent possible adverse effects.

• Help the client prevent and monitor for heat stroke/hyperthermia during times of high outdoor temperatures.

▲ In the event of temperature elevation above the adaptive range, institute measures to decrease temperature (e.g., get out of sun and into cool place, remove excess clothing, have client drink fluids). Keep physician informed if temperature does not stabilize below 104° F. Use emergency plan under physician's direction or when temperature indicators approach hyperthermia.
Hyperthermia is an acute and possibly life-threatening symptom. The client cannot stay at home safely.

▲ If the client is in hospice or is terminally ill, follow the client's wishes and physician's orders for determining management of fever. Keep the client comfortable and free of pain.
The goal of terminal care is to provide comfort and dignity during the dying process.

Client/Family Teaching

• Teach that fever enhances the immune system response in the presence of infection; the peak of beneficial effects occurs at an oral temperature of 104° F.
Fevers of <104° F enhance immune system functioning (Roberts, 1991).

• Recommend a liberal intake of nonalcoholic and noncaffeinated fluids.
Liberal fluid intake replaces fluid lost through perspiration and respiration. The presence of alcohol and caffeine in fluids can promote diuresis.

• Teach client the detrimental effects of shivering and to avoid activities that can cause shivering (e.g., blanket removal, lower room temperature, tepid water bath, ice packs).
External cooling measures result in shivering and discomfort (Styrt, Sugarman, 1990).

▲ Teach that the use of antipyretics is the most effective way to reduce an infection-related fever to <104° F.

• = **Independent**; ▲ = **Collaborative**

Antipyretics effectively reduce infection-related fevers (Clark, 1991).

- Teach client to avoid vigorous physical activity, wear light clothing, drink liberal amounts of fluids, and wear a hat to minimize sun exposure during periods of excessive outdoor heat.

Such methods reduce exposure to high environmental temperatures, which can cause heat stroke/hyperthermia.

WEB SITES FOR EDUCATION

MERLIN See the MERLIN web site for World Wide Web resources for client education.

REFERENCES   Beaudry M, VandenBosch T, Anderson J: Research utilization: once a day temperatures for afebrile patients, *Clin Nurs Spec* 10:21, 1995.

Brody GM: Hyperthermia and hypothermia in the elderly, *Clin Geriatr Med* 10:213, 1994.

Bull G, Morton J: Environment, temperature, and death rates, *Age Aging* 7:210, 1978.

Clark WG: Antipyretics. In Mackowiak PA, editor: *Fever: basic mechanisms and management,* New York, 1991, Raven.

Cunha BA: The clinical significance of fever patterns, *Infect Dis Clinics* 10:33, 1996.

El-Radhi AS et al: Recurrence rate of febrile convulsions related to the degree of pyrexia during the first attack, *Clin Pediatr* 25:311, 1986.

Harchelroad F: Acute thermoregulatory disorders, *Clin Geriatr Med* 9:621-639, 1993.

Holtzclaw BJ: The febrile response in critical care: state of the science, *Heart Lung* 21:482, 1992.

Holtzclaw BJ: *Clinical predictors and metabolic consequences of postoperative shivering after cardiac surgery,* paper presented at the meeting of the Fifth National Conference on Research for Clinical Practice, Chapel Hill, NC, April 23, 1993.

Klein NC, Cunha BA: Treatment of fever, *Infect Dis Clin* 10:211, 1996.

Kluger MJ: Fever: role of pyrogens and cryogens, *Physiol Rev* 71:93-127, 1991.

Kluger MJ et al: The adaptive value of fever, *Infect Dis Clin* 10:1, 1996.

Mackowiak PA: A critical appraisal of 98.6° F, the upper limit of body temperature and other legacies of Carl Reinhold August Wunderlich, *JAMA* 268:1578, 1992.

Morgan SP: A comparison of three methods of managing fever in the neurologic patient, *J Neurosci Nurs* 22:19, 1990.

Norman DC, Yoshikawa TT: Fever in the elderly, *Infect Dis Clin* 10:93, 1996.

Pernerstorfer T et al: Acetaminophen has greater antipyretic efficacy in endotoxemia: a randomized, double-blind, placebo-controlled trial, *Clin Pharmacol Ther* 66(1):51-57, 1999.

Powers JH, Scheld WM: Fever in neurological diseases, *Infect Dis Clin* 10:45, 1996.

Roberts NJ: The immunological consequences of fever. In Mackowiak PA, editor: *Fever: basic mechanisms and management,* New York, 1991, Raven.

Styrt B, Sugarman B: Antipyresis and fever, *Arch Intern Med* 150:1589, 1990.

Worfolk JB: Heat waves: their impact on the health of elders, *Geriatr Nurs* 21(2):70-77, 2000.

Hypothermia

Betty J. Ackley and Sandra K. Cunningham

NANDA   **Definition**   Body temperature below normal range

Defining Characteristics

Pallor; reduction in body temperature below normal range; shivering; cool skin; cyanotic nail beds; hypertension and then hypotension; piloerection; slow capillary refill; tachycardia

• = Independent; ▲ = Collaborative

Related Factors (r/t)

Exposure to cool or cold environment; medications causing vasodilation; malnutrition; inadequate clothing; illness or trauma; evaporation from skin in cool environment; decreased metabolic rate; damage to hypothalamus; consumption of alcohol; aging; inability or decreased ability to shiver; inactivity

NOC ## Outcomes (Nursing Outcomes Classification)

Suggested NOC Labels

Thermoregulation; Thermoregulation: Neonate

> **Example NOC Outcome**
>
> Accomplishes **Thermoregulation** as evidenced by the following indicators: Body temperature WNL*/Skin temperature IER†/Skin color changes not present/ Hydration adequate/Reported thermal comfort (Rate each indicator of **Thermoregulation:** 1 = extremely compromised, 2 = substantially compromised, 3 = moderately compromised, 4 = mildly compromised, 5 = not compromised [see Section I])

*Within Normal Limits
†In Expected Range

Client Outcomes

- Maintains body temperature within normal range
- Identifies risk factors of hypothermia
- States measures to prevent hypothermia
- Identifies symptoms of hypothermia and actions to take when hypothermia is present

NIC ## Interventions (Nursing Interventions Classification)

Suggested NIC Labels

Hypothermia Treatment; Temperature Regulation; Temperature Regulation: Inoperative; Vital Signs Monitoring

> **Example NIC Interventions—Temperature Regulation**
> - Institute a continuous core temperature monitoring device, as appropriate
> - Promote adequate fluid and nutritional intake

Nursing Interventions and Rationales

- ▲ Determine factors leading to hypothermic episode; see Related Factors.
  It is important to assess risk factors and precipitating events to prevent another incidence of hypothermia and direct treatment.
- • Remove client from cause(s) of hypothermic episode (e.g., cold environment, cold or wet clothing).
  The goal is to eliminate causative or contributing factors.
- ▲ Institute a low-reading, continuous core temperature monitoring device as appropriate, or take temperature hourly.
  The most accurate temperature reading is from a pulmonary artery catheter for the critically ill client (Aragon, 1999). If client is on the medical-surgical unit, an oral or axillary temperature is often best. Variations may occur with ear temperature measurement because of earwax, ear hairs, and position of the client. Rectal temperatures can be uncomfortable and embarrassing and also may not be accurate because of the presence of feces (Edwards,

• = Independent; ▲ = Collaborative

1999). Continual monitoring of the temperature with a rectal probe may be appropriate in some situations (Aragon, 1999).

▲ Monitor client's vital signs every hour and as appropriate. Note changes associated with hypothermia such as decreased pulse, irregular pulse rhythm, decreased respiratory rate, or initially increased then decreased blood pressure.

Decreased circulating volume during hypothermia results in decreased cardiac output and depressed oxygen delivery. Hypoxia, metabolic acidosis, and intrinsic irritability of a cold myocardium result in various dysrhythmias (Haskell et al, 1997; Aragon, 1999; Smith, Yamat, 2000).

• Monitor for signs of hypothermia (e.g., shivering, cool skin, piloerection, pallor, slow capillary refill, cyanotic nail beds, decreased mentation, coma).

This monitors the client's response to interventions and provides evidence of persistent hypothermia.

• Monitor for signs of coagulopathy (e.g., oozing of blood from any open areas, or from intravascular catheter sites or mucous membranes). Also note results of clotting studies as available.

Coagulopathy is a common occurrence during hypothermia in trauma clients (Aragon, 1999; Eddy, Morris, Cullinane, 2000).

• For mild to moderate hypothermia (core temperature 28° to 35° C with an onset of <12 hours), rewarm client passively:
  ▪ Set room temperature at 70° to 75° F
  ▪ Layer clothing and blankets and cover client's head; use insulated metallic blankets
  ▪ Keep the client dry
  ▪ Offer warm fluid with physician's order

▲ Allow client to rewarm at own pace. Passive rewarming is not encouraged for clients with temperatures <82.4° F (28° C).

Passive rewarming prevents heat loss via radiation and evaporation. Client's responses rely on ability to generate heat (Dexter, 1990). Gradual rewarming limits complications associated with hypothermia. Passive rewarming is a slow process and may increase risk of cardiac arrest in severe hypothermia (Edwards, 1999; Larach, 1995).

▲ For severe hypothermia (core temperature <28° C or not responding to passive rewarming), rewarm client actively.
  ▪ Use resistive heating with a carbon-fiber blanket
  ▪ Use radiant heat lights as available
  ▪ Administer heated and humidified oxygen through the ventilator as ordered
  ▪ Administer heated IV fluids at prescribed temperature

These methods increase heat gain via the four major mechanisms of heat transfer—radiation, conduction, convection, and evaporation (Giuffre, Heidenreich, Pruitt, 1994; Stevens, 1993). Resistive heating using a carbon-fiber blanket was shown to be much more effective to rewarm hypothermic subjects than metallic-foil blankets (Greif et al, 2000). Severe hypothermia is associated with acidosis, coma, ventricular fibrillation, apnea, thromocytopenia, platelet dysfunction, impaired clotting, and increased mortality for trauma clients (Eddy, Morris, Cullinane, 2000).

▲ For severe hypothermia, rewarm client using active core-rewarming techniques (e.g., peritoneal lavage, colonic lavage, bladder irrigations, continuous arteriovenous or venovenous rewarming, extracorporeal blood rewarming, and cardiopulmonary bypass) following physician's order.

• = Independent; ▲ = Collaborative

This type of rewarming increases heat gain via conduction (Gentilello, 1995). Active rewarming avoids peripheral dilation with decreased blood pressure and allows fluid deficits to be corrected (Edwards, 1999).

- Check blood pressure frequently when rewarming; watch for hypotension.
  As the body warms, formerly vasoconstricted vessels dilate, resulting in hypotension (Edwards, 1999).

▲ Administer IV fluids as ordered.
  Fluids are often needed to maintain adequate fluid volume. If client develops untreated fluid depletion, hypotension with decreased cardiac output and acute renal failure can result (Edwards, 1999).

▲ Request a social service referral to help client obtain the heat, shelter, and food needed to maintain body temperature.
  A preventive approach that includes adequate food and fluid intake, shelter, heat, and clothing decreases the risk of hypothermia.

▲ Encourage proper nutrition and hydration. Request a dietitian referral to identify appropriate dietary needs.
  Insufficient calorie and fluid intake predispose the client to hypothermia.

Geriatric

- Assess neurological signs frequently, watching for confusion and decreased level of consciousness.
  Older adults are less likely to shiver or complain of feeling cold. Early signs of hypothermia are subtle (Florez-Duquet, McDonald, 1998).

- Warm a hypothermic elderly client slowly, a rate of 1° F per hour.
  Slow warming avoids overheating and allows body to accommodate decreasing risk of complications (Miller, 1995).

Home Care Interventions

NOTE: Hypothermia is not a symptom that appears in the normal course of home care. When it occurs, it is a clinical emergency and the client/family should access emergency medical services immediately.

- Before a medical crisis, confirm that client or family has a thermometer and can read it. Instruct as needed.
  An accurate temperature is one indicator of the client's condition.

- Instruct client or family to take temperature when client displays cyanosis, pallor, or shivering.

- Monitor temperature every hour, as noted previously.

▲ If temperature of client begins dropping below normal range, apply layers of clothing or blankets, or adjust environmental heat to comfort level. Do not overheat. Contact physician.
  Passive rewarming is the only method of rewarming that is appropriate for home care under normal circumstances.

▲ If temperature continues dropping, activate emergency system and notify physician.
  Hypothermia is a clinically acute condition that may not be managed safely in the home.

▲ If client is in hospice care or is terminally ill, follow advance directives, client wishes, and physician's orders. Keep client free of pain.
  The goal of terminal care is to provide dignity and comfort during the dying process.

• = **Independent;** ▲ = **Collaborative**

Client/Family Teaching

- Teach client/family signs of hypothermia and method for taking a temperature (age-appropriate).
- Teach client methods to prevent hypothermia: wearing adequate clothing including a hat and mittens, heating environment to a minimum of 68° F, and ingesting adequate food and fluid.

  Simple measures such as layering clothes, wearing a hat, and avoiding extremes in temperature prevent significant heat loss (Laskowski-Jones, 2000).

- ▲ Teach client and family about medications such, as sedatives, opioids, and anxiolytics, that predispose client to hypothermia (as appropriate).

  If client has had hypothermia in the past, using alternative medications is an option if there is no contraindication (Miller, 1995).

WEB SITES FOR EDUCATION

MERLIN See the MERLIN web site for World Wide Web resources for client education.

REFERENCES   Aragon D: Temperature management in trauma patients across the continuum of care: the TEMP group, *AACN Clin Iss* 10(1):113-123, 1999.

Dexter WW: Hypothermia: safe and efficient methods of rewarming, *Postgrad Med* 88:55, 1990.

Eddy VA, Morris JA, Cullinane DC: Hypothermia, coagulopathy, and acidosis, *Surg Clin North Am* 80(3):845-854, 2000.

Edwards S: Hypothermia, *Prof Nurse* 14(4):253-259, 1999.

Florez-Duquet M, McDonald RB: Cold-induced thermoregulation and biological aging, *Physiol Rev* 78(2):339-358, 1998.

Gentilello LM: Advances in the management of hypothermia, *Surg Clin North Am* 75:243, 1995.

Giuffre M, Heidenreich T, Pruitt L: Rewarming cardiac surgery patients: radiant heat vs. forced warm air, *Nurs Res* 43:174, 1994.

Greif R et al: Resistive heating is more effective than metallic-foil insulation in an experimental model of accidental hypothermia: a randomized controlled trial, *Ann Emerg Med* 35(4):337-345, 2000.

Haskell RM et al: Hypothermia, *AACN Clin Issues Crit Care Nurs* 8(3):368-382, 1997.

Larach MG: Accidental hypothermia, *Lancet* 354:493, 1995.

Laskowski-Jones L: Responding to winter emergencies, *Nursing* 30(1)34-39, 2000.

Miller CA: *Nursing care of older adults,* ed 2, Glenview, Ill, 1995, Scott Foresman/Little, Brown.

Smith CE, Yamat RA: Avoiding hypothermia in the trauma patient, *Curr Op Anaesthesiol* 13:167-174, 2000.

Stevens T: Managing postoperative hypothermia, rewarming, and its complications, *Crit Care Nurs* 16:60, 1993.

Disturbed personal Identity

Gail B. Ladwig

NANDA   **Definition** The inability to distinguish between self and nonself

Defining Characteristics

Withdrawal from social contact; change in ability to determine relationship of body to environment; inappropriate or grandiose behavior (Carpenito, 1993)

• = Independent; ▲ = Collaborative

Related Factors (r/t)
Situational crisis; psychological impairment; chronic illness; pain

 Outcomes (Nursing Outcomes Classification)

Suggested NOC Labels
Identity

> **Example NOC Outcome**
> Able to distinguish between self and nonself as evidenced by: Verbalizes affirmations of personal identity/Exhibits congruent verbal and nonverbal behavior/Distinguishes self from environment and other human beings (Rate each indicator of **Identity:** 1 = never demonstrated, 2 = rarely demonstrated, 3 = sometimes demonstrated, 4 = often demonstrated, 5 = consistently demonstrated [see Section I])

Client Outcomes
- Shows interest in surroundings
- Responds to stimuli with appropriate affect
- Performs self-care and self-control activities appropriate for age
- Acknowledges personal strengths
- Engages in interpersonal relationships
- Verbalizes willingness to change lifestyle and use appropriate community resources

NIC **Interventions (Nursing Interventions Classification)**

Suggested NIC Labels
Decision-Making Support; Self-Esteem Enhancement

> **Example NIC Interventions—Decision-Making Support**
> - Inform client of alternative views or solutions
> - Facilitate client's articulation of goals for care

Nursing Interventions and Rationales
- Assess carefully for history of abuse.
  Series of clients fulfilling diagnostic criteria for dissociative identity disorder (DID), otherwise known as multiple personality disorder, in this study represents a significant component of a complex syndrome associated with a history of severe ongoing developmental trauma dating from early childhood (Middleton, Butler, 1998).
- Assess for any history of seizure disorder; adhere to diagnostic criteria for dissociative disorder from DSM IV and structured clinical interview.
  Misdiagnosis of persons with seizures and dissociative symptoms can be avoided by careful adherence to DSM dissociative disorder criteria, the use of video-EEG monitoring, and systematic assessment of dissociative symptoms with the SCID-D (Bowman, Coons, 2000).
- Avoid labeling of client with terms such as multiple personality disorder.
  In this study more patients attempted suicide after being diagnosed with MPD than before diagnosis in comparison study of other patients on a mood disorders unit (Fetkewicz, Sharma, Merskey, 2000).
- Offer reassurance to the client, and use therapeutic communication at frequent intervals.
  Client reassurance and communication are nursing skills that promote trust and orientation and reduce anxiety (Harvey, 1996).

• = **Independent;** ▲ = **Collaborative**

- Work with clients on setting personal goals.
  Social production function (SPF) basically asserts that people produce their own well-being by trying to optimize achievement of universal human goals (Ormel et al, 1997).
- Address clients by name. Let them know who is approaching and orient them to surroundings.
  These interventions help clients with loss of ego boundaries to identify boundaries between themselves and the environment (Haber et al, 1992).
- Have clients describe their perceptions of the environment as concretely as possible.
  These descriptions provide feedback that confirms the client's existence.
- Give clients permission to share their experiences; they have always lived in secrecy and they are not sure how much is safe to reveal or who believes their illness is an actual illness.
  An average of 6.8 years elapses between the time clients are first assessed and the time they receive an accurate diagnosis (Frye, 1990).
- Use touch only after a thorough assessment and as appropriate.
  Touch, which conveys caring, is an appropriate way of communicating unless it makes the person touched feel uncomfortable (Wells-Federman et al, 1995). Some clients may touch people to identify separateness from others; other clients experience fusion with others when they touch (Haber et al, 1992).
- Have all team members approach client in a consistent manner.
  Consistency promotes trust, which is necessary for establishing a therapeutic relationship that helps the client develop interpersonal relationships.
- Provide time for one-to-one interactions to establish a therapeutic relationship.
  Nursing presence, one-on-one interaction, connecting with the client's experience, going beyond the scientific data, and knowing what will work and when to act all support the nurse-client relationship and affirm their respective selves. As a result, the client grows in awareness of his own being (Doona, Chase, Haggerty, 1999).
- Encourage client to verbalize feelings about self and body image. Have client make a list of strengths.
  These verbalizations help the client recognize the self; listing strengths promotes self-exploration. In this study 48 women in a psychiatric outpatient clinic completed a survey that indicated a correlation with borderline personality and body weight/body image issues that are not necessarily a result of larger size (Sansone, Wiederman, Monteith, 2001).
- Hold client responsible for age-appropriate behavior; involve client in planning of self-care.
  Involving clients in care gives them a sense of control and helps the client gain ego strength (Preston, 1994).
- Give positive feedback when appropriate self-control is used.
  When presented with positive feedback, the boys in this study were able to relax defensive posture and offer more realistic self-assessment (Diener, Milich, 1997).
- ▲ Encourage participation in group therapy for building relationship skills and getting feedback from others with regard to behavior.
  Findings suggest that social skills training resulted in greater improvement in certain measures of social adjustment than supportive group therapy (Marder et al, 1996). An adaptive narcissistic client's need to depend on other people to feel whole suggests that group therapy could be a powerful tool for treating those who suffer profound wounds to self-esteem (Kurek-Ovshinsky, 1991).

• = **Independent;** ▲ = **Collaborative**

- Encourage client to use a daily diary to set achievable and realistic goals and monitor successes.

  Journal writing has been found to improve physical and mental health measurably (Wells-Federman et al, 1995).

Geriatric

- Monitor for signs of depression, grief, and withdrawal.

  The disturbed personal identity may mask underlying depression.

- Address clients by their full name preceded by the proper title (Mr., Mrs., Ms., Miss); use nickname or first name only if suggested by the client, and do not use terms of endearment (e.g., "honey").

  Calling a person honey, sweetie, or granny, etc., is demeaning and demoralizing and can increase feelings of loneliness by decreasing a sense of relatedness to self (Buchda, 1987).

- Practice reality orientation (RO) principles; ask specifically how the client feels about events that are happening.

  This evidence-based study indicated that there is some evidence that RO has benefits on both cognition and behavior for dementia sufferers (Spector et al, 2000). RO helps define ego boundaries.

- Ask client about important past experiences.

  Reconsideration of past experiences, missed opportunities, and mistakes allows older clients to reach ego integrity (Bulechek, McCloskey, 1992).

- ▲ If the client's symptoms are associated with a stroke, refer client for longer rehabilitation that includes physical programs that address psychological as well as neuromuscular issue.

  Clients who have had a stroke find their body unreliable, and their body appears separate from their self. These feelings may last a year or more (Ellis-Hill, Payne, Ward, 2000).

Multicultural

- Assess for the influence of cultural beliefs, norms, and values on the client's ethnic and racial identity.

  How the client self identifies himself or herself will be based on cultural perceptions (Leininger, 1996).

- Ask the client how they identify ethnically and/or racially and what they wish to be referred to as (e.g., Black vs. African-American, Hispanic vs. Latino).

  Ethnic/racial identity is part of a client's self-concept (Padilla, 1995). Biracial individuals may have unique ways of self-identification.

- Validate the client's feelings regarding their ethnic or racial identity.

  Validation lets the client know that the nurse has heard and understands what was said, and it promotes the nurse-client relationship (Stuart, Laraia, 2001; Giger, Davidhizar, 1995).

Home Care Interventions

- Assess client's immediate support system/family for relationship patterns and content of communication.

  Knowledge of relationship dynamics in the client's environment assists the nurse with individualizing care.

- Encourage family to provide support and feedback regarding client identity and ego boundaries.

  The family is a socially significant cultural group that generates behavior, defines roles, and promotes values.

- **= Independent; ▲ = Collaborative**

▲ If client is involved in counseling or self-help groups, monitor and encourage attendance. Help client identify value of group participation after each group encounter. *Discussion of group participation identifies group feedback and support and reinforces support for change.*

▲ If client is taking prescribed psychotropic medications, assess for understanding of side effects of and reasons for taking medication. Teach as necessary.

▲ Assess medications for effectiveness and side effects and monitor for compliance. *Clients with poor ego strength may have difficulty adhering to a medication regimen.*

Client/Family Teaching

• Teach stress reduction and relaxation techniques.
These techniques can be used when the client becomes anxious about the loss of self.

▲ Refer to community resources or other self-help groups appropriate for the client's underlying problem (e.g., Adult Children of Alcoholics, parent effectiveness group). *Group therapy provides an arena in which clients can experience the interdependent mode of adaptation without assaults to self-esteem (Kurek-Ovshinsky, 1991).*

▲ Refer to appropriate treatment as soon as signs of depression are noted. *Effective acute-phase depression treatment reduced somatic distress and improved self-rated overall health (Simon et al, 1998).*

• Be a role model for family members: talk to, not around, the client; give choices to the client when family members may be listening; always address the client by name; and do not interrupt when the client is attempting to communicate.
Role modeling helps to reinstate individualism and value for a client who has been treated by the family as a "nonperson" (Dolphin, 1984).

WEB SITES FOR EDUCATION

MERLIN   See the MERLIN web site for World Wide Web resources for client education.

REFERENCES   Bowman ES, Coons PM: The differential diagnosis of epilepsy, pseudoseizures, dissociative identity disorder, and dissociative disorder not otherwise specified, *Bull Menninger Clin* 64(2):164-180, 2000.

Buchda V: Loneliness in critically ill adults, *Dimens Crit Care Nurs* 6:335, 1987.

Bulechek G, McCloskey J: *Nursing interventions: essential nursing treatments*, ed 2, Philadelphia, 1992, WB Saunders.

Carpenito LJ: *Nursing diagnosis: application to clinical practice*, ed 5, Philadelphia, 1993, JB Lippincott.

Diener MB, Milich R: Effects of positive feedback on the social interactions of boys with attention deficit hyperactivity disorder: a test of the self-protective hypothesis, *J Clin Child Psychol* 26(3):256-265, 1997.

Dolphin N: Non-personhood: a nursing diagnosis in the psycho-social realm, *Home Healthc Nurse* 1(2):16-18, 1984.

Doona M, Chase S, Haggerty L: Nursing presence, *J Holistic Nurs* 17(1):54-69, 1999.

Ellis-Hill CS, Payne S, Ward C: Self-body split: issues of identity in physical recovery following a stroke, *Disabil Rehabil* 22(16):725-733, 2000.

Fetkewicz J, Sharma V, Merskey H: A note on suicidal deterioration with recovered memory treatment, *J Affect Disord* 58(2):155-159, 2000.

Frye B: Art and multiple personality disorder: an expressive framework for occupational therapy, *Am J Occup Ther* 44:1013, 1990.

Giger JN, Davidhizar RE: *Transcultural nursing*, ed 2, St Louis, 1995, Mosby.

Haber J et al: *Psychiatric nursing*, ed 4, St Louis, 1992, Mosby.

Harvey M: Managing agitation in critically ill patients, *Am J Crit Care* 5:7, 1996.

Kurek-Ovshinsky C: Group psychotherapy in an acute inpatient setting: techniques that nourish self-esteem, *Issues Ment Health Nurs* 12:81, 1991.

Leininger MM: *Transcultural nursing: theories, research and practices*, ed 2, Hilliard, Ohio, 1996, McGraw-Hill.

• = **Independent;** ▲ = **Collaborative**

Marder SR et al: Two-year outcome of social skills training and group psychotherapy for outpatients with schizophrenia, *Am J Psychiatry* 153(12):1585-1592, 1996.

Middleton W, Butler J: Dissociative identity disorder: an Australian series, *Aust NZ J Psychiatry* 32(6):794-804, 1998.

Ormel J et al: Quality of life and social production functions: a framework for understanding health effects, *Soc Sci Med* 45(7):1051-1063, 1997.

Padilla A: *Hispanic psychology: critical issues in theory and research,* Thousand Oaks, Calif, 1995, Sage.

Preston K: Rehabilitation nursing: a client-centered philosophy, *Am J Nurs* 94:66, 1994.

Sansone RA, Wiederman MW, Monteith D: Obesity, borderline personality symptomatology, and body image among women in a psychiatric outpatient setting, *Int J Eat Disord* 29(1):76-79, 2001.

Simon G et al: Impact of improved depression treatment in primary care on daily functioning and disability, *Psychol Med* 28(3):693-701, 1998.

Spector A et al: Reality orientation for dementia (Cochrane Review), *Cochrane Database Syst Rev* (4):CD001119, 2000.

Stuart GW, Laraia MT: Therapeutic nurse-patient relationship. In Stuart GW, Laraia MT, editors: *Principles and practice of psychiatric nursing,* St Louis, 2001, Mosby, p 30.

Wells-Federman C et al: The mind-body connection: the psychophysiology of many traditional nursing interventions, *Clin Nurse Spec* 9:59, 1995.

Functional urinary Incontinence

Mikel Gray

NANDA   **Definition** Inability of usually continent person to reach toilet in time to avoid unintentional loss of urine

Defining Characteristics

The relationship between functional limitations and urinary incontinence remains controversial (Hunskaar et al, 1999). While functional impairment clearly exacerbates the severity of urinary incontinence, the underlying factors that contribute to these functional limitations themselves contribute to abnormal lower urinary tract function and impaired continence.

Related Factors (r/t)

Cognitive disorders (delirium, dementias, severe or profound retardation); neuromuscular limitations impairing mobility or dexterity; impaired vision; psychological factors; weakened supporting pelvic structures; environmental barriers to toileting

NOC   ## Outcomes (Nursing Outcomes Classification)

Suggested NOC Labels

Urinary Continence, Urinary Elimination

> **Example NOC Outcome**
> Accomplishes **Urinary Continence** as evidenced by the following indicators: Recognizes urge to void/Responds in timely manner to urge/Voids in appropriate receptacle/Adequate time to reach toilet between urge and evacuation of urine/Underclothing dry during day/Underclothing or bedding dry during night (Rate each indicator of **Urinary Continence:** 1 = never demonstrated, 2 = rarely demonstrated, 3 = sometimes demonstrated, 4 = often demonstrated, 5 = consistently demonstrated [see Section I])

• = Independent; ▲ = Collaborative

Client Outcomes

- Eliminates or reduces incontinent episodes
- Eliminates or overcomes environmental barriers to toileting
- Uses adaptive equipment to reduce or eliminate incontinence related to impaired mobility or dexterity
- Uses portable urinary collection devices or urine containment devices when access to the toilet is not feasible

NIC ## Interventions (Nursing Interventions Classification)

Suggested NIC Labels

Urinary Habit Training; Urinary Incontinence Care

Example NIC Interventions—Urinary Habit Training
- Keep a continence specification record for 3 days to establish voiding pattern
- Establish interval for toileting of preferably not <2 hours

Nursing Interventions and Rationales

- Perform a focused history of the incontinence including duration, frequency and severity of leakage episodes, and alleviating and aggravating factors.
  The history provides clues to the causes, the severity of the condition, and its management.
- Complete a bladder log of diurnal and nocturnal urine elimination patterns and patterns of urinary leakage.
  The bladder log provides a more objective verification of urine elimination patterns as compared with the history (Resnick et al, 1994) and a baseline against which the results of management can be evaluated.
- ▲ Assess client for potentially reversible causes of acute/transient urinary incontinence (e.g., urinary tract infection [UTI], atrophic urethritis, constipation or impaction, sedatives or narcotics interfering with the ability to reach the toilet in a timely fashion, antidepressants or psychotropic medications interfering with efficient detrusor contractions, parasympatholytics, alpha adrenergic antagonists, polyuria caused by uncontrolled diabetes mellitus, or insipidus).
  Transient or acute incontinence can be eliminated by reversing the underlying cause (Urinary Incontinence Guideline Panel, 1996).
- Assess client for established/chronic incontinence: stress urinary incontinence, urge urinary incontinence, reflex, or extraurethral ("total") urinary incontinence. If present, begin treatment for these forms of urine loss.
  Functional incontinence often coexists with another form of urinary leakage, particularly among the elderly (Gray, 1992).
- Assess the home, acute care, or long-term care environment for accessibility to toileting facilities, paying particular attention to the following:
  - Distance of toilet from bed, chair, living quarters
  - Characteristics of the bed, including presence of side rails and distance of bed from the floor
  - Characteristics of the pathway to the toilet, including barriers such as stairs, loose rugs on the floor, and inadequate lighting
  - Characteristics of the bathroom, including patterns of use; lighting; height of toilet from floor; presence of hand rails to assist transfers to toilet; and breadth of door and its accessibility for wheelchair, walker, or other assistive device

• = Independent; ▲ = Collaborative

Functional continence requires access to the toilet; environmental barriers blocking this access can produce functional incontinence (Wells, 1992).

- Assess client for mobility, including ability to rise from chair and bed; ability to transfer to toilet and ambulate; and need for physical assistive devices such as a cane, walker, or wheel chair.
Functional continence requires the ability to gain access to a toilet facility, either independently or with the assistance of devices to increase mobility (Jirovec, Wells, 1990; Wells, 1992).

▲ Assess client for dexterity, including the ability to manipulate buttons, hooks, snaps, Velcro, and zippers needed to remove clothing. Consult physical or occupational therapist to promote optimal toilet access as indicated.
Functional continence requires the ability to remove clothing to urinate (Maloney, Cafiero, 1999; Wells, 1992).

- Evaluate cognitive status with a NEECHAM confusion scale (Neelan et al, 1992) for acute cognitive changes, a Folstein Mini-Mental Status Examination (Folstein, Folstein, McHugh, 1975), or other tool as indicated.
Functional continence requires sufficient mental acuity to respond to sensory input from a filling urinary bladder by locating the toilet, moving to it, and emptying the bladder (Maloney, Cafiero, 1999; Colling et al, 1992).

- Remove environmental barriers to toileting in the acute care, long-term care or home setting. Help the client remove loose rugs from the floor and improve lighting in hallways and bathrooms.

- Provide an appropriate, safe urinary receptacle such as a 3-in-1 commode, female or male hand-held urinal, no-spill urinal, or containment device when toileting access is limited by immobility or environmental barriers.
These receptacles provide access to a substitute toilet and enhance the potential for functional continence (Rabin, 1998; Wells, 1992).

▲ Assist the client with limited mobility to obtain evaluation for a physical therapist and to obtain assistive devices as indicated (Maloney, Cafiero, 1999); assist the client to select shoes with a nonskid sole to maximize traction when arising from a chair and transferring to the toilet.

- Assist the person to alter their wardrobe to maximize toileting access. Select loose-fitting clothing with stretch waist bands rather than buttoned or zippered waist; minimize buttons, snaps, and multilayered clothing; and substitute Velcro or other easily loosened systems for buttons, hooks, and zippers in existing clothing.

- Begin a prompted voiding program or patterned urge response toileting program for the elderly client with functional incontinence and dementia in the home or long-term care facility:
  - Determine the frequency of current urination using an alarm system or check and change device
  - Record urinary elimination and incontinent patterns on a bladder log to use as a baseline for assessment and evaluation of treatment efficacy
  - Begin a prompted toileting program based on the results of this program; toileting frequency may vary from every 1.5 to 2 hours, to every 4 hours
  - Praise the client when toileting occurs with prompting
  - Refrain from any socialization when incontinent episodes occur; change the client and make her or him comfortable

• = **Independent;** ▲ = **Collaborative**

Prompted voiding or patterned urge response toileting have been shown to markedly reduce or eliminate functional incontinence in selected clients in the long-term care facility and in the community setting (Colling et al, 1992; Eustice, Roe, Patterson, 2000).

Geriatric

- Institute aggressive continence management programs for the community-dwelling client in consultation with the patient and family.
  Uncontrolled incontinence can lead to institutionalization in an elderly person who prefers to remain in a home care setting (O'Donnell et al, 1992).
- Monitor elderly clients for dehydration in the long-term care facility, acute care facility, or home.
  Dehydration can exacerbate urine loss, produce acute confusion, and increase the risk of morbidity and morality, particularly in the frail elderly client (Colling, Owen, McCreedy, 1994).

Home Care Interventions

- Assess current strategies used to reduce urinary incontinence, including fluid intake, restriction of bladder irritants, prompted or scheduled toileting, and use of containment devices.
  Many elders and care providers use a variety of self-management techniques to manage urinary incontinence such as fluid limitation, avoidance of social contacts, and absorptive materials that may or may not be effective for reducing urinary leakage or beneficial to general health (Johnson, 2000).
- Teach the family general principles of bladder health, including avoidance of bladder irritants, adequate fluid intake, and a routine schedule of toileting (refer to care plan for **Impaired Urinary elimination**).
- Teach prompted voiding to the family and patient with mild to moderate dementia (refer to previous description) (Colling, 1996; McDowell et al, 1994).
- ▲ Advise the patient about the advantages of using disposable or reusable insert pads, pad-pant systems, or replacement briefs specifically designed for urinary incontinence (or double urinary and fecal incontinence) as indicated.
  Many absorptive products used by community-dwelling elders are not designed to absorb urine, prevent odor, and protect the perineal skin. Substitution of disposable or reusable absorptive devices specifically designed to contain urine or double incontinence are more effective than household products, particularly in moderate to severe cases (Shirran, Brazelli, 2000; Gallo, Staskin, 1997).
- Assist the family with arranging care in a way that allows the patient to participate in family or favorite activities without embarrassment.
  Careful planning can retain the dignity and integrity of family patterns.
- Teach principles of perineal skin care, including routine cleansing following incontinent episodes, daily cleaning and drying of perineal skin, and use of moisture barriers as indicated.
  Routine cleansing and daily cleaning with appropriate products help maintain integrity of perineal skin and prevent secondary cutaneous infections (Fiers, Thayer, 2000).
- ▲ Refer to occupational therapy for help in obtaining assistive devices and adapting the home for optimal toilet accessibility.
- ▲ Consider use of an indwelling catheter for continuous drainage in the patient who is both homebound and bed-bound and receiving palliative or end of life care (requires physician order).

- = **Independent**; ▲ = **Collaborative**

An indwelling catheter may increase patient comfort, ease care provider burden, and prevent urinary incontinence in bed-bound patients receiving end of life care.

▲ When an indwelling catheter is in place, follow prescribed maintenance protocols for managing the catheter, drainage bag, perineal skin, and urethral meatus. Teach infection control measures adapted to the home care setting.
Proper care reduces the risk of catheter-associated UTI.

Client/Family Teaching

- Work with the client, family, and their extended support systems to assist with needed changes in the environment and wardrobe and other alterations needed to maximize toileting access.
- Work with the client and family to establish a reasonable, manageable prompted voiding program using environmental and verbal cues, such as television programs, meals, and bedtime, to remind caregivers of voiding intervals.
- Teach the family to use an alarm system for toileting or to perform a check and change program and to maintain an accurate log of voiding and incontinent episodes.

WEB SITES FOR EDUCATION

MERLIN See the MERLIN web site for World Wide Web resources for client education.

REFERENCES   Colling JC: Noninvasive strategies to manage urinary incontinence among care-dependent persons, *J Wound Ostomy Continence Nurs* 23:302-308, 1996.

Colling JC et al: The effects of patterned urge response toileting (PURT) on urinary incontinence among nursing home residents, *J Am Geriatr Soc* 40:135-141, 1992.

Colling JC, Owen TR, McCreedy MR: Urine volumes and voiding patterns among incontinence nursing home residents, *Geriatr Nurs* 15:188-192, 1994.

Eustice S, Roe B, Patterson J: Prompted voiding for the management of urinary incontinence in adults, *Cochrane Database Syst Rev* CD002113, 2000.

Fiers S, Thayer D: Management of intractable incontinence. In Doughty DB, editor: *Urinary and fecal incontinence: nursing management,* St Louis, 2000, Mosby, pp 183-207.

Folstein MF, Folstein EF, McHugh P: Mini mental state: a practical method of grading the cognitive status of the patient for the clinician, *J Psychiatr Rev* 12:189-198, 1975.

Gallo M, Staskin DR: Patient satisfaction with a reusable undergarment for urinary incontinence, *J Wound Ostomy Continence Nurs* 24:226-236, 1997.

Gray ML: *Genitourinary disorders,* St Louis, 1992, Mosby.

Hunskaar S et al: Epidemiology and natural history of urinary incontinence. In Abrams P, Khoury S, Wein A: *Incontinence,* Plymbridge, 1999, Health Publications, p 213.

Jirovec MM, Wells TJ: Urinary incontinence in nursing home residents with dementia: the mobility-cognition paradigm, *Appl Nurs Res* 3:112-117, 1990.

Johnson ST: From incontinence to confidence, *Am J Nurs* 100(2):69-76, 2000.

Maloney C, Cafiero M: Implementing an incontinence program in long-term care settings: a multidisciplinary approach, *J Gerontol Nurs* 25:47-52, 1999.

McDowell BJ et al: Successful treatment using behavioral interventions of urinary incontinence in home-bound elder adults, *Geriatr Nurs* 15:303-307, 1994.

Neelan VJ et al: Use of the NEECHAM confusion scale to assess acute confusional states of hospitalized older patients. In: Funk SG et al, editors: *Key aspects of elder care: managing falls, incontinence and cognitive impairment,* New York, 1992, Springer.

O'Donnell BF et al: Incontinence and troublesome behaviors predict institutionalization in dementia, *J Geriatr Psych Neurol* 545-552, 1992.

Rabin JM: Clinical use of the FemAssist device in female urinary incontinence, *J Med Syst* 22:257-271, 1998.

- = **Independent**; ▲ = **Collaborative**

Resnick NM et al: Short term variability of self report of incontinence in older persons, *J Am Geriatr Soc* 42:202-207, 1994.

Shirran E, Brazelli M: Absorbent products for the containment of urinary and/or fecal incontinence, *Cochrane Database Syst Rev* CD0011406, 2000.

Urinary Incontinence Guideline Panel: *Urinary incontinence in adults: clinical practice guideline*, ed 2, Rockville, Md, 1996, Agency for Health Care Policy and Research.

Wells TJ: Managing incontinence through managing the environment, *Urol Nurs* 12:48-50, 1992.

Reflex urinary Incontinence

Mikel Gray

NANDA **Definition** Involuntary loss of urine at somewhat predictable intervals when a specific bladder volume is reached

An involuntary loss of urine caused by a defect in the spinal cord between the nerve roots at or below the first cervical segment and those above the second sacral segment; patterns of urine elimination occur at unpredictable intervals, and micturition may be elicited by tactile stimuli including stroking of inner aspect of thigh or perineum (Gray, 1992)

Defining Characteristics

Absent or diminished sensation or urge to void; incomplete emptying caused by dyssynergia of the striated sphincter mechanism, producing functional outlet obstruction of the bladder; may be associated with sweating, acute elevation in blood pressure and pulse in clients with spinal cord injury (see care plan for **Autonomic dysreflexia**)

Related Factors (r/t)

Paralyzing spinal disorder affecting spinal segments C1 to S2

NOC **Outcomes (Nursing Outcomes Classification)**

Suggested NOC Labels

Urinary Continence; Urinary Elimination

> **Example NOC Outcome**
> Accomplishes **Urinary Continence** as evidenced by the following indicators: Predictable pattern to passage of urine/Absence of UTI (<100,000 WBC)/ Underclothing dry during day/Underclothing or bedding dry during night (Rate each indicator of **Urinary Continence:** 1 = never demonstrated, 2 = rarely demonstrated, 3 = sometimes demonstrated, 4 = often demonstrated, 5 = consistently demonstrated [see Section I])

Client Outcomes

- Follows prescribed schedule for bladder evacuation
- Demonstrates successful use of triggering techniques to stimulate voiding
- Perineal skin remains intact
- Client remains clear of symptomatic urinary infection
- Demonstrates how to apply containment device or indwelling catheter or is able to provide caregiver with instructions to perform these procedures
- Demonstrates awareness of risk of autonomic dysreflexia and its prevention and management

• = Independent; ▲ = Collaborative

NIC   **Interventions (Nursing Interventions Classification)**
   Suggested NIC Labels
   Urinary Bladder Training; Urinary Catheterization: Intermittent

   Example NIC Interventions—Urinary Bladder Training
   ▪ Determine ability to recognize urge to void
   ▪ Keep a continence specification record for 3 days to establish voiding pattern

Nursing Interventions and Rationales

▲ Assess the client's neurological status, including the type of neurological disorder, the functional level of neurological impairment, its completeness (effect on motor and sensory function), and ability to perform bladder management, including intermittent catheterization, application of a condom catheter, etc.
The type of the neurological disorder and its functional level, completeness, and underlying disorder affect the severity of the urinary leakage, risk of striated sphincter dyssynergia, and subsequent management (Gray, 2000).

▲ Perform a focused assessment of the urinary system including perineal skin assessment, evaluation of the vaginal vault, reproduction of the sign of stress urinary incontinence (refer to care plan for **Stress urinary Incontinence**), and a neurological examination including reproduction of the bulbocavernosus reflex and testing of perineal sensation.
This focused physical examination will provide objective evidence of coexisting stress urinary incontinence and indirect evidence of bladder and urethral sensation (Gray, 2000).

• Complete a bladder log to determine the pattern of urine elimination, incontinent episodes, and current bladder management program.
The bladder log provides an objective record of urine elimination, confirming the accuracy of the historical report and a baseline for assessment and evaluation of treatment efficacy.

▲ Consult with the physician concerning current bladder function and the potential of the bladder to produce upper urinary tract distress (hydronephrosis, vesicoureteral reflux, febrile UTI, or compromised renal function).
Reflex incontinence is typically accompanied by detrusor striated sphincter dyssynergia, which increases the risk of upper urinary tract distress (Killorin et al, 1992; Gray et al, 1991).

▲ Determine a bladder management program in consultation with the client, family, and rehabilitation team.
The bladder management program affects the client and significant others; it is determined by holistic assessment that addresses potential of the bladder to create upper urinary tract distress, potential for continence and related complications, client and family preference, and perceived impact of the bladder management program on the client's lifestyle (Anson, Gray, 1993; Gray, Rayome, Anson, 1995).

▲ Counsel the client and family concerning the merits and potential risks associated with each bladder management program, including spontaneous voiding, intermittent self-catheterization, reflex voiding program with condom catheter containment, and indwelling catheterization in consultation with the rehabilitation team.
All bladder management programs carry some risk of urinary incontinence or serious urinary system complications. Spontaneous voiding and intermittent catheterization carry

• = **Independent;** ▲ = **Collaborative**

greater risk of urine loss as compared with condom catheter containment or indwelling catheter, but these strategies carry higher risk for serious urinary system complications, including upper urinary tract distress, when evaluated over a period of years (Gray, 2000; Anson, Gray, 1993; Gray, Rayome, Anson, 1995).

- Teach all clients with reflex incontinence to consume an adequate amount of fluids on a daily basis (30 ml/kg of body weight).
  Dehydration exacerbates urine loss and increases the risk of related complications, including constipation and urine infection (Pearson, 1993; Gray, Rayome, Anson, 1995).
- ▲ Teach the client with reflex urinary incontinence who is managed by spontaneous voiding to self-administer an alpha-adrenergic blocking medication as directed and to recognize and manage potential side effects.
  Clients who spontaneously urinate often take an alpha-adrenergic blocking drug to reduce urethral resistance to voiding (Perkash, 1995; Gray, 1996).
- ▲ Teach clean intermittent catheterization when this technique is selected for bladder management for reflex urinary incontinence. Include at least one family member or the client's spouse or significant other in this instruction.
  Intermittent catheterization has proved to be a safe and effective bladder management strategy for persons with reflex urinary incontinence. Inclusion of a family member, spouse, or significant other is particularly helpful for the client with limited upper extremity dexterity and reflex urinary incontinence (Anson, Gray, 1993; Chai et al, 1995; Gray, Rayome, Anson, 1995).
- ▲ Teach the client managed by intermittent catheterization to self-administer antispasmodic (parasympatholytic) medications as directed and to recognize and manage potential side effects.
  Persons who manage reflex incontinence by intermittent catheterization frequently require antispasmodic medications to manage the hyperreflexic detrusor contractions that produce urine loss (Gray, 1996).
- Teach the male client with reflex incontinence who cannot be managed effectively with spontaneous voiding, who does not choose to perform intermittent catheterization, or who cannot perform catheterization, to obtain, select, and apply a condom catheter with drainage bag. Include family in teaching. Help client and family choose a product that adheres to the penile shaft without allowing seepage of urine onto surrounding skin or clothing, a material and adhesive that does not produce hypersensitive reactions on the skin, and a leg bag that is easily concealed under clothing and does not cause irritation to the skin of the thigh.
  Many components of the condom catheter affect the product's ability to contain urinary leakage, protect underlying skin, and preserve the client's dignity (Watson, Kuhn, 1990; Watson, 1989).
- Teach the client who uses a condom catheter to remove the condom device, inspect the skin, cleanse the penis thoroughly, and reapply a new catheter every day.
  The risk of UTI increases if a condom catheter is worn for longer than 24 hours (Hirsh, Fainstein, Musher, 1979).
- Teach the client managed by a condom catheter to routinely inspect the skin with each catheter change for evidence of lesions caused by pressure from the containment device or by exposure to urine.
  Skin breakdown is a common complication associated with routine use of the condom catheter (Anson, Gray, 1993).

• = Independent; ▲ = Collaborative

▲ Teach the client managed by an intermittent or indwelling catheter to recognize signs of significant UTI and to promptly seek care when these signs occur. The following are signs of significant infection:
  ▪ Discomfort over the bladder or during urination
  ▪ Acute onset of urinary incontinence
  ▪ Fever
  ▪ Markedly increased spasticity of muscles below the level of the spinal lesion
  ▪ Malaise, lethargy
  ▪ Hematuria
  ▪ Autonomic dysreflexia (hyperreflexia) (National Institute on Disability and Rehabilitation Research, 1992)
    Intermittent catheterization is typically associated with asymptomatic bacteriuria, and the indwelling catheter is routinely associated with asymptomatic colonization. Antibiotic treatment of asymptomatic bacteriuria has not proven helpful, but prompt management of significant infection is necessary to prevent urosepsis or related complications (Stover, 1993; Waites, Cannupp, DeVivo, 1991).

Geriatric

▲ If having difficulties teaching elderly clients, refer them to a nurse who specializes in care of aging clients with urinary incontinence.

Home Care Interventions

▲ Instruct client in complications of reflex incontinence and when to report to physician or primary nurse.
  Early detection allows for early diagnosis and treatment before irreversible damage is done to the renal parenchyma (Gray, 2000).
▲ If client is taught intermittent self-catheterization, arrange for contingency care in the event client is unable to perform self-catheterization.
  Self-catheterization promotes client independence.
• Assess and instruct client and family in care of catheter and supplies in the home.
  Proper care of supplies decreases risk of infection.
• Assist the family with arranging care in a way that allows the client to participate in family or favorite activities without embarrassment.
  Careful planning can help client retain dignity and maintain the integrity of family patterns.
▲ If medications are ordered, instruct family or caregivers and client in medication administration, use, and side effects.
  Adherence to a medication regimen increases its chances of success and decreases the risk of losing the regimen as an option for care when other options are unacceptable.

Client/Family Teaching

• Teach signs of autonomic dysreflexia to all clients with a spinal injury, including its relationship to bladder fullness and management of the condition (refer to care plan for **Autonomic dysreflexia**).
  Teach the client and family/significant others the techniques of intermittent catheterization, indwelling catheter care and removal, and condom catheter management as appropriate.
▲ Teach the client and family/significant others techniques to clean intermittent catheters including washing with soap and water, allowing to air dry, and microwave cleaning techniques.

• = Independent; ▲ = Collaborative

REFERENCES   Anson C, Gray ML: Secondary complications after spinal cord injury, *Urol Nurs* 13:107-112, 1993.
Chai T et al: Compliance and complications of clean intermittent catheterization in the spinal cord injured patient, *Paraplegia* 33:161-163, 1995.
Gray ML: *Genitourinary disorders,* St Louis, 1992, Mosby.
Gray ML: *Urology nursing drug reference,* St Louis, 1996, Mosby.
Gray ML: Reflex urinary incontinence. In Doughty DB, editor: *Urinary and fecal incontinence: nursing management,* ed 2, St Louis, 2000.
Gray ML et al: Urethral pressure gradient in the prediction of upper urinary tract distress following spinal cord injury, *J Am Paraplegia Soc* 14:105-106, 1991.
Gray ML, Rayome RG, Anson C: Incontinence and clean intermittent catheterization following spinal cord injury, *Clin Nurs Res* 4:6-21, 1995.
Hirsh DD, Fainstein V, Musher DM: Do condom catheter collecting systems cause urinary tract infection? *JAMA* 242:340-341, 1979.
Killorin WK et al: Evaluative urodynamics and bladder management in the prediction of upper urinary infection in male spinal cord injury, *Paraplegia* 30:437-441, 1992.
National Institute on Disability and Rehabilitation Research: Prevention and management of urinary tract infections among people with spinal cord injuries, *J Am Paraplegia Soc* 15:194, 1992.
Pearson BD: Liquidate a myth: reducing liquid intake is not advisable for elderly with urine control problems, *Urol Nurs* 13:80-85, 1993.
Perkash I: Efficacy and safety of terazosin to improve voiding in spinal cord injury patients, *J Spinal Cord Med* 18:236-239, 1995.
Stover SL: Management of bacteriuria and infection in neurogenic bladder, *Rehabil Clin North Am* 4:343-362, 1993.
Waites KB, Cannupp KC, DeVivo MJ: Efficacy and tolerance of norfloxacin in treatment of complicated urinary tract infection in outpatients with neurogenic bladder secondary to spinal cord injury, *Urology* 38:589, 1991.
Watson R: A nursing trial of urinary sheath systems on male hospitalized patients, *J Adv Nurs* 14:467-470, 1989.
Watson R, Kuhn M: The influence of component parts on the performance of urinary sheath systems, *J Adv Nurs* 15:417-422, 1990.

Stress urinary Incontinence

Mikel Gray

NANDA   **Definition** Loss of <50 ml of urine occurring with increased abdominal pressure
NOTE: The restriction of the volume of urine loss to <50 ml may be exceeded by women and men with severe stress urinary incontinence caused by intrinsic sphincter deficiency. This is sometimes classified as "total urinary incontinence." However, in this book, "total urinary incontinence" will be used to refer exclusively to extraurethral incontinence, and all forms of stress urinary incontinence are reviewed under this diagnosis, regardless of severity.

Defining Characteristics

Observed urine loss with physical exertion (sign of stress urinary incontinence); reported loss of urine associated with physical exertion or activity (symptom of stress urinary incontinence); urine loss associated with increased abdominal pressure (urodynamic confirmation of stress urinary incontinence)

• = Independent; ▲ = Collaborative

Related Factors (r/t)

Urethral hypermobility (familial predisposition, multiple vaginal deliveries, delivery of large-for-gestational-age baby, forceps-assisted or breech delivery, obesity, changes in estrogen levels at climacteric, extensive abdominopelvic or pelvic surgery); intrinsic sphincter deficiency (multiple urethral suspensions in women, radical prostatectomy in men, uncommon complication of transurethral prostatectomy or cryosurgery of prostate, spinal lesion affecting sacral segments 2 to 4 or cauda equina, pelvic fracture)

NOC Outcomes (Nursing Outcomes Classification)

Suggested NOC Labels

Urinary Continence; Urinary Elimination

> **Example NOC Outcome**
>
> Accomplishes **Urinary Continence** as evidenced by the following indicators: No urine leakage with increased abdominal pressure (e.g., sneezing, laughing, lifting)/ Voids in appropriate receptacle/Adequate time to reach toilet between urge and evacuation of urine/Underclothing dry during day/Underclothing or bedding dry during night (Rate each indicator of **Urinary Continence:** 1 = never demonstrated, 2 = rarely demonstrated, 3 = sometimes demonstrated, 4 = often demonstrated, 5 = consistently demonstrated [see Section I])

Client Outcomes

- Reports relief from stress urinary incontinence, or reports a decrease in the incidence or severity of incontinent episodes
- Reduction in grams of urine loss measured objectively by a pad test
- Identifies containment devices that assist in the management of stress urinary incontinence

NIC Interventions (Nursing Interventions Classification)

Suggested NIC Labels

Urinary Incontinence Care; Pelvic Muscle Exercise

> **Example NIC Interventions—Urinary Incontinence Care**
> - Explain etiology of problem and rationale for actions
> - Modify clothing and environment to provide easy access to toilet

Nursing Interventions and Rationales

- Complete a history of urine loss including duration, severity, and frequency of symptoms; precipitating factors; and current management presence of symptoms of urge urinary incontinence.
  A history of stress urinary incontinence helps determine the likely cause of leakage and best treatment options.
- ▲ Perform a focused physical assessment, including perineal skin assessment, evaluation of the vaginal mucosa, reproduction of the sign of stress urinary incontinence, and observation of urethral hypermobility and related pelvic descent (prolapse).
  The physical evaluation provides information about the severity of urine loss and objective evidence of the condition and determines the presence of urethral hypermobility (Gray, Rayome, Moore, 1995).

- = Independent; ▲ = Collaborative

- Determine the client's current use of containment devices. Evaluate selection for ability to adequately contain urine loss, protect clothing, and control odor. Help client to identify containment devices designed to contain urinary leakage.
  Clients, particularly women, may select feminine hygiene pads for urine containment. These devices, designed to contain menstrual flow, are not well suited for containing urine loss (McClish et al, 1999).
- ▲ Review treatment options—including behavioral management; drug therapy; use of a pessary, vaginal device or urethral insert; and surgery—with the client and in close consultation with the physician, outlining the potential benefits, efficacy, and side effects of each treatment option.
  Multiple treatments have been used to manage stress urinary incontinence; behavioral management options should be offered initially (Urinary Incontinence Guideline Panel, 1996).
- Assess for signs of urge urinary incontinence (refer to care plan for **Urge urinary Incontinence**) and discuss the impact of this coexisting condition with the client suspected of having mixed urge and stress urinary leakage.
  Urge and stress urinary incontinence often coexist (Thom, 1998), and many options offered for stress urinary incontinence also have a beneficial effect on the frequency and severity of urge urinary incontinence (Urinary Incontinence Guideline Panel, 1996).
- Assess the client's pelvic muscle strength using pressure manometry, a digital evaluation technique, or a urine stop test.
  A baseline of pelvic muscle strength is needed for initial assessment and for evaluation of treatment efficacy (Brink et al, 1989, 1992; Sampselle, DeLancey, 1992; Worth, Dougherty, McKey, 1986).
- Begin a pelvic floor muscle rehabilitation program.
  Pelvic floor muscle rehabilitation is effective in the treatment of stress and mixed urinary incontinence (Hay-Smith, Bo, Berghmans, 2000; Bo, Talseth, Holme, 1999).
- Using biofeedback techniques, teach the patient undergoing pelvic muscle rehabilitation to identify, contract, and relax the periurethral muscles without contracting distant muscle groups (such as the abdominal muscles).
  Pelvic muscle rehabilitation is enhanced by the use of biofeedback (Berghmans et al, 1996; Bump et al, 1991).
- Incorporate principles of physiotherapy in a pelvic muscle exercise program, including the following:
  - A graded program beginning with 5 to 10 repetitions and advancing gradually to 35 to 50 repetitions every day or every other day
  - Sustained exercise sessions over a period of 3 to 6 months
  - Integration of the exercise program into activities of daily living (ADLs)
  - Repeated evaluations (no more than weekly) to encourage continued compliance with the muscle rehabilitation program, evaluate increases in pelvic muscle strength, and assess alleviation of stress urinary incontinence
  Pelvic muscle rehabilitation alleviates or cures stress urinary incontinence by a combination of factors, including biofeedback and strength training. The application of principles of physiotherapy maximize the value of the exercise program (Dougherty et al, 1992; Brink et al, 1992; Nygaard et al, 1996).
- Teach the patient to reeducate the pelvic muscles using weighted vaginal cones.
  Weighted vaginal cones have been shown to alleviate stress urinary incontinence (Fischer, Baessler, Linde, 1996; Kondo, Yamada, Niijima, 1995).

• = Independent; ▲ = Collaborative

▲ Begin transvaginal or transrectal electrical stimulation therapy with selected clients with stress urinary incontinence in consultation with the client and physician.
Electrical stimulation alleviates stress urinary incontinence, probably by strengthening the pelvic muscles and possibly via a biofeedback effect (Sand et al, 1995).

▲ Teach the patient to self-administer alpha-adrenergic medications, imipramine, and topical or oral estrogens as directed.
Pharmacotherapeutic agents alleviate or temporarily cure stress urinary incontinence in selected women (Radley et al, 2000; Gray, 1996).

▲ Refer the female client who wishes to employ a pessary, vaginal device, or urethral insert to manage stress urinary incontinence to a nurse specialist or gynecologist with expertise in the placement and maintenance of these devices.
Pessaries, vaginal devices, and urethral insert devices can alleviate or correct stress urinary incontinence; however, they may cause serious complications unless applied correctly and monitored closely (Frazer et al, 2000; Vierhout, Lose, 1997).

• Discuss potentially reversible or controllable risk factors with the client with stress urinary incontinence and assist him or her to formulate a strategy to alleviate or eliminate these conditions.
Although research supports a strong familial predisposition to stress urinary incontinence among women, other risk factors associated with the condition, including obesity and chronic coughing from smoking, are reversible (Skoner, Thompson, Caron, 1994; Mushkat, Bukovsky, Langer, 1996).

▲ Provide information about support groups such as the SIMON foundation or National Foundation for Continence.

▲ Refer the client with persistent stress urinary incontinence to a continence service, physician, or nurse who specializes in the management of this condition.
Complex stress urinary incontinence is best managed by a multidisciplinary approach (McDowell et al, 1992).

Geriatric

• Evaluate the elderly client's functional and cognitive status to determine the impact functional limitations exert on the frequency and severity of urine loss and plans for management.

Home Care Interventions

▲ Consider use of an indwelling catheter for continuous drainage in the client with severe stress urinary incontinence who is homebound, bed-bound, and receiving palliative or end of life care (requires physician order).
An indwelling catheter may increase patient comfort, ease caregiver burden, and prevent urinary incontinence in bed-bound patients receiving end of life care.

▲ When an indwelling catheter is in place, follow prescribed maintenance protocols for managing the catheter, drainage bag, and perineal skin and urethral meatus. Teach infection control measures adapted to the home care setting.
Proper care reduces the risk of catheter-associated urinary tract infection (UTI).

Client/Family Teaching

• Teach the client to perform pelvic muscle exercises using an audiotape or videotape if indicated.

• Teach the client the importance of avoiding dehydration and to consume 30 ml/kg of body weight daily.

• = **Independent**; ▲ = **Collaborative**

- Teach the client the importance of avoiding constipation by a combination of adequate fluid intake, dietary fiber, and exercise.
- Teach the client to apply and remove support devices such as the bladder neck support prosthesis.
- Teach the client to select and apply urine containment devices.

WEB SITES FOR EDUCATION

MERLIN See the MERLIN web site for World Wide Web resources for client education.

REFERENCES Berghmans LCM et al: Efficacy of biofeedback when included with pelvic muscle exercise treatment for stress urinary incontinence, *Neurourol Urodyn* 15:37-52, 1996.

Bo K, Talseth T, Holme I: Single blind, randomized controlled trial or pelvic floor exercises, electrical stimulation, vaginal cones, and no treatment of genuine stress urinary incontinence in women, *Br Med J* 318: 487-493, 1999.

Brink CA et al: A digital test for pelvic muscle strength in older women with urinary incontinence, *Nurs Res* 38:196-199, 1989.

Brink CA et al: Pelvic muscle exercise for elderly incontinence women. In Funk SG et al: *Key aspects of elder care: managing falls, incontinence and cognitive impairment,* New York, 1992, Springer.

Bump RC et al: Assessment of Kegel pelvic muscle exercise performance after brief verbal instruction, *Am J Obstet Gynecol* 165(2):322-327, 1991.

Dougherty MC et al: Variations in intravaginal pressure measurements, *Nurs Res* 40:282-285, 1991.

Dougherty MC et al: Graded exercise: effect of pressures developed by the pelvic muscles. In Funk SG et al: *Key aspects of elder care: managing falls, incontinence and cognitive impairment,* New York, 1992, Springer.

Fischer W, Baessler K, Linde A: Pelvic floor conditioning with vaginal weights—post partum and in urinary incontinence, *Zentrablatt fur Gynakologie* 118:18-28, 1996.

Frazer M et al: Mechanical devices for urinary incontinence in women, *Cochrane Database Syst Rev* 4, 2000.

Gray ML: *Urology nursing drug reference,* St Louis, 1996, Mosby.

Gray ML, Rayome RG, Moore KN: The urethral sphincter: an update, *Urol Nurs* 15:40-53, 1995.

Hay-Smith EJC, Bo K, Berghmans LCM: Pelvic floor muscle training for urinary incontinence in women, *Cochrane Database Syst Rev* 4, 2000.

Kondo A, Yamada Y, Niijima R: Treatment of stress incontinence by vaginal cones: short- and long-term results and predictive parameters, *Br J Urol* 76:464-466, 1995.

McClish DK et al: Use and costs of incontinence pads in female study volunteers, *J Wound Ostomy Contin Nurs* 26:207-208, 210-213, 1999.

McDowell B et al: An interdisciplinary approach to the assessment and behavioral treatment of urinary incontinence in geriatric outpatients, *J Am Geriatr Soc* 40:370, 1992.

Mushkat Y, Bukovsky I, Langer R: Female urinary stress incontinence—does it have familial prevalence? *Am J Obstet Gynecol* 174:617-619, 1996.

Nygaard IE et al: Efficacy of pelvic floor muscle exercise in women with stress, urge and mixed urinary incontinence, *Am J Obst Gynecol* 174:120-125, 1996.

Radley SC et al: Alpha adrenergic drugs for urinary incontinence in women, *Cochrane Database Syst Rev* 4, 2000.

Sampselle CM, DeLancey JOL: The urine stream interruption test and pelvic muscle function, *Nurs Res* 41:73-77, 1992.

Sand PK et al: Pelvic floor electrical stimulation in the treatment of genuine stress incontinence: a multicenter placebo controlled trial, *Am J Obstet Gynecol* 173:72-79, 1995.

Skoner MM, Thompson WD, Caron VA: Factors associated with risk of stress urinary incontinence in women, *Nurs Res* 43:301-306, 1994.

Thom D: Variation in estimates of urinary incontinence prevalence in the community: effects of differences in definition, population characteristics, and study type, *J Am Geriatr Soc* 46:473-480, 1998.

Urinary Incontinence Guideline Panel: *Urinary incontinence in adults: clinical practice guideline,* ed 2, Rockville, Md, Agency for Health Care Policy and Research, 1996.

Vierhout ME, Lose G: Preventive vaginal and intra-urethral devices in the treatment of female urinary stress incontinence, *Curr Opin Obstet Gynecol* 9(5):325-328, 1997.

• = Independent; ▲ = Collaborative

Worth AM, Dougherty MC, McKey PL: Development and testing of the circumvaginal muscle (CVM) rating scale, *Nurs Res* 35:166-168, 1986.

Total urinary Incontinence

Mikel Gray

NANDA   **Definition** Continuous and unpredictable loss of urine.
NOTE: In this book, the diagnosis total urinary incontinence will be used to refer to continuous urine loss from an extraurethral loss, and stress urinary incontinence will be used to refer to leakage from sphincter incompetence, regardless of severity.

Defining Characteristics
Continuous urine flow varying from dribbling incontinence superimposed upon an otherwise identifiable pattern of voiding to severe urine loss without identifiable micturition episodes

Related Factors (r/t)
Ectopia (ectopic ureter opens into the vaginal vault or cutaneously; bladder ectopia with exstrophy/epispadias complex); fistula (opening from bladder or urethra to vagina or skin that bypasses urethral sphincter mechanism, allowing continuous urine loss)

NOC   **Outcomes (Nursing Outcomes Classification)**
Suggested NOC Labels
Tissue Integrity: Skin and Mucous Membranes; Urinary Continence; Urinary Elimination

> **Example NOC Outcome**
> Maintains **Tissue Integrity: Skin and Mucous Membranes** as evidenced by the following indicators: Tissue lesion free/Skin intactness (Rate each indicator of **Tissue Integrity: Skin and Mucous Membranes:** 1 = extremely compromised, 2 = substantially compromised, 3 = moderately compromised, 4 = mildly compromised, 5 = not compromised [see Section I])

Client Outcomes
- Urine loss is adequately contained, clothing remains unsoiled, and odor is controlled
- Maintains intact perineal skin
- Maintains dignity, hides urine containment device in clothing, and minimizes bulk and noise related to the device

NIC   **Interventions (Nursing Interventions Classification)**
Suggested NIC Labels
Urinary Incontinence Care

> **Example NIC Interventions—Urinary Incontinence Care**
> - Provide proctective garments as needed
> - Cleanse genital skin area at regular intervals

• = Independent; ▲ = Collaborative

Nursing Interventions and Rationales

- Obtain a history of duration and severity of urine loss, previous method of management, and aggravating or alleviating features.

  The symptom of continuous incontinence may be caused by extraurethral leakage or other types of incontinence that have been inadequately evaluated and/or managed. The patient history will provide clues to the etiology of the urinary leakage (Gray, Haas, 2000).

- Perform a focused physical assessment, including inspection of the perineal skin, examination of the vaginal vault, reproduction of the sign of stress urinary incontinence (refer to care plan for **Stress urinary Incontinence**), and testing of bulbocavernosus reflex and perineal sensations.

  The physical examination will provide evidence supporting the diagnosis of extraurethral or another type of incontinence (stress, urge, or reflex), providing the basis for further evaluation and/or treatment (Gray, Haas, 2000).

- Complete a bladder log of urine elimination patterns and frequency and severity of urine loss.

  The bladder log provides further information, allowing the nurse to differentiate extraurethral from other forms of urine loss and providing the basis for further evaluation and treatment (Gray, Haas, 2000).

- Assist the patient to select and apply a urine containment device or devices. Review types of containment products with the patient, including advantages and potential complications associated with each type of product.

  Urine containment products include a variety of absorptive pads, incontinent briefs, underpads for bedding, absorptive inserts that fit into specially designed undergarments, and condom catheters. Careful selection of a containment product and education concerning its use maximizes its effectiveness in controlling urine loss for a particular individual (Shirran, Brazelli, 2000; McKibben, 1995).

- Evaluate disposable vs. reusable products for urine containment, considering factors of setting (home care vs. acute care vs. long-term care), preferences of the patient and caregiver(s), and immediate vs. long-term costs.

  The impact of routine use of urine containment devices is significant, regardless of the setting. Economic factors, as well as patient and caregiver preferences, have an impact on the success and ultimate cost of a reusable vs. disposable urine containment device (Shirran, Brazelli, 2000; Hu, Kaltreider, Igou, 1990; Cummings et al, 1995).

- Cleanse the skin with an incontinence cleansing product system or plain water when changing urinary containment devices or pads. Use soap and water on the perineum no more than once daily or every other day as necessary.

  Excessive cleansing of the perineal skin may exacerbate alterations in skin integrity, particularly among the elderly (Byers et al, 1995; Lindell, Olsson, 1990).

- Apply a skin moisturizer following cleansing.

  Moisturizers promote comfort and may reduce the risk of skin breakdown (Kemp, 1994).

- Apply a protective barrier or ointment to the perineal skin when incontinence is severe, when double fecal and urinary incontinence exist, or when the risk of a pressure ulcer is considered significant.

  A moisture barrier is indicated when the risk of altered skin integrity is complicated by coexisting factors of shear, fecal incontinence, or exposure to prolonged pressure (Fiers, Thayer, 2000; Kemp, 1994).

• = **Independent;** ▲ = **Collaborative**

▲ Consult the physician concerning use of an antifungal powder or ointment when perineal dermatitis is complicated by monilial infection. Teach the patient to use the product sparingly when applying to affected areas.

Antifungal powders or ointments provide effective relief from monilial rash; however, application of excessive amounts of the product retain moisture and diminish its effectiveness (Fiers, Thayer, 2000).

▲ Consult the physician concerning placement of an indwelling catheter when severe urine loss is complicated by urinary retention, when careful fluid monitoring is indicated, when perineal dryness is required to promote the healing of a stage 3 or 4 pressure ulcer, during periods of critical illness, or in the terminally ill client when use of absorbent products produces pain or distress.

Although not routinely indicated, the indwelling catheter provides an effective, transient management technique for carefully selected patients (Urinary Incontinence Guideline Panel, 1996; Treatment of Pressure Ulcers Guideline Panel, 1994).

▲ Refer the client with "intractable" or extraurethral incontinence to a continence service or specialist for further evaluation and management of urine loss.

The successful management of complex, severe urinary incontinence requires specialized evaluation and treatment from a health care provider with special expertise (Doughty, 1991; Gray, 1992).

Geriatric

• Provide privacy and support when changing incontinent device of elderly client.

Elderly, hospitalized clients frequently express feelings of shame, guilt, and dependency when undergoing urinary containment device changes (Biggerson et al, 1993).

• Employ meticulous infection control procedures when using an indwelling catheter.

Home Care Interventions

NOTE: The interventions identified are all applicable to the home care setting. Review the interventions for appropriateness to individual clients.

Client/Family Teaching

• Teach the family to obtain, apply, and dispose of or clean and reuse urine containment devices.

• Teach the family a routine perineal skin care regimen, including daily or every other day hygiene and cleansing with containment product changes.

• Teach the client and family to recognize and manage perineal dermatitis, ammonia contact dermatitis, and monilial rash.

• Teach the patient to maintain adequate fluid intake (30 ml/kg of body weight/day).

• Teach the client and family to recognize and manage urinary infection.

WEB SITES FOR EDUCATION

MERLIN   See the MERLIN web site for World Wide Web resources for client education.

REFERENCES   Biggersson AB et al: Elderly women's feelings about being incontinent, using napkins and being helped by nurses to change napkins, *J Clin Nurs* 2:165-171, 1993.

Byers PH et al: Effects of continence care cleansing regimens on skin integrity, *J Wound Ostomy Continence Nurs* 22:187-192, 1995.

Cummings V et al: Costs and management of urinary incontinence in long-term care, *J Wound Ostomy Continence Nurs* 22:193-198, 1995.

Doughty DB, editor: *Urinary and fecal incontinence: nursing management,* St Louis, 1991, Mosby.

• = **Independent**; ▲ = **Collaborative**

Fiers S, Thayer D: Management of intractable incontinence. In Doughty DB, editor: *Urinary and fecal incontinence: nursing management,* St Louis, 2000, Mosby, pp 183-207.

Gray ML: *Genitourinary disorders,* St Louis, 1992, Mosby.

Gray M, Haas J: Assessment of the patient with urinary incontinence. In Doughty DB, editor: *Urinary and fecal incontinence: nursing management,* St Louis, 2000, Mosby, pp 209-284.

Hu T, Kaltreider DL, Igou J: The cost-effectiveness of disposable vs. reusable diapers: a controlled experiment in a nursing home, *J Gerontol Nurs* 16:19-24, 36-37, 1990.

Kemp MG: Protecting the skin from moisture and associated irritants, *J Gerontol Nurs* 20:8-14, 1994.

Lindell ME, Olsson HM: Personal hygiene in external genitalia of health and hospitalized elderly women, *Health Care Women Int* 11:151-158, 1990.

McKibben E: Pad use in perspective, *Nurs Times* 91:60, 62, 1995.

Shirran E, Brazelli M: Absorbent products for the containment of urinary and/or fecal incontinence, *Cochrane Database Syst Rev* CD0011406, 2000.

Treatment of Pressure Ulcers Guideline Panel: *Treatment of pressure ulcer: clinical practice guideline,* Rockville, Md, 1994, Agency for Health Care Policy and Research.

Urinary Incontinence Guideline Panel: *Urinary incontinence in adults: clinical practice guideline,* ed 2, Rockville, Md, 1996, Agency for Health Care Policy and Research.

Urge urinary Incontinence

Mikel Gray

NANDA   **Definition** Involuntary passage of urine occurring soon after a strong sense of urgency to void

Defining Characteristics:

Diurnal urinary frequency (voids more often than every 2 hours while awake); urgency (subjective report of a precipitous or immediate need to urinate when urgency is perceived); nocturia (awakens more than once per night to urinate for persons <65 years of age; awakens more than twice per night if >65 years of age); symptom of urge urinary incontinence (urine loss associated with desire to urinate); enuresis (involuntary passage of urine while asleep); inability to reach toilet in time

Related Factors (r/t)

Inflammation of the bladder (calculi, tumor including transitional cell carcinomas and carcinoma in situ, inflammatory lesions of the bladder, urinary tract infection [UTI]); bladder outlet obstruction (see **Urinary retention**); stress urinary incontinence (mixed urinary incontinence; these conditions often coexist but relationship between them remains unclear); neurological disorders (disorders of the brain including cerebrovascular accident [CVA], brain tumor, normal pressure hydrocephalus, traumatic brain injury); idiopathic causes (implicated factors includes depression, sleep apnea/hypoxia)

NOC   **Outcomes (Nursing Outcomes Classification)**

Suggested NOC Labels

Urinary Continence, Urinary Elimination; Tissue Integrity: Skin and Mucous Membranes

• = Independent; ▲ = Collaborative

Example NOC Outcome
Accomplishes **Urinary Continence** as evidenced by the following indicators: Responds in timely manner to urge/Voids in appropriate receptacle/Adequate time to reach toilet between urge and evacuation of urine/Underclothing dry during day/Underclothing or bedding dry during night (Rate each indicator of **Urinary Continence:** 1 = never demonstrated, 2 = rarely demonstrated, 3 = sometimes demonstrated, 4 = often demonstrated, 5 = consistently demonstrated [see Section I])

Client Outcomes

- Reports relief from urge urinary incontinence or a decrease in the incidence or severity of incontinent episodes
- Identifies containment devices that assist in the management of urge urinary incontinence

 Interventions (Nursing Interventions Classification)

Suggested NIC Labels
Urinary Habit Training; Urinary Incontinence Care

Example NIC Interventions—Urinary Habit Training
- Keep a continence specification record for 3 days to establish voiding pattern
- Establish interval for toileting of preferably not <2 hours

Nursing Interventions and Rationales

- Perform a nursing history focusing on duration of urinary incontinence, diurnal frequency, nocturia, severity of symptoms, and alleviating and aggravating factors.
  A focused history helps determine the cause of urinary incontinence and guides its subsequent management.
- ▲ Complete a urinalysis, looking for the presence of nitrites, leukocytes, glucose, or hemoglobin (red blood cells).
  The presence of nitrites and leukocytes raise the suspicion of UTI, the presence of glucosuria raises the risk of undiagnosed or poorly controlled diabetes mellitus, and the presence of red blood cells in the absence of signs of infection raises a suspicion of a bladder tumor. Each condition may produce acute urinary incontinence requiring treatment of the underlying cause (Urinary Incontinence Guideline Panel, 1996).
- Complete a bladder log, including frequency of diurnal micturition and nocturia, patterns of incontinence, symptoms of accompanying urine loss, and the type and volume of fluids consumed.
  A bladder log provides a more objective record of diurnal urinary frequency, nocturia, and patterns of urgency and urge urinary incontinence when compared with a history (Resnick et al, 1994). Recording fluid consumption allows an evaluation of the volume of fluid consumed throughout a 24-hour period and the intake of bladder irritants.
- ▲ Review all medications the client is receiving, paying particular attention to sedatives, narcotics, diuretics, antidepressants, psychotropic drugs, or cholinergics. Consult physician concerning altering or eliminating these medications if they are suspected of affecting incontinence.
  The side effects of multiple medications may produce or exacerbate urge urinary incontinence (Urinary Incontinence Guideline Panel, 1996).

• = **Independent;** ▲ = **Collaborative**

- Assess the client for urinary retention (see care plan for **Urinary retention**).
  Urinary retention associated with bladder outlet obstruction may be a contributing cause of urge urinary incontinence (Rosier et al, 1995). Urinary retention, associated with poor detrusor contraction strength, has been described in frail, elderly clients (Resnick, Yalla, 1987). Regardless of its cause, retention significantly impacts the management of this condition (Gray, 2000).
- Assess the client for functional limitations (environmental barriers, limited mobility or dexterity, impaired cognitive function [see care plan for **Functional urinary Incontinence**]).
  Functional limitations impact the severity and management of urge urinary incontinence (Gray, 1992).
- ▲ Consult the physician concerning diabetic management and pharmacotherapy for UTI when indicated.
  In specific cases, urgency and an increased risk of urge urinary incontinence may be related to UTI (Molander et al, 2000) or polyuria from undiagnosed or poorly managed diabetes mellitus (Samsioe et al, 1999).
- ▲ Assess for signs and symptoms of atrophic vaginal changes in the perimenopausal or postmenopausal woman, including vaginal dryness, tenderness to touch, dryness of mucosa on touch with friability and discomfort with gentle palpation. Specifically query the woman with atrophic vaginitis concerning irritative lower urinary tract symptoms (diurnal frequency, nocturia episodes >2 per night, urgency, dysuria). Refer the woman with atrophic vaginal changes and bothersome lower urinary tract symptoms to a gynecologist, urologist, or women's health nurse practitioner for further evaluation and management.
  The relationship between atrophic vaginitis and urge urinary incontinence risk remains unclear. However, several studies have observed a relationship between systemic estrogen replacement and urinary incontinence (Molander et al, 2000; Brown et al, 1999). Nevertheless, the nature of this relationship remains unknown, and additional evidence suggests that local hormone replacement therapy may reduce irritative lower urinary tract symptoms and the risk of UTI (Eriksen, 1999).
- Establish bladder training (also called habit training or bladder retraining program) based on data gathered from the bladder log, physical assessment, and functional assessment.
  Bladder retraining has been shown effective in the management of urge, mixed stress, and urge urinary incontinence (Fantl et al, 1991; Wyman, Fantl, McClish, 1998).
- With the client, review the types of beverages consumed, focusing on the intake of bladder irritants including caffeine and alcohol.
  Caffeine increases urgency by a direct effect on detrusor smooth muscle (Lee, Wein, Levin, 1993; Creighton, Stanton, 1990), and alcohol acts as a bladder irritant via its sedative effect and its inhibitory effect on antidiuretic hormone secretion (Sinclair, Lambrecht, Smith 1990; Denays et al, 1994). A growing body of evidence supports limitation of caffeine as an effective means of reducing voiding frequency (Gray, 2001).
- With the client, review the volume of fluids consumed and gradually adjust the fluid intake to meet the Recommended Daily Allowance of 30 ml/kg of body weight/day (National Academy of Sciences, Food and Nutrition Board, 1980).
  Dehydration exacerbates symptoms of urgency, and excessive fluid intake increases the risk of urinary leakage. Increasing fluid intake in women with urinary incontinence may reduce the risk of UTI and slightly reduce the frequency of urine loss (Pearson, 1992; Pearson, 1993; Dougherty, 1999).

- = **Independent**; ▲ = **Collaborative**

- Teach techniques of urge suppression, including repeated, rapid contractions of the pelvic muscles and distraction techniques such as deep breathing or counting backward from 100 by factors of 7.
  Biofeedback techniques are effective in the management of urge urinary incontinence (Burgio, Engel et al, 1998; Wyman, Fantl, McClish, 1998).
- Begin transvaginal or transrectal electrical stimulation using a low Hertz frequency current (5 to 20 Hz) in consultation with the physician.
  Electrical stimulation is an effective treatment for urge urinary incontinence. In one randomized clinical trial, electrical stimulation was found to completely eliminate symptoms of urge urinary incontinence in 49% of a group of 121 subjects (Brubaker et al, 1997; Moore, Gray, Rayome, 1995).
- ▲ Teach the client to self-administer antispasmodic (anticholinergic) drugs as directed. Assist the client with determining and implementing a timed voiding schedule while taking these medications.
  The effectiveness of antispasmodic medications is enhanced when the patient voids on a timed schedule (before the occurrence of hyperactive detrusor contractions) (Gray, 1992, 1996).
- Assist the client to select, obtain, and apply a containment device for urine loss as indicated (see **Total urinary Incontinence**).
- ▲ Provide the client with information about incontinence support groups such as the National Association for Continence and the SIMON foundation.

Geriatric

- Assess functional and cognitive status of all elderly patients with urge urinary incontinence.
- ▲ Plan care in long-term or acute care facilities based on knowledge of the elderly client's established voiding patterns, paying particular attention to patterns of nocturia.
- ▲ Carefully monitor the elderly client for potential adverse effects of antispasmodic medications, including a severely dry mouth interfering with dentures, eating, or speaking; confusion; nightmares; constipation; mydriasis; or heat intolerance.
  Elderly persons are particularly susceptible to adverse effects associated with antispasmodic medications (Ghoneim, Hassouna, 1997).

Home Care Interventions

- Teach client and family to recognize foods and beverages that are likely to irritate the bladder.
- Teach the importance of avoiding dehydration or excessive fluid consumption and the paradoxical relationship between dehydration and symptoms of urgency.
- Teach the family and client to recognize and manage side effects of antispasmodic medications used to manage urge urinary incontinence.
- Teach family and client to identify and correct environmental barriers to toileting within the home.

WEB SITES FOR EDUCATION

Merlin   See the MERLIN web site for World Wide Web resources for client education.

REFERENCES   Brown JS et al: Prevalence of urinary incontinence and associated risk factors in postmenopausal women, *Obstet Gynecol* 94:66-70, 1999.
Brubaker L et al: Transvaginal electrical stimulation for female urinary incontinence, *Am J Obstet Gynecol* 177(3):536-540, 1997.

• = **Independent**; ▲ = **Collaborative**

Burgio KL et al: Behavioral vs drug treatment for urge urinary incontinence in older women: a randomized controlled trial, *JAMA* 280:1995-2000, 1998.

Creighton SM, Stanton SL: Caffeine: does it affect your bladder? *Br J Urol* 66:613-614, 1990.

Denays R et al: Bilateral cerebral mediofrontal hypoactivity in Tc-99m HMPAO SPECT imaging, *Clin Nucl Med* 19:873-876, 1994.

Dougherty MC: *Establishing goals and lifestyle management,* WOCN Continence Conference, Austin, Tex, Feb 1999.

Eriksen B: A randomized, open, parallel group study on the preventive effect of an estradiol-releasing vaginal ring (Estring) on recurrent urinary tract infections in postmenopausal women, *Am J Obstet Gynecol* 180:1072-1079, 1999.

Fantl JA et al: Efficacy of bladder training in older women with urinary incontinence, *JAMA* 265:609, 1991.

Ghoneim GM, Hassouna M: Alternatives for the pharmacologic management of urge and stress urinary incontinence in the elderly, *J Wound Ostomy Continence Nurs* 24:311-318, 1997.

Gray M: Urinary retention: management in the acute care setting, part 2, *Am J Nurs* 100:36-44, 2000.

Gray M: Caffeine and urinary continence, *J Wound Ostomy Continence Nurs* 28(2):66-69, 2001.

Gray ML: *Genitourinary disorders,* St Louis, 1992, Mosby.

Gray ML: *Urology nursing drug reference,* St Louis, 1996, Mosby.

Lee JG, Wein AJ, Levin RM: The effect of caffeine on the contractile response of the rabbit urinary bladder to field stimulation, *Gen Pharmacol* 24:1007-1011, 1993.

Molander U et al: A longitudinal cohort study of elderly women with urinary tract infection, *Maturitas* 34(2):127-131, 2000.

Moore KN, Gray ML, Rayome RG: Electric stimulation and urinary incontinence: research and alternatives, *Urol Nurs* 15(3):94-96, 1995.

National Academy of Sciences, Food and Nutrition Board: *Recommended daily allowances,* ed 9, Washington, DC, 1980, The Academy.

Pearson BD: Urine control by elders: noninvasive strategies. In Funk SG et al: *Key aspects of elder care: managing falls, incontinence and cognitive impairment,* New York, 1992, Springer.

Pearson BD: Liquidate a myth: reducing liquids is not advisable for elderly with urine control problems, *Urol Nurs* 13:86, 1993.

Resnick NM, Yalla SV: Detrusor hyperactivity with impaired contractile function: an unrecognized but common cause of incontinence in elderly patients, *JAMA* 257:3076-3081, 1987.

Resnick NM et al: Short term variability of self report of incontinence in older persons, *J Am Geriatr Soc* 42:202, 1994.

Rosier PF et al: Is detrusor instability in males related to the grade of obstruction? *Neurourol Urodyn* 14(6):625-633, 1995.

Samsioe G et al: Urogenital symptoms in women aged 50-59 years, *Gynecol Endocrinol* 13:113-117, 1999.

Sinclair J, Lambrecht L, Smith ET: Hepatic alcoholic dehydrogenase activity in chick hepatocytes towards the major alcohols present in commercial alcoholic beverages: comparison with activities in rat and human liver, *Comp Biochem Physiol B* 96(4):677-682, 1990.

Urinary Incontinence Guideline Panel: *Urinary incontinence in adults: clinical practice guideline,* ed 2, Rockville, Md, 1996, Agency for Health Care Policy and Research.

Wyman JF, Fantl JA, McClish DK: Comparative efficacy of behavioral interventions in the management of female urinary incontinence: continence program for women research group, *Am J Obstet Gynecol* 179:999-1007, 1998.

Risk for urge urinary Incontinence

Mikel Gray

NANDA **Definition** At risk for involuntary loss of urine associated with a sudden, strong sensation or urinary urgency

• = **Independent;** ▲ = **Collaborative**

Risk Factors

Effects of medications or bladder irritants including caffeine, alcohol, or aspartame; urinary tract infection (UTI); urethritis; tumors; lower ureteral or bladder calculi; detrusor muscle instability (overactive bladder)

NOC   ## Outcomes (Nursing Outcomes Classification)

Suggested NOC Labels

Urinary Continence; Urinary Elimination

> **Example NOC Outcome**
>
> Accomplishes **Urinary Continence** as evidenced by the following indicators: Responds in timely manner to urge/Voids in appropriate receptacle/Adequate time to reach toilet between urge and evacuation of urine/Underclothing dry during day/Underclothing or bedding dry during night (Rate each indicator of **Urinary Continence:** 1 = never demonstrated, 2 = rarely demonstrated, 3 = sometimes demonstrated, 4 = often demonstrated, 5 = consistently demonstrated [see Section I])

Client Outcomes

- Identifies risk factors for urge urinary incontinence
- Alters diet to minimize bladder irritants including alcohol, caffeine, and aspartame
- Describes and demonstrates mastery (by return demonstration) of urge suppression techniques

NIC   ## Interventions (Nursing Interventions Classification)

Suggested NIC Labels

Urinary Habit Training; Urinary Elimination Care

> **Example NIC Interventions—Urinary Habit Training**
> - Keep a continence specification record for 3 days to establish voiding pattern
> - Establish interval for toileting of preferably not <2 hours

Nursing Interventions and Rationales

- Perform a nursing history focusing on patterns of urine elimination, diurnal frequency, nocturia, urgency symptoms, alleviating and aggravating factors and a review of systems including neurological, gastrointestinal and reproductive systems as well as medical conditions including diabetes mellitus.
  A focused history and review of systems helps determine risk factors for urge urinary incontinence (Gray, 2000).
- ▲ Complete a urinalysis focusing on the presence of nitrites, leukocytes, glucose, or hemoglobin (red blood cells).
  The presence of nitrites and leukocytes raise the suspicion of UTI, the presence of glucosuria raises the risk of undiagnosed or poorly controlled diabetes mellitus, and the presence of red blood cells in the absence of signs of infection raises a suspicion of a bladder tumor. Each condition increases the risk of urgency symptoms and urge urinary incontinence (Urinary Incontinence Guideline Panel, 1996).
- Complete a bladder log, including frequency of diurnal micturition and nocturia, and the type and volume of fluids consumed.
  A bladder log provides a more objective record of diurnal urinary frequency, nocturia, and patterns of urgency when compared with a history (Resnick et al, 1994). Recording fluid

• = **Independent;** ▲ = **Collaborative**

consumption allows an evaluation of the volume of fluid consumed over a 24-hour period and the intake of bladder irritants.

- Review the types of beverages consumed with the client, focusing on the intake of bladder irritants, including caffeine and alcohol. Advise the client to reduce or eliminate intake of these substances to determine their effect on voiding frequency and symptoms of urgency.
Caffeine increases urgency by having a direct effect on detrusor smooth muscle (Lee, Wein, Levin, 1993; Creighton, Stanton, 1990), and alcohol acts as a bladder irritant via its sedative effect and its inhibitory effect on antidiuretic hormone secretion (Sinclair, Lambrecht, Smith 1990; Denays et al, 1994). A growing body of evidence supports limitation of caffeine as an effective means of reducing voiding frequency (Gray, 2001).

- Additional bladder irritants, including aspartame, carbonated drinks, decaffeinated coffee or tea, citrus juices, highly spiced foods, chocolates, or vinegar-containing foods may be eliminated from the diet and added back in singly to determine their impact on bothersome lower urinary tract symptoms and urgency.
Limited evidence supports the role of these substances as potential bladder irritants in clients at risk for urge urinary incontinence, but they do play a more significant role for those with interstitial cystitis (Bade, Peeters, Mensink, 1997; Interstitial Cystitis Association, 1999).

- With the client, review the volume of fluids consumed and gradually adjust the fluid intake to meet the Recommended Daily Allowance of approximately 30 ml/kg of body weight/day in the ambulatory adult (National Academy of Sciences, Food and Nutrition Board, 1980).
Dehydration exacerbates symptoms of urgency, and excessive fluid intake increases the risk of urgency and urinary leakage (Pearson, Larsen, 1992; Pearson, 1993; Dougherty, 1999).

▲ Review all medications the client is receiving, paying particular attention to sedatives, narcotics, diuretics, antidepressants, psychotropic drugs, and cholinergics. Consult physician concerning altering or eliminating these medications if they are suspected of affecting incontinence.
The side effects of multiple medications may produce or exacerbate urge urinary incontinence (Urinary Incontinence Guideline Panel, 1996).

- Assess the client for functional limitations—environmental barriers, limited mobility or dexterity, impaired cognitive function—and minimize these limitations as indicated (see care plan for **Functional urinary Incontinence**).
Functional limitations increase the time required for toileting and subsequent risk of urge urinary incontinence (Gray, 1992).

▲ Consult the physician concerning diabetic management and pharmacotherapy for UTI when indicated.
In specific cases, urgency and an increased risk of urge urinary incontinence may be related to UTI (Molander et al, 2000) or polyuria from undiagnosed or poorly managed diabetes mellitus (Samsioe et al, 1999).

▲ Assess for signs and symptoms of atrophic vaginal changes in the perimenopausal or postmenopausal woman, including vaginal dryness, tenderness to touch, dryness of mucosa on touch with friability and discomfort with gentle palpation. Specifically query the woman with atrophic vaginitis concerning irritative lower urinary tract symptoms (diurnal frequency, nocturia episodes >2 per night, urgency, dysuria). Refer the woman with atrophic vaginal changes and bothersome lower urinary tract

• = **Independent**; ▲ = **Collaborative**

symptoms to a gynecologist, urologist, or women's health nurse practitioner for
further evaluation and management.

*The relationship between atrophic vaginitis and urge urinary incontinence risk remains
unclear. However, several studies have observed a relationship between systemic estrogen
replacement and urinary incontinence (Molander et al, 2000; Brown et al, 1999). Nevertheless, the nature of this relationship remains unknown and additional evidence suggests
that local hormone replacement therapy may reduce irritative lower urinary tract symptoms and the risk of UTI (Eriksen, 1999).*

- Teach techniques of urge suppression including repeated, rapid contractions of the
  pelvic muscles and distraction techniques such as deep breathing or counting backward from 100 by factors of 7.
  *Urge suppression techniques reduce the risk of urine loss when a precipitous urge to urinate
  is experienced (Burgio et al, 1998; Wyman, Fantl, McClish, 1998).*

▲ Provide the client with information about incontinence support groups such as the
  National Association for Continence and the SIMON foundation.
  *These groups provide a variety of educational resources, including strategies for urinary
  incontinence prevention.*

Geriatric

- Assess functional and cognitive abilities of all elderly clients with irritative lower
  urinary tract symptoms or urge urinary incontinence.

▲ Advise men with bothersome lower urinary tract symptoms to see their physician or
  nurse practitioner because these symptoms may be related to prostate enlargement.

▲ Carefully monitor the elderly client for potential adverse effects of anticholinergic
  medications, including severe dry mouth interfering with dentures, eating or speaking
  or the occurrence of confusion, nightmares, constipation, mydriasis, or heat intolerance.
  *Elderly persons are particularly susceptible to adverse effects associated with anticholinergic
  medications (Ghoneim, Hassouna, 1997).*

Home Care Interventions

- Help the client and family to recognize and manage side effect of anticholinergic
  medications used to manage irritative lower urinary tract symptoms.
- Help the client and family to identify and correct environmental barriers to toileting
  within the home.

Client/Family Teaching

- Teach client and family to recognize foods and beverages that are likely to irritate
  the bladder.
- Teach the importance of avoiding dehydration or excessive fluid consumption and
  the paradoxical relationship between dehydration and symptoms of urgency.

WEB SITES FOR EDUCATION

MERLIN   See the MERLIN web site for World Wide Web resources for client education.

REFERENCES   Bade JJ, Peeters JM, Mensink HJ: Is the diet of patients with interstitial cystitis related to their disease? *Eur
Urol* 32:179-183, 1997.

Brown JS et al: Prevalence of urinary incontinence and associated risk factors in postmenopausal women,
Obstet Gynecol 94:66-70, 1999.

Burgio KL et al: Behavioral vs drug treatment for urge urinary incontinence in older women: a randomized
controlled trial, *JAMA* 280:1995-2000, 1998.

• = **Independent;** ▲ = **Collaborative**

Creighton SM, Stanton SL: Caffeine: does it affect your bladder? *Br J Urol* 66:613-614, 1990.

Denays R et al: Bilateral cerebral mediofrontal hypoactivity in Tc-99m HMPAO SPECT imaging, *Clin Nucl Med* 19:873-876, 1994.

Dougherty MC: Establishing goals and lifestyle management, WOCN Continence Conference, Austin Texas, Feb, 1999.

Eriksen B: A randomized, open, parallel group study on the preventive effect of an estradiol-releasing vaginal ring (Estring) on recurrent urinary tract infections in postmenopausal women, *Am J Obstet Gynecol* 180:1072-1079, 1999.

Ghoneim GM, Hassouna M: Alternatives for the pharmacologic manangement of urge and stress urinary incontinence in the elderly, *J Wound Ostomy Continence Nurs* 24(6):311-318, 1997.

Gray M: Urinary retention: management in the acute care setting, part 2, *Am J Nurs* 100:36-44, 2000.

Gray ML: *Genitourinary disorders,* St Louis, 1992, Mosby.

Gray ML: Evidence based report card: caffeine and urinary continence, *J Wound Ostomy Continence Nurs* 28(2):66-69, 2001.

Interstitial Cystitis Association: *Interstitial cystitis and diet,* Rockville, Md, 1999, The Association.

Lee JG, Wein AJ, Levin RM: The effect of caffeine on the contractile response of the rabbit urinary bladder to field stimulation, *Gen Pharmacol* 24:1007-1011, 1993.

Molander U et al: A longitudinal cohort study of elderly women with urinary tract infection, *Maturitas* 34(2):127-131, 2000.

National Academy of Sciences, Food and Nutrition Board: *Recommended daily allowances,* ed 9, Washington, DC, 1980, The Academy.

Pearson BD: Urine control by elders: noninvasive strategies. In Funk SG et al: *Key aspects of elder care: managing falls, incontinence and cognitive impairment,* New York, 1992, Springer.

Pearson BD: Liquidate a myth: reducing liquids is not advisable for elderly with urine control problems, *Urol Nurs* 13:86, 1993.

Resnick NM et al: Short term variability of self report of incontinence in older persons, *J Am Geriatr Soc* 42:202, 1994.

Samsioe G et al: Urogenital symptoms in women aged 50-59 years, *Gynecol Endocrinol* 13:113-117, 1999.

Sinclair J, Lambrecht L, Smith ET: Hepatic alcoholic dehydrogenase activity in chick hepatocytes towards the major alcohols present in commercial alcoholic beverages: comparison with activities in rat and human liver, *Comp Biochem Physiol B* 96:677-682, 1990.

Urinary Incontinence Guideline Panel: *Urinary incontinence in adults: clinical practice guideline,* ed 2, Rockville, Md, 1996, Agency for Health Care Policy and Research.

Wyman JF, Fantl JA, McClish DK: Comparative efficacy of behavioral interventions in the management of female urinary incontinence: continence program for women research group, *Am J Obstet Gynecol* 179:999-1007, 1998.

Disorganized Infant behavior

T. Heather Herdman and Mary A. Fuerst-DeWys

 Definition Disintegrated physiological and neurobehavioral responses to the environment

Defining Characteristics
Regulatory problems
Inability to inhibit startle; Irritability
State-organization system
Active awake (fussy, worried gaze); diffuse/unclear sleep, state-oscillation; quiet-awake (staring, gaze aversion); irritable or panicky crying
Attention-interaction system
Abnormal response to sensory stimuli (e.g., difficult to soothe, inability to sustain alert status)

• = Independent; ▲ = Collaborative

Motor system	Increased, decreased, or limp tone; finger splay, fisting, or hands to face; hyperextension of arms and legs; tremors, startles, twitches; jittery, jerky, uncoordinated movement; altered primitive reflexes
Physiological	Bradycardia, tachycardia, or arrhythmias; pale, cyanotic, mottled, or flushed color; "time-out signals" (e.g., gaze, grasp, hiccough, cough, sneeze, sigh, slack jaw, open mouth, tongue thrust); oximeter reading: desaturation; feeding intolerances (aspiration or emesis)

Related Factors (r/t)

Prenatal	Congenital or genetic disorders; teratogenic exposure
Postnatal	Malnutrition; oral/motor problems; pain; feeding intolerance; invasive/painful procedures; prematurity
Individual	Illness; immature neurological system, gestational age; postconceptual age
Environmental	Physical environment inappropriateness; sensory inappropriateness; sensory overstimulation; sensory deprivation
Caregiver	Cue misreading; cue-deficient knowledge; environmental stimulation contribution

NOC Outcomes (Nursing Outcomes Classification)

Suggested NOC Labels

Preterm Infant Organization; Newborn Adaptation; Growth; Nutritional Status: Food and Fluid Intake; Thermoregulation: Neonate; Vital Signs Status; Child Development: 2 Months, 4 Months, 6 Months; Muscle Function; Neurological Status; Sleep

> **Example NOC Outcome**
> Demonstrates **Preterm Infant Organization** as evidenced by the following indicators: O_2 saturation >85%/Skin color/Feeding tolerance/Muscle tone relaxed/Smooth synchronous movement/Posture flexed/Hands brought to mouth/Appropriate time-out signals/Self-consolability/Deep sleep/Quiet-alert/active alert (Rate each indicator of **Preterm Infant Organization:** 1 = extreme deviation, 2 = substantial deviation, 3 = moderate deviation, 4 = mild deviation, 5 = no deviation [see Section I])

Client Outcomes

Infant/child

- Vital signs stable
- Displays smooth and synchronous body movements
- Displays smooth transitions between sleep and wake states
- Demonstrates self-consoling behaviors
- Demonstrates ability to tolerate feedings
- Displays stable color

Parents/significant other

- Recognizes infant/child behaviors as a unique way of communicating needs and goals
- Recognizes infant behavior used to communicate stress, avoidance and approach, and regulation
- Recognizes and supports infant's/child's drive and behaviors used to self-regulate
- Demonstrates ways of being more responsive to infant/child cues and needs

• = Independent; ▲ = Collaborative

- Recognizes the way their interactions affect the infant's/child's responses and that allowing the infant/child to take lead in the interaction fosters adaptive communication patterns
- Structures and modifies the environment in response to infant/child behaviors
- Identifies appropriate positioning and handling techniques to enhance comfort and normal development and prevent abnormalities

NIC | Interventions (Nursing Interventions Classification)

Suggested NIC Labels

Developmental Care; Sleep Enhancement; Parent Education: Infant; Positioning

---

Example NIC Interventions—Developmental Care
- Teach parents to recognize infant states and cues
- Point out infant's self-regulatory activities (e.g., hand-to-mouth, sucking, use of visual or auditory stimulus)
- Provide time-out when infant exhibits signs of stress (e.g., finger splaying, poor color, lowered state, fluctuation of heart and respiratory rate)
- Teach parent(s) how to console infant using behavioral quieting techniques (e.g., hand on infant, positioning, swaddling)
- Avoid overstimulation by stimulating one sense at a time (e.g., avoid talking while handling, looking at infant while feeding)
- Provide boundaries that maintain flexion of extremities while still allowing room for extension (e.g., nesting, waddling, bunting, hammock, hat, clothing)
- Monitor stimuli (e.g., light, noise, handling, procedures) in infant's environment and reduce as appropriate

---

Nursing Interventions and Rationales

- Identify infant's/child's level of neurobehavioral organization as a unique way of communicating.
  The infant's principal method of communicating goals, needs, and limits for stress and stability is by behavior; therefore the infant's own behaviors provide a guide for individualizing care and interactions and promoting development (Als, 1982).
- Recognize behavior used to communicate stress, avoid, approach, and regulate.
  The ability to read and interpret infant/child behavior provides a framework for responding to an infant/child in a way that communicates both the infant's/child's importance and that he or she is able to affect his or her environment (Als, 1982; Blackburn, Vandenberg, 1991).
- Identify and support the infant's/child's self-regulatory coping behaviors used for mastery of the environment.
  A continuous interaction takes place between the infant and the environment; behaviors such as hand-to-mouth or hand-to-face, hand grasping, foot and leg bracing, sucking on fingers or fists, auditory and visual fixation, and postural changes are used to maintain or regain a balanced adaptation between the self and the environment. Supporting infant behaviors enhances the coregulatory fit between the infant and the environment (Als, 1986).
- Cluster caregiving whenever possible to allow for longer periods of uninterrupted sleep.

• = **Independent**; ▲ = **Collaborative**

Introduce one intervention at a time and observe infant responses. Take care to prevent overstimulation during clustering care (D'Apolito, 1991).

- Correlate the evidence of stress or disorganization to internal factors (e.g., pain, hunger, discomfort) or external factors (e.g., lights, noise, handling).
Noise is one of the common stresses in hospital intensive care units (ICUs), resulting in sensory overload with the potential for alteration in development (DePaul, Chambers, 1995; Elander, Hellstrom, 1995). Infant colic characterized by increased irritability, di-minished ability to be soothed, and excessive restlessness relects immature sleep-wake regu-lation (an internal factor) (Keefe et al, 1996). Intrauterine cocaine exposure can result in disorganized behavior patterns of infants (DeWys, McComish-Fry, 1992).

- Structure and modify care and environment.
A developmental care approach designed to reduce environmental and procedural stress and facilitate motor and sleep-wake organization results in improved behavioral organization during the preterm period (Newman, 1986; Becker et al, 1991; D'Apolito, 1991). Pat-terns of sound, light, and caregiving tasks should minimize stress, conserve energy, and protect the developing neonate from inappropriate environmental stimuli (Blackburn, Vandenberg, 1991; D'Apolito, 1991).

- Facilitate the use of developmentally supportive positioning and handling.
Developmentally correct positioning (e.g., supporting/positioning in flexion or with con-tainment, consoling infant, offering something to grasp) can be used to decrease stress, con-serve energy, and enhance sleep and normal development of the preterm infant (McGrath, Conliffe-Torres, 1996; D'Apolito, 1991).

- Facilitate Kangaroo Care/skin-to-skin contact to promote infant's adaptability to external environment.
Kangaroo Care provides an environment that supports autonomic stability and fosters improvement in basic physiologic functions (Ludington-Hoe, Swinth, 1996). Infants have been found to benefit with cardiorespiratory stabilization, improved oxygenation, thermo-regulation, increased weight gain, earlier feeding, easier breastfeeding, and decreased length of stay (Ludington-Hoe et al, 1999). Kangaroo Care reduces the amount of time spent in active sleep and increases time spent in quiet, regular sleep (Ludington, 1990).

- Identify techniques to assist development of state modulation and organization.
Providing care and stimulation contingent on the state of the infant is critical to state organization (Fajardo et al, 1990).

- Identify and support infant's/child's attention capabilities.
In organized attentive states, infants are able to focus attention and interact with their environments purposefully (Burns et al, 1994).

- Enhance normal developmental patterns through appropriate sensorimotor stimulation.
Healthy 33- to 34-week postconceptual age infants who received 15 minutes of auditory, visual, tactile, and vestibular stimulation each day were found to be better than others at state modulation. Their ability to maintain quiet-alertness enhances parent-infant interactions and feedings (White-Traut et al, 1993). Enhancing normal experiences through appropriate sensory stimulation, handling, and social interactions appropriate to an infant's developmental level can minimize secondary problems (Anderson, Auster-Liebhaber, 1984).

Multicultural

- Assess for the influence of cultural beliefs, norms, and values on the family's percep-tions of infant/child behavior.

• = Independent; ▲ = Collaborative

What the family considers normal infant/child behavior may be based on cultural perceptions (Leininger, 1996).

- Use a neutral, indirect style when addressing areas where improvement is needed (such as a need for verbal or oral stimulation) when working with Native American clients. *Using indirect statements such as "Other mothers have tried. . ." or "I had a client who tried 'X' and it seemed to work very well" will assist in avoiding resentment from the parent (Seiderman et al, 1996).*
- Acknowledge and praise parenting strengths noted. *This will increase trust and foster a working relationship with the parent (Seiderman et al, 1996).*
- Use therapeutic communication techniques that emphasize acceptance, offer the self, validate the client's concerns, and convey respect when discussing the infant/child behavior. *Validation lets the client know that the nurse has heard and understands what was said, and it promotes the nurse-client relationship (Stuart, Laraia, 2001; Giger, Davidhizar, 1995). Studies show that even when language is not a barrier, some ethnic clients may be reluctant to discuss their beliefs and practices because of fear of criticism or ridicule (Evans, Cunningham, 1996).*

Family teaching

- Assist families/support systems in recognizing and responding to infant's unique behavioral cues. *Demonstrating and modeling appropriate interactional skills is an integral component of family education and will improve family-infant interaction (McGrath, Conliffe-Torres, 1996). Assisting parents with recognizing infant states and state modulation and self-consoling strategies provides caregivers with greater sense of competence (Nursing Child Assessment Satellite Training, 1994).*

Home Care Interventions

- Assist families in structuring home environment *Patterns of sound, light, and caregiving tasks should minimize stress, conserve energy, and protect the developing neonate from inappropriate environmental stimuli (Blackburn, Vandenberg, 1991; D'Apolito, 1991).*
- Encourage families to teach friends/visitors to recognize and respond to infant's unique behavioral cues. *It is important for families to feel comfortable obtaining support from their regular support systems; therefore supportive persons need to be taught how to interact in the environment in a way that supports both the family and the infant. The ability to read and interpret infant behavior provides a framework for responding to infants in a way that communicates both the infant's/child's importance and the message that he or she is able to affect his or her environment (Als, 1982; Blackburn, Vandenberg, 1991).*

WEB SITES FOR EDUCATION

MERLIN See the MERLIN web site for World Wide Web resources for client education.

REFERENCES Als H: Toward a synactive theory of development: promise for the assessment and support of infant individuality, *Infant Ment Health J* 3:229, 1982.

Als H: A synactive model of neonatal behavioral organization: framework for the assessment and support of the neurobehavioral development of the premature infant and his parents in the environment of the neonatal intensive care unit, *Phys Occup Ther Pediatr* 6:3, 1986.

• = Independent; ▲ = Collaborative

Anderson J, Auster-Liebhaber J: Developmental therapy in the neonatal intensive care unit, *Phys Occup Ther Pediatr* 4:89, 1984.

Becker PT et al: Outcomes of developmentally supportive nursing care for very low birth weight infants, *Nurs Res* 40:150-155, 1991.

Blackburn S, Vandenberg K: Assessment and management of neonatal development. In Kenner C et al: *Comprehensive neonatal nursing: a physiologic approach,* Toronto, 1991, WB Saunders.

Burns M et al: Infant stimulation: modification of an intervention based on physiologic and behavioral cues, *J Obstet Gynecol Neonatal Nurs* 23:581, 1994.

D'Apolito K: What is an organized infant? *Neonatal Netw* 10(1):23-28, 1991.

DePaul D, Chambers SE: Environmental noise in the neonatal intensive care unit: implications for nursing practice, *J Perinat Neonat Nurs* 8:71, 1995.

DeWys M, McComish-Fry J: Infants states and cues: facilitating effective parent-infant interactions. In *Caring for infants: a resource manual for caring for infant trainers,* East Lansing, Mich, 1992, Michigan State University Board of Trustees.

Elander G, Hellstrom G: Reduction of noise levels in intensive care units for infants: evaluation of an intervention program, *Heart Lung* 24:376, 1995.

Evans CA, Cunningham BA: Caring for the ethnic elder, *Geriatr Nurs* 17(3):105-110, 1996.

Fajardo B et al: Effect of nursery environment on state regulation in very-low-birth-weight premature infants, *Infant Behav Dev* 13:287, 1990.

Giger JN, Davidhizar RE: *Transcultural nursing,* ed 2, St Louis, 1995, Mosby.

Keefe M et al: A longitudinal comparison of irritable and nonirritable infants, *Nurs Res* 45:4, 1996.

Leininger MM: *Transcultural nursing: theories, research and practices,* ed 2, Hilliard, Ohio, 1996, McGraw-Hill.

Ludington SM: Energy conservation during skin-to-skin contact between preterm infants and their mothers, *Heart Lung* 19(5 Pt 1):445-451, 1990.

Ludington-Hoe SM, Swinth JY: Developmental aspects of kangaroo care, *J Obstet Gynecol Neonatal Nurs* 25(8):691-703, 1996.

Ludington-Hoe SM et al: Birth-related fatigue in 34-36–week preterm neonates: rapid recovery with very early Kangaroo (skin-to-skin) care, *J Obstet Gynecol Neonatal Nurs* 28(1):94-103, 1999.

McGrath J, Conliffe-Torres S: Integrating family-centered developmental assessment and intervention into routine care in the neonatal intensive care unit, *Nurs Clin North Am* 31(2):367-386, 1996.

Newman L: Social and sensory environment of low birth weight infants in a special care nursery, *J Nerv Ment Dis* 169:448, 1986.

Nursing Child Assessment Satellite Training: *NCAST caregiver/parent-child interaction feeding manual,* Seattle, 1994, University of Washington School of Nursing.

Seiderman RY et al: Assessing American Indian families, *Am J Mat Child Nurs* 21(6):274-279, 1996.

Stuart GW, Laraia MT: Therapeutic nurse-patient relationship. In Stuart GW, Laraia MT, editors: *Principles and practice of psychiatric nursing,* St Louis, 2001, Mosby, p 30.

White-Traut R et al: Patterns of physiological and behavioral response of intermediate care preterm infants to intervention, *Pediatr Nurs* 19:625, 1993.

Risk for disorganized Infant behavior

T. Heather Herdman and Mary A. Fuerst-DeWys

NANDA   **Definition**   Risk for alteration in integrating and modulation of the physiological and neurobehavioral systems of functioning (i.e., autonomic, motor, state, organizational, self-regulatory, and attentional-interactional systems)

Risk Factors

Pain; invasive/painful procedures; lack of containment/boundaries; oral/motor problems; prematurity; environmental overstimulation

• = Independent; ▲ = Collaborative

NOC Outcomes, Client Outcomes, NIC Interventions, Nursing Interventions and Rationales, Home Care Interventions

See care plan for **Disorganized Infant behavior.**

WEB SITES FOR EDUCATION

Merlin See the MERLIN web site for World Wide Web resources for client education.

Readiness for enhanced organized Infant behavior

T. Heather Herdman and Mary A. Fuerst-DeWys

NANDA **Definition** A pattern of modulation of the physiological and behavioral systems of functioning (i.e., autonomic, motor, state-organizational, self-regulatory, and attentional-interactional systems) in an infant that is satisfactory but that can be improved, resulting in higher levels of integration in response to environmental stimuli

Defining Characteristics

Definite sleep-wake states; use of some self-regulatory behaviors; response to visual/auditory stimuli; stable physiologic measures

Related Factors (r/t)

Pain; prematurity

NOC **Outcomes (Nursing Outcomes Classification)**

Suggested NOC Labels

Preterm Infant Organization; Newborn Adaptation; Growth; Nutritional Status: Food and Fluid Intake; Thermoregulation: Neonate; Vital Signs Status; Child Development: 2 Months, 4 Months, 6 Months; Muscle Function; Neurological Status; Sleep

> **Example NOC Outcome**
> Demonstrates **Preterm Infant Organization** as evidenced by the following indicators: O_2 saturation >85%/Skin color/Feeding tolerance/Muscle tone relaxed/Smooth synchronous movement/Posture flexed/Hands brought to mouth/Appropriate time-out signals/Self-consolability/Deep sleep/Quiet-alert/Active-alert (Rate each indicator of **Preterm Infant Organizaiton:** 1 = extreme deviation, 2 = substantial deviation, 3 = moderate deviation, 4 = mild deviation, 5 = no deviation [see Section I])

Client Outcomes

Infant/child

- Vital signs stable
- Displays smooth and synchronous body movements
- Displays smooth transitions between sleep and wake states
- Demonstrates self-consoling behaviors
- Demonstrates ability to tolerate feedings
- Displays stable color

• = **Independent;** ▲ = **Collaborative**

Parents/significant other

- Recognizes infant/child behaviors as a unique way of communicating needs and goals
- Recognizes infant behavior used to communicate stress, avoidance and approach, and regulation
- Recognizes and supports infant's/child's drive and behaviors used to self-regulate
- Demonstrates ways of being more responsive to infant/child cues and needs
- Recognizes the way interactions affect the infant's/child's responses and that allowing the infant/child to take lead in the interaction fosters adaptive communication patterns
- Structures and modifies the environment in response to infant/child behaviors
- Identifies appropriate positioning and handling techniques to enhance comfort and normal development and prevent abnormalities

NIC   Interventions (Nursing Interventions Classification)

Suggested NIC Labels

Positioning; Developmental Care; Kangaroo Care; Nonnutritive Sucking; Sleep Enhancement; Environmental Management; Newborn Monitoring

> ### Example NIC Interventions—Developmental Care
> - Provide water mattress and sheepskin as appropriate
> - Use smallest diaper to avoid hip abduction
> - Time infant care and feeding around sleep/wake cycle
> - Cluster care to promote longest possible sleep interval and energy conservation
> - Promote parent participation in feeding
> - Use a pacifier for nonnutritive sucking if feeding via gavage and between feedings, as appropriate

Nursing Interventions and Rationales

- Identify infant's/child's level of neurobehavioral organization as a unique way of communicating.
  The infant's principal method of communicating goals, needs, and limits for stress and stability is by behavior; therefore the infant's own behaviors provide a guide for individualizing care and interactions and promoting development (Als, 1982).
- Recognize behavior used to communicate stress, avoid and approach, and regulate.
  The ability to read and interpret infant behavior provides a framework for responding to infants in a way that communicates both the infant's/child's importance and that he or she is able to affect his or her environment (Als, 1982; Blackburn, Vandenberg, 1991).
- Identify and support the infant's/child's self-regulatory coping behaviors used for mastery of the environment.
  A continuous interaction takes place between the infant and the environment; behaviors such as hand-to-mouth or hand-to-face, hand grasping, foot and leg bracing, sucking on fingers or fists, auditory and visual fixation, and postural changes are used to maintain or regain a balanced adaptation between the self and the environment. Supporting infant behaviors enhances the coregulatory fit between the infant and the environment (Als, 1986).

• = Independent; ▲ = Collaborative

- Cluster caregiving whenever possible to allow for longer periods of uninterrupted sleep. *Introduce one intervention at a time and observe infant responses. Take care to prevent overstimulation during clustering care (D'Apolito, 1991).*
- Correlate the evidence of stress or disorganization to internal factors (e.g., pain, hunger, discomfort) or external factors (e.g., lights, noise, handling).
  Noise is one of the common stresses in hospital intensive care units (ICUs), resulting in sensory overload with the potential for alteration in development (DePaul, Chambers, 1995; Elander, Hellstrom, 1995). Infant colic characterized by increased irritability, diminished ability to be soothed, and excessive restlessness relects immature sleep-wake regulation (an internal factor) (Keefe et al, 1996). Intrauterine cocaine exposure can result in disorganized behavior patterns of infants (DeWys, McComish-Fry, 1992).
- Structure and modify care and environment.
  A developmental care approach designed to reduce environmental and procedural stress and facilitate motor and sleep-wake organization results in improved behavioral organization during the preterm period (Newman, 1986; Becker et al, 1991; D'Apolito, 1991). Patterns of sound, light, and caregiving tasks should minimize stress, conserve energy, and protect the developing neonate from inappropriate environmental stimuli (Blackburn, Vandenberg, 1991; D'Apolito, 1991).
- Facilitate the use of developmentally supportive positioning and handling.
  Developmentally correct positioning (e.g., supporting/positioning in flexion or with containment, consoling infant, offering something to grasp) can be used to decrease stress, conserve energy, and enhance sleep and normal development of the preterm infant (McGrath, Conliffe-Torres, 1996; D'Apolito, 1991).
- Facilitate Kangaroo Care/skin-to-skin contact to promote infant's adaptability to external environment.
  Kangaroo Care provides an environment that supports autonomic stability and fosters improvement in basic physiologic functions (Ludington-Hoe, Swinth, 1996). Infants have been found to benefit with cardiorespiratory stabilization, improved oxygenation, thermoregulation, increased weight gain, earlier feeding, easier breastfeeding, and decreased length of stay (Ludington-Hoe et al, 1999). Kangaroo Care reduces the amount of time spent in active sleep and increases time spent in quiet, regular sleep (Ludington, 1990).
- Identify techniques to assist development of state modulation and organization.
  Providing care and stimulation contingent on the state of the infant is critical to state organization (Fajardo et al, 1990).
- Identify and support infant's/child's attention capabilities.
  In organized attentive states, infants are able to focus attention and interact with their environments purposefully (Burns et al, 1994).
- Enhance normal developmental patterns through appropriate sensorimotor stimulation.
  Healthy 33- to 34-week postconceptual-age infants who received 15 minutes of auditory, visual, tactile, and vestibular stimulation each day were found to be better than others at state modulation. Their ability to maintain quiet-alertness enhances parent-infant interactions and feedings (White-Traut et al, 1993). Enhancing normal experiences through appropriate sensory stimulation, handling, and social interactions appropriate to an infant's developmental level can minimize secondary problems (Anderson, Auster-Liebhaber, 1984).

• = Independent; ▲ = Collaborative

Multicultural

- Assess for the influence of cultural beliefs, norms, and values on the parent's/caregiver's perceptions of infant/child behavior.
  What the parent/caregiver considers normal infant/child behavior may be based on cultural perceptions (Leininger, 1996).
- Use a neutral, indirect style when addressing areas where improvement is needed (such as a need for verbal or oral stimulation) when working with Native American clients.
  Using indirect statements such as "Other mothers have tried. . ." or "I had a client who tried 'X' and it seemed to work very well" will assist in avoiding resentment from the parent (Seiderman et al, 1996).
- Acknowledge and praise parenting strengths and ability to respond to infant/child.
  This will increase trust and foster a working relationship with the parent (Seiderman et al, 1996).
- Use therapeutic communication techniques that emphasize acceptance, offer the self, validate the client's concerns, and convey respect when discussing the infant/child behavior.
  Validation lets the client know that the nurse has heard and understands what was said, and it promotes the nurse-client relationship (Stuart, Laraia, 2001; Giger, Davidhizar, 1995). Studies show that even when language is not a barrier, some ethnic clients may be reluctant to discuss their beliefs and practices because of the fear of criticism or ridicule (Evans, Cunningham, 1996).

Family teaching

- Assist families/support systems in recognizing and responding to infant's unique behavioral cues.
  Demonstrating and modeling appropriate interactional skills is an integral component of family education and will improve family-infant interaction (McGrath, Conliffe-Torres, 1996). Assisting parents in recognizing infant states and state modulation and self-consoling strategies provides caregivers with a greater sense of competence (Nursing Child Assessment Satellite Training, 1994).

Home Care Interventions

- Assist families in structuring home environment.
  Patterns of sound, light, and caregiving tasks should minimize stress, conserve energy, and protect the developing neonate from inappropriate environmental stimuli (Blackburn, Vandenberg, 1991; D'Apolito, 1991).
- Encourage families to teach friends/visitors to recognize and respond to infant's unique behavioral cues.
  It is important for families to feel comfortable obtaining support from their regular support systems; therefore supportive people need to be taught how to interact in the environment in a way that supports both the family and the infant. The ability to read and interpret infant behavior provides a framework for responding to infants in a way that communicates both the infant'/child's importance and the message that he or she is able to affect his or her environment (Als, 1982; Blackburn, Vandenberg, 1991).

WEB SITES FOR EDUCATION

MERLIN See the MERLIN web site for World Wide Web resources for client education.

REFERENCES   Als H: Toward a synactive theory of development: promise for the assessment and support of infant individuality, *Infant Ment Health J* 3:229, 1982.

• = Independent; ▲ = Collaborative

Als H: A synactive model of neonatal behavioral organization: framework for the assessment and support of the neurobehavioral development of the premature infant and his parents in the environment of the neonatal intensive care unit, *Phys Occup Ther Pediatr* 6:3, 1986.

Anderson J, Auster-Liebhaber J: Developmental therapy in the neonatal intensive care unit, *Phys Occup Ther Pediatr* 4:89, 1984.

Becker PT et al: Outcomes of developmentally supportive nursing care for very low birth weight infants, *Nurs Res* 40:150, 1991.

Blackburn S, Vandenberg K: Assessment and management of neonatal development. In Kenner C et al: *Comprehensive neonatal nursing: a physiologic approach,* Toronto, 1991, WB Saunders.

Burns M et al: Infant stimulation: modification of an intervention based on physiologic and behavioral cues, *J Obstet Gynecol Neonatal Nurs* 23:581, 1994.

D'Apolito K: What is an organized infant? *Neonatal Netw* 10(1):23-28, 1991.

DePaul D, Chambers SE: Environmental noise in the neonatal intensive care unit: implications for nursing practice, *J Perinat Neonat Nurs* 8:71, 1995.

DeWys M, McComish-Fry J: Infants states and cues: facilitating effective parent-infant interactions. In *Caring for infants: a resource manual for caring for infant trainers,* East Lansing, Mich, 1992, Michigan State University Board of Trustees.

Elander G, Hellstrom G: Reduction of noise levels in intensive care units for infants: evaluation of an intervention program, *Heart Lung* 24:376, 1995.

Evans CA, Cunningham BA: Caring for the ethnic elder, *Geriatr Nurs* 17(3):105-110, 1996.

Fajardo B et al: Effect of nursery environment on state regulation in very-low-birth-weight premature infants, *Infant Behav Dev* 13:287, 1990.

Giger JN, Davidhizar RE: *Transcultural nursing,* ed 2, St Louis, 1995, Mosby.

Keefe M et al: A longitudinal comparison of irritable and nonirritable infants, *Nurs Res* 45:4, 1996.

Leininger MM: *Transcultural nursing: theories, research and practices,* ed 2, Hilliard, Ohio, 1996, McGraw-Hill.

Ludington SM: Energy conservation during skin-to-skin contact between preterm infants and their mothers, *Heart Lung* 19(5 Pt 1):445-451, 1990.

Ludington-Hoe S, Swinth J: Developmental aspects of kangaroo care, *J Obstet Gynecol Neonatal Nurs* 25(8):691-703, 1996.

Ludington-Hoe S et al: Birth-related fatigue in 34-36–week preterm neonates: rapid recovery with very early Kangaroo (skin-to-skin) care, *J Obstet Gynecol Neonatal Nurs* 28(1):94-103, 1999.

McGrath J, Conliffe-Torres S: Integrating family-centered developmental assessment and intervention into routine care in the neonatal intensive care unit, *Nurs Clin North Am* 31(2):367-386, 1996.

Newman L: Social and sensory environment of low birth weight infants in a special care nursery, *J Nerv Ment Dis* 169:448, 1986.

Nursing Child Assessment Satellite Training: *NCAST caregiver/parent-child interaction feeding manual,* Seattle, 1994, University of Washington School of Nursing.

Seiderman RY et al: Assessing American Indian families, *MCN Am J Matern Child Nurs* 21(6):274-279, 1996.

Stuart GW, Laraia MT: Therapeutic nurse-patient relationship. In Stuart GW, Laraia MT, editors: *Principles and practice of psychiatric nursing,* St Louis, 2001, Mosby, p 30.

White-Traut R et al: Patterns of physiological and behavioral response of intermediate care preterm infants to intervention, *Pediatr Nurs* 19:625, 1993.

Ineffective Infant feeding pattern

Vicki E. McClurg and Virginia R. Wall

NANDA   **Definition** Impaired ability to suck or coordinate the suck-swallow response

Defining Characteristics

Inability to coordinate sucking, swallowing, and breathing; inability to initiate or sustain an effective suck

• = Independent; ▲ = Collaborative

Related Factors (r/t)

Prolonged NPO; anatomic abnormality; neurological impairment/delay; oral hypersensitivity; prematurity

NOC Outcomes (Nursing Outcomes Classification)

Suggested NOC Labels

Breastfeeding Establishment: Infant; Breastfeeding: Maintenance; Muscle Function; Nutritional Status: Food and Fluid Intake

> **Example NOC Outcome**
>
> Accomplishes **Breastfeeding Establishment: Infant** as evidenced by the following indicators: Proper alignment and latch on/Proper areolar grasp/Proper areolar compression/Correct suck and tongue placement/Swallowing a minimum of 5 to 10 minutes per breast/Minimum eight feedings per day/Six or more urinations per day/ Age appropriate weight gain (Rate each indicator of **Breastfeeding Establishment: Infant:** 1 = not adequate, 2 = slightly adequate, 3 = moderately adequate, 4 = substantially adequate, 5 = totally adequate [see Section I])

Client Outcomes

- Infant receives adequate nourishment, without compromising autonomic stability
- Infant progresses to a normal feeding pattern
- Family learns successful techniques for feeding the infant

NIC Interventions (Nursing Interventions Classification)

Suggested NIC Labels

Enteral Tube Feeding; Lactation Counseling; Nonnutritive Sucking; Tube Care: Umbilical Line

> **Example NIC Intervention—Nonnutritive Sucking**
> - Provide pacifier to encourage sucking during tube feeding and for 5 minutes following the tube feeding
> - Provide pacifier to encourage sucking at least every 4 hours for infants receiving long-term hyperalimentation
> - Instruct parents on the use of nonnutritive sucking

Nursing Interventions and Rationales

- Assess infant's oral reflexes (i.e., root, gag, suck, and swallow).
  These reflexes are necessary for successful oral feedings. Feeding by nipple or breast should be encouraged to aid in the growth and maturity of the gastrointestinal tract and for comfort and oral gratification (Lau et al, 2000).
- Determine infant's ability to coordinate suck, swallow, and breathing reflexes.
  As infants develop they become more able to coordinate breathing with sucking and swallowing (Shiao, 1997; Medoff-Cooper, McGrath, Bilker, 2000).
- ▲ Collaborate with other health care providers (e.g., physician, neonatal nutritionist, physical and occupational therapists, lactation specialists) to develop a feeding plan.
  Various health care providers contribute expertise to the care of an infant with special needs (Baker, Rasmussen, 1997; Caretto et al, 2000).
- ▲ Implement gavage feedings (or another alternative feeding method), using breast milk whenever possible, before infant's readiness for feedings by mouth.

- **= Independent; ▲ = Collaborative**

Even after a preterm infant develops the ability to suck and swallow, the infant may require too much energy to do so and gavage feedings may be necessary. Serious illness can interfere with a neonate's ability to suck, and calorie and nutrient needs are increased by the stress of illness (Lucas et al, 1997; Medoff-Cooper, McGrath, Bilker, 2000).

- Provide opportunities for nonnutritive sucking during gavage feedings (or other alternative feeding methods) and for 5 minutes before initiating oral feedings.
  Sucking helps calm infants, thus raising the oxygen level; may aid digestion and increase average daily weight gain; and may prepare infants for earlier nipple feedings and discharge (Pickler et al, 1996; Shiao, 1997).
- Evaluate the feeding environment and minimize sensory stimuli.
  Noxious stimuli must be kept to a minimum to decrease physiological stress on at-risk infants. The neonatal intensive care unit environment can interfere with normal development of the infant and breastfeeding success; therefore this environment must be modified to enhance attachment and normal development (Baker, Rasmussen, 1997; Brown, Heermann, 1997).
- Position preterm infant in a flexed feeding posture that is similar to the posture used for a full-term infant.
  The "total sucking pattern" of the full-term newborn combines strong physiological flexion and high rib cage position to provide support for the tongue and jaw, which is essential for effective nippling (Brown, Heermann, 1997; Brandon, Holditch-Davis, Beylea, 1999).
- Attempt to nipple feed baby only when infant is in a quiet-alert state.
  The infant must be able to find and grasp the nipple effectively and then be ready and eager to suck. The quiet-alert state was found to be optimal for feeding preterm infants (McCain, 1997; Brandt, Andrews, Kvale, 1998; Medoff-Cooper, McGrath, Bilker, 2000).
- Allow appropriate time for nipple feeding to ensure infant's safety without exceeding calorie expenditure.
  Nipple feeding can lead to nutritional deficits because of the increased metabolic demands placed on the at-risk infant by thermoregulation, work of respiration and feeding, and decreased ability to absorb nutrients (Shaio, 1997; Hill, Kurkowski, Garcia, 2000).
- Monitor infant's physiological condition during feeding.
  Cardiorespiratory stability is necessary for nipple feedings (Shaio, 1997).
- Determine infant's active feeding behaviors without prodding.
  Infants must be alert and eager to eat (rooting, latching on, and sucking readily) to ensure a successful feeding. Prodding compromises the infant's safety, interrupts learning, and may give an inaccurate picture of ability to take in adequate nutrients in preparation for discharge (Brandt, Andrews, Kvale, 1998; Shaio, 1997; Hill, Kurkowski, Garcia, 2000).
- Assess infant's ability to take in enough calories to sustain temperature and growth. Use electronic scale to estimate intake during breastfeeding sessions. Use nipple shield to increase milk intake during breastfeeding as needed.
  Calories are needed to sustain basal metabolic rate, activity, digestive and metabolic processes, and growth. Electronic scales are the only accurate way to estimate breast milk intake. Nipple shield use increases milk intake without decreasing total duration of breastfeeding for preterm infants (Meier et al, 1996, 2000; Shaio, 1997).
- Encourage family to participate in the feeding process.
  Nurses can promote the psychosocial development of the at-risk infant and family by encouraging the caregiving ability of the parents (Moran et al, 1999).

• = **Independent**; ▲ = **Collaborative**

▲ Refer to a neonatal nutritionist, physical or occupational therapist, or lactation specialist as needed.

Collaborative practice with others who are specially trained to meet the needs of this vulnerable population will help ensure feeding and parenting success (Baker, Rasmussen, 1997; Caretto et al, 2000).

Client/Family Teaching

- Provide anticipatory guidance for infant's expected feeding course.

  Knowing what to anticipate helps the family feel involved and enhances attachment (Jaeger, Lawson, Filteau, 1997; Huckabay, 1999; Caretto et al, 2000).

- Teach parents infant feeding methods.

  Parents should be involved in the feeding process as soon as possible to enhance attachment through positive feedback about their ability to nurture a child (Bruschweiler, 1998; Huckabay, 1999).

- Teach parents how to recognize infant cues.

  Parents' understanding of infant's cues may increase their involvement in caring for the infant by improving their perception of the infant's abilities (Brandt, Andrews, Kvale, 1998; Medoff-Cooper, McGrath, Bilker, 2000).

- Provide anticipatory guidance for the infant's discharge.

  Parents need assistance in assuming responsibility for infant care as the day of discharge approaches (Davis, Logsdon, Birkmer, 1996; Baker, Rasmussen, 1997; Elliott, Reimer, 1998).

WEB SITES FOR EDUCATION

MERLIN See the MERLIN web site for World Wide Web resources for client education.

REFERENCES   Baker BJ, Rasmussen TW: Organizing and documenting lactation support of NICU families, *J Obstet Gynecol Neonatal Nurs* 26:515, 1997.

Brandon DH, Holditch-Davis D, Beylea M: Nursing care and the development of sleeping and waking behaviors in preterm infants, *Res Nurs Health* 22(3):217-229, 1999.

Brandt KA, Andrews CM, Kvale J: Mother-infant interaction and breast-feeding outcome 6 weeks after birth, *J Obstet Gynecol Neonatal Nurs* 27:169, 1998.

Brown LD, Heermann JA: The effect of developmental care on preterm infant outcome, *Appl Nurs Res* 10(4):190-197, 1997.

Bruschweiler SN: Early emotional care for mothers and infants, *Pediatrics* 102(5 Suppl E):1278-1281, 1998.

Caretto V et al: Current parent education on infant feeding in the neonatal intensive care unit: the role of the occupational therapist, *Am J Occup Ther* 54(1):59-64, 2000.

Davis DW, Logsdon MC, Birkmer JC: Types of support expected and received by mothers after their infants' discharge from the NICU, *Issues Compr Pediatr Nurs* 19(4):263-273, 1996.

Elliott S, Reimer C: Postdischarge telephone follow-up program for breastfeeding preterm infants discharged from a special care nursery, *Neonatal Netw* 17(6):41-45, 1998.

Hill AS, Kurkowski TB, Garcia J: Oral support measures used in feeding the preterm infant, *Nurs Res* 49(1):2-10, 2000.

Huckabay LM: The effect on bonding behavior of giving a mother her premature baby's picture, *Sch Inq Nurs Pract* 13(4):349-362, 1999.

Jaeger MC, Lawson M, Filteau S: The impact of prematurity and neonatal illness on the decision to breast-feed, *J Adv Nurs* 25(4):729-737, 1997.

Lau C et al: Characterization of the developmental stages of sucking in preterm infants during bottle feeding, *Acta Paediatr* 89(7):846-852, 2000.

Lucas A et al: Breastfeeding and catch-up growth in infants born small for gestational age, *Acta Paediatr* 86:564, 1997.

• = **Independent**; ▲ = **Collaborative**

McCain GC: Behavioral state activity during nipple feedings for preterm infants, *Neonatal Netw* 16(5):43-47, 1997.

Medoff-Cooper B, McGrath JM, Bilker W: Nutritive sucking and neurobehavioral development in preterm infants from 34 weeks PCA to term, *MCN Am J Matern Child Nurs* 25(2):64-70, 2000.

Meier PP et al: Estimating milk intake of hospitalized preterm infants who breastfeed, *J Hum Lact* 12(1):21-26, 1996.

Meier PP et al: Nipple shields for preterm infants: effect on milk transfer and duration of breastfeeding, *J Hum Lact* 16(2):106-114, quiz 129-131, 2000.

Moran M et al: Maternal kangaroo (skin-to-skin) care in the NICU beginning 4 hours postbirth, *MCN Am J Matern Child Nurs* 24(2):74-79, 1999.

Pickler RH et al: Effects of nonnutritive sucking on behavioral organization and feeding performance in preterm infants, *Nurs Res* 45(3):132-135, 1996.

Shiao SY: Comparison of continuous vs. intermittent sucking in very-low-birth-weight infants, *J Obstet Gynecol Neonatal Nurs* 26:313, 1997.

Risk for Infection

Gail B. Ladwig

 Definition At increased risk for being invaded by pathogenic organisms

Risk Factors

Invasive procedures; insufficient knowledge regarding avoidance of exposure to pathogens; trauma; tissue destruction and increased environmental exposure; rupture of amniotic membranes; pharmaceutical agents (e.g., immunosuppressants); malnutrition; increased environmental exposure to pathogens; immunosuppression; inadequate acquired immunity; inadequate secondary defenses (e.g., decreased hemoglobin, leukopenia, suppressed inflammatory response); inadequate primary defenses (e.g., broken skin, traumatized tissue, decrease in ciliary action, stasis of body fluids, change in pH secretions, altered peristalsis); chronic disease

Related Factors (r/t)

See Risk Factors

 Outcomes (Nursing Outcomes Classification)

Suggested NOC Labels

Immune Status; Knowledge: Infection Control; Risk Control; Risk Detection

> **Example NOC Outcome**
> Demonstrates adequate **Immune Status** as evidenced by the following indicators: Recurrent infections not present/Skin and mucosa integrity/GI, Respiratory, GU/ Weight and body temperature IER* (Rate each indicator of **Immune Status:** 1 = extremely compromised, 2 = substantially compromised, 3 = moderately compromised, 4 = mildly compromised, 5 = not compromised [see Section I])

*In Expected Range

Client Outcomes

- Remains free from symptoms of infection
- States symptoms of infection of which to be aware
- Demonstrates appropriate care of infection-prone site
- Maintains white blood cell count and differential within normal limits

• = Independent; ▲ = Collaborative

- Demonstrates appropriate hygienic measures such as hand washing, oral care, and perineal care

NIC   **Interventions (Nursing Interventions Classification)**

Suggested NIC Labels

Immunization/Vaccination Administration; Infection Control; Infection Protection

> **Example NIC Interventions—Infection Control**
> - Wash hands before and after each patient care activity
> - Ensure aseptic handling of all IV lines
> - Ensure appropriate wound care technique

Nursing Interventions and Rationales

▲ Observe and report signs of infection such as redness, warmth, discharge, and increased body temperature.
With the onset of infection the immune system is activated and signs of infection appear.

▲ Assess temperature of neutropenic clients every 4 hours; report a single temperature of >38.5° C or three temperatures of >38° C in 24 hours.
Neutropenic clients do not produce an adequate inflammatory response; therefore fever is usually the first and often the only sign of infection (Wujcik, 1993).

• Use an electronic or mercury thermometer to assess temperature.
When temperature values have important consequences for treatment decisions, use mercury or electronic thermometers with established accuracy (Erickson et al, 1996).

▲ Note and report laboratory values (e.g., white blood cell count and differential, serum protein, serum albumin, and cultures).
Laboratory values are correlated with client's history and physical examination to provide a global view of the client's immune function and nutritional status and develop an appropriate plan of care for the diagnosis (Lehmann, 1991).

• Remove the granulocytopenic client from areas exposed to construction dust so that the client won't inhale fungal spores. Remove all plants and flowers from client's room.
Aspergillus, an organism that can cause fungal pneumonia, is commonly found in soil, water, and decomposing vegetation. This fungus can enter the hospital through an unfiltered air system, in dust stirred up during construction, or in food or ornamental plants (Calianno, 1999).

• Assess skin for color, moisture, texture, and turgor (elasticity). Keep accurate, ongoing documentation of changes.
Preventive skin assessment protocol, including documentation, assists in the prevention of skin breakdown. Intact skin is nature's first line of defense against microorganisms entering the body (Kovach, 1995).

• Carefully wash and pat dry skin, including skinfold areas. Use hydration and moisturization on all at-risk surfaces.
*Maintaining supple, moist skin is the best method of keeping skin intact. Dry skin can lead to inflammation, excoriations, and possible infection episodes (Kovach, 1995) (see care plan for **Risk for impaired Skin integrity**).*

• Encourage a balanced diet, emphasizing proteins to feed the immune system.
Immune function is affected by protein intake (especially arginine); the balance between omega-6 and omega-3 fatty acid intake; and adequate amounts of vitamins A, C, and E

• = **Independent;** ▲ = **Collaborative**

and the minerals zinc and iron. A deficiency of these nutrients puts the client at an increased risk of infection (Lehmann, 1991).

- Use strategies to prevent nosocomial pneumonia: assess lung sounds, sputum, and redness or drainage around stoma sites; use sterile water rather than tap water for mouth care of immunosuppressed clients; provide a clean manual resuscitation bag for each client; use sterile technique when suctioning; suction secretions above tracheal tube before suctioning; drain accumulated condensation in ventilator tubing into a fluid trap or other collection device before repositioning the client; assess patency and placement of nasogastric tubes; elevate the head of the client to $\geq 30°$ to prevent gastric reflux of organisms in the lung; institute feeding as soon as possible; assess for signs of feeding intolerance—no bowel sounds, abdominal distension, increased residual, emesis.

  Hospital-acquired pneumonia is the second most common nosocomial infection but has the highest mortality (30%) and morbidity rates. The strategies listed are used to prevent nosocomial pneumonia (Tasota et al, 1998). Once treatment for pneumonia has begun, it must continue for 48 to 72 hours, the minimum time to evaluate a clinical response (Ruiz et al, 2000).

- Encourage fluid intake.

  Fluid intake helps thin secretions and replace fluid lost during fever (Calianno, 1999).

- Encourage adequate rest to bolster the immune system.

  Chronic disease and physical and emotional stress increase the client's need for rest (Potter, Perry, 1993).

- Use proper hand washing techniques before and after giving care to client and any time hands become soiled, even if gloves are worn: Wet hands under running water; dispense a minimum of 3 to 5 ml of soap or detergent and thoroughly distribute it over all areas of both hands; vigorously wash all surfaces of hands and fingers for at least 10 to 15 seconds, including backs of hands and fingers and under nails; rinse to remove soap, and thoroughly dry hands; use a dry paper towel to turn the faucet off.

  Consistent and meticulous hand washing remains the most important contributing factor related to reduction of the frequency of nosocomial infections in the intensive care unit (ICU). Hand washing significantly decreases the number of pathogens on the skin and contributes to decreases in client's morbidity and mortality (Tasota et al, 1998). Ensure that all hospital staff members follow precautions to prevent the spread of infection. In a study in central India, a high percentage of staff did not wash hands at appropriate times (Chandra, Milind, 2001). When soap is used, the mechanical action of washing and drying removes most of the transient bacteria. Hands should remain in contact with the cleanser for 10 seconds, but 20 to 30 seconds is ideal (Gould, 1994a). Rinsing hands with tap water and drying them with towels can reduce methicillin-resistant Staphylococcus aureus (MRSA) contamination by 95% (Sarver-Steffensen, 1999).

- Hands should be thoroughly dried with paper towels after washing.

  Bacterial transfer occurs more readily between wet surfaces than dry ones (Marples, Towers, 1979). More microorganisms were removed with paper towels than with linen. After use of hot-air dryers, fecal organisms have been recovered from hands, and bacterial counts are significantly higher than when paper towels are used (Gould, 1994b).

- Follow Standard Precautions and wear gloves during any contact with blood, mucous membranes, nonintact skin, or any body substance except sweat. Use goggles, gloves, and gowns when appropriate.

• = Independent; ▲ = Collaborative

Wearing gloves does not obviate the need for scrupulous hand washing. The purpose of wearing gloves is either to protect the hands from becoming contaminated with dirt and microorganisms or to prevent the transfer of organisms that are already present on the hands (Smock, Shiel, 1994). The first and most important tier of the new Centers for Disease Control and Prevention (CDC) guidelines is Standard Precautions. Because client examination and medical history cannot reliably identify every client with blood-borne pathogens, Standard Precautions apply to all clients. You must assume all clients are carrying blood-borne pathogens such as human immunodeficiency virus (HIV) or Hepatitis B or C (HBV or HCV). Standard Precautions exceed Universal Precautions. Transmission of blood-borne pathogens takes place by parenteral, mucous membrane, or nonintact skin exposure to blood and other body substances. You must take precautions whenever contact is likely with blood, mucous membranes, nonintact skin, or any body substance except sweat (Medcom, 1999). This study indicates that when risk for infection is high, powder-free gloves should be considered because powder may promote wound infection (Dave, Wilcox, Kellett, 1999).

- Follow Transmission-Based Precautions for airborne-, droplet-, and contact-transmitted microorganisms:
    - **Airborne:** Isolate the client in a room with monitored negative air pressure, with the room door closed, and the client remaining in the room. Always wear appropriate respiratory protection when you enter the room. For tuberculosis, you should wear an approved particulate respirator mask. Limit the movement and transport of the client from the room to essential purposes only. If at all possible, have the client wear a surgical mask during transport.
    - **Droplet:** Keep the client in a private room, if possible. If not possible, maintain a spatial separation of 3 feet from other beds or visitors. The door may remain open. You should wear a mask when you must come within 3 feet of the client. Some hospitals may choose to implement a mask requirement for droplet precautions for anyone entering the room. Limit transport to essential purposes, and have the client wear a mask if possible.
    - **Transmission:** Place the client in a private room if possible or with someone who has an active infection from the same microorganism. Wear clean, nonsterile gloves when entering the room. When providing care, change gloves after contact with any infective material such as wound drainage. Remove the gloves and wash your hands before leaving the room and take care not to touch any potentially infectious items or surfaces on the way out. Wear a gown if you anticipate your clothing may have substantial contact with the client or other potentially infectious items. Remove the gown before leaving the room. Limit the transport of the client to essential purposes and take care that the client does not contact other environmental surfaces along the way. Dedicate the use of noncritical client care equipment to a single client. If use of common equipment is unavoidable, adequately clean and disinfect equipment before use with other clients.

Standard Precautions are based on the likely routes of transmission of pathogens. The second tier of the new CDC guidelines is Transmission-Based Precautions. This replaces many old categories of isolation precautions and disease-specific precautions with three simpler sets of precautions. These three sets of precautions are designed to prevent airborne transmission, droplet transmission, and contact transmission (Medcom, 1999).

- Sterile technique must be used when inserting urinary catheters. Catheters must be cared for at least every shift.

• = **Independent;** ▲ = **Collaborative**

The genitourinary (GU) tract is the most common site of nosocomial infections in the acute care setting. Catheterization and instrumentation of the urinary tract are implicated as precipitating factors in approximately 80% of cases (Tasota et al, 1998).

- Use careful technique when changing and emptying urinary catheter bags; avoid cross-contamination.
  Clients are most at risk for cross-infection during bag changing and emptying (Platt et al, 1983; Crow et al, 1993; Roe, 1993).

- Use alternatives to indwelling catheters whenever possible (external catheters, incontinence pads, bladder control techniques).
  The GU tract is the most common site of nosocomial infections in the acute care setting. Catheterization and instrumentation of the urinary tract are implicated as precipitating factors in approximately 80% of cases (Tasota et al, 1998).

- ▲ Provide well-designed site care for all peripheral, central venous, and arterial catheters: standardize insertion technique; select catheters with as few lumens as necessary; avoid use of femoral catheters in clients with fecal or urinary incontinence; use aseptic technique for insertion and care; stabilize cannula and tubing; maintain a sterile occlusive dressing (change every 72 hours per hospital policy); label insertion sites and all tubing with date and time of insertion, inspect every 8 hours for signs of infection, record and report; replace peripheral catheters per hospital policy (usually every 48 to 72 hours); when fever of unknown origin develops, obtain culture.
  More than 40% of bloodstream infections in ICUs are associated with short-term use of central venous catheters. Strict aseptic technique should be maintained. The risk of infection associated with use of triple-lumen catheters is as much as three times greater than the risk associated with single-lumen catheters. Clients with unexplained fever and signs of localized infection most likely have a catheter-related infection. The catheter should be removed and samples obtained for microbial culture (Tasota et al, 1998). Care in selection of site and catheter is important. The shortest catheter and smallest size should be used when possible. Accommodate the need to replace catheters before they occlude (Schmid, 2000).

- Use careful sterile technique wherever there is a loss of skin integrity.
  Use of sterile technique prevents infection in at-risk clients (Wujcik, 1993).

- Ensure client's appropriate hygienic care with hand washing; bathing; and hair, nail, and perineal care performed by either nurse or client.
  Hygienic care is important to prevent infection in at-risk clients (Wujcik, 1993).

- ▲ Recommend responsible use of antibiotics; use antibiotics sparingly.
  Clients infected with resistant strains of bacteria are more likely than control clients to have received previous antimicrobials, and hospital areas that have the highest prevalence of resistance also have the highest rates of antibiotic use. For these reasons, programs to prevent or control the development of resistant organisms often focus on the overuse or inappropriate use of antibiotics, for example, by restriction of widely used broad-spectrum antibiotics (e.g., third-generation cephalosporins) and vancomycin. Other approaches are to rotate antibiotics used for empiric therapy and to use combinations of drugs from different classes (Weber, Raasch, Rutala, 1999). Widespread use of certain antibiotics, particularly third-generation cephalosporins, has been shown to foster development of generalized beta-lactam resistance in previously susceptible bacterial populations. Reduction in the use of these agents (as well as imipenem and vancomycin) and concomitant increases in the use of extended-spectrum penicillins and combination therapy with aminoglycosides have been shown to restore bacterial susceptibility (Yates, 1999).

• = **Independent**; ▲ = **Collaborative**

Geriatric

- Recognize that geriatric clients may be seriously infected but have less obvious symptoms.
  The immune system declines with aging. The elderly may present with atypical manifestations of infections (Madhaven, 1994).
- Suspect pneumonia when the client has symptoms of fatigue or confusion.
  The only early indicators of pneumonia in an elderly client may be confusion and fatigue. An elderly client with pneumonia may not have such classic signs and symptoms as fever, cough, or an increased white blood cell (WBC) count, or lung consolidation may be masked by chronic pulmonary disease. Among all age groups, the elderly are at greatest risk because aging can impair normal pulmonary defense mechanisms. Once an older client develops pneumonia, his or her risk takes on deadly dimensions. Clients >65 years of age are five times more likely than those in any other age group to die of a bacterial nosocomial pneumonia (Calianno, 1999).
- Most clients develop nosocomial pneumonia by either aspirating contaminated substances or inhaling airborne particles. Refer to care plan for **Risk for Aspiration.**
- ▲ Foot care other than simple toenail cutting should be performed by a podiatrist.
- ▲ Observe and report if client has a low-grade temperature or new onset of confusion.
  The elderly can have infections with low-grade fevers. Be suspicious of any temperature rise or sudden confusion—these symptoms may be the only signs of infection (Madhaven, 1994).
- During the peak of the influenza epidemic, limit visits by relatives and friends.
  Hospital- and nursing home–acquired influenza A virus infection leads to high mortality in the elderly (Madhaven, 1994).
- ▲ Recommend that the geriatric client receive an annual influenza immunization and one-time pneumococcal vaccine.
  Among the many infections to which the aged are susceptible, pneumonia and influenza combined are responsible for the greatest mortality (Madhaven, 1994). Oseltamivir prophylaxis was very effective in protecting nursing home residents from ILI and in halting an outbreak of influenza B. A comparable nursing home in this study that did not use this treatment had double the cases (Parker, Loewen, Skowronski, 2001).
- Recognize that chronically ill geriatric clients have an increased susceptibility to infection; practice meticulous care of all invasive sites.

Home Care Interventions

- Assess home environment for general cleanliness, storage of food items, and appropriate waste disposal. Instruct as necessary in proper disposal and use of disinfecting agents.
  Presence of waste and inappropriate storage of food items can contribute to the presence of pathogens.
- Assess home care environment for appropriate disposal of used dressing materials.
  Used dressing materials may contain or be a primary medium for growth of pathogens.
- Role model all preventive behaviors in care of client (e.g., Universal Precautions). Do not visit client when you are ill.
  Demonstration is a more effective teaching strategy than verbalization.

• = **Independent;** ▲ = **Collaborative**

- Maintain the cleanliness of all irrigation and cleansing solutions. Change solutions when cleanliness has not been maintained—do not wait to finish bottle.
  Solutions exposed to contaminants provide a medium for growth of pathogens.
- Assess and teach clients about current medications and therapies that promote susceptibility to infection: corticosteroids, immunosuppressants, chemotherapeutic agents, and radiation therapy.
  Knowledge of risk factors promotes vigilance in assessment, prompt reporting, and early treatment.
- Assess client for knowledge of infections that have been drug resistant.
- ▲ Instruct client to complete any course of prophylactic antibiotic therapy unless experiencing adverse side effects.
  Prophylactic antibiotic therapy decreases the risk of infection.

Client/Family Teaching

- ▲ Teach client and family the symptoms of infection that should be promptly reported to a primary medical caregiver (e.g., redness; warmth; swelling; tenderness or pain; new onset of drainage or change in drainage from wound; increase in body temperature; hepatitis B virus [HBV]/acquired immunodeficiency syndrome [AIDS] symptoms: malaise, abdominal pain, vomiting or diarrhea, enlarged glands, rash; tuberculosis symptoms: cough, night sweats, dyspnea, changes in sputum, changes in breath sounds; insulin-dependent diabetes mellitus [IDDM] symptoms: sores or wounds that do not heal).
  A high prevalence of HBV/AIDS, an increasing incidence of tuberculosis, and the general risk of diabetes are related to increased rate of infection.
- ▲ Encourage high-risk persons, including health care workers, to have influenza vaccinations.
  Vaccinations help to prevent viral nosocomial pneumonia (Calianno, 1999).
- Assess whether client and family know how to read a thermometer; provide instructions if necessary. Chemical dot thermometers are easy to use and decrease risk of infection. Clients need to know that the instructions should be followed carefully and that electronic or mercury thermometers may be the best choice for accuracy.
  Chemical dot thermometers may underestimate the oral temperature by ≥0.4° C in about 50% of adults, thus lacking the sensitivity to screen for fever and providing many false readings. Conversely, they may overestimate axillary temperature by ≥0.4° C in about 50% of adults and some young children, thus lacking the specificity to rule out fever and providing many false–positive readings (Erickson et al, 1996).
- Instruct client and family about the need for good nutrition (especially protein) and proper rest to bolster immune function.
- If client has AIDS, discuss the continued need to practice safe sex, avoid unsterile needle use, and maintain a healthy lifestyle to prevent infection.
- ▲ Refer client and family to social services and community resources to obtain support in maintaining a lifestyle that increases immune function (e.g., adequate nutrition and rest, freedom from excessive stress).

WEB SITES FOR EDUCATION

MERLIN See the MERLIN web site for World Wide Web resources for client education.

• = Independent; ▲ = Collaborative

REFERENCES   Calianno C: *Nosocomial pneumonia,* Springnet, Springhouse, retrieved March 29, 1999, from the World Wide Web. Web site: www.springnet.com/ce/ce965a.htm

Chandra PN, Milind K: Lapses in measures recommended for preventing hospital-acquired infection, *J Hosp Infect* 47(3):218-222, 2001.

Crow R et al: *A study of patients with an indwelling urethral catheter and related nursing practice,* Nursing Practice Unit, 1993, University of Surrey.

Dave J, Wilcox MH, Kellett M: Glove powder: implications for infection control, *J Hosp Infect* 42(4):283-285, 1999.

Erickson R et al: Accuracy of chemical dot thermometers in critically ill adults and young children, *Image J Nurs Sch* 28:23, 1996.

Gould D: Making sense of hand hygiene, *Nurs Times* 90:63, 1994a.

Gould D: The significance of hand-drying in the prevention of infection, *Nurs Times* 90:33, 1994b.

Kovach T: The barrier defense: skin hydration as infection control, *J Pract Nurs* 45:13, 1995.

Lehmann S: Immune function and nutrition: the clinical role of the intravenous nurse, *J Intraven Nurs* 14:406, 1991.

Madhaven T: Infections in the elderly: current concepts in management, *Comprehen Ther* 20:465, 1994.

Marples RR, Towers A: A laboratory model for the contact transfer of microorganisms, *J Hygiene* 82:237, 1979.

Medcom: *Infection control and standard precautions,* retrieved on April 1, 1999, from the World Wide Web. Web site: www.medcominc.com/CE_Infection.htm

Parker R, Loewen N, Skowronski D: Experience with oseltamivir in the control of a nursing home influenza B outbreak, *Can Commun Dis Rep* 27(5):37-40, 2001.

Platt R et al: Reduction of mortality associated with nosocomial urinary tract infection, *Lancet* 1:893, 1983.

Potter P, Perry A: *Fundamentals of nursing: concepts, process and practice,* St Louis, 1993, Mosby.

Roe B: Catheter-associated urinary tract infection: a review, *J Clin Nurs* 2:197, 1993.

Ruiz M et al: Diagnosis of pneumonia and monitoring of infection eradication, *Drugs* 60(6):1289-1303, 2000.

Sarver-Steffensen J: When MRSA reaches into long-term care, *RN* 62(3):39-41, 1999.

Schmid MW: Risks and complications of peripherally and centrally inserted intravenous catheters, *Crit Care Nurs Clin North Am* 12(2):165-174, 2000.

Smock M, Shiel M: The role of surgeon and procedure gloves in infection control: a closer look at disposable gloves, *Prof Nurse* 9:324, 1994.

Tasota F et al: Protecting ICU patients from nosocomial infections, *Crit Care Nurse* 18(1):54-65, 1998.

Weber D, Raasch R, Rutala W: Nosocomial infections in the ICU: the growing importance of antibiotic-resistant pathogens, *Chest* 115(suppl):34S-41S, 1999.

Wujcik D: Infection control in oncology patients, *Nurs Clin North Am* 28:639, 1993.

Yates RR: New intervention strategies for reducing antibiotic resistance, *Chest* 115(suppl):24S-27S, 1999.

Risk for Injury

Betty J. Ackley

NANDA   **Definition**   At risk of injury as a result of the interaction of environmental conditions interacting with the individual's adaptive and defensive resources

NOTE: This nursing diagnosis overlaps with other diagnoses such as **Risk for Falls, Risk for Trauma, Risk for Poisoning, Risk for Suffocation, Risk for Aspiration** and, if the client is at risk of bleeding, **Ineffective Protection.** See care plans for these diagnoses if appropriate.

Risk Factors
External   Mode of transport or transportation; people or provider (e.g., nosocomial agents, staffing patterns, cognitive, affective and psychomotor factors); physical (e.g., design, struc-

• = Independent; ▲ = Collaborative

ture, and arrangement of community, building, and/or equipment); nutrients (e.g., vitamins, food types); biological (e.g., immunization level of community, microorganism); chemical (e.g., pollutants, poisons, drugs, pharmaceutical agents, alcohol, caffeine, nicotine, preservatives, cosmetics, and dyes)

Internal   Psychological (affective orientation); malnutrition; abnormal blood profile (e.g., leukocytosis/leukopenia); altered clotting factors; thrombocytopenia; sickle cell; thalassemia; decreased hemoglobin; immune-autoimmune dysfunction; biochemical, regulatory function (e.g., sensory dysfunction, integrative dysfunction, effector dysfunction, tissue hypoxia); developmental age (physiological, psychosocial); physical (e.g., broken skin, altered mobility)

Related Factors (r/t)

See Risk Factors.

NOC   Outcomes (Nursing Outcomes Classification)

Suggested NOC Labels

Risk Control; Parenting: Social Safety; Fetal Status: Intrapartum; Maternal Status: Intrapartum; Immune Status; Safety Behavior: Home Physical Environment; Safety Behavior: Personal: Safety Status: Falls Occurrence; Safety Status: Physical Injury

> ### Example NOC Outcome
> Accomplishes **Risk Control** as evidenced by the following indicators: Monitors environmental risk factors/Develops effective risk control strategies/Follows selected risk control strategies (Rate each indicator of **Risk Control:** 1 = never demonstrated, 2 = rarely demonstrated, 3 = sometimes demonstrated, 4 = often demonstrated, 5 = consistently demonstrated [see Section I])

Client Outcomes

- Remains free of injuries
- Explains methods to prevent injury

NIC   Interventions (Nursing Interventions Classification)

Suggested NIC Labels

Health Education; Behavior Modification; Patient Contracting; Self-Modification Assistance

> ### Example NIC Interventions—Health Education
> - Identify internal or external factors that may enhance or reduce motivation for healthy behavior
> - Determine current health knowledge and lifestyle behaviors of indivdual, family, or target group

Nursing Interventions and Rationales

- Thoroughly orient client to environment. Place call light within reach and show how to call for assistance; answer call light promptly.
- ▲ Avoid use of restraints. Obtain a physician's order if restraints are necessary. *Restrained elderly clients often experience an increased number of falls, possibly as a result of muscle deconditioning or loss of coordination (Tinetti, Liu, Ginter, 1992; Wilson, 1998). If the elderly are restrained and fall, they can sustain severe injuries, including strangulation, asphyxiation, or head injury from leading with their heads to get out of the*

• = Independent; ▲ = Collaborative

bed (DiMaio, Dana, Bix, 1986; Evans, Strumpf, 1990). Restraint-free extended care facilities were shown to have fewer residents with activities of daily living (ADLs) deficiencies and fewer residents with bowel or bladder incontinence than facilities that use restraints (Castle, Fogel, 1998).

- In place of restraints, use the following:
  - Alarm systems with ankle or wrist bracelets
  - Bed or wheelchair alarms
  - Increased observation of client
  - Locked doors to unit
  - Bed with wheels removed to keep bed low (NOTE: may not be acceptable with fire regulations)

  These are alternatives to restraints that can be helpful for preventing falls (Commodore, 1995; Wilson, 1998).

▲ If client is extremely agitated, consider using a special safety bed that surrounds client. If client has a traumatic brain injury, use the Emory cubicle bed.

  Special beds can be an effective alternative to restraints and can help keep the client safe during periods of agitation (Williams, Morton, Patrick, 1990).

- If client has a new onset of confusion (delirium), provide reality orientation when interacting with him or her. Have family bring in familiar items, clocks, and watches from home to maintain orientation. If client has chronic confusion with dementia, use validation therapy that reinforces feelings but does not confront reality.

  Reality orientation can help prevent or decrease the confusion that increases risk of injury when the patient becomes agitated. Validation therapy is more effective for clients with dementia (Fine, Rouse-Bane, 1995). (See Interventions for **Chronic Confusion**.)

- Ask family to stay with client to prevent client from accidentally falling or pulling out tubes.
- Remove all possible hazards in environment such as razors, medications, and matches.
- Place an injury-prone client in a room that is near the nurses' station.

  Such placement allows more frequent observation of the client.

- Help clients sit in a stable chair with armrests. Avoid use of wheelchairs and geri-chairs except for transportation as needed.

  Clients are likely to fall when left in a wheelchair or geri-chair because they may stand up without locking the wheels or removing the footrests. Wheelchairs do not increase mobility; people just sit in them the majority of the time (Lipson, Braun, 1993; Simmons et al, 1995).

- To ensure propulsion with legs or arms and ability to reach the floor, ensure that the chair or wheelchair fits the build, abilities, and needs of the client, eliminating footrests and minimizing problems with shearing.

  The seating system should fit the needs of the client so that the client can move the wheels, stand up from the chair without falling, and not be harmed by the chair or wheelchair. Footrests can cause skin tears and bruising, as well as postural alignment and sitting posture problems (Lipson, Braun, 1993).

- Avoid use of wheelchairs as much as possible because they can serve as a restraint device. Most people in wheelchairs do not move.

  Wheelchairs can be effective restraints. In one study, only 4% of residents in wheelchairs were observed to propel them independently and only 45% could propel them, even with

• = **Independent;** ▲ = **Collaborative**

cues and prompts. This study found that no residents could unlock the wheelchairs without help, wheelchairs were not fitted to residents, and residents were not trained in propulsion (Simmons et al, 1995).

▲ Refer to physical therapy for strengthening exercises and gait training to increase mobility. Refer to occupational therapy for assistance with helping clients perform ADLs.
   Gait training in physical therapy has been shown to effectively prevent falls (Galinda-Ciocon, Ciocon, Galinda, 1995; Wilson, 1998).

Pediatric

• Teach parents the need for close supervision of all young children playing near water. If child has epilepsy, recommend showers instead of tub baths, and no unsupervised swimming ever.
   Most drowning accidents involving children are preventable if basic safety measures are taken (Bolte, 2000).

Geriatric

• Encourage client to wear glasses and hearing aids and to use walking aids when ambulating.
• If client experiences dizziness because of orthostatic hypotension when getting up, teach methods to decrease dizziness, such as rising slowly, remaining seated several minutes before standing, flexing feet upward several times while sitting, sitting down immediately if feeling dizzy, and trying to have someone present when standing.
   The elderly develop decreased baroreceptor sensitivity and decreased ability of compensatory mechanisms to maintain blood pressure when standing up, resulting in postural hypotension (Aaronson, Carlon-Wolfe, Schoener, 1991; Matteson, McConnell, Linton, 1997).

Multicultural

• Acknowledge racial/ethnic differences at the onset of care.
   Acknowledgement of race/ethnicity issues will enhance communication, establish rapport, and promote treatment outcomes (D'Avanzo et al, 2001).
• Assess for the influence of cultural beliefs, norms, and values on the client's perceptions of risk for injury.
   What the client considers risky behavior may be based on cultural perceptions (Leininger, 1996).
• Assess whether exposure to community violence is contributing to risk for injury.
   Exposure to community violence has been associated with increases in aggressive behavior and depression (Gorman-Smith, Tolan, 1998). Minority students, especially African-American and Latino students in lower grades, may participate in and may more often be victims of school violence (Hill, Drolet, 1999).
• Use culturally relevant injury prevention programs whenever possible.
   The Make It Safe program is a bilingual, culturally sensitive educational presentation for Hispanic families that focuses on living and working safely in a rural environment (National Rural Health Association, 1998).
• Validate the client's feelings and concerns related to environmental risks.
   Validation lets the client know that the nurse has heard and understands what was said, and it promotes the nurse-client relationship (Stuart, Laraia, 2001; Giger, Davidhizar, 1995).

Home Care Interventions

• Assess home environment for threats to safety: clutter, inappropriate storage of chemicals, slippery floors, scatter rugs, unsafe stairs and stairwells, blocked entries,

• = **Independent;** ▲ = **Collaborative**

dim lighting, extension cords across pathways, unsafe electrical or gas connections, unsafe heating devices, unsafe oxygen placement, high beds without rails, excessively hot water, pets, and pet excrement.

Clients suffering from impaired mobility, impaired visual acuity, and neurological dysfunction, including dementia and other cognitive functional deficits, are at risk for injury from common hazards.

▲ Instruct client and family or caregivers in correcting identified hazards. Refer to occupational therapy services for assistance if needed. Notify landlord or code enforcement office of any structural building hazards.

▲ Refer to physical therapy services for client and family education in safe transfers and ambulation and for strengthening exercises for ambulation and transfers.

• Avoid extreme hot and cold around clients at risk for injury (e.g., heating pads, hot water for baths/showers).

Clients with decreased cognition or sensory deficits cannot discriminate extremes in temperature.

▲ Provide a signaling device for clients who wander or are at risk for falls. If client lives alone, provide a Lifeline or similar call device.

Orienting a vulnerable client to a safety net relieves anxiety of the client and caregiver and allows for rapid response to a crisis situation.

▲ Provide medical identification bracelet for clients at risk for injury from dementia, seizures, or other medical disorders.

Client/Family Teaching

• Teach how to safely ambulate at home, including using safety measures such as handrails in bathroom.

• If client has visual impairment, teach client and caregiver to label with bright colors such as yellow or red significant places in environment that must be easily located (e.g., stair edges, stove controls, light switches).

• Teach clients winter safety information:
  - Burn only untreated wood for heat
  - Keep portable space heaters at least 3 feet from anything that can burn
  - Install smoke alarms and carbon monoxide alarm near bedrooms
  - Check the chimney and flue each year
  - Avoid sitting in an idling car in winter when snow can obstruct the exhaust pipe
  - Follow safety guidelines for use of snow blowers

Winter presents many safety challenges both indoors and out. These safety tips can help increase safety (National Center for Injury Prevention and Control, 2000).

WEB SITES FOR EDUCATION

🖋MERLIN See the MERLIN web site for World Wide Web resources for client education.

REFERENCES Aaronson L, Carlon-Wolfe W, Schoener S: Pressures that fall on rising, *Geriatr Nurs* 12:67, 1991.
Bolte R: Drowning: a preventable cause of death, *Patient Care* 34(7):129-142, 2000.
Castle NG, Fogel B: Characteristics of nursing homes that are restraint free, *The Gerontologist* 38(2):181-188, 1998.
Commodore DI: Falls in the elderly population: a look at incidence, risks, healthcare costs, and preventive strategies, *Rehabil Nurs* 20:84, 1995.

• = **Independent;** ▲ = **Collaborative**

D'Avanzo CE et al: Developing culturally informed strategies for substance-related interventions. In Naegle MA, D'Avanzo CE, editors: *Addictions and substance abuse: strategies for advanced practice nursing,* St Louis, 2001, Mosby, pp 59-104.

DiMaio V, Dana S, Bix R: Death caused by restraint vests, *JAMA* 255:905, 1986.

Evans L, Strumpf N: Myths about elder restraint, *Image J Nurs Sch* 22:124, 1990.

Fine JI, Rouse-Bane S: Using validating techniques to improve communication with cognitively impaired older adults, *J Gerontol Nurs* 21:39, 1995.

Galinda-Ciocon DJ, Ciocon JO, Galinda DJ: Gait training and falls in the elderly, *J Gerontol Nurs* 21:11, 1995.

Giger JN, Davidhizar RE: *Transcultural nursing,* ed 2, St Louis, 1995, Mosby.

Gorman-Smith D, Tolan P: The role of exposure to community violence and developmental problems among inner city youth, *Dev Psychopatho* 10(1):101-116, 1998.

Hill SC, Drolet JC: School related violence among high school students in the United States 1993-1995, *J Sch Health* 69(7):264-272, 1999.

Leininger MM: *Transcultural nursing: theories, research and practices,* ed 2, Hilliard, Ohio, 1996, McGraw-Hill.

Lipson J, Braun S: *Toward a restraint-free environment: reducing the use of physical and chemical restraint in long-term care and acute settings,* Baltimore, 1993, Health Professions Press.

Matteson MA, McConnell ES, Linton AD: *Gerontological nursing,* ed 2, Philadelphia, 1997, WB Saunders.

National Center for Injury Prevention and Control: Winter safety, *Int J Trauma Nurs* 6(4):138-141, 2000.

National Rural Health Association: Make it safe: an injury prevention program for Hispanic farm workers and families at work and play, *Int Electronic J Health Ed,* 1(4):219-221, 1998.

Simmons S et al: Wheelchairs as mobility restraints: predictors of wheelchair activity in nonambulatory nursing home residents, *J Am Geriatr Soc* 43:384, 1995.

Stuart GW, Laraia MT: Therapeutic nurse-patient relationship. In Stuart GW, Laraia MT, editors: *Principles and practice of psychiatric nursing,* St Louis, 2001, Mosby, p 30.

Tinetti ME, Liu W-L, Ginter SF: Mechanical restraint use and fall-related injuries among residents of skilled nursing facilities, *Ann Intern Med* 116:369, 1992.

Williams LM, Morton GA, Patrick CH: The Emory cubicle bed: an alternative to restraints for agitated traumatically brain injured clients, *Rehabil Nurs* 15:30, 1990.

Wilson EB: Preventing patient falls, *AACN Clin Issues* 9(1):100-108, 1998.

Risk for perioperative-positioning Injury

Terri Foster and Pamela M. Emery

 Definition At risk for injury as a result of the environmental conditions found in the perioperative setting

Risk Factors

Disorientation; edema; emaciation; immobilization; muscle weakness; obesity; sensory/perceptual disturbances resulting from anesthesia (NANDA)

NOTE: The systems most frequently affected by surgical positioning are the neurological, musculoskeletal, integumentary, respiratory, and cardiovascular systems. Risk factors contributing to the incidence of injury related to surgical positioning include but are not limited to the client's age; height; weight; nutritional status; the presence of preexisting conditions such as diabetes, vascular disease, or impaired nerve function; physical mobility limitations such as arthritis, limited range of motion, implants/prosthesis, or malignancy; effects of anesthesia; staff's knowledge of the equipment; and the duration of the procedure. As a result of these factors, there may be a potential for impaired tissue perfusion, impaired skin integrity, or neuromuscular or joint injury related to surgical positioning.

• = Independent; ▲ = Collaborative

Complications of surgical positioning

Transient physiological reactions to surgical positioning include skin redness and/or bruising, lumbar backache, stiffness in the limbs and neck, and generalized muscle aches that usually resolve within 24 to 48 hours without treatment (Walsh, 1993). Lumbar back pain, previously considered a transient physiological reaction to positioning, may in some cases be persistent in nature (Clark et al, 1993).

More serious complications of surgical positioning include pressure ulcers, peripheral nerve injury, deep venous thrombosis, joint dislocation, compartment syndrome (impairment of microcirculation in soft tissue), and joint injury (Paschal, Strzelecki, 1992; Walsh, 1993). Because compartment syndrome is a reperfusion injury, its signs and symptoms may not be immediately apparent and may develop insidiously (Montgomery, Ready, 1991).

NOC ## Outcomes (Nursing Outcomes Classification)

Suggested NOC Labels

Muscle Function; Neurological Status; Risk Control; Tissue Perfusion: Peripheral; Circulation Status; Tissue Integrity: Skin and Mucous Membranes

> **Example NOC Outcome**
> Maintains **Tissue Perfusion: Peripheral** as evidenced by the following indicators: Peripheral edema not present/Localized extremity pain not present/Skin intact/ Muscle function intact/Sensation level normal/Distal peripheral pulses strong (Rate each indicator of **Tissue Perfusion: Peripheral:** 1 = extremely compromised, 2 = substantially compromised, 3 = moderately compromised, 4 = mildly compromised, 5 = not compromised [see Section I])

Client Outcomes

- Free of injury related to positioning during the surgical procedure
  NOTE: Nursing interventions are based on assessing the client preoperatively for the existence of or potential for injury to any of the previously mentioned systems based on observed or elicited risk factors.
- Physical mobility is unchanged or improved from preoperative status
- Cardiovascular status is unchanged or improved from preoperative status
- Peripheral sensory integrity is unchanged or improved from preoperative status

NIC ## Interventions (Nursing Interventions Classification)

Suggested NIC Labels

Positioning: Intraoperative; Skin Surveillance; Pressure Ulcer Prevention; Risk Identification

> **Example NIC Interventions—Positioning: Intraoperative**
> - Use an adequate number of personnel to transfer the client
> - Maintain client's proper body alignment

Nursing Interventions and Rationales

General interventions for any surgical patient

- Determine range of motion/mobility of the client's limbs.
  Clients with limited mobility/range of motion should be asked to position themselves under the nurse's guidance before induction of anesthesia so that the client can verify that a position of comfort has been obtained.

• = **Independent;** ▲ = **Collaborative**

- Monitor pressure being applied to the client intraoperatively by staff, equipment, and/or instruments.
  The staff's leaning on or equipment and/or instruments resting on a patient can cause redness and bruising and/or can lead to pressure ulcers.
- Keep linens on the OR table free of wrinkles.
  Wrinkled sheets can cause skin pressure (Fortunato, 2000).
- Maintain equipment in good working order: clean, operating, free of sharp edges.
  Equipment that is working properly leads to client safety and aids in improved exposure of the surgical site (Association of periOperatve Registered Nurses, 2001).
- Reassess the client after positioning and during the procedure for maintenance of proper alignment and skin integrity. Use of a simple snow sled (the roll-up thin, flexible plastic type) to reposition the patient up and down on the table can reduce shear or friction (Carris, Franczek, 1999).
  Changes in position can expose or damage body parts (e.g. shearing, friction, compression) that previously were protected (Association of periOperative Registered Nurses, 2001). Once the client has been positioned, lifting him or her slightly for a moment may allow skin to realign with the skeleton (Meeker, Rothrock, 1999).
- Do not allow extremities to extend beyond/off the OR table.
  Extremities allowed to hang freely can lead to compression or stretch injury (Spry, 1997).
- Avoid contact with metal when positioning the client.
  Contact with metal at any point during use of the electrosurgical unit may result in an electrical burn (Rothrock, 1996). Compression of soft tissue may predispose client to venous thrombosis (Paschal, Strzelecki, 1992).
- Any movement/positioning of the client should be done slowly.
  Slow movement allows the body time to adjust to circulatory and respiratory changes and allows the abdominal contents to reposition. It also allows the staff to have better control of the client's body (Fortunato, 2000; Spry, 1997).
- The OR table, cart, or bed should be locked before transfer/positioning of the client.
  An unlocked OR table, cart, or bed could lead to the client's sustaining a fall injury.
- Use a full-length silicone gel pad to prevent pressure injuries in procedures lasting longer than 3 hours.
  Use of a dry visco-elastic polymer pad (gel pad) intraoperatively reduced the probability of pressure sore development by half as compared to the standard operating table mattress (Nixon et al, 1998). The minimal cost of the dry visco-elastic polymer pads in comparison to the cost of pressure sore treatment and the personal cost to patients with regard to pain and discomfort supports their general use within the operating room suite practice.
- Prevent pooling of prep solutions, blood, irrigation, urine, and feces. Clean up as necessary.
  Pooling in areas of high pressure can increase the chances for the development of a more severe pressure sore (Meeker, Rothrock, 1999).
- Ensure privacy for the client during positioning, keeping the client covered as much as possible.
  The client should be kept warm during positioning to prevent hypothermia, which can lead to increased potential for infection and slower wound healing.

Supine position (dorsal recumbent)
- Pad all bony prominences (e.g., head, elbows, spinal column, sacrum, olecranon, and heels) and positioning devices.

• = **Independent;** ▲ = **Collaborative**

Bony prominences exert pressure on overlying tissue, which predisposes the client to the development of pressure ulcers (Blaylock, Gardner, 1994; Rothrock, 1996). Nerves that pass over or near bony prominences may be injured by compression (Spry, 1997).

- Support lumbar and popliteal areas.
  Maintaining normal lumbar concavity prevents muscle strain that can occur as a result of anesthetic agents and muscle relaxants affecting the paraspinal muscles (Spry, 1997). Support under the knees prevents muscle and ligament strain (Rothrock, 1996).
- Use a firm foam rubber support or padded footboard that extends beyond toes.
  A support or footboard prevents plantar flexion and protects the toes from the weight and pressure of draping materials (Spry, 1997).
- Use a padded footboard when Reverse Trendelenburg is required.
  Positioning aids help prevent skin injury from shearing forces (opposite parallel force between skin and subcutaneous tissue) (Rothrock, 1996).

  NOTE: Either of these two positions (Trendelenburg or Reverse Trendelenburg) may have adverse effects on both the circulatory system (i.e., increased blood pressure and intracranial pressure) and respiratory system (i.e., diaphragm movement is impeded), which in most circumstances are monitored and controlled by anesthesia personnel. Modifications of both positions may be suggested and implemented by the nurse in collaboration with the surgeon and anesthesiologist.

  Padded shoulder braces may be used in the Trendelenberg position. They should be placed at an equal distance from the head of the table, and a $1/2$-inch space allowed between the brace and the shoulder. The braces are placed over the acromion and spinous process of the scapula, avoiding the soft tissue areas of the neck.

  Incorrectly placed shoulder braces can cause injury to the brachial plexus; therefore their use is not recommended unless absolutely necessary (Spry, 1997). Allowing space between the shoulders and the braces prevents pressure from the braces to the shoulders (Fortunato, 2000).

- Position client's arms with palms down on armboards that are level with the table and at a <90-degree angle to the body.
  Hyperabduction may damage the brachial plexus, ulna, and pudendal nerves and may stretch the subclavian and axillary vessels (Association of periOperative Registered Nurses, 2001; Spry, 1997; Walsh, 1993). Positioning the arm in this manner decreases pressure on the postcondylar groove of the humerus (American Society of Anesthesiologists Task Force, 2000). Hyperabduction of the arm can cause the brachial plexus to be stretched and compressed between the clavicle and the first rib. This pressure/compression increases when the client's head is turned toward the opposite shoulder/arm. Another complication of hyperabduction of the arm is thrombosis. The palms-up position increases stretching of the brachial plexus (Meeker, Rothrock, 1999).
- Position arms at sides of the body with palms against the body or palms down, without flexing the elbow, and secure arms with a broad lift sheet, tucking the sheet under the client's arm.
  Tucking the arms prevents compression of the fingers if allowed to extend over the edge of the operating table, maintains proper alignment, and prevents compression of the ulnar nerve (Spry, 1997). The lift sheet should not be tucked under the sides of the mattress because the mattress weight and the client's torso could impair circulation (Fortunato, 2000).

• = **Independent**; ▲ = **Collaborative**

- Protect skin from direct contact with any metal surfaces.
  Faulty or improperly grounded electrosurgical units may seek an alternative pathway through any skin surface in contact with metal and could result in an electrical burn (Rothrock, 1996). Pressure on the skin against the metal may cause a compression injury (Spry, 1997).
- Lift rather than pull or slide client when positioning.
  Sliding and pulling increase the incidence of skin injury (dermal abrasion or soft tissue injury) from shearing and friction (Fortunato, 2000). Pressure and/or shearing cause decreased circulation.
  NOTE: There are now devices available that are very slippery, enabling a client to be pulled or slid using a blanket/sheet beneath them, without shearing forces.
- Maintain alignment of head with cervical, thoracic, and lumbar spine.
  Misalignment, flexion, and twisting may cause muscle and nerve damage, as well as airway interference. Proper alignment of the head and spine prevents neuromuscular strain (Meeker, Rothrock, 1999).
- Position client's legs parallel and uncrossed.
  Compression from crossed ankles may injure skin and peroneal and tibial nerves and may impede circulation (Spry, 1997).
- Place leg restraint strap (safety belt) loosely but securely over waist or mid-thigh at least 2 inches above knees, avoiding bony prominences by placing a blanket between the strap and the client.
  Clients may become disoriented and attempt to change position on the narrow operating table. Applying the strap at least 2 inches above the knees prevents hyperextension of the knees (Spry, 1997).
- The nurse's finger should be able to fit between the strap and the client (Fortunato, 2000).
- When placing a pillow under the client's knees, place it proximal to the popliteal space and examine the safety strap to make sure it is not too tight.
  The popliteal artery, common peroneal nerve, and tibial nerve could be compressed between the pillow and the safety strap, causing nerve damage, impaired circulation, or thrombosis (Meeker, Rothrock, 1999).
- Support the head with a headrest or pillow.
  Supporting the head prevents stretching of the neck muscles (Spry, 1997). Care should be taken when using a donut-type headrest because the portion of the head that rests on the donut supports the rest of the head, thus causing increased pressure to the areas providing the support (Meeker, Rothrock, 1999).
- When placing a pregnant client in the supine position, place a small roll under her right flank.
  In the supine position there is increased pressure to the inferior vena cava from the abdominal contents and the fetus, which can decrease the return of blood to the heart (Meeker, Rothrock, 1999).

Prone position (modification: kneeling, jackknife, or Kraske position)

- Provide an adequate number of personnel to accomplish "logroll" turning of the anesthetized client.
  Movement and positioning from the supine to the prone position may be safely undertaken by a minimum of four persons (Spry, 1997).

• = Independent; ▲ = Collaborative

- Place chest rolls from the acromioclavicular joint to the iliac crests.
  Chest rolls allow for lung expansion by lifting the chest off the OR table, thus removing abdominal pressure from the diaphragm, allowing it free movement, and they decrease pressure on female breast tissue (The Association of periOperative Registered Nurses, 2001; Meeker, Rothrock, 1999; Spry, 1997).
  NOTE: Some surgeons prefer to use a laminectomy frame.
- Place a bolster or pillow under the pelvis.
  Support of the pelvis decreases abdominal pressure on the inferior vena cava and male genitalia (Meeker, Rothrock, 1999).
- Place a bolster or pillow under client's ankles.
  A cushion prevents stretching of the anterior tibial nerve and prevents pressure on the toes, which can lead to plantar flexion and footdrop (Spry, 1997).
- Padding should be placed under client's knees.
  Padding the knees prevents undo pressure on the patellas (Spry, 1997).
- Guide client's arms down and forward to rest on armboards that are extended forward from the OR table, with elbows flexed and padded and hands placed palms down.
  This movement prevents shoulder dislocation and brachial plexus injury, and padding prevents ulnar and radial nerve compression (Meeker, Rothrock, 1995; Walsh, 1993).
- Place the head, turned to one side, on a padded headrest and protect the client's ears and eyes.
  Ear cartilage may be damaged if the ear folds or is bent. Corneal abrasions may occur if the eyes are not closed and secured during maneuvering and positioning (Spry, 1997). A padded headrest provides airway access (The Association of periOperative Registered Nurses, 2001).
- Avoid severe rotation of client's head to one side.
  Severe head rotation may stretch skeletal muscles and ligaments, causing postoperative pain and limited motion after surgery (Walsh, 1993).
- The breasts of female clients should be checked and positioned laterally and the genitals of male clients should be checked.
  Positioning female breasts laterally reduces pressure on them (Fortunato, 2000).
- Clients placed in the Kraske position should be observed for respiratory and circulatory changes.
  In the Kraske position, the client has restricted diaphragm movement and increased blood volume in the lungs and feet because of venous pooling, which can lead to a decrease in mean arterial blood pressure, decreased ventilation, and decreased cardiac output (Meeker, Rothrock, 1999; Spry, 1997).

Lateral position (lateral chest or kidney)

- Provide adequate personnel to properly position the client.
  Lateral positioning requires a four-person team to safely move the client from the supine position (Spry, 1997).
- Use a lift sheet to facilitate the turn.
  Lift sheets prevent skin injury resulting from shearing.
- Place a support under the head.
  A pillow or support keeps the head properly aligned with the cervical spine and thoracic vertebrae and lessens stretching of the brachial plexus (Meeker, Rothrock, 1999).
- Flex the bottom leg at the hip and knee.
  Flexing the bottom leg helps to stabilize the client (Meeker, Rothrock, 1999).

• = Independent; ▲ = Collaborative

- Place beanbags, sandbags, or bolsters against the back and abdomen.
  Additional positioning devices provide support and maintain body alignment (Meeker, Rothrock, 1999).
- Pad the lateral aspect of the bottom knee.
  Pressure of the fibula on the peroneal nerve can lead to footdrop (Spry, 1997).
- Place a pillow between the client's legs lengthwise so that the pillow also supports the foot.
  Pressing the bony prominences of one extremity against the other may cause injury to the peroneal and tibial nerves (Meeker, Rothrock, 1999; Walsh, 1993). Support of the feet and ankles is necessary to prevent footdrop and pressure injury to the malleolus (Spry, 1997).
- Pad the lower shoulder and bring it forward slightly; the lower arm is extended on a padded armboard.
  All bony prominences should be padded to prevent tissue breakdown (Walsh, 1993). Bringing the shoulder forward relieves pressure on the brachial plexus and improves chest expansion (Meeker, Rothrock, 1999).
- Place the upper arm on a padded raised armboard or over the lower arm with padding between the two arms.
  Raising the upper arm elevates the scapula and widens the intercostal spaces, which provides access to the upper thoracic cavity (Meeker, Rothrock, 1999).
- Place an axillary roll at the apex of the scapula in the axillary space of the dependent arm.
  A soft roll relieves pressure on the arm and possible compression to the brachial plexus from the humeral head, and facilitates chest expansion (Spry, 1997).
  NOTE: Some surgeons prefer the use of wide adhesive tape to secure the hips, arms, and legs. This practice would be contraindicated in clients with tape allergies or in the frail elderly with fragile skin. Some surgeons prefer to use a device known as the Montreal Positioning Device. When using this device, special care must be taken to pad the posts extremely well to prevent pressure injuries.

Lithotomy position
- Before placing the client in the lithotomy position, the stirrups should be checked to ensure that they are fastened securely in the sockets attached to the OR bed.
  If the stirrups are not fastened securely and slip, the client could sustain a dislocated hip, muscle or nerve injury, or a fracture (Meeker, Rothrock, 1999).
- Position the client's arms loosely secured across the abdomen, extended on padded armboards, or at the client's sides.
  Extreme care must be taken when positioning the client's arms at the sides in this position because the hand and fingers could get crushed or pinched in the OR table when raising and lowering the lower third of the table for the procedure (Meeker, Rothrock, 1999).
  NOTE: Some surgeons prefer to have the left arm positioned at the patient's side when they are doing a procedure such as a D & C with diagnostic laparoscopy. In this case, it is suggested that the arm is well padded and that, in the absence of a tape allergy, foam tape be used to tape the hands and fingers to the patient's thigh. Extreme care must be taken to ensure that the hands and fingers have not come loose before raising and lowering the lower third of the OR table.
- Pad the sacral area and provide a small lumbar roll. The client's buttocks should be even with the table edge once the lower portion of the OR table has been lowered.

• = Independent; ▲ = Collaborative

Bony prominences must be padded to prevent soft tissue damage. A lumbar roll helps maintain normal lumbar concavity (Association of periOperative Registered Nurses, 2001; Meeker, Rothrock, 1999). When the buttocks extends beyond the edge of the table it causes strain on the lumbosacral muscles and ligaments, and the client's body weight rests on the sacrum (Fortunato, 2000). The greatest amount of force is placed on the lower back muscles when the client is in the lithotomy position 9 (Anema et al, 2000).

- Stirrups should be positioned at equal height and adjusted according to the length of the patient's legs.
Positioning stirrups at equal height helps to prevent pressure at the knee and lumbar spine (Spry, 1997).
- Place client's legs in the stirrups simultaneously, using one hand to hold the foot and the other to hold the calf at the knee.
Raising the legs together requires two persons and helps prevent stress on hip joints and possible dislocation of the hips (Spry, 1997).
- Lower client's legs simultaneously and slowly, extending the legs fully.
Because 500 to 800 ml of blood goes from the visceral area to the extremities, hypotension can result. Slowly lowering the client's legs can decrease or prevent this hypotension. Fully extending the legs prevents abduction of the hips (Spry, 1997).
- Minimize the height of the legs.
The height of the lower legs should be only slightly above the level of the left atria. Perfusion is decreased when the legs are elevated (Lampert et al, 1997).
- Avoid acute flexion of the hips and thighs.
Acute flexion of the thigh increases intraabdominal pressure against the diaphragm, thus decreasing tidal volume (Meeker, Rothrock, 1999). Severe flexion may also strain the lumbar spine, damage the prosthetic hip joint, and cause nerve damage (Walsh, 1993). Excessive flexion of the hip and knee can cause venous obstruction (Anema et al, 2000). Excess flexion of the hip can stretch the sciatic nerve (Meeker, Rothrock, 1999).
- Avoid hyperabduction and excessive external rotation of the hip joint.
Lumbosacral plexus stretch injury may result from the plexus being stretched and compressed under the inguinal ligament or pubic ramus (Fowl, Skers, Kempczinski, 1992). Femoral myoneuropathy may result from excessive hip abduction and external rotation (Hakim, Katirji, 1993). Femoral, sciatic, and obturator nerves, along with the abductor muscles of the hip joint, are stretched when the legs are hyperabducted (Meeker, Rothrock, 1999).
- Select lithotomy leg holders with optimal body alignment and weight bearing in mind (e.g., combination knee-crutch-and-boot).
Product selection and evaluation should be based on identified needs and should promote client safety (Association of periOperative Registered Nurses, 2001). Boot stirrups distribute weight evenly and allow controlled and limited abduction (Meeker, Rothrock, 1999).
- Pad all bony prominences and surfaces that may contact the leg support system.
When using candy cane stirrups, the ankle strap presses on the distal sural and plantar nerves, which could cause neuropathies of the foot (Meeker, Rothrock, 1999). Pressure on the lateral aspect of the knee may damage the peroneal nerve (Paschal, Strzelecki, 1992). Pressure to the inner thigh can damage the femoral and obturator nerves (Spry, 1997). Knee crutch stirrups can put pressure on the posterior tibial, sural, and common peroneal nerves (Meeker, Rothrock, 1999).
- Avoid prolonged contact of the calf muscles with the leg supports, which can lead to compartment syndrome (Spry, 1997).

• = **Independent;** ▲ = **Collaborative**

Research has shown that intramuscular pressures in the leg are increased, especially in the anterior and lateral compartments, with the leg/legs in this position (Meyer et al, 2000).

NOTE: The Hemilithotomy position (one leg in the lithotomy position) is often used when operating to repair a fractured hip or femur. Studies have shown that the uninjured leg in the lithotomy holder can develop compartment syndrome because of elevated intramuscular pressures, decreased perfusion, and the length of the procedure. Therefore it has been suggested that the uninjured leg be supported at the heel rather than at the calf (Meyer et al, 2000).

- Assess the need for sequential compression stockings.

  Sequential compression stockings seem to closely resemble normal physiological conditions and could possibly decrease the risk of compartment syndrome (Anema et al, 2000). Flexing of the knee can impede venous return. It is recommended that clients have Ace bandages or antiembolitic stockings applied if the procedure will last longer than 2 hours (Meeker, Rothrock, 1999).

- To decrease the length of time the client is in the lithotomy position, evaluate the procedure to determine if any portion can be done in the supine position.

- Monitor the length of time the client remains in the lithotomy position.

  Most complications occur following procedures that exceed 5 hours (Fowl, Skers, Kempczinski, 1992). The increased practice of operative laparoscopy, especially in gynecology, has contributed to more prolonged procedures (Schwartz, Stahl, DeCherney, 1992). The potential for complications is directly proportional to the length of time a client is in the lithotomy position (Anema et al, 2000).

NOTE: If assessment reveals conditions that place the client at increased risk for injury in this position, attempting this position while the client is awake and can report any discomfort may help prevent positioning complications.

WEB SITES FOR EDUCATION

MERLIN See the MERLIN web site for World Wide Web resources for client education.

REFERENCES   American Society of Anesthesiologists Task Force on Prevention of Perioperative Peripheral Neuropathies: Practice advisory for the prevention of perioperative peripheral neuropathies, *Anesthesiology* 92(4):1168-1182, 2000 (report).

Anema JG et al: Complications related to the high lithotomy position during urethral reconstruction, *J Urol* 164:360-363, 2000.

Association of periOperative Registered Nurses: *AORN standards and recommended practices for perioperative nursing,* Denver, 2001, The Association.

Blaylock B, Gardner C: Measuring tissue interface pressures of two support surfaces used in the operating room, *Ostomy Wound Manage* 40:42-48, 1994.

Carris J, Franczek T: Patient positioning: snow fun in the OR, *Todays Surg Nurs* 21:47-48, 1999.

Clark A et al: Role of the surgical position in the development of postoperative low back pain, *J Spinal Disord* 6:238, 1993.

Emergency Care Research Institute (ECRI): *Surgery and anesthesia,* ed 9, 1996, p. 3.

Fortunato N: *Berry and Kohn's Operating Room Technique,* ed 9, St Louis, 2000, Mosby.

Fowl R, Skers D, Kempczinski R: Neurovascular lower extremity complications of the lithotomy position, *Ann Vasc Surg* 6:4, 1992.

Hakim M, Katirji M: Femoral myoneuropathy induced by the lithotomy position: a report of 5 cases with a review of literature, *Muscle Nerve* 16:891, 1993.

Lampert R et al: Compartment syndrome: a complication of the lithotomy position, *Dutch J Urol* 4:103-107, 1997.

• = **Independent;** ▲ = **Collaborative**

Meeker M, Rothrock J: *Alexander's care of the patient in surgery*, ed 11, St Louis, 1999, Mosby.

Meyer S et al: *Intramuscular and blood pressure in legs positioned in the hemi-lithotomy position on a fracture table*, 46th Annual Meeting of Orthopedics Research Society, Orlando, Fla, Mar 12-15, 2000.

Montgomery C, Ready L: Epidural opioid analgesia does not obscure diagnosis of compartment syndrome resulting from prolonged lithotomy position, *Anesthesiology* 75:541, 1991.

Nixon J et al: A sequential randomized controlled trial comparing a dry visco-elastic polymer pad and standard operating table mattress in the prevention of postoperative pressure sores, *Int J Nurs Stud* 35:193-203, 1998.

Paschal C, Strzelecki L: Lithotomy positioning devices, factors that contribute to patient injury, *AORN J* 55:1011, 1992.

Rothrock J: *Perioperative nursing care planning*, St Louis, 1996, Mosby.

Schwartz L, Stahl R, DeCherney A: Unilateral compartment syndrome after prolonged gynecologic surgery in the dorsal lithotomy position, *J Reprod Med* 38:6, 1992.

Spry C: *Essentials of perioperative nursing*, Gaithersburg, Md, 1997, Aspen.

Walsh J: Postoperative effects of O.R. positioning, *RN* 56:50, 1993.

Decreased Intracranial adaptive capacity

Pamela H. Mitchell

NANDA   **Definition** Intracranial fluid dynamic mechanisms that normally compensate for increases in intracranial volumes are compromised, resulting in repeated disproportionate increases in intracranial pressure (ICP) in response to a variety of noxious and non-noxious stimuli (Mitchell, 1993)

Defining Characteristics

Repeated increases in ICP of >10 mm Hg for more than 5 minutes following a variety of external stimuli; disproportionate increases in ICP following a single environmental or nursing maneuver stimulus; baseline ICP ≥10 mm Hg; elevated P_2 component of ICP waveform; wide-amplitude ICP waveform; volume-pressure response test variation (volume-pressure ratio 2, pressure-volume index of <10) (Rauch, Mitchell, Tyler, 1990; Mitchell, 1993; Mitchell et al, 1998)

Related Factors (r/t)

Decreased cerebral perfusion ≤50 to 60 mm Hg; sustained increase in ICP = 10 to 15 mm Hg; systemic hypotension with intracranial hypertension; brain injuries

NOC   ## Outcomes (Nursing Outcomes Classification)

Suggested NOC Labels

Neurological Status: Consciousness; Neurological Status

Example NOC Outcome
Satisfactory **Neurological Status** as evidenced by the following indicators: Neurological Function: consciousness/Intracranial pressure WNL*/Vital signs WNL/Neurological function: central motor control/Neurological function: cranial sensory-motor function/Neurological function: spinal sensory-motor function (Rate each indicator of **Neurological Status:** 1 = extremely compromised, 2 = substantially compromised, 3 = moderately compromised, 4 = mildly compromised, 5 = not compromised [see Section I])

*Within Normal Limits

• = **Independent**; ▲ = **Collaborative**

Client Outcomes

- Experiences fewer than five episodes of disproportionate increases in ICP (DIICP) in 24 hours
- Neurological status changes are not triggered by episodes of DIICP
- CPP remains ≥70 mm Hg in adults

NIC **Interventions (Nursing Interventions Classification)**

Suggested NIC Labels

Cerebral Edema Management; Cerebral Perfusion Promotion; Intracranial Pressure (ICP) Monitoring; Neurologic Monitoring: Cerebral Edema Management

> **Example NIC Interventions—Cerebral Edema Management**
> - Monitor for confusion, changes in mentation, complaints of dizziness, syncope
> - Allow ICP to return to baseline between nursing activities

Nursing Interventions and Rationales

- For episodes of disproportionate increases in intracranial pressure (DIICP), do the following:
  - Reverse stimulus if readily apparent.
  - Evaluate position of client. Head should be in midline without neck flexion to prevent intracranial trapping of jugular venous outflow.
    Positional changes of the head and neck are the most consistent triggers of sustained ICP elevations. Both lateral and rotational neck flexion will result in increased ICP until the neck position is restored to a neutral position (Yordy, Hanigan, 1985-1986; Mitchell, Ackerman, 1992; Williams, Coyne, 1993).
  - Return client to original position if a position change has triggered DIICP.
    No particular body position triggers DIICP unless combined with neck flexion; however, some individuals respond to passive turning to lateral or three-quarter prone positions. Routine physical therapy also does not trigger problematic increases in ICP (Lee, 1989; Mitchell, Ackerman, 1992; Brimioulle et al, 1997).
  - Stop suctioning if routine suctioning is triggering DIICP. Follow preventive protocol if future suctioning is indicated.
    A standard series of three suctioning passes can result in stair-step elevation of ICP with each successive pass, even with full hyperoxygenation and hyperinflation before suctioning. Brief hyperventilation may be protective against these increases (Kerr et al, 1993, 1997).
  - Have clients who can follow directions exhale through their mouth if they are doing a Valsalva's maneuver.
    If clients' nonvolitional movements such as posturing and unconscious straining are causing a Valsalva's maneuver, sedation or paralytics with sedation may be indicated (McClelland et al, 1995; Kerr et al, 1998).
  - Reduce environmental noise and painful or unexpected touching of client.
    All these factors have been shown to be potent noxious stimuli in individual adults and preterm infants but may not trigger DIICP in the majority of clients (Yordy, Hanigan, 1985-1986; Mitchell, Ackerman, 1992).
  - Elevate head of bed if the client maintains CPP when ICP is lowered by head elevation.
    Head elevation reduces the average ICP in groups of clients, but individuals may exhibit either no change or even increased ICP (Ropper, O'Rourke, Kennedy, 1982). In

• = **Independent;** ▲ = **Collaborative**

addition, when cerebral autoregulation is impaired, even a small systemic blood pressure drop with head elevation may decrease the CPP to an unacceptable level (March et al, 1990; Chesnut, 1997a). Optimal head position needs to be determined individually, depending on both ICP and CPP measurement (Simmons, 1997).

- For DIICP, if baseline ICP rises above 15 mm Hg or CPP (mean arterial blood pressure minus mean ICP) <70 mm Hg in adults for 5 minutes or more, do the following:
  - ▲ Initiate protocols for lowering ICP according to a collaborative plan with attending physician if ICP remains elevated or CPP decreases outside parameters—usually ICP >15 to 20 mm Hg or CPP <60 to 70 mm Hg for 10 or more minutes. *Current recommendations are to manage CPP to maintain pressure ≥70 mm Hg for adults based on observations from the Trauma Coma Data Bank indicating CPP as the crucial variable related to outcome (Lang, Chesnut, 1995). A recent small controlled study in clients with severe head injury demonstrated better control of both ICP and CPP variations with a standardized protocol consistent with the American Severe Head Injury Guidelines (McKinley, Parmley, Tonneson, 1999; Chesnut, 1997b).*
- The plan will vary by region and individual physician preference but may include the following (Ghajar et al, 1995):
  - ▲ Cerebrospinal fluid (CSF) drainage via ventriculostomy intermittently to maintain a given ICP level *CSF drainage will manage CPP by reducing ICP at least temporarily. It does not change adaptive capacity (intracranial compliance) (Chesnut, 1995).*
  - ▲ Addition of sedation (e.g., morphine, midazolam, propofol) and analgesia with or without paralysis (e.g., atracurium, pancuronium [Pavulon]) if body movements or fighting respirator continuously stimulate a CPP decrease *The short-acting agents allow rapid reversal of both sedation and paralysis for short periods to provide periodic neurological examination (McClelland et al, 1995).*
  - ▲ Bolus administration of osmotic diuretic or other hyperosmotic agent (mannitol, mannitol plus furosemide); may be followed with continuous administration if CPP is not maintained with bolus administration *Note that it is essential to keep serum osmolality <320 mOsm/L to prevent hyperosmolality-related seizures. These agents primarily reduce vascular volume and not cerebral edema. The older practice of keeping clients volume depleted in an attempt to prevent cerebral edema is no longer advocated (Chesnut, 1995).*
  - ▲ Control hyperventilation, maintaining PCO_2 of 30 to 35 mm Hg unless ICP continues to be refractory, in which case PCO_2 may be briefly decreased below 30 mm Hg if ICP is responsive *Older standards of early hyperventilation of clients to levels as low as 25 mm Hg have been shown to have poorer outcomes than in similar clients not hyperventilated. Prophylactic use of hyperventilation may induce cerebral ischemia. Although many clinicians continue to use extreme hyperventilation, major trauma centers recommend this only as a last resort in refractory intracranial hypertension (Chesnut, 1995).*
- To prevent DIICP in clients at risk (clients with elevated P_2 waveforms and ICP of <10 mm Hg; clients previously responsive to general stimuli), do the following:
  - ▪ Maintain 15- to 30-degree head elevation if CPP is maintained at >70 mm Hg.
  - ▲ Maintain systemic blood pressure adequate to keep CPP ≥70 mm Hg by body positioning and use of vasoactive protocols.

- • = Independent; ▲ = Collaborative

- ▪ Maintain adequate respiratory status; suction if needed but not prophylactically.
- ▲ If suctioning required, may use aerosolized lidocaine to reduce associated coughing. Preoxygenate, hyperventilate only very briefly, and limit number of catheter passes to one or two (Kerr et al, 1993, 1997).
- ▪ Use gentle touching and talking or family visitations.
These activities rarely stimulate DIICP (Schinner et al, 1995). Family voices and gentle stroking may help stabilize ICP (Treloar et al, 1991; Mitchell, Ackerman, 1992; Hepworth, Hendrickson, Lopez, 1994; Mitchell, Habermann, 1999).
- ▲ Use mechanical turning beds if manual repositioning is a stimulus to DIICP.
These beds keep the head and neck in a neutral alignment and have been shown not to alter ICP overall (Mitchell, 1993).
  - ▪ Avoid 90-degree hip flexion and use of the knee gatch of the bed.
Hip flexion may trap venous blood in the intraabdominal space, increasing abdominal and intrathoracic pressure, which in turn reduces venous outflow from the head (Vos, 1993).
  - ▪ Sequence nursing care to allow for recovery of baseline ICP between noxious activities such as suctioning, and position changes that involve neck flexion.
Several studies have shown stairstep increases in ICP when a stimulus to DIICP is repeated several times within a short time (Mitchell, Ackerman, 1992; Kerr et al, 1993).
- • With regard to general ICP monitoring:
  - ▪ Monitor ICP and CPP continuously with alarm settings on.
Secondary brain injury can result from even brief periods of hypoxia and hypotension. Data from the Traumatic Coma Data Bank and international studies have documented that even in well-attended intensive care units, periods of more than 5 minutes of systemic hypotension (systolic blood pressure of <90 mm Hg) or intracranial hypertension occur in 70% to 90% of clients (Miller, 1993; Jones et al, 1994).
  - ▲ Notify physician if nursing interventions and collaborative protocols do not maintain a CPP of ≥70 mm Hg and an ICP of <20 mm Hg for adults; values may be lower for infants.
  - ▲ Monitor neurological status and CPP, including level of arousal, ability to follow commands, response to painful stimuli if arousal is decreased, and brainstem signs (pupil response, respiratory pattern, symmetry of motor response, and vital signs). Notify physician of signs of neurological deterioration regardless of levels of ICP and CPP.
Brain shift and herniation will be manifested by these changes in neurological status and may occur at any level of ICP. If the client is sedated and paralyzed to control ICP, pupillary changes or changes in response to painful stimuli may be the only available sign of deterioration (Ross et al, 1989; Mitchell, Ackerman, 1992).

Home Care Interventions

NOTE: Clients experiencing potentially rapid changes in ICP are not candidates for home care. However, clients experiencing potentially gradual changes in ICP (i.e., clients with developmental delays resulting from genetic dysfunction) may be served by home care with the following considerations:

- • Identify baseline neurological data before discharge from institutional care.
Baseline data will help both to identify changes in status and to create an individualized care plan.

• = **Independent;** ▲ = **Collaborative**

- Evaluate neurological functioning at regular intervals.
  Neurological function improvements require long-term intervention.
- Instruct the caregiver about the client-specific changes that will indicate increased ICP. Examples include changes in speech articulation and eye coordination, decreased ability to focus, increased seizure activity, and decreased coping ability. The nurse is cautioned that changes will be specific to the disability of the client.
  Early reporting of status changes allows for early intervention in neurologically impaired clients.

WEB SITES FOR EDUCATION

MERLIN See the MERLIN web site for World Wide Web resources for client education.

REFERENCES   Brimioulle S et al: Effects of positioning and exercise on intracranial pressure in a neurosurgical intensive care unit, *Phys Ther* 77:1682, 1997.

Chesnut RM: Medical management of severe head injury: present and future, *New Horiz* 3:581, 1995.

Chesnut RM: Avoidance of hypotension: conditio sine qua non of successful severe head-injury management, *J Trauma* 42(5 suppl):s4, 1997a.

Chesnut RM: Guidelines for the management of severe head injury, *J Trauma* 42(5 suppl):519-522, 1997b.

Ghajar J et al: Survey of critical care management of comatose, head-injured patients in the United States, *Crit Care Med* 23:560, 1995.

Hepworth JT, Hendrickson SG, Lopez J: Time series analysis of physiological response during ICU visitation, *West J Nurs Res* 16:704, 1994.

Jones PA et al: Measuring the burden of secondary insults in head-injured patients during intensive care, *J Neurosurg Anesthesiol* 6:4, 1994.

Kerr ME et al: Head-injured adults: recommendations for endotracheal suctioning, *J Neurosci Nurs* 25:86, 1993.

Kerr ME et al: Effect of short-duration hyperventilation during endotracheal suctioning in severe head-injured adults, *Nurs Res* 46:195, 1997.

Kerr ME et al: Effect of neuromuscular blockers and opiates on the cerebrovascular response to endotracheal suctioning in adults with severe head injuries, *Am J Crit Care* 7:205, 1998.

Lang EW, Chesnut RM: Intracranial pressure and cerebral perfusion pressure in severe head injury, *New Horiz* 3:400, 1995.

Lee S: Intracranial pressure changes during positioning of patients with severe head injury, *Heart Lung* 18:411, 1989.

March K et al: Effects of backrest position on ICP and CPP, *J Neurosci Nurs* 22:375, 1990.

McClelland M et al: Continuous midazolam/atracurium infusions for the management of increased intracranial pressure, *J Neurosci Nurs* 27:96, 1995.

McKinley BA, Parmley CL, Tonneson AS: Standardized management of intracranial pressure: a preliminary clinical trial, *J Trauma* 46:271, 1999.

Miller JD: Head injury, *J Neurol Neurosurg Psychiatry* 56:440, 1993.

Mitchell PH: Decreased adaptive capacity. In Kinney MR, Packa DR, Dunbar SB, editors: *AACN's clinical reference for critical care nursing*, ed 3, St Louis, 1993, Mosby.

Mitchell PH, Ackerman LL: Secondary brain injury reduction. In Bulechek GM, McCloskey JC, editors: *Nursing interventions*, ed 2, Philadelphia, 1992, WB Saunders.

Mitchell PH, Habermann B: Rethinking physiological stability: touch and intracranial pressure, *Biol Res Nurs* 1(1):12-19, 1999.

Mitchell PH et al: Waveform predictors: adverse response to nursing care: ICPX A, *Acta Neurochirurgica Supplementum* 71:420, 1998.

Rauch ME, Mitchell PH, Tyler ML: Validation of risk factors for the nursing diagnosis of decreased intracranial adaptive capacity, *J Neurosci Nurs* 22:173, 1990.

Ropper AH, O'Rourke D, Kennedy SK: Head position, intracranial pressure, and compliance, *Neurology* 32:1288, 1982.

Ross DA et al: Brain shift, level of consciousness and restoration of consciousness in patients with acute intracranial hematoma, *J Neurosurg* 71:498, 1989.

• = **Independent**; ▲ = **Collaborative**

Schinner KM et al: Effects of auditory stimuli on intracranial pressure and cerebral perfusion pressure in traumatic brain injury, *J Neurosci Nurs* 27:348, 1995.

Simmons BJ: Management of intracranial hemodynamics in the adult: a research analysis of head positioning and recommendations for clinical practice and future research, *J Neurosci Nurs* 29:44, 1997.

Treloar DM et al: The effect of familiar and unfamiliar voice treatments on intracranial pressure in head-injured patients, *J Neurosci Nurs* 23(5):295, 1991.

Vos HR: Making headway with intracranial hypertension, *Am J Nurse* 93:28, 1993.

Williams A, Coyne SM: Effects of neck position on intracranial pressure, *Am J Crit Care* 2:68, 1993.

Yordy M, Hanigan WC: Cerebral perfusion pressure in the high-risk premature infant, *Pediatr Neurosci* 12:226, 1985-1986.

Deficient Knowledge

Suzanne Skowronski and Gail B. Ladwig

NANDA **Definition** Absence or deficiency of cognitive information related to a specific topic

Defining Characteristics

Verbalization of the problem; inaccurate follow-through of instruction; inaccurate performance of test; inappropriate or exaggerated behaviors (e.g., hysterical, hostile, agitated, apathetic)

Related Factors (r/t)

Lack of exposure; lack of recall; information misinterpretation; cognitive limitation; lack of interest in learning; unfamiliarity with information resources

NOC **Outcomes (Nursing Outcomes Classification)**

Suggested NOC Labels

Knowledge of: Diet, Disease Process, Energy Conservation, Health Behaviors, Health Resources, Infection Control, Medication, Personal Safety, Prescribed Activity, Substance Use Control, Treatment Procedure(s), Treatment Regimen

> **Example NOC Outcome**
> Demonstrates **Knowledge of Health Behaviors** as evidenced by the following indicators: Description of healthy nutritional practices/Benefits of exercise/Safe use of prescription and nonprescription drugs (Rate each indicator of **Knowledge of Health Behaviors:** 1 = no knowledge, 2 = limited knowledge, 3 = moderate knowledge, 4 = substantial knowledge, 5 = extensive knowledge [see Section I])

Client Outcomes

- Explains disease state, recognizes need for medications, understands treatments
- Explains how to incorporate new health regimen into lifestyle
- States an ability to deal with health situation and remain in control of life
- Demonstrates how to perform procedure(s) satisfactorily
- Lists resources that can be used for more information or support after discharge

NIC **Interventions (Nursing Interventions Classification)**

Suggested NIC Labels

Teaching: Disease Process; Teaching: Individual; Teaching: Infant Care

• = Independent; ▲ = Collaborative

Example NIC Interventions—Teaching: Disease Process
- Discuss therapy/treatment options
- Explain rationale for management/therapy/treatment recommendations

Nursing Interventions and Rationales

- Observe client's ability and readiness to learn (e.g., mental acuity, ability to see or hear, no existing pain, emotional readiness, absence of language or cultural barriers).
  Education in self-care must take into account physical, sensory, mobility, sexual, and psychosocial changes related to age (Bohny, 1997).

- Assess barriers to learning (e.g., perceived change in lifestyle, financial concerns, cultural patterns, lack of acceptance by peers or coworkers).
  The client brings to the learning situation a unique personality, established social interaction patterns, cultural norms and values, and environmental influences (Bohny, 1997).

- Determine client's previous knowledge of or skills related to his or her diagnosis and the influence on willingness to learn.
  New information is assimilated into previous assumptions and facts and may involve negotiating, transforming, or stalling.

- Involve clients in writing specific outcomes for the teaching session, such as identifying what is most important to learn from their viewpoint and lifestyle.
  Objectives put the content into focus, provide a forum for evaluation outcomes, and ensure continuity. Client involvement improves compliance with health regimen and makes teaching and learning a partnership.

- When teaching, build on client's literacy skills.
  In patients with low literacy skills, materials should be short and have culturally sensitive illustrations (Mayeaux et al, 1996). The National Adult Literacy Survey reported that 44 million Americans could not read or write well enough to meet the needs of everyday living and working (Quirk, 2000).

- Present material that is most significant to client first, such as how to give injections or change dressings; present additional material once client's most pressing educational needs have been met.
  Information building begins with explaining simple concepts and moves on to explanations of complex application situations.

- Determine client's understanding of common medical terminology, such as "empty stomach," "emesis," and "palpation."
  Clients are expected to read and understand labels on medicine containers, appointment slips, and informed consents, yet an estimated 40 million adults are functionally illiterate (Williams et al, 1995).

- Evaluate the readability of the material in pamphlets or written instructions.
  Nonadherence of older adults to new medication regimens appears to be a function of decreased cognitive ability and comprehension of instruction, poor communication, and increased physical limitations (Hayes, 1998).

- Use visual aids such as diagrams, pictures, videotapes, audiotapes, and interactive Internet web sites.
  Verbal reinforcement of personalized, written instructions appears to be the best tested intervention. Computer-generated, personalized instructions improved adherence when compared with handwritten instructions (Hayes, 1998). This evidence-based study suggested leaflets as a useful resource for information provision (Kubba, 2000).

• = **Independent**; ▲ = **Collaborative**

- Provide preadmission self-instruction materials to prepare client for postoperative exercises.
  Providing clients with preadmission information about exercises has been shown to increase positive feelings and the ability to perform prescribed exercises (Rice et al, 1992).
- Identify the primary family support person; be aware of that person's ability to learn and incorporate needed changes.
- Assess willingness of family to incorporate new information, immunizations, medical/dental care, and diet/behavior modifications in support of the client.
  Attention needs to be directed at family adjustment factors. For example, women recovering from alcohol abuse are at risk for relapse if their spouse continues to drink alcohol (Murphy, 1993), and modification of eating patterns plus social and partnership support have had more success than modification alone (Keller et al, 1997).
- Help client identify community resources for continuing information and support.
  Learning occurs through imitation, so persons who are currently involved in lifestyle changes can help the client anticipate adjustment issues. Community resources can offer financial and educational support. For example, role modeling and skill training have been used to monitor symptoms and solve asthma problems (Bartholomew et al, 2000).
- Evaluate client's learning through return demonstrations, verbalizations, or the application of skills to new situations.
  Presenting information along with examples of how to apply the information has been found more successful than providing information alone in a home care setting (Duffy, 1997).

Geriatric

- Adapt the teaching process for the physical constraints of the aging process (e.g., speak clearly, use a variety of audio-visual-psychomotor methods, provide examples, and allow time for client to repeat and review).
  Adults are capable of learning at any age. Age modifies but does not inhibit learning (Dellasega et al, 1994). Older adults need practice to use new technology (Westerman, Davies, 2000).
- Ensure that the client uses necessary reading aids (e.g., glasses, magnifying lenses, large-print text) or hearing aids.
  Visual and hearing deficits require amplification or clarification of sensory input.
- Use printed material, videotapes, lists, diagrams, and Internet addresses that the client can refer to at another time.
  These methods provide a reference that can be used in a less stressful setting, decreasing barriers to learning. This study demonstrated the effectiveness of printed material and a web-based format for education. The web-based format demonstrated two additional benefits when compared with printed material: increased social support and decreased anxiety (Scherrer-Bannerman et al, 2000).
- Assess client's previous knowledge and resistance or blocks to incorporating new information into the current lifestyle.
  The client brings to the learning situation a unique personality, established social interaction patterns, cultural norms and values, and environmental influences (Bohny, 1997).
- Repeat and reinforce information during several brief sessions.
  Understanding past information is essential to acquiring new knowledge. Brief sessions focus attention on essential information.
- Discuss healthy lifestyle changes that promote wellness for the older adult.
  It is never too late to stop smoking, lose weight, or modify dietary intake of fats and alcohol. Quality vs. quantity of life may be the key issue in teaching self-care health

• = **Independent;** ▲ = **Collaborative**

habits (Walker, 1992).

- Evaluate readability of the material.
  Nonadherence of older adults to new medication regimens appears to be a function of decreased cognitive ability, comprehension of instruction, poor communication, and increased physical limitations (Hayes, 1998).
- Consider health education programs using television and newspapers.
  There was a significant increase in stroke knowledge (52% more likely to know a risk factor and 35% know a symptom, p = 0.032) following this health education program as demonstrated through a telephone pretest and posttest (Becker et al, 2001).

Multicultural

- Acknowledge racial/ethnic differences at the onset of care.
  Acknowledgement of racial/ethnicity issues will enhance communication, establish rapport, and promote treatment outcomes (D'Avanzo et al, 2001).
- Assess for the influence of cultural beliefs, norms, and values on the client's knowledge base.
  The client's knowledge base may be influenced by cultural perceptions (Leininger, 1996).
- Use a neutral indirect style when addressing areas where improvement is needed when working with Native American clients.
  Using indirect statements such as "I had a client who tried 'X' and it seemed to work very well" will help avoid resentment from the client (Seiderman et al, 1996).
- Validate the client's feelings and concerns related to previous learning experiences.
  Validation lets the client know the nurse has heard and understands what was said. (Stuart, Laraia, 2001; Giger, Davidhizar, 1995).
- Approach individuals of color with respect, warmth, and professional courtesy.
  Instances of disrespect and lack of caring have special significance for individuals of color (D'Avanzo et al, 2001).

Home Care Interventions

NOTE: Because home care is an intermittent model of care having a goal of safety and optimal wellness of the client between visits, the importance of teaching (by nurse) and learning (by client) should not be understated. All of the previously mentioned interventions are applicable to the home setting.

- Select a space and time for teaching in which client and/or caregiver can focus on information to be learned.
  The home setting provides many distractions that may impair the ability of the client to learn.
- Consider the complexity of material or behaviors to be learned. Adjust care plan and respective teaching and learning experiences accordingly to build client confidence in ability to learn (and change).
  Confidence in ability to learn and change is part of readiness to learn.
- Assess for specific areas of learning that have the potential for strong emotional responses by the client or family/caregiver. Allow time for expression of feelings and encourage acceptance of need for learning.
  An individual's perception of barriers and benefits has consistently been most predictive of subsequent behavior. Clinicians should develop interventions that increase benefits and decrease barriers (Fenn, 1998).
- Document client's and caregivers' responses to learning.
  Clear documentation supports continuity in the learning experience.

• = Independent; ▲ = Collaborative

REFERENCES   Bartholomew LK et al: Watch, discover, think, and act: a model for patient education program development, *Patient Educ Couns* 39(2-3):269-280, 2000

Becker K et al: Community-based education improves stroke knowledge, *Cerebrovasc Dis* 11(1):34-43, 2001.

Bohny B: A time for self-care: role of the home healthcare nurse, *Home Healthc Nurse* 15(4):281-286, 1997.

D'Avanzo CE et al: Developing culturally informed strategies for substance-related interventions. In Naegle MA, D'Avanzo CE, editors: *Addictions and substance abuse: strategies for advanced practice nursing,* St Louis, 2001, Mosby, pp 59-104.

Dellasega D et al: Nursing process: teaching elderly clients, *J Gerontol Nurs* 31:20, 1994.

Duffy B: Using a creative teaching process with adult patients, *Home Healthc Nurse* 15(2):102-108, 1997.

Fenn M: Health promotion: theoretical perspectives and clinical applications, *Holistic Nurs Pract* 12(2):1-7, 1998.

Giger JN, Davidhizar RE: *Transcultural nursing,* ed 2, St Louis, 1995, Mosby.

Hayes K: Randomized trial of geragogy-based medication instruction in the emergency department, *Nurs Res* 47(4):211-218, 1998.

Keller C et al: Strategies for weight control success in adults, *Nurse Pract* 22(3):37-38, 40, 1997.

Kubba H: An evidence-based patient information leaflet about otitis media with effusion, *Clin Perform Qual Health Care* 8(2):93-99, 2000.

Leininger MM: *Transcultural nursing: theories, research and practices,* ed 2, Hilliard, Ohio, 1996, McGraw-Hill.

Mayeaux EJ et al: Improving patient education for patients with low literacy skills, *Am Physician* 53(1):205-211, 1996.

Murphy SP: Coping strategies of abstainers from alcohol 3 years to post treatment, *Image J Nurs Sch* 25:32, 1993.

Quirk PA: Screening for literacy and readability: implications for the advanced practice nurse, *Clin Nurse Spec* 14(1):26-32, 2000.

Rice VH et al: Preadmission self-instruction effects on preadmission and postoperative indicators in CABG patients partial replication and extension, *Res Nurs Health* 15:253, 1992.

Scherrer-Bannerman A et al: Waiting list, *J Telemed Telecare,* 6 Suppl 2:S72-S74, 2000.

Seiderman RY et al: Assesing American Indian families, *Am J Mat Child Nurs* 21(6):274-279, 1996.

Stuart GW, Laraia MT: Therapeutic nurse-patient relationship. In Stuart GW, Laraia MT, editors: *Principles and practice of psychiatric nursing,* St Louis, 2001, Mosby, p 30.

Walker S: Wellness for elders, *Holistic Nurs Pract* 38:7, 1992.

Westerman SJ, Davies DR; Acquisition and application of new technology skills: the influence of age, *Occup Med (Lond)* 50(7):478-482, 2000.

Williams M et al: Inadequate functional health literacy among patients at two public hospitals, *JAMA* 274:1677, 1995.

Risk for Loneliness

Gail B. Ladwig, Marty Martin

NANDA   **Definition** At risk for experiencing vague dysphoria

Risk Factors

Affectional deprivation; social isolation; cathectic deprivation; physical isolation

Related Factors (r/t)

See Risk Factors

NOC   **Outcomes (Nursing Outcomes Classification)**

Suggested NOC Labels

Loneliness; Social Interaction Skills; Social Involvement; Social Support

• = Independent; ▲ = Collaborative

> **Example NOC Outcome**
> Demonstrates **Social Involvement** as evidenced by interaction with close friends, neighbors, family members and work groups (Rate **Social Involvement:** 1 = none, 2 = limited, 3 = moderate, 4 = substantial, 5 = extensive [see Section I])

Client Outcomes

- Maintains one or more meaningful relationships (growth enhancing vs. codependent or abusive in nature)—relationships allowing self-disclosure—and demonstrates a balance between emotional dependence and independence
- Participates in ongoing positive and relevant social activities and interactions that are personally meaningful
- Demonstrates positive use of time alone when socialization is not possible

NIC   Interventions (Nursing Interventions Classification)

Suggested NIC Labels

Family Integrity Promotion; Socialization Enhancement; Visitation Facilitation

> **Example NIC Interventions—Socialization Enhancement**
> - Encourage involvement in already established relationships
> - Use role playing to practice improved communication skills and techniques

Nursing Interventions and Rationales

- Establish a therapeutic relationship by being emotionally present and authentic.
  Being emotionally present and authentic fosters growth in relationships and decreases isolation (Jordan, 2000).
- Assess client's perception of loneliness. (Is the person alone by choice or is the aloneness imposed by others?)
  *Social isolation is perceived by others, loneliness is not. See care plan for **Social isolation**, an important nursing diagnosis because it is often a precursor to loneliness (Buchda, 1987).*
- Assist client with identifying loneliness as a feeling and the causes related to loneliness.
  Loneliness was the number one fear identified. Chi Square analysis showed that homeless who did not stay in shelters were significantly longer-term residents (p <0.0001) of the community and reported fear of loneliness significantly more frequently (Reichenbach, McNamee, Seibel, 1998).
- Assess client's social support system.
  Use a social support tool or validated assessment tool if possible (e.g., UCLA Loneliness Scale for adolescents [Mahon, Yarcheski, Yarcheski, 1995]).
- Assess client's ability and/or inability to meet physical, psychosocial, spiritual, and financial needs and how unmet needs further challenge ability to be socially integrated (e.g., loss of job leading to inability to afford usual and familiar social interaction, fatigue; lack of energy necessary for social interaction and personal engagement; impaired skin integument and its relationship to real and/or perceived social isolation). NOTE: See care plan for **Disturbed Body image** if loneliness is associated with impaired skin integument.
  Assessment of overall human needs gives direction to the care and treatment of nursing diagnostic categories such as loneliness (O'Brien, Pheiffer, 1993). A tool that measures the sense of belonging is important in addressing the relationship between social support and

• = Independent; ▲ = Collaborative

physical illness (particularly cardiac disease) and mortality (Case et al, 1992; House, Landis, Umberson, 1988).

- Use active listening skills including assessment and clarification of client's verbal and nonverbal responses and interactions.
  Using therapeutic observation and listening skills helps to accurately assess and validate this diagnosis. Clients are often unable to identify the problems or factors that directly contribute to their sense of isolation (O'Brien, Pheiffer, 1993).

- Evaluate client's desire for social interaction in relation to actual social interaction.
  The concept of loneliness involves a discrepancy between the client's desired and achieved level of social interaction (Christian, Dluhy, O'Neill, 1989).

- Assess client's interpersonal skills and address deficits and behaviors that are blocking communication.

- Encourage client to be involved in meaningful social relationships that are characteristic of both giving and receiving support.
  It is important to recognize that the positive relevance of social relationships is related to the content and quality of relationships (Gulick, 1994).

- Explore ways to increase client's support system and participation in groups and organizations.
  Studies indicate that people with smaller support systems have higher levels of loneliness than those with larger support systems (Mahon, 1982). Peer support is helpful for clients in the mental health system (Lynch, 2000).

- Encourage client to develop closeness in at least one relationship.
  Dependence and independence should be balanced in healthy relationships. Previous research has indicated that the development of a balanced level of emotional dependence and the ability to self-disclose are important factors in reducing the risk for loneliness (Mahon, 1982; Mahon, Yarcheski, 1992).

Adolescents

- See References for assessment tool.
- Evaluate the depth and level of character traits, shyness, and self-esteem, particularly of younger and middle adolescent clients.
- Evaluate the family stability of younger and middle adolescent clients and advocate and encourage healthy, growth-producing relationships with family and support systems.
  This study showed a fear of intimacy and loneliness among adolescents who were taught during childhood not to trust strangers (Terrell, Terrell, Von Drashek, 2000).

- For older adolescents, encourage close relationships with peers and involvement with groups and organizations.
  Research indicates that younger adolescents are at a higher risk for loneliness if they are shy or have low self-esteem. Younger adolescents rely more on parental relationships. An expanded set of relationships becomes increasingly important in alleviating loneliness as adolescents mature (Mahon, Yarcheski, 1992).

- Consider use of pets to cope with loneliness.
  In this study of homeless youths, participants identified pets as companions that provide unconditional love and decrease feelings of loneliness (Rew, 2000).

Geriatric

- Identify community support systems specific to elderly populations.
  Aging is often accompanied by significant losses of family members and other social support systems, which may lead to loneliness and depression. A study of residents of a nursing

• = **Independent;** ▲ = **Collaborative**

facility showed that social relationships with other residents was a strong predictor of decreased depression and loneliness (Fessman, Lester, 2000).

- Consider a retirement village.
  In this study of 323 residents in 25 retirement villages, participants reported that isolation and loneliness decreased when clients relocated to a retirement village (Buys, 2001).
- Encourage support by friends and family when the decision to stop driving must be made.
  In this study, increased loneliness and isolation affected the older driver, although an enhanced sense of responsibility was evident among friends and family. Findings suggest that the support offered by friends and family played a significant role in the decision to stop driving (Johnson, 1998).
- Assess client's adaptive sensory functions or any other health deviations that may limit or decrease his or her ability to interact with others.
- ▲ Assess client's potential or actual hearing loss or hearing impairment and make appropriate referrals if a problem is identified.
  Research shows that hearing loss is one of the most prevalent chronic health problems of the elderly in the United States (Christian, Dluhy, O'Neill, 1989). Because of the nature of this sensory deprivation, communication barriers are increased and human intimacy and self-esteem are negatively affected (Chen, 1994). In addition, it is important to note that hearing impairments often go unnoticed and may not be obvious as are more visibly recognized handicaps (Chen, 1994).
- Encourage physical activity such as aerobics or stretching and toning in a group.
  These activities decreased loneliness in former sedentary adults (n = 174, median age = 65.5 years) (McAuley et al, 2000).
- Encourage positive use of solitude to prevent loneliness (e.g., reading, listening to music, enjoying nature).
  The positive use of solitude and a decreased dependence on external stimuli may be particularly important for older individuals, who often find themselves alone without external stimuli or social support.
- Provide reading materials for clients who are able to read.
  Older people who enjoyed reading for pleasure were rarely lonely (Rane-Szotak, Herth, 1994).

Home Care Interventions

- ▲ If the client is experiencing somatic complaints, evaluate client complaints to ensure physical needs are being met, then identify relationship between somatic complaints and loneliness.
  Loneliness precipitates somatic complaints and sleeplessness.
- Help client to identify periods when loneliness is greatest (e.g., certain times of day, anniversaries of past special events). With client permission, refer for services of visiting volunteers.
  The only agenda of visiting volunteers is to meet the social needs of the client. Long-term friendships sometimes develop from volunteer experiences.
- To keep older people independent, interventions to prevent loneliness should be explored.
  Study shows that extreme loneliness predicts admission to the nursing home (PSL Consulting Group, 1999).
- Identify alternatives to eating alone.
  Clients are often susceptible to loneliness at mealtimes. Loneliness may contribute to nutritional deficiencies or excesses.
- Identify alternatives to being alone (e.g., telephone contact).

- **• = Independent; ▲ = Collaborative**

- Provide opportunities for the client to contribute to the social well-being of others. Homebound clients can contribute via the telephone.
  Contributing to society enhances self-esteem and decreases loneliness. Loss of meaning contributes to loneliness.
- Support religious beliefs.
  Belief in a Supreme Being provides a feeling of ever-present help and prevents loneliness. If clients have regrets about their life, they may be separated from their usual source of religious comfort.
- Discuss the meaning of death and fears associated with dying alone. Explore the possibility of significant others being with the client at time of death.
  In later stages of life, individuals give significant thought to death and the meaning of their life. If they perceive their life as undesirable, they may fear death.

Client/Family Teaching

- Encourage positive use of solitude to prevent loneliness (e.g., reading, listening to music, enjoying nature).
  A positive use of solitude plays a strong role in preventing or alleviating loneliness. The mentioned activities are flow activities—self-directed, independent activities that enhance well-being and decrease feelings of loneliness (Rane-Szotak, Herth, 1994).
- Include the family in all client teaching activities, and give them accurate information regarding the illness severity.
  The family can also experience loneliness. Clients and families often have grossly different perceptions of the severity and threats of illness. The family often perceives the person to be much more ill than the ill person does. A realistic understanding of the person, family, and significant others will decrease the emotional threats of illness (Buchda, 1987).
- Give family members something to do such as holding a hand, applying lotion, or assisting with feeding.
  Facilitation of an individual's sense of relatedness to significant others can reduce loneliness for critically ill clients. Providing a specific task increases the quality of the interaction (Buchda, 1987).
- Encourage family members to express caring by telling the client where they will be and sending messages when they cannot be present.
  Keeping the client informed is a way of expressing caring and helps reduce loneliness (Buchda, 1987). If people could spare a smile or a word for others who might be perceived as lonely, even if in doing so they selfishly think "there but for the grace of God go I," such a small gesture might just make the day of a lonely person a little less of an ordeal (Killeen, 1998). Everyone is lonely to some degree, no matter how much they pretend they are not: it is part of the human condition. Loneliness is such an innate part of the human psyche that it cannot be solved like a puzzle; it can only be alleviated and made less painful. This can only be achieved by increasing humankind's awareness of this distressing condition that everyone has to endure in some way, shape or form, sometime during their lives, about which there is nothing to be embarrassed (Killeen, 1998).

Multicultural

- Acknowledge racial/ethnic differences at the onset of care.
  Acknowledgment of racial/ethnicity issues will enhance communication, establish rapport, and promote treatment outcomes (D'Avanzo et al, 2001).
- Assess for the influence of cultural beliefs, norms, and values on the client's perception of social activity and relationships.

• = Independent; ▲ = Collaborative

What the client considers normal social interaction may be based on cultural perceptions (Leininger, 1996).

- Approach individuals of color with respect, warmth, and professional courtesy.
  Instances of disrespect and lack of caring have special significance for individuals of color and may impede efforts to increase social outlets (D'Avanzo et al, 2001).
- Assess the use of personal space needs, communication styles, acceptable body language, eye contact, perception of touch, and use of paraverbals when communicating with the client.
  Nurses need to consider these when interpreting verbal and nonverbal messages (Siantz, 1991). Native Americans may consider avoidance of direct eye contact as a sign of respect and asking questions to be rude and intrusive (Seiderman et al, 1996).
- Use a family-centered approach when working with Latino, Asian, African-American, and Native American clients.
  Latinos may perceive family as source of support, solver of problems, and a source of pride. Asian Americans may regard the family as the primary decision maker and influence on individual family members (D'Avanzo et al, 2001).
- Promote a sense of ethnic attachment.
  Older Korean clients with strong ethnic attachments had lower levels of loneliness than those without strong attachments (Kim, 1999).
- Validate the client's feelings regarding isolation and loneliness.
  Validation lets the client know that the nurse has heard and understands what was said, and it promotes the nurse-client relationship (Stuart, Laraia, 2001; Giger, Davidhizar, 1995).

WEB SITES FOR EDUCATION

Merlin See the MERLIN web site for World Wide Web resources for client education.

REFERENCES   Buchda V: Loneliness in critically ill adults, *Dimens Crit Care Nurs* 6:335, 1987.

Buys LR: Life in a retirement village: implications for contact with community and village friends, *Gerontology* 47(1):55-59, 2001.

Case R et al: Living alone after myocardial infarction: impact on prognosis, *JAMA* 267:515, 1992.

Chen H: Hearing in the elderly, relation of healing loss, loneliness, and self-esteem, *J Gerontol Nurs* 20:22, 1994.

Christian E, Dluhy E, O'Neill R: Sounds of silence, *J Gerontol Nurs* 15:4, 1989.

D'Avanzo CE et al: Developing culturally informed strategies for substance-related interventions. In Naegle MA, D'Avanzo CE, editors: *Addictions and substance abuse: strategies for advanced practice nursing*, St Louis, 2001, Mosby, pp 59-104.

Fessman N, Lester D: Loneliness and depression among elderly nursing home patients, *Int J Aging Hum Dev* 51(2):137-141, 2000.

Giger JN, Davidhizar RE: *Transcultural nursing*, ed 2, St Louis, 1995, Mosby.

Gulick E: Social support among persons with multiple sclerosis, *Res Nurs Health* 17:195, 1994.

House J, Landis K, Umberson D: Social relationships and health, *Science* 241:540, 1988.

Johnson J: Older rural adults and the decision to stop driving: the influence of family and friends, *J Community Health Nurs* 15(4):205-216, 1998.

Jordan JV: The role of mutual empathy in relational/cultural therapy, *J Clin Psychol* 56(8):1005-1016, 2000.

Killeen C: Loneliness: an epidemic in modern society, *J Adv Nurs* 28(4):762-770, 1998.

Kim O: Mediation effect of social support between ethnic attachment and loneliness in older Korean immigrants, *Res Nurs Health* 22(2):169-175, 1999.

Leininger MM: *Transcultural nursing: theories, research and practices*, ed 2, Hilliard, Ohio, 1996, McGraw-Hill.

Lynch K: The long road back, *J Clin Psychol* 56(11):1427-1432, 2000.

Mahon NE: The relationship of self-disclosure, interpersonal dependency, and life changes to loneliness in young adults, *Nurs Res* 31:343, 1982.

• = **Independent;** ▲ = **Collaborative**

Mahon NE, Yarcheski A: Alternate explanations of loneliness in adolescents: a replication and extension study, *Nurs Res* 41:151, 1992.

Mahon NE, Yarcheski T, Yarcheski A: Validation of the revised UCLA loneliness scale for adolescents, *Res Nurs Health* 18:263, 1995.

McAuley E et al: Social relations, physical activity, and well-being in older adults, *Prev Med* 31(5):608-617, 2000.

O'Brien ME, Pheiffer W: Physical and psychosocial nursing care for patients with HIV infection, *Nurs Clin North Am* 28:303, 1993.

PSL Consulting Group: *Loneliness may foreshadow nursing home admission*, doctor's guide, retrieved on March 31, 1999, from the World Wide Web. Web site: www.pslgroup.com/dg/56afe.htm

Rane-Szotak D, Herth K: A new perspective on loneliness in later life, *Issues Ment Health Nurs* 16:583, 1994.

Reichenbach E, McNamee M, Seibel L: The community health nursing implications of the self-reported health status of a local homeless population, *Public Health Nurs* 15(6):398-405, 1998.

Rew L: Friends and pets as companions: strategies for coping with loneliness among homeless youth, *J Child Adolesc Psychiatr Nurs* 13(3):125-132, 2000.

Seiderman RY et al: Assessing American Indian families, *MCN Am J Matern Child Nurs* 21(6):274-279, 1996.

Siantz ML: How can we be more aware of culturally specific body language and use this awareness therapeutically? *J Psychosocial Nurs Ment Health Serv* 29(11):38-41, 1991.

Stuart GW, Laraia MT: Therapeutic nurse-patient relationship. In Stuart GW, Laraia MT, editors: *Principles and practice of psychiatric nursing*, St Louis, 2001, Mosby, p 30.

Terrell F, Terrell IS, Von Drashek SR: Loneliness and fear of intimacy among adolescents who were taught not to trust strangers during childhood, *Adolescence* 35(140):611-617, 2000.

Impaired Memory

Betty J. Ackley

NANDA   **Definition** Inability to remember or recall bits of information or behavioral skills; impaired memory may be attributed to pathophysiological or situational causes that are either temporary or permanent

Defining Characteristics

Inability to recall factual information; inability to recall recent or past events; inability to learn or retain new skills or information; inability to determine whether a behavior was performed; observed or reported experiences of forgetting; inability to perform a previously learned skill; forgets to perform a behavior at a scheduled time

Related Factors (r/t)

Fluid and electrolyte imbalance; neurological disturbances; excessive environmental disturbances; anemia; acute or chronic hypoxia; decreased cardiac output

NOC   **Outcomes (Nursing Outcomes Classification)**

Suggested NOC Labels

Cognitive Orientation; Memory; Neurological Status: Consciousness

> **Example NOC Outcome**
> Improves **Memory** as evidenced by the following indicators: Recalls immediate information accurately/Recalls recent information accurately/Recalls remote information accurately (Rate each indicator of **Memory:** 1 = never demonstrated, 2 = rarely demonstrated, 3 = sometimes demonstrated, 4 = often demonstrated, 5 = consistently demonstrated [see Section I])

• = **Independent;** ▲ = **Collaborative**

Client Outcomes

- Demonstrates use of techniques to help with memory loss
- States has improved memory

NIC Interventions (Nursing Interventions Classification)

Suggested NIC Labels

Memory Training

> **Example NIC Interventions—Memory Training**
> - Stimulate memory by repeating patient's last expressed thought, as appropriate
> - Provide opportunity to use memory for recent events, such as questioning patient about a recent outing

Nursing Interventions and Rationales

- Assess neurological function; use an assessment tool such as the metamemory in adulthood (MIA) questionnaire or the Mini-Mental State Examination (MMSE). *The MIA is reliable and nonthreatening and has been validated to be effective (McDougall, Balyer, 1998). The MMSE can help determine whether the client has memory loss only or also has delirium or dementia and needs to be referred for further treatment (Breitner, Welsh, 1995).*

▲ Determine whether onset of memory loss is gradual or sudden. If memory loss is sudden, refer client to a physician for evaluation. *Acute onset of memory loss may be associated with neurological disease, electrolyte disturbances, hypoxia, hypothyroidism, mental illness, or many other physiological factors (Vinson, 1989; Breitner, Welsh, 1995; Elliott, 2000).*

- Determine amount and pattern of alcohol intake. *Alcohol intake has been associated with blackouts; clients may function but not remember their actions. Long-term alcohol use causes Korsakoff's syndrome with associated memory loss (Vinson, 1989). Heavy alcohol use by adolescents can impair brain function, including memory (Brown et al, 2000).*

▲ Note client's current medications and intake of any mind-altering substances such as benzodiazepines, marijuana, cocaine, or glucocorticoids. *Benzodiazepines can produce memory loss for events that occur after taking the medication; information is not stored in long-term memory (Mejo, 1992; Fluck et al, 1998). In adolescents, excessive marijuana use has been shown to result in selective short-term memory deficits that continue at least 6 weeks after discontinuing intake of the drug (Schwartz et al, 1989). Cocaine abuse has been shown to decrease memory (Butler, Frank, 2000). Glucocorticoid therapy can cause a mild decrease in memory function that is usually reversible once a person is off the medications (Wolkowitz et al, 1997). Clients receiving long-term prednisone performed significantly worse on memory tasks than matched control subjects (Keenan, 1996).*

- Note client's current level of stress. Ask if there has been a recent traumatic event. *Post-traumatic stress and anxiety-inducing general life factors can cause memory problems (Mejo, 1992). Elevated cortisol levels associated with stress have been shown to impair memory (Lupien et al, 1994, 1997; Greendale et al, 2000).*

▲ If stress is associated with memory loss, refer to a stress reduction clinic. If not available, suggest that client meditate, exercise, receive massages, or take whatever actions necessary to relieve the stress. *Nonpharmacological therapy for treatment of stress syndromes is preferable and less likely to aggravate memory loss than commonly used antianxiety medications (Mejo, 1992).*

• = Independent; ▲ = Collaborative

▲ If signs of depression such as weight loss, insomnia, or sad affect are evident, refer client for psychotherapy.

Depression is commonly associated with memory loss (Mejo, 1992). Depression can result in source memory errors, in which case the client is not sure if he or she did something or just thought about doing it (Elias, 2001).

▲ Perform a nutritional assessment. If nutritional status is marginal, confer with a dietitian and primary care practitioner to evaluate if client needs supplementation with foods or vitamins. Teach client the need to eat a healthy diet with adequate intake of whole grains, fruits, and vegetables to decrease cerebrovascular infarcts.

Moderate, long-term deficiencies of nutrients may lead to loss of memory. This condition may be preventable or diminished through diet (Cataldo, DeBruyne, Whitney, 1999). Adequate levels of vitamin E may help protect memory (Miller, 2000).

▲ Question client about cholesterol level. If high, refer to physician or dietitian for help in lowering.

One study demonstrated that individuals who were prescribed statin medications that lowered cholesterol had a substantially lowered risk of developing dementia (Jick et al, 2000).

• Encourage client to use a calendar for appointments, keep reminder lists, place a string around finger or rubber band around wrist as reminders, or enlist someone else to remind him or her of important events.

Using reminders can serve as cues for memory-impaired clients.

• Help client set up a medication box that reminds client to take medication at needed times; assist client with refilling the box at intervals if necessary.

Medication boxes are effective because clients will know whether medication has been taken when corresponding compartments are empty.

• If safety is an issue with certain activities (e.g., client forgets to turn off stove after use or forgets emergency telephone numbers), suggest alternatives such as using a microwave or whistling teakettle for heating water and programming emergency numbers in telephone so that they are readily available.

These measures can increase client safety (Agostinelli et al, 1994).

▲ Refer client to a memory clinic (if available), a neuropsychologist, or an occupational therapist.

Memory clinics can help the client learn ways to improve memory. Clinics may be more effective if work is done in groups because of increased support, reinforcement, and motivation (McDougall, 1999). Neuropsychologists have expertise in working with the memory impaired, as do many occupational therapists (Robinson, 1992).

• Suggest clients use cues, including alarm watches, electronic organizers, calenders, lists, or pocket computers, to trigger certain actions at designated times.

Cues can help remind clients of certain actions (Wilson, Moffat, 1992); these external cognitive strategies can be effective (McDougall, 1999).

• For clients with memory impairments associated with dementia, see care plan for **Chronic Confusion.**

Geriatric

• Assess for signs of depression.

Depression is the most important affective variable for memory loss in the older adult (Byers, 1993; McDougall, 1999). Cognitive impairment is not an inevitable consequence of aging, even in very old age (Snowdon, 1997).

• = Independent; ▲ = Collaborative

▲ Evaluate all medications that client is taking to determine whether they are causing the memory loss.
Many medications can cause memory loss in the elderly, including anticholinergics, H2-receptor antagonists, beta-blockers, digitalis, benzodiazepines, barbiturates, and even mild opiates (DeMaagd, 1995; Sjogren, Thomsen, Olsen, 2000).

• Recommend that elderly clients maintain a positive attitude and active involvement with the world around them, as well as good nutrition.
Findings from the Nun Study demonstrated that it is possible to maintain good cognitive function until extreme old age if elderly persons maintain active involvement with their environment and are able to avoid having vascular disease with infarction of brain tissue. Cognitive impairment is not an inevitable consequence of aging and disease (Snowdon, 1997).

• Encourage the elderly to believe in themselves and to work to improve their memory.
Elderly clients may be able to improve their memory function up to 50% if they use appropriate strategies and invest the energy and time (Keen, 1998). New research has shown that there is formation of new neurons in the brain, a process called neurogenesis, throughout the lifespan, and stimulation of the brain is necessary for this formation (Eriksson et al, 1998).

▲ Refer client to a memory class that focuses on helping older adults learn memory strategies.
Research has demonstrated that classes that focus on memory strategies can improve memory (McDougall, Bayler, 1998).

• Help family develop a memory aid booklet or wallet that contains pictures and labels from client's life.
Using memory aids helps clients with dementia make more factual statements and stay on topic and decreases the number of confused, erroneous, and repetitive statements made (Bourgeois, 1992).

• Help family label items such as the bathroom or sock drawer to increase recall.
A supportive environment that includes orientation can help increase the client's awareness (Green, Gildemeister, 1994).

Multicultural

• Assess for the influence of cultural beliefs, norms, and values on the family or caregiver's understanding of impaired memory.
What the family considers normal and abnormal health behavior may be based on cultural perceptions (Leininger, 1996).

• Use bias-free instruments when assessing memory in the culturally diverse client.
Use of the MMSE without modification for ethnic bias resulted in younger Hispanics being categorized as more severely impaired than others (Mulgrew et al, 1999).

• Inform client's family or caregiver of meaning of and reasons for common behavior observed in client with impaired memory.
An understanding of impaired memory behavior will enable the client family/caregiver to provide the client with a safe environment.

• Validate family members' feelings regarding the impact of client's behavior on family lifestyle.
Validation lets the client know that the nurse has heard and understands what was said, and it promotes the nurse-client relationship (Stuart, Laraia, 2001; Giger, Davidhizar, 1995).

• = Independent; ▲ = Collaborative

Home Care Interventions

- Identify a checking-in support system (e.g., Lifeline or significant others).
  Checking in ensures client safety.
- Keep furniture placement and household patterns consistent.
  Change increases risk of impaired memory and decreased functioning.

Client/Family Teaching

- When teaching client, determine what the client knows about memory techniques and then build on that knowledge.
  New material is organized in terms of what knowledge already exists, and efficient teaching should attempt to take advantage of what is already known in order to graft on new material (Wilson, Moffat, 1992).
- When teaching a skill to client, set up a series of practice attempts. Begin with simple tasks so that client can be positively reinforced and progress to more difficult concepts.
  Distributed practice with correct recall attempts can be a very effective teaching strategy. Widely distribute practice over time if possible (Wilson, Moffat, 1992).
- Teach clients to use memory techniques such as repeating information they want to remember, making mental associations to remember information, and placing items in strategic places so that they will not be forgotten.
  These methods increase recall of information the client thinks is important. The internal methods of increasing memory can be effective, especially if used along with external methods such as calenders, lists, and other methods (McDougall, 1999).

WEB SITES FOR EDUCATION

Merlin See the MERLIN web site for World Wide Web resources for client education.

REFERENCES Agostinelli B et al: Targeted interventions: use of the Mini-Mental State Exam, *J Gerontol Nurs* 20:15, 1994.

Bourgeois MS: *Conversing with memory impaired individuals using memory aids: a memory aid workbook,* Gaylord, Mich, 1992, Northern Speech Services.

Breitner JC, Welsh KA: Diagnosis and management of memory loss and cognitive disorders among elderly persons, *Psychiatr Serv* 46:29, 1995.

Brown et al: Neurocognitive functioning of adolescents: effects of protracted alcohol use, *Alcohol Clin Exp Res* 24(2):164-171, 2000.

Butler LF, Frank EM: Neurolinguistic function and cocaine abuse, *J Med Speech Lang Pathol* 8(3):199-212, 2000.

Byers PH: Older adults' metamemory: coping, depression, and self-efficacy, *Appl Nurs Res* 6:28, 1993.

Cataldo CB, DeBruyne LK, Whitney EN: *Nutrition and diet therapy: principles and practice,* ed 5, Belmont, Calif, 1999, Wadsworth.

DeMaagd G: High-risk drugs in the elderly population, *Geriatr Nurs* 16:198, 1995.

Elias J: Why caregiver depression and self-care abilities should be part of the PPS case mix methodology, *Home Healthc Nurs* 19(1):23-30, 2001.

Elliott B: Case report. Diagnosing and treating hypothyroidism, *Nurs Pract* 25(3):92-94, 99-105, 2000.

Eriksson PS et al: Neurogenesis in the adult human hippocampus, *Nature Med* 4(11):1313-1317, 1998.

Fluck E et al: Does the sedation resulting from sleep deprivation and lorazepam cause similar cognitive deficits? *Pharmacol Biochem Behav* 59(4):909-915, 1998.

Giger JN, Davidhizar RE: *Transcultural nursing,* ed 2, St Louis, 1995, Mosby.

Green PM, Gildemeister JE: Memory aging research and memory support in the elderly, *J Neurosci Nurs* 26:241, 1994.

Greendale GA et al: Higher basal cortisol predicts verbal memory loss in postmenopausal women: Rancho Bernardo Study, *J Am Geriatr Soc* 48(12):1655-1658, 2000.

• = **Independent;** ▲ = **Collaborative**

Jick H et al: Statins and risk of dementia, *Lancet* 356(9242):1627-1631, 2000.

Keen C: Elderly should ignore stereotypes about memory loss, 1998. Web site: www.napa.ufl.edu/98news/eldermem.htm

Keenan PA: Chronic prednisone use causes memory loss, *Neurology* 47:1396-1402, 1996.

Leininger MM: *Transcultural nursing: theories, research and practices,* ed 2, Hilliard, Ohio, 1996, McGraw-Hill.

Lupien SJ et al: Basal cortisol levels and cognitive deficits in human aging, *J Neurosci* (5 Pt 1):2893-2903, 1994.

Lupien SJ et al: Stress-induced declarative memory impairment in healthy elderly subjects: relationship to cortisol reactivity, *J Clin Endocrinol Metab* 82(7):2070-2075, 1997.

McDougall GJ: Cognitive interventions among older adults, *Annu Rev Nurs Res* 17:219-240, 1999.

McDougall GJ, Balyer J: Decreasing mental frailty in at-risk elders, *Geriatr Nurs* 19(4):220-224, 1998.

Mejo SL: Anterograde amnesia linked to benzodiazepines, *Nurse Pract* 17:44, 1992.

Miller JW: Vitamin E and memory: is it vascular protection? *Nutr Rev* 58(4):109-111, 2000.

Mulgrew CL et al: Cognitive functioning and impairment among rural elderly Hispanics and non-Hispanic whites as assessed by the Mini-Mental State Exam, *J Gerontol B Psychol Sci Soc Sci* 54B(4):223-230, 1999.

Robinson S: Occupational therapy in a memory clinic, *Brit J Occup Ther* 55:394, 1992.

Schwartz RH et al: Short-term memory impairment in cannabis-dependent adolescents, *Am J Dis Child* 143(8):1214-1220, 1989.

Sjogren P, Thomsen AB, Olsen AK: Impaired neuropsychological performance in chronic nonmalignant pain patients receiving long-term oral opioid therapy, *J Pain Symptom Manage* 19(2):100-108, 2000.

Snowdon DA: Aging and Alzheimer's disease: lessons from the nun study, *Gerontologist* 37(2):150-156, 1997.

Stuart GW, Laraia MT, editors: *Principles and practice of psychiatric nursing,* St Louis, 2001, Mosby, p 30.

Vinson DC: Acute transient memory loss, *Am Fam Physician* 39:249, 1989.

Wilson BA, Moffat N: *Clinical management of memory problems,* San Diego, 1992, Singular.

Wolkowitz OM et al: Glucocorticoid medication, memory and steroid psychosis in medical illness, *Ann NY Acad Sci* 823:81-96, 1997.

Impaired bed Mobility

Brenda Emick-Herring

NANDA   **Definition** Limitation of independent movement from one bed position to another

Defining Characteristics

Impaired ability to turn from side to side; impaired ability to move from supine to sitting or sitting to supine; impaired ability to "scoot" or reposition self in bed; impaired ability to move from supine to prone or prone to supine; impaired ability to move from supine to long sitting or long sitting to supine

Related Factors (r/t)

Intolerance to activity; decreased strength and endurance; pain or discomfort; perceptual or cognitive impairment; neuromuscular impairment; musculoskeletal impairment; depression; severe anxiety

Suggested functional level classifications

0	Completely independent
1	Requires use of equipment or device
2	Requires help from another person
3	Requires help from another person and equipment device
4	Dependent—does not participate in activity

• = Independent; ▲ = Collaborative

Outcomes (Nursing Outcomes Classification)

Suggested NOC Labels

Joint Movement: Active; Self-Care: Activities of Daily Living (ADLs); Mobility Level

> **Example NOC Outcome**
> Demonstrates **Joint Movement: Active** as evidenced by self-initiated movement of the following joints: Fingers/Thumb/Wrist/Elbow/Shoulder/Ankle/Knee/Hip (Rate each indicator of **Joint Movement: Active:** 1 = no motion, 2 = limited motion, 3 = moderate motion, 4 = substantial motion, 5 = full motion [see Section I])

Client Outcomes

- Demonstrates optimal independence in positioning, exercising, and performing functional activities in bed
- Demonstrates ability to direct others on how to do bed positioning, exercising, and functional activities

NIC **Interventions (Nursing Interventions Classification)**

Suggested NIC Labels

Bed Rest Care

> **Example NIC Interventions—Bed Rest Care**
> - Position in proper alignment
> - Teach bed exercises as appropriate

Nursing Interventions and Rationales

▲ Perform accurate physical assessment to determine client's risk for increased intracranial pressure (ICP), respiratory abnormalities, aspiration, pressure ulcer formation, muscle tone abnormalities, and pain levels.
These conditions warrant certain bed positions to prevent complications (Mitchell, Ozuna, Lipe, 1981; Palmer, Wyness, 1988; Feldman et al, 1992; Panel for the Prediction and Prevention of Pressure Ulcers in Adults, 1992).

- Employ critical thinking and priority setting to decide the most therapeutic bed positions and frequency of turns based on client's history, risk profile, and preventative needs.
Positioning for one condition may negatively impact another. For example, elevation of head of bed is therapeutic for persons with increased ICP, tube feedings, and difficulty breathing but is contraindicated in persons with intravascular volume deficit, cervical traction, abnormal tone, reflexive posturing, and high risk for pressure ulcers (Mitchell, Ozuna, Lipe, 1981; Feldman et al, 1992; Arbour, 1998).

- If client has increased intracranial pressure, refer to care plan for **Decreased Intracranial adaptive capacity.**

- If client is dysphagic, assist to sit upright during and after feedings or ingestion of pills. Refer to care plan for **Impaired Swallowing.**
Sitting upright helps prevent aspiration of food, liquids, and pills in clients with dysphasia (Emick-Herring, Wood, 1990).

- Position client in an upright position at intervals as tolerated by condition. If possible, move client from bed to a "stretcher chair"—a stretcher that turns into a chair—to get out of bed and into a more vertical position.

- = Independent; ▲ = Collaborative

Being vertical reduces the work of the heart, changes intravascular pressure, and stimulates the neural reflexes. It improves lung ventilation and aeration at the base of the lungs, improves diaphragmatic movement, enhances symmetrical body alignment and awareness of the surroundings, and reduces abnormal posturing in the severely brain injured (Palmer, Wyness, 1988; Murphy, 1997). A review of studies on the effects of bed rest demonstrated that generally there are few indications for bed rest and that bed rest may delay recovery or cause harm to the client (Allen, Glasziou, Del Mar, 1999).

- Maintain the head of the bed at the lowest degree of elevation consistent with medical conditions and other restrictions to prevent pressure ulcer formation.
  Sacral shearing risk is high when the head of the bed is elevated past 30 degrees. Skin may stick to linens if clients slide down, causing skin to pull away from underlying tissue and potentially stretch or tear arteries, thereby reducing local blood flow (Maklebust, 1991; Panel for the Prediction of Pressure Ulcers in Adults, 1992). A 30-degree laterally inclined position puts less pressure on tissue than the 90-degree side lying position (Defloor, 2000).

- Position the bed flat at intervals, unless contraindicated for a medical reason.
  This helps maintain body alignment, which is a means of normalizing tone; prevents trunk and pelvic shortening in clients with hemiparesis; helps prevent forward head flexion in the elderly and those with Parkinson's disease or stroke; is the start position for most bed mobility tasks; and is the position of most clients' beds at home (Wilson, 1988; Kumagai, 1998).

- Prevent complications of immobility.
  The inability to be upright disturbs many body systems (Olson, 1967; Rubin, 1988; Murphy, 1997).

- Assess risk for pressure ulcer development and place client on foam, static air, alternating gel, or water mattress.
  Pressure-reducing devices such as these help prevent pressure ulcers caused by prolonged periods of lying in bed (Panel for the Prediction and Prevention of Pressure Ulcers in Adults, 1992).

- Encourage client to take deep breaths and cough at intervals.
  This prevents atelectasis and possible pneumonia (Carroll, 1996).

- Ensure that client receives adequate fiber and fluid, and recognize that he or she may need a stool softener to prevent constipation. Refer to care plan for **Constipation.**
  Immobility leads to constipation; however, increased fiber and fluids can help prevent constipation (Wong, Kadakia, 1999).

- Apply antiembolic stocking and sequential compression device to legs and encourage client to move lower extremities as tolerated. Refer to care plan for **Ineffective Tissue perfusion.**
  Immobility is a cause of deep vein thrombosis and pulmonary emboli, which can result from 3 or more days of bed rest (Ecklund, 1995).

- Encourage fluid intake of 2000 to 3000 ml/day as tolerated by medical condition.
  Increased fluids help flush mobilized calcium and bacteria from the body to prevent kidney stones and urinary infection (McCourt, 1993).

▲ Take scrupulous care of indwelling foley catheter if present, and detect and report signs of urinary tract infection as early as possible.
  Loss of weight bearing on bones and presence of an indwelling catheter can lead to increased urinary calculi and infection (Olson, 1967; McConnell, 1984; Rubin, 1988; Murphy, 1997).

• = Independent; ▲ = Collaborative

- Use the following interventions during bed mobility activities:
  - Place positioning devices such as pillows or foam wedges between bony prominences.
  - Use lifting devices such as a trapeze or bed linen to move (rather than drag) individuals in bed who cannot assist with position changes.
  - Avoid positioning persons directly on the trochanter bone when in side-lying position.

  These interventions protect against external mechanical forces (e.g., pressure, friction, and shear). Note, however, that use of a trapeze may be contraindicated in persons with cardiac disease and stroke because of their isotonic effect. Trapeze use is discouraged with persons with hemiplegia because movement and gripping with the sound arm elicits an "associated reaction" of abnormal tone and flexion in the hemiplegic side (Bobath, 1978; Panel for the Prediction and Prevention of Pressure Ulcers in Adults, 1992; Borgman-Gainer, 1996).

- Allow and encourage client bed mobility, repositioning, and self-care activities to prevent contractures and disuse syndromes.

  Chronic spasticity, immobility, and muscle atrophy related to connective tissue changes contribute to contractures (Finocchiaro, Herzfeld, 1998). Bed mobility prevents lymph fluid accumulation, which impedes movement, in the upper extremities of persons with dense hemiplegia (Borgman, Passarella, 1991). Leg and foot contractures may elicit discomfort in sitting or lying positions and may interfere with positioning options during sexual activity (Pires, 1984).

- Explain the importance of exhaling when pulling self up in bed or rolling, or during any other activity that may precipitate breath holding or straining.

  This prevents the Valsalva's maneuver and increased intraabdominal and intrathoracic pressure, which elevate blood pressure and impair myocardial and cerebral perfusion (Borgman-Gainer, 1996; Rodriguez, 1998).

- ▲ Assess pain level and administer adequate analgesics before bed repositioning, mobility, or self-care activities. Develop a specific preventative analgesic schedule with clients if chronic pain is experienced.

  Nurses must be willing to accept clients' definition and self-rating of pain and believe their need for analgesics (McCaffery, Pasero, 1999).

- Assist clients to splint an incision, wound, or other painful abdominal area with a pillow as they change positions, cough, or do functional activities.

- ▲ Administer antispasmodic medications as prescribed to help control muscle spasms that interfere with movement.

  Spasticity is a primary cause of contractures and is painful. A therapeutic level is one that prevents spasms but does not produce muscle weakness (Finocchiaro, Herzfeld, 1998).

- ▲ Refer clients to a dietitian, or provide dietary information to promote normal body weight.

  Excessive weight places extra work and stress on body parts during bed mobility activities and may prevent tolerance to prone positioning.

Exercising

- Perform passive range-of-motion (ROM) at least twice a day to those body parts that clients cannot actively range or move spontaneously. Support body parts above and below the joint being ranged (e.g. hold the forearm and hand while ranging the wrist).

• = Independent; ▲ = Collaborative

Passive ROM maintains joint and muscle movement and prevents contracture. Muscles get stronger only by working, so progress clients to active ROM, self-movement, and functional activities as soon as possible. Adequate support of the joint allows for true range of movement and detection of ease or resistance to movement (Wilson, 1988; Borgman-Gainer, 1996).

- Range hemiplegics' affected upper extremity with the shoulder in slight external rotation.
  Spasticity often pulls hemiplegic shoulders into retraction, which prevents normal gliding movement. External rotation prevents soft tissue from becoming pinched between the head of the humerus and the acromion, thus it reduces shoulder pain (Borgman, Passarella, 1991).

- Perform ROM slowly and rhythmically. Do not range beyond the point of pain in those with sensation; range only to the point of resistance in those with poor sensation and mental awareness.
  Fast, jerky ROM may create discomfort, thereby increasing abnormal tone. Slow, rhythmical movements may relax and lengthen tight (spastic) muscles so they can be ranged further. Slow joint movement with gentle stretch may also potentiate muscle relaxation. NOTE: This is not the case for those with rigidity, as in Parkinson's disease (Palmer, Wyness, 1988).

- ▲ Reinforce clients' self-initiated practice of exercise programs, developed by physical or occupational therapists. Exercises may include muscle setting, active strengthening, contraction of muscles against resistance, and weight lifting as appropriate.
  Clients will need to initiate exercise programs at home; allowing them to do so early on encourages self-responsibility and ownership. Active exercise and weight lifting helps maintain muscle tone and strength. Isometric (muscle setting) exercises shorten muscle fibers without actually moving limbs or joints. Progressive resistive exercises cause muscles to work against gentle force and gravity, which stimulates muscle lengthening (Wilson, 1988; Borgman-Gainer, 1996; Finocchiaro, Herzfeld, 1998).

- Assess and intervene for misalignment, asymmetry, abnormal tone (flaccidity and spasticity), synergistic flexor or extensor patterns, abnormal posture, inability to shift weight, poor coordination, reduced sensation, and excessive effort while moving in bed.
  Therapeutic bed positioning and moving can counteract such problems; enhance sensation; and restore more normal tone, posture, and functioning (Bobath, 1978; Johnston, Olson, 1980; Gee, Passarella, 1985; Palmer, Wyness, 1988; Ossman, Campbell, 1990; Kumagai, 1998).

- Use manual guidance and verbal cueing during bed positioning and mobility to facilitate more normal alignment, tone, posture, and movement. Wait for clients to respond and do as much of the activity as they can.
  Clients need the opportunity to feel more normal tone, posture, and movements so they do not relearn abnormal patterns (Bobath, 1978; Gee, Passarella, 1985; Passarella, Lewis, 1987; Ossman, Campbell, 1990).

Positioning

Use the following measures for persons with neurological problems, especially hemiplegia, and persons with joint pain, inflammation, orthopedic problems, and the elderly. NOTE: Refer to the article by Ossman and Campbell (1990) for detailed sketches and instructions on positioning hemiplegics and to the article by Kumagai (1998) on positioning paralyzed clients.

• = Independent; ▲ = Collaborative

- Position head and neck in neutral alignment.

  Head, neck and trunk alignment influences muscle tone in the extremities; therefore positioning should begin proximally and proceed distally to normalize tone (Bobath, 1978).

- Use a flat pillow when clients are supine if head/neck flexion occurs. Place a small towel or pillow behind the head and/or between the shoulder blades if extension occurs.

  This prevents flexor or extensor tone and contractures of the head and neck (Bobath, 1978; Palmer, Wyness, 1988).

- Place a sandbag under the pillow on one or both sides of the head when a client is supine, and one or two pillows under the head in the side-lying position to prevent lateral head flexion.

  Lateral head flexion, extension, or rotation may occlude the internal jugular vein, preventing cerebral ventricular outflow and thus contributing to high ICP (Palmer, Wyness, 1988).

- Change the position of clients' shoulders and arms frequently. Abduct the shoulders of persons with high paraplegia or quadriplegia horizontally (to 90 degrees) twice a day. The shoulders of hemiplegics should not be positioned out past 90 degrees.

  Positioning paralyzed clients' arms in the horizontal plane provides full range of motion (Pires, 1989). Too much abduction may be contraindicated in hemiplegia because of spasticity around the scapula. Normal gliding movements are thus impaired so soft tissue can become pinched and painful (Borgman, Passarella, 1991).

- Position elbows so they are extended or only slightly flexed with the wrist and fingers in extension (except for clients with increased ICP).

  Extension counteracts flexor patterns (Bobath, 1978). However, arm extension increases cerebral ventricular fluid pressure in clients with acute head injury, thus worsening their increased ICP (Mitchell, Ozuna, Lipe, 1981).

- ▲ Apply resting forearm, wrist, and hand splints as ordered. On a routine schedule, check underlying skin for evidence of pressure and poor circulation. Strictly adhere to on/off orders.

  Splints are used to maintain hands and wrists in neutral position or to immobilize inflamed joints as a means of controlling pain. The efficacy of splinting to inhibit spasticity is questionable (Mathiowetz, Bolding, Trombly, 1983).

- ▲ Use hard cones in hands as ordered to help prevent contractures. Soft hand rolls should not be used for persons with spastic hands.

  Soft rolls may elicit flexor patterns in the wrists and hands. Instead, a hard cone is suggested because it may inhibit the long flexors of the hand (Jamieson, Dayhoff, 1980).

- Prevent external and internal rotation of the hips unless clients have a hip fracture, or have had a surgical hip pinning or replacement.

  Neutral alignment of the hip and leg is obtained by placing a thin pillow or folded pad under the weak pelvic girdle, hip, and upper thigh. A pillow or folded pad should not be positioned under the knee. Persons with hip pinning and the like need legs in abduction to stabilize the new prosthesis in the joint; therefore an abductor splint or pillows are used (Hoeman, 1996).

• = **Independent**; ▲ = **Collaborative**

▲ Position the leg and knees so that the toes point toward the ceiling; apply resting leg splints, boots, or high top tennis shoes. Assess underlying skin as mentioned.
These strategies help prevent foot and ankle plantar flexion by promoting neutral ankle alignment. Footboards are undesirable for persons with spasticity because pressure on the ball of the foot stimulates plantar flexion (Bobath, 1978; Palmer, Wyness, 1988; Borgman-Gainer, 1996).

• Assist clients to lie prone or semiprone as part of the routine turn schedule (may be contraindicated in those with cardiopulmonary disturbances or increased intracranial pressure).
The prone-lying position promotes drainage and mobilization of respiratory secretions from dependent lobes of the lung to improve lung aeration, thus oxygenation. It also enhances hip and trunk extension and is therapeutic for persons with lower extremity amputations, paraplegia, quadriplegia, and brain injury (Palmer, Wyness, 1988; Kumagai, 1998).

• Position hemiplegics on both the unaffected and affected sides. Position the affected shoulder well forward, moving it from the shoulder, not the arm.
Weight bearing relaxes tone in the hemiplegic side; protraction of the shoulder reduces its tone and prevents lying on the humerus. Moving the affected shoulder vs. the arm prevents shoulder pain (Bobath, 1978; Borgman, Passarella, 1991).

• Put a flat pad between the ribs and hip if trunk shortening occurs as hemiplegics lie on their affected side.
This helps elongate the trunk into neutral alignment (Bobath, 1978).

• Use assistive devices (e.g., hydraulic or mechanical lift, friction reducer, or commercial repositioner) for severely dependent patients who need to be turned or moved up in bed. Do not use manual lifting such as the two person under-axilla techniques.
Manual lifting often causes overexertion back stress and injuries to staff and may be uncomfortable to clients (Owen, Welden, Kane, 1999).

Bed mobility—rolling

• Recognize components of normal movement with bed mobility activities (e.g. rolling, bridging, scooting, long sitting, and sitting upright). Most movements start with client supine, flat in bed.
Normal movements are bilateral, segmental, well timed, and effortless. They involve set positions, segmental action, weight bearing and shifting, trunk centering, and stabilization against gravity (Gee, Passarella, 1985; Borgman, Passarella, 1991; Kumagai, 1998).

• Assist client into the set position for rolling. For hemiplegics this includes:
  ▪ Moving the shoulder and arm on the side to which client will turn outward with palm facing up
  ▪ Flexing the knees with the feet flat on the bed

• For persons with bilateral paralysis this includes:
  ▪ Crossing the outside leg over the other leg, or manually flexing the outside leg
  ▪ Stretching the arms out in front of the chest with the hands clasped together if possible
Set positions are those normal postures assumed to prepare the body for purposeful movements. Set positions and bilateral activity are often lost with neurological insult. Relearning these in bed prepares clients for bilateral activity as mobilization progresses to sitting, transfers, and standing (Gee, Passarella, 1985; Kumagai, 1998).

• = Independent; ▲ = Collaborative

- Instruct and guide client to roll over segmentally. Start the roll by lifting and turning the head in the direction of the turn, then moving the shoulders/arms/trunk, as the hips and knees follow. Be prepared to assist the affected shoulder and leg of hemiplegics.
  This follows normal segmental patterns for rolling (Bobath, 1978; Ossman, Campbell, 1990; Kumagai, 1998).
  NOTE: For guidelines on how to assist the person with paraplegia or quadriplegia with rolling, refer to Kumagai (1998). For safety, always logroll a client with known or suspected spinal cord injury.

Bed mobility—bridging

- Help client to use bridging to move laterally or up in bed, or during functional activities such as using the bedpan, pulling up pants, or straightening bed linens.
  Bridging is a bilateral activity that prepares the legs and feet for weight bearing while the hips are extended (Gee, Passarella, 1985).
- Reinforce the set position for bridging (e.g., the knees flexed and the feet flat on the bed close to the buttocks). Assistance may be needed to keep the legs from externally rotating.
  The hips can be lifted off the bed when the knees are flexed; the closer the feet are to the buttocks, the higher the hips can be lifted (Gee, Passarella, 1985). Lower extremity pain, limited range of motion, fractures, etc., may limit knee flexion.
- Help client rest his or her arms and hands alongside the trunk.
- Help lift or guide the pelvis as indicated.
  It may be difficult for persons with hemiplegia, obesity, or pain to extend their hips (Gee, Passarella, 1985).

Bed mobility—scooting laterally

- Communicate which direction client is to move.
  Help client to bridge as described previously. Remind client to place both feet flat on the bed and close to the buttocks.
- Support client's pelvis to the extent needed as he or she moves over toward the side of the bed.
  The lower body is moved first in lateral scooting.
- Lower client's pelvis down supine to the same starting position. Instruct client to lift head and shoulders forward off the bed, then assist to move upper trunk over to the side of the bed. If client has hemiplegia, support the affected shoulder from the scapula.
  The upper body and head move after the lower body does.
- Repeat above movements until client is on the desired side of the bed.

Bed mobility—scooting up

- Assist client to bridge, then move pelvis and buttocks up toward the head of the bed.
- Guide client's buttocks back to the same starting position.
- Ask client to tuck the chin and lift head and shoulders off the bed, then lay back down, straightening the trunk.
  This elongates the trunk and moves client up in bed bit by bit.
- To move their shoulders up in bed, persons with hemiplegia can clasp hands together, outstretch them above the chest, then actively lower them toward the knees. Or, they can move the affected shoulder blade forward with the sound hand, lift their upper body and head forward, then lay back down.

• = Independent; ▲ = Collaborative

Both methods help protract the affected shoulder forward to move and elongate the trunk while shifting upward. They also promote bilateral activity and sensory stimulation to the hemiplegic arm (Gee, Passarella, 1985; Ossman, Campbell, 1990).

- Remind client to move feet up toward buttocks each time before moving the lower body. Client should repeatedly raise the lower then the upper body and head until he or she is far enough up in bed.

Bed mobility—side-lying to sitting upright

- Assess whether client is over to one side of the bed far enough; if not, help client to move over.
  This will reduce the risk of sliding off the edge of the bed while sitting up.
- Plan the bed and furniture arrangement so that persons with hemiplegia can sit up using their affected side.
  Weight bearing on the affected side is a means of increasing tone and promotes bilateral activity and sensory stimulation (Bobath, 1978).
- Assist or cue client into side-lying position (on their affected side if hemiplegic).
- Instruct client to lower legs slowly over the edge of the bed with knees flexed and close to chest. If client has recently had back or neck surgery or back pain, legs should instead be lowered slowly off the bed at the same time he or she pushes up with arms, keeping spine straight.
  Hanging legs over the edge of the bed reduces the amount of weight to be shifted and managed while sitting up. However, in cases of back surgery or pain, legs are moved in unison with the body because the weight of freely hanging legs would aggravate back pain.
- Ask client to lift his or her head off the bed.
- Ensure that the bottom shoulder of hemiplegics is positioned forward before sitting up. If not, move it forward from the shoulder blade (not by pulling on the distal arm).
  This allows the elbow to take weight as the body moves upright (Ossman, Campbell, 1990; Bobath, 1978).
- Instruct client to bear weight on the bottom arm and elbow while at the same time pushing against the mattress with the palm of other hand to sit up. Alternatively, instead of pushing up onto the elbow, client is guided forward diagonally while pushing with the palm of his or her hand to sit himself or herself up (Kumagai, 1998).
- Help client sit up by placing one of your hands under the bottom shoulder blade to keep it well forward and pushing down on the opposite iliac crest with your other hand. Shift the client's weight; do not lift it. Encourage client to initiate and complete as much of the pushing and weight shifting as possible.
  Protraction of the shoulder helps prevent abnormal tone and pain during movement. The shoulder and pelvis are key points of control for guiding client's movements (Gee, Passarella, 1985; Ossman, Campbell, 1990). The nurse's weight shifts from the front foot (the one near the head of the bed) to the back foot using leverage, not strength (Gee, Passarella, 1985).
- Assist clients to achieve a stable sitting posture with weight on both legs and buttocks. Hips and knees should flex to 90 degrees. If possible, feet should be flat on the floor.
  Weight needs to shift so it is centered and distributed onto both sides of the body in a bilateral manner (Bobath, 1978).

• = Independent; ▲ = Collaborative

Bed mobility—long sitting

- Assess client's ability for 100-degree straight leg raises; if this ability is absent, avoid long sitting position.
  Straight leg raise function indicates hamstring tone. If hamstring muscles are too tight and long sitting is attempted, back extensor muscles will be overstretched and person will lose passive stability of the trunk (Kumagai, 1998).
- Cue client to start from the set position (flat and supine in bed).
- Instruct client to grasp the side rails of the bed and pull himself or herself up to a sitting position. If hand function is poor, teach client to raise head and trunk up by pushing against the mattress with flexed forearms until sitting upright. The legs remain in extension as client sits up in bed.
- Assist quadriplegics and high paraplegics with the wrist extension method in the following manner:
  - Remind client to wedge hands under hips and tuck chin.
  - Stand to the side and face client.
  - Support client from the scapula when raising trunk off the bed as he or she comes up onto elbows.
  - Support the trunk and scapulas from behind as client shifts weight side to side.
  - Move behind client to avoid getting in his or her way as client unweights one arm and throws the other straightened arm back into an extended, locked position.
  - Kneel on the bed behind client to support upper trunk as weight is shifted onto the locked arm.
  - Repeat the sequence for the remaining arm.
  - Help client with hand and arm positioning if necessary.
  - Support client's trunk (still kneeling from behind) as he or she shifts back and forth to bring extended arms closer to the body so that client can support self sitting erect.
  Physical and occupational therapists teach the wrist extension method to persons with high-level quadriplegia or paraplegia; nurses may have to reinforce principles and assist client as he or she practices outside of therapy (Kumagai, 1998).
  NOTE: Refer to Kumagai (1998) for further information and sketches on how to assist quadriplegic or paraplegic clients with rolling to the semiprone and upright sitting position.

Geriatric

- Develop appropriate strategies for positioning and bed mobility based on client's multiple chronic and disabling conditions.
  The number of comorbid conditions in the elderly is high (Hoeman, 1996).
- Assess the family caregivers' strength, health history, and cognitive status to predict ability and risk for helping clients with positioning and bed mobility tasks. Help family explore and develop other options if helping clients would place them at too high a risk.
  Caregivers of elderly clients are often themselves frail elderly persons with chronic health problems. They would be at high risk for injury when helping clients with bed mobility, exercise, and ROM activities (McAnaw, 2001).
- Prevent failure by assessing client's stamina and energy level during exercising and bed mobility activities; give assistance or rest breaks as needed.

• = Independent; ▲ = Collaborative

Elderly clients may have less energy reserves and may fatigue easily because of respiratory and circulatory impairments (McAnaw, 2001).

- Spread out bed activities, exercise programs, and ADLs rather than clumping them together.
- Anticipate that day-to-day abilities may fluctuate based on factors such as chronic disease, pain, restful sleep, constipation, nutritional intake, and mood.
- Incorporate memory aids and strategies (e.g., written schedules, directions, sketches, or notes), timers, audiotaped instructions, etc., so that clients with cognitive decline can function independently.

Home Care Interventions

- Encourage use of client's regular bed in the home unless contraindicated for specific medical reasons.
  Emotionally, persons may benefit from sleeping in their own bed, with their partner. Note that most of the bed activities described above did not require side rails or head elevation. Foam wedges or blocks can add elevation if necessary.
- Place indented or grooved-out areas in wood pieces under each leg of the bed and set bed against the walls in a corner of the room.
  Such actions may prevent injury from bed movements because regular beds do not have brakes.
- Suggest rearranging furniture at home to make it accessible to meet sleeping, toileting, and living needs.
  Converting an existing room on a main level into a suite for living and sleeping purposes and decorating it so it is cozy yet functional may be emotionally soothing and prevent an institutional look (Yearns, 1995).
- Discuss the psychological and physical benefits of allowing clients to be as self-sufficient as possible in bed mobility and repositioning, even though it may be time consuming.
  Caregivers may try to help or save time by "doing for" their loved one. Discussion about prevention of helplessness, complications of disuse, and promoting self-esteem may change the caregiver's approach.
- Prepare family members for potential regression in self-care during transition from hospital to home environment.
  Relocation anxiety may interfere with independence. Confidence building, coaching, written instructions, sketches, instructional videotapes of proper techniques, and referrals may be needed (Theuerkauf, 1996).
- Offer emotional support and suggest community resources and social supports to help with adjustment issues.
  The home environment may trigger the reality of loss and change experienced with impaired physical mobility (Hoeman, 1996).
- See the Home Care Interventions section of the care plan for **Impaired physical Mobility.**

Client/Family Teaching

- Use various sensory modalities to teach client, family, and caregivers correct techniques for ROM, exercising, repositioning, and bed mobility activities.
- Give information visually (demonstrations, sketches, instructional videos, written instructions).
- Give tactile stimulation (manual guidance, hand-on-hand technique, return demonstrations, note taking).

• = **Independent;** ▲ = **Collaborative**

- Give auditory information (verbal instructions, instructional audiotapes, verbal repeating of instructions, self-talk during motor activity, reading aloud written instructions).
  Developmentally, motor activities are first learned by trial and error, then by feeling normal movement, and last by repeated practice. Providing various sensory stimulation helps motor learning and memory retention (Bobath, 1978).
- Schedule time with family and caregivers for client education and practice sessions in addition to sharing information informally. Suggest that family members come prepared with their questions and wearing appropriate clothing and shoes for practice.
  Practice—repetition promotes learning and retention.
- Teach caregivers proper body mechanics and use of assistive devices (if applicable) while assisting clients with bed mobility activities.
  This prevents injury and discomfort.

WEB SITES FOR EDUCATION

MERLIN See the MERLIN web site for World Wide Web resources for client education.

REFERENCES Allen C, Glasziou P, Del Mar C: Bed rest: a potentially harmful treatment needing more careful evaluation, *Lancet* 354(9186):1229-1233, 1999.

Arbour R: Aggressive management of intracranial dynamics, *Crit Care Nurs* 18(3):30-40, 1998.

Bobath B: *Adult hemiplegia: evaluation and treatment,* London, 1978, William Heinemann Medical Books.

Borgman-Gainer F: Independent function: movement and mobility. In Hoeman S, editor: *Rehabilitation nursing: process and application,* ed 2, St Louis, 1996, Mosby.

Borgman MF, Passarella PM: Nursing care of the stroke patient using Bobath principles: an approach to altered movement, *Nurs Clin North Am* 26(4):1019-1103, 1991.

Carroll P: Tradition or science? spotting the difference in respiratory care *RN* 59(5):26-30, 1996

Defloor T: The effect of position and mattress on interface pressure, *Appl Nurs Res* 13(1):2-11, 2000.

Ecklund MM: Optimizing the flow of care for prevention and treatment of deep vein thrombosis and pulmonary embolism, *AACN Clin Issues* 6(4):558-601, 1995.

Emick-Herring B, Wood P: A team approach to neurologically based swallowing disorders, *Rehab Nurs* 15:126-132, 1990.

Feldman Z et al: Effect of head elevation on intracranial pressure, cerebral perfusion pressure, and cerebral blood flow in head-injured patients, *J Neurosurg* 76(2):207-211, 1992.

Finocchiaro D, Herzfeld S: Neurological deficits associated with spinal cord injury. In Chin PA, Finocchiaro D, Rosebrough A: *Rehabilitation nursing practice,* New York, 1998, McGraw-Hill, pp 278-307.

Gee ZL, Passarella PM: *Nursing care of the stroke patient: a therapeutic approach,* Pittsburgh, 1985, AREN.

Hoeman SP: Coping with chronic, disabling, or developmental disorders. In Hoeman SP: *Rehabilitation nursing: process and application,* ed 2, St Louis, 1996, Mosby, pp 188-224.

Jamieson S, Dayhoff NE: A hard hand-positioning device to decrease wrist and finger hypertonicity: a sensorimotor approach for the patient with nonprogressive brain damage, *Nurs Res* 29:285-289, 1980.

Johnston K, Olson E: Application of Bobath principles for nursing care of the hemiplegic patient, *Assoc Rehab Nurs J* 5:8-11, 1980.

Kumagai KAS: Physical management of the neurologically involved client: techniques for bed mobility and transfers. In Chin PA, Finocchiaro D, Rosebrough A, editors: *Rehabilitation nursing practice,* New York, 1998, McGraw-Hill, pp 524-601.

Maklebust J: Pressure ulcer update, *RN* 54(12):56-63, 1991.

Mathiowetz V, Bolding DJ, Trombly CA: Immediate effects of positioning devices on the normal and spastic hand measured by electromyography, *Am J Occup Ther* 37:247-254, 1983.

McAnaw MB: Normal changes with aging. In Maas ML et al, editors: *Nursing care of older adults: diagnoses, outcomes & interventions,* St Louis, 2001, Mosby, pp 281-283.

McCaffery M, Pasero C: Pain: clinical manual, ed 2, St Louis, 1999, Mosby.

McConnell J: Preventing urinary tract infections, *Geriatr Nurs* 5(8):361-362, 1984.

• = **Independent;** ▲ = **Collaborative**

McCourt A, editor: *The specialty practice of rehabilitation nursing: a core curriculum*, ed 3, Skokie, Ill, 1993, Rehabilitation Nursing Foundation, pp 130-135.

Mitchell PH, Ozuna J, Lipe HP: Moving the patient in bed: effects on intracranial pressure, *Nurs Res* 30(4):212-218, 1981.

Murphy JB: Dysmobility and immobility. In Ham RJ, Sloane PD, editors: *Primary care geriatrics: a case-based approach*, ed 3, St Louis, 1997, Mosby, pp 278-293.

Olson EV: The hazards of immobility, *Am J Nurs* 67:781-797, 1967.

Ossman NJ, Campbell M: *Therapist guide: adult positions, transitions, and transfers—reproducible instruction cards for caregivers*, Tucson, 1990, Communication Skill Builders.

Owen BD, Welden N, Kane J: What are we teaching about lifting and transferring patients? *J Res Nurs Health* 22(1):3-13, 1999.

Palmer M, Wyness MA: Positioning and handling: important considerations in the care of the severely head-injured patient, *J Neurosurg Nurs* 20(1):42-49, 1988.

Panel for the Prediction and Prevention of Pressure Ulcers in Adults: *Pressure ulcers in adults: prediction and prevention—quick reference guide for clinicians*, AHCPR Publications No. 920050, Rockville, Md, 1992, Agency for Health Care Policy and Research, Public Health Service, U.S. Department of Health and Human Services.

Passarella PM, Lewis N: Nursing application of Bobath principles in stroke care, *J Neurosurg Nurs* 19(2):106-109, 1987.

Pires M: Spinal cord injuries: coping with devastating damage. In Ursevich PR, editor: *Coping with neurologic problems proficiently*, ed 2, Nursing '84 Skillbook series, Springhouse, Penn, 1984, Springhouse, pp 99-123.

Pires M: *Spinal cord injury part II: specific nursing interventions*, Independent Study Module, Evanston, Ill, 1989, Rehabilitation Nursing Foundation, p 9.

Rodriguez L: Medical-surgical complications in the rehabilitation client. In Chin PA, Finocchiaro D, Rosebrough A, editors: *Rehabilitation nursing practice*, New York, 1998, McGraw-Hill, pp 661-667.

Rubin M: The physiology of bedrest, *Am J Nurs* 88:50, 55, 57-58, 1988.

Theuerkauf A: Self-care and activities of daily living. In Hoeman SP, editor: *Rehabilitation nursing: process and application*, ed 2, St Louis, 1996, Mosby, pp 156-187.

Wilson G: Progressive mobilization. In Sine RD et al, editors: *Basic rehabilitation techniques: a self-instructional guide*, ed 3, Gaithersburg, Md, 1988, Aspen, pp 69-112.

Wong PWK, Kadakia S: How to deal with chronic constipation: a stepwise method of establishing and treating the course of the problem, *Postgrad Med* 106(6):199-200, 203-204, 207-210, 1999.

Yearns MH: Modest home makeovers to improve farmhouse accessibility: how our AgrAgbility team used this fast, affordable alternative to remodeling with the Miller family, *Technol Disabil* 4:49-60, 1995.

Impaired physical Mobility

Teepa Snow and Betty J. Ackley

 Definition A limitation in independent, purposeful physical movement of the body or of one or more extremities

Defining Characteristics

Postural instability during performance of routine activities of daily living (ADLs); limited ability to perform gross motor skills; limited ability to perform fine motor skills; uncoordinated or jerky movements; limited range of motion; difficulty turning; decreased reaction time; movement-induced shortness of breath; gait changes (e.g., decreased walking speed, difficulty initiating gait, small steps, shuffles feet, exaggerated lateral postural sway); engages in substitutions for movement (e.g., increased attention to other's activity, controlling behavior, focus on preillness/predisability); slowed movement; movement-induced tremor

• = Independent; ▲ = Collaborative

Related Factors (r/t)

Medications; prescribed movement restrictions; discomfort; lack of knowledge regarding value of physical activity; body mass index >30; sensoriperceptual impairments; neuromuscular impairment; pain; musculoskeletal impairment; intolerance to activity/decreased strength and endurance; depressive mood state or anxiety; cognitive impairment; decreased muscle strength, control, and/or mass; reluctance to initiate movement; sedentary lifestyle or disuse or deconditioning; selective or generalized malnutrition; loss of integrity of bone structures; developmental delay; joint stiffness or contractures; limited cardiovascular endurance; altered cellular metabolism; lack of physical or social environmental supports; cultural beliefs regarding age-appropriate activity

Suggested functional level classifications

0	Completely independent
1	Requires use of equipment or device
2	Requires help from another person for assistance, supervision, or teaching
3	Requires help from another person and equipment device
4	Dependent—does not participate in activity

NOC Outcomes (Nursing Outcomes Classification)

Suggested NOC Labels

Ambulation: Walking; Ambulation: Wheelchair; Joint Movement: Active; Mobility Level; Self-Care: Activities of Daily Living (ADLs); Transfer Performance

> **Example NOC Outcome**
>
> Accomplishes **Ambulation: Walking** as evidenced by the following indicators: Walks with effective gait/Walks at moderate pace/Walks up and down steps/Walks moderate distance (Rate each indicator of **Ambulation: Walking:** 1 = dependent—does not participate, 2 = requires assistive person and device, 3 = requires assistive person, 4 = indepndent with assistive device, 5 = completely independent [see Section I])

Client Outcomes

- Increases physical activity
- Meets mutually defined goals of increased mobility
- Verbalizes feeling of increased strength and ability to move
- Demonstrates use of adaptive equipment (e.g., wheelchairs, walkers) to increase mobility

NIC Interventions (Nursing Interventions Classification)

Suggested NIC Labels

Exercise Therapy: Ambulation; Exercise Therapy: Joint Mobility; Positioning

> **Example NIC Interventions—Exercise Therapy: Ambulation**
> - Assist client to use footwear that facilitates walking and prevents injury
> - Instruct in availability of assistive devices, if appropriate

Nursing Interventions and Rationales

▲ Screen for mobility skills in the following order: (1) bed mobility; (2) supported and unsupported sitting; (3) transition movements such as sit to stand, sitting down, and transfers; and (4) standing and walking activities. Use a physical activity tool if available to evaluate mobility.

• = Independent; ▲ = Collaborative

Screening mobility skills helps provide baselines of performance that can guide mobility-enhancement programming and allows nursing staff to integrate movement and practice opportunities into daily routines and regular and customary care. There are many tools available to measure physical activity; selection of the appropriate tool depends on the setting and situation (Halfmann, Keller, Allison, 1997).

- Observe client for cause of impaired mobility. Determine whether cause is physical or psychological.
  *Some clients choose not to move because of psychological factors such as an inability to cope or depression. See interventions for **Ineffective Coping** or **Hopelessness**.*
- Monitor and record client's ability to tolerate activity and use all four extremities; note pulse rate, blood pressure, dyspnea, and skin color before and after activity. See care plan for **Activity intolerance.**
- ▲ Before activity observe for and, if possible, treat pain. Ensure that client is not oversedated.
  Pain limits mobility and is often exacerbated by movement.
- ▲ Consult with physical therapist for further evaluation, strength training, gait training, and development of a mobility plan.
  Techniques such as gait training, strength training, and exercise to improve balance and coordination can be very helpful for rehabilitating clients (Tempkin, Tempkin, Goodman, 1997).
- Obtain any assistive devices needed for activity, such as walking belts, walkers, canes, crutches, or wheelchairs, before the activity begins.
  Assistive devices can help increase mobility.
- If client is immobile, perform passive range of motion (ROM) exercises at least twice a day unless contraindicated; repeat each maneuver three times.
  Passive ROM exercises help maintain joint mobility, prevent contractures and deformities, increase circulation, and promote a feeling of comfort and well-being (Kottke, Lehmann, 1990; Bolander, 1994).
- ▲ If client is immobile, consult with physician for a safety evaluation before beginning an exercise program; if program is approved, begin with the following exercises:
  - Active ROM exercises using both upper and lower extremities (e.g., flexing and extending at ankles, knees, hips)
  - Chin-ups and pull-ups using a trapeze in bed (may be contraindicated in clients with cardiac conditions)
  - Strengthening exercises such as gluteal or quadriceps sitting exercises
  These exercises help reverse weakening and atrophy of muscles.
- Help client achieve mobility and start walking as soon as possible if not contraindicated.
  The longer a client is immobile, the longer it takes to regain strength, balance, and coordination (Bolander, 1994). A study has shown that bed rest for primary treatment of medical conditions or after healthcare procedures is associated with worse outcomes than early mobilization (Allen, Glasziou, Del Mar, 1999).
- Use a walking belt when ambulating the client.
  The client can walk independently with a walking belt, but the nurse can rapidly ensure safety if the knees buckle.
- ▲ Apply any ordered brace before mobilizing client.
  Braces support and stabilize a body part, allowing increased mobility.

• = **Independent;** ▲ = **Collaborative**

- Increase independence in ADLs and discourage helplessness as client gets stronger.
  Providing unnecessary assistance with transfers and bathing activities may promote dependence and a loss of mobility (Mobily, Kelley, 1991).
- If client does not feed or groom self, sit side-by-side with client, put your hand over client's hand, support client's elbow with your other hand, and help client feed self; use the same technique to help client comb hair.
  This feeding technique increases client mobility, range of motion, and independence, and clients often eat more food (Pedretti, 1996).

Geriatric

- Help the mostly immobile client achieve mobility as soon as possible, depending on physical condition.
  In the elderly, mobility impairment can predict increased mortality and dependence; however, this can be prevented by physical exercise (Hirvensalo, Rantanen, Heikkinen, 2000).
- For a client who is mostly immobile, minimize cardiovascular deconditioning by positioning client as close to the upright position as possible several times daily.
  The hazards of bed rest in the elderly are multiple, serious, quick to develop, and slow to reverse. Deconditioning of the cardiovascular system occurs within days and involves fluid shifts, fluid loss, decreased cardiac output, decreased peak oxygen uptake, and increased resting heart rate (Resnick, 1998).
- If client is mostly immobile, encourage him or her to attend a low-intensity aerobic chair exercise class that includes stretching and strengthening chair exercises.
  Chair exercises have been shown to increase flexibility and balance (Mills, 1994).
- Initiate a walking program in which client walks with or without help every day as part of daily routine.
  Walking programs have been shown to be effective in improving ambulatory status and decreasing disability and the number of falls in the elderly (Koroknay et al, 1995).
- ▲ Evaluate client for signs of depression (flat affect, insomnia, anorexia, frequent somatic complaints) or cognitive impairment (use Mini-Mental State Exam [MMSE]). Refer for treatment or counseling as needed.
  Multiple studies have demonstrated that depression and decreased cognition in the elderly correlate with decreased levels of functional ability (Resnick, 1998).
- Watch for orthostatic hypotension when mobilizing elderly clients. If relevant, have client flex and extend feet several times after sitting up, then stand up slowly with someone watching.
  Orthostatic hypotension as a result of cardiovascular system changes, chronic diseases, and medication effects is common in the elderly (Matteson, McConnell, Linton, 1997).
- Be very careful when getting a mostly immobile client up. Be sure to lock the bed and wheelchair and have sufficient personnel to protect client from falls.
  The most important preventative measure to reduce the risk of injurious falls for nonambulatory residents involves increasing safety measures while transferring, including careful locking of equipment such as wheelchairs and beds before moves (Thapa et al, 1996). Elderly clients most commonly sustain the most serious injuries when they fall.
- Help clients assume the prone position three times per week for 20 minutes each time. If clients are unable to do so, help them turn partially over and assume the position gradually.

• = **Independent;** ▲ = **Collaborative**

The prone position helps prevent hip deformities that can interfere with balance and walking. This position may be contraindicated in some clients, such as morbidly obese clients, respiratory or cardiac clients who cannot lie flat, and neurological clients.

- Do not routinely assist with transfers or bathing activities unless necessary.
  The nursing staff may contribute to impaired mobility by helping too much. Encourage client independence (Mobily, Kelley, 1991).
- Use gestures and nonverbal cues when helping clients move if they are anxious or have difficulty understanding and following verbal instructions.
  Nonverbal gestures are part of a universal language that can be understood when the client is having difficulty with communication.
- Recognize that wheelchairs are not a good mobility device and often serve as a mobility restraint.
  Wheelchairs can be very effective restraints. In one study, only 4% of residents in wheelchairs were observed to propel them independently; only 45% could propel them, even with cues and prompts; no residents could unlock them without help; the wheelchairs were not fitted to residents; and residents were not trained in propulsion (Simmons et al, 1995).
- Ensure that chairs fit clients. Chair seat should be 3 inches above the height of the knee. Provide a raised toilet seat if needed.
  Raising the height of a chair can dramatically improve the ability of many older clients to stand up. Low, deep, soft seats with armrests that are far apart reduce a person's ability to get up and down without help.
- If client is mainly immobile, provide opportunities for socialization and sensory stimulation (e.g., television and visits). See **Deficient Diversional activity.**
  *Immobility and a lack of social support and sensory input may result in confusion or depression in the elderly (Mobily, Kelley, 1991). See interventions for **Acute Confusion** or **Hopelessness** as appropriate.*

Home Care Interventions

- ▲ Assess home environment for factors that create barriers to physical mobility. Refer to occupational therapy services if needed to assist client in restructuring home and daily living patterns.
- ▲ Refer to home health aide services to support client and family through changing levels of mobility. Reinforce need to promote independence in mobility as tolerated.
  Providing unnecessary assistance with transfers and bathing activities may promote dependence and a loss of mobility (Mobily, Kelley, 1991).
- Assess skin condition at every visit. Establish a skin care program that enhances circulation and maximizes position changes.
  Impaired mobility decreases circulation to dependent areas. Decreased circulation and shearing place the client at risk for skin breakdown.
- Provide support to client and family/caregivers during long-term impaired mobility.
  *Long-term impaired mobility may necessitate role changes within the family and precipitate caregiver stress (see care plan for **Caregiver role strain**).*

Client/Family Teaching

- Teach client to get out of bed slowly when transferring from the bed to the chair.
- Teach client relaxation techniques to use during activity.
- Teach client to use assistive devices such as a cane, a walker, or crutches to increase mobility.

• = **Independent;** ▲ = **Collaborative**

- Teach family members and caregivers to work with clients during self-care activities such as eating, bathing, grooming, dressing, and transferring rather than having client be a passive recipient of care.
  Maintaining as much independence as possible helps maintain mobility skills (Lipson, Braun, 1993).
- Develop a series of contracts with mutually agreed on goals of increased activity. Include measurable landmarks of progress, consequences for meeting or not meeting goals, and evaluation dates. Sign the contracts with the client.
  Using a series of evolving contracts to modify behavior toward increasing activity, help the client learn skills to change behavior (Boehm, 1992).

WEB SITES FOR EDUCATION

$Merlin$ See the MERLIN web site for World Wide Web resources for client education.

REFERENCES   Allen C, Glasziou P, Del Mar C: Bed rest: a potentially harmful treatment needing more careful evaluation, *Lancet* 354(9186):1229-1233, 1999.

Boehm S: Patient contracting. In Bulechek G, McCloskey JC: *Nursing interventions: essential nursing treatments,* ed 2, Philadelphia, 1992, WB Saunders.

Bolander VB: Meeting mobility needs. In *Sorensen and Luckmann's basic nursing: a psychophysiologic approach,* Philadelphia, 1994, WB Saunders.

Halfmann PL, Keller C, Allison M: Pragmatic assessment of physical activity, *Nurse Pract Forum* 8(4):160-164, 1997.

Hirvensalo M, Rantanen T, Heikkinen E: Mobility difficulties and physical activity as predictors of mortality and loss of independence in the community-living older population, *J Am Geriatr Soc* 48(5):493-498, 2000.

Koroknay VJ et al: Maintaining ambulation in the frail nursing home resident: a nursing administered walking program, *J Gerontol Nurs* 21:18, 1995.

Kottke FJ, Lehmann JF: *Krusen's handbook of physical medicine,* ed 4, Philadelphia, 1990, WB Saunders.

Lipson J, Braun S: *Toward a restraint-free environment: reducing the use of physical and chemical restraint in long term care and acute settings,* Baltimore, 1993, Health Professions Press.

Matteson MA, McConnell ES, Linton AD: *Gerontological nursing,* Philadelphia, 1997, WB Saunders.

Mills EM: The effect of low-intensity aerobic exercise on muscle strength, flexibility, and balance among sedentary elderly persons, *Nurs Res* 43:207, 1994.

Mobily PR, Kelley LS: Iatrogenesis in the elderly: factors of immobility, *J Gerontol Nurs* 17:5, 1991.

Pedretti LW: *Occupational therapy: practice skills for physical dysfunction,* ed 4, St Louis, 1996, Mosby.

Resnick B: Predictors of functional ability in geriatric rehabilitation patients, *Rehabil Nurs* 23(1):21-28, 1998.

Simmons S et al: Wheelchairs as mobility restraints: predictors of wheelchair activity in nonambulatory nursing home residents, *J Am Geriatr Soc* 43:384-388, 1995.

Tempkin T, Tempkin A, Goodman H: Geriatric rehabilitation, *Nur Pract Forum* 8(2):59-63, 1997.

Thapa P et al: Injurious falls in nonambulatory nursing home residents: a comparative study of circumstances, incidence, and risk factors, *J Am Geriatr Soc* 44:273-278, 1996.

Impaired wheelchair Mobility

Brenda Emick-Herring

NANDA   **Definition** Limitation of independent movement within the environment using a device equipped with wheels

• = **Independent**;   ▲ = **Collaborative**

Defining Characteristics

Impaired ability to operate a manual or power wheelchair on even or uneven surface; impaired ability to operate manual or power wheelchair on an incline or decline; impaired ability to operate wheelchair on curbs

Related Factors (r/t)

Intolerance to activity; decreased strength and endurance; pain or discomfort; perceptual or cognitive impairment; neuromuscular impairment; musculoskeletal impairment; depression; severe anxiety; amputation

Suggested functional level classifications

0   Completely independent
1   Requires use of equipment or device
2   Requires help from another person for assistance, supervision, or teaching
3   Requires help from another person and equipment or device
4   Dependent—does not participate in activity

 Outcomes (Nursing Outcomes Classification)

Suggested NOC Labels

Ambulation: Wheelchair

> **Example NOC Outcome**
>
> Demonstrates **Ambulation: Wheelchair** as evidenced by the following indicators: Propels wheelchair safely/Tranfers to and from wheelchair/Maneuvers curbs, doorways, ramps (Rate each indicator of **Ambulation: Wheelchair:** 1 = dependent—does not participate, 2 = requires assistive person and device, 3 = requires assistive person, 4 = independent with assistive device, 5 = completely independent [see Section I])

Client Outcomes

- Demonstrates optimal independence in operating and moving a wheelchair or other device equipped with wheels
- Demonstrates the ability to direct others in operating and moving a wheelchair or other device equipped with wheels
- Demonstrates therapeutic positioning, pressure relief, and safety principles while operating and moving wheelchair or other device equipped with wheels

NIC   Interventions (Nursing Interventions Classification)

Suggested NIC Labels

Positioning: Wheelchair; Exercise Therapy: Muscle Control

> **Example NIC Interventions—Positioning: Wheelchair**
> - Select the appropriate wheelchair for the patient
> - Monitor for patient's inability to maintain correct posture in wheelchair

Nursing Interventions and Rationales

- Assist or remind client to don appropriate equipment (e.g., braces, corsets, shells, splints, orthosis, immobilizers, and abdominal binders) in bed before wheelchair mobility; loosen or remove equipment after client returns to bed.
  To provide stabilization and alignment of necessary body parts; the abdominal binder helps prevent postural hypotension, supports abdominal contents, and increases vital capacity in persons with high paraplegia or quadriplegia.

• = Independent; ▲ = Collaborative

▲ Obtain referrals for physical therapy, occupational therapy, or a Wheelchair Seating Clinic to ensure that the wheelchair cushion fits the build, abilities, postural support, and pressure prevention needs of client. The seating system should fit the needs of the client so that the client can propel the wheels, safely and ably use the hands to complete ADLs/self care/job/recreational activities, reach the floor with the feet, stand up from the chair without falling, and not be harmed by the wheelchair legs and foot rests.

Wheelchair seating and cushion systems are the basis of postural support for clients. Poor posture (slouching, side leaning, and sliding down) can cause deformities, discomfort, overuse of physical restraints, and trunk compression, which affects arousal, respiratory, circulatory, digestive, urinary, swallowing and speech functioning. An individualized seating system promotes independence, safety, comfort, and prevention of medical complications such as pressure ulcers from developing (Rader, Jones, Miller, 1999; Cooper et al 2000; Minkel, 2000).

• Remove leg and foot rests from wheelchairs of client who can actively move the wheelchair short distances by himself or herself.

Foot rests can cause skin tears and bruising, as well as postural alignment problems. There is less pressure on sacral and buttock tissue sitting upright with feet on the floor than with feet on foot rests (Defloor, Grypdonck, 1999; Rader, Jones, Miller, 1999).

• Use wheelchairs with solid backs and firm, contoured seats rather than sling-type upholstered wheelchairs.

Standard wheelchair seats and backs often sag; a solid seat and backrest improves posture, stability, function, and comfort (Gee, Passarella, 1985; Sussman, Bates-Jensen, 1998; Rader, Jones, Miller, 1999; Saur, 1999).

▲ Obtain referrals for physical therapy, occupational therapy, or a Seating Clinic to individualize wheelchair cushion systems for clients.

Cushions have numerous purposes such as relieving pressure (thick air cushions can be placed over a firm seat or a cutout seat board to prevent ischial and sacral pressure for example); providing postural control, balance, and stability; and minimizing shock impact and repetitive vibration, which causes fatigue, pain, improper body mechanics over time. Special postural supports and back cushions may be necessary for those with fixed or flexion deformities or unique spinal curvatures. For example, adjustable-angle foot plates are available for fixed ankle deformities or tight calves (Gee, Passarella, 1985; Sussman, Bates-Jensen, 1998; Defloor, Grypdonck, 1999; Saur, 1999; Cooper et al, 2000).

• Deliberately and frequently help client to position self in wheelchair in good alignment so that hips, knees, and ankles are in 90-degree flexion and hips and pelvis are fully back in the chair. Avoid allowing the client to slide down and slouch in the wheelchair.

Nurses need to specifically assess clients' sitting posture and reposition them to correct poor posture and joint alignment (Dowswell, Dowswell, Young, 2000).

• Consistently instruct client to unlock wheelchair brakes, place feet on foot plates with heels securely against heel loops, and fasten safety restraints and seat belts (across the top of the thighs) before propelling chair.

Practicing and sequencing will help habituate steps of the safety plan. Securing feet on foot plates helps prevent foot, ankle, and skin injuries. Soft waist restraints may be needed to prevent clients from falling or getting out of the chair by themselves. Wheelchair seat belts

• = **Independent;** ▲ = **Collaborative**

help stabilize and hold the pelvis in place and should be strapped over thighs, not the abdomen (Rader, Jones, Miller, 1999).

- Verbally reinforce and demonstrate placement of hand(s) on manual wheelchair rim(s) and propel wheelchair by: (1) pushing forward on both wheel rims to go straight ahead, (2) pushing the right rim to turn left and vice versa, and (3) pulling backward on both wheels to back up (Wilson, Kerr, 1988).
- Guide or instruct client with unilateral leg and arm functioning to propel the wheelchair by: (1) raising that foot plate and putting foot flat on the floor, (2) getting a lower wheelchair if whole foot doesn't reach the floor, (3) placing sound hand on the rim, (4) pushing as described above with the sound hand, and (5) "walking" the chair forward by extending the knee, then putting the heel then the entire foot on the floor and flexing the knee. NOTE: A hemi, one-arm drive wheelchair is recommended for persons with hemiplegia.
  The sound foot propels the chair by repeating the process (Wilson, Kerr, 1988).
- Suggest that client back wheelchair or wheeled device into an elevator, or if entering face first, instruct to turn chair around to face the elevator doors.
  This allows client to see the control panel, floor monitor display, and opening of doors. Client should exit by facing forward rather than backing out (Minor, Minor, 1995).
- Model or verbally cue clients to go backward through self-closing doors. Nurses should use this approach when transporting client.
  Repetition (and practice) helps clients remember instructions. A backward approach lets clients control the opening and closure of doors (Younker Rehabilitation Center, 1990).
- Reinforce concept of descending a curb backward ("popping a wheelie") if balance, trunk control, strength, and timing are adequate. Client needs to lean slightly forward and guide both wheels off curb at the same time.
  Compared with a forward curb decent, there is less risk with a backward descent of client losing control and falling forward out of the wheelchair. If someone is helping the client, backing down the curb places less stress on the helper (Minor, Minor, 1995).
- Reinforce principles of ascending curbs in a forward position by popping a wheelie or having an assistant tilt the chair back, placing the front wheels over the curb, and rolling the back wheels up. If surface is soft (muddy, sandy) go up curb backward via a wheelie.
  The front casters will not roll on soft surfaces. A backward approach will require less energy and prevent getting stuck or injured from falling forward (Younker Rehabilitation Center, 1990).
- During wheelies, hold the wheelchair until all four wheels are on the ground and client has balance and control of the wheelchair.
  Releasing your grip too soon may affect client's balance and cause injury.
- When client experiences unilateral neglect, agnosia, somatognosia, or proprioception deficits, cue client and reinforce team intervention strategies for propelling the chair, entering doorways, and detecting and avoiding obstacles.
  Too often nurses move the wheelchair or obstacle when clients run into doorways, furniture, etc., instead of cueing clients to detect and solve the problem. Scanning, self-talk, self-questioning about what could be wrong, and manual guiding are some cognitive strategies nurses should employ.

• = **Independent**; ▲ = **Collaborative**

- Implement precautionary measures to prevent skin breakdown in areas of high risk, including leather gloves, use of friction coated or projection hand rims, wheelchair cushions (not donut-type), firm seat, and proper placement of heels against the heel straps on wheelchair foot rests.

  Persons without finger flexor function use palm action against the projection rims to propel a wheelchair. They are at risk for sores and calluses on the hands. Friction-coated projection rims are less invasive and slippery than aluminum hand rims. Tissues over bony prominences including the sacrum, buttocks, and heels are at high risk for pressure or shearing (Maklebust, 1991; Perez, 1993).

- For client with loss of sensory and motor functioning, emphasize importance of weight shifts every 15 minutes. Reinforce side leans (leaning toward opposite side of chair), forward leans (leaning forward as arms lie alongside thighs; a safety belt is advised) if balance and trunk control are present, push ups (placing hands on the armrests and pushing to lift buttocks off the seat), and rear tilts (wheelchair is tilted backward by another person from 45 to 65 degrees). Client may also sit with the back of the wheelchair reclined (150-degrees) with legs on leg/foot rests to lower tissue pressure.

  Weight shifts, push-ups, and reclined positioning should be used by clients for intermittent pressure relief to prevent ulcers related to capillary occlusion from great force on a small bony area (Panel for the Prediction and Prevention of Pressure Ulcers in Adults, 1992; McCourt, 1993; Pellow, 1999; Minkel, 2000).

- ▲ Support clients and request referrals as needed to help clients cope and adjust to issues related to physical disability, loss of independence, and use of a wheelchair.

  Clients may experience depression and anxiety with physical loss, especially with the inability to walk. Value systems of clients and nurses with regard to wheelchair use may vary greatly and create tension. Need for a wheelchair may symbolize weakness, disability, and loss of autonomy to clients, whereas it may symbolize increased independence and functioning to professionals (Minkel, 2000).

- ▲ Physical therapists, occupational therapists, or physicians may recommend an electric vs. a manual wheelchair for a client who will need to use, or has used, a wheelchair long term. Client may resist the idea and need psychosocial support as he or she faces this issue.

  Shoulder/wrist pain and injury may result from overuse of a manual wheelchair. An electric wheelchair may be prescribed to protect the integrity of the shoulder joints. However, it may signify further loss of independence and greater disability to clients.

Geriatric

- Alternate wheelchair mobility with stationary rest periods when resting pulse rate, respiratory patterns, and blood pressure reading suggest compromised activity tolerance.

  Pulmonary changes produce decreased lung reserve capacity (McCourt, 1993).

- ▲ Do not place an elderly client in a standard wheelchair; rather, consult an occupational therapist or physical therapist for proper evaluation of wheelchair seating and back systems.

  Elderly clients' lumbar spine tends to flatten, and hip flexion is often less than 90 degrees. A wheelchair with a reclining back offers support at the appropriate angle and may be more comfortable (Sussman, Bates-Jensen, 1998); however, compared with standard wheelchairs, reclining wheelchairs are heavier, harder to propel, and may limit indepen-

• = **Independent;** ▲ = **Collaborative**

dence. Hamstring muscles may tighten and shorten behind the knees, preventing feet from reaching foot rests or the floor. Elderly clients may move to get comfortable or do a task, which may inadvertently result in poor posture and sliding down in the chair. Nurses may unnecessarily restrain such clients.

- Emphasize the importance of placing both feet either on foot plates or on the floor when wheelchair is stationary; that is, do not leave only one foot up on foot plate.
  Tight hamstrings and a posterior pelvic tilt are common in the elderly. These abnormalities are accentuated when the feet are not on an equal level and may create discomfort (Gee, Passarella, 1985).

▲ Assess for side effects of medications and potential need for dosage readjustments related to increasing physical activity.
  Antidepressants and benzodiazepines can cause postural hypotension and dizziness; antihypertensive and cardiac medications often create hypotension, dizziness, and may alter cardiac output; and diuretics cause postural hypotension (Skidmore-Roth, 2001; Radwanski, Hoeman, 1996).

- Allow client to move at his or her own speed. Avoid rushing.
  The elderly normally move more slowly than younger people because of diminished ROM and strength, stiff joints, cardiopulmonary compromise, and discomfort (Radwanski, Hoeman, 1996).

Home Care Interventions

- Assess client and obtain complete history with reference to reasons for impairment.
  Complete understanding of the client problem promotes accurate determination of client needs and individualizes care.

- Assess home environment for all barriers to wheelchair access.
  If client resides alone, assess support system for emergency and contingency care (e.g., Lifeline). Impaired mobility may pose a life threat during a crisis (e.g., falls, fire).

- Assess for skin breakdown. Establish a skin care program to enhance circulation and decrease risk of skin breakdown.
  Impaired mobility decreases circulation to dependent areas, placing the client at risk for skin breakdown.

▲ Refer to home health aide services as appropriate for assistance with ADLs and attention to skin care.
  Mobility impairments may serve as a barrier to self-care.

▲ Provide support to clients with long-term impairments and their caregivers. Refer to medical social services or mental health/support group services as necessary.
  Long-term impairment may necessitate role changes and create anger and frustration. Counseling and support groups provide validation of feelings and alternative methods of problem solving.

- Ensure that client has information on advocacy, options for disability access, and related issues (e.g., education, personnel, and equipment availability) under the Americans with Disabilities Act.
  Information creates the potential for independence.

- Assess and help develop a plan for client accessibility to key spaces and functions (e.g., toileting upright, sleeping, bathing, and preparing and eating meals).
  The ability to perform these activities is critical for staying in one's own home (Yearns, Huntoon, 1997).

• = **Independent**; ▲ = **Collaborative**

- Rearrange room functions, furniture, and cupboards so that toileting, sleeping, bathing, and preparing and eating meals can take place on one level of the home.
- ▲ Request a physical therapy referral to teach client how to build endurance and propel wheelchair on carpet, over doorway thresholds, and on other irregular surfaces, plus how to get back into wheelchair if he or she falls (or intentionally moves) onto the floor.
- Remind clients and family to remove as many wheelchair parts as possible when lifting the chair into the car. Check that armrests or other parts of chair or device are fastened securely before picking them or the chair up. Check temperature of wheelchair or wheeled device in case the surface is excessively hot or cold.
  Prevention is important. Removing parts reduces the weight that needs to be lifted, locking parts into place prevents dropping them, and checking temperature of chair and parts prevents skin from being burned or chilled from inadvertent exposure (Younker Rehabilitation Center, 1990).
- Ensure that traffic patterns are wide enough for a wheelchair or wheeled device to get around.
  Having adequate space prevents damage to skin (especially on knuckles of hands), wheelchair, walls, woodwork, and furniture (Yearns, Huntoon, 1997).
- Familiarize yourself with literature on universal design concepts to make simple and economic changes such as replacing door hardware with fold-back hinges or doorway encasement removal if doorways are too narrow and removing or replacing doorway thresholds if existing ones are too high.
  A branch of the universal design literature deals with ways to modify existing homes (and appliances) to make them more accessible.
- Explain that a 5-foot turning space is necessary to maneuver a wheelchair in key areas of the home (bathroom, kitchen), doorways need to be 32 to 36 inches wide, ramps or paths ascending to an entrance should slope 1 inch per foot, and one outside entrance should have space enough to open the door and accommodate the wheelchair or wheeled device (Yearns, Huntoon, 1997).
- Investigate and share community resources and written information for locating wheelchair parts and services to repair and preventatively tune up devices if client is not able to do it himself or herself (an annual tune-up is wise).

Client/Family Teaching

- Suggest that client test-drive wheelchairs and try out cushions and postural supports before purchasing them.
  Equipment is very expensive, and different makes and models have different advantages and disadvantages (Minkel, 2000).
- ▲ Teach or secure social services referral to educate clients on financial coverage/regulations of third-party payors and HCFA for durable medical equipment. Realize that light and ultra light wheelchairs may be easier to propel and may be more comfortable and adjustable than heavier models. They initially are expensive, but over time they cost less to operate than heavier chairs.
  It is important to recognize the advantages, cost, and durability of different wheelchair models before deciding on a purchase (Cooper et al, 2000).
- Supervise and reinforce client's and family's correct performance of pressure relief techniques (which should be performed every 15 minutes).

• = Independent; ▲ = Collaborative

Pressure relief techniques prevent prolonged pressure to the ischial tuberosities and sacrum during chair sitting (McCourt, 1993; Minkel, 2000).

- Teach client to prevent carpal tunnel syndrome by not putting pressure on the elbows. Client should redistribute pressure along the entire forearm, especially when doing weight shifts and pressure relief techniques. Rest, splints, assistance with transfers, and temporary use of an electric wheelchair may help treat upper extremity tendonitis.

  Persons who are dependent on manual wheelchairs overwork their arms during transfers, repositioning, ADLs, and when propelling the chair. They are at risk for numerous painful syndromes (Dove, 1995).

- Teach client the importance of using seatbelts or chair tiedowns when riding in motor vehicles. If unable to use seat belts or tiedown systems, clients in wheelchairs should be transported in large, heavy vehicles.

  Clients need protection for abrupt vehicle maneuvers. They should be restrained with a seatbelt system and/or with a wheelchair tiedown for greater safety. If neither is available, they are more safely transported in large, heavy vehicles (Shaw, 2000).

WEB SITES FOR EDUCATION

MERLIN See the MERLIN web site for World Wide Web resources for client education.

REFERENCES Cooper RA et al: Long-term rehab: advanced seating systems, parts I and II, *Rehab Manage* 13(2-3):58, 60-61, 62-64, 2000.

Defloor T, Grypdonck MH: Sitting posture and prevention of pressure ulcers, *Appl Nurs Res* 12(3):136-143, 1999.

Dove C: *Complications of spinal cord injury.* Lecture for the Greater Iowa Chapter of the Association Rehabilitation Nurses, July 20, 1995, Cedar Rapids, Iowa.

Dowswell G, Dowswell T, Young J: Adjusting stroke patients' poor position: an observational study, *J Adv Nurs* 32(2):286-291, 2000.

Gee ZL, Passarella PM: *Nursing care of the stroke patient: a therapeutic approach,* Pittsburgh, 1985, America Rehabilitation Educational Network.

Maklebust J: Pressure ulcer update, *RN* 34(12):56, 1991.

McCourt A: *The specialty practice of rehabilitation nursing: a core curriculum,* ed 3, Skokie, Ill, 1993, Rehabilitation Nursing Foundation.

Minkel JL: Seating and mobility considerations for people with spinal cord injury, *Phys Ther* 80(7):701-709, 2000.

Minor MAD, Minor SD: *Patient care skills,* ed 3, Norwalk, Conn, 1995, Appleton & Lange.

Panel for the Prediction and Prevention of Pressure Ulcers in Adults: *Pressure ulcers in adults: prediction and prevention,* Clinical Practice Guideline No. 3, AHCPR Pub. No. 92-0047, Rockville, Md, 1992, U.S. Department of Health and Human Services, Public Health Service.

Pellow TR: A comparison of interface pressure readings to wheelchair cushions and positioning: a pilot study, *Can J Occup Ther* 66(3):140-149, 1999.

Perez E: Pressure ulcers: updated guidelines for treatment and prevention, *Geriatrics* 48(1):39, 1993.

Rader J, Jones D, Miller LL: Individualized wheelchair seating: reducing restraints and improving comfort and function, *Top Geriatr Rehabil* 15(2):43-47, 1999.

Radwanski MB, Hoeman SP: Geriatric rehabilitation nursing. In Hoeman SP, editor: *Rehabilitation nursing: process and application,* ed 2, St Louis, 1996, Mosby.

Shaw G: Wheelchair rider risk in motor vehicles: a technical note, *J Rehabil Res Dev* 37(1):89-100, 2000.

Skidmore-Roth L: *Mosby's nursing drug reference,* St Louis, 2001, Mosby.

Saur T: Long-term rehab: seating and positioning in the newly injured, *Rehab Manage* 12(6):70, 72-73, 1999.

Sussman C, Bates-Jensen BM, editors: *Wound care: a collaborative practice manual for physical therapists and nurses,* Gaithersburg, Md, 1998, Aspen.

• = **Independent;** ▲ = **Collaborative**

Wilson G, Kerr VL: Wheelchairs: selection, uses, adaptation, and maintenance. In Sine RD et al, editors: *Basic rehabilitation techniques: a self-instructional guide,* ed 3, Gaithersburg, Md, 1988, Aspen.

Yearns MH, Huntoon R: *A home for all ages: convenient, comfortable, and attractive,* Handout for 47th Annual Conference of the National Council on the Aging, HDFS-H-294, March 1997.

Younker Rehabilitation Center: *Wheelchair mobility class: do's and don'ts,* Physical Therapy Patient Teaching Sheet, No. 105, 1990. (Available from Younker Rehabilitation Center, Iowa Health System, 1200 Pleasant, Des Moines, IA 50309.)

Nausea

Betty J. Ackley

 Definition An unpleasant wave-like sensation in the back of the throat, epigastrium, or throughout the abdomen that may or may not lead to vomiting

Defining Characteristics

Usually precedes vomiting, but may be experienced after vomiting or when vomiting does not occur; accompanied by pallor, cold and clammy skin, increased salivation, tachycardia, gastric stasis, and diarrhea; accompanied by swallowing movements affected by skeletal muscles; reports "nausea" or "sick to stomach"

Related Factors (r/t)

Chemotherapy; postsurgical anesthesia; irritation to the gastrointestinal system; stimulation of neuropharmacologic mechanisms

 Outcomes (Nursing Outcomes Classification)

Suggested NOC Labels

Comfort Level; Hydration; Nutritional Status: Nutrient Intake; Nutritional Status: Food and Fluid Intake

> ### Example NOC Outcome
> Improves **Comfort Level** as evidenced by the following indicators: Reported satisfaction with symptom control/Reported physical well-being (Rate each indicator of **Comfort Level:** 1 = none, 2 = limited, 3 = moderate, 4 = substantial, 5 = extensive [see Section I])

Client Outcomes

- States relief of nausea
- Explains methods can use to decrease nausea and vomiting

 Interventions (Nursing Interventions Classification)

Suggested NIC Labels

Distraction; Medication Administration; Progressive Muscle Relaxation; Simple Guided Imagery; Therapeutic Touch

> ### Example NIC Interventions
> - Encourage the client to choose the distraction technique(s) desired, such as music, engaging in conversation or tellng a detailed account of event or story, guided imagery, or humor
> - Advise client to practice the distraction technique before it is needed, if possible

• = Independent; ▲ = Collaborative

Nursing Interventions and Rationales

- Determine cause of nausea and vomiting (e.g., medication effects, viral illness, food poisoning, extreme anxiety, pregnancy).
  The cause of nausea and vomiting often determines the treatment.
- Keep a clean emesis basin and tissues within client's reach.
- Provide oral care after client vomits.
  Oral care helps remove the taste and smell of vomitus, thus reducing the stimulus for further vomiting.
- Stay with client to give support, place hand on shoulder, and hold the emesis basin.
  Human support can be helpful and comforting to an uncomfortable client (Morse, Bottorff, Hutchinson, 1994).
- Provide distraction from sensation of nausea using soft music, television, and videos per client preference.
  Distraction can help direct attention away from the sensation of nausea. Music therapy has been shown to decrease nausea and vomiting (Ezzone et al, 1998).
- Maintain a quiet, well-ventilated environment.
  Odors from a kitchen or bathroom can trigger nausea (Pervan, 1990; Quinton, 1998).
- Avoid sudden movement of client; allow client to lie still.
  Movement can trigger further nausea and vomiting.
- After vomiting is controlled and nausea abates, begin feeding client small amounts of clear fluids such as clear soda or preferably ginger ale, and then crackers; progress to a soft diet.
  Ginger root (found in some ginger ales) has been shown to be more effective than a placebo for treatment of postoperative nausea and vomiting (Hawthorn, 1995; Thompson, 1999).
- Remove cover of food tray before bringing it into client's room.
  The sudden, concentrated food odors that come when the cover is removed in front of the client can trigger nausea (Pervan, 1990; Hawthorn, 1995, Quinton, 1998).

Nausea in pregnancy

- Recommend that the woman eat dry crackers or dry toast in bed before arising, then get up slowly. Also advise to chew gum or suck hard candies, eat small frequent meals, avoid foods with offensive odors, and avoid preparing food or shopping when nauseated.
  These are traditional strategies for alleviating nausea (Whitney et al, 2001).
- Recommend that she sit down when experiencing nausea.
  Sitting down reduces nausea up to 80% of the time (Dilorio, van Lier, 1989).
- Determine if the woman is receiving adequate rest.
  Fatigue predisposes to morning sickness (Rhodes, Johnson, McDaniel, 1995).
- ▲ Discuss with client possibility of using transcutaneous electrical stimulation in the form of ReliefBand Device (Woodside Biomedical) to help relieve nausea.
  The results of a systmatic review of the studies showed that the results of using P6 acupressure are generally positive (Jewell, Young, 2000).

Nausea following surgery

- ▲ Alleviate postoperative pain using ordered analgesic agents. (Refer to care plan for **Acute Pain**.)
  The pain sensation is known to be a factor in the development of postoperative nausea and vomiting (Thompson, 1999).

• = **Independent;** ▲ = **Collaborative**

▲ If nausea is associated with the use of opioids, consult with primary care practitioner for possible use of alternative pain medication.

Opioids can cause nausea in the postoperative client (Thompson, 1999).

• Ensure that nauseated client is not hypotensive. Check blood pressure and note signs of postural hypotension.

Postural hypotension can be caused by deficient fluid volume following surgery and can result in nausea (Thompson, 1999).

▲ Consult with primary care practitioner for use of nonpharmacologic techniques such as acupuncture, electroacupuncture, acupoint stimulation, transcutaneous electrical nerve stimulation, or acupressure as an adjunct for controlling postoperative nausea and vomiting. Give the treatment soon after surgery.

A systematic review of literature on these nonpharmacological techniques demonstrated that they were equivalent to commonly used antiemetic drugs in preventing vomiting following surgery, especially within 6 hours of surgery in adults. These techniques were not of benefit in children (Lee, Done, 1999). Acupressure with sea bands can be taught to clients, is harmless, and may provide relief from postoperative nausea and vomiting (Mann, 1999).

• Use relaxation and distraction techniques for nausea: encourage the client to take slow, deep breaths.

Deep breaths can serve as a distraction technique and can help rid the body of the anesthetic agent (Thompson, 1999).

Nausea following chemotherapy

▲ Consult with physician regarding need for antiemetic medications.

There are antiemetic drugs that can be very effective for clients with nausea from chemotherapy (Goebel, 1996; Glick, Griffith, Mortimer, 1998).

▲ Recognize that opioids used to treat pain may also result in nausea, but generally it is short in duration (Aparasu, 1999).

▲ Consult with primary care provider on the use of transcutaneous electrical nerve stimulation as an adjunct for controlling chemotherapy-induced nausea and vomiting.

Antiemetic medications may stop vomiting, but not nausea (Roscoe et al, 2000). Transcutaneous electric nerve stimulation, using the ReliefBand, was shown to be an effective adjunct to medications for controlling nausea in gynecologic oncology clients (Pearl et al, 1999).

• Help the client learn how to use acupressure for nausea, applying pressure bilaterally at P6 and ST36 acupressure points on the back of the wrist and by the knee.

Finger acupressure may be effective to relieve chemotherapy-induced nausea (Dibble et al, 2000).

• Offer the nauseated client a 10-minute foot massage.

Foot massage was shown to be an effective way to decrease nausea, pain, and anxiety in a group of oncology clients (Grealish, Lomasney, Whiteman, 2000).

▲ For clients who continue to experience nausea after antiemetic drugs or other treatments, consult with the primary care practitioner regarding the possibility of using acupuncture to control nausea and vomiting.

Acupuncture has been shown to effectively control chemotherapy-induced nausea and vomiting in adults (Kaplan, LaRiccia, Pian-Smith, 1999; Acupuncture, 2000).

Geriatrics

▲ Administer antiemetic drugs carefully; watch for side effects.

Elderly clients have increased risk of side effects, such as extrapyramidal effects or sedation, from antiemetic drugs (Johnson, Moroney, Gay, 1997).

• = Independent; ▲ = Collaborative

Home Care Interventions

- Assist the client and family with identifying and avoiding irritants in the home setting that exacerbate nausea (e.g., strong odors from food, plants, perfume, and room deodorizers).

Client/Family Teaching

- Teach client techniques to use when uncomfortable, including relaxation techniques, guided imagery, hypnosis, and music therapy (Jablonski, 1993; Pervan, 1993; Rhodes, Johnson, McDaniel, 1995).

  Guided imagery has been shown to effectively decrease nausea associated with chemo-therapy (Troesch, 1993). Behavioral interventions for nausea such as hypnosis, progressive muscle relaxation training, systematic desensitization, biofeedback, and distractions have also been shown to be effective (Dodd, 1993). Music therapy has been shown to be helpful for decreasing nausea and vomiting in clients receiving high-dose chemotherapy (Ezzone et al, 1998).

WEB SITES FOR EDUCATION

MERLIN See the MERLIN web site for World Wide Web resources for client education.

REFERENCES   Acupuncture: National Institutes of Health consensus development conference statement, *Dermatol Nurs* 12(2):126-133, 2000.

Aparasu R et al: Opioid-induced emesis among hospitalized nonsurgical patients: effect on pain and quality of life, *J Pain Symptom Manage* 8(4):280-288, 1999.

Dibble SL et al: Acupressure for nausea: results of a pilot study, *Onc Nurs Forum* 27(1):41-47, 2000.

Dilorio CK, van Lier DJ: Nausea and vomiting in pregnancy. In Funk SG et al, editors: *Key aspects of comfort: management of pain, fatigue, and nausea,* New York, 1989, Springer.

Dodd MJ: Side effects of cancer chemotherapy, *Annu Rev Nurs Res* 11:77-103, 1993.

Ezzone S et al: Music as an adjunct to antiemetic therapy, *Oncol Nurs Forum* 25(9):1551-1556, 1998.

Glick JH, Griffith RS, Mortimer JE: Cancer treatment, chemotherapy: helping the patient cope, *Patient Care* 32(1):49-54, 1998.

Goebel C: Prevention and control of nausea and vomiting for patients with cancer, *Home Healthc Nurs* 14:15, 1996.

Grealish L, Lomasney A, Whiteman B: Foot massage: a nursing intervention to modify the distressing symptoms of pain and nausea in patients hospitalized with cancer, *Cancer Nurs* 23(3):237-243, 2000.

Hawthorn J: *Understanding and management of nausea and vomiting,* Oxford, 1995, Blackwell Science.

Jablonski RS: Nausea: the forgotten symptom, *Holistic Nurs Pract* 7:64, 1993.

Jewell D, Young G: Interventions for nausea and vomiting in early pregnancy, *Cochrane Library* (2):CD000145, 2000.

Johnson MH, Moroney CE, Gay CF: Relieving nausea and vomiting in patients with cancer: a treatment algorithm, *Oncol Nurs Forum* 24(1):51-58, 1997.

Kaplan G, LaRiccia PJ, Pian-Smith M: Acupuncture: another therapeutic choice? *Patient Care* 33(11):149-176, 1999.

Lee A, Done ML: The use of nonpharmacologic techniques to prevent postoperative nausea and vomiting: a meta-analysis, *Anesth Analg* 88(6):1362-1369, 1999.

Mann E: Using acupuncture and acupressure to treat postoperative emesis, *Prof Nurs* 14(10):691-694, 1999.

Morse JM, Bottorff JL, Hutchinson S: The phenomenology of comfort, *J Adv Nurs* 20:189, 1994.

Pearl ML et al: Transcutaneous electrical nerve stimulation as an adjunct for controlling chemotherapy-induced nausea and vomiting in gynecologic oncology patients, *Cancer Nurs* 22(4):307-311, 1999.

Pervan V: Practical aspects of dealing with cancer therapy–induced nausea and vomiting, *Semin Oncol Nurs* 6:3, 1990.

Pervan V: Understanding anti-emetics, *Nurs Times* 89(10):36-37, 1993.

Quinton D: Anticipatory nausea and vomiting in chemotherapy, *Prof Nurse* 13(10):663-666, 1998.

Rhodes VA, Johnson MH, McDaniel RW: Nausea, vomiting, and retching: the management of the symptom experience, *Semin Oncol Nurs* 11:256, 1995.

• = Independent; ▲ = Collaborative

Roscoe J et al: Nausea and vomiting remain a significant clinical problem: trends over time in controlling chemotherapy-induced nausea and vomiting in 1413 patients treated in community clinical practices, *J Pain Symptom Manage* 20(2):113-121, 2000.

Thompson HJ: The management of post-operative nausea and vomiting, *J Adv Nurs* 29(5):1130-1136, 1999.

Troesch LM et al: The influence of guided imagery on chemotherapy-related nausea and vomiting, *Oncol Nurs Forum* 20:1179, 1993.

Whitney EN et al: *Nutrition for health and health care,* ed 2, Belmont, Calif, 2001, Wadsworth.

Unilateral Neglect

Betty J. Ackley and Leslie Kalbach

NANDA   **Definition** Lack of awareness and attention to one side of the body

Defining Characteristics

Consistent inattention to stimuli on an affected side; does not look toward affected side; inadequate positioning and/or safety precautions with regard to the affected side; inadequate self-care; leaves food on plate on the affected side

Related Factors (r/t)

Effects of disturbed perceptual abilities (e.g., hemianopsia [one-sided blindness], neurological illnesses, trauma)

NOTE: Because the right hemisphere is dominant in directing attention, unilateral neglect is more common if neurological pathology occurs in the right hemisphere of the brain, which results in left-sided neglect (Katz et al, 2000). Also, unilateral neglect frequently occurs with parietal lesions (Herman, 1992; Kalbach, 1991).

NOC   **Outcomes (Nursing Outcomes Classification)**

Suggested NOC Labels

Body Image; Body Positioning: Self-Initiated; Self-Care: Activities of Daily Living

> **Example NOC Outcome**
> Improves **Body Image** as evidenced by the following indicators: Willingness to touch affected body part/Adjustment to changes in body function/Willingness to use strategies to enhance appearance and function (Rate each indicator of **Body Image:** 1 = never positive, 2 = rarely positive, 3 = sometimes positive, 4 = often positive, 5 = consistently positive [see Section I])

Client Outcomes

- Demonstrates techniques that can be used to minimize unilateral neglect
- Cares for both sides of the body appropriately and keeps affected side free from harm

NIC   **Interventions (Nursing Interventions Classification)**

Suggested NIC Labels

Unilateral Neglect Management

> **Example NIC Interventions—Unilateral Neglect Management**
> - Provide realistic feedback about patient's perceptual deficit
> - Touch unaffected shoulder when initiating conversation

• = Independent; ▲ = Collaborative

Nursing Interventions and Rationales

- Monitor client for signs of unilateral neglect (e.g., not washing, shaving, or dressing one side of the body; sitting or lying inappropriately on affected arm or leg; failing to respond to stimuli on the contralateral side of lesion; eating food on only one side of plate; or failing to look to one side of the body).
  Looking, listening, touching, and searching deficits occur on the affected side of the body and may or may not be associated with a loss of vision, sensation, or motion on the affected side (Kalbach, 1991; Herman, 1992).

▲ If available, use the "star cancellation test" to evaluate presence of unilateral neglect.
  The star cancellation test consists of a series of big and little stars and words scattered on a page. When directed to cross out all the little stars, clients with unilateral neglect will miss stars on one side of the paper (Halligan, Marshall, Wade, 1989; Taylor, Ashburn, Ward, 1994).

- Provide a safe, well-lighted, and clutter-free environment. Place call light on unaffected side. Keep side rails up when client is in bed. Cue client to environmental hazards when mobile.
  Cognitive impairment may accompany neglect; therefore safety is of paramount importance.

- Nursing interventions for clients with unilateral neglect should be implemented in the following stages as client progresses:
  Stage I: Focus attention mainly on nonneglected side.
  - Set up environment so that most activity is on unaffected side.
  - Keep client's personal items within view and on unaffected side.
  - Position client's bed so that activity is on unaffected side.
  The initial priority is client safety (Kalbach, 1991).
  Stage II: Help client develop an awareness of neglected side.
  - Gradually focus client's attention on affected side.
  - Gradually move personal items and activity to affected side.
  - Stand on client's affected side when assisting with ambulation or activities of daily living (ADLs).
  The goal now is for the client to develop an awareness of the neglected side (Kalbach, 1991).
  Stage III: Help client develop ability to compensate for neglect.
  - Encourage client to bathe and groom affected side first.
  - Focus touch and talking on affected side; use a positive approach (e.g., "Mary, turn your head to the left and you'll see your grandchildren" [Carnevali, Patrick, 1993]).
  - Use constant and positive reminders to keep client scanning entire environment.
  - Use bright yellow or red stickers on outer margins in reading or writing exercises. Have client look for the sticker before reading or writing.
  - Use cues and anchors to promote attention to the neglected side and help the client develop compensatory mechanisms to deal with the neglect syndrome (Riddoch, Humphreys, 1983; Kalbach, 1991; Cooke, 1992).

▲ Refer to a rehabilitation nurse specialist, neuropsychologist, or occupational therapist for continued help in dealing with unilateral neglect. Helpful therapy can include visual stimuli, visuomotor imagery, videotaping, use of specific devices (Bon Saint Com's device), and eye-patching techniques.

• = Independent; ▲ = Collaborative

Monocular patching with lateralized visual stimulation may significantly reduce neglect in daily activities (Butter, Kirsch, 1992). The device that associates exploratory reconditioning with voluntary trunk rotation can improve unilateral neglect (Wiart et al, 1997). The neuropsychologist can help to ameliorate symptoms of unilateral neglect (Riddoch, Humphreys, Bateman, 1995). Videotaping can help clients perceive their own performance and improve function on some tasks (Tham, Tegner, 1997).

Home Care Interventions
- Many of the listed interventions may be adapted for use in the home care setting.

Client/Family Teaching
- Explain pathology and symptoms of unilateral neglect.
- Teach client how to scan regularly to check the position of body parts and to regularly turn head from side to side for safety when ambulating.
- Teach caregivers positive cueing (reminders to help client remember to interact with entire environment).

WEB SITES FOR EDUCATION

 See the MERLIN web site for World Wide Web resources for client education.

REFERENCES Butter CM, Kirsch N: Combined and separate effects of eye patching and visual stimulation on unilateral neglect following stroke, *Arch Phys Med Rehab* 73:1133, 1992.

Carnevali DL, Patrick M: *Nursing management for the elderly,* ed 3, Philadelphia, 1993, JB Lippincott.

Cooke D: Remediation of unilateral neglect: what do we know? *Aust Occup Ther J* 39:19, 1992.

Halligan PW, Marshall JC, Wade DT: Visuospatial neglect: underlying factors and test sensitivity, *Lancet* 2(8668):908, 1989.

Herman EW: Spatial neglect: new issues and their implications for occupational therapy practice, *Am J Occup Ther* 46:207, 1992.

Kalbach LR: Unilateral neglect: mechanisms and nursing care, *J Neurosci Nurs* 23:125, 1991.

Katz N et al: Relationships of cognitive performance and daily function of clients following right hemisphere stroke: predictive and ecological validity of the LOTCA Battery, *Occup Ther J Res* 20(1):3-17, 2000.

Riddoch MF, Humphreys GW: The effect of cueing on unilateral neglect, *Neuropsychologist* 21:589, 1983.

Riddoch MF, Humphreys GW, Bateman A: Cognitive deficits following stroke, *Physiotherapy* 81:465, 1995.

Taylor D, Ashburn A, Ward CD: Asymmetrical trunk posture, unilateral neglect and motor performance following stroke, *Clin Rehab* 8:48, 1994.

Tham K, Tegner R: Video feedback in the rehabilitation of patients with unilateral neglect, *Arch Phys Med Rehabil* 78(4):410-413, 1997.

Wiart et al: Unilateral neglect syndrome rehabilitation by trunk rotation and scanning training, *Arch Phys Med Rehabil* 78(4):424, 1997.

Noncompliance

Betty J. Ackley

NANDA **Definition** Behavior of person and/or caregiver that fails to coincide with a health-promoting or therapeutic plan agreed on by the person (and/or family and/or community) and health-care professional; in the presence of an agreed-on, health-promoting,

• = Independent; ▲ = Collaborative

or therapeutic plan, person's or caregiver's behavior is fully or partially nonadherent and may lead to clinically ineffective or partially ineffective outcomes

Defining Characteristics

Behavior indicative of failure to adhere (directly observed or verbalized by patient or significant others) (critical); objective tests (e.g., physiological measures, detection of markers); evidence of development of complications; evidence of exacerbation of symptoms; failure to keep appointments; failure to progress

Related Factors (r/t)

Healthcare plan

Duration; significant others; cost; intensity; complexity

Indivdual factors

Personal and developmental abilities; health beliefs, cultural influences, spiritual values; individual's value system; knowledge and skill relevant to the regimen behavior; motivational forces

Health system   Satisfaction with care; credibility of provider; access and convenience of care; financial flexibility of plan; client-provider relationships; provider reimbursement of teaching and follow-up; provider continuity and regular follow-up; individual health coverage; communcation and teaching skills of the provider

Network   Involvement of members in health plan; social value regarding plan; perceived beliefs of significant others

NOTE: The nursing diagnosis **Noncompliance** is judgmental and places blame on the client (Bakker, Kastermans, Dassen, 1995; Ward-Collins, 1998). The author recommends use of the diagnosis **Ineffective Therapeutic regimen management** in place of the diagnosis **Noncompliance.** The diagnosis **Ineffective Therapeutic regimen management** has interventions that are developed by both the health care providers and the client. It is a more respectful and efficacious nursing diagnosis than **Noncompliance.**

`NOC`   Outcomes (Nursing Outcomes Classification)

Suggested NOC Labels

Adherence Behavior; Compliance Behavior; Pain Level; Symptom Control Behavior; Treatment Behavior; Illness or Injury

> **Example NOC Outcome**
> Demonstrates **Adherence Behavior** as evidenced by the following indicators: Describes strategies to maximize health/Describes strategies to eliminate unhealthy behavior/Provides rationale for adopting a regimen/Reports using strategies to eliminate unhealthy behavior (Rate each indicator of **Adherence Behavior:** 1 = never demonstrated, 2 = rarely demonstrated, 3 = sometimes demonstrated, 4 = often demonstrated, 5 = consistently demonstrated [see Section I])

Client Outcomes

- Describes consequence of continued noncompliance with treatment regimen
- States goals for health and the means by which to obtain them
- Communicates an understanding of disease and treatment
- Lists treatment regimens and expectations and agrees to follow through
- Lists alternative ways to meet goals
- Describes the importance of family participation to help achieve goals

• = **Independent;** ▲ = **Collaborative**

NIC	**Interventions (Nursing Interventions Classification)**

Suggested NIC Labels

Health System Guidance; Self-Modification Assistance

> **Example NIC Interventions—Health System Guidance**
> - Inform client of appropriate community resources and contact persons
> - Inform client how to access emergency services by telephone and vehicle, as appropriate

Nursing Interventions and Rationales

- Ask client why he or she has not complied with the prescribed treatment. Have client "tell their story." Listen nonjudgmentally.
  Compliance assessment should begin with a nonthreatening discussion with the client (Kluckowski, 1992; London, 1998).
- Make client an active partner in own health care management. Recognize that client has absolute control over whether he or she follows health care regime. Always treat client with respect, and develop mutual outcomes for treatment.
  If client feels respected and is involved in decision making, compliance will increase. Many clients report that how they are treated by health professionals has a great impact on whether or not they follow advice (Lannon, 1997).
- Observe for cause of noncompliance (see Related Factors). Recognize that noncompliance is very common.
  Rates of noncompliance are estimated at 50% (Kluckowski, 1992; Dunbar-Jacob et al, 2000).
- Recognize that behavioral change comes slowly, and often in stages (Prochaska, 1994).
    Precontemplation—change is not contemplated; unaware of problem or risk
    Contemplation—aware that problem exists; no specific plans or commitment to change
    Preparation—plan to take action within the next 30 days
    Action—now taking action to improve health; often behavior not consistently carried out
    Maintenance—consistently engages in healthful behavior for more than 6 months
  Individuals tend to cycle through the stages of change, often not in a linear progression, and may go through the cycle several times. The most important thing is unconditional acceptance of the person, understanding of the behavior, and subtle encouragement when asked. Make information available, but do not preach or force information on clients (Samuelson, 1998).
- If client is in denial: provide information, communicate unconditional positive regard, avoid distancing yourself, and look for opportunities for authentic contact with your client, being present psychologically and physically.
  The most important thing you can do for someone who appears to be in denial is to take the time to genuinely connect (Robinson, 1999).
- Determine client's and family's knowledge of illness and treatment. Teach them about the illness and purpose of the treatment regimen if necessary.
  Knowledge is power, and with it comes increased control; the more control clients have, the more likely they are to comply with the prescribed regimen (Kluckowski, 1992).
- Observe whether locus of control is internal or external. Recognize that people with external locus of control are more likely to be noncompliant because they don't

• = **Independent;** ▲ = **Collaborative**

believe they can help themselves. They believe that it's a matter of luck or destiny that they are ill.

Clients with an internal locus of control are more compliant (Warren, 1992; Muscari, 1998).

▲ Monitor client for signs of depression that may cause noncompliance. Refer for treatment if appropriate.

Depression can cause increased incidence of "source memory errors," resulting in client being unable to remember if he or she did something or just thought about doing it, which can be very serious when it involves taking needed medications (Elias, 2001). Depression can also cause apathy, in which case the client doesn't care whether he or she takes needed actions for health.

• Monitor client's ability to follow directions, solve problems, concentrate, and read.

Clients with cognitive impairments or who are illiterate may not be able to follow directions and the prescribed treatment regimen.

• Avoid using threats, pressure, and inappropriate fear arousal to increase compliance.

These measures are unethical and generally ineffective. If clients are "browbeaten" and attempts are made to shame, induce guilt, or embarrass the client, the noncompliant client will only dig deeper in his or her resolve not to change (Samuelson, 1998).

• Determine whether client's support system helps or hinders therapy. Bring family members and significant others into the educational process as desired by the client.

A positive social support system is associated with increased compliance (Warren, 1992). Schizophrenic clients who have little family support are more likely to be noncompliant than those with family support, especially if there is a history of substance abuse and difficulty recognizing own symptoms (Olfson et al, 2000).

• Develop a therapeutic relationship based on active listening.

Good communication has been shown to increase compliance (Crane, Kirby, Kooperman, 1996). Compliance is increased when the client feels that the health care provider is interested in and genuinely cares about the client (Warren, 1992).

• Listen to client's descriptions of abilities; encourage client to use these abilities in self-care.

• When dealing with complex health care regimens, start client with small behavioral changes (e.g., have chemotherapy client rinse mouth with a saliva substitute twice daily). When one step has been accomplished, add another step.

The client is often overwhelmed by what is expected and needs help with managing behavioral changes (Boehm, 1992).

• Work with client to develop cues that trigger needed health care behaviors (e.g., checking blood sugar before putting on makeup each morning), including weekends, holidays, and vacations.

Associating cues with desired behaviors increases the frequency of these behaviors. Compliance often decreases when the client no longer has a usual routine.

• Work with client to develop an instruction and reminder sheet that fits medications and treatments into the client's lifestyle.

Visual reminders help increase compliance.

• Observe noncompliant client for possibility of secondary gain such as increased attention if client continues to be ill and noncompliant.

Adolescent clients may use noncompliance as a passive form of manipulation to control their relationships with others to avoid school, work, or the legal system. Also, sometimes

• = Independent; ▲ = Collaborative

the illness has become part of the client's self-concept and identity and therefore meets needs (Muscari, 1998).

▲ For a chronically ill client, develop a multidisciplinary team to provide care, including a nurse, physician, pharmacist, dietitian, and additional therapists as needed. Have team meetings to ensure continuity of care.
Multidisciplinary team care has been shown to increase compliance (Warren, 1992).

• Consider allowing client to take own medications while in the hospital if appropriate.
Clients who learned to take medications successfully in the hospital were less likely to be readmitted in a group of mental health clients (DeProspero, Riffle, 1997).

• Develop a mutually agreed on written contract with client regarding needed health care behaviors; give reinforcement as client meets defined goals.
A client contract that helps the client analyze behaviors and choose behavioral strategies can be very effective in changing health care behaviors (Boehm, 1992; Simons, 1999).

▲ Consult with primary care practitioner regarding the possibility of simplifying the health care regimen so that it more easily fits into client's lifestyle (e.g., taking medications one time per day vs. four times per day).
Complex regimens and inconvenient dose scheduling decrease compliance (Crane, Kirby, Kooperman, 1996).

Geriatric

▲ If client has sensory and coordination deficits, use a medication organizer and have the home health nurse or family place client's medications in daily compartments.
A medication organizer used along with a written schedule of when medications should be taken can increase compliance in the elderly (Park et al, 1992).

• Help client feel like a partner in managing health care condition; use caring, encouragement, written goals, and a "power with" relationship with nurse.
These methods have been shown to increase self-efficacy and empower both teenagers and elderly clients to manage their condition (Resnick, 1996; Muscari, 1998).

▲ Ask clients if they can afford medications. Refer for financial help from social worker or case manager if needed.
The cost of the therapeutic regimen may be a source of noncompliance, especially in the elderly (De Geest, 1998).

▲ Monitor client for signs of depression associated with noncompliance (e.g., refusing to eat or take medications). Refer client for treatment of depression as needed.
Noncompliance in the elderly may be a form of indirect self-destructive behavior that is associated with depression and leads to suicide (Meisekothen, 1993). One study demonstrated that depressed clients were three times more likely than nondepressed clients to be noncompliant (DiMatteo, Lepper, Croghan, 2000).

• Use repetition, verbal cues, and memory aids such as pictures, schedule, or reminder sheet when teaching the health care regimen.
There may be age-related memory deficits that necessitate an increased use of measures that cue the client to perform needed health care behaviors (De Geest, 1998; Dunbar-Jacob et al, 2000).

Multicultural

• Assess for the influence of cultural beliefs, norms, and values on the client's ability to modify health behavior.
What the client considers normal and abnormal health behavior may be based on cultural perceptions (Leininger, 1996).

• = Independent; ▲ = Collaborative

- Discuss with the client those aspects of their health behavior/lifestyle that will remain unchanged by their health status.
  Aspects of the client's life that are meaningful and valuable to him or her should be understood and preserved without change (Leininger, 1996).
- Negotiate with the client regarding the aspects of health behavior that will need to be modified.
  Give and take with the client will lead to culturally congruent care (Leininger, 1996).
- Assess the role of fatalism on the client's ability to modify health behavior
  Fatalistic perspectives, which involve the belief that you cannot control your own fate, may influence health behaviors in some African American and Latino populations (Phillips, Cohen, Moses, 1999; Harmon, Castro, Coe, 1996).
- Validate the client's feelings regarding the impact of health status on current lifestyle.
  Validation lets the client know that the nurse has heard and understands what was said, and it promotes the nurse-client relationship (Stuart, Laraia, 2001; Giger, Davidhizar, 1995).

Home Care Interventions

NOTE: Because the home care nurse enters the client's home as a guest, the ability of the nurse to establish a supportive, therapeutic relationship is especially important.

- Before providing any care, review the home health care Bill of Rights with the client, including the right to refuse treatment.
  Identifying the rights of the client demonstrates respect of the health care system and its representatives for client wishes.
- If included in agency policies and procedures, also review patient responsibilities with client (which is often part of printed Bill of Rights).
  Reviewing responsibilities helps client define roles of mutual respect and partnership with the health care provider.
- When client is noncompliant, redefine personal and health priorities (contract for services) with client to determine alternative motivational strategies or health actions to meet health goals.
  For clients to carry out desired health actions, they must perceive actions as beneficial to self and the cost of the health action as not being greater than the benefit (Rosenstock, 1974).
- ▲ If noncompliant behavior continues and client chooses not to cooperate with medical regimen, home health care cannot continue to provide services.
  Reimbursement guidelines and agency policies do not support the continued use of health care resources when the client makes an informed decision to not follow the prescribed regimen.
- If care is to be terminated, identify all possible alternatives for the client and assist with making an informed choice about future health actions.
  Some regulatory guidelines require health care providers to give written notice of discontinuance of care using established time frames. Noncompliance and a plan for termination of care notwithstanding, it remains the goal and ethical responsibility of home health care providers to promote optimal wellness, independence, and safety.
- Respect the wishes of terminally ill clients to refuse selected aspects of medical regimen.
  With terminally ill clients, do not terminate care. Provide those aspects of care that client and family or caregivers will accept. The goal of hospice care is to provide comfort and dignity in the dying process.

• = **Independent;** ▲ = **Collaborative**

Client/Family Teaching

▲ Teach clients about medication side effects (e.g., mental changes, sexual dysfunction) so that they understand them and feel comfortable discussing them.

Many medications can cause side effects such as changes in mental function and impotence, which can lead to noncompliance.

• Teach clients to control their "self-talk" by giving themselves positive messages that will be used to promote desired behaviors, such as taking medications and controlling food intake.

Self-talk has been shown to be a common motivating method for behavior changes (McSweeney, 1993).

WEB SITES FOR EDUCATION

MERLIN See the MERLIN web site for World Wide Web resources for client education.

REFERENCES   Bakker RH, Kastermans MC, Dassen TW: An analysis of the nursing diagnosis in effective management of therapeutic regimen compared to noncompliance and Orem's self-care deficit theory of nursing, *Nurs Diagn* 6(4):161-166, 1995.

Boehm S: Patient contracting. In Bulechek GM, McCloskey JC, editors: *Nursing interventions: essential nursing treatments,* Philadelphia, 1992, WB Saunders.

Crane K, Kirby B, Kooperman D: Patient compliance for psychotropic medications, *J Psychosoc Nurs* 34(1):8-15, 1996.

De Geest S: Compliance issues with the geriatric population, *Nurs Clin North Am* 33(3):467-478, 1998.

DeProspero T, Riffle WA: Improving patients' drug compliance, *Psychiatr Serv* 48(11):1468, 1997.

DiMatteo MR, Lepper HS, Croghan TW: Depression is a risk factor for noncompliance with medical treatment: meta-analysis of the effects of anxiety and depression on patient adherence, *J Psychosoc Nurs Ment Health Serv* 38(5):37-44, 2000.

Dunbar-Jacob et al: Adherence in chronic disease, *Annu Rev Nurs Res* 18:48-90, 2000.

Elias JW: Why caregiver depression and self-care abilities should be part of the PPS case mix methodology, *Home Healthc Nurse* 19(1):23-30, 2001.

Giger JN, Davidhizar RE: *Transcultural nursing,* ed 2, St Louis, 1995, Mosby.

Harmon MP, Castro FG, Coe K: Acculturation and cervical cancer: knowledge, beliefs, and behaviors of Hispanic women, *Women Health* 24(3):37-57, 1996.

Kluckowski JC: Solving medication noncompliance in home care, *Caring* 11:34-40, 1992.

Lannon SL: Using a health promotion model to enhance medication compliance, *J Neurosci* 29(3):170-178, 1997.

Leininger MM: *Transcultural nursing: theories, research and practices,* ed 2, Hilliard, Ohio, 1996, McGraw-Hill.

London F: Improving compliance: what you can do, *RN* 98(1):43-46, 1998.

McSweeney JC: Making behavior changes after a myocardial infarction, *West J Nurs Res* 15(4):441-445, 1993.

Meisekothen LM: Noncompliance in the elderly: a pathway to suicide, *J Am Acad Nurs Pract* 5(2):67-71, 1993.

Muscari ME: Rebels with a cause, *Am J Nurs* 98(12):26-30, 1998.

Olfson M et al: Predicting medication noncompliance after hospital discharge among patients with schizophrenia, *Psychiatr Serv* 51(2):216-222, 2000.

Park DC et al: Medication adherence behaviors in older adults: effects of external cognitive supports, *Psychol Aging* 7(2):252-256, 1992.

Phillips JM, Cohen MZ, Moses G: Breast cancer screening and African American women: fear, fatalism, and silence, *Oncol Nurs Forum* 26(3):561-571, 1999.

Prochaska JO et al: *Changing for good: a revolutionary six stage program for overcoming bad habits and moving your life positively forward,* New York, 1994, Avon Books, p 304.

Resnick B: Motivation in geriatric rehabilitation, *Image* 28(1):41-45, 1996.

Robinson AW: Getting the heart of denial, *Am J Nurs* 99(5):38-42, 1999.

Rosenstock I: Health belief model and preventive behavior. In Becker M, editor: *The health belief model and personal health behavior,* Thorofare, NJ, 1974, CB Slack.

• = **Independent;** ▲ = **Collaborative**

Samuelson M: Stages of change: from theory to practice, *Art Health Promotion* 2(5):1-12, 1998.

Simons MR: Patient contracting. In Bulechek GM, McCloskey JC: *Nursing interventions: effective nursing treatments,* ed 3, Philadelphia, 1999, WB Saunders.

Stuart GW, Laraia MT: Therapeutic nurse-patient relationship. In Stuart GW, Laraia MT, editors: *Principles and practice of psychiatric nursing,* St Louis, 2001, Mosby, p 30.

Ward-Collins D: Noncompliant: isn't there a better way to say it? *Am J Nurs* 98(5):27-32, 1998.

Warren JJ: Ethical concerns about noncompliance in the chronically ill patient, *Prog Cardiovasc Nurs* 7(4):10-14, 1992.

Imbalanced Nutrition: less than body requirements

Carroll A. Lutz

NANDA **Definition** Intake of nutrients insufficient to meet metabolic needs

Defining Characteristics

Body weight ≥20% under ideal weight; pale conjunctival and mucus membranes; weakness of muscles required for swallowing or mastication; sore, inflamed buccal cavity; satiety immediately after ingesting food; reported or evidence of lack of food; reported inadequate food intake less than RDA (Recommended Dietary Allowance); reported altered taste sensation; perceived inability to ingest food; misconceptions; loss of weight with adequate food intake; aversion to eating; abdominal cramping; poor muscle tone; abdominal pain with or without pathology; lack of interest in food; capillary fragility; diarrhea and/or steatorrhea; excessive loss of hair; hyperactive bowel sounds; lack of information; misinformation

Related Factors (r/t)

Inability to ingest or digest food or absorb nutrients because of biological, psychological, or economic factors

NOC **Outcomes (Nursing Outcomes Classification)**

Suggested NOC Labels

Nutritional Status; Nutritional Status: Food and Fluid Intake; Nutritional Status: Nutrient Intake; Weight Control

Example NOC Outcome

Demonstrates improved **Nutritional Status** as evidenced by the following indicators: Food and fluid intake/Body mass index/Weight/Biochemical measures (Rate each indicator of **Nutritional Status:** 1 = extremely compromised, 2 = substantially compromised, 3 = moderately compromised, 4 = mildly compromised, 5 = not compromised [see Section I])

Client Outcomes

- Progressively gains weight toward desired goal
- Weight is within normal range for height and age
- Recognizes factors contributing to underweight
- Identifies nutritional requirements
- Consumes adequate nourishment
- Free of signs of malnutrition

• = **Independent;** ▲ = **Collaborative**

| NIC | **Interventions (Nursing Interventions Classification)** |

Suggested NIC Labels

Nutrition Management; Eating Disorders Management; Electrolyte Management: Hypophosphatemia; Enteral Tube Feeding; Feeding; Nutrition Therapy; Nutritional Counseling; Nutritional Monitoring; Swallowing Therapy; Weight Gain Assistance; Weight Management

> **Example NIC Interventions—Nutrition Management**
> - Ascertain client's food preferences
> - Provide client with high-protein, high-calorie, nutritious finger foods and drinks that can be readily consumed, as appropriate

Nursing Interventions and Rationales

▲ Determine healthy body weight for age and height. Refer to dietitian for complete nutrition assessment if 10% under healthy body weight or if rapidly losing weight. Legal intervention may be necessary.

Early diagnosis and a holistic team treatment of eating disorders are desirable. Of women who ran 15 to 30 miles per week, 20% to 25% had increased risk of eating disorders (Estok, Rudy, 1996). In the developed world, protein-calorie malnutrition (PCM) most often accompanies a disease process. Surveys of hospitalized children in this country revealed that 20% to 40% had PCM (Baker, 1997). Over the short term, patients involuntarily committed for treatment of eating disorders progressed as well as those seeking treatment voluntarily (Watson, Bowers, Andersen, 2000).

- Compare usual food intake to USDA Food Pyramid, noting slighted or omitted food groups.

Milk consumption has decreased among children while intake of fruit juices and carbonated beverages has increased. A higher incidence of bone fractures in teenage girls has been associated with a greater consumption of carbonated beverages (Wyshak, 2000). Possibly also related is the substitution of soda for milk. Omission of entire food groups increases risk of deficiencies.

- If client is a vegetarian, evaluate if obtaining sufficient amounts of vitamin B_{12} and iron.

Strict vegetarians may be at particular risk for vitamin B_{12} and iron deficiencies. Special care should be taken when implementing vegetarian diets for pregnant women, infants, children, and the elderly. A dietitian can usually furnish a balanced vegetarian diet (with adequate substitutes for omitted foods) for inpatients and can provide instruction for outpatients.

- Assess client's ability to obtain and use essential nutrients.

Cases of vitamin D deficiency rickets have been reported among dark-skinned infants and toddlers who were exclusively breast fed and were not given supplemental vitamin D. The children resided in northern (Fitzpatrick et al, 2000), mid-south (Kreiter et al, 2000), and southern (Shah et al, 2000) states, indicating that the presence of natural sunlight does not eliminate the risk of disease.

- Observe client's ability to eat (time involved, motor skills, visual acuity, ability to swallow various textures).

Poor vision was associated with lower protein and energy (calorie) intakes in home care clients independent of other medical conditions (Payette et al, 1995).

• = **Independent;** ▲ = **Collaborative**

NOTE: If client is unable to feed self, refer to Nursing Interventions and Rationales for **Feeding Self-care deficit.** If client has difficulty swallowing, refer to Nursing Interventions and Rationales for **Impaired Swallowing.**

- If client lacks endurance, schedule rest periods before meals and open packages and cut up food for client.
  Nursing assistance with activities of daily living (ADLs) will conserve the client's energy for activities the client values. Clients who take longer than 1 hour to complete a meal may require assistance (Evans, 1992).
- ▲ Evaluate client's laboratory studies (serum albumin, serum total protein, serum ferritin, transferrin, hemoglobin, hematocrit, vitamins, and minerals).
  An abnormal value in a single diagnostic study may have many possible causes, but serum albumin less than 3.2 g/dl was shown to be highly predictive of mortality in hospitals, and serum cholesterol of less than 156 mg/dl was the best predictor of mortality in nursing homes (Morley, 1997).
- Maintain a high index of suspicion of malnutrition as a contributing factor in infections.
  Impaired immunity is a critical adjunct factor in malnutrition-associated infections in all age groups in all populations of the world (Chandra, 1997).
- Be alert for food-nutrient-drug interactions.
  Individuals at greatest risk are those who are malnourished, consume alcohol, receiving many drugs long term for chronic diseases, or take medications with meals or through a feeding tube (Lutz, Przytulski, 2001). Case reports still appear in medical journals describing scurvy in persons with alcoholism (Garg, Draganescu, Albornoz, 1998).
- Assess for recent changes in physiological status that may interfere with nutrition.
  The consequences of malnutrition can lead to a further decline in the patient's condition that then becomes self-perpetuating if not recognized and treated. Extreme cases of malnutrition can lead to septicemia, organ failure, and death (Arrowsmith, 1997). Diarrhea in patients receiving warfarin has been suggested as possibly causing lower intake and/or malabsorption of vitamin K (Black, 1994; Smith, Aljazairi, Fuller, 1999).
- If the client is pregnant, ensure that she is receiving adequate amounts of folic acid by eating a balanced diet and taking prenatal vitamins as ordered.
  All women of childbearing potential are urged to consume 400 μg of synthetic folic acid from fortified foods or supplements in addition to food folate from a varied diet (National Academy of Sciences, 1998).
- ▲ Observe client's relationship to food. Attempt to separate physical from psychological causes for eating difficulty.
  It may be difficult to tell if the problem is physical or psychological. Refusing to eat may be the only way the client can express some control, and it may also be a symptom of depression (Evans, 1992).
- Provide companionship at mealtime to encourage nutritional intake.
  Mealtime usually is a time for social interaction; often clients will eat more food if other people are present at mealtimes.
- Consider six small nutrient-dense meals vs. three larger meals daily to reduce the feeling of fullness.
  Eating small, frequent meals reduces the sensation of fullness and decreases the stimulus to vomit (Love, Seaton, 1991).
- Weigh client weekly under same conditions.

• = Independent; ▲ = Collaborative

▲ Monitor food intake; specify proportion of served food that is eaten (25%, 50%); consult with dietitian for actual calorie count.

• Monitor state of oral cavity (gums, tongue, mucosa, teeth).

• Provide good oral hygiene before and after meals.

Good oral hygiene enhances appetite; the condition of the oral mucosa is critical to the ability to eat. The oral mucosa must be moist, with adequate saliva production to facilitate and aid in the digestion of food (Evans, 1992).

▲ If a client has anorexia and dry mouth from medication side effects, offer sips of fluids throughout the day.

Although artificial salivas are available, more often than not clients preferred water to the more expensive products (Ganley, 1995).

• Determine relationship of eating and other events to onset of nausea, vomiting, diarrhea, or abdominal pain.

• Determine time of day when the client's appetite is the greatest. Offer highest calorie meal at that time.

Clients with liver disease often have their largest appetite at breakfast time.

• Offer small volumes of light liquids as an appetizer before meals.

Small volumes of liquids (up to 240 ml) stimulate the gastrointestinal tract, which enhances peristalsis and motility (Rogers-Seidel, 1991).

▲ Administer antiemetics as ordered before meals.

Antiemetics are more effective when given before nausea occurs.

• Prepare the client for meals. Clear unsightly supplies and excretions. Avoid invasive procedures before meals.

A pleasant environment helps promote intake.

• If food odors trigger nausea, remove food covers away from client's bedside.

Trapped odors diffuse into air away from client.

• If vomiting is a problem, discourage consumption of favorite foods.

If favorite foods are consumed and then vomited, the client may later reject them.

• Work with client to develop a plan for increased activity.

Immobility leads to negative nitrogen balance that fosters anorexia.

• If client is anemic, offer foods rich in iron and vitamins B_{12}, C, and folic acid.

Heme iron in meat, fish, and poultry is absorbed more readily than nonheme iron in plants. Vitamin C increases the solubility of iron. Vitamin B_{12} and folic acid are necessary for erythropoiesis.

▲ If the client is lactose intolerant (genetically or following diarrhea), suggest cheeses (natural or processed) with less lactose than fluid milk. Encourage client to identify the extent of the intolerance.

When lactose intake is limited to the equivalent of 240 ml of milk or less a day, symptoms are likely to be negligible and the use of lactose-digestive aids unnecessary (Suarez, Savaiano, Levitt, 1995).

• For the agitated client, offer finger foods (sandwiches, fresh fruit) and fluids that can be ingested while pacing.

If a client cannot be still, food can be consumed while he or she is in motion.

Geriatric

▲ Assess for protein-energy malnutrition.

Protein-energy malnutrition in older persons is rarely recognized and even more rarely treated appropriately (Morley, 1997). Clients in institutions are susceptible to protein-

• = **Independent;** ▲ = **Collaborative**

calorie malnutrition (PCM) or protein-energy malnutrition when they are unable to feed themselves. When followed for 6 months in a long-care hospital, 84% of patients had an intake below estimated energy expenditure and 30% were below estimated basal metabolic rate (BMR) (Elmstahl et al, 1997). Patients admitted to a geriatric rehabilitation unit had an average of four nutritional problems. The primary nutrition problem was protein-energy malnutrition, which was associated with an increased length of stay (Keller, 1997). Nutritional risk independently increased the likelihood of death in cognitively impaired older adults (Keller, Ostbye, 2000).

▲ Interpret laboratory findings cautiously.
Compromised kidney function makes reliance on urine samples for nutrient analyses less reliable in the elderly than in younger persons.

▲ Offer high protein supplements based on individual needs and capabilities. Give client a choice of supplements to increase personal control. If client is unwilling to drink a glass of liquid supplement, offer 30 ml per hour in a medication cup and serve it like medicine.
Patients with decreased kidney function may not be able to excrete the waste products from protein metabolism. Often the elderly will take medications when they will not take food. The supplement is then served as a medicine.

• Offer liquid energy supplements.
Energy supplementation has been shown to produce weight gain and reduce falls in frail elderly living in the community. It also has been shown to decrease mortality in hospitalized older persons and to decrease morbidity and mortality in hip fracture patients. When given liquid preloads 60 minutes before the next meal, older persons consistently ate a greater total energy load (Morley, 1997). Inadequate kilocaloric intake has been correlated with increased mortality in the elderly (Elmstahl et al, 1997; Incalzi et al, 1996).

▲ Unless medically contraindicated, permit self-selected seasonings and foods.
Older persons rate flavor as the most important determinant of their food choice. Ability to taste declines in most but not all aging clients. Usually salt receptors are most affected and sweet receptors least affected. Blindfolded older subjects have about one half the ability of younger subjects to recognize blended foods, which predominantly results from a decline in olfactory sense (Morley, 1997). In hospitalized patients permitted their preferred food, ice cream, ad libitum, protein-energy malnutrition was reversed (Winograd, Brown, 1990).

• Play relaxing dinner music during mealtime.
On a nursing home ward for demented patients, the patients ate more calmly and spent more time with dinner when music was played (Ragneskog et al, 1996). Selections with a slow tempo, at or below the human heart rate, have usually been used to dampen environmental noises that might otherwise startle clients. Fewer incidents of agitated behaviors occurred during the weeks that music was played compared with weeks without music (Denney, 1997).

▲ Assess components of bone health: calcium intake, vitamin D status, and regular exercise.
The Adequate Intake (AI) for calcium for adults aged 19 to 50 years is 1000 mg. For those >50 years of age the amount is 1200 mg (National Academy of Sciences, 1998). Milk and milk products are the best animal sources of calcium, followed by sardines, clams, oysters, and salmon. In milk, calcium is combined with lactose, which increases absorption (although only 28% of the available calcium in milk is absorbed). Besides lactose, another advantageous component in milk is the protein the osteoblasts need to rebuild the bone

• = **Independent;** ▲ = **Collaborative**

matrix. In sum, milk is such an important source of calcium that it is virtually impossible to obtain adequate dietary calcium without milk or dairy products (Lutz, Przytulski, 2001). In the absence of adequate exposure to sunlight, the AI for vitamin D is set at 5 mg/day for persons 31 to 50 years of age, 10 mg for those 51 to 70 years of age, and 15 mg for persons ≥71 years of age (National Academy of Sciences, 1998). An 80-year-old person requires almost twice as much time in the sun to produce the same amount of vitamin D as a 20-year-old person does (Ryan, Eleazer, Egbert, 1995). Even among institutionalized elderly, prevalence of vitamin D deficiency showed significant seasonal variation (Liu et al, 1997). The USDA Modified Food Guide Pyramid for People Over 70 Years of Age specifies calcium, vitamin D, and vitamin B_{12} supplementation (Russell, Rasmussen, Lichtenstein, 1999). Exercise not only increases bone density but also increases muscle mass and improves balance (Nelson et al, 1994).

- Instruct in wise use of supplements.

  Milk-alkali syndrome has occurred in women ingesting 4 to 12 g of calcium carbonate daily (Beall, Scofield, 1995).

- Consider social factors that may interfere with nutrition (e.g., lack of transportation, inadequate income, lack of social support).

  Nutritional deficiencies are seen in at least one third of the elderly in industrialized countries (Chandra, 1997). In most surveys, poverty was found to be the major social cause of food insecurity and weight loss, but friendship networks play an important role in maintaining adequate food intake (Morley, 1997).

- Assess for psychological factors that impact nutrition. Watch for signs of depression.

  In persons with depression, 90% of the elderly lose weight, compared with 60% of younger persons (Morley, 1997).

▲ Consider the effects of medications on food intake. Appetite-stimulating drugs may have a role in some cases.

  The side effects of drugs are a major cause of weight loss in older persons (Morley, 1997). Compared with a placebo, megestrol acetate improved appetite and promoted weight gain in geriatric patients (Yeh et al, 2000).

▲ Provide appropriate food textures for chewing ease. Insert dentures (if needed) before meals. Assess fit of dentures. Refer for dental consultation if needed.

  The bony structure of jaws changes over time, requiring adjustment of dentures. The most common feeding difficulties among geriatric rehabilitation clients involved dentures (lack of or ill fitting) and oral infections (Keller, 1997).

  NOTE: If client unable to feed self, refer to Nursing Interventions and Rationales for **Feeding Self-care deficit.**

Multicultural

- Assess for dietary intake of essential nutrients.

  Studies have shown that black women have calcium intakes of <75% of the RDA (Zablah et al, 1999). Hispanics with type II diabetes also often have inadequate protein nutritional status (Castenada, Bermudez, Tucker, 2000). Mexican-American women have a higher prevalence of iron deficiency anemia than non-Hispanic white females (Frith-Terhune et al, 2000). Rural black men had low caloric intakes coupled with high fat intakes but nutrient deficiencies (Vitolins et al, 2000).

- Assess for the influence of cultural beliefs, norms, and values on the client's nutritional knowledge.

• = **Independent;** ▲ = **Collaborative**

What the client considers normal dietary practices may be based on cultural perceptions (Leininger, 1996).

- Discuss with the client those aspects of their diet that will remain unchanged.
  Aspects of the client's life that are meaningful and valuable to them should be understood and preserved without change (Leininger, 1996).
- Negotiate with the client regarding the aspects of his or her diet that will need to be modified.
  Give and take with the client will lead to culturally congruent care (Leininger, 1996).
- Validate the client's feelings regarding the impact of current lifestyle, finances, and transportation on ability to obtain nutritious food.
  Validation lets the client know that the nurse has heard and understands what was said, and it promotes the nurse-client relationship (Stuart, Laraia, 2001; Giger, Davidhizar, 1995).

Client/Family Teaching

- Foster client's/family's input into care plan.
  Extrinsic motivations, such as pressure from others, may be less effective than intrinsic motivations, such as beliefs, on promoting healthful behaviors (Patterson et al, 1995).
- Help client/family identify area to change that will make the greatest contribution to improved nutrition.
  Change is difficult. Multiple changes may be overwhelming.
- Build on the strengths in the client's/family's food habits. Adapt changes to their current practices.
  Accepting the client's/family's preferences shows respect for their culture.
- Select appropriate teaching aids for the client's/family's background.
- Implement instructional follow-up to answer client's/family's questions.
- ▲ Suggest community resources as suitable (food sources, counseling, Meals on Wheels, Senior Centers).
- Teach client and family how to manage tube feedings or parenteral therapy at home.

WEB SITES FOR EDUCATION

MERLIN   See the MERLIN web site for World Wide Web resources for client education.

REFERENCES   Arrowsmith H: Malnutrition in hospital: detection and consequences, *Br J Nurs* 6:1131, 1997.

Baker SS: Protein-energy malnutrition in the hospitalized pediatric patient. In Walker WA, Watkins JB, editors: *Nutrition in pediatrics*, Hamilton, Ontario, 1997, BC Decker.

Beall D, Scofield, R: Milk-alkali syndrome associated with calcium carbonate consumption, *Medicine* 74:89-96, 1995.

Black J: Diarrhoea, vitamin K and warfarin, *Lancet* 344:1373, 1994 (letter).

Castenada C, Bermudez OI, Tucker KL: Protein nutritional status and functions are associated with type II diabetes in Hispanic elders, *Am J Clin Nutr* 72(1):89-95, 2000.

Chandra RK: Nutrition and the immune system: an introduction, *Am J Clin Nutr* 66:460S, 1997.

Denney A: Quiet music: an intervention for mealtime agitation? *J Gerontol Nurs* 23:16, 1997.

Elmstahl S et al: Malnutrition in geriatric patients: a neglected problem? *J Adv Nurs* 26:851, 1997.

Estok PJ, Rudy EB: The relationship between eating disorders and running in women, *Res Nurs Health* 19:377-387, 1996.

Evans NJ: Feeding. In Bulechek GM, McCloskey JC, editors: *Nursing interventions: essential nursing treatments*, ed 2, Philadelphia, 1992, WB Saunders.

• = Independent; ▲ = Collaborative

Fitzpatrick S et al: Vitamin D-deficient rickets: a multifactorial disease, *Nutr Rev* 58:218-222, 2000.

Frith-Terhune AL et al: Iron deficiency anemia: higher prevalence in Mexican American than in non-Hispanic white females in the third National Health and Nutrition Examination Survey, 1988-1994, *Am J Clin Nutr* 72(4):963-968, 2000.

Ganley BJ: Effective mouth care for head and neck radiation therapy patients, *Medsurg Nurs* 4:133-141, 1995.

Garg K, Draganescu JM, Albornoz MA: A rash imposition from a lifestyle omission, *Postgrad Med* 104:183, 1998.

Giger JN, Davidhizar RE: *Transcultural nursing*, ed 2, St Louis, 1995, Mosby.

Incalzi RA et al: Energy intake and in-hospital starvation: a clinically relevant relationship, *Arch Intern Med* 156:425-429, 1996.

Keller HH: Nutrition problems and their association with patient outcomes in a geriatric rehabilitation setting, *J Nutr Elderly* 17(2):1, 1997.

Keller HH, Ostbye T: Do nutrition indicators predict death in elderly Canadians with cognitive impairment? *Can J Public Health* 91:220-224, 2000.

Kreiter SR et al: Nutritional rickets in African American breast-fed infants, *J Pediatr* 137:153-157, 2000.

Leininger MM: *Transcultural nursing: theories, research and practices,* ed 2, Hilliard, Ohio, 1996, McGraw-Hill.

Liu BA et al: Seasonal prevalence of vitamin D deficiency in institutionalized older adults, *J Am Geriatr Soc* 45:598-603, 1997.

Love CC, Seaton H: Eating disorders: highlights of nursing assessment and therapeutics, *Nurs Clin N Am* 26:677-697, 1991.

Lutz CA, Przytulski KR: *Nutrition and diet therapy,* ed 3, Philadelphia, 2001, FA Davis.

McCloskey JC, Bulechek GM: *Nursing interventions classification (NIC),* ed 3, St Louis, 2000, Mosby.

Morley JE: Anorexia of aging: physiologic and pathologic, *Am J Clin Nutr* 66:760, 1997.

National Academy of Sciences: *Dietary reference intakes,* Washington, DC, 1998, National Academy Press.

Nelson ME et al: Effects of high-intensity strength training on multiple risk factors for osteoporotic fractures, *JAMA* 272(24):1909-1914, 1994.

Patterson RE et al: Diet-cancer related beliefs, knowledge, norms, and their relationship to healthful diets, *J Nutr Educ* 27:86-92, 1995.

Payette H et al: Predictors of dietary intake in a functionally dependent elderly population in the community, *Am J Public Health* 85:677-683, 1995.

Ragneskog H et al: Dinner music for demented patients: analysis of video-recorded observations, *Clin Nurs Res* 5:262, 1996.

Rogers-Seidel FF editor: *Geriatric nursing care plans,* St Louis, 1991, Mosby.

Russell RM, Rasmussen H, Lichtenstein AH: Modified food guide pyramid for people over 70 years of age, *J Nutr* 129:751, 1999.

Ryan C, Eleazer P, Egbert J: Vitamin D in the elderly, *Nutr Today* 30:228-233, 1995.

Shah M et al: Nutritional rickets still afflict children in north Texas, *Tex Med* 96:64-68, 2000.

Smith JK, Aljazairi A, Fuller SH: INR elevation associated with diarrhea in a patient receiving warfarin, *Ann Pharmacother* 33:301-304, 1999.

Stuart GW, Laraia MT: Therapeutic nurse-patient relationship. In Stuart GW, Laraia MT, editors: *Principles and practice of psychiatric nursing,* St Louis, 2001, Mosby, p 30.

Suarez FL, Savaiano DA, Levitt MD: A comparison of symptoms after consumption of milk or lactose-hydrolyzed milk by people with self-reported severe lactose intolerance, *N Engl J Med* 333:1-4, 1995.

Vitolins MZ et al: Ethnic and gender variation in the dietary intake of rural elders, *J Nutr Elderly* 19(3):15-29, 2000.

Watson T, Bowers WA, Andersen AE: Involuntary treatment of eating disorders, *Am J Psychiatry* 175:1806-1810, 2000.

Winograd CH, Brown EM: Aggressive oral refeeding in hospitalized patients, *Am J Clin Nutr* 52:967-968, 1990.

Wyshak G: Teenaged girls, carbonated beverage consumption, and bone fractures, *Arch Pediatr Adolesc Med* 154:610-613, 2000.

Yeh S et al: Improvement in quality-of-life measures and stimulation of weight gain after treatment with megesterol acetate oral suspension in geriatric cachexia: results of a double-blind, placebo-controlled study, *J Am Geriatr Soc* 48:485-492, 2000.

Zablah EM et al: Barriers to calcium intake in African American women, *J Hum Nutr* 12(2):123-132, 1999.

• = **Independent;** ▲ = **Collaborative**

Imbalanced Nutrition: more than body requirements

Carroll A. Lutz

NANDA   **Definition** Intake of nutrients that exceeds metabolic needs

Defining Characteristics

Triceps skin fold >25 mm in women; triceps skin fold >15 mm in men; body weight ≥20% over ideal for height and frame; eating in response to external cues (e.g., time of day, social situation); eating in response to internal cues other than hunger (e.g., anxiety); reported or observed dysfunctional eating pattern pairing food with other activities; sedentary activity level; weight 10% over ideal for height and frame; concentrating food intake at the end of the day

Related Factors (r/t)

Excessive intake in relation to metabolic need; deficient knowledge related to desirability of nutritional supplements

NOC   ## Outcomes (Nursing Outcomes Classification)

Suggested NOC Labels

Weight Control; Nutritional Status: Nutrient Intake; Nutritional Status: Food and Fluid Intake Management

> **Example NOC Outcome**
> Demonstrates **Weight Control** as evidenced by the following indicators: Demonstrates progress toward target weight/Balances exercise with caloric intake/Maintains recommended eating pattern/Controls preoccupation with food (Rate each indicator of **Weight Control:** 1 = never demonstrated, 2 = rarely demonstrated, 3 = sometimes demonstrated, 4 = often demonstrated, 5 = consistently demonstrated [see Section I])

Client Outcomes

- States pertinent factors contributing to weight gain
- Identifies behaviors that remain under client's control
- Claims ownership for current eating patterns
- Designs dietary modifications to meet individual long-term goal of weight control, using principles of variety, balance, and moderation
- Accomplishes desired weight loss in a reasonable period (1 to 2 pounds/week)
- Incorporates appropriate activities requiring energy expenditure into daily life
- Uses sound scientific sources to evaluate need for nutritional supplements

NIC   ## Interventions (Nursing Interventions Classification)

Suggested NIC Labels

Weight Management; Eating Disorders Management; Nutrition Management; Nutritional Counseling, Weight Reduction Assistance

> **Example NIC Interventions—Weight Management**
> - Determine client's motivation for changing eating habits
> - Develop with the client a method to keep a daily record of intake

• = Independent; ▲ = Collaborative

Nursing Interventions and Rationales

▲ Obtain a thorough history. Refer to dietitian if client has a medical condition.
The most appropriate clients for the nursing intervention of weight management are adults with no major health problems who require diet therapy. If a patient has a medical condition necessitating diet therapy, the assistance of a dietitian may be required (Crist, 1992).

▲ Evaluate client's physiological status in relation to weight control. Refer as appropriate.
Nondieting approaches focus on changing disturbed thoughts, emotions, and body image associated with obesity to help obese persons to accept themselves and resolve issues that may hinder long-term weight maintenance (Foreyt, Walker, Poston II, 1998).

• Assess dietary intake through 24-hour recall or questions regarding usual intake of food groups.
Information may not be completely accurate. Permits appraisal of client's knowledge about diet also.

• Determine client's knowledge of a nutritious diet and need for supplements.
This information is useful for developing an individualized teaching plan based on client's current state.

• Calculate body mass index (BMI) (use this formula: weight in kg divided by height in m^2 [kg/(m)^2]; or use this alternate formula: weight in lb multiplied by 705, divided by height in inches, divided again by height in inches).
A normal BMI is 20 to 25, 26 to 29 is overweight, and a BMI of ≥ 30 is defined as obesity.

• Compute the waist to hip ratio (WHR).
A WHR >0.85 in women and >1.0 in men indicates increased risk of problems related to obesity (Lutz, Przytulski, 2001).

▲ Define client's healthy body weight with client, considering physiological, experiential, and cultural factors.
Overweight has been viewed as an individual problem, and treatment oriented toward an individual victim-blame model, with little consideration of personal context or the influence of cultural values on behavior (Allan, 1994). Children have been included in weight management programs but their growth factor has not been factored into the equation, potentially risking future growth-related health problems. These potential risks may require the direct attention of dietitians and physicians (Crist, 1992).

• Determine client's motivation to lose weight, whether for appearance or health benefits.
Female peripheral fat pattern (gynecoid), predominant in most women, is associated with virtually no impairment of health (Allan, 1994). Often a healthier body weight is only a 5% to 10% reduction from initial body weight (Nonas, 1998).

▲ Observe for situations that indicate a nutritional intake of more than body requirements.
Such observations help gain a clear picture of the client's dietary habits. Overfeeding of post-trauma patients that was attributed to the lack of an interdisciplinary plan of care has been documented (Klein, Henry, 1999).

• Suggest client keep a diary of food intake and circumstances surrounding its consumption (methods of preparation, duration of meal, social situation, overall mood, activities accompanying consumption).

• = **Independent;** ▲ = **Collaborative**

Self-monitoring helps the client assess adherence to self-determined performance criteria and progress toward desired goals. Self-monitoring serves an important role in the maintenance of internal standards of behavior (Fleury, 1991).

- Adopt a weight loss plan that incorporates the client's culture and preferences.
  Dramatic weight loss was achieved in Hawaii with a culturally appropriate methodology (Shintani et al, 1991).
- Advise client to measure food periodically.
  Measuring food alerts client to normal portion sizes. Estimating amounts can be extremely inaccurate.
- ▲ Review client's current exercise level. With client and primary health care provider, design a long-term exercise program.
  A health risk appraisal should be performed on all previously sedentary individuals beginning a program of exercise (Grubbs, 1993). Exercise is important for increased energy expenditure, for maintenance of lean body mass, and as part of a total change in lifestyle (Lutz, Przytulski, 2001). In one study, 80% of the weight lost by exercisers was fat; whereas 40% of the weight loss by dieters was lean tissue (Pritchard, Nowson, Wark, 1997). Loss of lean tissue is undesirable because muscle tissue is estimated to be as much as 70 times as metabolically active as fat tissue (Rippe, Hess, 1998). Women consuming an energy-restricted diet in addition to performing aerobic and strength training exercise lost more weight than the other study groups and slightly increased their lean muscle tissue (Rippe, Hess, 1998).
- Establish a reasonable goal for client's body weight and for weight loss (e.g., 1 to 2 pounds/week).
  Height and weight tables have been criticized because they are based on middle-class white men (Allan, 1994). Because subjects in one study achieved comparable weight loss on liquid formula diets of 420, 600, or 800 calories/day, choosing the higher energy diets may minimize adverse side effects (Foster et al, 1992).
- Initiate a client contract that involves rewarding and reinforcing progressive goal attainment.
  Patient contracts provide a unique opportunity for patients to learn to analyze their behavior in relationship to the environment and to choose behavioral strategies that will facilitate learning. A series of written contracts provides a history of progress toward desired behaviors (Boehm, 1992).
- Weigh client twice a week under the same conditions.
  It is important to most clients and their progress to have the tangible reward that the scale shows. Monitoring twice a week keeps the client on the program by not allowing him or her to eat out of control for a couple of days and then fast to lose weight (Crist, 1992).
- Instruct client regarding adequate nutritional intake. A total plan permits occasional treats.
  Permanent lifestyle changes must occur for weight loss to be long lasting. Eliminating all treats is not sustainable. Numerous studies have demonstrated that fewer than 5% of persons who lose weight through energy restriction alone are able to maintain this weight loss for 2 years or more (Rippe, Hess, 1998). During energy restriction, a client should consume 72 to 80 g of high biological value protein per day to minimize risk of ventricular arrhythmias (Nonas, 1998).
- Familiarize client with the following behavior modification techniques (Lutz,

• = **Independent;** ▲ = **Collaborative**

Przytulski, 2001):

Self-monitor

- Keep a food and exercise diary
- Graph weight weekly

Stimulus control

- Limit food intake to one site in the home
- Sit down at the table to eat
- Plan food intake for each day
- Rearrange schedule to avoid inappropriate eating
- Save or reschedule everyday activities for times when you are hungry
- Avoid boredom; keep a list of activities on the refrigerator
- At a party: eat before you go, sit away from the snack foods, and substitute lower calorie beverages for alcoholic ones
- Decide beforehand what to order in a restaurant

Slow down eating

- Drink a glass of water before each meal; take sips of water between bites of food
- Swallow food before putting more food on the utensil
- Try to be the last one to finish eating
- Pause for a minute during your meal, and attempt to increase the number of pauses

Reward yourself

- Chart your progress
- Make an agreement with yourself or significant other for a meaningful reward
- Do not reward yourself with food

Cognitive strategies

- View exercise as a means of controlling hunger
- Practice relaxation techniques
- Imagine yourself ordering a side salad, diet dressing, low-fat milk, and a small hamburger at a fast-food restaurant
- Visualize yourself enjoying a fresh apple in preference to apple pie

- Encourage client to adopt an exercise program that involves 45 minutes of exercise five times/week.

  As exercise time increases beyond 30 minutes, there is an increased reliance on fat stores for energy (Grubbs, 1993). Moderately intense physical activity for 30 to 45 minutes 5 to 7 days/week can expend the 1500 to 2000 calories/week that appear to be necessary to maintain weight loss. Cross-sectional and longitudinal studies illustrate that persons who increase their physical activity also increase their resting metabolic rate (Rippe, Hess, 1998).

- Assess for use of nonprescription diet aids.

  Ingestion of an herbal supplement (containing Ma-huang, the main plant source of ephedrine) for weight loss caused mania in a client with no history of psychiatric illness (Capwell, 1995). Clinicians should be aware that ostensibly harmless herbal remedies may have potent ingredients that are not subjected to the same scrutiny that the FDA devotes to prescription drugs (Woolf, 1994).

- Observe for overuse of particular nutrients.

  Almost all nutrients given in quantities beyond a certain threshold will reduce immune responses (Chandra, 1997). Daily ingestion of 500 ml of tonic water containing 40 mg of quinine hydrochloride caused photosensitivity. Other conditions associated with tonic water

• = Independent; ▲ = Collaborative

are disseminated intravascular coagulation, recurrent dermatitis, fixed drug eruption, and toxic epidermal necrolysis (Wagner et al, 1994). Clients who are consuming excessive amounts of some nutrients may also be consuming less than adequate amounts of others.

Geriatric

- Assess fluid intake. Recommend routine drinks of water whether thirsty or not.
  Thirst sensation becomes dulled in the elderly.
- Observe for socioeconomic factors that influence food choices (e.g., funds, cooking facilities).
  Food choices in today's food markets are greatly enhanced, even for those on a limited budget (Love, Seaton, 1991).
- Suggest a variety of seasonings.
  The ability to taste sweet, bitter, sour, and salty declines in most, but not all, older persons (Morley, 1997).
- Encourage social involvement in activities other than eating.
  Energy needs decrease an estimated 5% per decade after the age of 40.
- Recommend weight reduction changes judiciously.
  Weight reduction should be pursued if it is needed to treat current problems, such as diabetes mellitus or hypertension, but not to prevent new ones (Feldman, 1988).

Multicultural

- Assess for the influence of cultural beliefs, norms, and values on the client's nutritional knowledge.
  What the client considers normal dietary practices may be based on cultural perceptions (Leininger, 1996).
- Assess for the influence of cultural beliefs, norms, and values on the client's ideal of acceptable body weight and body size.
  Ideal body weight and size may be based on cultural perceptions (Leininger, 1996). African-American women report more satisfaction than other women with body size (Miller et al, 2000). Overweight Hispanic women with high levels of binge eating and depression preferred a slimmer body ideal (Fitzgibbon et al, 1998).
- Discuss with client those aspects of his or her diet that will remain unchanged, and work with client to adapt cultural core foods.
  Aspects of the client's life that are meaningful and valuable to them should be understood and preserved without change (Leininger, 1996). Core foods are those foods which are universal, staple, important, and consistently used in the culture (Sanjur, 1995).
- Negotiate with the client regarding the aspects of his or her diet that will need to be modified.
  Give and take with the client will lead to culturally congruent care (Leininger, 1996).
- Validate the client's feelings regarding the impact of current lifestyle, finances, and transportation on ability to obtain and prepare nutritious food.
  Validation lets the client know that the nurse has heard and understands what was said, and it promotes the nurse-client relationship (Stuart, Laraia, 2001; Giger, Davidhizar, 1995).

Client/Family Teaching

- Foster client's/family's input into care plan.
  Extrinsic motivations (such as pressure from others) may be less effective than intrinsic motivations (such as beliefs) on promoting healthful behaviors (Patterson et al, 1995).

• = **Independent**; ▲ = **Collaborative**

- Provide the client and family with information regarding the treatment plan options.
  Because the purpose is to obtain a permanent change in weight management, the decision regarding treatment plans should be left up to the client and family (Crist, 1992).
- Inform the client about the health risks associated with obesity.
- Guide the client toward changes that will make a major impact on health.
  Even modest weight loss contributes to diabetes and hypertension control.
- Inform the client/family of the disadvantages of trying to lose weight by dieting alone.
  Resting metabolic rate is decreased as much as 45% with extreme calorie restriction. The decrease persists after the diet period has ended, leading to the "yo-yo effect." With a reduced-calorie diet alone, as much as 25% of the weight lost can be lean body mass rather than fat. Resting energy expenditure is positively related to lean body mass (Grubbs, 1993).
- Teach the importance of exercise in a weight control program.
  A physically conditioned person uses more fat for energy at rest and with exercise than a sedentary person does (Grubbs, 1993). The majority of patients will benefit from establishing walking as a cornerstone of their physical activity program (Rippe, Crossley, Ringer, 1998).
- Teach stress reduction techniques as alternatives to eating.
  The client needs to substitute healthy for unhealthy behaviors.

WEB SITES FOR EDUCATION

MERLIN See the MERLIN web site for World Wide Web resources for client education.

REFERENCES Allan JD: A biomedical and feminist perspective on women's experiences with weight management, *West J Nurs Res* 16:524-543, 1994.

Boehm S: Patient contracting. In Bulechek GM, McCloskey JC, editors: *Nursing interventions: essential nursing treatments,* ed 2, Philadelphia, 1992, WB Saunders.

Capwell R: Ephedrine-induced mania from an herbal diet supplement, *Am J Psychiatry* 152:647, 1995 (letter).

Chandra RK: Nutrition and the immune system: an introduction, *Am J Clin Nutr* 66:460S, 1997.

Crist J: Weight management. In Bulechek GM, McCloskey JC, editors: *Nursing interventions: essential nursing treatments,* ed 2, Philadelphia, 1992, WB Saunders.

Feldman EB: *Essentials of clinical nutrition,* Philadelphia, 1988, FA Davis.

Fitzgibbon ML et al: Correlates of binge eating in Hispanic, black and white women, *Int J Eat Disord* 24(1):43-52, 1998.

Fleury J: Empowering potential: a theory of wellness motivation, *Nurs Res* 40:288, 1991.

Foreyt JP, Walker S, Poston II C: The role of the behavioral counselor in obesity treatment, *J Am Diet Assoc* 98(suppl 2):S27, 1998.

Foster GD et al: A controlled comparison of three very-low-calorie diets: effects on weight, body composition and symptoms, *Am J Clin Nutr* 55:811, 1992.

Giger JN, Davidhizar RE: *Transcultural nursing,* ed 2, St Louis, 1995, Mosby.

Grubbs L: The critical role of exercise in weight control, *Nurse Pract* 18:20-29, 1993.

Klein CJ, Henry SM: Acute nutrition interventions help identify indicators of quality in a trauma service, *Nutr Clin Pract* 14:85-92, 1999.

Leininger MM: *Transcultural nursing: theories, research and practices,* ed 2, Hilliard, Ohio, 1996, McGraw-Hill.

Love CC, Seaton, H: Eating disorders: highlights of nursing assessment and therapeutics, *Nurs Clin North Am* 26:677-697, 1991.

Lutz CA, Przytulski, KR: *Nutrition and diet therapy,* ed 3, Philadelphia, 2001, FA Davis.

Miller KJ et al: Comparisons of body image by race/ethnicity and gender in a university population, *Int J Eat Disord* 27(3):310-316, 2000.

Morley JE: Anorexia of aging: physiologic and pathologic, *Am J Clin Nutr* 66:760, 1997.

• = Independent; ▲ = Collaborative

Nonas CA: A model for chronic care of obesity through dietary treatment, *J Am Diet Assoc* 98(suppl 2):S16, 1998.

North American Nursing Diagnosis Association (NANDA): *Nursing diagnoses: definitions and classification, 1999-2000*, Philadelphia, 1999, The Association.

Patterson RE et al: Diet-cancer related beliefs, knowledge, norms, and their relationship to healthful diets, *J Nutr Educ* 27:86-92, 1995.

Pritchard JE, Nowson CA, Wark, JD: A worksite program for overweight middle-aged men achieves lesser weight loss with exercise than with dietary change, *J Am Diet Assoc* 97:37, 1997.

Rippe JM, Crossley S, Ringer, R: Obesity as a chronic disease: modern medical and lifestyle management, *J Am Diet Assoc* 98(suppl 2):S9, 1998.

Rippe JM, Hess S: The role of physical activity in the prevention and management of obesity, *J Am Diet Assoc* 98(suppl 2):S31, 1998.

Sanjur D: *Hispanic foodways, nutrition, & health*, Needham Heights, Mass, 1995, Allyn & Bacon.

Shintani TT et al: Obesity and cardiovascular risk intervention through the ad libitum feeding of traditional Hawaiian diet, *Am J Clin Nutr* 53:1647S, 1991.

Stuart GW, Laraia MT: Therapeutic nurse-patient relationship. In Stuart GW, Laraia MT, editors: *Principles and practice of psychiatric nursing*, St Louis, 2001, Mosby, p 30.

Wagner G et al: "I'll have mine with a twist of lemon": quinine photosensitivity from excessive intake of tonic water, *Br J Dermatol* 131:734-735, 1994 (letter).

Woolf G et al: Acute hepatitis associated with the Chinese herbal product Jin Bu Huan, *Ann Intern Med* 121:729-735, 1994.

Risk for imbalanced Nutrition: more than body requirements

J. Keith Hampton, Gail B. Ladwig, and Carroll A. Lutz

NANDA   **Definition** At risk for an intake of nutrients that exceeds metabolic needs

Risk Factors

Reported use of solid food as major food source before 5 months of age; concentrating food intake at end of day; reported or observed obesity in one or both parents; reported or observed higher baseline weight at beginning of each pregnancy; rapid transition across growth percentiles in infants or children; pairing food with other activities; observed use of food as reward or comfort measure; eating in response to internal cues other than hunger, such as anxiety; eating in response to external cues, such as time of day, social situation; dysfunctional eating patterns

NOC   **Outcomes (Nursing Outcomes Classification)**

Suggested NOC Labels

Nutritional Status: Food and Fluid Intake; Nutritional Status: Nutrient Intake; Weight Control

> **Example NOC Outcome**
> Demonstrates **Weight Control** as evidenced by the following indicators: Demonstrates progress toward target weight/Balances exercise with caloric intake/Maintains recommended eating pattern/Controls preoccupation with food (Rate each indicator of **Weight Control:** 1 = never demonstrated, 2 = rarely demonstrated, 3 = sometimes demonstrated, 4 = often demonstrated, 5 = consistently demonstrated [see Section I])

• = Independent; ▲ = Collaborative

Client Outcomes

- Explains concept of a balanced diet
- Compares current eating pattern with a recommended healthy one
- Designs dietary modifications to meet individual long-term goal of weight control, using principles of variety, balance, and moderation
- Identifies role of exercise in weight control
- Uses sound scientific sources to evaluate need for nutritional supplements

NIC   Interventions (Nursing Interventions Classification)

Suggested NIC Labels

Nutrition Management; Nutritional Counseling; Weight Management

> **Example NIC Interventions—Weight Management**
> - Determine client's motivation for changing eating habits
> - Develop with the client a method to keep a daily record of intake

Nursing Interventions and Rationales

- Observe for the presence of risk factors (see Risk Factors).
- Assess nutritional intake, including the use of supplements.
  Clients may not volunteer information on supplements because they do not consider them pertinent. However, almost all nutrients given in quantities beyond a certain threshold will reduce immune responses (Chandra, 1997).
- Determine client's knowledge of nutrition.
  Inform client of the health risks associated with overconsumption of nutrients. Fetal abnormalities have been related to vitamin A intake. Women who are, or who might become, pregnant should avoid consuming daily supplements containing more than 8000 IU of vitamin A and should consume liver and liver products only in moderation because they contain large amounts of vitamin A (Oakley, Erickson, 1995). The hazard is related to preformed vitamin A in animal products, not the provitamin A, carotene, in plants. A client consuming more than ten times the RDA for vitamin A for 6 years developed fatal liver toxicity (Kowalski, 1994).
- Discuss wise selection, use, and discontinuation of supplements.
  Choosing calcium supplements that have been tested and found free of lead is recommended. Researchers found 38% (Ross, Szabo, Tebbett, 2000) and 66% (Scelfo, Flegal, 2000) of calcium products tested contained lead. Rebound scurvy has occurred in clients who suddenly discontinued megadoses (ten times the RDA) of vitamin C. The body cannot adjust quickly enough and continues to absorb a meager proportion of the now-smaller dose (DePaola, Faine, Palmer, 1999). Even without megadose supplements, however, plasma vitamin C levels fall to deficiency levels within 1 to 3 weeks of removal of vitamin-rich fruits and vegetables from the diet (Johnston, 1999).
- Establish a plan with the client, using techniques listed in the care plan for **Imbalanced Nutrition: more than body requirements.**
  Intervening when the client is at risk allows relatively small changes in lifestyle to be effective. Lifestyle modification is one of the main predictors of success for weight management programs (Coulston, 1998).

Geriatric

- Give client credit for making enough wise choices to have lived to an advanced age.
  Studies show nutrition practices are related to health in certain ways. They are not predictive for individuals.

• = Independent; ▲ = Collaborative

- Encourage varying suppliers of foodstuffs in the unlikely event of contamination.
  Hypervitaminosis D was caused by inadvertent overfortification of milk from a home-delivery dairy. The two fatalities occurred in 72- and 86-year-old persons (Blank et al, 1995).

Multicultural

- Assess for the influence of cultural beliefs, norms, and values on the client's nutritional knowledge.
  What the client considers normal dietary practices may be based on cultural perceptions (Leininger, 1996).
- Assess for the influence of cultural beliefs, norms, and values on the client's ideal of acceptable body weight and body size.
  Ideal body weight and size may be based on cultural perceptions (Leininger, 1996). African-American women report more satisfaction than other women with body size (Miller et al, 2000). Overweight Hispanic women with high levels of binge eating and depression preferred a slimmer body ideal (Fitzgibbon et al, 1998).
- Discuss with the client those aspects of their diet that will remain unchanged, and work with client to adapt cultural core foods.
  Aspects of the client's life that are meaningful and valuable to them should be understood and preserved without change (Leininger, 1996). Core foods are those foods that are universal, staple, important, and consistently used in the culture (Sanjur, 1995).
- Negotiate with the client regarding the aspects of his or her diet that will need to be modified.
  Give and take with the client will lead to culturally congruent care (Leininger, 1996).
- Assess whether the client's concerns about the amount of food eaten is contributing to early feeding of solid foods in infants.
  Some cultures may add semisolid food within the first month of life because of concerns that the infant is not getting enough to eat and the perception that "big is healthy" (Higgins, 2000; Bentley et al, 1999).
- Assess for the influence of family on patterns of eating.
  Women are the keepers and transmitters of culture in families. Female family members can play a dominant role in how infants and children are fed (Pillitteri, 1999).
- Validate the client's feelings regarding the impact of current lifestyle, finances, and transportation on his or her ability to obtain and prepare nutritious food.
  Validation lets the client know that the nurse has heard and understands what was said, and it promotes the nurse-client relationship (Stuart, Laraia, 2001; Giger, Davidhizar, 1995).

Client/Family Teaching

- Analyze client's nutritional pattern and suggest lower calorie substitutes for high calorie dishes.
  Ice milk contains 185 calories/cup, compared with 270 calories/cup for ice cream. Low calorie Italian dressing may be had for 5 calories/tbsp, compared with 80 calories/tbsp for the regular dressing.
- Demonstrate the use of food labels to make healthful choices. Alert the client/family to focus on serving size, total fat, and simple carbohydrate.
  The standardized food label in bold type simplifies the search for information. Fats and sugars contribute the least to a healthful diet and the most to excessive calorie intake.

- = **Independent;** ▲ = **Collaborative**

REFERENCES Bentley M et al: Infant feeding practices of low-income, African-American, adolescent mothers: an ecological, multigenerational perspective, *Soc Sci Med* 49(8):1085-1100, 1999.

Blank S et al: An outbreak of hypervitaminosis D associated with the overfortification of milk from a home-delivery dairy, *Am J Public Health* 85:656-659, 1995.

Chandra RK: Nutrition and the immune system: an introduction, *Am J Clin Nutr* 66:460S, 1997.

Coulston AM: Obesity as an epidemic: facing the challenge, *J Am Diet Assoc* 98(suppl 2):S6, 1998.

DePaola DP, Faine MP, Palmer CA: Nutrition in relation to dental medicine. In Shils ME et al, editors: *Modern nutrition in health and disease,* ed 9, Philadelphia, 1999, Lippincott Williams & Wilkins.

Fitzgibbon ML et al: Correlates of binge eating in Hispanic, black and white women, *Int J Eat Disord* 24(1):43-52, 1998.

Giger JN, Davidhizar RE: *Transcultural nursing,* ed 2, St Louis, 1995, Mosby.

Higgins B: Puerto Rican cultural beliefs: influence on infant feeding practices in western New York, *J Transcultural Nurs* 11(1):19-30, 2000.

Johnston CS: Biomarkers for establishing a tolerable upper intake level for vitamin C, *Nutr Rev* 57:71, 1999.

Kowalski T et al: Vitamin A hepatotoxicity: a cautionary note regarding 25,000 IU supplements, *Am J Med* 97:523-528, 1994.

Leininger MM: *Transcultural nursing: theories, research and practices,* ed 2, Hilliard, Ohio, 1996, McGraw-Hill.

Miller KJ et al: Comparisons of body image by race/ethnicity and gender in a university population, *Int J Eat Disord* 27(3):310-316, 2000.

North American Nursing Diagnosis Association (NANDA): *NANDA nursing diagnoses: definitions and classification, 1999-2000,* Philadelphia, 1999, The Association.

Oakley GP, Erickson JD: Vitamin A and birth defects, *N Engl J Med* 333:1414-1415, 1995.

Pillitteri A: Nutritional needs of the newborn. In Pillitteri A, editor: *Maternal & child health nursing: care of the childbearing & childrearing family,* Philadelphia, 1999, JB Lippincott, pp 654-666.

Ross EA, Szabo NJ, Tebbett, IR: Lead content of calcium supplements, *JAMA* 284:1425-1429, 2000.

Sanjur D: *Hispanic foodways, nutrition, & health,* Needham Heights, Mass, 1995, Allyn & Bacon.

Scelfo GM, Flegal AR: Lead in calcium supplements, *Environ Health Perspect* 108:309-319, 2000.

Stuart GW, Laraia MT: Therapeutic nurse-patient relationship. In Stuart GW, Laraia MT, editors: *Principles and practice of psychiatric nursing,* St Louis, 2001, Mosby, p 30.

Impaired Oral mucous membrane

Betty J. Ackley

NANDA **Definition** Disruptions of the lips and soft tissues of the oral cavity

Defining Characteristics

Purulent drainage or exudates; gingival recession, pockets deeper than 4 mm; enlarged tonsils beyond what is developmentally appropriate; smooth atrophic, sensitive tongue; geographic tongue; mucosal denudation; presence of pathogens; difficult speech; self-report of bad taste; gingival or mucosal pallor; oral pain/discomfort; xerostomia (dry mouth); vesicles, nodules, or papules; white patches/plaques, spongy patches, or white curd-like exudate; oral lesions or ulcers; halitosis; edema; hyperemia; desquamation; coated tongue; stomatitis; self-report of difficult eating or swallowing; self-report of

• = Independent; ▲ = Collaborative

diminished or absent taste; bleeding; macroplasia; gingival hyperplasia; fissures, cheilitis; red or bluish masses (e.g., hemangiomas)

Related Factors (r/t)

Chemotherapy; chemical (e.g., alcohol, tobacco, acidic foods, regular use of inhalers); depression; immunosuppression; aging-related loss of connective, adipose, or bone tissue; barriers to professional care; cleft lip or palate; medication side effects; lack of or decreased salivation; chemical trauma (e.g., acidic foods, drugs, noxious agents, alcohol); pathological conditions—oral cavity (radiation to head or neck); NPO for more than 24 hours; mouth breathing; malnutrition or vitamin deficiency; dehydration; infection; ineffective oral hygiene; mechanical (e.g., ill-fitting dentures, braces, tubes [endotracheal/nasogastric], surgery in oral cavity); decreased platelets; immunocompromised; impaired salivation; radiation therapy; barriers to oral self-care; diminished hormone levels (women); stress; loss of supportive structures

NOC   Outcomes (Nursing Outcomes Classification)

Suggested NOC Labels

Oral Health; Tissue Integrity: Skin and Mucous Membranes

Example NOC Outcome

Demonstrates **Oral Health** as evidenced by the following indicators: Cleanliness of mouth/Moisture of oral mucosa and tongue/Color of mucous membranes/Oral mucosa integrity (Rate each indicator of **Oral Health:** 1 = extremely compromised, 2 = substantially compromised, 3 = moderately compromised, 4 = mildly compromised, 5 = not compromised [see Section I])

Client Outcomes

- Maintains intact, moist oral mucous membranes that are free of ulceration and debris
- Describes or demonstrates measures to regain or maintain intact oral mucous membranes

NIC   Interventions (Nursing Interventions Classification)

Suggested NIC Labels

Oral Health Restoration

Example NIC Intervention—Oral Health Restoration

- Use a soft toothbrush for removal of dental debris
- Instruct client to avoid commercial mouthwashes

Nursing Interventions and Rationales

- ▲ Inspect oral cavity at least once daily and note any discoloration, lesions, edema, bleeding, exudate, or dryness. Refer to a physician or specialist as appropriate.
  Oral inspection can reveal signs of oral disease, symptoms of systemic disease, drug side effects, or trauma of the oral cavity (White, 2000).
- • Assess for mechanical agents such as ill-fitting dentures or chemical agents such as frequent exposure to tobacco that could cause or increase trauma to oral mucous membranes.
  Irritative and causative agents for stomatitis should be eliminated (Rhodes, McDaniel, Johnson, 1995).

• = Independent; ▲ = Collaborative

- Monitor client's nutritional and fluid status to determine if adequate. Refer to the care plan for **Deficient Fluid volume** or **Imbalanced Nutrition: less than body requirements** if applicable.
  Dehydration and malnutrition predispose clients to impaired oral mucous membranes.
- Encourage fluid intake up to 3000 ml per day if not contraindicated by client's medical condition (Rhodes, McDaniel, Johnson, 1995).
  Fluids help increase moisture in the mouth, which protects the mucous membranes from damage and helps the healing process.
- Determine client's mental status. If client is unable to care for self, oral hygiene must be provided by nursing personnel. The nursing diagnosis **Bathing/Hygiene Self-care deficit** is then also applicable.
- Determine client's usual method of oral care and address any concerns regarding oral hygiene.
  Whenever possible, build on client's existing knowledge base and current practices to develop an individualized plan of care.
- If client does not have a bleeding disorder and is able to swallow, encourage to brush teeth with a soft pediatric-sized toothbrush using a fluoride-containing toothpaste after every meal and to floss teeth daily.
  The toothbrush is the most important tool for oral care. Brushing the teeth is the most effective method for reducing plaque and controlling periodontal disease (Buglass, 1995; Stiefel et al, 2000; Roberts, 2000).
- Use tap water or normal saline to provide oral care; do not use commercial mouthwashes containing alcohol or hydrogen peroxide. Also, do not use lemon-glycerin swabs.
  Alcohol dries the oral mucous membranes. Hydrogen peroxide can damage oral mucosa and is extremely foul tasting to clients (Tombes, Gallucci, 1993; Winslow, 1994). Lemon-glycerin swabs can result in decreased salivary amylase and oral moisture, as well as erosion of tooth enamel (Stiefel et al, 2000; Roberts, 2000).
- Use foam sticks to moisten the oral mucous membranes, clean out debris, and swab out the mouth of the edentulous client. Do not use to clean the teeth or else the platelet count is very low, and the client is prone to bleeding gums.
  Studies have shown that foam sticks are probably not effective for removing plaque from teeth (Roberts, 2000). However, they are useful for cleansing the oral cavity of the client who is edentulous (Curzio, McCowan, 2000).
- If client's oral cavity is dry, the keep inside of the mouth moist with frequent sips of water and salt water rinses ($1/2$ tsp salt in 8 oz of warm water) or artificial saliva.
  Moisture promotes the cleansing effect of saliva and helps avert mucosal drying, which can result in erosions, fissures, or lesions (Rhodes, McDaniel, Johnson, 1995). Sodium chloride rinses have been shown to be effective for the prevention and treatment of stomatitis (Feber, 1994).
- Keep lips well lubricated using petroleum jelly or a similar product (Yeager et al, 2000).
- ▲ For clients with stomatitis, increase frequency of oral care up to every hour while awake if necessary.
  Increasing the frequency of oral care has been shown to be effectively decrease stomatitis (Armstrong, 1994).
- Provide scrupulous oral care to critically ill clients.

- **= Independent; ▲ = Collaborative**

Cultures of the teeth of critically ill clients have yielded significant bacterial colonization, which can cause nosocomial pneumonia (Scannapieco, Stewart, Mylotte, 1992).

▲ If mouth is severely inflamed and it is painful to swallow, contact the physician for a topical anesthetic agent or analgesic order. Modification of oral intake (e.g., soft or liquid diet) may also be necessary to prevent friction trauma. The nursing diagnosis **Imbalanced Nutrition: less than body requirements** may apply.

▲ If whitish plaques are present in the mouth or on the tongue and can be rubbed off readily with gauze, leaving a red base that bleeds, suspect a fungal infection and contact the physician for follow-up.

Oral candidiasis (moniliasis) is extremely common secondary to antibiotic therapy, steroid therapy, HIV infection, diabetes, or immunosuppressive drugs and should be treated with oral or systemic antifungal agents (Fauci et al, 1998; Epstein, Chow, 1999).

• If client is unable to swallow, keep suction nearby when providing oral care.

• Refer to **Impaired Dentition** if the client has problems with the teeth.

Geriatric

▲ Carefully observe oral cavity and lips for abnormal lesions such as white or red patches, masses, ulcerations with an indurated margin, or a raised granular lesion.

Malignant lesions are more common in elderly persons than in younger persons (especially if there is a history of smoking or alcohol use), and many elderly persons rarely visit a dentist (Aubertin, 1997).

• Ensure that dentures are removed and scrubbed at least once daily, removed and rinsed thoroughly after every meal, and removed and kept in an appropriate solution at night.

This is an evidence-based protocol for denture care (Curzio, McCowan, 2000). Denture plaque-containing candidiasis can cause denture-induced stomatitis, which is more common with unhealthy lifestyles and poor oral hygiene than otherwise (Sakki et al, 1997; Nikawa, Hamada, Yamamoto, 1998).

Home Care Interventions

▲ If dryness is a side effect of client's medication(s), instruct client in the use of artificial saliva. Monitor sodium intake in hypertensive clients (Humphrey, 1994). Use alternatives to sodium chloride rinses.

Frequent sodium chloride rinses place the client at risk for exacerbation of hypertension or heart failure.

• Instruct client to avoid alcohol- or hydrogen peroxide–based commercial products for mouth care and to avoid other irritants to the oral cavity (e.g., tobacco, spicy foods).

Oral irritants can further damage the oral mucosa and increase the client's discomfort.

• Instruct client in ways to soothe the oral cavity (e.g., cool beverages, Popsicles, viscous lidocaine) (Jaffe, Skidmore-Roth, 1993).

• If client often breathes by mouth, add humidity to room unless contraindicated.

▲ If necessary, refer for home health aide services to support family in oral care and observation of the oral cavity.

Client/Family Teaching

• Teach client how to inspect the oral cavity and monitor for signs and symptoms of infection, complications, and healing.

• Teach how to implement a personal plan of oral hygiene including a schedule of care.

Encouragement and reinforcement of oral care are important to oral outcomes (Armstrong, 1994).

• = Independent; ▲ = Collaborative

WEB SITES FOR EDUCATION

ᶮₑᵣₗᵢₙ See the MERLIN web site for World Wide Web resources for client education.

REFERENCES   Armstrong TS: Stomatitis in the bone marrow transplant patient, *Cancer Nurs* 17(5):403-410, 1994.
Aubertin MA: Oral cancer screening in the elderly: the home healthcare nurse's role, *Home Healthc Nurs* 15(9):594-604, 1997.
Buglass EA: Oral hygiene, *Br J Nurs* 4(9):516-519, 1995.
Curzio J, McCowan M: Getting research into practice: developing oral hygiene standards, *Br J Nurs* 9(7):434-438, 2000.
Epstein JB, Chow AW: Oral complications associated with immunosuppression and cancer therapies, *Infect Dis Clin North Am* 13(4):901-923, 1999.
Fauci AS et al, editors: *Harrison's principles of internal medicine*, New York, 1998, McGraw-Hill.
Feber T: Mouth care for patients receiving oral irradiation, *Prof Nurse* 10(10):666-670, 1994.
Humphrey C: *Home care nursing handbook*, ed 2, Gaithersburg, Md, 1994, Aspen.
Jaffe MS, Skidmore-Roth L: *Home health care nursing care plans*, ed 2, St Louis, 1993, Mosby.
Nikawa H, Hamada T, Yamamoto T: Denture plaque—past and recent concerns, *J Dent* 26(4):299-304, 1998.
Rhodes VA, McDaniel RW, Johnson MH: Patient education: self care guide, *Semin Oncol Nurs* 11(4):298-304, 1995.
Roberts J: Developing an oral assessment and intervention tool for older people: 2, *Br J Nurs* 9(18):2033-2040, 2000.
Sakki TK et al: The association of yeasts and denture stomatitis with behavioral and biologic factors, *Oral Surg Oral Med Oral Pathol Oral Radiol Endontics* 84(6):624-629, 1997.
Scannapieco FA, Stewart EM, Mylotte JM: Colonization of dental plaque by respiratory pathogens in medical intensive care patients, *Crit Care Med* 20(6):740-745, 1992.
Stiefel KA et al: Improving oral hygiene for the seriously ill patient: implementing research-based practice, *Medsurg Nurs* 9(1):40-43, 46, 2000.
Tombes MB, Gallucci B: The effects of hydrogen peroxide rinses on the normal oral mucosa, *Nurs Res* 42(6):332-337, 1993.
White R: Nurse assessment of oral health: a review of practice and education, *Br J Nurs* 9(5):260-266, 2000.
Winslow EH: Don't use H_2O_2 for oral care, *Am J Nurs* 94(3):19, 1994.
Yeager KA et al: Implementation of an oral care standard for leukemia and transplantation patients, *Cancer Nurs* 23(1):40-47, 2000.

Acute Pain

Chris Pasero and Margo McCaffery

NANDA   **Definition** Pain is whatever the experiencing person says it is, existing whenever the person says it does (McCaffery, 1968); an unpleasant sensory and emotional experience arising from actual or potential tissue damage or described in terms of such damage (International Association for the Study of Pain); sudden or slow onset of any intensity from mild to severe with an anticipated or predictable end and a duration of <6 months (NANDA)

Defining Characteristics

Subjective   Pain is always subjective and cannot be proved or disproved. A client's report of pain is the most reliable indicator of pain (Acute Pain Management Guideline Panel, 1992). A

• = Independent; ▲ = Collaborative

client with cognitive ability who can speak or point should use a pain rating scale (e.g., 0 to 10) to identify the current level of pain intensity (self-report) and determine a comfort/function goal (McCaffery, Pasero, 1999).

Objective   Expressions of pain are extremely variable and cannot be used in lieu of self-report. Neither behavior nor vital signs can substitute for the client's self-report (McCaffery, Ferrell, 1991, 1992; McCaffery, Pasero, 1999). However, observable responses to pain are helpful in clients who cannot or will not use a self-report pain rating scale. Observable responses may be loss of appetite and inability to deep breathe, ambulate, sleep, or perform activities of daily living (ADLs). Clients may show guarding, self-protective behavior, self-focusing or narrowed focus, distraction behavior ranging from crying to laughing, and muscle tension or rigidity. In sudden and severe pain, autonomic responses such as diaphoresis, blood pressure and pulse changes, pupillary dilation, or increases or decreases in respiratory rate and depth may be present.

Related Factors (r/t)

Actual or potential tissue damage (mechanical [e.g., incision or tumor growth], thermal [e.g., burn], or chemical [e.g., toxic substance])

NOC   **Outcomes (Nursing Outcomes Classification)**

Suggested NOC Labels

Pain Level, Pain Control, Comfort Level; Pain: Disruptive Effects

> **Example NOC Outcome**
> States/demonstrates decreased **Pain Level** as evidenced by the following indicators: Reported pain/Frequency of pain/Length of pain episodes/Facial expressions of pain/Fewer pain behaviors (Rate each indicator of **Pain:** 1 = severe, 2 = substantial, 3 = moderate, 4 = slight, 5 = none [see Section I])

Client Outcomes

- Uses a pain rating scale to identify current level of pain intensity and determines a comfort/function goal (if client has cognitive abilities)
- Describes how unrelieved pain will be managed
- Reports that the pain management regimen relieves pain to a satisfactory level with acceptable or manageable side effects
- Performs activities of recovery with a reported acceptable level of pain (if pain is above the comfort/function goal, takes action that decreases pain or notifies a member of the health care team)
- States an ability to obtain sufficient amounts of rest and sleep
- Describes a nonpharmacological method that can be used to control pain

NIC   **Interventions (Nursing Interventions Classification)**

Suggested NIC Labels

Pain Management, Analgesic Administration; Conscious Sedation; Patient-Controlled Analgesia (PCA) Assistance

> **Example NIC Interventions—Pain Management**
> - Ensure that client receives attentive analgesic care
> - Perform a comprehensive assessment of pain to include location, characteristics, onset/duration, frequency, quality, intensity or severity, and precipitating factors

• = Independent; ▲ = Collaborative

Nursing Interventions and Rationales

▲ Determine whether client is experiencing pain at the time of the initial interview. If so, intervene at that time to provide pain relief.

The intensity, character, onset, duration, and aggravating and relieving factors of pain should be assessed and documented during the initial evaluation of the patient (American Pain Society Quality of Care Committee, 1995; JCAHO, 2000).

• Ask client to describe past experiences with pain and effectiveness of methods used to manage pain, including experiences with side effects, typical coping responses, and how he or she expresss pain.

A number of concerns (barriers) may affect patients' willingness to report pain and use analgesics (Ward et al, 1993).

• Describe adverse effects of unrelieved pain.

Numerous pathophysiological and psychological morbidity factors may be associated with pain (McCaffery, Pasero, 1999; Page, Ben-Eliyahu, 1997; Puntillo, Weiss, 1994).

• Tell client to report location, intensity (using a pain rating scale), and quality when experiencing pain.

The intensity of pain and discomfort should be assessed and documented after any known pain-producing procedure, with each new report of pain, and at regular intervals (American Pain Society Quality of Care Committee, 1995; JCAHO, 2000).

▲ Determine client's current medication use.

To aid in planning pain treatment, obtain a medication history (Acute Pain Management Guideline Panel, 1992).

▲ Explore the need for both opioid (narcotic) and non-opioid analgesics.

Pharmacological interventions are the cornerstone of pain management (Acute Pain Management Guideline Panel, 1992; McCaffery, Pasero, 1999).

▲ Obtain a prescription to administer a non-opioid (acetaminophen, Cox-2 inhibitor, or a nonsteroidal antiinflammatory drug [NSAID]), unless contraindicated, around the clock (ATC).

NSAIDs act mainly in the periphery to inhibit the initiation of pain impulses (Dahl, Kehlet, 1991). Unless contraindicated, all patients with acute pain should receive a non-opioid ATC (Acute Pain Management Guideline Panel, 1992). The analgesic regimen should include a non-opioid, even if pain is severe enough to require the addition of an opioid (Jacox et al, 1994; McCaffery, Pasero, 1999).

▲ Obtain a prescription to administer opioid analgesia if indicated, especially for severe pain.

Opioid analgesics are indicated for the treatment of moderate to severe pain (Jacox et al, 1994; McCaffery, Pasero, 1999).

▲ Administer opioids orally or intravenously, not intramuscularly. Use a preventive approach to keep pain at or below an acceptable level. Provide PCA and intraspinal routes of administration when appropriate and available.

The least invasive route of administration capable of providing adequate pain control is recommended. The intramuscular (IM) route is avoided because of unreliable absorption, pain, and inconvenience. The intravenous (IV) route is preferred for rapid control of severe pain. For ongoing pain, give analgesia ATC. PRN dosing is appropriate for intermittent pain (Jacox et al, 1994; McCaffery, Pasero, 1999).

• Discuss client's fears of undertreated pain, overdose, and addiction.

A number of concerns may affect clients' willingness to report pain and use opioid analgesics (Ward et al, 1993). Because of the many misconceptions regarding pain and its treat-

• = **Independent;** ▲ = **Collaborative**

ment, education about the ability to control pain effectively and correction of myths about the use of opioids should be included as part of the treatment plan (Jacox et al, 1994; McCaffery, Pasero, 1999). Addiction is extremely unlikely after patients use opioids for acute pain (Acute Pain Management Guideline Panel, 1992).

▲ When opioids are administered, assess pain intensity, sedation, and respiratory status at regular intervals.

Opioids may cause respiratory depression because they reduce the responsiveness of carbon dioxide chemoreceptors located in the respiratory centers of the brain. Because even more opioid is required to produce respiratory depression than is required to produce sedation, patients with clinically significant respiratory depression are usually also sedated. Respiratory depression can be prevented by assessing sedation and decreasing the opioid dose when the patient is arousable but has difficulty staying awake (McCaffery, Pasero, 1999; Pasero, McCaffery, 1994).

• Review client's flow sheet and medication records to determine overall degree of pain relief, side effects, and analgesic requirements during the past 24 hours.

Systematic tracking of pain appears to be an important factor in improving pain management (Faries et al, 1991; JCAHO, 2000).

▲ Administer supplemental opioid doses as needed to keep pain ratings at or below an acceptable level.

A PRN order for supplementary opioid doses between regular doses is an essential backup (American Pain Society, 1999).

▲ Obtain prescriptions to increase or decrease opioid doses as needed; base prescriptions on client's report of pain severity and response to the previous dose in terms of relief, side effects, and ability to perform the activities of recovery.

Increase or decrease the dose of opioid based on assessment of the patient's response. Patients' responses, and therefore their requirements, vary widely, so it is less important to focus on the amount given than on the response (McCaffery, Pasero, 1999; Pasero, McCaffery, 1994).

▲ When client is able to tolerate oral analgesics, obtain a prescription to change to the oral route; use an equianalgesic chart to determine initial dose. (See Appendix E for an equianalgesic chart.)

The oral route is preferred because it is the most convenient and cost-effective (Jacox et al, 1994). Use of equianalgesic doses when switching from one opioid or route of administration to another will help to prevent loss of pain control from underdosing and side effects from overdosing (McCaffery, Pasero, 1999).

• In addition to use of analgesics, support client's use of nonpharmacological methods to control pain, such as distraction, imagery, relaxation, massage, and heat and cold application.

Cognitive-behavioral strategies can restore the clients' sense of self-control, personal efficacy, and active participation in own care (Jacox et al, 1994).

▲ Teach and implement nonpharmacological interventions when pain is relatively well controlled with pharmacological interventions.

Nonpharmacological interventions should be used to supplement, not replace, pharmacological interventions (Acute Pain Management Guideline Panel, 1992).

• Plan care activities around periods of greatest comfort whenever possible.

Pain diminishes activity (Jacox et al, 1994; McCaffery, Pasero, 1999).

• = **Independent;** ▲ = **Collaborative**

▲ Ask client to describe appetite, bowel elimination, and ability to rest and sleep. Administer medications and treatments to improve these functions. Obtain a prescription for a peristaltic stimulant to prevent opioid-induced constipation.
Because there is great individual variation in the development of opioid-induced side effects, these side effects should be monitored and, if their development is inevitable (e.g., constipation), prophylactically treated. Opioids cause constipation by decreasing bowel peristalsis (Jacox et al, 1994; McCaffery, Pasero, 1999).

Geriatric

- Always take the elderly client's reports of pain seriously and ensure that the pain is relieved.
In spite of what many professionals and clients believe, pain is not an expected part of normal aging (McCaffery, Pasero, 1999).
- When assessing pain, speak clearly, slowly, and loudly enough for client to hear; repeat information as needed. Be sure client can see well enough to read pain scale (use enlarged scale) and written materials.
- Handle client's body gently. Allow client to move at own speed.
▲ Use acetaminophen and NSAIDs with low side-effect profiles such as choline and magnesium salicylates (Trilisate) and diflunisal (Dolobid), and watch for side effects, such as GI disturbances and bleeding problems.
Elderly people are at increased risk for gastric and renal toxicity from NSAIDs (Griffin et al, 1991; Acute Pain Management Guideline Panel, 1992).
▲ Avoid or use with caution drugs with a long half-life, such as the NSAID piroxicam (Feldene), the opioids methadone (Dolophine) and levorphanol (Levo-Dromoran), and the benzodiazepine diazepam (Valium).
The higher prevalence of renal insufficiency in the elderly than in younger persons can result in toxicity from drug accumulation (American Pain Society, 1999; Acute Pain Management Guideline Panel, 1992; McCaffery, Pasero, 1999).
▲ Use opioids with caution in the elderly client.
The elderly are more sensitive to the analgesic effects of opioid drugs because they experience a higher peak effect and a longer duration of pain relief. Reduce the initial recommended adult starting opioid dose by 25% to 50%, especially if the client is frail and debilitated; then increase the dose if safe and necessary (Acute Pain Management Guideline Panel, 1992).
▲ Avoid the use of opioids with toxic metabolites, such as meperidine (Demerol) and propoxyphene (Darvon, Darvocet), in elderly clients.
Meperidine's metabolite, normeperidine, can produce CNS irritability, seizures, and even death; propoxyphene's metabolite, norpropoxyphene, can produce both CNS and cardiac toxicity. Both of these metabolites are eliminated by the kidneys, making meperidine and propoxyphene particularly poor choices for elderly clients, many of whom have at least some degree of renal insufficiency (Acute Pain Management Guideline Panel, 1992; McCaffery, Pasero, 1999).

Multicultural

▲ Assess pain in a culturally diverse client using a self-report 0 to 10 numerical pain rating scale or the Wong Baker Faces pain rating scale (see Appendix E). Have scale translated into client's native language if necessary.
Inadequate pain management is widespread, especially among minority groups, and a major reason is the failure to assess pain properly. The more cultural differences between

• = **Independent;** ▲ = **Collaborative**

patient and nurse, the more difficult it is for the nurse to assess and treat pain. Self-report of pain is the single most reliable indicator of pain, regardless of culture (McCaffery, 1999; McCaffery, Pasero, 1999).

▲ Administer analgesics on a preventive basis to keep pain ratings at or below an acceptable level.
   Regardless of the patient's cultural background, pain rated at ≥4 on a 0 to 10 pain rating scale interferes significantly with daily function. Perceived quality of life appears to be comparable across cultures, with pain ratings of >6 interfering markedly with a person's ability to enjoy life (McCaffery, 1999; McCaffery, Pasero, 1999).

• Assess for the influence of cultural beliefs, norms, and values on the client's perception and experience of pain.
   The client's experience of pain may be based on cultural perceptions (Leininger, 1996).

• Assess for the role of fatalism on the client's beliefs regarding their current state of comfort.
   Fatalistic perspectives, which involve the belief that you cannot control your own fate, may influence health behaviors in some African American and Latino populations (Phillips, Cohen, Moses, 1999; Harmon, Castro, Coe, 1996).

• Incorporate folk health care practices and beliefs into care whenever possible.
   Incorporating folk health care beliefs and practices into pain management care increased compliance with the treatment plan (Juarez, Ferrell, Borneman, 1998).

• Use a family-centered approach when working with Latino, Asian American, African-American, and Native American clients.
   Involving family in pain management care increased compliance with the treatment regimen (Juarez, Ferrel, Borneman, 1998).

• Use culturally relevant pain scales (e.g., the Oucher scale) to assess pain in the client.
   Culturally diverse clients may express pain differently than clients from the majority culture. The Oucher scale has African-American and Hispanic versions and is used to assess pain in children (Beyer, Denyes, Villarruel, 1992).

• Ensure that directions for medications are available in the client's language of choice and are understood by client and caregiver.
   Bilingual instructions for medications increased compliance with the pain management plan (Juarez, Ferrell, Borneman, 1998).

• Validate the client's feelings and emotions regarding current health status.
   Validation lets the client know the nurse has heard and understands what was said, and it promotes the nurse-client relationship. (Stuart, Laraia, 2001; Giger, Davidhizar, 1995).

Home Care Interventions

• Review with client and caregivers the cause(s) of pain and the medical regimen specific to the cause. Assess client knowledge and teach disease process as necessary.
   Compliance with the medical regimen for diagnoses involving pain improves the likelihood of successful management (Humphrey, 1994).

▲ Develop a full medication profile, including medications prescribed by all physicians and all over-the-counter medications. Assess for drug interactions. Instruct client to refrain from mixing medications without physician approval.
   Pain medications may significantly impact or be impacted by other medications and may cause severe side effects. Some combinations of drugs are specifically contraindicated (Jacox et al, 1994).

• = Independent; ▲ = Collaborative

- Assess client and family knowledge of side effects and safety precautions associated with pain medications (e.g., use caution when operating machinery when opioids are initiated or dose has been increased).

  The cognitive effects of opioids usually subside within a week of initial dosing or dose increases (McCaffery, Pasero, 1999). The use of long-term opioid treatment does not appear to affect neuropsychological performance. Pain itself may deteriorate performance of neuropsychological tests more than oral opioid treatment (Sjogren et al, 2000).

▲ If administering medication using highly technological methods, assess home for necessary resources (e.g., electricity), and ensure that there will be responsible caregivers available to assist client with administration.

  Some routes of medication administration require special conditions and procedures to be safe and accurate (McCaffery, Pasero, 1999).

- Assess knowledge base of client and family for highly technological medication administration. Teach as necessary. Be sure clients know when, how, and who to contact if analgesia is unsatisfactory.

  Appropriate instruction in the home increases the accuracy and safety of medication administration (McCaffery, Pasero, 1999).

Client/Family Teaching

NOTE: To avoid the negative connotations associated with the words *drugs* and *narcotics,* use the words *pain medicine* when teaching clients.

- Provide written materials on pain control such as the Agency for Health Care Policy and Research (AHCPR) pamphlet, *Pain Control: Patient Guide.*
- Discuss the various discomforts encompassed by the word *pain,* and ask client to give examples of previously experienced pain. Explain pain assessment process and purpose of the pain rating scale.
- Teach client to use the pain rating scale to rate intensity of past or current pain. Ask client to set a comfort/function goal by selecting a pain level on the rating scale that makes it easy to perform recovery activities (e.g., turn, cough, deep breathe). If pain is above this level, client should take action that decreases pain or notify a member of the health care team. (See Appendix E for information on teaching clients to use the pain rating scale.)
▲ Demonstrate medication administration and use of supplies and equipment. If PCA is ordered, determine client's ability to press appropriate button. Remind client and staff that the PCA button is for patient-only use.
- Reinforce importance of taking pain medications to keep pain under control.
- Reinforce that taking opioids for pain relief is not addiction and that addiction is very unlikely to occur.
- Demonstrate use of appropriate nonpharmacological approaches for controlling pain, such as heat, cold, distraction techniques, relaxation breathing, visualization, rocking, stroking, music, and television.

WEB SITES FOR EDUCATION

᯽ Merlin See the MERLIN web site for World Wide Web resources for client education.

REFERENCES   Acute Pain Management Guideline Panel: *Acute pain management operative or medical procedures and trauma: clinical practice guideline,* Agency for Health Care Policy and Research Pub No 92-0032, Rockville, Md, 1992, Public Health Service, U.S. Department of Health and Human Services.

• = **Independent;** ▲ = **Collaborative**

American Pain Society: *Principles of analgesic use in the treatment of acute pain and cancer pain,* ed 4, Glenview, Ill, 1999, The Society.

American Pain Society Quality of Care Committee: Quality improvement guidelines for the treatment of acute pain and cancer pain, *JAMA* 274:1874, 1995.

Beyer J, Denyes M, Villarruel A: The creation, validation, and continuing development of the Oucher: a measure of pain intensity in children, *J Pediatr Nurs* 7(5):335, 1992.

Dahl JB, Kehlet H: Non-steroidal anti-inflammatory drugs: rationale for use in severe postoperative pain, *Br J Anaesth* 66:703, 1991.

Faries JE et al: Systematic pain records and their impact on pain control, *Cancer Nurs* 14:306, 1991.

Giger JN, Davidhizar RE: *Transcultural nursing,* ed 2, St Louis, 1995, Mosby.

Griffin MR et al: Nonsteroidal anti-inflammatory drug use and increased risk for peptic ulcer disease in elderly persons, *Ann Intern Med* 11(4):257, 1991.

Jaurez G, Ferrell B, Borneman T: Influence of culture on cancer pain management in Hispanic clients, *Cancer Practice* 6(5):262-269, 1998.

Joint Commission on Accreditation of Healthcare Organizations (JCAHO): *2000 Hospital accreditation standards,* Oakbrook, Ill, 2000, The Organization.

Harmon MP, Castro FG, Coe K: Acculturation and cervical cancer: knowledge, beliefs, and behaviors of Hispanic women, *Women Health* 24(3):37-57, 1996.

Humphrey C: Home care nursing handbook, ed 2, Gaithersburg, Md, 1994, Aspen.

Jacox A et al: *Management of cancer pain: clinical practice guideline no 9,* Agency for Health Care Policy and Research Pub No 94-0592, Rockville, Md, 1994, Public Health Service, U.S. Department of Health and Human Services.

Leininger MM: *Transcultural nursing: theories, research and practices,* ed 2, Hilliard, Ohio, 1996, McGraw-Hill.

McCaffery M: *Nursing practice theories related to cognition, bodily pain and man-environment interactions,* Los Angeles, 1968, University of California at Los Angeles Students' Store.

McCaffery M: Culturally sensitive pain assessment, *Am J Nurs* 99(8):18, 1999.

McCaffery M, Ferrell BR: How would you respond to these patients in pain? *Nursing* 21(6):34-37, 1991.

McCaffery M, Ferrell BR: How vital are vital signs? *Nursing* 22(1):42-46, 1992.

McCaffery M, Pasero C: *Pain: clinical manual,* St Louis, 1999, Mosby.

Page GG, Ben-Eliyahu S: The immune-suppressive nature of pain, *Semin Oncol Nurs* 13(1):10-15, 1997.

Pasero C, McCaffery M: Avoiding opioid-induced respiratory depression, *Am J Nurs* 94:25, 1994.

Phillips JM, Cohen MZ, Moses G: Breast cancer screening and African American women: fear, fatalism, and silence, *Oncol Nurs Forum* 26(3):561-571, 1999.

Puntillo K, Weiss SJ: Pain: its mediators and associated morbidity in critically ill cardiovascular surgical patients, *Nurs Res* 43(3):1, 1994.

Sjogren P et al: Neuropsychological performance in cancer patients: the role of oral opioids, pain and performance status, *Pain* 86:237-245, 2000.

Stuart GW, Laraia MT: Therapeutic nurse-patient relationship. In Stuart GW, Laraia MT, editors: *Principles and practice of psychiatric nursing,* St Louis, 2001, Mosby, p 30.

Ward S et al: Patient-related barriers to management of cancer pain, *Pain* 52:319, 1993.

Chronic Pain

Chris Pasero and Margo McCaffery

NANDA   **Definition** Pain is whatever the experiencing person says it is, existing whenever the person says it does (McCaffery, 1968); an unpleasant sensory and emotional experience arising from actual or potential tissue damage or described in terms of such damage (International Association for the Study of Pain); sudden or slow onset of any intensity from mild to severe, constant or recurring, without an anticipated or predictable end and a duration >6 months (NANDA); a state in which an individual experiences pain

 = **Independent;** ▲ = **Collaborative**

that persists for a month beyond the usual course of an acute illness or a reasonable duration for an injury to heal, is associated with a chronic pathologic process, or recurs at intervals for months or years (Bonica, 1990)

Defining Characteristics

Subjective   Pain is always subjective and cannot be proved or disproved. The client's report of pain is the most reliable indicator of pain (Acute Pain Management Guideline Panel, 1992). Clients with cognitive abilities who can speak or point should use a pain rating scale (e.g., 0 to 10) to identify their current level of pain intensity (self-report) and determine a comfort/function goal (McCaffery, Pasero, 1999).

Objective   Expressions of pain are extremely variable and cannot be used in lieu of self-report. Neither behavior nor vital signs can substitute for the client's self-report (McCaffery, Ferrell, 1991, 1992; McCaffery, Pasero, 1999). However, observable responses to pain are helpful in its assessment, especially in clients who cannot or will not use a self-report pain rating scale. Observable responses may be loss of appetite or the inability to ambulate, perform activities of daily living (ADLs), work, or sleep. Clients may show guarding, self-protective behavior, self-focusing or narrowed focus, distraction behavior ranging from crying to laughing, and muscle tension or rigidity. In sudden severe pain, autonomic responses such as diaphoresis, blood pressure and pulse changes, pupillary dilation, and increase or decrease in respiratory rate and depth may be present but are usually not present with chronic pain that is relatively stable. Clients with chronic, cancer, or nonmalignant pain may experience threats to self-image; a perceived lack of options for coping; and worsening helplessness, anxiety, and depression. Chronic pain may affect almost every aspect of the client's daily life, including concentration, work, and relationships.

Related Factors (r/t)

Actual or potential tissue damage; tumor progression and related pathology; diagnostic and therapeutic procedures; nerve injury (neuropathic pain)

NOTE: The cause of chronic nonmalignant pain may not be known because pain is a new science and an area of diverse types of problems.

NOC   Outcomes (Nursing Outcomes Classification)

Suggested NOC Labels

Pain Level; Pain Control; Comfort Level; Pain: Disruptive Effects

> **Example NOC Outcome**
> States/demonstrates decreased **Pain Level** as evidenced by the following indicators: Reported pain/Frequency of pain/Length of pain episodes/Facial expressions of pain/Fewer pain behaviors (Rate each indicator of **Pain Level:** 1 = severe, 2 = substantial, 3 = moderate, 4 = slight, 5 = none [see Section I])

Client Outcomes

- Uses pain rating scale to identify current level of pain intensity, determines a comfort/function goal, and maintains a pain diary (if client has cognitive abilities)
- Describes the total plan for drug and nondrug pain relief, including how to safely and effectively take medicines and integrate nondrug therapies
- Demonstrates ability to pace self, taking rest breaks before they are needed

• = **Independent;** ▲ = **Collaborative**

- Functions on an acceptable ability level with minimal interference from pain and medication side effects (if pain is above the comfort/function goal, takes action that decreases pain or notifies a member of the health care team)

NIC **Interventions (Nursing Interventions Classification)**

Suggested NIC Labels

Pain Management, Analgesic Administration

Example NIC Interventions—Pain Management
- Ensure that client receives attentive analgesic care
- Perform a comprehensive assessment of pain to include location, characteristics, onset/duration, frequency, quality, intensity or severity, and precipitating factors

Nursing Interventions and Rationales

▲ Determine whether client is experiencing pain at time of initial interview. If so, intervene at that time to provide pain relief.

The intensity, character, onset, duration, and aggravating and relieving factors of pain should be assessed and documented during the initial evaluation of the patient (American Pain Society Quality of Care Committee, 1995; JCAHO, 2000).

- Ask client to describe past and current experiences with pain and effectiveness of the methods used to manage the pain, including experiences with side effects, typical coping responses, and how he or she expresses pain.

A number of concerns (barriers) may affect client's willingness to report pain and use analgesics (Ward et al, 1993).

- Describe the adverse effects of unrelieved pain.

Numerous pathophysiological and psychological morbidity factors may be associated with pain (McCaffery, Pasero, 1999; Page, Ben-Eliyahu, 1997; Puntillo, Weiss, 1994).

- Tell client to report pain location, intensity, and quality when experiencing pain.

The intensity of pain and discomfort should be assessed and documented after any known pain-producing procedure, with each new report of pain, and at regular intervals (American Pain Society Quality of Care Committee, 1995; JCAHO, 2000).

- Ask client to maintain a diary of pain ratings, timing, precipitating events, medications, treatments, and what works best to relieve pain.

Systematic tracking of pain appears to be an important factor in improving pain management (Faries et al, 1991; JCAHO, 2000).

▲ Determine client's current medication use.

To aid in planning pain treatment, obtain a medication history (Acute Pain Management Guideline Panel, 1992).

▲ Explore need for medications from the three classes of analgesics: opioids (narcotics), non-opioids (acetaminophen, Cox-2 inhibitors, and nonsteroidal antiinflammatory drugs [NSAIDs]), and adjuvant medications. For chronic neuropathic pain, consider adjuvant medications that are analgesic, such as anticonvulsants and antidepressants.

Some types of pain respond to non-opioid drugs alone. However, if pain is not responding, consider increasing the dosage or adding an opioid. At any level of pain, analgesic adjuvants may be useful (American Pain Society, 1999). Analgesic combinations may enhance pain relief (McCaffery, Pasero, 1999).

- = **Independent;** ▲ = **Collaborative**

▲ The oral route is preferred. If client is receiving parenteral analgesia, use an equianalgesic chart to convert to an oral or another noninvasive route as smoothly as possible. (See Appendix E for an equianalgesic chart.)

The least invasive route of administration capable of providing adequate pain control is recommended. The oral route is the most preferred because it is the most convenient and cost effective. Avoid the intramuscular (IM) route because of unreliable absorption, pain, and inconvenience (Jacox et al, 1994).

▲ Obtain a prescription to administer a non-opioid, unless contraindicated, around the clock (ATC).

NSAIDs act mainly in the periphery to inhibit the initiation of pain signals (Dahl, Kehlet, 1991). The analgesic regimen should include a non-opioid drug ATC, even if pain is severe enough to require the addition of an opioid (American Pain Society, 1999).

▲ For persistent cancer pain, obtain a prescription to administer opioid analgesics.

When pain persists or increases, an opioid such as codeine or hydrocodone should be added to the non-opioid (Jacox et al, 1994). If this is not effective, switch to morphine or other single-entity opioids.

▲ Establish ATC dosing and administer supplemental opioid doses as needed to keep pain ratings at or below an acceptable level.

A prn order for a supplementary opioid dose between regular doses is an essential backup (American Pain Society, 1999).

▲ Ask client to describe appetite, bowel elimination, and ability to rest and sleep. Administer medications and treatments to improve these functions. Always obtain a prescription for a peristaltic stimulant to prevent opioid-induced constipation.

Because there is great individual variation in the development of opioid-induced side effects, they should be monitored and, if their development is inevitable (e.g., constipation), prophylactically treated. Opioids cause constipation by decreasing bowel peristalsis (Jacox et al, 1994; McCaffery, Pasero, 1999).

▲ Explain pain management approach that has been ordered, including therapies, medication administration, side effects, and complications.

One of the most important steps toward improved control of pain is a better client understanding of the nature of pain, its treatment, and the role client needs to play in pain control (Jacox et al, 1994).

• Discuss client's fears of undertreated pain, addiction, and overdose.

A number of concerns (barriers) may affect patients' willingness to report pain and use analgesics (Ward et al, 1993). Because of the many misconceptions regarding pain and its treatment, education about the ability to control pain effectively and correction of myths about the use of opioids should be included as part of the treatment plan (McCaffery, Pasero, 1999). Opioid tolerance and physical dependence are expected with long-term opioid treatment and should not be confused with addiction (Jacox et al, 1994).

• Review client's pain diary, flow sheet, and medication records to determine overall degree of pain relief, side effects, and analgesic requirements for an appropriate period (e.g., one week).

Systematic tracking of pain appears to be an important factor in improving pain management (Faries et al, 1991; JCAHO, 2000).

▲ Obtain prescriptions to increase or decrease analgesic doses when indicated. Base prescriptions on the client's report of pain severity and the comfort/function goal

• = Independent; ▲ = Collaborative

and response to previous dose in terms of relief, side effects, and ability to perform the daily activities and the prescribed therapeutic regimen.

Opioid doses should be adjusted individually to achieve pain relief with an acceptable level of adverse effects (Jacox et al, 1994; McCaffery, Pasero, 1999).

▲ If opioid dose is increased, monitor sedation and respiratory status for a brief time.

Patients receiving long-term opioid therapy generally develop tolerance to the respiratory depressant effects of these agents (Jacox et al, 1994; McCaffery, Pasero, 1999).

• In addition to the use of analgesics, support the client's use of nonpharmacological methods to control pain, such as distraction, imagery, relaxation, massage, and heat and cold application.

Cognitive-behavioral strategies can restore clients' sense of self-control, personal efficacy, and active participation in their own care (Jacox et al, 1994).

• Teach and implement nonpharmacological interventions when pain is relatively well controlled with pharmacological interventions.

Nonpharmacological interventions should be used to supplement, not replace, pharmacological interventions (Acute Pain Management Guideline Panel, 1992).

• Plan care activities around periods of greatest comfort whenever possible.

Pain diminishes activity (Jacox et al, 1994; McCaffery, Pasero, 1999).

▲ Ask clients to describe their appetite, bowel elimination, and ability to rest and sleep. Administer medications and treatments directed toward improving these functions.

Because there is great individual variation in the development of opioid-induced side effects, clinicians should monitor and, if development is inevitable, prophylactically treat them (Jacox et al, 1994).

▲ Explore appropriate resources for management of pain on a long-term basis (e.g., hospice, pain care center).

Most patients with cancer or chronic nonmalignant pain are treated for pain in outpatient and home care settings. Plans should be made to ensure ongoing assessment of the pain and the effectiveness of treatments in these settings (Jacox et al, 1994).

• If client has progressive cancer pain, assist client and family with handling issues related to death and dying.

Peer support groups and pastoral counseling may increase the client's and family's coping skills and provide needed support (Jacox et al, 1994).

• If client has chronic nonmalignant pain, assist client and family with minimizing effects of pain on interpersonal relationships and daily activities such as work and recreation.

Pain reduces clients' options to exercise control, diminishes psychological well-being, and makes them feel helpless and vulnerable. Therefore clinicians should support active client involvement in effective and practical methods to manage pain (Hitchcock, Ferrell, McCaffery, 1994; Jacox et al, 1994).

Geriatric

• Always take an elderly client's reports of pain seriously and ensure that the pain is relieved.

In spite of what many professionals and clients believe, pain is not an expected part of normal aging (McCaffery, Pasero, 1999).

• When assessing pain, speak clearly, slowly, and loudly enough for client to hear; repeat information as needed. Be sure client can see well enough to read pain scale (use enlarged scale) and written materials.

• = **Independent;** ▲ = **Collaborative**

- Handle client's body gently. Allow client to move at own speed.
▲ Use NSAIDs with caution and avoid ATC NSAID dosing.
  Opioids ATC are preferable to chronic NSAID administration in the elderly client because of an increased risk for NSAID adverse effects (American Geriatric Society Panel on Chronic Pain in Older Persons, 1998).
▲ Use acetaminophen and NSAIDs with low side effect profiles such as choline and magnesium salicylates (Trilisate) and diflunisal (Dolobid). Watch for side effects such as GI disturbances and bleeding problems.
  Elderly clients are at increased risk for gastric and renal toxicity from NSAIDs (Griffin et al, 1991; Acute Pain Management Guideline Panel, 1992).
▲ Avoid or use with caution drugs with a long half-life, such as the NSAID piroxicam (Feldene), the opioids methadone (Dolophine) and levorphanol (Levo-Dromoran), and the benzodiazepine diazepam (Valium).
  A higher prevalence of renal insufficiency in the elderly than in younger persons can result in toxicity from drug accumulation (American Pain Society, 1999; Acute Pain Management Guideline Panel, 1992; McCaffery, Pasero, 1999).
▲ In an elderly client, avoid the use of opioids with toxic metabolites, such as meperidine (Demerol) and propoxyphene (Darvon, Darvocet).
  Meperidine's metabolite, normeperidine, can produce CNS irritability, seizures, and even death; propoxyphene's metabolite, norpropoxyphene, can produce both CNS and cardiac toxicity. Both of these metabolites are eliminated by the kidneys, making meperidine and propoxyphene particularly poor choices for elderly clients, many of whom have at least some degree of renal insufficiency (Acute Pain Management Guideline Panel, 1992; McCaffery, Pasero, 1999).

Multicultural

▲ Assess pain in a culturally diverse client using a self-report 0 to 10 numerical pain rating scale or the Wong Baker Faces pain rating scale (see Appendix E). Use a scale that has been translated into client's native language if necessary.
  Inadequate pain management is widespread, especially among minority groups, and a major reason is the failure to assess pain properly. The more cultural differences between patient and nurse, the more difficult it is for the nurse to assess and treat pain. Self-report of pain is the single most reliable indicator of pain, regardless of culture (McCaffery, 1999; McCaffery, Pasero, 1999).
▲ Administer analgesics on a preventive basis to keep pain ratings at or below an acceptable level.
- Assess for the influence of cultural beliefs, norms, and values on the client's perception and experience of pain.
  The client's experience of pain may be based on cultural perceptions (Leininger, 1996).
- Assess for the role of fatalism on the client's beliefs regarding their current state of comfort.
  Fatalistic perspectives, which involve the belief that you cannot control your own fate, may influence health behaviors in some African American and Latino populations (Phillips, Cohen, Moses, 1999; Harmon, Castro, Coe, 1996).
- Incorporate folk health care practices and beliefs into care whenever possible.
  Incorporating folk health care beliefs and practices into pain management care increased compliance with the treatment plan (Juarez, Ferrell, Borneman, 1998).

• = Independent; ▲ = Collaborative

- Use a family-centered approach when working with Latino, Asian American, African-American, and Native American clients.
  Involving family in pain management care increased compliance with the treatment regimen (Juarez, Ferrel, Borneman, 1998).
- Use culturally relevant pain scales (e.g., the Oucher scale) to assess pain in the client.
  Culturally diverse clients may express pain differently than clients from the majority culture. The Oucher scale has African-American and Hispanic versions and is used to assess pain in children (Beyer, Denyes, Villarruel, 1992).
- Ensure that directions for medications are available in the client's language of choice and are understood by client and caregiver.
  Bilingual instructions for medications increased compliance with the pain management plan (Juarez, Ferrell, Borneman, 1998).
- Validate the client's feelings and emotions regarding current health status.
  Validation lets the client know the nurse has heard and understands what was said, and it promotes the nurse-client relationship (Stuart, Laraia, 2001; Giger, Davidhizar, 1995).

Home Care Interventions

- Review with client and caregivers the cause(s) of pain and the medical regimen specific to the cause. Assess client knowledge and teach disease process as necessary.
  Compliance with the medical regimen for diagnoses involving pain improves the likelihood of successful management (Humphrey, 1994).
- ▲ Develop a full medication profile, including medications prescribed by all physicians and all over-the-counter medications. Assess for drug interactions. Instruct client to refrain from mixing medications without physician approval.
  Pain medications may significantly impact or be impacted by other medications and may cause severe side effects. Some combinations of drugs are specifically contraindicated (Jacox et al, 1994).
- Assess client and family knowledge of side effects and safety precautions associated with pain medications (e.g., use caution when operating machinery when opioids are initiated or dose has been increased).
  The cognitive effects of opioids usually subside within a week of initial dosing or dose increases (McCaffery, Pasero, 1999). The use of long-term opioid treatment does not appear to affect neuropsychological performance. Pain itself may deteriorate performance of neuropsychological tests more than oral opioid treatment (Sjogren et al, 2000).
- ▲ Collaborate with health care team on an ongoing basis (including client and family) to determine optimal pain control profile. Identify the most effective interventions and the medication administration routes most acceptable to the family and client.
  Success in pain control is partially dependent on the acceptability of the suggested intervention. Acceptability promotes compliance. Dosages vary among routes and will need to be adjusted accordingly to avoid breakthrough or transitional pain (Bohnet, 1995).
- ▲ If administering medication using highly technological methods, assess home for necessary resources (e.g., electricity), and ensure that there will be responsible caregivers available to assist client with administration.
  Some routes of medication administration require special conditions and procedures to be safe and accurate (McCaffery, Pasero, 1999).
- ▲ Assess knowledge base of client and family for highly technological medication administration including the use of PCA pump. Teach as necessary.

- **= Independent; ▲ = Collaborative**

Appropriate instruction in the home increases the accuracy and safety of medication administration (McCaffery, Pasero, 1999).
▲ Support the client and family in the use of opioid analgesics.
Well-intentioned friends and family may create added stress by expressing judgment or fears regarding the use of opioid analgesics (McCaffery, Pasero, 1999).

Client/Family Teaching

NOTE: To avoid the negative connotations associated with the words *drugs* and *narcotics*, use the words *pain medicine* when teaching clients.

• Provide written materials regarding pain control, such as the Agency for Health Care Policy and Research pamphlet, *Managing Cancer Pain: Patient Guide.*
• Discuss the various discomforts encompassed by the word *pain* and ask clients to give examples of pain they have experienced. Explain the pain assessment process and the purpose of the pain rating scale that will be used. Teach clients to use the pain rating scale to rate the intensity of current or past pain. Ask them to set a pain relief goal by selecting a pain rating on the scale; if pain goes above this level, they should take action that decreases pain or notify a member of the health care team. (See Appendix E for information on teaching clients to use the pain rating scale.)
▲ Discuss the total plan for drug and nondrug treatment, including the medication plan for ATC administration and supplemental doses, the maintenance of a pain diary, and the use of supplies and equipment.
▲ Reinforce the importance of taking pain medications to keep pain under control.
• Reinforce that taking opioids for pain relief is not an addiction.
▲ Explain to clients with chronic neuropathic pain the process of taking adjuvant analgesics (e.g., tricyclic antidepressants); a low dose is used initially and is increased gradually. Emphasize that pain relief is delayed and the drugs must be taken daily. Reassure the client that although the medicine is an antidepressant, it is used for analgesia and not depression. Comparable teaching should take place when an anticonvulsant is prescribed for analgesia.
▲ Emphasize to clients with chronic nonmalignant pain the importance of participating in therapeutic regimens other than medication (e.g., physical therapy, group therapy).
• Emphasize to clients the importance of pacing themselves and taking rest breaks before they are needed.
• Demonstrate the use of appropriate nonpharmacological approaches for controlling pain.

WEB SITES FOR EDUCATION

ᶴMᴇʀʟɪɴ See the MERLIN web site for World Wide Web resources for client education.

REFERENCES   Acute Pain Management Guideline Panel: *Acute pain management operative or medical procedures and trauma: clinical practice guideline,* Agency for Health Care Policy and Research Pub No 92-0032, Rockville, Md, 1992, Public Health Service, U.S. Department of Health and Human Services.

American Geriatric Society Panel on Chronic Pain in Older Persons: The management of chronic pain in older persons: clinical practice guidelines, *J Am Geriatr Soc* 46:635-651, 1998.

American Pain Society: *Principles of analgesic use in the treatment of acute pain and cancer pain,* ed 4, Glenview, Ill, 1999, The Society.

American Pain Society Quality of Care Committee: Quality improvement guidelines for the treatment of acute pain and cancer pain, *JAMA* 274:1874, 1995.

Beyer J, Denyes M, Villarruel A: The creation, validation, and continuing development of the Oucher: a measure of pain intensity in children, *J Pediatr Nurs* 7(5):335, 1992.

• = Independent; ▲ = Collaborative

Bohnet N: Chronic pain management in the home care setting, *J Wound Ostomy Cont Nurs* 22:135, 1995.

Bonica JJ: Definitions and taxonomy of pain. In Bonica JJ, editor: *The management of pain*, Philadelphia, 1990, Lea & Febiger.

Dahl JB, Kehlet H: Non-steroidal anti-inflammatory drugs: rationale for use in severe postoperative pain, *Br J Anaesth* 66:703, 1991.

Faries JE et al: Systematic pain records and their impact on pain control, *Cancer Nurs* 14:306, 1991.

Giger JN, Davidhizar RE: *Transcultural nursing*, ed 2, St Louis, 1995, Mosby.

Griffin ME et al: Nonsteroidal anti-inflammatory drug use and increased risk for peptic ulcer disease in elderly persons, *Ann Intern Med* 11:257, 1991.

Harmon MP, Castro FG, Coe K: Acculturation and cervical cancer: knowledge, beliefs, and behaviors of Hispanic women, *Women Health* 24(3):37-57, 1996.

Hitchcock LS, Ferrell BR, McCaffery M: The experience of chronic nonmalignant pain, *J Pain Symptom Manage* 9:312, 1994.

Humphrey C: *Home care nursing handbook*, ed 2, Gaithersburg, Md, 1994, Aspen.

Jacox A et al: *Management of cancer pain: clinical practice guideline no 9*, Agency for Health Care Policy and Research Pub No 94-0592, Rockville, Md, 1994, Public Health Service, U.S. Department of Health and Human Services.

Juarez G, Ferrell B, Borneman T: Influence of culture on cancer pain management in Hispanic clients, *Cancer Practice* 6(5):262-269, 1998.

Joint Commission on Accreditation of Healthcare Organizations (JCAHO): *2000 Hospital accreditation standards*, Oakbrook, Ill, 2000, The Organization.

Leininger MM: *Transcultural nursing: theories, research and practices*, ed 2, Hilliard, Ohio, 1996, McGraw-Hill.

McCaffery M: *Nursing practice theories related to cognition, bodily pain, and man-environment interactions*, Los Angeles, 1968, University of California at Los Angeles Students' Store.

McCaffery M: Culturally sensitive pain assessment, *Am J Nurs* 99(8):18, 1999.

McCaffery M, Ferrell BR: How would you respond to these patients in pain? *Nursing* 21(6):34-37, 1991.

McCaffery M, Ferrell BR: How vital are vital signs? *Nursing* 22(1):42-46, 1992.

McCaffery M, Pasero C: *Pain: clinical manual*, St Louis, 1999, Mosby.

Page GG, Ben-Eliyahu S: The immune-suppressive nature of pain, *Semin Oncol Nurs* 13(1):10-15, 1997.

Phillips JM, Cohen MZ, Moses G: Breast cancer screening and African American women: fear, fatalism, and silence, *Oncol Nurs Forum* 26(3):561-571, 1999.

Puntillo K, Weiss SJ: Pain: its mediators and associated morbidity in critically ill cardiovascular surgical patients, *Nurs Res* 43:31, 1994.

Sjogren P et al: Neuropsychological performance in cancer patients: the role of oral opioids, pain and performance status, *Pain* 86:237-245, 2000.

Stuart GW, Laraia MT: Therapeutic nurse-patient relationship. In Stuart GW, Laraia MT, editors: *Principles and practice of psychiatric nursing*, St Louis, 2001, Mosby, p 30.

Ward S et al: Patient-related barriers to management of cancer pain, *Pain* 52:319, 1993.

Impaired Parenting

Peggy A. Wetsch and Mary Markle

NANDA   **Definition** Inability of the primary caretaker to create, maintain, or regain an environment that promotes the optimum growth and development of the child

Defining Characteristics

Infant/child   Poor academic performance; frequent illness; runaway; incidence of physical and psychological trauma or abuse; frequent accidents; lack of attachment; failure to thrive; behavioral disorders; poor social competence; lack of separation anxiety; poor cognitive development

Parental   Inappropriate child care arrangements; rejection of or hostility to child; statements of inability to meet child's needs; inflexibility in meeting needs of child or situation; poor

• = Independent; ▲ = Collaborative

or inappropriate caretaking skills; regularly punitive; inconsistent care; child abuse; inadequate child health maintenance; unsafe home environment; verbalization of inability to control child; negative statements about child; verbalization of role inadequacy or frustration; inappropriate visual, tactile, auditory stimulation; abandonment; insecure or lack of attachment to infant; inconsistent behavior management; child neglect; little cuddling; maternal-child interaction deficit; poor parent-child interaction

Related Factors (r/t)

Social
Lack of access to resources; social isolation; lack of resources; poor home environment; lack of family cohesiveness; inadequate child care arrangements; lack of transportation; unemployment or job problems; role strain or overload; marital conflict, declining satisfaction; lack of value of parenthood; change in family unit; low socioeconomic class; unplanned or unwanted pregnancy; presence of stress (e.g., financial, legal, recent crisis, cultural move); lack of or poor parental role model; single parent; lack of social support network; father of child not involved; history of being abusive; history of being abused; financial difficulties; maladaptive coping strategies; poverty; poor problem-solving skills; inability to put child's needs before own; low self-esteem; relocations; legal difficulties

Knowledge
Lack of knowledge about child health maintenance; lack of knowledge about parenting skills; unrealistic expectations for self, infant, partner; limited cognitive functioning; lack of knowledge about child development; inability to recognize and act on infant cues; low educational level or attainment; poor communication skills; lack of cognitive readiness for parenthood; preference for physical punishment

Physiological
Physical illness

Infant/child
Premature birth; illness; prolonged separation from parent; not desired gender; attention deficit hyperactivity disorder; difficult temperament; separation from parent at birth; lack of goodness of fit (temperament) with parental expectations; unplanned or unwanted child; handicapping condition or developmental delay; multiple births; altered perceptual abilities

Psychological
History of substance abuse or dependencies; disability; depression; difficult labor and/or delivery; young age, especially adolescent; history of mental illness; high number of or closely spaced pregnancies; sleep derivation or disruption; lack of or late prenatal care; separation from infant/child

NOTE: It is important to reaffirm that adjustment to parenting in general is a normal maturational process that elicits nursing behaviors to prevent potential problems and to promote health.

NOC Outcomes (Nursing Outcomes Classification)

Suggested NOC Labels

Child Development: 2 Months; 4 Months; 6 Months; 2 Years; 3 Years; 4 Years; 5 Years; Middle Childhood (6-11 Years); Adolescence (12-17 Years); Parent-Infant Attachment; Parenting; Parenting: Social Safety; Role Performance; Safety Behavior: Home Physical Environment; Social Support

> **Example NOC Outcome**
> Accomplishes **Parenting** as evidenced by: Provides for child's needs/Interacts positively with child/Has realistic expectations of parental role (Rate each indicator of **Parenting:** 1 = not adequate, 2 = slightly adequate, 3 = moderately adequate, 4 = substantially adequate, 5 = totally adequate [see Section I])

• = **Independent;** ▲ = **Collaborative**

Client Outcomes

- Affirms desire to develop constructive parenting skills to support infant/child growth and development
- Initiates appropriate measures to develop a safe, nurturing environment
- Acquires and displays attentive, supportive parenting behaviors
- Identifies strategies to protect child from harm and/or neglect and initiates action when indicated

NIC   Interventions (Nursing Interventions Classification)

Suggested NIC Labels

Abuse Protection: Child; Attachment Promotion; Developmental Enhancement; Family Integrity Promotion; Parenting Promotion

> **Example NIC Interventions—Parenting Promotion**
> - Assist parents to have realistic expectations appropriate to developmental and ability level of child
> - Assist parents with role transition and expectations of parenthood

Nursing Interventions and Rationales

- Use active listening to explore parent's understanding of developmental needs and expectations of child and self within the context of cultural perspectives and influences.
  Interviewing with empathy while reserving judgment allows parent to more freely express frustrations and disappointments regarding negative feelings, needs, and parenting skills. Unrealistic expectations may be present when parent does not discern what is normal for the child (Denehy, 1992; Herman-Staab, 1994; Mrazek, Mrazek, Klinnert, 1995).
- Examine characteristics of parenting style and behaviors, including the following:
  - Emotional climate at home
  - Attribution of negative traits to child
  - Failure to support child's increases in autonomy
  - Type of interaction with infant/child
  - Competition with child for spousal/significant other attention
  - Lack of knowledge/concern about health maintenance or behavioral problems
  - Other behaviors or concerns
  Children are at risk for neglect, abuse, and other negative psychosocial outcomes in families with dysfunctions (Mrazek, Mrazek, Klinnert, 1995).
- ▲ Institute abuse/neglect protection measures if evidence of inability to cope with family stressors or crisis, signs of parental substance abuse, or significant level of social isolation apparent.
  Risk of abuse/neglect is higher in families with high levels of stress, substance abuse, or lack of social support systems (Devlin, Reynolds, 1994).
- For mothers with toddlers, assess maternal depression, perceptions of difficult temperament in toddler, and low maternal self-efficacy.
  Self-efficacy is defined as one's judgment of how effectively one can execute a task or manage a situation that may contain novel, unpredictable, and stressful elements. A cyclic relationship among depression, perceived difficult temperament, and self-efficacy has been identified. Negative feelings about oneself and one's child are likely to negatively influence the parent-child relationship (Gross et al, 1994).

• = Independent; ▲ = Collaborative

- Appraise parent's resources and availability of social support systems. Determine single mother's particular sources of support, especially availability of her own mother and partner. Encourage use of healthy, strong support systems.
  Before adequate interventions and education can be initiated, understanding of the current support system and concerns must occur. The mother's partner and her mother are often important sources of support (Zacharia, 1994).
- Model age- and cognitively appropriate caregiver skills by doing the following:
  - Communicating with child at an appropriate cognitive level of development
  - Giving child tasks and responsibilities appropriate to age or functional age/level
  - Instituting safety considerations such as assistive equipment
  - Encouraging child to perform activities of daily living (ADLs) as appropriate
  These activities illustrate parenting and child-rearing skills and behaviors for parents and family (McCloskey, Bulechek, 1992).

Multicultural

- Assess for the influence of cultural beliefs, norms, and values on the client's perception of parenting.
  What the client considers normal parenting may be based on cultural perceptions (Leininger, 1996).
- Acknowledge racial/ethnic differences at the onset of care.
  Acknowledgement of racial/ethnicity issues will enhance communication, establish rapport, and promote treatment outcomes (D'Avanzo et al, 2001).
- Approach individuals of color with respect, warmth, and professional courtesy.
  Instances of disrespect have special significance for individuals of color (D'Avanzo et al, 2001).
- Give rationale when assessing black individuals about sensitive issues.
  Blacks may expect white caregivers to hold negative and preconceived ideas about them. Giving rationale for questions will help alleviate this perception (D'Avanzo et al, 2001).
- Acknowledge that value conflicts from acculturation stresses may contribute to increased anxiety and significant conflict with children.
  Challenges to traditional beliefs and values are anxiety provoking. Less acculturated parents may experience conflict with their more acculturated children as the children demand greater independence and freedom (True, 1995).
- Use a neutral, indirect style when addressing areas where improvement is needed (such as a need for verbal stimulation) when working with Native American clients.
  Using indirect statements such as "Other mothers have tried. . ." or "I had a client who tried 'X' and it seemed to work very well" will help to avoid resentment from the parent (Seiderman et al, 1996).
- Acknowledge and praise parenting strengths noted.
  This will increase trust and foster a working relationship with the parent (Seiderman et al, 1996).
- Validate the client's feelings regarding parenting.
  Validation lets the client know that the nurse has heard and understands what was said, and it promotes the nurse-client relationship (Stuart, Laraia, 2001; Giger, Davidhizar, 1995).
- Facilitate modeling and role-playing to help family improve parenting skills.

• = Independent; ▲ = Collaborative

It is helpful for families and the client to practice parenting skills in a safe environment before trying them in real-life situations (Rivera-Andino, Lopez, 2000).

Client/Family Teaching

- Explain individual differences in child temperaments and compare and contrast with reality of parents' expectations. Help parents determine and understand the implications of their child's temperament.
  Promoting parental understanding of temperament facilitates development of more realistic expectations (McClowry, 1992; Melvin, 1995).
- Discuss sound disciplinary techniques, which include catching children being good, active listening, conveying positive regard, ignoring minor transgressions, giving good directions, use of praise, and use of time-out.
  Disciplinary methods are subject to a variety of opinions. Proper discipline provides children with security, and clearly enforced rules help them learn self-control and social standards. Parenting classes can be beneficial when parent has had little formal or informal preparation (Herman-Staab, 1994).
- Foster acquisition of positive parenting skills.
  Parents may feel powerless. Helping them develop necessary skills or gain knowledge maintains the integrity of the parental role, and parents are then unlikely to use maladaptive coping styles (Baker, 1994).
- Plan parental education directed toward the following age-related parental concerns:

Birth to 2 years	Transition, sleep, aggression
3 to 5 years	Transition, parent-child relationship, sleep
6 to 10 years	School, parent-child relationship, divorce
11 to 18 years	Parent-child relationship, divorce, school

  Parents with children of any age may seek basic information about a variety of concerns, which can be anticipated and addressed by providing ongoing information and support (Jones, Maestri, McCoy, 1993).
- ▲ Initiate referrals to community agencies, parent education opportunities, stress management training, and social support groups.
  The parent needs support to manage angry or inappropriate behaviors. Use of support systems and social services can provide an opportunity to decrease feelings of inadequacy (Campbell, 1992; Baker, 1994).
- ▲ Provide information regarding available telephone counseling services.
  Telephone counseling services can provide confidential advice and support to families who might not otherwise have access to help in dealing with behavioral problems and parenting concerns (Jones, Maestri, McCoy, 1993).
- Refer to care plan for **Delayed Growth and development** for additional teaching interventions.

WEB SITES FOR EDUCATION

MERLIN See the MERLIN web site for World Wide Web resources for client education.

REFERENCES Baker NA: Avoid collisions with challenging families, *MCN Am J Matern Child Nurs* 19:97, 1994.
Campbell JM: Parenting classes: focus on discipline, *J Commun Health Nurs* 9:197, 1992.

• = **Independent**; ▲ = **Collaborative**

D'Avanzo CE et al: Developing culturally informed strategies for substance-related interventions. In Naegle MA, D'Avanzo CE, editors: *Addictions and substance abuse: strategies for advanced practice nursing*, St Louis, 2001, Mosby, pp 59-104.

Denehy JA: Intervention related to parent-infant attachment, *Nurs Clin North Am* 27:425, 1992.

Devlin BK, Reynolds E: Child abuse: how to recognize it, how to intervene, *Am J Nurs* 94:26, 1994.

Giger JN, Davidhizar RE: *Transcultural nursing*, ed 2, St Louis, 1995, Mosby.

Gross D et al: A longitudinal model of maternal self-efficacy, depression, and difficult temperament during toddlerhood, *Res Nurs Health* 17:207, 1994.

Herman-Staab B: Screening, management and appropriate referral for pediatric behavior problems, *Nurs Pract* 19:40, 1994.

Jones LC, Maestri BO, McCoy K: Why parents use the warm line, *MCN Am J Matern Child Nurs* 18:258, 1993.

Leininger MM: *Transcultural nursing: theories, research and practices*, ed 2, Hilliard, Ohio, 1996, McGraw-Hill.

McCloskey JC, Bulechek GM, editors: *Nursing interventions classification (NIC)*, St Louis, 1992, Mosby.

McClowry SG: Temperament theory and research, *Image* 24:319, 1992.

Melvin N: Children's temperament: intervention for parents, *J Pediatr Nurs* 10:152, 1995.

Mrazek DA, Mrazek P, Klinnert M: Clinical assessment of parenting, *J Am Acad Child Adolesc Psychiatry* 34:272, 1995.

Rivera-Andino J, Lopez L: When culture complicates care, *RN* 63(7):47-49, 2000.

Seiderman RY et al: Assessing American Indian families, *MCN Am J Matern Child Nurs* 21(6):274-279, 1996.

Stuart GW, Laraia MT: Therapeutic nurse-patient relationship. In Stuart GW, Laraia MT, editors: *Principles and practice of psychiatric nursing*, St Louis, 2001, Mosby, p 30.

True RH: Mental health issues of Asian/Pacific island women. In Adams DL, editor: *Health issues for women of color: a cultural diversity perspective*, Thousand Oaks, Calif, 1995, Sage, pp 102-105.

Zacharia R: Perceived social support and social network of low-income mothers of infants and preschoolers: pre- and postparenting program, *J Commun Health Nurs* 11:11, 1994.

Risk for impaired Parenting

Peggy A. Wetsch and Mary Markle

 Definition Risk for inability of the primary caretaker to create, maintain, or regain an environment that promotes the optimum growth and development of the child

Risk Factors

Social Marital conflict/declining satisfaction; history of being abused; poor problem-solving skills; role strain/overload; social isolation; legal difficulties; lack of access to resources; lack of value of parenthood; relocation; poverty; poor home environment; lack of family cohesiveness; lack of or poor parental role model; father of child not involved; history of being abusive; financial difficulties; low self-esteem; lack of resources; unplanned or unwanted pregnancy; inadequate child care arrangements; maladaptive coping strategies; low socioeconomic class; lack of transportation; change in family unit; unemployment or job problems; single parent; lack of social support network; inability to put child's needs before own; stress

Knowledge Low educational level or attainment; unrealistic expectations of child; lack of knowledge about parenting skills; poor communication skills; preference for physical punishment; inability to recognize and act on infant cues; low cognitive functioning; lack of

• = Independent; ▲ = Collaborative

knowledge about child health maintenance; lack of knowledge about child development; lack of cognitive readiness for parenthood

Physiological Physical illness

Infant/child Multiple births; handicapping condition or developmental delay; illness; altered perceptual abilities; lack of goodness of fit (temperament) with parental expectations; unplanned or unwanted child; premature birth; not gender desired; difficult temperament; attention deficit hyperactivity disorder; prolonged separation from parent; separation from parent at birth

Psychological Separation from infant/child; large number of closely spaced children; disability; sleep deprivation or disruption; difficult labor and/or delivery; young age (especially adolescent); depression; history of mental illness; lack of or late prenatal care; history of substance abuse or dependence

NOTE: It is important to reaffirm that adjustment to parenting in general is a normal maturational process that elicits nursing behaviors to prevent potential problems and to promote health.

Related Factors (r/t)

Lack of available role models; ineffective role models; physical and psychosocial abuse of nurturing figure; lack of support from significant others; unmet social, emotional, or maturational needs of parenting figures; interruption in bonding process (e.g., maternal, paternal); unrealistic expectations for self, infant, or partner; perceived threat to own physical and emotional survival; mental or physical illness; presence of stressor (e.g., finances, legal issues, recent crisis, cultural move); lack of knowledge; limited cognitive functioning; lack of role identity; absent or inappropriate response of child to relationship; multiple pregnancies

NOC ## Outcomes (Nursing Outcomes Classification)

Suggested NOC Labels

Abuse Recovery: Emotional; Caregiver Stressors; Coping; Parent-Infant Attachment; Parenting; Risk Control: Unintended Pregnancy

> **Example NOC Outcome**
> Accomplishes **Parenting** as evidenced by the following indicators: Provides for child's needs/Interacts positively with child/Has realistic expectations of parental role (Rate each indicator of **Parenting:** 1 = not adequate, 2 = slightly adequate, 3 = moderately adequate, 4 = substantially adequate, 5 = totally adequate [see Section I])

Client Outcomes

- Successfully establishes a nurturing parenting role
- Affirms desire to acquire and maintain constructive parenting skills to support infant/child growth and development
- Maintains appropriate measures to develop a safe, nurturing environment
- Displays attentive, supportive parenting behaviors
- Has knowledge of strategies to protect child from harm and/or neglect

NIC ## Interventions (Nursing Interventions Classification)

Suggested NIC Labels

Abuse Protection: Child; Attachment Promotion; Developmental Enhancement; Family Integrity Promotion; Parenting Promotion

• = Independent; ▲ = Collaborative

> **Example NIC Interventions—Parenting Promotion**
> - Assist parents to have realistic expectations appropriate to developmental and ability level of child
> - Assist parents with role transition and expectations of parenthood

Nursing Interventions and Rationales

NOTE: Management of a risk diagnosis necessitates approaches using primary and secondary prevention. Primary prevention interventions, which include such activities as safety instruction and focus on thwarting the development of disease or conditions. Early detection through screening, monitoring, and surveillance is secondary prevention (Shortridge, Valanis, 1992).

- Conduct risk identification noting presence of history of abuse, parental/family stressors, strength and adequacy of social support systems, established coping styles, and other related factors (see Related Factors).
  Identification of a family at risk signals special teaching and referral needs (McCloskey, Bulechek, 1992).
- Monitor parent-infant interactions that may signal interrupted or inadequate attachment or other parenting issues.
  Early detection can lead to early intervention, which can prevent or limit problems (McCloskey, Bulechek, 1992).
- Refer to care plan for **Impaired Parenting** for other interventions as appropriate to situation.

Multicultural

- Assess for the influence of cultural beliefs, norms, and values on the client's perception of parenting.
  What the client considers normal parenting may be based on cultural perceptions (Leininger, 1996).
- Acknowledge racial/ethnic differences at the onset of care.
  Acknowledgement of racial/ethnicity issues will enhance communication, establish, rapport, and promote treatment outcomes (D'Avanzo et al, 2001).
- Approach individuals of color with respect, warmth, and professional courtesy.
  Instances of disrespect have special significance for individuals of color (D'Avanzo et al, 2001).
- Give rationale when assessing black individuals about sensitive issues.
  Many blacks expect white caregivers to hold negative and preconceived ideas about them. Giving rationale for questions will help alleviate this perception (D'Avanzo et al, 2001).
- ▲ Acknowledge that value conflicts from acculturation stresses may contribute to increased anxiety and significant conflict with children.
  Challenges to traditional beliefs and values are anxiety provoking. Less acculturated parents may experience conflict with their more acculturated children as the children demand greater independence and freedom (True, 1995).
- ▲ Use a neutral, indirect style when addressing areas where improvement is needed (such as a need for verbal stimulation) when working with Native American clients.
  Using indirect statements such as "Other mothers have tried. . ." or "I had a client who tried 'X' and it seemed to work very well" will assist in avoiding resentment from the parent (Seiderman et al, 1996).

• = Independent; ▲ = Collaborative

▲ Acknowledge and praise parenting strengths noted.
This will increase trust and foster a working relationship with the parent (Seiderman et al, 1996).

▲ Validate the client's feelings regarding parenting.
Validation lets the client know that the nurse has heard and understands what was said, and it promotes the nurse-client relationship (Stuart, Laraia, 2001; Giger, Davidhizar, 1995).

▲ Facilitate modeling and role-playing to help family to improve parenting skills.
It is helpful for families and the client to practice parenting skills in a safe environment before trying them in real-life situations (Rivera-Andino, Lopez, 2000).

Client/Family Teaching

▲ Initiate referrals to an appropriate community agency for early follow-up if actual problem is identified.

• Refer to care plan for **Impaired Parenting** for additional teaching interventions.

WEB SITES FOR EDUCATION

$\int_{\text{MERLIN}}$ See the MERLIN web site for World Wide Web resources for client education.

REFERENCES   D'Avanzo CE et al: Developing culturally informed strategies for substance-related interventions. In Naegle MA, D'Avanzo CE, editors: *Addictions and substance abuse: strategies for advanced practice nursing,* St Louis, 2001, Mosby, pp 59-104.

Giger JN, Davidhizar RE: *Transcultural nursing,* ed 2, St Louis, 1995, Mosby.

Leininger MM: *Transcultural nursing: theories, research and practices,* ed 2, Hilliard, Ohio, 1996, McGraw-Hill.

McCloskey JC, Bulechek GM, editors: *Nursing interventions classification (NIC),* St Louis, 1992, Mosby.

Rivera-Andino J, Lopez L: When culture complicates care, *RN* 63(7):47-49, 2000.

Seiderman RY et al: Assessing American Indian families, *MCN Am J Matern Child Nurs* 21(6):274-279, 1996.

Shortridge L, Valanis B: The epidemiological model applied in community health nursing. In Stanhope M, Lancaster J, editors: *Community health nursing: process and practice for promoting health,* ed 3, St Louis, 1992, Mosby.

Stuart GW, Laraia MT: Therapeutic nurse-patient relationship. In Stuart GW, Laraia MT, editors: *Principles and practice of psychiatric nursing,* St Louis, 2001, Mosby, p 30.

True RH: Mental health issues of Asian/Pacific island women. In Adams DL, editor: *Health issues for women of color: a cultural diversity perspective,* Thousand Oaks, Calif, 1995, Sage, pp 102-105.

Risk for Peripheral neurovascular dysfunction

Betty J. Ackley

NANDA   **Definition** At risk for a disruption in circulation, sensation, or motion of an extremity

Risk Factors

Trauma; fractures; mechanical compression (e.g., tourniquet, cast, brace, dressing, restraints); orthopedic surgery; immobilization; burns; vascular obstruction

NOC   **Outcomes (Nursing Outcomes Classification)**

Suggested NOC Labels

Tissue Perfusion: Peripheral; Circulation Status; Risk Detection; Neurological Status: Spinal Sensory/Motor Function; Muscle Function; Joint Movement: Active

• = Independent; ▲ = Collaborative

> **Example NOC Outcome**
> **Tissue Perfusion: Peripheral** will be intact as evidenced by the following indicators:
> Distal peripheral pulses strong/Sensation level normal/Skin color normal/Muscle
> function intact/Skin intact/Peripheral edema not present/Localized extremity pain
> not present (Rate each indicator of **Tissue Perfusion: Peripheral:** 1 = extremely
> compromised, 2 = substantially compromised, 3 = moderately compromised,
> 4 = mildly compromised, 5 = not compromised [see Section I])

Client Outcomes

- Maintains circulation, sensation, and movement of an extremity within own normal limits
- Explains signs of neurovascular compromise and ways to prevent venous stasis

 Interventions (Nursing Interventions Classification)

Suggested NIC Labels

Circulatory Care; Exercise Therapy: Joint Mobility; Peripheral Sensation Management

> **Example NIC Interventions—Peripheral Sensation Management**
> - Monitor for paresthesia: numbness, tingling, hyperesthesia, and hypoesthesia
> - Monitor for thrombophlebitis and deep vein thrombosis

Nursing Interventions and Rationales

▲ Perform neurovascular assessment q ___ hr(s) or q ___ min(s). Use the five Ps of assessment:

- **Pain**—Assess severity (on scale of 1 to 10), quality, radiation, and relief by medications.
  Pain that is unrelieved by medication can be an early symptom of compartment syndrome or may indicate that client needs more effective pain medication (Dykes, 1993).

- **Pulses**—Check the pulses distal to the injury. Check uninjured side first to establish a baseline for a bilateral comparison.
  An intact pulse generally indicates a good blood supply to the extremity (Dykes, 1993), although compartment syndrome may be present even if the pulse is intact (Gulli, Templeman, 1994).

- **Pallor**—Check color and temperature changes below the fracture site. Check capillary refill.
  A cold, pale, or bluish extremity indicates arterial insufficiency or arterial damage, and physician should be notified. A reddened warm extremity may indicate infection (Feldman, 1998). Normal capillary refill is 3 seconds or less (Dykes, 1993).

- **Paresthesia** (change in sensation)—Check by lightly touching the skin proximal and distal to the injury. Ask if client has any unusual sensations such as hypersensitivity, tingling, prickling, decreased feeling, or numbness accompanied by a lack of sensation.
  Changes in sensation are indicative of nerve compression and damage and can also indicate compartment syndrome (Dykes, 1993; Gulli, Templeman, 1994).

- **Paralysis**—Ask client to do appropriate range of motion exercises in the unaffected and then the affected extremity.

▲ Monitor client for symptoms of compartment syndrome evidenced by decreased sensation, weakness, loss of movement, pain with passive movement, pain greater than

• = **Independent;** ▲ = **Collaborative**

expected, pulselessness, and tension in the skin that surrounds the muscle compartment. The symptoms are not always present and can be difficult to assess.
Compartment syndrome is characterized by increased pressure within the muscle compartment, which compromises circulation, viability, and function of tissues (Gulli, Templeman, 1994; Tumbarello, 2000).

▲ Monitor appropriate application and function of corrective device (e.g., cast, splint, traction) q ___ hr(s).
An improperly applied device can cause nerve damage, circulatory impairment, or pressure ulcers.

• Position extremity in correct alignment with each position change; check q h to ensure appropriate alignment.

▲ Get client out of bed and mobilize as soon as possible after consultation with physician.
Immobility is a risk factor for deep vein thrombosis (DVT); early ambulation can help prevent clot formation (Launius, Graham, 1998).

▲ Monitor for signs of DVT, especially in high-risk populations, including persons >40 years of age; persons with immobility or obesity; persons taking estrogen or oral contraceptives; persons with a history of trauma, surgery, or previous DVT; and persons with a cerebrovascular accident (CVA), varicose veins, malignancy, or cardiovascular disease.
There are identified risk factors that increase the incidence of DVT and have been validated using a DVT risk scale (Autar, 1996; Hyers, 1999).

▲ Apply thigh-high graduated compression elastic stockings if ordered, removing daily to give skin care. Also request an order for intermittent pneumatic compression devices and medications as appropriate.
These stockings can be helpful for preventing DVT. If DVT risk is high, consult with physician regarding need for intermittent pneumatic compression of the calves or subcutaneous administration of heparin (Brock, 1994; Ecklund, 1995). A combination of an anticoagulant and mechanical methods to prevent DVT have been shown to be more effective in postoperative clients (Hyers, 1999).

▲ Watch for and report signs of DVT evidenced by pain, deep tenderness, swelling in the calf and thigh, and redness in the involved extremity. Take serial leg measurements of the thigh and leg circumferences. In some clients there is a palpable, tender venous cord that can be felt in the popliteal fossa. Do not rely on Homans' sign.
Thrombosis with clot formation is usually first detected as edema of the involved leg and then as pain. Leg measurement discrepancies greater than 2 cm warrant further investigation. Homans' sign is not reliable (Herzog, 1992). Unfortunately, symptoms of DVT will not be found on exam of 25% of the clients, even though a DVT is present (Eftychiou, 1996).

• Help client perform prescribed exercises q ___ hr(s).

• Provide a nutritious diet and adequate fluid replacement.
Good nutrition and sufficient fluids are needed to promote healing and prevent complications.

Geriatric

• Use heat and cold therapies cautiously; elderly clients often have decreased sensation and circulation.

Home Care Interventions

• Assess knowledge base of client and family following any institutional care. Teach disease process and care as necessary.

• = Independent; ▲ = Collaborative

Length of time for institutional care and teaching may have been very short and insuffi-cient for learning.
- If risk is related to fractures and cast care, teach family to complete a neurovascular as-sessment; it may be as often as q 4 h but is more commonly two to three times per day.
  A risk requiring monitoring more often than q 4 h for longer than 24 hours indicates a need for institutionally based care.
- If fracture is peripheral, position the limb for comfort, and change position fre-quently, avoiding dependent positions for extended periods.
  Changes in position enhance circulation.
- ▲ Refer to physical therapy services as necessary to establish exercise program and safety in transfers or mobility within limitations of physical status.
- Establish an emergency plan.
  A preset plan will save valuable time in the event of emergency.

Client/Family Teaching
- Teach client and family to recognize signs for neurovascular dysfunction and report signs immediately to the appropriate person.
- Emphasize proper nutrition to promote healing.
- ▲ If necessary, refer client to rehabilitation facility for proper use of assistive devices and measures to improve mobility without compromising neurovascular function.

WEB SITES FOR EDUCATION

MERLIN See the MERLIN web site for World Wide Web resources for client education.

REFERENCES Autar R: Nursing assessment of clients at risk of deep vein thrombosis (DVT): the Autar DVT scale, *J Adv Nurs* 23:763-770, 1996.
Brock JC: Compression stockings: do they prevent DVT? *Am J Nurs* 11:25, 1994.
Dykes PC: Minding the five P's of neurovascular assessment, *Am J Nurs* 93(6):38-39, 1993.
Ecklund MM: Optimizing the flow of care for prevention and treatment of deep vein thrombosis and pul-monary embolism, *AACN Clin Issues* 6(4):588-601, 1995.
Eftychiou V: Clinical diagnosis and management of the patient with deep venous thromboembolism and acute pulmonary embolism, *Nurse Pract* 21:50, 1996.
Feldman CB: Caring for feet: patients and nurse practitioners working together, *Nurse Pract* Forum 9(2):87-93, 1998.
Gulli B, Templeman D: Compartment syndrome of the lower extremity, *Orthop Clin North Am* 25(4):677-680, 1994.
Herzog JA: Deep vein thrombosis in the rehabilitation client, *Rehabil Nurs* 17(4):196-197, 1992.
Hyers TM: Venous thromboembolism, *Am J Resp Crit Care Med* 159:1-4, 1999.
Launius BK, Graham BD: Understanding and prevention deep vein thrombosis and pulmonary embolism, *AACN Clin Issues* 9(1):91-99, 1998.
Tumbarello C: Acute extremity compartment syndrome, *J Trauma Nurs* 7(2):30-38, 2000.

Risk for Poisoning

Catherine Vincent; revised by Gail B. Ladwig and Mary Markle

 Definition At accentuated risk of accidental exposure to, or ingestion of, drugs or dan-gerous products in doses sufficient to cause poisoning

• = Independent; ▲ = Collaborative

Risk Factors
External   Unprotected contact with heavy metals or chemicals; medicines stored in unlocked cabinets accessible to children or confused persons; presence of poisonous vegetation; presence of atmospheric pollutants, paint, lacquer, etc., in poorly ventilated areas or without effective protection; flaking, peeling paint or plaster in presence of young children; chemical contamination of food and water; availability of illicit drugs potentially contaminated by poisonous additives; large supplies of drugs in house; dangerous products placed or stored within reach of children or confused persons

Internal   Verbalization that occupational setting is without adequate safeguards; reduced vision; lack of safety or drug education; lack of proper precautions; insufficient finances; cognitive or emotional difficulties

Related Factors (r/t)
See Risk Factors

NOC   Outcomes (Nursing Outcomes Classification)
Suggested NOC Labels
Safety Behavior: Home Physical Environment; Knowledge: Medication; Risk Control; Risk Control: Drug Use, Risk Detection

> **Example NOC Outcome**
> Accomplishes **Risk Control** as evidenced by: Monitors environmental risk factors/ Develops effective risk control strategies (Rate each indicator of **Risk Control:** 1 = never demonstrated, 2 = rarely demonstrated, 3 = sometimes demonstrated, 4 = often demonstrated, 5 = consistently demonstrated [see Section I])

Client Outcomes
- Averts inadvertent ingestion of or exposure to toxins or poisonous substances
- Explains and undertakes appropriate safety measures to prevent ingestion of or exposure to toxins or poisonous substances

NIC   Interventions (Nursing Interventions Classification)
Suggested NIC Labels
Environmental Management: Safety

> **Example NIC Interventions—Environmental Management: Safety**
> - Identify safety hazards in the environment (i.e., physical, biological, and chemical)
> - Modify or remove hazards from the environment when possible

Nursing Interventions and Rationales
NOTE: Management of a risk diagnosis necessitates approaches using primary and secondary prevention. Primary prevention interventions, which include such activities as safety instruction, focus on thwarting the development of the disease or condition. Secondary prevention is early detection through screening, monitoring, and surveillance (Shortridge, Valanis, 1992).
- Identify risk factors, noting special circumstances in which preventive or protective measures are indicated.
  Identification of family at risk signals special teaching and referral needs (McCloskey, Bulechek, 1996).

• = Independent; ▲ = Collaborative

▲ Evaluate lead exposure risk and consult health care provider regarding lead screening measures as indicated (public/ambulatory health).

Lead poisoning is one of the most common and preventable types of childhood poisoning today. Assessment of exposure risk and blood level testing are important preventive measures (U.S. Department of Health and Human Services, 1994; Agency Toxic Substance & Disease Registry, 1995b).

▲ Properly label medications, using large print for the visually impaired. Supply "Mr. Yuk" labels for families with children.

Implementing poisoning prevention program strategies benefits the client and family (Jones, 1993).

▲ Detect possible interactions and cumulative or other adverse effects among prescribed medications, self-administered over-the-counter products, culturally based home treatments, and foods.

Serious consequences may occur if interactions are not identified (Weitzel, 1992).

• Complete an exposure history in work environment if toxic exposure occurs (occupational concerns).

Early exposure detection and treatment and prevention of sequelae are important in the work setting (Agency Toxic Substance & Disease Registry, 1995a).

Home Care Interventions

▲ Prepour medications for clients who are at risk of ingesting too much of a given medication because of mistakes in preparation. Delegate this task to family or caregivers if possible.

Elderly clients who live alone are at greatest risk.

▲ Identify poisonous substances in the immediate surroundings of the home such as garage or barn: include paints and thinners, fertilizers, rodent and bug control substances, animal medications, gasoline, and oil. Label with name, poison warning sign, and poison control center number. Lock out of the reach of children.

Poisonous substances of equal danger exist in areas other than the internal home setting. Curious children are at risk for ingestion when exploring.

▲ Identify risk of toxicity from environmental activities such as spraying trees or roadside shrubs. Contact local departments of agriculture or transportation to get Material Substance Data Sheets (MSDSs) or to prevent the activity in desired areas.

Very young children, women of childbearing age or who are pregnant, and the elderly are at greatest risk.

• Avoid carbon monoxide poisoning. Use a carbon monoxide detector in the home, have chimney professionally cleaned each year, have furnace professionally inspected each year, ensure that all combustion equipment is properly vented, and install a chimney screen and cap to prevent small animals from moving into the chimney.

Many deaths each year are attributed to carbon monoxide poisoning. Take these precautions to protect child and family (Promark Interactive, 1998).

Client/Family Teaching

▲ Counsel client and family members regarding medication safety:
  ▪ Avoid sharing prescriptions
  ▪ Read and follow labeling instructions on all products; adjust dosage for age
  ▪ Avoid excessive amounts and/or frequency of doses ("If a little does some good, a lot should do more")

• = Independent; ▲ = Collaborative

Each year, thousands of adverse drug events occur, including poisoning. Poisoning is a major cause of morbidity and mortality.

▲ Advise family to post first aid charts and poison center instructions in an accessible location. Poison control center phone numbers should be posted close to the phone. Poison control should always be called immediately before initiating any first aid measures. *Rapid initiation of proper treatment reduces mortality and morbidity and decreases emergency room visits and inpatient admissions (Jones, 1993). Consultation with a poison control center is necessary for assessing and treating poisoned clients (Larsen, Cummings, 1998).*

• Encourage client/family to take first aid and other types of safety-related programs. *These programs raise participants' level of emergency preparation.*

▲ Initiate referrals to peer group interventions, peer counseling, and other types of substance abuse prevention/rehabilitation programs when substance abuse is identified as a risk factor.
Clients with substance abuse problems are at risk for contact with tainted substances or for overdose. The peer pressure factor is extremely strong for adolescents; rehabilitation programs providing nonpunitive and skill-focused approaches are most effective (Anderson, 1996).

Infant/child

• Provide guidance for parents/caregivers regarding age-related safety measures including the following:
  ▪ Storing potentially harmful substances in the original containers
  ▪ Avoiding storage of medications or toxic substances in food containers
  ▪ Placing poisonous houseplants out of the reach of infants and children
  ▪ Preventing access to poisonous outdoor plants
  ▪ Locking up cleaning agents, disinfectants, and other hazardous materials
  ▪ Using extreme caution with pesticides and gardening materials close to children's play areas
  ▪ Keeping perfume and makeup out of reach of children
  Infants have a high level of hand-to-mouth behavior and will ingest anything. Young children may inadvertently ingest poisonous materials, particularly if those materials are thought to be food or beverage (Jones, 1993; Mitchell et al, 1995).

• Review the necessity of keeping prescription and over-the-counter medications secure and out of the reach of children. Lock cupboard if toddler is prone to climbing.
  Once infants learn to crawl, they explore and are persistent. When children begin to walk, climb, and develop the concept of object and object permanence, they can reach most heights, open cupboards, and unscrew lids. Many toxic substances are not protected with safety caps alone (Kuhn, 1992; Liebelt, Shannon, 1993; Corbett, 1995).

• Recommend placement of perfumes, ointments, creams, and talcum powder out of infant's/child's reach.
  Even in small quantities, many common over-the-counter remedies and products can be lethal to infants and young children (Liebelt, Shannon, 1993; Morelli, 1993).

• Emphasize avoiding eating or drinking out of containers with the "Mr. Yuk" label (directed at children).
  Prevent overdosing or inadvertent poisoning resulting from inappropriate medication use (Kuhn, 1992). Many deaths and disabling sequelae in children following poisoning could be prevented if more attention were given to implementing preventive measures at home. Medications and chemicals should always be safely packed and stored (Chan, 1998).

• = Independent; ▲ = Collaborative

▲ Advise families with young children to prepare a first aid kit for poisoning. Keep syrup of ipecac on hand at all times (two doses per child) and any other supplies recommended by the local poison control center.
Ipecac induces vomiting; other items will be used to neutralize effects. The steady decline in syrup of ipecac used by poisoned victims from a peak of 15% in 1985 to 2.3% in 1995 is of concern. It is important that the recommended treatment protocols are followed carefully (Marchbanks et al, 1999).

▲ Teach appropriate use of ipecac. Do not administer to a client who has a decreased level or impending loss of consciousness or who has ingested a corrosive substance or hydrocarbon. Contact poison control about appropriateness of administration.
There is a high aspiration potential with these clients. Ipecac may delay the administration or reduce the effectiveness of activated charcoal, oral antidotes, and whole bowel irrigation (Krenzelok, McGuigan, Lheur, 1997).

Community

• Propane-fueled ice-resurfacing machines should not be used in indoor ice arenas.
Outbreak of acute respiratory illness among adolescent ice hockey players was attributed to the high level of nitrogen dioxide that resulted from poor ventilation and a malfunctioning ice-resurfacing machine (Rosenlund, Bluhm, 1999).

Geriatric

• Caution client and family to avoid storing medications with similar appearances close to one another (e.g., nitroglycerin ointment near toothpaste or denture creams).
Confusion and visual impairment can place the older person at risk of incorrectly identifying of contents (Weitzel, 1992).

• Remind older persons to store medications out of reach when young children come to visit.
Children are inquisitive and may ingest medicines in containers without safety caps (Cudney, Hunter, 1992).

Multicultural

• Assess housing for pathways of lead poisoning.
Minority individuals are more likely to reside in older and substandard housing. About 74% of privately owned, occupied housing units in the United States built before 1980 contain lead-based paint (Centers for Disease Control and Prevention, 2001).

WEB SITES FOR EDUCATION

MERLIN See the MERLIN web site for World Wide Web resources for client education.

REFERENCES   Agency Toxic Substance & Disease Registry: Lead toxicity, *Am Assoc Occup Health Nurs J* 43:428, 1995a.
Agency Toxic Substance & Disease Registry: Taking an exposure history, *Am Assoc Occup Health Nurs J* 43:380, 1995b.
Anderson NLR: Decisions about substance abuse among adolescents in juvenile detention, *Image J Nurs Sch* 28:65, 1996.
Centers for Disease Control and Prevention: Sources and pathways of lead exposure. In *Preventing lead poisoning in young children,* Atlanta, 2001, The Center.
Chan T: Childhood poisoning: the scope for prevention, *Vet Hum Toxicol* 40(6):361-363, 1998.
Corbett JV: Pharmacopeia: accidental poisoning with iron supplements, *MCN Matern Child Nurs* 20:234, 1995.
Cudney SA, Hunter MM: Danger! grandparents' drugs may be lethal to children: redesigning medicine packages may prevent tragedy, *Geriatr Nurs* 13:222, 1992.

• = **Independent;** ▲ = **Collaborative**

Jones NE: Childhood residential injuries, *MCN Matern Child Nurs* 18:1168, 1993.

Krenzelok E, McGuigan M, Lheur P: Position statement: ipecac syrup—American Academy of Clinical Toxicology; European Association of Poisons Centres and Clinical Toxicologists, *J Toxicol Clin Toxicol* 35(7):699-709, 1997.

Kuhn MM: Drug overdose: salicylates, *Crit Care Nurse* 12:16, 1992.

Larsen LC, Cummings D: Oral poisonings: guidelines for initial evaluation and treatment, *Am Fam Physician* 57(1):85-92, 1998.

Liebelt E, Shannon MW: Small doses, big problems: a selected review of highly toxic common medications, *Pediatr Emerg Care* 9:292, 1993.

Marchbanks B et al: Trends in ipecac use: a survey of poison center staff, *Vet Hum Toxicol* 41(1):47-48, 1999.

McCloskey JC, Bulechek GM editors: *Nursing interventions classification (NIC)*, ed 2, St Louis, 1996, Mosby.

Mitchell A et al: Acute organophosphate pesticide poisoning in children, *MCN Matern Child Nurs* 20:261, 1995.

Morelli J: Pediatric poisoning: the 10 most toxic prescription drugs, *Am J Nurs* 93:26, 1993.

Promark Interactive, 1998, retrieved from World Wide Web on April 2, 1999. Web site: www.kidssafe.com/p15.htm#pois

Rosenlund M, Bluhm G: Health effects resulting from nitrogen dioxide exposure in an indoor ice arena, *Arch Environ Health* 54(1):2-7, 1999.

Shortridge L, Valanis B: The epidemiological model applied in community health nursing. In Stanhope M, Lancaster J, editors: *Community health nursing: process and practice for promoting health*, ed 3, St Louis, 1992, Mosby.

U.S. Department of Health and Human Services, U.S. Public Health Service: Put prevention into practice: lead screening in children, *J Am Acad Nurs Pract* 6: 379, 1994.

Weitzel EA: Medication management. In McCloskey JC, Bulechek GM, editors: *Nursing interventions classification (NIC)*, ed 2, St Louis, 1992, Mosby.

Post-trauma syndrome

Gail B. Ladwig and Judith S. Rizzo

NANDA   **Definition** Sustained maladaptive response to a traumatic, overwhelming event

Defining Characteristics

Avoidance; repression; difficulty in concentrating; grief; intrusive thoughts; neurosensory irritability; palpitations; enuresis (in children); anger and/or rage; intrusive dreams; nightmares; aggression; hypervigilant; exaggerated startle response; hopelessness; altered mood states; shame; panic attacks; alienation; denial; horror; substance abuse; depression; anxiety; guilt; fear; gastric irritability; detachment; psychogenic amnesia; irritability; numbing; compulsive behavior; flashbacks; headaches

Related Factors (r/t)

Events outside the range of the usual human experience; physical and psychosocial abuse; tragic occurrence involving multiple deaths; epidemics; sudden destruction of one's home or community; being held prisoner of war or criminal victimization (torture); wars; rape; natural and/or manmade disasters; serious accidents; witnessing mutilation, violent death, or other horrors; serious threat or injury to self or loved ones; industrial and motor vehicle accidents; military combat

NOC   ## Outcomes (Nursing Outcomes Classification)

Suggested NOC Labels

Abuse Cessation; Protection; Abuse Recovery: Emotional, Sexual; Coping; Impulse Control; Self-Mutilation Restraint

• = Independent; ▲ = Collaborative

> **Example NOC Outcome**
> Demonstrates **Abuse Recovery** as evidenced by: Resolution of trauma-induced psychoneurotic behaviors, conduct disorders, and learning difficulties (Rate indicator of **Abuse Recovery:** 1 = none, 2 = limited, 3 = moderate, 4 = substantial, 5 = extensive [see Section I])

Client Outcomes

- Returns to pretrauma level of functioning as quickly as possible
- Acknowledges the traumatic event and begins to work with the trauma by talking about the experience and expressing feelings of fear, anger, anxiety, guilt, and helplessness
- Identifies support systems and available resources and is able to connect with them
- Returns to and strengthens coping mechanisms used in previous traumatic event
- Acknowledges event and perceives it without distortions
- Assimilates the event and moves forward to set and pursue life goals

NIC   Interventions (Nursing Interventions Classification)

Suggested NIC Labels

Counseling; Support System Enhancement

> **Example NIC Interventions—Counseling**
> - Encourage expression of feelings
> - Assist client to identify strengths and reinforce these

Nursing Interventions and Rationales

- Observe for reaction to traumatic event in all clients regardless of age.
  Groups at risk are those who have a history of emotional problems, are domestic violence victims, have lost a friend or family member by homicide, are homeless, are sexual assault victims (especially those abused as children), and have previous involvement with a traumatic event. Give serious attention to childhood loss (Irwin, 1994). Posttraumatic stress disorder (PTSD) is the expected outcome of youths exposed to suicide, loss, and abuse (Brent, 1995). In a survey of 5877 persons, 1703 reported a traumatic event, and combat was reported as the worst trauma. Men who have faced combat are likely to have lifetime PTSD, delayed PTSD symptom onset, and unresolved symptoms and are likely to be unemployed, fired, divorced, and physically abusive spouses (Prigerson, Maciejewski, Rosenheck, 2001).
- Observe the severity of the client's response and its effect on current functioning.
  The first few days following an event, expect a roller coaster of emotions. A return to normal can take up to 6 to 8 weeks, and for some it can take months (NOVA, 1988).
- Provide a safe and therapeutic environment, enabling the client to regain control.
  Safety and empowerment are vital to recovery, as are treating the person with dignity and sensitivity and being able to tolerate high emotional arousal. Intervention must strike a balance between protection of the victim and confrontation about the reality of the event. A study showed that victims found the confrontational aspects of intervention, such as viewing the body and returning to the site, to be helpful (Winje, Ulvik, 1995).
- Remain with client and provide support during periods of overwhelming emotions.
  Being able to withstand a client's strong emotions can be difficult for an unskilled nurse. The client may initially be in shock and appear dazed or confused.

• = Independent; ▲ = Collaborative

- Use touch with client's permission (e.g., hand on shoulder, holding hand).
  In a study of personal space invasion in the nurse-client relationship, anxiety scores of the experimental group showed a definite downward trend, indicating that the intrusion of a nurse into a client's space had a calming rather than a stimulating effect (Ricci, 1981).
- For clients who are uncomfortable with physical touch, consider the use of Therapeutic Touch techniques. (See care plan for **Disturbed Energy field.**)
  Therapeutic Touch, when provided by the nurse, can promote feelings of comfort, peace, calm, and security (Hayes, Cox, 1999).
- Use planned communication to assist client with describing the event and expressing feelings.
  A debriefing model for groups has shown to be effective for traumatized clients (Mitchell, 1988; NOVA, 1988). These models can be modified for individuals.
- Provide opportunities for verbally emotional expression through activities.
- Avoid pressuring clients to express emotions if they are not ready to do so.
- Explore and enhance available support systems.
  Social supports clearly benefit the client. Social support was the most important factor in predicting adaptive coping among family members of the seriously mentally ill (Solomon, Draine, 1995). Support systems decrease isolation, encourage communication, and provide diversional activities. Nurses should help traumatized children by strengthening their social relationships and enhancing their ability to self-soothe and process information, which helps them process traumatic memories (Burgess, Hartman, Clements, 1995).
- ▲ Assist client with regaining previous sleeping and eating habits.
  Disrupted sleep is the most prevalent symptom following a traumatic event (Schwartz, Kettley, Rizzo, 1992). Consider short-term drug treatment such as short-acting benzodiazepine for the first few days following a traumatic event. Imipramine, fluoxetine, clonidine, and carbamazepine have shown promise (Marshall, Kleine, 1995).
- ▲ Consider use of medication.
  This evidence-based study indicated that medications can be effective for treating PSST. The largest trials showing efficacy have been with selective serotonin reuptake inhibitors (SSRIs) (Stein et al, 2000).
- Help client use positive cognitive restructuring to reestablish feelings of self-worth.
  In two studies of 159 and 138 motor vehicle accidents, cognitive strategies to control intrusive negative thoughts play a major role in reducing posttraumatic stress in victims (Steil, Ehlers, 2000). In one study, cognitive behavioral interventions were shown to be more effective than other interventions for reducing occupational stress (van der Klink et al, 2001).
- Provide the means for clients to express feelings through therapeutic drawing.
  The inclusion of expressive techniques such as therapeutic drawing can be used to facilitate the emotional work of chronic trauma issues (Glaister, McGuinness, 1992).
- Normalize symptoms; help client to understand that his or her feelings and thoughts are a result of the trauma and do not indicate mental illness.
  Many symptoms of a trauma response are mistaken for mental illness, when actually they are normal responses to an abnormal event (Forster, 1994).
- Encourage client to return to normal routine as quickly as possible.
  Nurses can help traumatized children and adolescents relearn flexible responses to begin processing traumatic memories.

• = Independent; ▲ = Collaborative

Geriatric

- Use environmental assessment skills to identify elderly clients who are traumatized by disaster, loss, or both.
  The elderly who live alone are at greatest risk. Early intervention can minimize the response.
- Observe client for concurrent losses that may affect coping skills.
  As the elderly grow older, the number of losses are multiplied and compounded.
- Allow client more time to establish trust and express anger, guilt, and shame about the trauma.
- Review past coping skills and give client positive reinforcement for successfully dealing with other life crises.
  Clients who have adjusted positively to aging and can put events into proper perspective may adjust to loss more positively.
- ▲ Monitor client for clinical signs of depression and anxiety; refer to physician for medication if appropriate.
  Depression in the elderly is underestimated in this country.
- Instill hope.
  The therapeutic technique of reminiscence can renew hope (Forbes, 1994). The energy generated by hope can help elderly cope, overcome obstacles, and maintain normal functioning.

Multicultural

- Assess for the influence of cultural beliefs, norms, and values on the client's ability to cope with a traumatic experience.
  What the client views as healthy coping may be based on cultural perceptions (Leininger, 1996).
- Acknowledge racial and ethnic differences at onset of care.
  Acknowledgement of race/ethnicity issues will enhance communication, establish rapport, and promote positive treatment outcomes (D'Avanzo et al, 2001).
- Use a family-centered approach when working with Latino, Asian, African-American, and Native American clients.
  Latinos may perceive family as a source of support, solver of problems, and a source of pride. Asian Americans may regard family as the primary decision maker and influence on individual family members (D'Avanzo et al, 2001).
- When working with Asian-American clients, provide opportunities by which the family can save face.
  Asian-American families may avoid situations and discussion of issues that will bring shame on the family unit (D'Avanzo et al, 2001).
- Validate the client's feelings regarding the trauma.
  Validation lets the client know that the nurse has heard and understands what was said, and it promotes the nurse-client relationship (Stuart, Laraia, 2001; Giger, Davidhizar, 1995).

Home Care Interventions

- ▲ Assess family support and response to client's coping mechanisms. Refer family for medical social services or other counseling as necessary.
  Persons who have not shared the client's traumatic experience may have unrealistic expectations about recovery and recovery time. Support may be denied if the client's response to the trauma does not stay within support system expectations.
- Provide a stable routine of day-to-day activities consistent with pretrauma experience. Do not force a new routine on client.

- **= Independent; ▲ = Collaborative**

Resuming a pretrauma routine can be reassuring to the client and can help place the trauma in perspective. Imposing an undesired routine can further isolate the client.

▲ If client is receiving medications, assess client's self-medicating ability. Assign a responsible person to administer medications if necessary.
Crisis creates a feeling of helplessness. The client may be unable to make the simplest decisions (Spradley, 1990).

▲ Assess the impact of the trauma on significant others (e.g., a father may have to take over his partner's parenting responsibility after she has been raped and injured). Provide empathy and caring to significant others. Refer for additional services as necessary.
Traumatic events can pose a crisis for significant others as well as the involved client.

Client/Family Teaching

• Explain to client and family what to expect the first few days after the traumatic event and in the future.
Knowing what to expect can minimize much of the anxiety that accompanies a traumatic response.

• Teach positive coping skills and avoidance of negative coping skills such as alcohol use.

• Teach stress reduction methods such as deep breathing, visualization, meditation, and physical exercise. Encourage use especially when intrusive thoughts or flashbacks occur.
After a traumatic event, it is tempting for clients to maladaptively cope with their overwhelming emotions, which can establish unhealthy patterns for the future.

• Encourage other healthy living habits of proper diet, adequate sleep, regular exercise, family activities, and spiritual pursuits.

▲ Refer client to peer support groups.
Peer support decreases sense of social isolation, enhances knowledge, and increases coping skills (Solomon, Draine, 1995).

▲ Refer clients who have been in accidents to counseling for posttraumatic stress disorder (PTSD).
It is estimated that PTSD occurs in at least 25% of traffic accident victims who sustain physical injuries. This percentage is probably greater in clients with chronic whiplash complaints. This case report shows that improvement of PTSD symptoms can have a beneficial effect on coping with the chronic whiplash complaints (Jaspers, 1998).

▲ Refer clients who have suffered traumatic brain injury (TBI) for counseling for PTSD.
This study highlights the significant number of clients who experience an acute trauma response after TBI and raises the possibility that those with acute stress disorder denote those for whom an early intervention may prevent long-term psychopathology (Harvey, Bryant, 1998).

• Instruct family in ways to be helpful to and supportive of the traumatized person. Emphasize the importance of listening and being there. Also emphasize that there are no magic phrases capable of easing the person's emotional suffering.

• Consider use of complementary and alternative therapies.
This literature review of research-based studies suggests the use of humanistic treatments (complementary and alternative medicine) for clients who have catastrophic illness or injuries (Halstead, 2001).

WEB SITES FOR EDUCATION

MERLIN   See the MERLIN web site for World Wide Web resources for client education.

• = **Independent;** ▲ = **Collaborative**

REFERENCES Brent D: Risk factors for adolescent suicide and suicidal behavior, mental and substance abuse disorders, family environmental factors, and life stress, *Suicide Life Threat Behav* 25(suppl):52, 1995.

Burgess A, Hartman C, Clements P: Biology of memory and childhood trauma, *J Psychosoc Nurs Ment Health Serv* 33:16, 1995.

D'Avanzo CE et al: Developing culturally informed strategies for substance-related interventions. In Naegle MA, D'Avanzo CE, editors: *Addictions and substance abuse: strategies for advanced practice nursing,* St Louis, 2001, Mosby, pp 59-104.

Forbes S: Hope: an essential human need in the elderly, *J Gerontol Nurs* 20:5, 1994.

Forster K: Traumatic stress reactions and the psychiatric emergency, *Psychiatr Ann* 24:603, 1994.

Giger JN, Davidhizar RE: *Transcultural nursing,* ed 2, St Louis, 1995, Mosby.

Glaister JA, McGuinness T: The art of therapeutic drawing: helping chronic trauma survivors, *J Psychosoc Nurs Ment Health Serv* 30(5):9-17, 1992.

Halstead LS: The John Stanley Coulter lecture: the power of compassion and caring in rehabilitation healing, *Arch Phys Med Rehabil* 82(2):149-154, 2001.

Harvey AG, Bryant R: Acute stress disorder after mild traumatic brain injury, *J Nerv Ment Dis* 186(6):333-337, 1998.

Hayes J, Cox C: The experience of therapeutic touch from a nursing perspective, *Br J Nurs* 8(18):1249-1254, 1999.

Irwin J: Proneness to dissociation and traumatic childhood, *J Nerv Ment Dis* 182:456, 1994.

Jaspers J: Whiplash and posttraumatic stress disorder, *Disabil Rehabil* 20(11):397-404, 1998.

Leininger MM: *Transcultural nursing: theories, research and practices,* ed 2, Hilliard, Ohio, 1996, McGraw-Hill.

Marshall R, Kleine D: Pharmacotherapy in the treatment of posttraumatic stress disorder, *Psychiatr Ann* 25:588-597, 1995.

Mitchell J: Stress: development and functions of a critical incident stress debriefing team, *J Emerg Med Serv* 13:43, 1988.

National Organization for Victim Assistance (NOVA): *Coordinating a community crisis response, National Organization for Victim Assistance (NOVA) training manual,* Washington, DC, 1988, The Organization.

Prigerson HG, Maciejewski PK, Rosenheck RA: Combat trauma: trauma with highest risk of delayed onset and unresolved posttraumatic stress disorder symptoms, unemployment, and abuse among men, *J Nerv Ment Dis* 189(2):99-108, 2001.

Ricci MS: An experiment with personal space invasion in the nurse-patient relationship and its effect on anxiety, *Issues Ment Health Nurs* 3:203, 1981.

Schwartz J, Kettley J, Rizzo J: *Predictors of vulnerability after trauma,* unpublished manuscript, 1992.

Solomon P, Draine J: Adaptive coping among family members of persons with serious mental illness, *Psychiatr Serv* 46:1156, 1995.

Spradley B: *Community health nursing, concepts and practice,* ed 3, Glenview, Ill, 1990, Scott Foresman/Little, Brown.

Steil R, Ehlers A: Dysfunctional meaning of posttraumatic intrusions in chronic PTSD, *Behav Res Ther* 38(6):537-558, 2000.

Stein DJ et al: Pharmacotherapy for posttraumatic stress disorder (Cochrane Review), *Cochrane Database Syst Rev* 4:CD002795, 2000.

Stuart GW, Laraia MT: Therapeutic nurse-patient relationship. In Stuart GW, Laraia MT, editors: *Principles and practice of psychiatric nursing,* St Louis, 2001, Mosby, p 30.

van der Klink JJ et al: The benefits of interventions for work-related stress, *Am J Public Health* 91(2), 2001.

Winje D, Ulvik A: Confrontations with reality: crises intervention services for traumatized families after a school bus accident in Norway, *J Trauma Stress* 8(3):429-444, 1995.

Risk for Post-trauma syndrome

Gail B. Ladwig

NANDA **Definition** A risk for sustained maladaptive response to a traumatic, overwhelming event

• = Independent; ▲ = Collaborative

Risk Factors

Exaggerated sense of responsibility; perception of event; survivor's role in the event; occupation (e.g., police, fire, rescue, corrections, emergency room staff, mental health worker); displacement from home; inadequate social support; nonsupportive environment; diminished ego strength; duration of the event

NOC Outcomes (Nursing Outcomes Classification)

Suggested NOC Labels

Abuse Cessation; Abuse Protection; Abuse Recovery; Aggression Control; Anxiety Control; Coping; Grief Resolution; Sleep

> **Example NOC Outcome**
> Demonstrates **Abuse Recovery** as evidenced by the following indicator: Resolution of trauma induced psychoneurotic behaviors, conduct disorders, and learning difficulties (Rate indicator of **Abuse Recovery:** 1 = none, 2 = limited, 3 = moderate, 4 = substantial, 5 = extensive [see Section I])

Client Outcomes

- Identifies symptoms associated with posttraumatic stress disorder (PTSD) and seeks help
- Identifies event in realistic, cognitive terms
- States that he or she is not to blame for the event

NIC Interventions (Nursing Interventions Classification)

Suggested NIC Labels

Counseling; Support System Enhancement

> **Example NIC Interventions—Counseling**
> - Encourage expression of feelings
> - Assist client to identify strengths and reinforce these

Nursing Interventions and Rationales

- Assess for PTSD in patients with chronic illness and anxiety.
  PTSD has emerged as the most common anxiety disorder in women. There are also high rates of PTSD in chronically ill and psychiatric patients (McFarlane, 2000).
- Consider the use of the Stanford Acute Stress Reaction Questionnaire to evaluate anxiety and dissociation symptoms after traumatic events
  This test was developed to assess dissociative and anxiety symptoms that research suggests trauma victims experience after the traumatic event (Cardena, et al, 2000).
- Provide peer support to contact co-workers to remind them that others in the organization are concerned about their welfare; allow opportunity to discuss the incident and assess for the need for further post-trauma services.
  The purpose of peer support in a post-trauma program is to ensure that each person involved in potentially traumatic incidents will receive the support and services necessary to make a successful recovery. Without the availability of peers, some individuals will certainly be overlooked. Peer supporters are not counselors. Their tasks include contacting co-workers to remind them that others in the organization are concerned about their welfare, allowing the opportunity to discuss the incident and assessing for the need for further post-trauma services (Post Trauma Resources, 1998).

• = Independent; ▲ = Collaborative

- Provide post-trauma debriefings. Effective post-trauma coping skills are taught and each participant creates a plan for his or her recovery. During the debriefing, the facilitators assess participants to determine their needs for further services in the form of post-trauma counseling. For maximum effectiveness, the debriefing should occur within 2 to 5 days of the incident.

  A debriefing is a specially designed group meeting that provides the opportunity to discuss the traumatic incident experiences and post-trauma consequences (Post Trauma Resources, 1998). The need for debriefing remains acute to accelerate recovery from traumatic events before harmful stress reactions have a chance to damage the performance, careers, health, and families of personnel responding to emergencies (Hayes, 1997).

▲ Provide post-trauma counseling. Counseling sessions are extensions of debriefings and include continued discussion of the traumatic event, post-trauma consequences, and the further development of coping skills.

  Immediate post-trauma responses cannot be prevented. Long-term problems can develop if post-trauma consequences are not managed. With immediate and effective responses to duty-related trauma, most of these long-term problems can be prevented (Post Trauma Resources, 1998).

- Instruct the client to use the following critical incident stress management techniques: Things To Try: Critical Incident Stress Debriefing (CISD)
  - Within the first 24 to 48 hours, periods of appropriate physical exercise alternated with relaxation will alleviate some of the physical reactions.
  - Structure your time—keep busy.
  - You're normal and having normal reactions—don't label yourself crazy.
  - Talk to people—talk is the most healing medicine.
  - Be aware of numbing the pain with overuse of drugs or alcohol; you don't need to complicate the stress with a substance abuse problem.
  - Reach out—people do care.
  - Maintain as normal a schedule as possible.
  - Spend time with others.
  - Help your co-workers as much as possible by sharing feelings and checking out how they are doing.
  - Give yourself permission to feel rotten and share your feelings with others.
  - Keep a journal—write your way through those sleepless hours.
  - Do things that feel good to you.
  - Realize those around you are under stress.
  - Don't make any big life changes.
  - Do make as many daily decisions as possible to give you a feeling of control over your life (i.e., if someone asks you what you want to eat, answer them even if you're not sure).
  - Get plenty of rest.
  - Reoccurring thoughts, dreams, or flashbacks are normal—don't try to fight them; they'll decrease over time and become less painful.
  - Eat well-balanced and regular meals (even if you don't feel like it).

  The Critical Incident Stress Debriefing (CISD) process is specifically designed to prevent or mitigate the development of PTSD among emergency services professions. CISD represents an integrated "system" of interventions that is designed to prevent and/or mitigate the adverse psychological reactions that so often accompany emergency services, public safety, and disaster

• = Independent; ▲ = Collaborative

response functions. CISD interventions are especially directed towards the mitigation of post-traumatic stress reactions (International Critical Incident Stress Foundation, 1999).

▲ Assess for history of life-threatening illness such as cancer and provide appropriate counseling.

People with histories of cancer can now be considered to be at risk for PTSD. The physical and psychological impact of having a life-threatening disease, of undergoing cancer treatment, and of living with recurring threats to physical integrity and autonomy constitute traumatic experiences for many cancer clients (National Cancer Institute, 1999).

• Provide protection for children who have witnessed violence or who have had traumatic injuries. Help the child to acknowledge the event and to express grief over the event.

Child witnesses to violent events are at risk for PTSD. Prevention measures during the first stage focus on protection and advocacy, while second stage interventions help the child acknowledge and tolerate the realities of the violent event (Rollins, 1997). This study supports the need for psychological evaluation and treatment for children who have had disfiguring traumatic injuries (Rusch et al, 2000).

Geriatric

• Carefully assess elderly client's response to traumatic events (e.g., natural disasters) and use the critical incident stress techniques described previously to prevent symptoms associated with PTSD.

Older adults appeared to be especially vulnerable to PTSD. Nurses who are aware of the effects of natural disasters, particularly flooding, may be better able to identify vulnerable populations and understand the health needs of other survivors (Keene, 1998).

Home Care Interventions

▲ Assess client's ability to meet primary needs of shelter, nourishment, and safety. Refer to medical social services, state departments of human services, or other organizations as appropriate.

Clients in need of primary life requirements are unable to master higher level coping.

• Identify other losses or stressors that may affect coping ability (e.g., role or relationship changes, deaths).

Presence of other stressors can compound the risk of trauma response and ineffective coping.

▲ Assess family's response to client risk. Refer family to medical social services or mental health services or support groups as necessary. Provide nursing support.

Client support systems may not understand or be able to cope with the risk involved in selected occupations or the response to selected traumatic events in the client's experience. This is a barrier to the provision of immediate and ongoing support to the client.

▲ If the client is on medication, assess effectiveness and compliance. Identify who administers the medication.

Clients with diminished ego strength may have difficulty adhering to a medication regimen.

• Assist clients in the home to identify and establish daily patterns that have meaning for them.

Daily patterns provide the client and support system with structure, stability, and a point of reference for perspective development.

• With clients who are displaced from the home, identify internal values that can be maintained while displaced, such as respite, contact with specific persons, and honesty.

Maintaining internal values reinforces ego strength, supports dignity, and promotes hope. Caution: Hope should not be misconstrued to mean that a client displaced from home can return home if this is not possible.

• = **Independent;** ▲ = **Collaborative**

▲ Encourage client to verbalize feelings of risk and trauma to therapeutic staff or other supportive persons. Refer to medical social services or mental health/support group services as appropriate.
Venting validates client feelings, fears, and needs. Professional support systems may be a necessary substitute for inadequate personal support systems on a temporary basis.

• See care plan for **Post-trauma syndrome.**

Client/Family Teaching

• Instruct the family and friends to use the following critical incident stress management techniques (International Critical Incident Stress Foundation, 1999):
For Family Members and Friends:
   ▪ Listen carefully.
   ▪ Spend time with the traumatized person.
   ▪ Offer your assistance and a listening ear, even if they have not asked for help.
   ▪ Help them with everyday tasks like cleaning, cooking, caring for the family, and minding children.
   ▪ Give them some private time.
   ▪ Don't take their anger or other feelings personally.
   ▪ Don't tell them that they are "lucky it wasn't worse"; traumatized people are not consoled by those statements. Instead, tell them that you are sorry such an event has occurred and you want to understand and assist them.
• Teach the client and family to recognize symptoms of PTSD and to seek treatment when the following occur:
   ▪ Relives the traumatic event by thinking or dreaming about it frequently.
   ▪ Is unsettled or distressed in other areas of his or her life such as in school, at work, or in personal relationships.
   ▪ Avoids any situation that might cause him or her to relive the trauma.
   ▪ Demonstrates a certain amount of generalized emotional numbness.
   ▪ Shows a heightened sense of being on guard.
▲ Refer clients with history of substance abuse and PTSD for appropriate counseling.
This study suggests that women with PTSD and substance abuse can be helped when provided with a treatment designed for them (Najavits, et al, 1998).

Multicultural

• Assess for the influence of cultural beliefs, norms, and values on the client's ability to cope with traumatic experience.
What the client views as healthy coping may be based on cultural perceptions (Leininger, 1996).
• Acknowledge racial ethnic differences at onset of care.
Acknowledgement of race/ethnicity issues will enhance communication, establish rapport, and promote positive treatment outcomes (D'Avanzo et al, 2001).
• Use a family centered approach when working with Latino, Asian, African-American, and Native American clients.
Latinos may perceive family as a source of support, solver of problems and a source of pride. Asian Americans may regard family as the primary decision maker and influence on individual family members (D'Avanzo et al, 2001).
• Provide opportunities by which the family and individual can save face when working with Asian American clients.
Some Asian American families may avoid situations and discussion of issues that will bring shame on the family unit (D'Avanzo et al, 2001).

• = Independent; ▲ = Collaborative

- Assure client of confidentiality.
  Many Indo-Chinese women will not discuss traumatic events like rape if they think that other staff members, their families, their husbands, or their community may find out (Mollica, Lavelle, 1988).
- Validate the client's feelings regarding the trauma and allow the client to tell the trauma story.
  Validation lets the client know that the nurse has heard and understands what was said, and it promotes the nurse-client relationship (Stuart, Laraia, 2001; Giger, Davidhizar, 1995). Through the trauma story, the clinician can bridge the disrupted social connection that exists between the client, his or her family, and the community (Mollica, Lavelle, 1988).

WEB SITES FOR EDUCATION

See the MERLIN web site for World Wide Web resources for client education.

REFERENCES Cardena E et al: Psychometric properties of the Stanford Acute Stress Reaction Questionnaire (SASRQ): a valid and reliable measure of acute stress, *J Trauma Stress* 13(4):719-734, 2000.

D'Avanzo CE et al: Developing culturally informed strategies for substance-related interventions. In Naegle MA, D'Avanzo CE, editors: *Addictions and substance abuse: strategies for advanced practice nursing,* St Louis, 2001, Mosby, pp 59-104.

Giger JN, Davidhizar RE: *Transcultural nursing,* ed 2, St Louis, 1995, Mosby.

Hayes L: Jail suicide and the need for debriefing, *Crisis* 18(4):150-151, 1997.

International Critical Incident Stress Foundation: *Critical incident stress information, signs & symptoms,* retrieved April 2, 1999, from the World Wide Web. Web site: www.icisf.org

Keene EP: Phenomenological study of the North Dakota flood experience and its impact on survivors' health, *Int J Trauma Nurs* 4(3):79-84, 1998.

Leininger MM: *Transcultural nursing: theories, research and practices,* ed 2, Hilliard, Ohio, 1996, McGraw-Hill.

McFarlane AC: Traumatic stress in the 21st century, *Aust N Z J Psychiatry* 34(6):919-928, 2000.

Mollica RF, Lavelle J: Southeast Asian refugees. In Comas-Diaz L, Griffith EEH, editors: *Clinical guidelines in cross-cultural mental health,* New York, 1988, John Wiley & Sons.

Najavits LM et al: Seeking safety: outcome of a new cognitive-behavioral psychotherapy for women, *J Trauma Stress* 11(3):437-456, 1998.

National Cancer Institute: *Posttraumatic stress disorder,* retrieved February 15, 1999, from the World Wide Web. Web site: cancernet.nci.nih.gov/clinpdq/supportive/Post-traumatic_stress_disorder_Physician.html#3

Post Trauma Resources: *Traumatic stress in law enforcement.* Originally published in *South Carolina Trooper* 1998; retrieved February 21, 1999, from the World Wide Web. Web site: www.posttrauma.com/publicsaart.html

Rollins JA: Minimizing the impact of community violence on child witnesses, *Crit Care Nurs Clin North Am* 9(2):211-220, 1997.

Rusch MD et al: Psychological adjustment in children after traumatic disfiguring injuries: a 12-month follow-up, *Plast Reconstr Surg* 106(7):1451-1458, 2000.

Stuart GW, Laraia MT: Therapeutic nurse-patient relationship. In Stuart GW, Laraia MT, editors: *Principles and practice of psychiatric nursing,* St Louis, 2001, Mosby, p 30.

Powerlessness

Gail B. Ladwig and Jill M. Barnes

NANDA **Definition** Perception that one's own actions will not significantly affect an outcome; a perceived lack of control over a current situation or immediate happening

• = **Independent;** ▲ = **Collaborative**

Defining Characteristics

Low   Expressions of uncertainty about fluctuating energy levels; passivity

Moderate   Nonparticipation in care or decision-making when opportunities are provided; resentment, anger, and guilt; reluctance to express true feelings; passivity; dependence on others that may result in irritability; fearing alienation from caregivers; expressions of dissatisfaction and frustration because of inability to perform previous tasks/activities; expression of doubt regarding role performance; does not monitor progress; does not defend self-care practices when challenged; inability to seek information regarding care

Severe   Verbal expressions of having no control over self-care, or influence over situation, or influence over outcome; apathy; depression regarding physical deterioration that occurs despite patient compliance with regimens

Related Factors (r/t)

Health care environment; interpersonal interactions; lifestyle of helplessness; illness-related regimen

NOC **Outcomes (Nursing Outcomes Classification)**

Suggested NOC Labels

Health Beliefs; Health Beliefs: Perceived Ability to Perform; Health Beliefs: Perceived Control; Health Beliefs: Perceived Resources; Participation: Health Care Decisions

Example NOC Outcome

Accomplishes **Health Beliefs: Perceived Control** as evidenced by the following indicators: Perceived responsibility for health decisions/Beliefs that own decisions and actions control health outcomes (Rate each indicator of **Health Beliefs: Perceived Control:** 1 = very weak belief, 2 = weak belief, 3 = moderate belief, 4 = strong belief, 5 = very strong belief [see Section I])

Client Outcomes

- States feelings of powerlessness and other feelings related to powerlessness (e.g., anger, sadness, hopelessness)
- Identifies factors that are uncontrollable
- Participates in planning care; makes decisions regarding care and treatment when possible
- Asks questions about care and treatment
- Verbalizes hope for the future

NIC **Interventions (Nursing Interventions Classification)**

Suggested NIC Labels

Self-Esteem Enhancement; Self-Responsibility Facilitation

Example NIC Interventions—Self-Responsibility Facilitation
- Encourage independence, but assist client when unable to perform
- Assist clients to identify areas in which they could readily assume more responsibility

Nursing Interventions and Rationales

- Observe for factors contributing to powerlessness (e.g., immobility, hospitalization, unfavorable prognosis, no support system, misinformation about situation, inflexible routine).

• = Independent; ▲ = Collaborative

Powerlessness can be experienced by people suffering from acute or chronic illness, as well as those attempting health promotion (Kubsch, Wichowski, 1997). Correctly identifying the actual or perceived problem is essential to providing appropriate support measures.

- Assess for noncompliance.
  Noncompliance can be an assertion of the need for control (Gibson, Kenrick, 1998).
- Assess client's locus of control related to his or her health.
  An external locus of control can lead a client to believe that he or she has no power over a situation (Gibson, Kenrick, 1998).
- Establish a therapeutic relationship with client by spending one-to-one time with him or her, assigning the same caregiver, and keeping commitments (e.g., saying, "I will be back to answer your questions in the next hour").
  Sharing feelings often leads to the realization that feelings are shared and this can lead to solidarity and reduce powerlessness (de Schepper, Francke, Abu-Saad, 1997). Consistency of caregivers minimizes the amount of disruption in a client's daily routine (Tolley, 1997). The trust and consistency fostered by a therapeutic relationship provides the client with a secure environment in which to deal with problems and develop adaptation skills (Johnson, 1993).
- Allow client to express hope, which may range from "I hope my coffee will be hot," to "I hope I will die with my significant other here." Listen to client's priorities.
  Hope is a way of coping with a stressful situation and motivates the client to continue living. Motivation is necessary in the change process.
- Allow the client to share feelings.
  Sharing feelings often leads to the realization that feelings are shared, and this realization can lead to solidarity and reduce powerlessness (de Schepper, Francke, Abu-Saad, 1997).
- Allow time for questions (15 to 20 minutes each shift); have client write down questions.
  Allowing time for questions encourages the client to take some control of the situation (Roberts, White, 1990).
- Have client assist in planning of care if possible (e.g., determining what time to bathe, taking pain medication before uncomfortable procedures, expressing food and fluid preferences). Document specifics in care plan.
  Allowing patients to participate more fully in their care provides a sense of control (Gibson, Kenrick, 1998). Allowing clients to make some decisions can increase their self-esteem and maintain their dignity (Kasten, 1998).
- Keep items client uses and needs, such as urinal, tissues, phone, and television controls, within reach.
  Well-being can be affected much more by choices related to activities of daily living (ADLs) like eating, sleeping, and grooming as opposed to larger, occasional events (Tolley, 1997). Client is able to participate in own care if care devices are accessible. Participation in care enhances a sense of control.
- When dealing with possible long-term deficits, work with the client to set small, attainable goals.
  Clients with spinal cord injuries focus hope on small gains and take one step at a time. One client stated, "Every little step I took was more important to me than what I had in the end" (Morse, Doberneck, 1995).
- Have client write goals (e.g., dangle legs at bedside 10 minutes for 2 days, then sit in chair 10 minutes for 2 days, then walk to window) and plans to achieve them.
  Active participation enhances a feeling of power.

• = Independent; ▲ = Collaborative

- Give praise for accomplishments.
  Giving praise assists clients in developing positive feelings and enhances self-concept (Meddaugh, Peterson, 1997). Positive reinforcement encourages repetition of behavior.
- Help clients identify factors not under their control.
  Identifying items within client's control encourages the client to take some control of the situation.
- Keep interactions with client focused on client, not on family or physician. Actively listen to client.
  For teens, this will support their developing ego. Directly focusing on the client also aids in practicing decision-making skills and increases their investment in adapting behavior (Hennessy-Harstad, 1999). It is important to convey the message that the client is unique and valued. Letting the client know that the schedule is tailored to meet his or her needs instead of tailored to the institution helps the client maintain a sense of self (Tolley, 1997). The client can use a lot of energy by holding in unacceptable or frightening feelings. By listening to the client and allowing these feelings to be expressed, the energy is released and can be used in other ways (Clark, 1993).
- Acknowledge subjective concerns or fears.
  All feelings are personal and have meaning for the client.
- Allow client to take control of as many ADLs as possible; keep client informed of all care that will be given.
  Providing opportunity for control is an important intervention for people experiencing powerlessness (Kasten, 1998). Clients are more amenable to therapy if they know what to expect and can perform some tasks independently.
- Develop contract with client that states client's and nurse's responsibilities and privileges.
  Contracting can encourage clients to assume responsibility and increase motivation (Kubsch, Wichowski, 1997). A contract helps give a situation structure and clarifies what may or may not happen and who has responsibility for the client's care.
- See the care plans for **Hopelessness** and **Spiritual distress.**

Geriatric

- Explore feelings of powerlessness—the feeling that client's behavior will not affect outcomes.
  Powerlessness can exhibit as apathy, depression, expressions of no control, nonparticipation, indecisiveness, and passivity (Meddaugh, Peterson, 1997). Quadriplegics and clients >60 years of age had higher incidences of feelings of powerlessness than others (p <0.5) (Richmond et al, 1992).
- Establish therapeutic relationships by listening; give the client choices and accept his or her statement of limitations.
  Allowing clients to make choices increases their autonomy and may make them feel good about their decision-making skills (Meddaugh, Peterson, 1997). "Power with" interactions occur when the staff listens to clients: "In therapy, my therapist listened to me. She would not push me if I couldn't do it. She would switch and we would do something else." This factor helped motivate people in a geriatric rehabilitation unit (Resnick, 1996).
- Encourage positive use of solitude—reading, listening to music, enjoying nature—to prevent loneliness.
  A positive use of solitude, with decreased dependence on external stimuli, may be particularly important for older individuals, who often find themselves increasingly alone without external stimuli or social support (Rane-Szostak, Herth, 1994).

• = **Independent;** ▲ = **Collaborative**

- Provide reading materials for clients who are able to read.
  Older people who enjoyed reading for pleasure were rarely lonely (Rane-Szostak, Herth, 1994).

Multicultural

- Assess for the influence of cultural beliefs, norms, and values on the client's feelings of powerlessness.
  The client's expressions of powerlessness may be based on cultural perceptions (Leininger, 1996).
- Assess the role of fatalism on the client's expression of powerlessness.
  Fatalistic perspectives, which involve the belief that you cannot control your own fate, may influence health behaviors in some African-American and Latino populations (Phillips, Cohen, Moses, 1999; Harmon, Castro, Coe, 1996).
- Encourage spirituality as a source of support to decrease powerlessness.
  African-Americans and Latinos may identify spirituality, religiousness, prayer, and church-based approaches as coping resources (Samuel-Hodge et al, 2000; Bourjolly, 1998; Mapp, Hudson, 1997).
- Validate the client's feelings regarding the impact of health status on current lifestyle.
  Validation lets the client know that the nurse has heard and understands what was said, and it promotes the nurse-client relationship (Stuart, Laraia, 2001; Giger, Davidhizar, 1995).

Home Care Interventions

NOTE: All of the mentioned nursing interventions are applicable in the home care setting.

- Include an initial and ongoing assessment and evaluation of potential abuse and neglect. Photograph evidence of abuse or neglect when possible.
  Assault is the single major cause of injury to women (Attala, 1996). Chronic abuse and neglect by spouse or other family among the elderly is often hidden until home care is actively involved.
- ▲ If neglect or abuse is suspected, identify an emergency plan that addresses the problem immediately and includes a report to the appropriate authorities.
  Client safety is a nursing priority. Reporting is a legal requirement of health care workers.
- Develop a written contract with client that designates what care will be given and responsibility for care elements. Focus should be on care that is controlled by the client.
  A written contract reassures the client that control of care as designated will be honored.
- Empower clients by allowing them to guide specifics of care such as wound care procedures and dressing and grooming details. Confirm client knowledge before empowering and document in chart that client is able to guide procedures. Document in home and in chart preferred approach to procedures. Orient family and caregivers to client role.
  Empowering the client as described motivates the client to actively learn and participate in care. Client values self and perceives power secondary to level of knowledge. Accurate documentation of client knowledge and abilities supports teamwork with health care team and avoids conflict.

Client/Family Teaching

- Explain all procedures, treatments, and expected outcomes.
  By increasing knowledge and adapting new behaviors, clients learn what they have some control over their health (Hennessy-Harstad, 1999). With knowledge comes power; the

• = Independent; ▲ = Collaborative

health care professional must ensure that the client has a sound knowledge base in order to make informed decisions (Meddaugh, Peterson, 1997). Clients are more amenable to therapy if they know what to expect.

- Provide written instructions for treatments and procedures for which the client will be responsible.

  A written record provides a concrete reference so that the client and family can clarify any verbal information that was given. People tend to forget half of what they hear within a few minutes, so it is important for nurses to supplement oral instructions with written material (Wong, 1992).

- Teach stress reduction, relaxation, and imagery. Many cassette tapes are available on relaxation and meditation. Assist the client with relaxation based on the client's preference indicated in the initial assessment.

  These techniques can restore power in the client by allowing the client to learn how to control the autonomic nervous system and other physiological mechanisms (Johnson, Dahlen, Roberts, 1997). Relaxation techniques, desensitization, and guided imagery can help clients to cope, increase their control, and allay anxiety (Narsavage, 1997). Such techniques are useful in combating depression, hopelessness, powerlessness, and poor self-image (Anderson, 1992). Individuals experiencing a sense of powerlessness can use imagery to develop a much needed sense of control (Stephens, 1993).

- Teach cognitive activities, such as using "self-talk"—telling self that the situation is under own control and things can change.

  Self-motivation techniques such as self-talk facilitate lasting behavior change (McSweeney, 1993).

- Help client practice assertive communication techniques.

  Clients with conditions such as quadriplegia need to be assertive so that they can direct their care and be as independent as possible (Bach, McDaniel, 1993).

- Role play (e.g., say, "Tell me what you are going to ask your doctor").

  Role playing is the most commonly used technique in assertiveness training. It deconditions the anxiety that arises from interpersonal encounters.

- ▲ Refer to support groups, pastoral care, or social services.

  There is an assignment of power in the imparting of advice (Bonhote, Romano-Egan, Cornwell, 1999). These services help decrease levels of stress, increase levels of self-esteem, and reassure clients that they are not alone.

WEB SITES FOR EDUCATION

MERLIN See the MERLIN web site for World Wide Web resources for client education.

REFERENCES Anderson SB: Guillain-Barré syndrome: giving the patient control, *J Neurosci Nurs* 24:158, 1992.

Attala JM: Detecting abuse against women in the home, *Home Care Provider* 1:1, 1996.

Bach C, McDaniel R: Quality of life in quadriplegic adults: a focus group study, *Rehabil Nurs* 18:364, 1993.

Bonhote K, Romano-Egan J, Cornwell C: Altruism and creative expressions in a long-term older adult psychotherapy group, *Issues Ment Health Nurs* 20(6):603-617, 1999.

Bourjolly JN: Differences in religiousness among black and white women with breast cancer, *Soc Work Health Care* 28(1):21-39, 1998.

Clark S: Challenges in critical care nursing: helping patients and families cope, *Crit Care Nurs* 13(4 suppl):1-22, 1993.

de Schepper AM, Francke AL, Abu-Saad HH: Feelings of powerlessness in relation to pain: ascribed causes and reported strategies, *Cancer Nurs* 20(6):422-429, 1997.

• = Independent; ▲ = Collaborative

Gibson JM, Kenrick M: Pain and powerlessness: the experience of living with peripheral vascular disease, *J Adv Nurs* 27(4):737-745, 1998.

Giger JN, Davidhizar RE: *Transcultural nursing*, ed 2, St Louis, 1995, Mosby.

Harmon MP, Castro FG, Coe K: Acculturation and cervical cancer: knowledge, beliefs, and behaviors of Hispanic women, *Women Health* 24(3):37-57, 1996.

Hennessy-Harstad EB: Empowering adolescents with asthma to take control through adaptation, *J Pediatr Health Care* 13:273-277, 1999.

Johnson BS: *Adaptation and growth: psychiatric-mental health nursing*, Philadelphia, 1993, JB Lippincott.

Johnson LH, Dahlen R, Roberts SL: Supporting hope in congestive heart failure patients, *Dimens Crit Care Nurs* 16(2):65-78, 1997.

Kasten AA: Case study: clinical opportunities and challenges related to diagnosis of and interventions for loss of control, *Nurs Diagn* 9(3):90:119-121, 1998.

Kubsch S, Wichowski HC: Restoring power through nursing intervention, *Nurs Diagn* 8(1):7-15, 1997.

Leininger MM: *Transcultural nursing: theories, research and practices*, ed 2, Hilliard, Ohio, 1996, McGraw-Hill.

Mapp I, Hudson R: Stress and coping among African American and Hispanic parents of deaf children, *Am Ann Deaf* 142(1):48-56, 1997.

McSweeney J: Making behavior changes after a myocardial infarction, *West J Nurs Res* 15:441, 1993.

Meddaugh D, Peterson B: Removing powerlessness from the nursing home, *Nurs Homes* 46(8):32-34, 36, 1997.

Morse J, Doberneck B: Delineating the concept of hope, *Image J Nurs Sch* 27:277, 1995.

Narsavage GL: Promoting function in clients with chronic lung disease by increasing their perception of control, *Holistic Nurs Pract* 12(1):17-26, 1997.

Phillips JM, Cohen MZ, Moses G: Breast cancer screening and African American women: fear, fatalism, and silence, *Oncol Nurs Forum* 26(3):561-571, 1999.

Rane-Szostak D, Herth K: A new perspective on loneliness in later life, *Issues Ment Health Nurs* 16:583, 1994.

Resnick B: Motivation in geriatric rehabilitation, *Image J Nurs Sch* 28:41, 1996.

Richmond T et al: Powerlessness in acute spinal cord injury patients: a descriptive study, *J Neurosci Nurs* 24:146, 1992.

Roberts S, White BS: Powerlessness and personal control model applied to the myocardial infarction patient, *Prog Cardiovasc Nurs* 5:84, 1990.

Samuel-Hodge CD et al: Influences on day-to-day self-management of type 2 diabetes among African-American women: Spirituality, the multi-caregiver role, and other social context factors, *Diabetes Care* 23(7):928-933, 2000.

Stephens R: Imagery: a strategic intervention to empower clients, part II—a practical guide, *Clin Nurs Spec* 7:235, 1993.

Stuart GW, Laraia MT: Therapeutic nurse-patient relationship. In Stuart GW, Laraia MT, editors: *Principles and practice of psychiatric nursing*, St Louis, 2001, Mosby, p 30.

Tolley M: Power to the patient, *J Gerontol Nurs* 23(10):7-12, 1997.

Wong M: Self-care instructions: do patients understand educational materials? *Focus Crit Care* 19:47, 1992.

Risk for Powerlessness

Gail B. Ladwig

 Definition At risk for perceived lack of control over a situation and/or one's ability to significantly affect an outcome

Related Factors (r/t)

Physiological Chronic or acute illness (hospitalization, intubation, ventilator, suctioning); acute injury or progressive debilitating disease process (e.g., multiple sclerosis); aging (e.g., decreased physical strength, decreased mobility); dying

• = Independent; ▲ = Collaborative

Psychosocial Lack of knowledge of illness or healthcare system; lifestyle of dependency with inadequate coping patterns; absence of integrality (e.g., essence of power); decreased self-esteem; low or unstable body image

NOC **Outcomes (Nursing Outcomes Classification)**

Suggested NOC Labels

Health Beliefs; Health Beliefs: Perceived Ability to Perform; Health Beliefs: Perceived Control; Health Beliefs: Perceived Resources; Participation: Health Care Decisions

> **Example NOC Outcome**
>
> Accomplishes **Health Beliefs: Perceived Control** as evidenced by the following indicators: Perceived responsibility for health decisions/Beliefs that own decisions and actions control health outcomes (Rate each indicator of **Health Beliefs: Perceived Control:** 1 = very weak belief, 2 = weak belief, 3 = moderate belief, 4 = strong belief, 5 = very strong belief [see Section I])

Client Outcomes

- States feelings of powerlessness and other feelings related to powerlessness (e.g., anger, sadness, hopelessness)
- Identifies factors that are uncontrollable
- Participates in planning care; makes decisions regarding care and treatment when possible
- Asks questions about care and treatment
- Verbalizes hope for the future

NIC **Interventions (Nursing Interventions Classification)**

Suggested NIC Labels

Self-Esteem Enhancement; Self-Responsibility Facilitation

> **Example NIC Interventions—Self-Responsibility Facilitation**
> - Encourage independence, but assist patient when unable to perform
> - Assist patients to identify areas in which they could readily assume more responsibility

Nursing Interventions and Rationales, Home Care Interventions, Client/Family Teaching, Web Sites for Education

See the care plan for **Powerlessness.**

Ineffective Protection

Betty J. Ackley

NANDA **Definition** Decrease in the ability to guard self from internal or external threats such as illness or injury

Defining Characteristics

Maladaptive stress response; neurosensory alteration; impaired healing; deficient immunity; altered clotting; dyspnea; insomnia; weakness; restlessness; pressure ulcers; perspiring; itching; immobility; chilling; fatigue; disorientation; cough; anorexia

 = Independent; ▲ = Collaborative

Related Factors (r/t)

Abnormal blood profiles (e.g., leukopenia, thrombocytopenia, anemia, coagulation); extremes of age; inadequate nutrition; alcohol abuse; drug therapies (e.g., antineoplastic, corticosteroid, immune, anticoagulant, thrombolytic); treatments (e.g., surgery, radiation); diseases such as cancer and immune disorders

NOC   Outcomes (Nursing Outcomes Classification)

Suggested NOC Labels

Immune Status; Abuse Protection; Coagulation Status; Endurance

Example NOC Outcome

Has sufficient **Immune Status** as evidenced by the following indicators: Recurrent infections not present/Tumors not present/Gastrointestinal status IER*/Respiratory status IER/Weight IER/Body temperature IER/Absolute WBC† values WNL‡ (Rate each indicator of **Immune Status:** 1 = extremely compromised, 2 = substantially compromised, 3 = moderately compromised, 4 = mildly compromised, 5 = not compromised [see Section I])

*In Expected Range
†White Blood Cell
‡Within Normal Limits

Client Outcomes

- Remains free of infection
- Remains free of any evidence of new bleeding
- Explains precautions to take to prevent infection
- Explains precautions to take to prevent bleeding

NIC   Interventions (Nursing Interventions Classification)

Suggested NIC Labels

Bleeding Precautions; Infection Control; Infection Protection

Example NIC Interventions—Infection Control
- Monitor for systemic and localized signs and symptoms of infection
- Inspect skin and mucous membranes for redness, extreme warmth, or drainage

Nursing Interventions and Rationales

▲ Take temperature, pulse, and blood pressure (e.g., q __ hr[s]).
Changes in vital signs can indicate the onset of bleeding or infection.

▲ Observe nutritional status (e.g., weight, serum protein and albumin, muscle mass size, usual food intake). Work with dietitian to increase nutritional status if needed. All clients diagnosed with human immunodeficiency virus (HIV) should have a dietary consult.
Early assessment of nutrition, good management of nutrition, and psychological support are essential for meeting the needs of the neutropenic client (Rust, Simpson, Lister, 2000). Good nutrition is needed to maintain immune function and support formation of clotting elements. Most people who die of AIDS actually die of starvation. Malnutrition is almost universal among persons with AIDS because of malabsorption (Woznicki, D'Alessandro, 1997).

• Observe sleep pattern; if altered, see Nursing Interventions and Rationales for **Disturbed Sleep pattern.**

• = Independent; ▲ = Collaborative

- Determine the amount of stress in client's life. If stress is uncontrollable, see Nursing Interventions and Rationales for **Ineffective Coping.**
  Uncontrolled stress depresses immune system function (Carter, 1993).

Prevention of infection

- ▲ Monitor for and report any signs of infection (e.g., fever, chills, flushed skin, drainage, edema, redness, and pain) and notify the physician promptly.
  The immune system is stimulated with the onset of infection, resulting in classic signs of infection. In the neutropenic client, antibiotics must be given promptly because a delay increases morbidity and mortality (Quadri, Brown, 2000).
- ▲ If immune system is depressed, notify physician of elevated temperature, even in the absence of other symptoms of infection.
  Clients with depressed immune function are unable to mount the usual immune responses to the onset of infection; fever may be the only sign of infection. A neutropenic client with fever represents an absolute medical emergency (Burney, 2000; Quadri, Brown, 2000).
- If white blood cell count is severely decreased (absolute neutrophil count <1000 per mm^3), initiate the following precautions:
  - Take vital signs every 4 hours.
  - Complete a head-to-toe assessment twice daily, including inspection of oral mucosa, invasive sites, wounds, urine, and stool; monitor for onset of new complaints of pain.
  - ▲ Avoid any invasive procedures including catheterization, injections, or rectal or vaginal procedures.
    Infection can invade when a treatment damages the skin or mucous membranes, which are natural barriers against infection (Flyge, 1993).
  - ▲ Administer granulocyte growth factor therapy as ordered.
    These myeloid growth factors for granulocytes are more useful for preventing than for treating neutropenic infections in cancer patients (Glaspy, 2000).
  - Take meticulous care of all invasive sites (Fenelon, 1998).
  - Provide frequent oral care.
    The effects of chemotherapy or radiation leave the mouth inflamed; combined with immunosuppression this can result in stomatitis. Good oral care can help prevent this complication (Dose, 1995).
  - Have client wear a mask when leaving room.
  - Limit and screen visitors to minimize exposure to contagion.
  - Enforce careful hand washing for everyone entering the client's room.
    Infection in the neutropenic client can be reduced by careful washing of health care workers' hands (Fenelon, 1998).
  - Help client bathe daily.
- Serve client well-cooked food only; avoid all raw foods, including salads. Avoid serving processed meats, cheeses, yogurt, and beer or wine. Have client drink sterile or boiled water only, and make ice cubes out of sterile water (Fenelon, 1998; Rust, Simpson, Lister, 2000).
  There is a lack of data validating that neutropenic diets make a difference in diminishing rates of infection. Most centers use guidelines that recommend specific dietary restrictions during a period of immunosuppression (Rust, Simpson, Lister, 2000; Smith, Besser, 2000).

• = Independent; ▲ = Collaborative

▲ Ensure that client is well nourished. If appetite is suppressed, institute a dietary referral. Keep track of serum albumin levels, as well as transferrin and prealbumin levels.

It is essential that the nurse ensure adequate nutrition for the neutropenic client. If the client can't eat, and the gastrointestinal system is temporarily damaged, it may be necessary for the client to receive total parenteral nutrition. The visceral proteins levels (albumin, transferrin, and prealbumin) are an indirect measure of nutritional status (Rust, Simpson, Lister, 2000).

▪ Help client to cough and practice deep breathing regularly. Maintain appropriate activity level.

▲ Obtain a private room for client. Take ordered precautions including use of protective isolation or laminar air flow room if available and appropriate. Recognize that cotton cover gowns may not be effective in decreasing infection.

A private room is always necessary for neutropenic clients. There is no standardization of infection prevention practices nationwide for bone marrow transplant clients (Poe et al, 1994). A client with an absolute neutrophil count of <1000 per mm^3 is severely neutropenic, has an impaired immune function, and is extremely prone to infection. Precautions should be taken to limit exposure to pathogens (Wujcik, 1993). A pilot study investigating the routine use of cotton cover gowns in the care of neutropenic clients found that the rate of infection were no different than if cover gowns were not used (Kenny, Lawson, 2000).

▲ Watch for signs of sepsis, including change in mental status, fever, shaking, chills, and hypotension. If present, notify the physician promptly.

Change in mental status, fever, shaking, chills, and hypotension are indicators of sepsis (Flyge, 1993).

• See care plan for **Risk for Infection** for more interventions regarding prevention of infection.

Prevention of bleeding

▲ Monitor client's risk for bleeding; evaluate clotting studies and platelet counts.

Laboratory studies give a good indication of the seriousness of the bleeding disorder.

• Watch for hematuria, melena, hematemesis, hemoptysis, epistaxis, bleeding from mucosa, petechiae, and ecchymoses.

These areas of bleeding can be detected in a bleeding disorder (Ellenberger, Hass, Cundiff, 1993; Paschall, 1993).

▲ Give medications orally or intravenously (IV) only; avoid giving them intramuscularly, subcutaneously, or rectally (Shuey, 1996). Apply pressure for a longer time than usual to invasive sites such as venipuncture or injection sites.

Additional pressure is needed to stop bleeding of invasive sites of clients with bleeding disorders.

• Take vital signs frequently; watch for changes associated with fluid-volume loss.

Excessive bleeding causes a decreased blood pressure and increased pulse and respiratory rates.

• Monitor menstrual flow if relevant; have client use pads instead of tampons.

Menstruation can be excessive in clients with bleeding disorders. Tampons can increase trauma to the vagina.

• Have client use a moistened toothette instead of a toothbrush, or a very soft child's toothbrush. Have client use alcohol-free dental products and avoid flossing.

These actions help prevent trauma to the oral mucosa, which could result in bleeding (Shuey, 1996).

• = **Independent;** ▲ = **Collaborative**

- Ask client either to not shave or to use an electric razor only.
  This helps to prevent any unnecessary trauma that could result in bleeding (Shuey, 1996).
- ▲ To decrease risk of bleeding, avoid administering salicylates or nonsteroidal antiin-flammatory drugs (NSAIDs) if possible.
  Salicylates and NSAIDs can cause gastrointestinal bleeding; salicylates interfere with platelet function and can increase bleeding.

Home Care Interventions

- ▲ For terminally ill clients, teach and institute all of the mentioned noninvasive pre-cautions that will maintain quality of life. Discuss with client, family, and physician the consequences of contracting infection. Determine which precautions do not maintain quality of life and should not be used (e.g., physical assessment twice daily, multiple vital sign assessments).
  Multiple assessments and other invasive procedures are recovery-based, cure-focused ac-tivities. The client and physician must agree on an approach to care for the client's re-maining life.

Client/Family Teaching

Depressed immune function

- Teach precautions to take to decrease the chance of infection (e.g., avoiding un-cooked fruits or vegetables, using appropriate self-care, ensuring a safe environment).
- Teach client and family how to take a temperature. Encourage family to take client's temperature between 3 pm and 7 pm at least once daily.
  The client's temperature is more likely to be elevated in the evening hours because the cir-cadian rhythm peaks during this time (Samples et al, 1985).
- ▲ Teach client and family to notify physician of elevated temperature, even in the absence of other symptoms of infection.
  Clients with depressed immune function are unable to mount the usual immune response to the onset of infection; fever may be the only present sign of infection (Wujcik, 1993).
- Teach client to avoid crowds and contact with persons who have infections.
- Teach the need for good nutrition, avoidance of stress, and adequate rest to maintain immune system function.
  Client education to increase nutrition, manage stress, and perform self-care can reduce the risk of neutropenic infection (Carter, 1993).

Bleeding disorder

- ▲ Teach client to wear a Medic-Alert bracelet and notify all health care personnel of the bleeding disorder.
- Teach client and family the signs of bleeding, precautions to take to prevent bleed-ing, and action to take if bleeding begins.
- ▲ Caution client to avoid taking over-the-counter medications without permission of physician.
  Medications containing salicylates can increase bleeding.
- Teach client to wear loose-fitting clothes and avoid physical activity that might cause trauma.

WEB SITES FOR EDUCATION

MERLIN See the MERLIN web site for World Wide Web resources for client education.

• = Independent; ▲ = Collaborative

REFERENCES   Burney KY: Tips for timely management of febrile neutropenia, *Oncol Nurs Forum* 27(4):617-618, 2000.

Carter LW: Influences of nutrition and stress on people at risk for neutropenia: nursing implications, *Oncol Nurs Forum* 20(8):1241-1249, 1993.

Dose AM: The symptom experience of mucositis, stomatitis, and xerostomia, *Semin Oncol Nurs* 11:248, 1995.

Ellenberger BJ, Hass L, Cundiff L: Thrombotic thrombocytopenia purpura: nursing during the acute phase, *Dimens Crit Care Nurs* 12:58-62, 1993.

Fenelon L: Strategies for prevention of infection in short-duration neutropenia, *Infect Control Hosp Epidemiol* 19(8):590-592, 1998.

Flyge HA: Meeting the challenge of neutropenia, *Nursing* 23(7):60-64, 1993.

Glaspy JA: Hematologic supportive care of the critically ill cancer patient, *Semin Oncol* 27(3):375-383, 2000.

Kenny H, Lawson E: The efficacy of cotton cover gowns in reducing infection in nursing neutropenic patients: an evidence-based study, *Int J Nurs Pract* 6(3):135-139, 2000.

Paschall FE: Thrombotic thrombocytopenic purpura: the challenges of a complex disease process, *AACN Clin Issues* 4:655-660, 1993.

Poe SS et al: A national survey of infection prevention practices on bone marrow transplant units, *Oncol Nurs Forum* 21(10):1687-1690, 1994.

Quadri TL, Brown AE: Infectious complications in the critically ill patient with cancer, *Semin Oncol* 27(3):335-346, 2000.

Rust DM, Simpson JK, Lister J: Nutritional issues in patients with severe neutropenia, *Semin Oncol Nurs* 16(2), 152-162, 2000.

Samples JF et al: Circadian rhythms: basis for screening for fever, *Nurs Res* 34:377, 1985.

Shuey KM: Platelet-associated bleeding disorders, *Semin Oncol Nurs* 12(1):15-27, 1996.

Smith LH, Besser SG: Dietary restrictions for patients with neutropenia: a survey of institutional practices, *Oncol Nurs Forum* 27(3):515-520, 2000.

Woznicki D, D'Alessandro G: Nutrition against AIDS, *Health Priorities* (Internet) 9(2), 1997. Web site: www.acsh.org/publications/priorities/0902/nutrition.html

Wujcik D: Infection control in oncology patients, *Nurs Clin North Am* 28:639, 1993.

Rape-trauma syndrome

Nancee B. Radtke and Gail B. Ladwig

 Definition   Sustained maladaptive response to a forced, violent sexual penetration against the victim's will and consent

Defining Characteristics

Disorganization; change in relationships; confusion; physical trauma (e.g., bruising, tissue irritation); suicide attempts; denial; guilt; paranoia; humiliation; embarrassment; aggression; muscle tension and/or spasms; mood swings; dependence; powerlessness; nightmares and sleep disturbances; sexual dysfunction; revenge; phobias; loss of self-esteem; inability to make decisions; dissociative disorders; self-blame; hyperalertness; vulnerability; substance abuse; depression; helplessness; anger; anxiety; agitation; shame; shock; fear

Related Factors (r/t)

Rape

NOC   Outcomes (Nursing Outcomes Classification)

Suggested NOC Labels

Abuse Cessation; Protection; Abuse Recovery: Emotional, Sexual; Coping; Impulse Control; Self-Mutilation Restraint

• = **Independent;** ▲ = **Collaborative**

> **Example NOC Outcome**
> Demonstrates **Abuse Recovery** as evidenced by: Resolution of trauma-induced psychoneurotic behaviors, conduct disorders, and learning difficulties (Rate each indicator of **Abuse Recovery:** 1 = none, 2 = limited, 3 = moderate, 4 = substantial, 5 = extensive [see Section I])

Client Outcomes

- Shares feelings, concerns, and fears
- Recognizes that the rape or attempt was not own fault
- States that no matter what the situation, no one has the right to assault another
- Identifies behaviors and situations within own control to prevent or reduce risk of recurrence
- Describes treatment procedures and reasons for treatment
- Reports absence of physical complications or pain
- Identifies support people and is able to ask them for help in dealing with this trauma
- Functions at same level as before crisis, including sexual functioning
- Recognizes that it is normal for full recovery to take a year

NIC Interventions (Nursing Interventions Classification)

Suggested NIC Labels
Counseling; Support System Enhancement

> **Example NIC Interventions—Counseling**
> - Encourage expression of feelings
> - Help client to identify strengths, and reinforce these

Nursing Interventions and Rationales

- Observe client's responses, including anger, fear, self-blame, sleep pattern disturbances, and phobias.
- Monitor client's verbal and nonverbal psychological state (e.g., crying, wringing hands, avoiding interactions or eye contact with staff).
  The most depressed victims are those most concerned with being stigmatized and blamed for the crime (Frable, Blackstone, Sherbaum, 1990).
- Stay with (or have a trusted person stay with) client initially. If a law enforcement interview is permitted, provide support by staying with client.
  Early crisis intervention involves helping client decide whom to tell about the rape and regain the control after the assault.
- Explain each part of treatment. Discuss the importance of a pelvic examination. If it is the client's first examination, explain instruments and let client know when and where you will touch.
  Do not wait for the client to ask questions; explain everything you are doing, why it must be done, and when and where you will touch. Eye contact is very important because it helps the client feel worthy and alive (Ruckman, 1992).
- Observe for signs of physical injury. Ask questions such as, "Did he push you?" "Did he hit you?" "Did he choke you?" and "Do you feel sore anywhere?" Instruct client to return for additional photos if bruises become more pronounced in a few days.
  It is important to carefully document that force was used and sexual contact was not consensual. Sore areas are not visible in photos.

• = Independent; ▲ = Collaborative

- Encourage client to verbalize feelings.
  Listening to clients helps them gain self-control by feeling acceptance from others (Ruckman, 1992).
- Provide privacy so that client can express feelings. Limit the number of nurses present, escort to treatment room as soon as possible, do not question in triage area, close curtains and door, and avoid other interruptions during contact with client (e.g., telephone calls, leaving the room, outside stimuli such as radios).
- Document a one- or two-sentence summary of what happened; getting the details of the sequence of events is the police officer's job.
  If some details that are not in the nurse notes were told to police, the defense attorney may attempt to make this look like a discrepancy in facts, causing reasonable doubt and resulting in an acquittal (Ledray, 1992).
- ▲ Enlist the help of supportive counselors who are experienced with rape trauma; refer client to a rape crisis counselor, mental health clinic, or psychotherapist.
  After physical needs are met, the client should be placed in the care of a counselor who can maintain a relationship long after discharge from the emergency department (Ruckman, 1992).
- ▲ Provide an interdisciplinary approach such as the Sexual Assault Nurse Examiner (SANE) to minimize trauma for the victim; gather necessary evidence; and provide a caring, supportive, and healing environment.
  Evidence Based Practice indicates that this model brings quality care to women (Selig, 2000). Comparing a baseline group of 130 sexual assault victims with 39 clients who were evaluated after the SANE approach was implemented indicated that the SANE approach increased clinical interaction and completeness of evaluation and information gathered (Derhammer et al, 2000).
- Instead of asking client if she wants you to call the community rape crisis center, describe the center and how the staff will be available after client goes home.
  Clients want control but may have difficulty making decisions during the initial visit to the emergency department. Involvement of social service agencies will help to guarantee a timely follow-up home visit (Jones, 1994).
- Explain collection of specimens for evidence; provide items for self-care after examination (e.g., for cleansing the vaginal and rectal area).
  A card with the victim's name and date is held next to the injury in each picture for identification; direct quotes rather than summaries or paraphrases should be used. Most states provide sexual assault evidence collection kits, which prevent any inconsistencies in the collection of evidence that will be used in court.
- Explain that client's undergarments may need to be kept for evidence; instruct client to put other clothing in a paper bag once at home and to not wash it until it is known if it will be needed for evidence.
  Do not place clothes in plastic because moisture may accumulate and cause deterioration. Observe for seminal fluid on body with a Wood's lamp, which shows seminal fluid as fluorescent yellow and violet colors in a dark room (Ledray, 1992).
- ▲ Discuss the possibility of pregnancy and sexually transmitted diseases (STDs) and the treatments available.
  Administering a urine pregnancy test is routine before giving medications to prevent pregnancy or treat STDs. Most clients prefer to prevent pregnancy rather than face the possibility of terminating it in the future. The risk of human immunodeficiency virus (HIV)

• = **Independent;** ▲ = **Collaborative**

exposure is a special concern to rape victims; the nurse should bring up this issue and inform the client of locations and schedules for HIV testing.

- Explain that it is the client's choice whether to report the rape.
  The first step in evidence collection is obtaining a signed consent from the client to do an examination and release collected evidence to police.
- Encourage client to report the rape.
  It is important for rape victims to recognize they are victims of a crime that is not their fault (Ledray, 1992). Reporting is an issue separate from prosecution; if victims report, they will not be forced to appear as a witness.
- Discuss client's support system. Involve support system if appropriate and client grants permission. Unsupportive and victim-blaming attitudes by significant others are common responses.
  Research indicates that significant others are coping with their own responses to trauma and may be incapable of supporting the victim (Mackey et al, 1992).
- ▲ Obtain blood alcohol level if indicated.

Geriatric

- Build a trusting relationship with client.
  Recognize the attitudes and values of an older generation; stigmatization may cause victim to view self with disgust and shame (Delorey, Wolf, 1993).
- Explain reporting and encourage client to report.
  Embarrassment may prevent reporting; respect client's choice. Older rape victims have reported having a greater fear of people finding out about their rape than younger women (Tyra, 1993). Timely reporting within 72 hours is necessary to document injuries (Adams, Girardin, Faugno, 2000).
- Observe for psychosocial distress (e.g., memory impairment, sleep disturbances, regression, changes in bodily functions).
  Exacerbation of a chronic illness may be a major consequence of sexual assault.
- Identify and obtain treatment for new injuries related to the assault and the immediate effects on the client's existing health problems (e.g., cardiovascular disease, arthritis, respiratory disease).
  A review of the client's current medications may add to the nurse's understanding of relevant health problems.
- Modify the rape protocol to promote comfort for geriatric clients. Consider positioning female clients with pillows rather than stirrups and consider using a smaller speculum.
  Aging results in decreased muscle tone and thinning of the vaginal wall.
- Assess for mobility limitations and cognitive impairment.
  Elicit information from family or caregivers to verify level of functioning before sexual assault.
- Respect client's need for privacy.
  Older clients may be reluctant to have their children or younger family members present during examination and treatment; give clients a choice.
- Consider arrangements for temporary housing.
  Most sexual assaults of older clients occur in the home.
  NOTE: Older age increases the powerlessness of a person, especially if isolated as a result of living alone. Physical injury can have a much greater effect on older victims, and they may experience a compound reaction because they are older. Sexual violence against an older female is a reflection of antiage and antiwoman attitudes. Of older

• = **Independent;** ▲ = **Collaborative**

sexually assaulted females, 43% are beaten, 7% are stabbed, 60% are severely injured, and 10% are murdered (Delorey, Wolf, 1993).

Male rape

- Reactions to male rape are often either disbelief or an assumption that males who are raped are gay.
  Most females are aware of the possibility that they may be raped, but many males are not. The care required is very similar to the care of females who have been raped (Laurent, 1993). Approximately 10% of rape victims who go to rape crisis centers are men (Dunn, Gilchrist, 1993).

Multicultural

- Assess for the influence of cultural beliefs, norms, and values on the client's ability to cope with the trauma of the rape experience.
  What the client views as healthy coping may be based on cultural perceptions (Leininger, 1996).
- Acknowledge racial and ethnic differences at onset of care.
  Acknowledgement of race/ethnicity issues will enhance communication, establish rapport, and promote positive treatment outcomes (D'Avanzo et al, 2001).
- Use a family-centered approach when working with Latino, Asian, African-American, and Native American clients.
  Latinos may perceive family as a source of support, solver of problems and a source of pride. Asian Americans may regard family is the primary decision maker and influence on individual family members (D'Avanzo et al, 2001).
- Provide opportunities by which the family and individual can save face when working with Asian American clients.
  Asian American families may avoid situations and discussion of issues that will bring shame on the family unit (D'Avanzo et al, 2001).
- Assure client of confidentiality.
  Many Indo-Chinese women will not discuss rape if they think that other staff members, their families, their husbands, or their community may find out (Mollica, Lavelle, 1988).
- Validate the client's feelings regarding the rape and allow the client to tell his or her rape story.
  Validation lets the client know that the nurse has heard and understands what was said, and it promotes the nurse-client relationship (Stuart, Laraia, 2001; Giger, Davidhizar, 1995). Through the trauma story, the clinician can bridge the disrupted social connection that exists between the client, family, and community (Mollica, Lavelle, 1988).

Home Care Interventions

- Interact with client nonjudgmentally; it supports the client's self-worth.
  Rape victims usually experience a loss of self-worth.
- Assist the client with realistically assessing the home setting for safety and/or selecting a safe environment in which to live.
  Rape clients may be unable to make a realistic assessment of home safety both immediately after the rape and during long-term recovery.
- ▲ Ensure that client has support system in place for long-term support. Instruct family that recovery may take a long time. Refer for medical social work services to assist in setting up a support system if necessary. Refer for counseling if necessary.
  The long-term response to rape (up to 4 years) requires ongoing support for the client to reorganize and reintegrate.
- Make sure that physical symptoms from the rape or other physical conditions are followed up.

• = **Independent;** ▲ = **Collaborative**

Stress response to rape can precipitate reemergence of other physical conditions that may be ignored because of the rape.

Client/Family Teaching

▲ Provide information on prophylactic antibiotic therapy, hepatitis B vaccine, and tetanus prophylaxis for nonimmunized clients with trauma.
   Prophylactic antibiotic therapy should be prescribed if the assailant is known to be infected, the victim has signs or symptoms of infection, or prophylaxis is requested (Hampton, 1995).

• Discharge instructions should be written for client.
   Anxiety can hamper comprehension and retention of information; repeat instructions and provide them in a written form.

• Give instructions to significant others.
   Significant others need many of the same supportive and caring interventions as the client; suggest that they too might benefit from counseling.

▲ Explain purpose of "morning after pill."
   The morning after pill—norgestrel (Ovral)—prevents pregnancy and is only used in emergencies. It must be taken within 72 hours (3 days) of sexual contact for it to work. It will not cause a miscarriage if client is already pregnant, but it could harm the baby.

▲ Explain potential for common side effects related to treatment with norgestrel, such as breast swelling or nausea and vomiting. (Call the emergency department if client vomits within 1 hour of taking pill because pill may need to be taken again.) The menstrual period may take 3 to 30 days to start; if menstruation has not started in 30 days, contact physician.

▲ Explain potential for severe side effects related to treatment with norgestrel, such as severe leg or chest pain, trouble breathing, coughing up blood, severe headache or dizziness, and trouble seeing or talking.

• Advise client to call or return if new problems develop.
   Physical injuries may not be recognized because of client's emotional numbness during the initial examination or because client may have forgotten or not understood some of the instructions.

• Teach relaxation techniques.

• Discuss practical lifestyle changes within client's control to reduce the risk of future attacks.
   A client's financial situation may limit some options such as moving to another home. Provide other alternatives such as keeping doors locked, checking car before getting in, not walking alone at night, keeping someone informed of whereabouts, asking someone to check if client has not arrived within reasonable amount of time, keeping lights on in entryway, having keys in hand when approaching car or house, having a remote-key entry car or garage.

▲ Teach client to use self-defense techniques to surprise attacker and get an opportunity to run for help. Refer client to self-defense school.

• Teach client appropriate outlets for anger.

• Encourage significant other to direct anger at event and attacker, not at the client.

• Emphasize vulnerability of client and ensure that reactions are appropriate for the victim of sexual assault.
   Females are at higher risk for depression than males, and the risk is significantly higher between the ages of 18 and 44 (Mackey et al, 1992).

• = **Independent**; ▲ = **Collaborative**

NOTE: Post-traumatic stress disorder (PTSD) has a high probability of being a psychological sequelae to rape. Research demonstrated two effective treatments for improvement of PTSD in rape victims—prolonged exposure and stress inoculation training (Foa, Steketee, Roghbaum, 1991). Prolonged exposure involves reliving the rape scene by imagining it as vividly as possible, describing it aloud in the present tense, taping this description, and listening to the tape at least once daily. Stress inoculation training uses breathing exercises to diminish anxiety and instruction in coping skills, thought stopping, cognitive restructuring, self-dialogue, and role-playing. Research suggests that a combination of both treatments may provide the optimal effect.

WEB SITES FOR EDUCATION

MERLIN See the MERLIN web site for World Wide Web resources for client education.

REFERENCES Adams JA, Girardin B, Faugno D: Signs of genital trauma in adolescent rape victims examined acutely, *J Pediatr Adolesc Gynecol* 13(2):88, 2000.

D'Avanzo CE et al: Developing culturally informed strategies for substance-related interventions. In Naegle MA, D'Avanzo CE, editors: *Addictions and substance abuse: strategies for advanced practice nursing*, St Louis, 2001, Mosby, pp 59-104.

Delorey C, Wolf KA: Sexual violence and older women, *Clin Issues Perinatal Women Health Nurs* 4:173, 1993.

Derhammer F et al: Using a SANE interdisciplinary approach to care of sexual assault victims, *Jt Comm J Qual Improv* 26(8):488-496, 2000.

Dunn SF, Gilchrist VJ: Sexual assault, *Primary Care* 20(2):359-373, 1993.

Frable D, Blackstone T, Sherbaum C: Marginal and mindful: deviants in social interaction, *J Pers Soc Psychol* 59:140, 1990.

Giger JN, Davidhizar RE: *Transcultural nursing*, ed 2, St Louis, 1995, Mosby.

Hampton H: Care of the woman who has been raped, *N Engl J Med* 322:234, 1995.

Jones J: Elder abuse and neglect: responding to a national problem, *Ann Emerg Med* 23:845, 1994.

Laurent C: Male rape, *Nurs Times* 89(6):18-19, 1993.

Ledray L: The sexual assault nurse clinician: a 15-year experience in Minneapolis, *J Emerg Nurs* 18(3):217-222, 1992.

Leininger MM: *Transcultural nursing: theories, research and practices*, ed 2, Hilliard, Ohio, 1996, McGraw-Hill.

Mackey T et al: Factors associated with long-term depressive symptoms of sexual assault victims, *Arch Psychiatr Nurs* 6:10, 1992.

Mollica RF, Lavelle J: Southeast Asian refugees. In Comas-Diaz L, Griffith EEH, editors: *Clinical guidelines in cross-cultural mental health*, New York, 1988, John Wiley & Sons.

Ruckman LM: Rape: how to begin the healing, *Am J Nurs* 92:48, 1992.

Selig C: Sexual assault nurse examiner and sexual assault response team (SANE/SART) program, *Nurs Clin North Am* 35(2):311-319, 2000.

Stuart GW, Laraia MT: Therapeutic nurse-patient relationship. In Stuart GW, Laraia MT, editors: *Principles and practice of psychiatric nursing*, St Louis, 2001, Mosby, p 30.

Tyra PA: Older women: victims of rape, *J Gerontol Nurs* 19(5):7-12, 1993.

Rape-trauma syndrome: compound reaction

Nancee B. Radtke and Gail B. Ladwig

NANDA **Definition** Forced violent sexual penetration against the victim's will and consent resulting in a trauma syndrome that includes an acute phase of disorganization of the victim's lifestyle and a long-term process or reorganization of lifestyle

• = Independent; ▲ = Collaborative

Defining Characteristics

Change in lifestyle (e.g., changes in residence, dealing with repetitive nightmares and phobias, seeking family support, seeking social network support in long-term phase); emotional reaction (e.g., anger, embarrassment, fear of physical violence and death, humiliation, revenge, self-blame in acute phase); multiple physical symptoms (e.g., gastrointestinal irritability, genitourinary discomfort, muscle tension, sleep pattern disturbance in acute phase); reactivated symptoms of such previous conditions (i.e., physical illness, psychiatric illness in acute phase); reliance on alcohol and/or drugs (acute phase)

Related Factors (r/t)

Rape

NOC Outcomes (Nursing Outcomes Classification)

Suggested NOC Labels

Abuse Cessation; Protection; Abuse Recovery: Emotional, Sexual; Coping; Impulse Control; Self-Mutilation Restraint

> **Example NOC Outcome**
> Demonstrates **Abuse Recovery** as evidenced by: Resolution of trauma-induced psychoneurotic behaviors, conduct disorders, and learning difficulties (Rate each indicator of **Abuse Recovery:** 1 = none, 2 = limited, 3 = moderate, 4 = substantial, 5 = extensive [see Section I])

Client Outcomes

- Shares feelings, concerns, and fears
- Recognizes that the rape or attempt was not own fault
- States that no matter what the situation, no one has the right to assault another
- Identifies behaviors and situations within own control to prevent or reduce risk of recurrence
- Describes treatment procedures and reasons for treatment
- Reports absence of physical complications or pain
- Identifies support people and is able to ask them for help in dealing with this trauma
- Functions at same level as before crisis, including sexual functioning
- Recognizes that it is normal for full recovery to take a year

NIC Interventions (Nursing Interventions Classification)

Suggested NIC Labels

Counseling; Support System Enhancement

> **Example NIC Interventions—Counseling**
> - Encourage expression of feelings
> - Help client to identify strengths, and reinforce these

Nursing Interventions and Rationales

See care plans for **Rape-trauma syndrome, Powerlessness, Ineffective Coping, Dysfunctional Grieving, Anxiety, Fear, Risk for self-directed Violence,** and **Sexual dysfunction.**

• = Independent; ▲ = Collaborative

Geriatric

- A new subgroup of rape victims resides in nursing homes. Treatment is necessary.
  Nursing home victims can suffer both compound and silent rape trauma (Burgess, Dowdell, Prentky, 2000).

Risk for compound reaction

See care plan for **Rape-trauma syndrome.**

Multicultural

- Assess for the influence of cultural beliefs, norms, and values on the client's ability to cope with the trauma of the rape experience.
  What the client views as healthy coping may be based on cultural perceptions (Leininger, 1996).
- Provide opportunities by which the family and individual can save face when working with Asian American clients
  Asian American families may avoid situations and discussion of issues that will bring shame on the family unit (D'Avanzo et al, 2001).
- Assure client of confidentiality.
  Many Indo-Chinese women will not discuss rape if they think that other staff members, their families, their husbands, or their community may find out (Mollica, Lavelle, 1988).
- Validate the client's feelings regarding the rape and allow the client to tell his or her rape story.
  Validation lets the client know that the nurse has heard and understands what was said, and it promotes the nurse-client relationship (Stuart, Laraia, 2001; Giger, Davidhizar, 1995). Through the trauma story, the clinician can bridge the disrupted social connection that exists between the client, family, and community (Mollica, Lavelle, 1988).

Home Care Interventions

- ▲ If client has pursued psychiatric counseling, monitor and encourage attendance.
  Reliving the rape experience and the accompanying feelings is painful. Client may need additional support to continue.
- ▲ If client is receiving medications, assess client knowledge base of its purpose, side effects, and interactions with medications for other diagnoses. Monitor for effectiveness, side effects, and interactions.
  Ongoing stress may leave client overwhelmed and less able to cope with impact of changing medical status.
- Establish an emergency plan including hotlines. Contract with the client to use the emergency plan. Role-play using the hotlines.
  Having an emergency plan reassures the client and decreases the risk of suicide.
- For other home care and hospice considerations, see care plan for **Rape-trauma syndrome.**

Client/Family Teaching

- Teach client what reactions to expect during the acute and long-term phases: acute phase—anger, fear, self-blame, embarrassment, vengeful feelings, physical symptoms, muscle tension, sleeplessness, stomach upset, genitourinary discomfort; long-term phase—changes in lifestyle or residence, nightmares, phobias, seeking of family and social network support.
  Of assessed rape victims, 16.5% were diagnosed with posttraumatic stress disorder (PTSD) an average of 17 years after the assault (Mackey et al, 1992).
- ▲ Encourage psychiatric consultation if client is suicidal, violent, or unable to continue activities of daily living (ADLs).

• **= Independent; ▲ = Collaborative**

Rape victims are four times more likely than the general population to attempt suicide, which is an 8.7% higher rate than that of nonrape victims (Mackey et al, 1992).

▲ Discuss any of client's current stress-relieving medications that may result in substance abuse.

The initial response to trauma is for the noradrenergic system to maintain the arousal state, increase vigilance, and be protective to prevent subsequent trauma. Following massive trauma, neurotransmitters are depleted at the synapse level, which is associated with long-term depression and numbing. This depletion also leaves the client with a different threshold, increasing vulnerability to subsequent stress (Mackey et al, 1992).

WEB SITES FOR EDUCATION

$\frac{\$}{}$ ᶠᴹᴱᴿᴸᴵᴺ See the MERLIN web site for World Wide Web resources for client education.

REFERENCES   Burgess AW, Dowdell EB, Prentky RA: Sexual abuse of nursing home residents, *J Psychosoc Nurs Ment Health Serv* 38(6):10-18, 2000.

D'Avanzo CE et al: Developing culturally informed strategies for substance-related interventions. In Naegle MA, D'Avanzo CE, editors: *Addictions and substance abuse: strategies for advanced practice nursing*, St Louis, 2001, Mosby, pp 59-104.

Giger JN, Davidhizar RE: *Transcultural nursing*, ed 2, St Louis, 1995, Mosby.

Leininger MM: *Transcultural nursing: theories, research and practices*, ed 2, Hilliard, Ohio, 1996, McGraw-Hill.

Mackey T et al: Factors associated with long-term depressive symptoms of sexual assault victims, *Arch Psychiatr Nurs* 6(1):10-25, 1992.

Mollica RF, Lavelle J: Southeast Asian refugees. In Comas-Diaz L, Griffith EEH, editors: *Clinical guidelines in cross-cultural mental health*, New York, 1988, John Wiley & Sons.

Stuart GW, Laraia MT: Therapeutic nurse-patient relationship. In Stuart GW, Laraia MT, editors: *Principles and practice of psychiatric nursing*, St Louis, 2001, Mosby, p 30.

Rape-trauma syndrome: silent reaction

Nancee B. Radtke and Gail B. Ladwig

NANDA   **Definition** Forced violent sexual penetration against the victim's will and consent resulting in a trauma syndrome that includes an acute phase of disorganization of the victim's lifestyle and a long-term process or reorganization of lifestyle

Defining Characteristics

Increased anxiety during interview (e.g., blocking of associations, long periods of silence, minor stuttering, physical distress); sudden onset of phobic reactions; no verbalization about the rape; abrupt changes in relationships with males; increased nightmares; pronounced changes in sexual behavior

Related Factors (r/t)

Rape

NOC   **Outcomes (Nursing Outcomes Classification)**

Suggested NOC Labels

Abuse Cessation; Protection; Abuse Recovery: Emotional, Sexual; Coping; Impulse Control; Self-Mutilation Restraint

• = Independent; ▲ = Collaborative

> **Example NOC Outcome**
> Demonstrates **Abuse Recovery** as evidenced by: Resolution of trauma-induced psychoneurotic behaviors, conduct disorders, and learning difficulties (Rate each indicator of **Abuse Recovery:** 1 = none, 2 = limited, 3 = moderate, 4 = substantial, 5 = extensive [see Section I])

Client Outcomes

- Resumes previous level of relationships with significant others
- States improvement in sleep and fewer nightmares
- Expresses feelings about and discusses the rape
  Nondisclosure about a sexual assault may arise out of self-protection, but this defensive coping style acts as a pressure cooker and is associated with more intense depressive symptoms (Mackey et al, 1992).
- Returns to usual pattern of sexual behavior
  Women who are sexually active after the assault report lower levels of depression (Mackey et al, 1992). However, being sexually active cannot be construed to mean that the client has adjusted to or resolved the sexual trauma.
- Remains free of phobic reactions
- See care plan for **Rape-trauma syndrome.**

NIC | Interventions (Nursing Interventions Classification)

Suggested NIC Labels

Counseling; Support System Enhancement

> **Example NIC Interventions—Counseling**
> - Encourage expression of feelings
> - Help client to identify strengths, and reinforce these

Nursing Interventions and Rationales

- See care plan for **Rape-trauma syndrome, Powerlessness, Ineffective Coping, Dysfunctional Grieving, Anxiety, Fear, Risk for self-directed Violence, Sexual dysfunction,** or **Impaired verbal Communication.**
- Observe for disruptions in relationships with significant others.
  Poorly adjusted clients may elicit nonsupportive behavior from others or perceive actions of others in a negative way.
- Monitor for signs of increased anxiety (e.g., silence, stuttering, physical distress, irritability, unexplained crying spells).
- Focus on client's coping strengths.
- Observe for changes in sexual behavior.
  More than 80% of sexually active victims reported some sexual dysfunction as a result of the assault (Mackey et al, 1992). Some victims engage in sexual intimacy to prove to themselves and their partners that they are normal or unaffected by the assault.
- Identify phobic reactions to objects in environment (e.g., strangers, doorbells, being with groups of people, knives).
- Provide support by listening when client is ready to talk.
  In one study, delayed disclosure of childhood rape was very common and long delays were typical. Close friends are the most common confidants (Smith et al, 2000).

• = Independent; ▲ = Collaborative

- Be nonjudgmental when feelings are expressed. Explain that anger is normal and needs to be verbalized. Reassure client with phrases such as, "I'm sorry this happened to you."
- Remain with anxious client even if client is silent. Use gentle speech and actions; move slowly.
- Evaluate somatic complaints.
  Women are at higher risk for depression than men (Mackey et al, 1992).

Geriatric

- A new subgroup of rape victims resides in nursing homes. Treatment is necessary.
  Nursing home victims can suffer both compound and silent rape trauma (Burgess, Dowdell, Prentky, 2000)
- See care plan for **Rape-trauma syndrome.**

Multicultural

- Assess for the influence of cultural beliefs, norms, and values on the client's ability to cope with the trauma of the rape experience.
  What the client views as healthy coping may be based on cultural perceptions (Leininger, 1996).
- Provide opportunities by which the family and individual can save face when working with Asian American clients.
  Asian American families and individuals may avoid situations and discussion of issues that will bring shame on the family unit (D'Avanzo et al, 2001).
- Assure client of confidentiality.
  Many Indo-Chinese women will not discuss rape if they think that other staff members, their families, their husbands, or their community may find out (Mollica, Lavelle, 1988).
- Allow the client to tell his or her rape story without probing.
  Through the rape story, the clinician can bridge the disrupted social connection that exists between the client, family, and community (Mollica, Lavelle, 1988).

Home Care Interventions

See care plan for **Rape trauma syndrome.**

Client/Family Teaching

- Reassure clients they are not bad and are not at fault. Avoid questions beginning with "why."
  "Why" questions may sound judgmental and feed into self-blame.
- ▲ Refer client to sexual assault counselor.
  Long-term counseling may be necessary.
- Offer information about testing, treatment, and procedures for pregnancy, hepatitis B, and sexually transmitted diseases (STDs). Do not wait for victim to request information.
- See care plan for **Rape-trauma syndrome.**

WEB SITES FOR EDUCATION

Merlin See the MERLIN web site for World Wide Web resources for client education.

REFERENCES   Burgess AW, Dowdell EB, Prentky RA: Sexual abuse of nursing home residents, *J Psychosoc Nurs Ment Health Serv* 38(6):10-18, 2000.
D'Avanzo CE et al: Developing culturally informed strategies for substance-related interventions. In Naegle MA, D'Avanzo CE, editors: *Addictions and substance abuse: strategies for advanced practice nursing,* St Louis, 2001, Mosby, pp 59-104.

• = **Independent**; ▲ = **Collaborative**

Leininger MM: *Transcultural nursing: theories, research and practices,* ed 2, Hilliard, Ohio, 1996, McGraw-Hill.

Mackey et al: Factors associated with long-term depressive symptoms of sexual assault victims, *Arch Psychiatr Nurs* 6:10, 1992.

Mollica RF, Lavelle J: Southeast Asian refugees. In Comas-Diaz L, Griffith EEH, editors: *Clinical guidelines in cross-cultural mental health,* New York, 1988, John Wiley & Sons.

Smith DW et al: Delay in disclosure of childhood rape: results from a national survey, *Child Abuse Negl* 24(2):273-287, 2000.

Relocation stress syndrome

Betty J. Ackley

NANDA   **Definition**   Physiological and/or psychosocial disturbances that result from a transfer from one environment to another

NOTE: Recent research on the nursing diagnosis of relocation stress syndrome may indicate that the nursing diagnosis is not valid, or may not be valid when applied to group moves of clients (Mallick, Whipple, 2000). More research is needed in this area to validate this nursing intervention.

Defining Characteristics

Temporary and/or permanent move; voluntary and/or involuntary move; aloneness, alienation, loneliness; depression; anxiety (e.g., separation); sleep disturbance; withdrawal; anger; loss of identity, self-worth, or self-esteem; increased verbalization of needs, unwillingness to move, or concern over relocation; increased physical symptoms/illness (e.g., gastrointestinal disturbance, weight change); dependency; insecurity; pessimism; frustration; worry; fear

Related Factors (r/t)

Unpredictability of experience/isolation from family/friends; passive coping; language barrier; decreased health status; impaired psychosocial health; past, concurrent, and recent losses; feeling of powerlessness; lack of adequate support system/group; lack of predeparture counseling

NOC   **Outcomes (Nursing Outcomes Classification)**

Suggested NOC Labels

Psychosocial Adjustment: Life Change; Child Adaptation to Hospitalization; Depression Level; Loneliness; Coping; Depression Control; Anxiety Control; Quality of Life; Coping

> **Example NOC Outcome—Anxiety Control**
> Demonstrates **Anxiety Control** as evidenced by the following indicators: Seeks information to reduce anxiety/Plans coping strategies for stressful situations/Uses effective coping strategies/Uses relaxation techniques to reduce anxiety/Maintains social relationships/Reports adequate sleep/Reports absence of physical manifestations of anxiety (Rate each indicator of **Anxiety Control:** 1 = never demonstrated, 2 = rarely demonstrated, 3 = sometimes demonstrated, 4 = often demonstrated, 5 = consistently demonstrated [see Section I])

• = Independent; ▲ = Collaborative

Client Outcomes

- Recognizes and knows the name of at least one staff member
- Expresses concerns about move when encouraged to do so during individual contacts
- Carries out activities of daily living (ADLs) in usual manner
- Maintains previous mental and physical health status (e.g., nutrition, elimination, sleep, social interaction)

NIC   Interventions (Nursing Interventions Classification)

Suggested NIC Labels

Anxiety Reduction; Coping Enhancement; Discharge Planning; Hope Instillation; Self-Responsibility Facilitation

> **Example NIC Interventions—Anxiety Reduction**
> - Stay with patient to promote safety and reduce fear
> - Provide objects that symbolize safeness

Nursing Interventions and Rationales

- Obtain a history, including reason for the move, client's usual coping mechanisms, history of losses, and family support for the client.
  A history helps determine the amount of support needed and appropriate interventions to decrease relocation stress (Manion, Rantz, 1995).
- ▲ If client is an adolescent, try not to move in the middle of the school year, find a newcomers club for adolescent to join, and refer for counseling if needed.
  An adolescent who is relocating can experience emotional, social, and cognitive dysfunctions. The interventions listed can be helpful (Puskar, Dvorsak, 1991).
- Observe the following procedures if client is being transferred to a nursing home or adult foster care:
  - Allow client to have a choice of placement and arrange a preadmission visit if possible.
    Having some control over the event strengthens problem-solving coping strategies (Oleson, Shadick, 1993; Nypaver, Titus, Brugler, 1996) and may help decrease mortality (Thorson, Davis, 2000).
  - If client cannot choose placement, arrange for a visit or phone call by a member of the staff to welcome client and show a videotape or at least provide pictures of the new care facility.
  - Have a familiar person accompany client to the new facility.
    This lessens client and family anxiety, confusion, and dissatisfaction (Manion, Rantz, 1995).
  - Validate the caregiver's feelings of difficulty with putting a loved one in a different environment.
    This is a distressing experience, and caregivers feel responsible. Validating their feelings will help establish a trusting relationship (Dellasega, Mastrian, 1995).
- Identify previous routines for ADLs. Try to maintain as much continuity with previous schedule as possible.
  Continuity of routines has been shown to be a crucial factor in positively influencing adjustment to a new environment (Manion, Rantz, 1995).
- Bring in familiar items from home (e.g., pictures, clocks, afghans).
- Establish the way the client would like to be addressed (Mr., Mrs., Miss, first name, nickname).
  Calling clients by their desired name shows respect.

• = Independent; ▲ = Collaborative

- Thoroughly orient client to the new environment and routines; repeat directions as needed.
  The stress of the move may interfere with client's ability to remember directions (Harkulich, 1992).
- Spend one-to-one time with client. Allow client to express feelings and convey acceptance of them; emphasize that the client's feelings are real and individual and that it is acceptable to be sad or angry about moving.
  Expressing feelings can help the client adjust to the situation.
- Assign the same staff to client; maintain consistency in personnel client interacts with.
  Consistency hastens adjustment (Harkulich, 1992).
- Ask client to state one positive aspect of the new living situation each day.
  Helping the client to focus on the positive aspects of the move can help change attitude and reframe the situation in a positive fashion.
- ▲ Monitor client's health status and provide appropriate interventions for problems with social interaction, nutrition, sleep, new onset of infection, or elimination problems.
  Stress from the transfer can cause physiological and psychological disturbances (Barnhouse, Brugler, Harkulich, 1992; Lander, Brazill, Ladrigan, 1997). Clients who moved showed decreased natural killer cell immunity one month after moving than was shown in a control group of elderly who did not move (Lutgendorf et al, 1999).
- If client is being transferred within a facility, have staff members from the new unit visit client before transfer.
  Once client is transferred, have previous staff make occasional visits until client is comfortable in new surroundings.
- Watch for coping problems (e.g., withdrawal, regression, or angry behavior) and intervene immediately.
  Failure to cope in a timely manner may cause a permanent pattern of impaired adjustment (Oleson, Shadick, 1993).
- Allow client to grieve for loss of old situation; explain that it is normal to feel sadness over change and loss.
- Allow client to participate in care as much as possible and make decisions when possible (e.g., where to place bed, choice of roommate, bathing routines). Make an effort to accommodate the client.
  Having choices helps prevent feelings of powerlessness that may lead to depression.

Geriatric

- Monitor need for transfer, and transfer only when necessary.
  Elderly clients often adapt poorly to transfer; they can lose normal functioning in areas such as self-care (Lander, Brazill, Ladrigan, 1997), and relocation may even cause death (Rantz, Egan, 1987; Thorson, Davis, 2000).
- Protect client from injuries such as falls.
  An increase in the number of accidents in frail elderly can happen with relocation (Lander, Brazill, Ladrigan, 1997).
- After the transfer, determine client's mental status. Document and observe for any new onset of confusion.
  Confusion can follow relocation because of the overwhelming stress and sensory overload.
- Use reality orientation if needed (e.g., "Today is . . ." "The date is . . ." "You are at . . . facility"). Repeat information as needed, and provide clock or calendar.
  Reality orientation can be helpful to prevent new onset of confusion (Manion, Rantz, 1995).

- **= Independent; ▲ = Collaborative**

Client/Family Teaching

- Teach family members about relocation stress syndrome. Encourage them to monitor for signs of the syndrome. Acceptance of the new living situation begins within 6 to 8 weeks after institutionalization, and adjustment is usually complete within 3 to 6 months (Manion, Rantz, 1995).
- Help significant others learn how to support client with the move by setting up a schedule of visits, arranging for holidays, bringing familiar items from home, and establishing a system for contact when client needs support.

WEB SITES FOR EDUCATION

 See the MERLIN web site for World Wide Web resources for client education.

REFERENCES   Barnhouse AH, Brugler CJ, Harkulich JT: Relocation stress syndrome, *Nurs Diagn* 3(4):166-167, 1992.

Dellasega C, Mastrian K: The process and consequences of institutionalizing an elder, *West J Nurs Res* 17(2):123-140, 1995.

Harkulich JT: Relocation stress. In Gettrust K, Brabeck PD, editors: *Nursing diagnosis in clinical practice: guides for care planning*, Albany, NY, 1992, Delmar.

Lander SM, Brazill AL, Ladrigan PM: Intrainstitutional relocation: effects on residents' behavior and psychosocial functioning, *J Gerontol Nurs* 23(4):35-41, 1997.

Lutgendorf SK et al: Sense of coherence moderates the relationship between life stress and natural killer cell activity in healthy older adults, *Psychol Aging* 14(4):552-563, 1999.

Mallick MJ, Whipple TW: Validity of the nursing diagnosis of relocation stress syndrome, *Nurs Res* 49(2):97-100, 2000.

Manion PD, Rantz MJ: Relocation stress syndrome: a comprehensive plan for long-term care admissions, *Geriatr Nurs* 16(3):108-112, 1995.

Nypaver JM, Titus M, Brugler CJ: Patient transfer to rehabilitation: just another move? relocation stress syndrome, *Rehabil Nurs* 21(2):94-97, 1996.

Oleson M, Shadick KM: Application of Moos' and Schaefer's model to nursing care of elderly persons relocating to a nursing home, *J Adv Nurs* 18:479-485, 1993.

Puskar KR, Dvorsak KG: Relocation stress in adolescents: helping teenagers cope with a moving dilemma, *Pediatr Nurs* 17(3):295-297, 1991.

Rantz M, Egan K: Reducing death from translocation syndrome, *Am J Nurs* 87(9):1351-1352, 1987.

Thorson JA, Davis RE: Relocation of the institutionalized aged, *J Clin Psychol* 56(1):131-138, 2000.

Risk for Relocation stress syndrome

Betty J. Ackley

NANDA   **Definition** At risk for physiological and/or psychosocial disturbances that result from a transfer from one environment to another

Risk Factors

Moderate to high degree of environmental change (e.g., physical, ethnic, cultural) temporary and/or permanent move; voluntary and/or involuntary move; lack of adequate support system/group; feelings of powerlessness; moderate mental competence (e.g., alert enough to experience changes); unpredictability of experiences; decreased psychosocial or physical health status; lack of predeparture counseling; passive coping; past, current, recent losses

- = Independent; ▲ = Collaborative

NOC **Outcomes (Nursing Outcomes Classification)**

Suggested NOC Labels

Psychosocial Adjustment: Life Change; Child Adaptation to Hospitalization; Loneliness; Coping; Anxiety Control; Quality of Life; Coping

Example NOC Outcome

Demonstrates **Anxiety Control** as evidenced by the following indicators: Seeks information to reduce anxiety/Plans coping strategies for stressful situations/Uses effective coping strategies/Uses relaxation techniques to reduce anxiety/Maintains social relationships/Reports adequate sleep/Reports absence of physical manifestations of anxiety (Rate each indicator of **Anxiety Control:** 1 = never demonstrated, 2 = rarely demonstrated, 3 = sometimes demonstrated, 4 = often demonstrated, 5 = consistently demonstrated [see Section I])

Client Outcomes

- Recognizes and knows the name of at least one staff member
- Expresses concerns about move when encouraged to do so during individual contacts
- Carries out activities of daily living (ADLs) in usual manner
- Maintains previous mental and physical health status (e.g., nutrition, elimination, sleep, social interaction)

NIC **Interventions (Nursing Interventions Classification)**

Suggested NIC Labels

Anxiety Reduction; Coping Enhancement; Discharge Planning; Hope Instillation; Self-Responsibility Facilitation

Example NIC Interventions—Anxiety Reduction

- Stay with patient to promote safety and reduce fear
- Provide objects that symbolize safeness

Nursing Interventions and Rationales and Client/Family Teaching

Refer to care plan for **Relocation stress syndrome.**

WEB SITES FOR EDUCATION

$\int_{MERLIN}$ See the MERLIN web site for World Wide Web resources for client education.

Ineffective Role performance

Gail B. Ladwig

NANDA **Definition** Patterns of behavior and self-expression that do not match the environmental context, norms, and expectations

Defining Characteristics

Change in self-perception of role; role denial; inadequate external support for role enactment; inadequate adaptation to change or transition, system conflict; change in usual

• = **Independent;** ▲ = **Collaborative**

patterns of responsibility; discrimination; domestic violence; harassment uncertainty; altered role perceptions; role strain; inadequate self-management; role ambivalence; pessimistic attitude; inadequate motivation; inadequate confidence; inadequate role competency and skills; inadequate knowledge; inappropriate developmental expectations; role conflict; role confusion; powerlessness; inadequate coping; anxiety or depression; role overload; change in other's perception or role; role dissatisfaction; inadequate opportunities for role enactment

Related Factors (r/t)

Social   Inadequate or inappropriate linkage with the health care system; job schedule demands; young age; developmental level; lack of rewards; poverty; family conflict; inadequate support system; inadequate role socialization (e.g., role model, expectations responsibilities); low socioeconomic status; stress and conflict; domestic violence; lack of resources

Knowledge   Inadequate role preparation (e.g., role transition, skill, rehearsal, validation); lack of knowledge about role, role skills; role transition; lack of opportunity for role rehearsal; developmental transitions; unrealistic role expectations; education attainment level; lack of or inadequate role model

Physiological   Inadequate/inappropriate linkage with health care system; substance abuse; mental illness; body image alteration; physical illness; cognitive deficits; health alterations (e.g., physical health, body image, self-esteem, mental health, psychosocial health, cognitive, learning style, neurological health); depression; low self-esteem; pain; fatigue

NOTE: There is typology of roles: sociopersonal (friendship, family, marital, parenting, community), home management intimacy (sexuality, relationship building), leisure/exercise/recreation, self-management, socialization (developmental transitions), community contributor, and religious.

NOC   ## Outcomes (Nursing Outcomes Classification)

Suggested NOC Labels

Coping; Psychosocial Adjustment: Life Change

> **Example NOC Outcome**
> Demonstrates **Coping** as evidenced by: Identifies effective and ineffective coping patterns/Modifies lifestyle as needed (Rate each indicator of **Coping:** 1 = never demonstrated, 2 = rarely demonstrated, 3 = sometimes demonstrated, 4 = often demonstrated, 5 = consistently demonstrated [see Section I])

Client Outcomes

- Identifies realistic perception of role
- States personal strengths
- Acknowledges problems contributing to inability to carry out usual role
- Accepts physical limitations regarding role responsibility and considers ways to change lifestyle to accomplish goals associated with role performance
- Demonstrates knowledge of appropriate behaviors associated with new or changed role
- States knowledge of change in responsibility and new behaviors associated with new responsibility
- Verbalizes acceptance of new responsibility

NIC   ## Interventions (Nursing Interventions Classification)

Suggested NIC Labels

Role Enhancement

• = **Independent;** ▲ = **Collaborative**

Nursing Interventions and Rationales

- Observe client's knowledge of behaviors associated with role.
  Ability to perform perceived roles is easily hampered by illness. It is important to note whether or not the client feels capable of functioning in the usual role.

- Allow client to express feelings regarding the role change.
  The client may experience disappointment and feelings of grief because of a role change. It is therapeutic for the client to express these feelings.

- Ask client direct questions regarding new roles and how the health care system can help him or her continue in roles.
  To maintain self-esteem, it is important to accurately assess the client's needs and ways to meet them. Direct questions help elicit factual information.

- Assist new parents to adjust to changes in workload associated with childbirth.
  Expectant parents in this study anticipated increase in workload after childbirth. Work increases were greater for women than men (Gjerdingen, 2000).

- Reinforce client's strengths, have client identify past coping skills, and support the continued use of these skills.
  Behavioral change is facilitated by a personal sense of control. If people believe that they can take action to solve a problem instrumentally, they become more inclined to do so and feel more committed to this decision (Schwarzer, Fuchs, 1995).

- Have client make a list of strengths that are needed for the new role. Acknowledge which strengths client has and which strengths need to be developed. Work with client to set goals for desired role.
  In setting valued goals, people adapt their world to self-generated needs and projects rather than adapting themselves to a given world (Nuttin, 1992). Focusing on strengths helps the client to positively enhance behaviors associated with role performance.

- Have client list problems associated with the new role and identify ways of overcoming them (e.g., if pain is worse late in day, have client complete necessary role tasks early in day).
  There are many ways to accomplish tasks; help the client recognize this and make the appropriate accommodations.

- Provide parents with coping skills when the role change is associated with a critically ill child.
  Mothers who received the Creating Opportunities for Parent Empowerment (COPE) program: (1) provided more support for their child during intrusive procedures; (2) provided more emotional support to their child; (3) reported less negative mood state and less parental stress related to their child's emotions and behaviors; and (4) reported fewer post-traumatic stress symptoms and less parental role change 4 weeks following hospitalization. Results indicate the need to educate parents regarding their children's responses as they recover from critical illness and how they can assist their children in coping with the stressful experience (Melnyk et al, 1997).

- Assist families with life beyond the hospital when living with the illness of a child. Teach family members to value the small things children do, connect with other families, locate community resources, and understand the short- and long-term needs of the child.

- = Independent; ▲ = Collaborative

Family-focused activities can help families cope better with the hospital experience. To promote optimal healing, health care providers must recognize that a family's life goes on after the hospital stay. Many stresses make life difficult for families. Most families are resilient, but many can benefit from help with managing the transition from hospital to home (Worthington, 1995).

- Support client's religious practices.
  Research suggests that religion plays a role in helping clients cope with illness and the outcomes of illness (Koenig, Larson, Larson, 2001).
- Identify ways to compensate for physical disabilities (e.g., have a ramp built to provide access to house, put household objects within client's reach from wheelchair).
  Helping clients to help themselves by modifying the environment enhances self-esteem and fosters a sense of power because they remain able to function in their role.
- See care plans for **Readiness for enhanced family Coping, Impaired Home maintenance, Impaired Parenting, Risk for Loneliness, Readiness for enhanced community Coping,** and **Ineffective Sexuality patterns.**

Geriatric

- Support client's religious beliefs and activities and provide appropriate spiritual support persons.
  The findings from this study suggest that religious coping is a common behavior that is inversely related to depression in hospitalized elderly men (Koenig et al, 1992).
- Encourage the use of humor by family caregivers to describe their role reversal.
  This study suggested that humor is a useful communication tool for family caregivers that releases nervous energy (Bethea, Travis, Pecchioni, 2000).
- Explore community needs after assessing client's strengths. Suggest functional activities (e.g., being a foster grandparent or a mentor for small businesses).
  If physical strength is declining, activities that require less physical prowess and more mental expertise are sometimes appropriate (Ringsven, Bond, 1991).
- ▲ Refer to family counseling as needed for adjustment to role changes.
  The family needs to be helped as a system because a change in one person's role affects the entire family.

Multicultural

- Assess for the influence of cultural beliefs, norms, values, and expectations on the individual's role.
  The individual's role may be based on cultural perceptions (Leininger, 1996).
- Assess for conflicts between the caregiver's cultural role obligations and competing factors like employment.
  Conflicts between cultural expectations and competing factors can increase role stress (Jones, 1996).
- Negotiate with the client regarding the aspects of their role that can be modified and still honor cultural beliefs.
  Give and take with the client will lead to culturally congruent care (Leininger, 1996).
- Encourage family to use support groups or other service programs to assist with role changes.
  Studies indicate that minority families of clients with dementia use few support programs even though these programs could have a positive impact on caregiver well-being (Cox, 1999).

• = Independent; ▲ = Collaborative

- Validate the individual's feelings regarding the impact of role changes on family and personal lifestyle.
  Validation lets the client know that the nurse has heard and understands what was said (Stuart, Laraia, 2001; Giger and Davidhizar, 1995).

Home Care Interventions

- Determine the anticipated duration of role change.
  Knowing the anticipated duration of role change helps the client and significant others determine the acceptability of role change, role conflict, and changes in communication patterns.
- Assess family's ability to physically or psychologically assume responsibilities of decrease or change in client's role function.
  The health, abilities, or other role expectations of caregivers or significant others may prohibit the assumption of responsibilities once held by the client.
- ▲ Offer a referral to medical social services to assist with assessing the short- and long-term impacts of role change.
  Social workers may assist clients with life care planning (Rice, Hicks, Wiehe, 2000). Collaboration with specialists provides the client with greater resources for adaptation. Terminally ill clients may see the transition of role responsibilities as a task that must be completed before dying. Resolution of role transition will reassure the client, allow remaining energy to be focused elsewhere, and may give client permission to die.

Client/Family Teaching

- Teach significant others about health care changes to expect when the client returns home.
  All spouses, male and female, expressed uncertainty about their roles and what their partner could do after discharge (McSweeney, 1993).
- Help client identify resources for assistance in caring for a disabled or aging parent (e.g., adult day care).
  There are varying levels of assistance for the aging clients. Clients and their families need help with identifying these levels.
- ▲ Refer to appropriate community agencies to learn skills for functioning in the new or changed role (e.g., vocational rehabilitation, parenting classes, hospice, respite care).
  As one person changes, other family members need to alter their patterns of communication and behavior to maintain balance. Family members also need assistance with developing these new skills (Barry, 1994).

WEB SITES FOR EDUCATION

MERLIN See the MERLIN web site for World Wide Web resources for client education.

REFERENCES   Barry P: Mental health and mental illness, ed 5, Philadelphia, 1994, JB Lippincott.
Bethea LS, Travis SS, Pecchioni L: Family caregivers' use of humor in conveying information about caring for dependent older adults, *Health Commun* 12(4):361-376, 2000.
Cox C: Race and caregiving: patterns of service use by African American and white caregivers of persons with Alzheimer's, *J Gerontol Soc Work* 32(2):5-19, 1999.
Giger JN, Davidhizar RE: *Transcultural nursing*, ed 2, St Louis, 1995, Mosby.
Gjerdingen D: Expectant parents' anticipated changes in workload after the birth of their first child, *J Fam Pract* 49(11):993-997, 2000.
Jones PS: Asian American women caring for elderly parents, *J Fam Nurs* 2(1):56-75, 1996.

• = **Independent;** ▲ = **Collaborative**

Koenig HG, Larson DB, Larson SS: Religion and coping with serious medical illness, *Ann Pharmacother* 35(3):352-359, 2001.

Koenig H et al: Religious coping and depression among elderly, hospitalized medically ill men, *Am J Psychiatry* 149(12):1693-1700, 1992.

Leininger MM: *Transcultural nursing: theories, research and practices,* ed 2, Hilliard, Ohio, 1996, McGraw-Hill.

McSweeney J: Making behavior changes after a myocardial infarction, *West J Nurs Res* 5:441, 1993.

Melnyk B et al: Helping mothers cope with a critically ill child: a pilot test of the COPE intervention, *Res Nurs Health* 20(1):3-14, 1997.

Nuttin J: Motivation, intention, and volition. In Fleury J, editor: The application of motivational theory to cardiovascular risk reduction, *Image J Nurs Sch* 24:229, 1992.

Rice J, Hicks PB, Wiehe V: Life care planning: a role for social workers, *Soc Work Health Care* 31(1):85-94, 2000.

Ringsven M, Bond D: *Gerontology and leadership skills for nurses,* Albany, NY, 1991, Delmar.

Schwarzer R, Fuchs R: Self-efficacy and health behaviors. In Conner M, Norman P: *Predicting health behaviour: research and practice with social cognition models,* Buckingham, 1995, Open University Press.

Stuart GW, Laraia MT: Therapeutic nurse-patient relationship. In Stuart GW, Laraia MT, editors: *Principles and practice of psychiatric nursing,* St Louis, 2001, Mosby, p 30.

Worthington R: Effective transitions for families: life beyond the hospital, *Pediatr Nurs* 21(1):86-87, 1995.

Bathing/hygiene Self-care deficit

Linda S. Williams

NANDA   **Definition**   Impaired ability to perform or complete bathing/hygiene activities for oneself

Defining Characteristics

Inability to: wash body or body parts; obtain or get to water source; regulate temperature or flow of bath water; get bath supplies; dry body; get in and out of bathroom
Impaired physical mobility-functional level classification:

0   Completely independent
1   Requires use of equipment or device
2   Requires help from another person for assistance, supervision, or teaching
3   Requires help from another person and equipment or device
4   Dependent—does not participate in activity

Related Factors (r/t)

Decreased or lack of motivation; weakness and tiredness; severe anxiety; inability to perceive body part or spatial relationship; perceptual or cognitive impairment; pain; neuromuscular impairment; musculoskeletal impairment; environmental barriers

NOC   **Outcomes (Nursing Outcomes Classification)**

Suggested NOC Labels

Self-Care: Activities of Daily Living (ADLs); Self-Care: Bathing; Self-Care: Hygiene

> **Example NOC Outcome**
> Able to perform **Self-Care: Activities of Daily Living (ADLs)** as evidenced by:
> Bathing/ Hygiene (Rate each indicator of **Self-Care: Activities of Daily Living [ADLs]:** 1 = dependent—does not participate, 2 = requires assistive person and device, 3 = requires assistive person, 4 = independent with assistive device, 5 = completely independent [see Section I])

• = Independent; ▲ = Collaborative

Client Outcomes

- Remains free of body odor and maintains intact skin
- States satisfaction with ability to use adaptive devices to bathe
- Bathes with assistance of caregiver as needed without anxiety
- Explains and uses methods to bathe safely and with minimal difficulty

NIC Interventions (Nursing Interventions Classification)

Suggested NIC Labels

Bathing; Self-Care Assistance: Bathing/Hygiene

> **Example NIC Interventions—Self-Care Assistance: Bathing/Hygiene**
> - Monitor client's ability for independent self-care
> - Provide assistance until client is fully able to assume self-care

Nursing Interventions and Rationales

- Assess client's ability to bathe self through direct observation (in usual bathing setting only) and from client/caregiver report, noting specific deficits and their causes.
  Use of observation of function and report of function provide complementary assessment data for goal and intervention planning (Reuben et al, 1992).
- If in a typical bathing setting for the client, assess via direct observation using physical performance tests for ADLs.
  Observation of bathing performed in an atypical bathing setting may result in false data for which use of a physical performance test compensates to provide more accurate ability data (Guralnik, 1994).
- Ask client for input on bathing habits and cultural bathing preferences.
  Creating opportunities for guiding personal care honors long-standing routines, increases control, prevents learned helplessness, and preserves self-esteem (Miller, 1997). Cultural preferences are respected (Freeman, 1997).
- Develop a bathing care plan based on client's own history of bathing practices that addresses skin needs, self-care needs, client response to bathing and equipment needs.
  Bathing is a healing rite and should not be routinely scheduled with a task focus. It should be a comforting experience for the client that enhances health (Rader, Hoeffer, McKenzie, 1996).
- Individualize bathing by identifying function of bath (e.g., odor or urine removal), frequency required to achieve function, and best bathing form (e.g., towel bathing, tub, or shower) to meet client preferences, preserve client dignity, make bathing a soothing experience, and reduce client aggression.
  Individualized bathing produces a more positive bathing experience and preserves client dignity. Client aggression is increased with shower (especially) and tub bathing. Towel bathing increases privacy and eliminates need to move client to central bathing area; therefore it is a more soothing experience than either showering or tub bathing (Rader, Hoeffer, McKenzie 1996; Hoeffer et al, 1997; Miller, 1997).
- ▲ Request referrals for occupational and physical therapy.
  Collaboration and correlation of activities with interdisciplinary team members increases the client's mastery of self-care tasks (Schemm, Gitlin, 1998).
- Plan activities to prevent fatigue during bathing and seat client with feet supported.
  Energy conservation increases activity tolerance and promotes self-care.
- ▲ Provide medication for pain 45 minutes before bathing if needed.
  Pain relief promotes participation in self-care.

• = Independent; ▲ = Collaborative

- Consider environmental and human factors that may limit bathing ability, such as bending to get into tub, reaching required for bathing items, grasping force needed for faucets, and lifting of self. Adapt environment by placing items within easy reach, lowering faucets, and using a handheld shower.
  Environmental factors affect task performance. Function can be improved based on engineering principles that adapt environmental factors to the meet the client's capabilities (Rogers et al, 1998).
- Use any necessary adaptive bathing equipment (e.g., long-handled brushes, soap-on-a-rope, washcloth mitt, wall bars, tub bench, shower chair, commode chair without pan in shower).
  Adaptive devices extend the client's reach, increase speed and safety, and decrease exertion.
- Provide privacy: have only one caregiver providing bathing assistance, encourage a traffic-free bathing area, and post privacy signs.
  The client perceives less privacy if more than one caregiver participates or if bathing takes place in a central bathing area in a high-traffic location that allows staff to enter freely during care (Miller, 1997).
- Keep client warmly covered.
  Clients, especially elderly clients, who are prone to hypothermia may experience evaporative cooling during and after bathing, which produces an unpleasant cold sensation (Miller, 1997).
- Allow client to participate as able in bathing. Smile and provide praise for accomplishments in a relaxed manner.
  The client's expenditure of energy provides the caregiver the opportunity to convey respect for a well-done task, which increases the client's self-esteem. Smiling and being relaxed are associated with a calm, functional client response (Maxfield et al, 1996).
- Inspect skin condition during bathing.
  Observation of skin allows detection of skin problems.
- Use or encourage caregiver to use an unhurried, caring touch.
  The basic human need of touch offers reassurance and comfort.
- If client is bathing alone, place assistance call light within reach.
  A readily available signaling device promotes safety and provides reassurance for the client.

Geriatric

- Provide same type of bathrobe and bathing articles, such as scented dusting powder and bath oil, that client used previously.
  Use of sensory channels to stimulate memory may help foster understanding of bathing and self-care (Danner et al, 1993).
- Assess for grieving resulting from loss of function.
  Grief resulting from loss of function can inhibit relearning of self-care.
- Arrange bathing environment to promote sensory comfort: reduce noise of voices and water and decrease glare from tiles, white walls, and artificial lights.
  Noise discomfort can result from high-echo tiled walls, loud voices, and running water. Glare can cause visual discomfort, especially in clients with visual changes or cataracts (Miller, 1997).
- When bathing a cognitively impaired client, have all bathing items ready for client's needs before bathing begins.
  Injury often occurs when cognitively impaired client is left alone to obtain forgotten items (Sloane et al, 1995).

• = **Independent;** ▲ = **Collaborative**

- Bathe elderly clients before bedtime to improve sleep.
  An evening bath helps elderly clients sleep better (Kanda, Tochihara, Ohnaka, 1999).
- Bathe cognitively impaired clients before bedtime.
  Bathing a cognitively impaired client in the evening helps improve symptoms of dementia (Deguchi et al, 1999).
- Limit bathing to once or twice a week; provide a partial bath at other times.
  Frequent bathing promotes skin dryness. Reducing frequency of bathing decreases aggressive behavior in cognitively impaired clients (Hoeffer et al, 1997).
- Allow client or caregiver adequate time to complete the bathing activity.
  Significant aging increases the time required to complete a task; therefore elderly individuals with a self-care deficit require more time to complete a task.
- Avoid soap or use only mild soap on genital and axillary areas; rinse well.
  Soap can alter skin pH and thus skin defenses, and it may increase skin dryness that results from decreased oil and perspiration production in the elderly (Skewes, 1997).
- Use tepid water: test water temperature before use with a thermometer.
  Hot water promotes skin dryness and may burn a client with decreased sensation.
- Use a gentle touch when bathing; avoid vigorous scrubbing motions.
  Aging skin is thinner, more fragile, and less able to withstand mechanical friction than younger skin.
- Add hydrating bath oils to tub bath water 15 minutes after client immerses in water.
  Client's skin is coated with oil rather than being hydrated if bath oil is placed in water before client's skin is moistened with water (Skewes, 1997).

Home Care Interventions

- ▲ Based on functional assessment and rehabilitation capacity, refer for home health aide services to assist with bathing and hygiene.
  Support by home health aides preserves the energy of the client and provides respite for caregivers.
- Cue cognitively impaired clients in steps of hygiene.
  Cognitively impaired clients can successfully participate in many activities with cueing, and participation in self-care can enhance their self-esteem.
- Respect the preference of terminally ill clients to refuse or limit hygiene care.
  Maintaining hygiene, even with assistance, may require excessive energy demands from terminally ill clients. Pain on touch or movement may be intractable and not resolved by medication.
- If a terminally ill client requests hygiene care, make an extra effort to meet request and provide care when client and family will most benefit (e.g., before visitors, at bedtime, in the early morning).
  When desired, improved hygiene greatly boosts the morale of terminally ill clients.
- Maintain temperature of home at a comfortable level when providing hygiene care to terminally ill clients.
  Terminally ill clients may have difficulty with thermoregulation, which will add to the energy demand or decrease comfort during hygiene care.

Client/Family Teaching

- Teach client and family how to use adaptive devices for bathing, and teach bathing techniques that promote safety (e.g., getting into tub before filling it with water, emptying water before getting out, using an antislip mat, wall-grab bars, tub bench).
  Adaptive devices can provide independence, safety, and speed (Schemm, Gitlin, 1998).

• = **Independent;** ▲ = **Collaborative**

- Teach client and family an individualized bathing routine that includes a schedule, privacy, skin inspection, soap or lubricant, and chill prevention.
  Teaching methods to meet client's needs increases the client's satisfaction with the bathing experience.

WEB SITES FOR EDUCATION

 See the MERLIN web site for World Wide Web resources for client education.

REFERENCES

Danner C et al: Cognitively impaired elders: using research findings to improve nursing care, *J Gerontol Nurs* 19:5, 1993.

Deguchi A et al: Improving symptoms of senile dementia by a night time spa bathing, *Arch Gerontol Geriatr* 29(3):267-273, 1999.

Freeman E: International perspectives on bathing, *J Gerontol Nurs* 23(5):40-44, 1997.

Guralnik JM: A short physical performance battery assessing lower extremity function: association with self-reported disability and prediction of mortality and nursing home admission, *J Gerontol Med Sci* 49:M85-M94, 1994.

Hoeffer B et al: Reducing aggressive behavior during bathing cognitively impaired nursing home residents, *J Gerontol Nurs* 23(5):16-23, 1997.

Kanda K, Tochihara Y, Ohnaka T: Bathing before sleep in the young and in the elderly, *Eur J Appl Physiol* 80:71-75, 1999.

Maxfield MC et al: Training staff to prevent aggressive behavior of cognitively impaired elderly patients during bathing and grooming, *J Gerontol Nurs* 22(1):37-43, 1996.

Miller M: Physically aggressive resident behavior during hygienic care, *J Gerontol Nurs* 23(5):24-39, 1997.

Rader J, Hoeffer B, McKenzie D: Individualizing the bathing process, *J Gerontol Nurs* 22(3):32-38, 1996.

Reuben DB et al: The predictive validity of self-report and performance-based measures of function and health, *J Gerontol Med Sci* 47:M106, 1992.

Rogers WA et al: Functional limitations to daily living tasks in the aged: a focus group analysis, *Hum Factors* 40(1):111-125, 1998.

Schemm RL, Gitlin LN: How occupational therapists teach older patients to use bathing and dressing devices in rehabilitation, *Am J Occup Ther* 52(4):276-282, 1998.

Skewes S: Bathing: it's a tough job! *J Gerontol Nurs* 23(5):45-49, 1997.

Sloane P et al: Bathing the Alzheimer's patient in long term care: results and recommendation from three studies, *Am J Alzheimers Dis* 10(4):3-11, 1995.

Dressing/grooming Self-care deficit

Linda S. Williams

NANDA **Definition** Impaired ability to perform or complete dressing and grooming activities for self

Defining Characteristics

Impaired ability to put on or take off necessary items of clothing; impaired ability to fasten clothing; impaired ability to obtain or replace articles of clothing; inability to clothe upper body; inability to clothe lower body; inability to choose clothing; inability to use assistive devices; inability to use zippers; inability to remove clothes; inability to put on socks; inability to maintain appearance at a satisfactory level; inability to pick up clothing; inability to put on shoes

- = **Independent;** ▲ = **Collaborative**

Related Factors (r/t)

Decreased or lack of motivation; pain; severe anxiety; perceptual or cognitive impairment; weakness or tiredness; neuromuscular impairment; musculoskeletal impairment; discomfort; environmental barriers

NOTE: See suggested Functional Level Classification in care plan for **Impaired physical Mobility.**

NOC   Outcomes (Nursing Outcomes Classification)

Suggested NOC Labels

Self-Care: Activities of Daily Living (ADLs); Self-Care: Dressing, Self-Care: Grooming; Self-Care: Hygiene

Example NOC Outcome

Able to perform **Self-care: Activities of Daily Living (ADLs)** as evidenced by: Gets clothes from closet and puts on upper body, lower body/Shampoos, combs, brushes hair/Applies makeup (Rate each indicator of **Self-care: Activities of Daily Living [ADLs]:** 1 = dependent—does not participate, 2 = requires assistive person and device, 3 = requires assistive person, 4 = independent with assistive device, 5 = completely independent [see Section I])

Client Outcomes

- Dresses and grooms self to optimal potential
- Uses adaptive devices to dress and groom
- Explains and uses methods to enhance strengths during dressing and grooming
- Dresses and grooms with assistance of caregiver as needed

NIC   Interventions (Nursing Interventions Classification)

Suggested NIC Labels

Dressing; Haircare; Self-Care Assistance: Dressing/Grooming

Example NIC Interventions—Self-Care Assistance: Dressing/Grooming
- Be available for assistance in dressing as necessary
- Reinforce efforts to dress, groom self

Nursing Interventions and Rationales

- Observe client's ability to dress and groom self through direct observation and from client/caregiver report, noting specific deficits and their causes.
  Use of both observation and report of function provides complementary assessment data for goal and intervention planning (Reuben et al, 1992).
- Consider environmental and human factors that may limit dressing/grooming ability, such as reaching for clothes or grooming aids in closets or drawers. Help client arrange clothing and grooming devices within easy reach. Installing turntables and closet rods or drawers between eye and hip level is helpful.
  Environmental factors affect task performance. Function can be improved based on engineering principles that adapt environmental factors to meet the client's capabilities (Rogers et al, 1998).
- Identify and include client's strengths in dressing and grooming to individualize dressing process.

• = Independent; ▲ = Collaborative

Incorporating the client's strengths into a dressing and grooming program increases self-care independence (Vogelpohl et al, 1996).

- Ask client for input on clothing choices and how to increase the ease of dressing.
Providing the client with opportunities for guiding own care increases control and prevents learned helplessness (LeSage et al, 1989).

▲ Request referrals for occupational and physical therapy.
Collaboration and correlation of activities with interdisciplinary team members increases the client's mastery of self-care tasks.

▲ Provide medication for pain 45 minutes before dressing and grooming if needed.
Pain relief promotes participation in self-care.

- Plan activities to prevent fatigue while dressing and grooming.
Energy conservation increases activity tolerance and promotes self-care.

- Provide privacy and limit people/caregivers in room.
Privacy conveys respect and increases dressing ability (Beck et al, 1997).

- Select larger-sized clothing, clothing with elastic waistbands, wide sleeves and pant legs, dresses that open down the back for wheelchair-bound women; and Velcro fasteners or larger buttons.
Simplifying clothing facilitates dressing for those with impaired mobility (Matteson, McConnell, 1997).

- Use adaptive dressing and grooming equipment as needed (e.g., long-handled brushes, grasping devices, Velcro closures, zipper pulls, button hooks, elastic shoe-laces, large buttons, soap-on-a-rope, suction holders).
Adaptive devices increase speed and safety and decrease exertion.

- Lay clothing out in the order that it will be put on by the client. Dress bottom half, then top half of body.
Simplifying dressing tasks increases self-care ability (Beck et al, 1997).

- Encourage client to dress appropriately for time of day.

- Perform dressing and grooming activities in a consistent sequence each day.
An established routine of waking and dressing provides a sense of normalcy and increases motivation to perform self-care. Prolonged repetition promotes increased relearning of self-care tasks (Giles, Shore, 1989). Use verbal prompting to complete dressing task and provide positive reinforcement immediately for accomplished steps of task (Vogelpohl et al, 1996).

- Encourage participation; guide client's hand through task if necessary.
Experiencing the normal process of a task through guided practice facilitates optimal re-learning (Beck et al, 1997).

Geriatric

- Assess for grieving resulting from loss of function.
Grief resulting from loss of function can inhibit relearning of self-care tasks.

- Frequently assess client's pain; provide pain relief as needed before dressing and grooming activities.
Elderly people have twice the incidence of pain of younger people. They often have more than one pain source, which commonly includes arthritis (Acute Pain Management Guideline Panel, 1992).

- Assess tasks client can complete.
Assessing what the client can do decreases caregiver responsibility and allows caregiver to give positive reinforcement to client.

• = Independent; ▲ = Collaborative

- Allow client or caregiver adequate time to complete dressing (e.g., do not insist that client is dressed at an early hour).
  Significant aging increases the time required to complete a task; elderly clients with a self-care deficit require more time than others to complete a task (Matteson, McConnell, 1997).

Home Care Interventions

- ▲ Based on functional assessment and rehabilitation capacity, refer for home health aide services to assist with dressing and grooming.
  Support by home health aides preserves the energy of the client and provides respite for caregivers.
- Cue cognitively impaired clients in steps of dressing and grooming.
  Cognitively impaired clients can participate successfully in many activities with cueing, and participation in self-care can enhance their self-esteem.
- Respect the preference of the terminally ill client to refuse dressing and limit grooming.
  Dressing and grooming, even with assistance, may require excessive energy demands from the terminally ill. Pain on touch or movement may be intractable and not resolved by medication.
- If terminally ill clients request dressing and grooming, make an extra effort to meet request and provide care when client and family will most benefit (e.g., before visitors, in early morning).
  When desired, dressing and grooming are a great boost to the morale of terminally ill clients and their families.
- Maintain the temperature of the home at a comfortable level when dressing terminally ill client.
  Terminally ill clients may have difficulty with thermoregulation, which will add to the energy demand or decrease comfort during hygiene activities.

Client/Family Teaching

- Teach client to dress the affected side first, then the unaffected side.
  Dressing the affected side first allows for easier manipulation of clothing.
- Teach the simplest step in a task until mastered, and then proceed to more complicated steps. Give praise.
  Simplifying dressing and grooming tasks that consist of many small steps promotes mastery (Beck et al, 1997).
- Teach client how to use adaptive devices for dressing and grooming.
  Adaptive devices can provide independence and safety and promote speed.
- Teach client and family to select clothes appropriate for the season, temperature, and weather.
  Clients with altered sensation need to understand the factors that influence body temperature and the environment.

WEB SITES FOR EDUCATION

MERLIN See the MERLIN web site for World Wide Web resources for client education.

REFERENCES   Acute Pain Management Guideline Panel: *Acute pain management: operative or medical procedures and trauma,* Clinical Practice Guideline, Rockville, Md, 1992, Agency for Health Care Policy and Research, Pub No 92-0032, Public Health Service, U.S. Department of Health and Human Services.

• = Independent; ▲ = Collaborative

Beck C et al: Improving dressing behavior in cognitively impaired nursing home residents, *Nurs Res* 46(3):126-132, 1997.

Giles G, Shore M: A rapid method for teaching severely brain injured adults how to wash and dress, *Arch Phys Med Rehabil* 70:156, 1989.

LeSage J et al: Learned helplessness, *J Gerontol Nurs* 15:9, 1989.

Matteson M, McConnell E: *Gerontological nursing,* Philadelphia, 1997, WB Saunders.

Reuben DB et al: The predictive validity of self-report and performance-based measures of function and health, *J Gerontol Med Sci* 47:M106, 1992.

Rogers WA et al: Functional limitations to daily living tasks in the aged: a focus group analysis, *Hum Factors* 40(1):111-125, 1998.

Vogelpohl TS et al: "I can do it!" dressing: promoting independence through individualized strategies, *J Gerontol Nurs* 22(3):39-42, 1996.

Feeding Self-care deficit

Linda S. Williams

NANDA   **Definition** Impaired ability to perform or complete feeding activities

Defining Characteristics

Inability to swallow food; inability to prepare food for ingestion; inability to handle utensils; inability to chew food; inability to use assistive device; inability to get food onto utensils; inability to open containers; inability to ingest food safely; inability to manipulate food in mouth; inability to bring food from a receptacle to the mouth; inability to complete a meal; inability to ingest food in a socially acceptable manner; inability to pick up cup or glass; inability to ingest sufficient food

Related Factors (r/t)

Weakness or tiredness; severe anxiety; neuromuscular impairment; pain; perceptual or cognitive impairment; discomfort; environmental barriers; decreased or lack of motivation; musculoskeletal impairment

NOTE: See suggested Functional Level Classification in the care plan **Impaired physical Mobility.**

NOC   **Outcomes (Nursing Outcomes Classification)**

Suggested NOC Labels

Self-Care: Activities of Daily Living (ADLs); Self-Care: Eating

> **Example NOC Outcome**
> Able to perform **Self-care: Activities of Daily Living (ADLs)** as evidenced by:
> Opens containers/Handles utensils/Completes a meal (Rate each indicator of **Self-care: Activities of Daily Living [ADLs]:** 1 = dependent—does not participate, 2 = requires assistive person and device, 3 = requires assistive person, 4 = independent with assistive device, 5 = completely independent [see Section I])

Client Outcomes

- Feeds self
- States satisfaction with ability to use adaptive devices for feeding
- Provides assistance with feeding when necessary (caregiver)

• = Independent; ▲ = Collaborative

NIC **Interventions (Nursing Interventions Classification)**
Suggested NIC Labels
Feeding; Self-Care Assistance: Feeding

> **Example NIC Interventions—Self-Care Assistance: Feeding**
> - Provide adaptive devices to facilitate client's feeding self (e.g., long handles, handle with large circumference, or small strap on utensils) as needed
> - Provide frequent cueing and close supervision as appropriate

Nursing Interventions and Rationales
- Observe for cause of inability to feed self independently (see Related Factors).
  Self-care requires multisystem competence. Restorative program planning is specific to problems that interfere with self-care (Phaneuf, 1996).
- Assess client's ability to feed self. Test gag reflex bilaterally, and note specific deficits.
  Functional assessment provides ADLs task analysis data for matching client's ability to feed self with caregiver's level of assistance (Van Ort, Phillips, 1995).
- Ask client for input on methods to facilitate eating and feeding (e.g., cultural foods, other food and fluid preferences) and provide four entrée choices, including ethnic choice.
  When clients are given a choice, their food intake increases (Kayser-Jones, 1997).
- ▲ Request referral for occupational and physical therapy; request a dietician.
  Collaboration and correlation of activities with interdisciplinary team members increases the client's mastery of self-care tasks.
- Ensure that client has dentures, hearing aids, and glasses in place.
  Adaptive devices increase opportunity for self-care.
- Use any necessary adaptive feeding equipment (e.g., rocker knives, plate guards, suction mats, built-up handles on utensils, scoop dishes, large-handled cups).
  Adaptive devices increase independence.
- Seat client at table using name card and place mat with meal in visual range next to role model who can eat, if applicable.
  Familiar feeding patterns and cues increase self-feeding (Van Ort, Phillips, 1995).
- Help client into sitting position; ensure that client's head is flexed slightly forward and shoulders are supported while eating and for 1 hour after a meal.
  Gravity assists with swallowing, and aspiration is decreased when sitting upright.
- Prepare meal items before client begins eating.
  Preparing items for the client conserves energy for hand-to-mouth activities.
- Provide small portions of favorite foods, one entrée at a time, at proper serving temperature.
  Food intake is increased when meal appeals to client and is simplified (Kayser-Jones, Schell, 1997).
- Provide consistency in caregiver and meal activities.
  Assigning caregivers to clients rather than dining areas allows caregiver to learn client's needs and promotes a positive attitude between caregiver and client (Kennedy-Holzapfel et al, 1996).
- Caregiver should sit beside client (on client's unaffected side) at eye level.
  Sitting at eye level with client increases eye contact and promotes a relaxed atmosphere that increases consumed food (Kennedy-Holzapfel et al, 1996).

• = Independent; ▲ = Collaborative

- Caregiver should sit at a half circle table if interacting with a group of clients and should remain with clients until meal is completed.
  Environmental strategies that reduce interruptions and distractions increase food intake (Van Ort, Phillips, 1995).
- Encourage participation; guide client's hand through task if needed; provide cues and pantomime desired behaviors.
  Experiencing the normal process of a task through guided practice facilitates optimal re-learning (Tappen, 1994).
- Allow client to participate in feeding as able; provide verbal prompting; provide praise for all feeding attempts; increase tasks as able.
  The client should be an active participant in feeding instead of a passive recipient of food (Osburn, Marshall, 1993).
- Plan activities to prevent fatigue before meals.
  Energy conservation increases activity tolerance and promotes self-care.
- ▲ Provide medication for pain before meals if needed.
  Pain relief promotes participation in self-care.
- Provide client with a pleasant social meal environment. Keep the environment free of toileting devices and odors, avoid painful procedures before meals, remove lids from tray, and provide clean utensils for separate courses.
  Attention to the aesthetics of feeding increases food intake (Kayser-Jones, Schell, 1997).
- Do not mix different foods together when assisting client with eating.
  Mixing foods together decreases client dignity and reduces appeal of food, decreasing food intake (Kayser-Jones, Schell, 1997).
- Play slow-tempo, quiet music during meals.
  Agitated behaviors may communicate anxiety from a noisy, overwhelming environment; quiet music can mask this, resulting in relaxed and smiling clients (Denney, 1997).
- Encourage client to keep food on the unaffected side of mouth with a rocking motion to deposit the food.
  Keeping food away from the affected side of the mouth prevents pocketing of food (Donahue, 1990).
- Be prepared to intervene if choking occurs; have suction equipment readily available and know the Heimlich maneuver.
  Dysphagia increases the risk of choking (Donahue, 1990).
- Provide oral hygiene after eating and check for pocketing of food.
  Aspiration can occur from food left in the mouth.

Geriatric

- Allow client with dentures adequate time to chew.
  Chewing with dentures takes four times longer to reach a certain level of mastication than chewing with natural teeth.
- Choose soft foods rather than liquids, or use dietary thickeners.
  Choking occurs more easily with clear liquids than with solid or soft foods.
- Assess for intolerance to food texture and, if found, reverse food texture pattern as tolerated, progressing finally to texture stage of thick liquids.
  Dementia clients lose ability to tolerate texture-pattern reverses from regular to soft to mechanical soft to mechanical soft with chopped meat to puree to thick liquids, and pocketing of food is seen, along with statements of choking and spitting of food (Boylston et al, 1995).

• = Independent; ▲ = Collaborative

- Provide finger foods for clients with Alzheimer's disease and place in hands as needed to cue.

  Finger foods attract patient attention and increase involvement in meal. They are easier to handle than utensils and, as a result, weight is maintained (Slotesz, Dayton, 1995). Finger foods can be nutritious and can allow independence and the choice of what and when to eat (Kennedy-Holzapfel et al, 1996).

Home Care Interventions

- ▲ Based on functional assessment and rehabilitation capacity, refer for home health aide services to assist with feeding.

  Support by home health aides preserves the energy of the client and provides respite for caregivers.

- Cue cognitively impaired client when feeding.

  Cognitively impaired clients can participate successfully in many activities with cueing. Participation in self-care can enhance the self-esteem of cognitively impaired clients.

- Respect the preference of terminally ill clients to refuse nutrition or assistance with eating. Refer to care plans for **Imbalanced Nutrition: less than body requirements** and **Impaired Swallowing.**

- If terminally ill client requests nutrition, take special care to provide foods and assistive devices that protect the client from aspiration, minimize energy requirements, and meet the client's taste preferences.

  Terminally ill clients have altered taste and other sensations, which impacts their willingness to eat or to invest time or energy in eating.

Client/Family Teaching

- Teach client how to use adaptive devices.

  Adaptive devices increase independence.

- Teach client with hemianopsia to turn head so that the plate is in the line of vision.

  Compensation for hemianopsia is done by turning head to place items in line of vision (Needham, 1993).

- Teach visually impaired client to locate foods according to numbers on a clock.

- Teach caregiver-feeding techniques that prevent choking (e.g., sitting beside client on the unaffected side, feeding client slowly, checking food temperature, providing fluid between bites, establishing a method to communicate readiness for next bite, limiting conversation while chewing).

WEB SITES FOR EDUCATION

See the MERLIN web site for World Wide Web resources for client education.

REFERENCES   Boylston E et al: Increase oral intake in dementia patients by altering food texture, *Am J Alzheimers Dis* 10(6):37-39, 1995.

Denney A: Quiet music: an intervention for mealtime agitation, *J Gerontol Nurs* 23(7):16-23, 1997.

Donahue P: When it's hard to swallow: feeding techniques for dysphagia management, *J Gerontol Nurs* 16:6, 1990.

Kayser-Jones J: Inadequate staffing at mealtime: implications for nursing and health policy, *J Gerontol Nurs* 23(8):4-21, 1997.

Kayser-Jones J, Schell E: The mealtime experience of a cognitively impaired elder: ineffective and effective strategies, *J Gerontol Nurs* 23(7):33, 1997.

Kennedy-Holzapfel S et al: Feeder position and food and fluid consumed by nursing home residents, *J Gerontol Nurs* 22(4):6-12, 1996.

Needham J: *Gerontological nursing: a restorative approach,* Albany, NY, 1993, Delmar.

• = **Independent;** ▲ = **Collaborative**

Osburn C, Marshall M: Self-feeding performance in nursing home residents, *J Gerontol Nurs* 19:7, 1993.

Phaneuf C: Screening elders for nutritional deficits, *Am J Nurs* 96:58, 1996.

Slotesz KS, Dayton JH: The effects of menu modification to increase dietary intake and maintain the weight of Alzheimer's residents, *Am J Alzheimers Dis* 10(6):20-23, 1995.

Tappen R: The effect of skill training on functional abilities of nursing home residents with dementia, *Res Nurs Health* 17:159, 1994.

Van Ort S, Phillips L: Nursing interventions to promote functional feeding, *J Gerontol Nurs* 21:6, 1995.

Toileting Self-care deficit

Linda S. Williams

NANDA **Definition** Impaired ability to perform or complete own toileting activities

Defining Characteristics
Inability to get to toilet or commode; inability to sit on or rise from toilet or commode; inability to manipulate clothing for toileting; inability to carry out proper toilet hygiene; inability to flush toilet or commode

Related Factors (r/t)
Environmental barriers; weakness or tiredness; decreased or lack of motivation; severe anxiety; impaired mobility status; impaired transfer ability; musculoskeletal impairment; neuromuscular impairment; pain; perceptual or cognitive impairment

NOTE: See suggested Functional Level Classification in care plan for **Impaired physical Mobility.**

NOC **Outcomes (Nursing Outcomes Classification)**
Suggested NOC Labels
Self-Care: Activities of Daily Living (ADLs); Self-Care: Toileting

> **Example NOC Outcome**
> Able to perform **Self-care: Activities of Daily Living (ADLs)** as evidenced by: Recognizes and responds to a full bladder and urge to have a bowel movement/Gets to and from toilet (Rate each indicator of **Self-care: Activities of Daily Living [ADLs]:** 1 = dependent—does not participate, 2 = requires assistive person and device, 3 = requires assistive person, 4 = independent with assistive device, 5 = completely independent [see Section I])

Client Outcomes
- Remains free of incontinence and impaction with no urine or stool on skin
- States satisfaction with ability to use adaptive devices for toileting
- Explains and uses methods to be safe and independent in toileting

NIC **Interventions (Nursing Interventions Classification)**
Suggested NIC Labels
Environmental Management; Self-Care Assistance: Toileting

> **Example NIC Interventions—Self-Care Assistance: Toileting**
> - Assist client to toilet/commode/bedpan/fracture pan/urinal at specified intervals
> - Institute a toileting schedule as appropriate

• = **Independent;** ▲ = **Collaborative**

Nursing Interventions and Rationales

- Observe cause of inability to toilet independently (see Related Factors).
  Self-care requires multisystem competence. Restorative program planning is specific to problems that interfere with self-care.
- Assess ability to toilet; note specific deficits.
  Functional assessment provides analysis data for ADLs tasks for use in goal and intervention planning.
- Ask client for input on toileting methods and timing and how to better provide toileting activity assistance.
  Providing the client with opportunities for guiding own care increases control and prevents learned helplessness (LeSage et al, 1989).
- Assess client's usual bowel and bladder toileting patterns and the terminology used for toileting.
  Individuals develop a unique pattern of toileting over time for faster, normal elimination.
- ▲ Request referral for occupational and physical therapy for help in working with client to transfer from bed to commode.
  Collaboration and correlation of activities with interdisciplinary team members increases the client's mastery of self-care tasks.
- Use any necessary assistive toileting equipment (e.g., raised toilet seat, suction mats, spill-proof urinals, support rails next to toilet, toilet safety frames, Sanifems [allows a woman to void standing], fracture bedpans, long-handled toilet paper holders).
  Adaptive devices promote independence and safety.
- Provide privacy.
  Privacy can prevent suppression of elimination resulting from embarrassment about noise and odor.
- Develop toileting schedule using clocks, written schedules, or verbal prompting as cues for client.
  Toileting schedules convey that continence is valued. Toileting rounds reduce incontinence (Matteson, McConnell, 1997).
- Schedule toileting to occur when defecation urge is strongest or voiding is likely (e.g., in the morning, every 2 hours, after meals, at bedtime). Assist client until self-care ability increases.
  The defecation urge is strongest in the morning or within 1 hour after meals or warm beverages. Approximately 50 to 75 ml of urine is produced hourly, and the urge to void occurs when 200 ml has accumulated. Therefore a 2-hour schedule can reduce incontinence.
- Allow client to participate as able in toileting, and provide praise for accomplishments. Increase tasks as client is able, and work with client to aim toward independence in toileting.
  Client's expenditure of energy provides caregiver the opportunity to convey respect for a well done task, which increases self-esteem.
- Obtain a bedside commode if necessary and adapt it for client's needs; avoid bedpans if possible. If client is acutely ill, provide bedpan at appropriate intervals.
  A sitting position uses gravity and is more conducive to normal elimination than a lying position.
- Make assistance call button readily available to client and answer call light promptly.
  To decrease incontinence, the client needs rapid access to toileting facilities.
- Assess and remove physical barriers to toilet, such as cluttered walkways.

• = Independent; ▲ = Collaborative

Environmental assessment identifies barriers that can increase incontinence episodes (Penn et al, 1996).

- Keep toilet paper and hand-washing items within easy reach of client.
- Inspect skin condition.
  Observation of skin allows detection of skin problems.
- Provide prompt skin care and linen changes after incontinence episodes.
  The presence of urine or stool on the skin leads to skin breakdown.

Geriatric

- Monitor clients with dementia for behavioral toileting cues (e.g., pacing, restlessness, fidgeting) and assist with prompt toileting, or use an individualized scheduled toileting for memory impaired elderly.
  Assisting clients promptly when toileting cues are observed can reduce toileting accidents and the resulting upsetting client reactions that occur (Hutchinson, Leger-Krall, Wilson, 1996). An individual toileting schedule helps prevent incontinence in moderately cognitively impaired elders (Jirovec, Templin, 2001).
- Assess client's mobility status and speed of movement.
  Elderly women with slower mobility have more incontinent episodes than others (Wyman, Eiswick, 1993).
- Reassure client that call light will be answered promptly.
  The elderly cannot respond quickly to the urge to void because of limited functional ability and environmental barriers; they are also unable to delay voiding because of decreased muscle tone and neurological changes (Palmer, 1994).
- Provide a small footstool in front of toilet or commode.
  Intraabdominal pressure is increased by elevating knees above the hips, which facilitates elimination in elderly persons with weak abdominal muscles.
- Assess client's functional ability to manipulate clothing for toileting. If necessary, modify clothing with Velcro fasteners and elastic waists.
  Delays caused by having to manipulate zippers and buttons may cause functional incontinence (Penn et al, 1996).
- Avoid use of indwelling or condom catheters if possible.
  An indwelling urinary catheter is a source of infection and keeps the bladder empty, which reduces bladder capacity and decreases the opportunity for independent toileting.

Home Care Interventions

- ▲ Based on functional assessment and rehabilitation capacity, refer for home health aide services to assist with toileting.
  Support by home health aides preserves the energy of the client and provides respite for caregivers.
- Cue cognitively impaired clients in steps of toileting.
  Cognitively impaired persons can participate successfully in many activities with cueing, and participation in self-care can enhance their self-esteem.
- ▲ Avoid the use of medications that place undue toileting stress on the client who is terminally ill.
- ▲ Provide pain medication for terminally ill clients 20 to 45 minutes before toileting in anticipation of possible pain (e.g., in coordination with a bowel stimulation program). See care plan for **Constipation.**
  Pain from touch or movement may be intractable and not resolved by medication, but medication may decrease the pain enough to allow limited movement and passing of stool.

• = **Independent;** ▲ = **Collaborative**

▲ Consider use of an indwelling catheter when terminally ill clients are in too much pain to move and hygiene and skin integrity are difficult to maintain.
The goal of hospice care is to promote comfort and dignity in the dying process.

Client/Family Teaching

• Teach client and family how to toilet client with adaptive and safety devices.
Adaptive devices can provide independence and safety and promote speed.

▲ Prepare client for toileting needs by teaching the action of medications such as diuretics.
Medications that promote elimination require prompt responses to toileting needs.

• Help the visually impaired client to develop a plan for locating bathrooms in new environments.
Clients with visually impairments may find locating bathrooms in unfamiliar settings difficult, causing a toileting self-care deficit (Matteson, McConnell, 1997).

WEB SITES FOR EDUCATION

MERLIN See the MERLIN web site for World Wide Web resources for client education.

REFERENCES Hutchinson S, Leger-Krall S, Wilson HS: Toileting: a biobehavioral challenge in Alzheimer's dementia care, *J Gerontol Nurs* 22(10):18-27, 1996.

Jirovec MM, Templin T: Predicting success using individualized scheduled toileting for memory-impaired elders at home, *Res Nurs Health* 24:1-8, 2001.

LeSage J et al: Learned helplessness, *J Gerontol Nurs* 15:9, 1989.

Matteson M, McConnell E: *Gerontological nursing,* Philadelphia, 1997, WB Saunders.

Palmer M: Level 1: basic assessment and management of urinary incontinence in nursing homes, *Nurs Pract Forum* 5:152, 1994.

Penn C et al: Assessment of urinary incontinence, *J Gerontol Nurs* 22:8, 1996.

Wyman J, Eiswick R: Influence of functional, urological, and environmental characteristics on urinary incontinence in community-dwelling older women, *Nurs Res* 42:270, 1993.

Chronic low Self-esteem

Helen Kelley and Judith R. Gentz

NANDA **Definition** Long-standing negative self-evaluations/feelings about self or self-capabilities

Defining Characteristics

Rationalizes away/rejects positive feedback and exaggerates negative feedback about self (long-standing or chronic); self-negating verbalization (long-standing or chronic); hesitant to try new things/situations (long-standing or chronic); expressions of shame/guilt (long-standing or chronic); evaluates self as unable to deal with events (long-standing or chronic); lack of eye contact; nonassertive/passive; frequent lack of success in work or other life events; excessively seeks reassurance; overly conforming, dependent on others' opinions; indecisive

Related Factors (r/t)

To be developed

• = Independent; ▲ = Collaborative

NOC **Outcomes (Nursing Outcomes Classification)**
Suggested NOC Labels
Self-Esteem

> ### Example NOC Outcome
> Demonstrates **Self-Esteem** as evidenced by: Verbalizations of acceptance of self and limitations/Open communication (Rate each indicator of **Self-Esteem:** 1 = never positive, 2 = rarely positive, 3 = sometimes positive, 4 = often positive, 5 = consistently positive [see Section I])

Client Outcomes

- Demonstrates improved ability to interact with others (e.g., maintains eye contact, expresses feelings)
- Verbalizes increased self-acceptance through use of positive self-statements
- Identifies personal strengths
- Sets small, achievable goals
- Attempts independent decision-making

NIC **Interventions (Nursing Interventions Classification)**
Suggested NIC Labels
Self-Esteem Enhancement

> ### Example NIC Interventions—Self-Esteem Enhancement
> - Encourage client to identify strengths
> - Assist client in setting realistic goals to achieve higher self-esteem

Nursing Interventions and Rationales

- Actively listen to and respect the client.
  An attentive attitude conveys acceptance (Norris, 1992).
- Assist client with identifying and confronting problems of not valuing self or enduring abuse from others.
  Tolerance of abusive or violent behavior may be developed over time (Norris, 1992).
- Assess existing strengths and coping abilities, and provide opportunities for their expression and recognition.
  Self-esteem is enhanced by the ability to perform competently (Coopersmith, 1981).
- Reinforce the personal strengths and positive self-perceptions that client identifies.
  This is effective in enhancing global self-worth (Manus, Killeen, 1995).
- Identify and limit client's negative self-assessments.
  Limitations disrupt the pattern of negative distortion (Mynatt, 1998).
- Encourage realistic and achievable goal setting; recognize the value of attempts and accomplishments.
  Reframe failures as opportunities to learn and change tactics (Mynatt, 1998).
- Demonstrate and promote effective communication techniques.
  Effective communication increases the opportunity to receive positive validation from others (Maynard, 1993).
- Encourage independent decision-making by reviewing options and their possible consequences with client.
  Autonomy enhances self-esteem (Crouch, Straub, 1983).

• = Independent; ▲ = Collaborative

- Assist client to challenge negative perceptions of self and performance.
  Reduction in negative thinking is correlated with increase in self-esteem (Peden et al, 2000).
- Use failure as an opportunity to provide valuable feedback (Grainger, 1991).
- Promote a positive environment and activities that enhance self-esteem.
  Self-esteem is positively correlated with the ability to meet self-care requirements (Connelly, 1993; Bailey, 1992).
- Assist client with evaluating the impact of family and peer group on feelings of self-worth.
  Peer group and family may be factors in reinforcing feeling of guilt, blame, and shame (Bennett, 1995).
- Support socialization and communication skills.
  Socialization increases opportunities for support and validation from others (Maynard, 1993).
- Help client to identify a range of feelings in response to situations.
  Shame is decreased when acceptance of all feelings occurs (Merritt, 1997).
- Help client to increase sense of belonging.
  A sense of belonging reduces vulnerability to depression, effecting self-esteem (Hagerty, Williams, 1999).

Geriatric

- Support client in identifying and adapting to functional changes.
  Accurate evaluation allows client to establish realistic expectations of self.
- Use reminiscence therapy to identify patterns of strength and accomplishment.
  Identifying strengths and accomplishments counteracts pervasive negativity.
- Encourage participation in peer group activities.
  Withdrawal and social isolation are detrimental to feelings of self-worth.
- Encourage activities in which client can support/help others.
  Helping others increases self-esteem in older adults. (Krause, Shaw, 2000).

Multicultural

- Assess for the influence of cultural beliefs, norms, and values on the client's sense of self esteem.
  How the client values self may be based on cultural perceptions (Leininger, 1996).
- Validate the client's feelings regarding ethnic or racial identity.
  Validation lets the client know that the nurse has heard and understands what was said, and it promotes the nurse-client relationship (Stuart, Laraia, 2001; Giger, Davidhizar, 1995). Individuals with strong ethnic affiliation have higher levels of self-esteem than others (Phinney, 1995).

Home Care Interventions

- Assess client's immediate support system/family for relationship patterns and content of communication.
  Knowledge of client relationships helps the nurse to individualize care.
- Encourage family to provide support and feedback regarding client value or worth.
  The family is a socially significant cultural group that generates behavior, defines roles, and promotes values.
- ▲ Refer to medical social services to assist the family in pattern changes that could benefit the client.
  The best nursing plan may be to access specialty services for the client and family.
- ▲ If client is involved in counseling or self-help groups, monitor and encourage attendance. Help client identify value of group participation after each group encounter.
  Discussion about group participation clarifies and reinforces group feedback and support.

- = **Independent;** ▲ = **Collaborative**

▲ If client is taking prescribed psychotropic medications, assess for knowledge of medication side effects and reasons for taking medication. Teach as necessary.
Understanding the medical regimen supports compliance.

▲ Assess medications for effectiveness and side effects and monitor client for compliance.
Clients with poor ego strength may have difficulty adhering to a medication regimen. Clients who experience negative side effects are less likely than others to adhere to medication regimen.

Client/Family Teaching

▲ Refer to community agencies for psychotherapeutic counseling.

▲ Refer to psychoeducational groups on stress reduction and coping skills.

▲ Refer to self-help support groups specific to needs.

WEB SITES FOR EDUCATION

 See the MERLIN web site for World Wide Web resources for client education.

REFERENCES Bailey BJ: Meditators of depression in adults with diabetes, *Clin Nurs Res* 5:28, 1992.
Bennett LA: Accountability for alcoholism in American families, *Soc Sci Med* 40:15, 1995.
Connelly CE: An empirical study of a model of self-care in chronic illness, *Clin Nurs Spec* 7:247, 1993.
Coopersmith S: *The antecedents of self-esteem*, Palo Alto, Calif, 1981, Consulting Psychologist Press.
Crouch MA, Straub V: Enhancement of self-esteem in adults, *Fam Comm Health* 6:65, 1983.
Giger JN, Davidhizar RE: *Transcultural nursing*, ed 2, St Louis, 1995, Mosby.
Grainger RD: Dealing with feelings of guilt and shame, *Am J Nurs* 9:12, 1991.
Hagerty B, Williams R: The effects of sense of belonging, social support, conflict and loneliness on depression, *Nurs Res* 48:4, 1999.
Krause N, Shaw BA. Giving social support to others: socioeconomic status and self-esteem in late life, *J Gerontol B Psychol Sci Soc Sci* 55:11, 2000.
Leininger MM: *Transcultural nursing: theories, research and practices*, ed 2, Hilliard, Ohio, 1996, McGraw-Hill.
Manus HE, Killeen MR: Maintenance of self-esteem by obese children, *J Child Adolescent Psych Nurs* 8:17, 1995.
Maynard C: Psychoeducational approach to depression in women, *J Psychosoc Nurs Ment Health Serv* 31:12, 1993.
Merritt P: Guilt and shame in recovering addicts: a personal account, *J Psychosoc Nurs Ment Health Serv* 35:7, 1997.
Mynatt S: Increasing resiliency to substance abuse in recovering women with comorbid depression, *J Psychosoc Nurs Ment Health Serv* 36:1, 1998.
Norris J: Nursing interventions for self-esteem disturbance, *Nurs Diagn* 3:48, 1992.
Peden A et al: Reducing negative thinking and depressive symptoms in college women, *J Nurs Scholarsh* 32:2, 2000.
Phinney JS: Ethnic identity and self-esteem. In Padilla A, editor: *Hispanic psychology: critical issues in theory and research*, Thousand Oaks, Calif, 1995, Sage.
Stuart GW, Laraia MT: Therapeutic nurse-patient relationship. In Stuart GW, Laraia MT, editors: *Principles and practice of psychiatric nursing*, St Louis, 2001, Mosby, p 30.

Situational low Self-esteem

Helen Kelley and Judith R. Gentz

NANDA **Definition** Development of a negative perception of self-worth in response to a current situation (specify)

Defining Characteristics

Verbally reports current situational challenge to self-worth; self-negating verbalizations; indecisive, nonassertive behavior; evaluation of self as unable to deal with situations or events; expressions of helplessness and uselessness

• = **Independent;** ▲ = **Collaborative**

Related Factors (r/t)

Developmental changes (specify); disturbed body image; functional impairment (specify); loss (specify); social role changes (specify); lack of recognition/rewards; behavior inconsistent with values; failures/rejections

NOC   Outcomes (Nursing Outcomes Classification)

Suggested NOC Labels

Decision Making; Self-Esteem

> **Example NOC Outcome**
>
> Demonstrates **Self-Esteem** as evidenced by: Verbalizations of acceptance of self and limitations/Open communication (Rate each indicator of **Self-Esteem:** 1 = never positive, 2 = rarely positive, 3 = sometimes positive, 4 = often positive, 5 = consistently positive [see Section I])

Client Outcomes

- States effect of life events on feelings about self
- Recognizes personal strengths
- Acknowledges presence of guilt and does not blame self if an action was related to another person's appraisal
- Seeks help when necessary
- Self-perceptions are accurate given physical capabilities
- Separation of self-perceptions from societal stigmas

NIC   Interventions (Nursing Interventions Classification)

Suggested NIC Labels

Self-Esteem Enhancement

> **Example NIC Interventions—Self-Esteem Enhancement**
> - Encourage client to identify strengths
> - Assist client in setting realistic goals to achieve higher self-esteem

Nursing Interventions and Rationales

- Actively listen to, demonstrate respect for, and accept client.
  Clarification of thoughts and feelings promotes self-acceptance (LeMone, 1991).
- Assist in the identification of problems and situational factors that contribute to problems.
  Identification validates problems.
- Use statements such as, "No one can make you feel guilty without your consent," to help client recognize that no one else can control client's feelings.
- Mutually identify strengths, resources, and previously effective coping strategies.
  Acknowledgment of competence enhances self-esteem (Miller, 1983) and reinforces previously intact self-esteem (Anderson, 1995).
- Have client list strengths.
- Accept client's own pace in working through grief or crisis situations.
  Pressuring the client to prematurely resolve feelings increases the client's sense of inadequacy (Kus, 1985). Maladjustment to loss or change can have detrimental effects on the entire concept of self (Drench, 1994).
- Accept the client's own defenses in dealing with the crisis.

- = **Independent;** ▲ = **Collaborative**

Denial protects the self-concept by distorting reality in a self-enhancing way (Russell, 1993).

- Assess for unhealthy coping mechanisms such as substance abuse.
Low self-esteem in adolescents has been linked to health risk behaviors (Modrcin-Talbott et al, 1998).

▲ Assess client for symptoms of depression and potential for suicide or violence. If present, immediately notify appropriate personnel of symptoms. See care plans for **Risk for other-directed Violence** and/or **Risk for self-directed Violence.**
Safety measures and psychiatric interventions are essential when there is a risk of violence. Coping attempts may be ineffective during time of crisis.

▲ Provide information about support groups of people who have common experiences or interests.
Support groups provide an opportunity to both give and receive support and understanding. Social support is a significant predictor of self-esteem (Dirsken, 2000).

- Support problem-solving strategies but discourage decision-making when in crisis.
Crisis is a time of increased tension and disorganization.

- Explore constructive outlets for frustration.
Exploration expands strategies for coping.

- Encourage objective appraisal of self and life events and challenge negative or perfectionistic expectations of self.
A positive adjustment to illness may be the result of the ability to lower ideal self-expectations (Heidrich, Ward, 1992).

- Validate confusion when feeling ill but looking well.
Validation will decrease shame and guilt, and invites further verbalization (Gordon et al, 1998).

- Acknowledge the presence of societal stigma. Teach management tools.
Health promotion requires modification of stigmas (O'Brien, 1998).

- Validate the impact of past experiences on self-esteem and work on corrective measures.
Family dysfunction, child abuse, and other childhood stressors may lead to low self-esteem. (Harter, 2000).

- See care plan for **Chronic low Self-esteem.**

Multicultural

- Assess for the influence of cultural beliefs, norms, and values on the client's sense of self-esteem.
How the client values self may be based on cultural perceptions (Leininger, 1996).

- Validate the client's feelings regarding ethnic or racial identity.
Validation lets the client know that the nurse has heard and understands what was said, and it promotes the nurse-client relationship (Stuart, Laraia, 2001; Giger, Davidhizar, 1995). Individuals with strong ethnic affiliation have higher levels of self-esteem than others (Phinney, 1995).

Home Care Interventions

- Establish an emergency plan and contract with the client for its use.
Having an emergency plan is reassuring to the client. Establishing a contract validates the worth of the client and provides a caring link between the client and society.

- Access supplies that support client's success at independent living.

- See care plan for **Chronic low Self-esteem.**

- **= Independent; ▲ = Collaborative**

Client/Family Teaching

- Assess person's support system (family, friends, community) and involve if desired.
- Educate client and family regarding the grief process.
  Understanding this process normalizes responses of sadness, anger, guilt, and helplessness.
- Teach client and family that the crisis is temporary.
  Knowing that the crisis is temporary provides a sense of hope for the future.
- ▲ Refer to appropriate community resources or crisis intervention centers.
- ▲ Refer to resources for handicap and/or disability services.
- ▲ Refer to illness-specific consumer support groups.
- ▲ Refer to self-help support groups specific to needs.

WEB SITES FOR EDUCATION

 See the MERLIN web site for World Wide Web resources for client education.

REFERENCES   Anderson K: The effect of chronic obstructive pulmonary disease on quality of life, *Res Nurs Health* 18:547, 1995.

Dirsken SR: Predicting well being among breast cancer survivors, *J Adv Nurs* 32:4, 2000.

Drench ME: Changes in body image secondary to disease and injury, *Rehabil Nurs* 19:31, 1994.

Giger JN, Davidhizar RE: *Transcultural nursing*, ed 2, St Louis, 1995, Mosby.

Gordon P et al: The meaning of disability: how women with chronic illness view their experiences, *J Rehabil* 64:3, 1998.

Harter SL: Psychosocial adjustment of adult children of alcoholics, *Clin Psychol Rev* 20:3, 2000.

Heidrich SM, Ward SE: The role of the self in adjustment to cancer in elderly women, *Oncol Nurs Forum* 19:1491, 1992.

Kus RJ: Crisis intervention. In Bulechek GM, McCloskey JC, editors: *Nursing interventions: treatments for nursing diagnoses,* Philadelphia, 1985, WB Saunders.

Leininger MM: *Transcultural nursing: theories, research and practices,* ed 2, Hilliard, Ohio, 1996, McGraw-Hill.

LeMone P: Analysis of a human phenomenon: self-concept, *Nurs Diagn* 2:126, 1991.

Miller JF: *Coping with chronic illness: overcoming powerlessness,* Philadelphia, 1983, FA Davis.

Modrcin-Talbott MA et al: A study of self-esteem among well adolescents: seeking a new direction, *Issues Compr Pediatr Nurs* 21:4, 1998.

O'Brien SM: Health promotion and schizophrenia: the year 2000 and beyond, *Holistic Nurs Pract* 12:2, 1998.

Phinney JS: Ethnic identity and self-esteem. In Padilla A, editor: *Hispanic psychology: critical issues in theory and research,* Thousand Oaks, Calif, 1995, Sage.

Russell GC: The role of denial in clinical practice, *J Adv Nurs* 18:938, 1993.

Stuart GW, Laraia MT: Therapeutic nurse-patient relationship. In Stuart GW, Laraia MT, editors: *Principles and practice of psychiatric nursing,* St Louis, 2001, Mosby, p 30.

Risk for situational low Self-esteem

Judith R. Gentz

NANDA   **Definition**   At risk for developing negative perception of self-worth in response to a current situation (specify)

Risk Factors

Developmental changes (specify); disturbed body image; functional impairment (specify); loss (specify); social role changes (specify); history of learned helplessness; history of abuse, neglect, or abandonment; unrealistic self-expectations; behavior incon-

• = Independent; ▲ = Collaborative

sistent with values; lack of recognition/rewards; failures/rejections; decreased power/control over environment; physical illness (specify)

NOC **Outcomes (Nursing Outcomes Classification)**

Suggested NOC Labels

Decision-Making; Self-Esteem

Example NOC Outcome

Demonstrates **Self-Esteem** as evidenced by: Verbalizations of acceptance of self and limitations/Open communication (Rate each indicator of **Self-Esteem:** 1 = never positive, 2 = rarely positive, 3 = sometimes positive, 4 = often positive, 5 = consistently positive [see Section I])

Client Outcomes

- Accurate self-appraisal
- Ability to self-validate
- Ability to make decisions independent of primary peer group
- Recognizes effects of media on self-appraisal
- Recognizes influence of substances on self-esteem
- Identifies strengths and healthy coping skills
- Recognizes life events and change as influencing self-esteem

NIC **Interventions (Nursing Interventions Classification)**

Suggested NIC Labels

Self-Esteem Enhancement

Example NIC Interventions—Self-Esteem Enhancement

- Encourage client to identify strengths
- Help client to set realistic goals to achieve higher self-esteem

Nursing Interventions and Rationales

- Help client to identify environmental factors which increase risk for low self-esteem.
  Identification is early stage of problem solving process.
- Help client to identify current behaviors resulting from low self-esteem.
  Low self-esteem increases risk for unhealthy behaviors (Mcgee, Williams, 2000).
- Encourage creative problem solving through writing exercises.
  Using creative writing, allowing clients to "tell their story." Giving positive feedback can increase self-esteem (Chandler, 1999).
- Encourage client to maintain highest level of functioning, including work schedule.
  Positive self-esteem is maintained at higher levels in working individuals than in non-working individuals (VanDongen, 1998).
- Encourage client to verbalize thoughts and feelings about the current situation.
  Allowing the client to clarify thoughts and feelings promotes self-acceptance (LeMone, 1991).
- Help the client to identify what has helped maintain positive self-esteem thus far.
  Identifying what works empowers the client and encourages positive outcomes.
- Help the client to identify the resources and social support network available to them at this time.
  Resourcefulness and social support are significant predictors of self-esteem (Dirksen, 2000).

• = **Independent;** ▲ = **Collaborative**

- Encourage the client to find a self-help or therapy group that focuses on self-esteem enhancement.
  Improved self-esteem of such group members is reported (Hakim-Larson, Mruk, 1997).
- Encourage the client to create a sense of competence through short-term goal setting and goal achievement.
  Sense of competence is related to global self-esteem (Willoughby et al, 2000).
- Educate female clients about self-esteem differences between genders, and encourage exploration.
  Females tend to have lower self-esteem than males no matter what domain is measured (Bolognini et al, 1996).
▲ Assess the client for symptoms of depression and anxiety. Refer to specialist as needed.
  Prompt and effective treatment can prevent exacerbation of symptoms or safety risks.
- Teach client a systematic problem-solving process.
  Crisis provides an opportunity for effective change in coping skills.
- See care plans for **Disturbed personal Identity** and **Situational low Self-esteem.**

Geriatric

- Help the client to identify age-related and/or developmental factors which may be affecting self-esteem.
  Self-esteem levels vary with the normal aging process and tend to decrease with older age (Dietz, 1996).
- Assist the client in life review and identifying positive accomplishments.
  Life review is a developmental task that increases a person's sense of peace and serenity.
- Help client to establish a peer group and structured daily activities.
  Social isolation and lack of structure increase a client's sense of feeling lost and worthless.

Home Care Interventions

- Assess current environmental stresses and identify community resources.
  Accessing resources to help decrease environmental stress will increase the client's ability to cope.
- Encourage family members to acknowledge and validate the client's strengths.
  Validation allows the client to increase self-reliance and to trust personal decisions.
- Assess the need for establishing an emergency plan.
  Openly assessing safety risks increases the client's sense of limits, boundaries, and safety.
- See care plans for **Situational low Self-esteem** and **Chronic low Self-esteem.**

Client/Family Teaching

▲ Refer the client/family to community-based self-help and support groups.
▲ Refer to educational classes on stress management, relaxation training, etc.
▲ Refer to community agencies that offer support and environmental resources.

WEB SITES FOR EDUCATION

MERLIN See the MERLIN web site for World Wide Web resources for client education.

REFERENCES   Bolognini M et al: Self-esteem and mental health in early adolescence: developmental and gender differences, *J Adolescence* 3:19, 1996.
Chandler GE: A creative writing program to enhance self-esteem and self-efficacy in adolescence, *J Child Adolesc Psychiatr Nurs* 2:12, 1999.
Dietz BE: The relationship of aging to self-esteem: the relative effects of maturation and role accumulation, *Int J Aging Hum Dev* 3:43, 1996.
Dirksen SR: Predicting well being among breast cancer survivors, *J Adv Nurs* 4:32, 2000.

• = Independent; ▲ = Collaborative

Hakim-Larson J, Mruk C: Enhancing self-esteem in community mental health setting, *Am J Orthopsychiatry* 4:67, 1997.

LeMone P: Analysis of a human phenomenon: self-concept, *Nurs Diagn* 2:126, 1991.

Mcgee R, Williams S: Does low self-esteem predict health compromising behaviours among adolescents? *J Adolesc* 5:23, 2000.

VanDongen CJ: Self-esteem among persons with severe mental illness, *Issues Ment Health Nurs* 1:19, 1998.

Willoughby C et al: Measuring the self-esteem of adolescents with mental health problems: theory meets practice, *Can J Occup Ther* 4:67, 2000.

Self-mutilation

Gail B. Ladwig

NANDA   **Definition**   Deliberate self-injurious behavior causing tissue damage with the intent of causing nonfatal injury to attain relief of tension

Defining Characteristics

Cuts/scratches on body; picking at wounds; self-inflicted burns (e.g., eraser, cigarette); ingestion/inhalation of harmful substances/objects; biting; abrading; severing; insertion of object(s) into body orifice(s); hitting; constricting a body part

Related Factors (r/t)

Psychotic state (command hallucinations); inability to express tension verbally; childhood sexual abuse; violence between parental figures; family divorce; family alcoholism; family history of self-destructive behaviors; adolescence; peers who self-mutilate; isolation from peers; perfectionism; substance abuse; eating disorders; sexual identity crisis; low or unstable self-esteem; low or unstable body image; labile behavior (mood swings); history of inability to plan solutions or see long-term consequences; use of manipulation to obtain nurturing relationship with others; chaotic/disturbed interpersonal relationships; emotionally disturbed; battered child; feels threatened with actual or potential loss of significant relationship (e.g., loss of parent/parental relationship); experiences dissociation or depersonalization; mounting tension that is intolerable; impulsivity; inadequate coping; irresistible urge to cut/damage self; needs quick reduction of stress; childhood illness or surgery; foster, group, or institutional care; incarceration; character disorder; borderline personality disorder; developmentally delayed or autistic individual; history of self-injurious behavior; feelings of depression, rejection, self-hatred, separation anxiety, guilt, depersonalization; poor parent-adolescent communication; lack of family confidant

NOC   **Outcomes (Nursing Outcomes Classification)**

Suggested NOC Labels

Aggression Control; Impulse Control; Risk Detection; Self-Mutilation Restraint

> **Example NOC Outcome**
> Accomplishes **Self-mutilation Restraint** as evidenced by: Restrains from gathering means for self-mutilation and seeks help when feeling urge to injure self (Rate each indicator of **Self-mutilation Restraint:** 1 = never demonstrated, 2 = rarely demonstrated, 3 = sometimes demonstrated, 4 = often demonstrated, 5 = consistently demonstrated [see Section I])

• = Independent; ▲ = Collaborative

Client Outcomes

- Injuries are treated
- States appropriate ways to cope with increased psychological or physiological tension
- Expresses feelings
- Seeks help when having hallucinations
- Uses appropriate community agencies when caregivers are unable to attend to emotional needs

NIC   Interventions (Nursing Interventions Classification)

Suggested NIC Labels

Anger Control Assistance; Behavior Management: Self-Harm; Environmental Management

> **Example NIC Interventions—Behavior Management: Self-Harm**
> - Anticipate trigger situations that may prompt self-harm and intervene to prevent
> - Teach and reinforce effective coping behaviors and appropriate expression of feelings

Nursing Interventions and Rationales

- ▲ Provide medical treatment for injuries. Use careful aseptic technique when caring for wounds.
  A significant impediment to wound healing is infection. Treatment of chronic wounds should be directed toward the main etiologic factors responsible for the wound. Moreover, factors that may impede healing must be identified and, if possible, corrected for healing to occur (Stadelmann, Digenis, Tobin, 1998).
- • Assess for risk of suicide.
  This study of suicide attempters showed that individuals who mutilate themselves are at greater risk for suicide than those who do not (Stanley et al, 2001). Refer to the care plan for **Risk for Suicide.**
- • Assess for signs of depression, anxiety, and impulsivity.
  These behaviors are identified in clients with a history of self-mutilation (Stanley et al, 2001).
- • Establish trust.
  Establishing trust appears to the most critical component of assess and treating the client who self-mutilates (Dallam, 1997).
- • Secure a written or verbal contract from client to notify staff when experiencing the desire to self-mutilate.
  This study indicated reduced repetition of self-harm when there is an emergency contact card in addition to standard care (Hawton et al, 1998).
- ▲ Use a collaborative approach for care.
  A collaborative approach to care is more helpful to the client (Clarke, Whittaker, 1998).
- ▲ Refer for medication such as clozapine.
  In this study of seven subjects known to have a personality disorder and severe self-mutilation, there was a statistically significant reduction in incidents of self-mutilation with the use of medication (Chengappa et al, 1999).
- ▲ Consider partial hospitalization with individual and group therapy.
  Psychoanalytically oriented partial hospitalization is superior to standard psychiatric care for clients with borderline personality disorder. These clients had a decrease in self-mutilation (Bateman, Fonagy, 1999).
- • Refer to care plan for **Risk for Self-mutilation** for additional information.

• = **Independent;** ▲ = **Collaborative**

Home Care Interventions and Client/Family Teaching

See care plan for **Risk for Self-mutilation.**

WEB SITES FOR EDUCATION

 See the MERLIN web site for World Wide Web resources for client education.

REFERENCES   Bateman A, Fonagy P: Effectiveness of partial hospitalization in the treatment of borderline personality disorder: a randomized controlled trial, *Am J Psychiatry* 156(10):1563-1569, 1999.

Chengappa KN et al: Clozapine reduces severe self-mutilation and aggression in psychotic patients with borderline personality disorder, *J Clin Psychiatry* 60(7):477-484, 1999.

Clarke L, Whittaker M: Self-mutilation: culture, contexts and nursing responses, *J Clin Nurs* 7(2):129-137, 1998.

Dallam SJ: The identification and management of self-mutilating patients in primary care, *Nurse Pract* 22(5):151-153, 159-165, 1997.

Hawton K et al: Deliberate self-harm: systematic review of efficacy of psychosocial and pharmacological treatments in preventing repetition, *BMJ* 317(7156):441-447, 1998.

Stanley B et al: Are suicide attempters who self-mutilate a unique population? *Am J Psychiatry* 158(3):427-432, 2001.

Stadelmann WK, Digenis AG, Tobin GR: Impediments to wound healing, *Am J Surg* 176(2A suppl):39S, 1998.

Risk for Self-mutilation

Gail B. Ladwig

NANDA   **Definition** At risk for deliberate self-injurious behavior causing tissue damage with the intent of causing nonfatal injury to attain relief of tension

Risk Factors

Psychotic state (command hallucinations); inability to express tension verbally; childhood sexual abuse; violence between parental figures; family divorce; family alcoholism; family history of self-destructive behaviors; adolescence; peers who self-mutilate; isolation from peers; perfectionism; substance abuse; eating disorders; sexual identity crisis; low or unstable self-esteem; low or unstable body image; history of inability to plan solutions or see long-term consequences; use of manipulation to obtain nurturing relationship with others; chaotic/disturbed interpersonal relationships; emotionally disturbed and/or battered child; feels threatened with actual or potential loss of significant relationship; loss of parent/parental relationships; experiences dissociation or depersonalization; experiences mounting tension that is intolerable; impulsivity; inadequate coping; experiences irresistible urge to cut/damage self; needs quick reduction of stress; childhood illness or surgery; foster, group, or institutional care; incarceration; character disorders; borderline personality disorders; loss of control of problem-solving situations; developmentally delayed or autistic individual; history of self-injurious behavior; feelings of depression, rejection, self-hatred, separation anxiety, guilt, and depersonalization

NOC   ## Outcomes (Nursing Outcomes Classification)

Suggested NOC Labels

Aggression Control; Impulse Control; Risk Detection; Self-Mutilation Restraint

• = Independent; ▲ = Collaborative

Example NOC Outcome
Accomplishes **Self-Mutilation Restraint** as evidenced by: Restrains from gathering means for self-mutilation/Seeks help when feeling urge to injure self (Rate each indicator of **Self-Mutilation Restraint:** 1 = never demonstrated, 2 = rarely demonstrated, 3 = sometimes demonstrated, 4 = often demonstrated, 5 = consistently demonstrated [see Section I])

Client Outcomes

- States appropriate ways to cope with increased psychological or physiological tension
- Expresses feelings
- Seeks help when having hallucinations
- Uses appropriate community agencies when caregivers are unable to attend to emotional needs

NIC ## Interventions (Nursing Interventions Classification)

Suggested NIC Labels

Anger Control Assistance; Behavior Management: Self-Harm; Environmental Management

Example NIC Interventions—Behavior Management: Self-Harm
- Anticipate trigger situations that may prompt self-harm and intervene to prevent
- Teach and reinforce effective coping behaviors and appropriate expression of feelings

Nursing Interventions and Rationales

- Assessment data may have to be gathered at different times; allowing a family member or trusted friend to be present during the assessment may be helpful. *Self-mutilation sometimes occurs if clients have been victims of sadistic ritual abuse. They may react intensely and irrationally to routine office visits. Rather than postponing treatment, use of the listed interventions may be helpful (Young, 1993).*
- Assess for family history of substance abuse. *Self-mutilation and heavy use of mental health services have been correlated with having an alcoholic parent (Rose, Peabody, Strategies, 1991).*
- Monitor client's behavior using 15-minute checks at irregular times so that client does not notice a pattern. *When there is lack of control, client safety is an important issue and close observation is essential. Not following a pattern prevents clients from being self-abusive when they know a caregiver will not be present.*
- Monitor clients with obsessive-compulsive disorder for possible self-mutilation. *Clients with high levels of obsessive-compulsive symptoms may self-mutilate (McKay, Kulchycky, Danyko, 2000).*
- Secure a written or verbal contract from client to notify staff when experiencing the desire to self-mutilate. *This study indicated reduced repetition of self-harm when there is an emergency contact card in addition to standard care (Hawton et al, 1998). Discussing feelings of self-harm with a trusted person provides relief for the client. A contract gets the subject out in the open and places some of the responsibility for safety with the client.*

• = **Independent;** ▲ = **Collaborative**

- Help the client identify cues that precede impulsive behavior.
  Often, supposedly impulsive events are preceded by tension and unrecognized impulse control (Gallop, 1992).
- Give praise when client identifies urges and delays self-destructive behavior.
  Delaying destructive behavior and increasing awareness of urges to be self-destructive should both be acknowledged as progress (Gallop, 1992).
- Monitor for presence of hallucinations. Ask specific questions such as, "Do you hear voices that other people do not hear?"
  Brief, reversible psychotic episodes tend to occur as a response to stress (First et al, 1993). An accurate assessment of the client's contact with reality is important in planning care. Acknowledging that the client may hear something that others do not may open up communication and help establish trust.
- ▲ Assure client that he or she will not be alone and will be safe during hallucinations. Provide referrals for medication.
  Hallucinations can be very frightening; therefore clients need reassurance that they will not be left alone. Significantly reduced rates of further self-harm were observed for depot flupentixol versus placebo in multiple repeaters (Hawton et al, 1998).
- Be extremely cautious about touching client when he or she is experiencing an abreaction (reenactment of precipitating trauma). Sometimes physically holding a client is necessary to prevent self-injury.
  Touch may be interpreted as coming from an abuser and could result in aggressive acting out. Even well-intentioned or consoling touching may further upset the client. A therapist who is attempting to be consoling should always ask abreacting clients whether they may be touched. Clients may initially refuse, but they generally appreciate the offer. An offer may be repeated several times and clients may eventually agree to be touched or held. If clients must be held to prevent self-injury, explain why it is necessary before touching them (Fike, 1990).
- Assess client who has issues with gender for possible self-mutilation.
  This study suggested that clients attending gender dysphoria clinics were at risk for self-mutilation (Wylie, 2000).
- If self-mutilation does occur, care for the wounds in a matter-of-fact way.
  This approach does not promote inappropriate attention-getting behavior and may decrease repetition of behavior.
- When client is experiencing extreme anxiety, use one-to-one staffing.
  The presence of a trusted individual may calm fears about personal safety.
- Reinforce alternative ways of dealing with anxiety such as exercise, engaging in unit activities, or talking about feelings.
  The 12-month effects of exercise training on psychological outcomes in adults 50 to 65 years of age were evaluated (N = 357). Participants were randomly assigned to assessment-only control or to higher intensity group, higher intensity home, or lower intensity home exercise training. Exercisers showed reductions in perceived stress and anxiety in relation to controls (p < .04). Regardless of program assignment, greater exercise participation was significantly related to less anxiety and fewer depressive symptoms, independent of changes in fitness or body weight (p < .05) (King, Taylor, Haskell, 1993).
- Keep environment safe; remove all harmful objects from the area. Use of unbreakable glass is recommended for client at risk for self-injury.
  Client safety is a nursing priority. Putting a hand through a window was the most fre-

• = Independent; ▲ = Collaborative

quent self-injuring behavior in this study. Unbreakable glass would eliminate this type of injury (Callias, Carpenter, 1994).

- Assess client with history of previous assaults. Listen to and acknowledge feelings of anger, observe for increased motor activity, and prepare to intervene if client becomes aggressive.
  In this study, those who assaulted had significantly more previous assaults (p = .04) and more difficulty verbalizing angry feelings appropriately on their units (p < .01) than control group members. Before the assault, assaultive clients were more verbally hostile (p = .037) and showed more increased motor activity (p = .001) than controls (Lanza et al, 1996).

- If client is unable to control behavior, provide interactive supervision, not isolation.
  Isolation and deprivation take away individuals' coping abilities and place them at risk for self-harm. Implementing seclusion for clients who have injured themselves in the past may actually facilitate self-injury. "Despite finding themselves lodged within spartan rooms cleared of artifacts, having had personal clothing removed, and having been searched, clients showed an extraordinary 'morbid resourcefulness' for inflicting injury" (Burrow, 1992).

▲ Refer for medication such as clozapine
  In this study of seven subjects known to have a personality disorder and severe self-mutilation, there was a statistically significant reduction in incidents of self-mutilation with use of medication (Chengappa et al, 1999).

- Involve client in planning of care and emphasize that client can make choices.
  Problem solving is a way to gain better emotional control by assisting clients with seeing the connection between problems and emotions (Miller, Eisner, Allport, 1994).

- Emphasize that client must comply with the rules of the unit. Give positive reinforcement for compliance and minimize attention paid to disruptive behavior.
  It is important to reinforce appropriate behavior to encourage repetition.

▲ Involve the client in group therapy.
  Group members learn to identify patterns of behavior that were acquired as a result of painful past events. The past is not trivialized but acknowledged as leading to patterns that now influence all interactions (Gallop, 1992).

▲ Use group therapy to exchange information about methods of coping with loneliness, self-destructive impulses, and interpersonal relationships, as well as housing, employment, and health care system issues directly and noninterpretively.
  Data suggest that an important component of effective group treatment for a seriously ill person with borderline personality disorder is the meaningful exchange of information. The degree of structure may be a necessary condition for positive outcomes (Nehls, 1992). Individuals with multiple personality disorder/dissociative disorder (MPD/DD) often are estranged from abusive families and have difficulty with social connection. Group therapy can be a useful and successful adjunct to individual psychotherapy for relatively stable clients with MPD/DD. The group's focus should be here and now, supportive and psychoeducative (Dallam, Manderino, 1997).

- Concentrate on client's strengths. Have client visualize the word "Stop!" when negative self-talk begins, then replace the negativity with an affirmation or positive statement.
  Individuals with borderline personality disorder commonly engage in self-talk that is invalid and self-deprecating (Miller, Eisner, Allport, 1994).

▲ Refer to protective services if there is evidence of abuse.
  It is the nurse's legal responsibility to report abuse.

• = Independent; ▲ = Collaborative

Geriatric

- Provide back rubs when elderly client experiences symptoms of anxiety.
  In this study of elderly residents in a long-term care facility, there was a statistically significant difference in the mean anxiety (STAI) score between the back massage group and the no intervention group (Fraser, Kerr, 1993).

Home Care Interventions

- Assess the family and caregiving situation for ability to protect the client.
  Client safety between home visits is a nursing priority.
- ▲ Establish an emergency plan, including when to use hotlines and 911. Develop a contract with the client for use of the emergency plan. Role-play access to the emergency resources with the client and caregivers.
  Having an emergency plan reassures the client and caregivers and promotes client safety. Contracting gives guided control to the client and enhances self-esteem.
- Assess the home environment for harmful objects. Have family remove or lock objects as able.
  Client safety is a nursing priority.
- ▲ If client behaviors intensify, refer for mental health intervention.
  The degree of disturbance and the ability to manage care safely at home determines the level of services needed to protect the client.
- ▲ Refer for homemaker or psychiatric home health aide services for respite and client reassurance.
  Responsibility for a person at high risk for self-mutilation provides high caregiver stress. Respite decreases caregiver stress. The presence of caring individuals is reassuring to both the client and caregivers, especially during periods of client anxiety.
- ▲ If client is on psychotropic medications, assess client and family knowledge of medication administration and side effects. Teach as necessary.
  Knowledge of the medical regimen promotes compliance.
- ▲ Evaluate the effectiveness and side effects of medications.
  Accurate clinical feedback improves physician ability to prescribe an effective medical regimen specific to client needs.

Client/Family Teaching

- Suggest feasible activities for the client and significant others (simple tasks like washing dishes, taking out the garbage). Performance of complex previous tasks such as bill paying may not be possible until therapy is complete. Client and family need to know this is a temporary situation.
  The education of clients with multiple personality disorder and their significant others is both critical and practical. Teaching helps to reduce anxiety and gives clients and families strategies for coping with their distress (Fike, 1990).
- Teach stress reduction techniques such as imagery and controlled breathing (e.g., breathing in on "re" and out on "lax"); teach client to sustain the breathing-out phase.
  Imagery is effective for helping clients adjust to the demands of chronic illness (Stephens, 1993).
- ▲ Provide client and family with phone numbers of appropriate community agencies for therapy and counseling.
  Continuous follow-up care may be necessary; therefore the method to access this care must be given to the client.

• = **Independent;** ▲ = **Collaborative**

- Give client positive things on which to focus by referring to appropriate agencies for job-training skills or education.
  Alternative coping skills and the means to access them are essential for continued good mental health.

WEB SITES FOR EDUCATION

See the MERLIN web site for World Wide Web resources for client education.

REFERENCES Burrow S: The deliberate self-harming behavior of clients within a British special hospital, *J Adv Nurs* 17:138, 1992.

Callias M, Carpenter M: Self-injurious behavior in a state psychiatric hospital, *Hosp Comm Psychiatry* 45:170, 1994.

Chengappa KN et al: Clozapine reduces severe self-mutilation and aggression in psychotic patients with borderline personality disorder, *J Clin Psychiatry* 60(7):477-484, 1999.

Dallam S, Manderino MA: "Free to be" peer group supports patients with MPD/DD, *J Psychosoc Nurs Ment Health Serv* 35(5):22-27, 1997.

Fike ML: Considerations and techniques in the treatment of persons with multiple personality disorder, *Am J Occup Ther* 44:999, 1990.

First MB et al: Changes in mood, anxiety, and personality disorders, *Hosp Comm Psychiatry* 44(11):1034-1036, 1043, 1993.

Fraser J, Kerr J: Psychophysiological effects of back massage on elderly institutionalized, *J Adv Nurs* 18(2):238-245, 1993.

Gallop R: Self-destructive and impulsive behavior in the client with a borderline personality disorder: rethinking hospital treatment and management, *Arch Psychiatr Nurs* 6:178, 1992.

Hawton K et al: Deliberate self-harm: systematic review of efficacy of psychosocial and pharmacological treatments in preventing repetition, *BMJ* 317(7156):441-447, 1998.

King A, Taylor C, Haskell W: Effects of differing intensities and formats of 12 months of exercise training on psychological outcomes in older adults, *Health Psychol* 12(4):292-300, 1993.

Lanza M et al: The relationship of behavioral cues to assaultive behavior, *Clin Nurs Res* 5(1):6-25, discussion pp 26-27, 1996.

McKay D, Kulchycky S, Danyko S: Borderline personality and obsessive-compulsive symptoms, *J Personal Disord* 14(1):57-63, 2000.

Miller C, Eisner W, Allport C: Creative coping: a cognitive-behavioral group for borderline personality disorder, *Arch Psychiatr Nurs* 8:280, 1994.

Nehls N: Group therapy for people with borderline personality disorder: interventions associated with positive outcomes, *Issues Ment Health Nurs* 13:255, 1992.

Rose SM, Peabody CG, Strategies B: Undetected abuse among intensive case management clients, *Hosp Comm Psychiatry* 42:5, 1991.

Stephens R: Imagery: a strategic intervention to empower clients, part II—a practical guide, *Clin Nurs Spec* 7:235, 1993.

Wylie KR: Suction to the breasts of a transsexual male, *J Sex Marital Ther* 26(4):353-356, 2000.

Young W: Sadistic ritual abuse: an overview in detection and management, *Primary Care* 20:447, 1993.

Disturbed Sensory perception (specify: visual, auditory, kinesthetic, gustatory, tactile, olfactory)

Betty J. Ackley

NANDA **Definition** Change in the amount or patterning of incoming stimuli accompanied by a diminished, exaggerated, distorted, or impaired response to such stimuli

- = **Independent;** ▲ = **Collaborative**

Defining Characteristics

Poor concentration; auditory distortions; change in usual response to stimuli; restlessness; reported or measured change in sensory acuity; irritability; disoriented in time, inplace, or with people; change in problem-solving abilities; change in behavior pattern; altered communication patterns; hallucinations; visual distortions

Related Factors (r/t)

Altered sensory perception; excessive environmental stimuli; psychological stress; altered sensory reception, transmission, and/or integration/insufficient environmental stimuli; biochemical imbalances for sensory distortion (e.g., illusions, hallucinations); electrolyte imbalance; biochemical imbalance

NOC **Outcomes (Nursing Outcomes Classification) for Disturbed Sensory Perception: Visual**

Suggested NOC Labels

Body Image; Cognitive Orientation; Sensory Function: Vision; Vision Compensation Behavior

> **Example NOC Outcome**
> Uses **Vision Compensation Behavior** as evidenced by the following indicators: Uses adequate light for activity being performed/Wears eyeglasses correctly/Uses low-vision assistive devices/Uses computer assistive devices/Uses support services for low-vision (Rate each indicator of **Vision Compensation Behavior:** 1 = never demonstrated, 2 = rarely demonstrated, 3 = sometimes demonstrated, 4 = often demonstrated, 5 = consistently demonstrated [see Section I])

NOC **Outcomes (Nursing Outcomes Classification) for Disturbed Sensory Perception: Auditory**

Suggested NOC Labels

Cognitive Orientation; Communication: Receptive Ability; Distorted Thought Control; Hearing Compensation Behavior

> **Example NOC Outcome**
> Uses **Hearing Compensation Behavior** as evidenced by the following indicators: Reminds others to use techniques that advantage hearing/Eliminates background noise/Uses sign language/Uses lip reading/Uses hearing assistive devices/Uses hearing aid(s) correctly/Uses support services for hearing impaired (Rate each indicator of **Hearing Compensation Behavior:** 1 = never demonstrated, 2 = rarely demonstrated, 3 = sometimes demonstrated, 4 = often demonstrated, 5 = consistently demonstrated [see Section I])

Client Outcomes

- Demonstrates understanding by a verbal, written, or signed response
- Demonstrates relaxed body movements and facial expressions
- Explains plan to modify lifestyle to accommodate visual or hearing impairment
- Remains free of physical harm resulting from decreased balance or a loss of vision, hearing, or tactile sensation
- Maintains contact with appropriate community resources

• = Independent; ▲ = Collaborative

NIC   **Interventions (Nursing Interventions Classification)**

Suggested NIC Labels

Communication Enhancement: Visual Deficit; Communication Enhancement: Hearing Deficit; Cognitive Stimulation; Environmental Management

> **Example NIC Interventions—Communication Enhancement: Visual Deficit**
> - Identify yourself when you enter the patient's space
> - Build on patient's remaining vision, as appropriate

Nursing Interventions and Rationales

Visual—loss of vision

- Identify name and purpose when entering client's room.
  Identification when entering the room helps the client feel secure and decreases social isolation.
- Orient to time, place, person, and surroundings. Provide a radio or talking books.
  These actions help client remain oriented and provide sensory stimulation.
- Keep doors completely open or closed. Keep furniture out of path to bathroom, and do not rearrange furniture.
  These steps help maintain a safe environment for the client (Beaver, Mann, 1995).
- Feed client at mealtimes if blindness is temporary.
- Keep side rails up using half or three-quarter rails, and maintain bed in a low position. Explain this precaution to client.
- Converse with and touch client frequently during care if frequent touch is within client's cultural norm.
  Appropriate touch can decrease social isolation.
- Walk client by having client grasp nurse's elbow and walk partly behind nurse. Walk a frightened or confused client by having client put both hands on nurse's shoulders; nurse backs up in desired direction while holding client around the waist.
  These methods help the client feel secure and ensure safety.
- Keep call light button within client's reach, and check location of call light button before leaving the room.
- ▲ For blind client, consider referring to a clinic for use of a blind mobility aid device that utilizes ultrasound.
  These devices can be helpful to the blind client to increase acuity to the environment and movement of objects in the environment (Bitjoka, Pourcelot, 1999).
- Ensure access to eyeglasses or magnifying devices as needed.
- Pay attention to client's emotional needs. Encourage expression of feelings and expect grieving behavior.
  Blind people grieve the loss of vision and experience a loss of identity and control over their lives (Vader, 1992).
- ▲ Refer to optometrist, ophthalmologist, or specialist in vision loss for vision care if needed.
  Treatment of diabetic retinopathy can greatly reduce the incidence of blindness (Winslow, 1994). Many clients with eye disorders need frequent medical care to maintain vision.

Auditory-hearing loss

- Keep background noise to a minimum. Turn off television and radio when communicating with client.
  Background noise significantly interferes with hearing in the hearing-impaired client (Jupiter, Spiver, 1997).

• = **Independent;** ▲ = **Collaborative**

- Stand or sit directly in front of client when communicating. Make sure adequate light is on nurse's face, avoid chewing gum or covering mouth or face with hands while speaking, establish eye contact, and use nonverbal gestures.
  These measures make it easier to read lips and see nonverbal communication, which is a large component of all communication (Jupiter, Spiver, 1997).
- Speak distinctly in lower voice tones if possible. Do not over-enunciate or shout at client.
  In many kinds of hearing loss, clients lose the ability to hear higher-pitched tones but can still hear lower-pitched tones. Over-enunciating makes it difficult to read lips. Shouting makes the words less clear and may be painful (Jupiter, Spiver, 1997).
- If necessary, provide a communication board or personnel who know sign language.
  Alternative forms of communication help decrease social isolation.
- Try inserting the earpieces of the stethoscope into the client's ears, and talking into diaphragm.
  Stethoscopes magnify sound and can help some clients hear better.
- ▲ Refer to appropriate resources such as a speech and hearing clinic; audiologist; or ear, nose, and throat physician. Refer children early for help.
  Hearing loss can be treated with medical or surgical interventions or use of a hearing aid. Research demonstrates the positive effects of early diagnosis and intervention on the social and cognitive development of hearing impaired children (Meadow-Orland et al, 1997).
- Encourage client to wear hearing aid, but understand if he or she chooses to leave hearing aid out.
  Hearing aids amplify all noise, and loud noises in the environment can be amplified to an unbearable volume (Committee on Disabilities, 1997).
- Observe emotional needs and encourage expression of feelings.
  Hearing impairments may cause frustration, anger, fear, and self-imposed isolation (Taylor, 1993)
- For **Disturbed Sensory perception: kinesthetic and tactile,** see care plan for **Risk for Injury.** For **Disturbed Sensory perception: olfactory and gustatory,** see care plan for **Imbalanced Nutrition: less than body requirements.**

Geriatric

- Keep environment quiet, soothing, and familiar. Use consistent caregivers.
  These measures are comforting to the elderly and help decrease confusion.
- Avoid providing extremely hot or cold foods or using hot bath water if client has decreased sensation in mouth, hands, or feet.
- If client has a sensory deprivation, encourage family to provide sensory stimulation with music, voices, photographs, touch, and familiar smells.
- If client has a hearing or vision loss, work with client to ensure contact with others and to strengthen the social network.
  Severe loneliness can accompany hearing or vision loss in the elderly as a result of self-imposed isolation (Christian, Dluhy, O'Neill, 1989; Foxall et al, 1992).

Home Care Interventions

- The listed interventions are applicable in the home care setting.

Client/Family Teaching

Low vision

- Teach client how to use a lighted magnification device to increase the ability to read text or see details.

- **= Independent;** ▲ **= Collaborative**

- Teach client to put a yellow or green transparency over text to make the text more visible. An alternative method is to highlight the text with a green or yellow highlighter.
- Put red or yellow identifiers on important items that need to be seen, such as a red strip at the edge of steps, red behind a light switch, or a red dot on a stove or washing machine to indicate how far to turn knob.
  Color cues can improve the legibility of the environment and increase the ability to target objects quickly (Cooper, 1999).
- Use a watch or clock that verbally tells time and a phone with large numbers and emergency numbers programmed in.
- Teach blind client how to feed self; associate food on plate with hours on a clock so that client can identify location of food.
- Use low-vision aids including magnifying devices, a closed-circuit television that magnifies print, a special lens for close and distant vision, and guides for writing checks and envelopes.
- Increase lighting in the home, and decrease glare where light reflects on shiny surfaces. Use motion lights that come on automatically when a person enters the room. Use non-glare wax on the floor.
  Visual acuity can be improved by taking steps to overcome age-related changes to vision (Smith, 1998). Illumination can increase mobility in clients with age-related macular degeneration (Kuyk, Elliott, 1999).
- ▲ Refer to low-vision clinics and rehabilitation centers.
  Clients with vision loss should be referred to clinics early, before vision is gone, for help dealing with the loss (Brown, 1998).

Hearing loss

- Suggest installation of devices such as ring signalers for the telephone and doorbell, sensors that detect an infant's cry, alarm clocks that vibrate the bed, and closed caption decoders for television sets. Other helpful devices include telephone amplifiers, speaker phones, pocket talker personal listening system, and FM and infrared amplification systems that connect directly to a TV or audio output jack. Also available is a telecommunication device—a typewriter keyboard with an alphanumeric display that allows the hearing impaired person to send typed messages over the telephone line, and software and modems are available that allow a home computer to be used in this fashion. Use of a hearing ear dogs—dogs specially trained to alert their owners to specific sound—may also be helpful.
  These devices and the dogs can be helpful to increase communication and safety for the hearing impaired client (Committee on Disabilities, 1997; Jupiter, Spiver, 1997).
- Teach family how to provide appropriate stimuli in the home environment to prevent disturbed sensory perception.
- ▲ Refer to hearing clinics.

WEB SITES FOR EDUCATION

MERLIN See the MERLIN web site for World Wide Web resources for client education.

REFERENCES   Beaver KA, Mann WC: Overview of technology for low vision, *Am J Occup Ther* 49:913, 1995.
Bitjoka L, Pourcelot L: New blind mobility aid devices based on the ultrasonic Doppler effect, *Int J Rehabil Res* 22(3):227-231, 1999.

• = Independent; ▲ = Collaborative

Brown B: Five easy steps to helping your low vision patient, *J Ophthal Nurs Technol* 17(1):7-12, 1998.

Christian E, Dluhy N, O'Neill R: Sounds of silence: coping with hearing loss and loneliness, *J Gerontol Nurse* 15:4, 1989.

Committee on Disabilities: Issues to consider in deaf and hard-of-hearing patients, *Am Fam Physician* 56(8):2057-2063, 1997.

Cooper BA: The utility of functional colour cues: seniors' views, *Scand J Caring Sci* 13(3):186-192, 1999.

Foxall MJ et al: Predictors of loneliness in low vision adults, *West J Nurs Res* 14:86, 1992.

Jupiter T, Spiver V: Perception of hearing loss and hearing handicap on hearing aid use by nursing home residents: geriatric nursing, *Am J Care Aging* 18(5):201-208, 1997.

Kuyk T, Elliott JL: Visual factors and mobility in persons with age-related macular degeneration, *J Rehabil Res Dev* 36(4):303-312, 1999.

Meadow-Orland KP et al: Support services for parents and their children who are deaf or hard of hearing, *Am Ann Deaf* 142(4):278-293, 1997.

Smith SD: Aging, physiology, and vision, *Nurse Pract Forum* 9(1):19-22, 1998.

Taylor KS: Geriatric hearing loss: management strategies for nurses, *Geriatr Nurs* 14:74, 1993.

Vader LA: Vision and vision loss, *Nurs Clin North Am* 27:705, 1992.

Winslow EH: Research for practice: laser treatment prevents blindness, *Am J Nurs* 94(3):19, 1994.

Sexual dysfunction

Gail B. Ladwig

NANDA **Definition** Change in sexual function that is viewed as unsatisfying, unrewarding, inadequate

Defining Characteristics

Change of interest in self and others; conflicts involving values; inability to achieve desired satisfaction; verbalization of problem; alteration in relationship with significant other; alteration in achieving sexual satisfaction; actual or perceived limitation imposed by disease or therapy; seeking confirmation of desirability; alteration in achieving perceived sex role

Related Factors (r/t)

Misinformation or lack of knowledge; vulnerability; value conflict; psychosocial abuse (e.g., harmful relationships); physical abuse; lack of privacy; ineffectual or absent role models; altered body structure of function (e.g., pregnancy, recent childbirth, drugs, surgery, anomalies, disease process, trauma, radiation); lack of significant other; biopsychosocial alterations of sexuality

 Outcomes (Nursing Outcomes Classification)

Suggested NOC Labels

Abuse Recovery: Sexual; Child Development: Adolescence (12-17 Years); Physical Aging Status; Risk Control: Sexually Transmitted Diseases (STD); Sexual Functioning

> **Example NOC Outcome**
> Demonstrates **Sexual Functioning** as evidenced by: Expresses comfort with sexual expression/Expresses comfort with body/Expresses sexual interest (Rate each indicator of **Sexual Functioning:** 1 = never demonstrated, 2 = rarely demonstrated, 3 = sometimes demonstrated, 4 = often demonstrated, 5 = consistently demonstrated [see Section I])

• = Independent; ▲ = Collaborative

Client Outcomes

- Identifies individual cause of sexual dysfunction
- Identifies stressors that contribute to dysfunction
- Discusses alternative, satisfying, and acceptable sexual practices for self and partner
- Discusses with partner concerns about body image and sex role

NIC Interventions (Nursing Interventions Classification)

Suggested NIC Labels

Sexual Counseling

> **Example NIC Interventions—Sexual Counseling**
> - Provide privacy and ensure confidentiality
> - Discuss modifications in sexual activity, as appropriate

Nursing Interventions and Rationales

- Gather client's sexual history, noting normal patterns of functioning and client's vocabulary.

  Sexual problems can result from biological, intrapersonal, and interpersonal distress. Generally, several of these factors combine to produce sexual dysfunction. Nurses can prevent some sexual dysfunctions from developing by being prepared and willing to empathetically discuss sexuality with their clients and provide them with accurate information. Sexuality and sexual behavior must be assessed on an individual basis (Fontaine, 1991).

- Determine client's and partner's current knowledge and understanding.

  For patients, self-identity and communication were the predominant themes that emerged from the data. A lack of information related to issues of sexual functioning was the most prominent subcategory (Steinke, Patterson-Midgley, 1998). If unsure of a client's sexuality, use the term partner, *which helps avoid making any assumptions or judgments about a relationship. A sexual relationship may be heterosexual or homosexual, and nurses must not lose sight of this (Taylor, 1994).*

- Observe for stress, anxiety, and depression as possible causes of dysfunction.

  Sexual dysfunction can be attributed to many psychological factors. Sexual problems are common in chronic-pain patients. Patients who reported symptoms of depression and distress had more sexual problems than others (Monga et al, 1998). Recognition of sexual dysfunction associated with depression and its treatment is critical for client satisfaction and medication compliance (Clayton, 2001).

- Observe for grief related to loss (e.g., amputation, mastectomy, ostomy).

  *A change in body image often precedes sexual dysfunction (see care plan for **Disturbed Body image**). The trauma of being diagnosed and treated for breast cancer can impact greatly on women's psychosexual functioning and intimate relationships. Survivors of breast cancer report that issues of body image, sexuality, and partner communication are rarely addressed by traditional health care providers (Anllo, 2000).*

- Explore physical causes such as diabetes, arteriosclerotic heart disease, arthritis, drug or medication side effects, or smoking (males).

  Researchers have shown that sexual difficulties often occur as a result of cardiovascular disease. In fact, at least 25% to 50% of men and women who have suffered a previous myocardial infarction (MI) never regain their earlier frequency of sexual activity, and some do not resume any sexual activity at all (Papadopoulos, 1991). In this research study, women with arthritis and a high degree of morning stiffness worried more about their

• = Independent; ▲ = Collaborative

bodies and reported significantly more problems with sexuality than others (Gutweniger et al, 1999).

- Provide privacy and be verbally and nonverbally nonjudgmental.
  Privacy is important to ensure confidentiality. To facilitate communication, it is also vital that the nurse clarify personal values and remain nonjudgmental.
- Provide privacy to allow sexual expression between client and partner (e.g., private room, "Do Not Disturb" sign for a specified length of time).
  The hospital setting has little opportunity for privacy, so the nurse must ensure that it is available.
- Explain the need for client to share concerns with partner.
  Regardless of sexual function and activities, maintaining the relationship is important for meeting intimacy needs (Lemone, 1991).
- Validate client's feelings, let client know that he or she is normal, and correct misinformation.
  A sensitive nurse who has an understanding of sexual health and functioning and the conditions that interfere with them can direct those who need help toward treatment (Lewis, 1992).

Geriatric

- Discuss with client and partner their present role adjustments.
  This discussion assists client and partner with coping.
- Teach about normal changes that occur with aging: Female—reduction in vaginal lubrication, decrease in the degree and speed of vaginal expansion, reduction in duration and resolution of orgasm. Male—increase in time required for erection, increase in erection time without ejaculation, less firm erection, decrease in volume of seminal fluid, increase in time before another erection can occur (12 to 24 hours).
  The older adult experiences a number of physiological changes; however, these changes are gradual and vary from person to person (Shell, Smith, 1994).
- ▲ Suggest the following to enhance sexual functioning: Female—use water-based vaginal lubricant, increase foreplay time, avoid direct stimulation of the clitoris if painful (clitoris may be exposed because of atrophy of the labia), practice Kegel exercises (alternately contracting and relaxing the muscles in the pelvic area), urinate immediately after coitus to prevent irritation of the urethra and bladder, and consult with a physician about use of systemic estrogen therapy or topical estrogen cream. Male—have female partner try a new coital position by bending her knees and placing a pillow under her hips to elevate pelvis (will more easily accommodate a partially erect penis); massage penis down using pressure at base, which puts pressure on major blood vessel and keeps blood in the penis; ask the female partner to push the penis into the vagina herself and flex her vaginal muscles that have been strengthened by Kegel exercises. If one of the partners has a protruding abdomen, experiment to find a position that allows the penis to reach the vagina (e.g., have woman lie on her back with legs apart and knees sharply bent while the man places himself over her with his hips under the angle formed by the raised knees). Consult with a physician about use of penis self-injection with phentolamine/papaverine, which will elicit an erection that lasts about 1 hour.
  These gender-specific sexual interventions for the elderly may help maintain sexual functioning (Shell, Smith, 1994).

• = **Independent;** ▲ = **Collaborative**

- Assess the possibility of erectile dysfunction.
  Erectile dysfunction occurs in men of any age but is more common in older men. Sexual functioning can almost always be restored, but many men never seek help (Lewis, 1992). Erectile dysfunction affects the lives of up to 30 million American men and their partners (Mayo Foundation for Medical Education and Research, 2001).
- Explore with client and partner various sexual gratification alternatives (e.g., caressing, sharing feelings).
  There are many satisfying alternatives for expressing sexual feelings. The many losses associated with aging leave the elderly with special needs for love and affection.
- Discuss the difference between sexual function and sexuality.
  All individuals possess sexuality from birth to death, regardless of the changes that occur over the lifespan.
- ▲ If prescribed, teach how to use nitroglycerin before sexual activity.
  Pain inhibits satisfying sexual activity.
- See care plan for **Ineffective Sexuality pattern.**

Multicultural

- Assess for the influence of cultural beliefs, norms, and values on the client's perceptions of normal sexual functioning.
  What the client considers normal sexual functioning may be based on cultural perceptions (Leininger, 1996).
- Discuss with the client those aspects of sexual health/lifestyle that remain unchanged by his or her health status.
  Aspects of the client's life that are valuable to him or her should be understood and preserved without change (Leininger, 1996),
- Validate the client's feelings and emotions regarding the changes in sexual behavior.
  Validation lets the client know the nurse has heard and understands what was said, and it promotes the nurse-client relationship (Giger, Davidhizar, 1995; Stuart, Laraia, 2001).

Home Care Interventions

- Help the client and significant other to identify a place and time in the home and daily living for privacy to share sexual or relationship activity. If necessary, help client to communicate the need for privacy to other family members. Consider periodic escapes to desirable surroundings.
  The home setting can be one that affords little, if any, privacy without conscious effort on the part of members of the home.
- ▲ Confirm that physical reasons for dysfunction have been addressed. Encourage participation in support groups or therapy if appropriate.
  Clients often express embarrassment at continuing medical intervention or participation in groups once they are back in the community and know that peers may judge their activities.
- Reinforce or teach client about sexual functioning, alternative sexual practices, and necessary sexual precautions. Update teaching as client status changes.
  If the client and/or significant other have received information during an institutional stay, other stressors may have made the information a temporarily low priority or may have impaired learning. Depending on the cause for dysfunction, the client may experience changing status or feelings about the problem.

• = Independent; ▲ = Collaborative

Client/Family Teaching

- Teach the importance of resting before sexual activity. For some clients, mornings are the best time for sexual activity.
  Clients may have a more satisfying experience if they are not tired.
- Teach the client to resume intimate physical contact by using mutual touching 3 to 6 weeks after a MI.
  Sexual activity after a MI should not be demanding; therefore mutual touching is recommended (Papadopoulos, 1991).
- Teach client to begin vigorous sexual activity after a MI when client can walk rapidly for 10 minutes and then climb two flights of stairs in 10 seconds.
  If this can be done without shortness of breath or other symptoms, then the client is ready to begin preestablished levels of sexual activity (Papadopoulos, 1991). MI patients often have unanswered questions about resuming sexual activity after this life-threatening event (Steinke, Patterson-Midgley, 1996).
- ▲ Teach client to take prescribed pain medications before sexual activity.
  Pain inhibits satisfying sexual activity.
- Teach possible need for modifying positions (e.g., side-to-side, limited resting on arms, heavier person on bottom).
  Changes in position can enhance satisfaction and comfort.
- ▲ Refer to appropriate community resources, such as a clinical specialist, family counselor, or sexual counselor. If appropriate, include both partners in the discussion.
  A high percentage of women report a need for more information after a cancer surgery that affected their sexual response. They also express a need for partners to be included in the discussions (Corney et al, 1992). Changes in the sexual relationship were described in the context of the effects of having interstitial cystitis and the centrality of maintaining relationships. Participation in support groups has a healing potential related to the woman's desire to maintain independence and to help others with the disease (Webster, 1997).
- Teach vaginal dilation to prevent stenosis. Inform client to expect a bit of spotting after first session of intercourse.
  Clients with gynecological cancer and surgery, particularly cervical cancer, can reduce the number of physical problems if this information is taught (Laurent, 1994).
- ▲ Teach how drug therapy affects sexual response (e.g., the possible side effects and the need to report them).
  Some drugs used to treat multiple sclerosis (MS) may impair sexual functioning. Antispastic drugs (e.g., methantheline, baclofen) may reduce libido, and tranquilizing drugs (e.g., diazepam, barbiturates) may interfere with emission and ejaculation in men. Tricyclic antidepressant drugs (e.g., imipramine, amitriptyline) may interfere with erection in men and with vaginal lubrication, clitoral engorgement, and orgasm in women (Dupont, 1995).
- ▲ Teach the importance of diabetic control and its effect on sexuality to clients with insulin-dependent diabetes.
  Sexual functioning may be changed by alterations in glucose levels, infections that affect comfort during sexual intercourse, changes in vaginal lubrication and penile erection, and changes in sexual desire and arousal (Lemone, 1993).
- ▲ Refer for medical advice for erectile dysfunction that lasts longer than 2 months or is recurring.
  Erectile dysfunction can be treated, and underlying causes need to be investigated (Mayo Foundation for Medical Education and Research, 2001).

- **= Independent; ▲ = Collaborative**

- Teach the following interventions to decrease the likelihood of erectile dysfunction: limit or avoid the use of alcohol, stop smoking, exercise regularly, reduce stress, get enough sleep, deal with anxiety or depression, and see doctor for regular checkups and medical screening tests.

  These interventions may prevent erectile dysfunction (Mayo Foundation for Medical Education and Research, 2001).

▲ Refer for medication to treat erectile dysfunction if necessary

  The oral agent sildenafil is now widely used, but not without concern about specific health risks (Mulhall, 2000).

- Teach specifics if client has a stoma: do not substitute the stoma for an anus.

  If a stoma is abused in this way, it can become traumatized and need further surgery. (Taylor, 1994).

- See geriatric interventions if there is a problem with erection associated with stoma surgery.

WEB SITES FOR EDUCATION

MERLIN   See the MERLIN web site for World Wide Web resources for client education.

REFERENCES   Anllo LM: Sexual life after breast cancer, *J Sex Marital Ther* 26(3):241-248, 2000.

Clayton AH: Recognition and assessment of sexual dysfunction associated with depression, *J Clin Psychiatry* 62(suppl 3):5-9, 2001.

Corney R et al: The care of patients undergoing surgery for gynecological cancer: the need for information, emotional support and counseling, *J Adv Nurs* 17:667, 1992.

Dupont S: Multiple sclerosis and sexual functioning: a review, *Clin Rehab* 9:135, 1995

Fontaine K: Unlocking sexual issues, *Nurs Clin North Am* 26:737, 1991.

Giger JN, Davidhizar RE: *Transcultural nursing*, ed 2, St Louis, 1995, Mosby.

Gutweniger S et al: Body image of women with rheumatoid arthritis, *Clin Exp Rheumatol* 17(4):413-417, 1999.

Laurent C: Talking treatment: therapy for cervical cancer has left some women with severe sexual problems, *Nurs Times* 90:14, 1994.

Leininger MM: *Transcultural nursing: theories, research and practices*, ed 2, Hilliard, Ohio, 1996, McGraw-Hill.

Lemone P: Human sexuality in adults with insulin-dependent diabetes mellitus, *Image* 25:101, 1993.

Lemone P: *Transforming: patterns of sexual function in adults with insulin-dependent diabetes mellitus*, Birmingham, 1991, University of Alabama.

Lewis JH: Treatment options for men with sexual dysfunction, *J ET Nurs* 19:131, 1992.

Mayo Foundation for Medical Education and Research: *Erectile dysfunction*, retrieved from the World Wide Web March 24, 2001. Web site: www.mayohealth.org/home?id=DS00162

Mulhall JP: Current concepts in erectile dysfunction, *Am J Manag Care* 6(12 suppl):S641-S643, 2000.

Papadopoulos C: Sex and the cardiac patient, 1991, *Med Aspects Hum Sexuality* 24:55, 1991. In Quadagno D et al: Cardiovascular disease and sexual functioning, *Appl Nurs Res* 8:143, 1995.

Shell J, Smith C: Sexuality and the older person with cancer, *Oncol Nurs Forum* 21:553, 1994.

Steinke EE, Patterson-Midgley P: Sexual counseling of MI patients: nurses' comfort, responsibility, and practice, *Dimens Crit Care Nurs* 15(4):216-223, 1996.

Steinke EE, Patterson-Midgley PE: Perspectives of nurses and patients on the need for sexual counseling of MI patients, *Rehabil Nurs* 23(2):64-70, 1998.

Stuart GW, Laraia MT: Therapeutic nurse-patient relationship. In Stuart GW, Laraia MT, editors: *Principles and practice of psychiatric nursing*, St Louis, 2001, Mosby, p 30.

Taylor P: Beating the taboo, *Nurs Times* 90:51, 1994.

Webster DC: Recontextualizing sexuality in chronic illness: women and interstitial cystitis, *Health Care Women Int* 18(6):575-589, 1997.

• = Independent; ▲ = Collaborative

Ineffective Sexuality patterns

Gail B. Ladwig

NANDA   **Definition** Expressions of concern regarding own sexuality

Defining Characteristics

Reported difficulties, limitations, or changes in sexual behaviors or activities

Related Factors (r/t)

Lack of significant other; conflicts with sexual orientation or variant preferences; fear of pregnancy or of acquiring a sexually transmitted disease; impaired relationship with significant other; ineffective or absent role models; knowledge/skill deficit about alternative responses to health-related transitions, altered body function or structure, illness or medical treatment; lack of privacy

NOC   **Outcomes (Nursing Outcomes Classification)**

Suggested NOC Labels

Abuse Recovery: Sexual; Child Development: Adolescence (12-17 Years); Risk Control: Role Performance; Self-Esteem; Sexually Transmitted Diseases (STDs); Sexual Functioning

> ### Example NOC Outcome
>
> Demonstrates **Sexual Functioning** as evidenced by: Expresses comfort with sexual expression/Expresses comfort with body/Expresses sexual interest (Rate each indicator of **Sexual Functioning:** 1 = never demonstrated, 2 = rarely demonstrated, 3 = sometimes demonstrated, 4 = often demonstrated, 5 = consistently demonstrated [see Section I])

Client Outcomes

- States knowledge of difficulties, limitations, or changes in sexual behaviors or activities
- States knowledge of sexual anatomy and functioning
- States acceptance of altered body structure or functioning
- Describes acceptable alternative sexual practices
- Identifies importance of discussing sexual issues with significant other
- Describes practice of safe sex with regard to pregnancy and avoidance of STDs

NIC   **Interventions (Nursing Interventions Classification)**

Suggested NIC Labels

Sexual Counseling

> ### Example NIC Interventions—Sexual Counseling
> - Provide privacy and ensure confidentiality
> - Discuss modifications in sexual activity, as appropriate

Nursing Interventions and Rationales

- After establishing rapport or a therapeutic relationship, give client permission to discuss issues dealing with sexuality. Ask client specifically, "Have you been or are you concerned about functioning sexually because of your health status?"
  Sexual problems can result from biological, intrapersonal, and interpersonal distress. Generally, several of these factors combine to produce sexual dysfunction. Nurses can prevent

• = Independent; ▲ = Collaborative

some sexual dysfunctions from developing by being prepared and willing to empathetically discuss sexuality with their clients and provide them with accurate information. Sexuality and sexual behavior must be assessed on an individual basis (Fontaine, 1991). Of 96 patients surveyed after a myocardial infarction, 71% believed that staff should address sexuality in the hospital setting (Steinke, Patterson-Midgley, 1996).

- Determine client's and partner's current knowledge and understanding.
  One of the most important nursing interventions is giving practical information (Laurent, 1994).
- Discuss alternative sexual expressions for altered body functioning or structure. Closeness and touching are other forms of expression, and some clients choose masturbation for sexual release.
  Masturbation is one of the most common sexual expressions, but at the same time it is one of the least acknowledged (Fontaine, 1991).
- If mutual masturbation is a choice of expression, provide latex gloves.
  Latex gloves prevent possible exposure to infection through cuts on hands (Tucker et al, 1996).
- Discuss modifying positions to accommodate the altered physical state; instruct in the use of pillows for comfort.
  Modified positions can enable and enhance sexual satisfaction otherwise impeded by physical disability.
- Encourage client to discuss concerns with his or her partner.
  If unsure of a client's sexuality, use the term partner to avoid making any assumptions or judgments about the relationship. A sexual relationship may be heterosexual or homosexual, and nurses must not lose sight of this (Taylor, 1994). Communication between partners plays a direct key role in facilitating condom use and forms the basis for maintaining emotional intimacy (Parish et al, 2001).
- Provide the client privacy for sexual expression (e.g., closed door when significant other visits, "Do Not Disturb" sign on door).
  The hospital environment needs to allow for sexual expression between partners.

Geriatric

- Help client redefine sexuality in broader terms such as sharing, communication, and intimacy.
  Sexuality is a primary part of being human and does not cease after age 65. Elderly persons need to continue to view themselves as masculine or feminine (Shell, Smith, 1994).
- ▲ Explore possible changes in sexuality related to menopause
  Evidence from existing research suggests a decline in sexual interest, frequency of sexual intercourse, and vaginal lubrication in association with menopause. Findings for variables such as capacity for orgasm, satisfaction with sex partner, and vaginal pain or discomfort are few and mixed (McCoy, 1998).
- Allow client to verbalize feelings regarding loss of sexual partner or significant other. Acknowledge problems such as disapproval of children, lack of available partner for women, and environmental variables that make forming new relationships difficult.
  Many individuals face loneliness when they lose a partner, and the loss of interpersonal intimacy is a sensitive problem. After a loss of this magnitude, elderly persons often find that forming new relationships is difficult. Privacy is also a problem (Shell, Smith, 1994).
- Provide a milieu that allows for discussion of sexual issues and a higher level of sexual satisfaction. Allow couples to room together and bring in double beds from

• = Independent; ▲ = Collaborative

home. Place signs on the door to ensure privacy.

Environmental variables have an impact on elderly people's ability to freely express sexuality (Shell, Smith, 1994).

- Provide clients with the following information:
  - Exercise, such as walking, swimming, cycling, and riding a stationary bike, will help control flabby thighs and weak musculature and make people feel more sexually attractive.
  - Overindulgence in food or alcohol can affect sexual activity (see care plan for **Imbalanced Nutrition: less than body requirements**).
  - Resting and sleeping on a firm mattress may augment sexual desire.
  - Femininity and masculinity are still important.
  - Pay attention to cleanliness, skin care, and clothing.
  - Change environment.
  - Experiment with position changes.

  Because the majority of the elderly population maintains sexual interest, desire, and functioning, these interventions may be helpful during the rehabilitation process. Older adults may exercise aerobically 3 to 5 times a week for 15 to 30 minutes depending on physical status and treatment regimen (Steinke et al, 1986).
- See care plan for **Sexual dysfunction.**

Culturally appropriate interventions

- Assess for the influence of cultural beliefs, norms, and values on the client's perceptions of normal sexual behavior.

  What the client considers normal sexual behavior may be based on cultural perceptions (Leininger, 1996).
- Discuss with the client those aspects of his or her sexual health/lifestyle that remain unchanged by their health status.

  Aspects of the client's life that are valuable to him or her should be understood and preserved without change (Leininger, 1996).
- Validate the client's feelings and emotions regarding the changes in sexuality patterns.

  Validation lets the client know the nurse has heard and understands what was said and promotes the nurse-client relationship (Stuart, Laraia, 2001; Giger, Davidhizar, 1995).

Home Care Interventions

- Help the client and significant other to identify a place and time in the home and daily living for privacy in sharing sexual or relationship activity. If necessary, help client to communicate the need for privacy to other family members. Consider periodic escapes to desirable surroundings.

  The home setting can be one that affords little, if any, privacy without a conscious effort made by members of the home.
- ▲ Confirm that physical reasons for dysfunction have been addressed. Encourage participation in support groups or therapy if appropriate.

  Clients express embarrassment at continuing medical intervention or participation in groups once they are back in the community and know that peers may judge their activities. However, 22 female psychiatric outpatients with experience of childhood sexual abuse took part in a 2-year group therapy, and at the end of the 2 years, group members evaluated their relationships as having improved (Lundquist, Ojehagen, 2001).
- Reinforce or teach about sexual functioning, alternative sexual practices, and necessary sexual precautions. Update teaching as client status changes.

• = **Independent;** ▲ = **Collaborative**

If the client or significant other has received information during an institutional stay, other stressors may have made the information a temporarily low priority or may have impaired learning. Depending on the cause for dysfunction, the client may experience changing status or feelings about the problem.

Client/Family Teaching

▲ Refer to appropriate community agencies (e.g., certified sex counselor, Reach to Recovery, Ostomy Association).

There may be needs that either are beyond the nurse's skill and ability to address or are related to a particular situation (e.g., presence of an ostomy that requires intervention from specialized sources) (Lewis, 1992). Sexuality concerns should be addressed with all clients undergoing ostomy placement (Sprunk, Alteneder, 2000).

• Provide information regarding self-care (e.g., Beauty and Cancer [Noyes, Mellodey, 1988]) and positioning (e.g., Sexuality and Cancer: For the Woman Who has Cancer and Her Partner [Schover, 1988]).

Couples may hesitate to change their routines. Providing this kind of information in a sensitive way often gives permission to change (Shell, Smith, 1994).

▲ Discuss contraceptive choices. Refer to appropriate health professional (e.g., gynecologist, nurse practitioner).

Specialists may be needed for complex situations.

• Teach safe sex, which includes using latex condoms, washing with soap immediately after sexual contact, not ingesting semen, avoiding oral-genital contact, not exchanging saliva, avoiding multiple partners, abstaining from sexual activity when ill, and avoiding recreational drugs and alcohol when engaging in sexual activity. Contrary to previously published information, the use of a spermicide containing nonoxynol-9 (N-9) should not be recommended as a preventative strategy for HIV infection.

Accurate information regarding safe sex is essential for sexually active clients (Tucker et al, 1996). In a study of 1000 women it was determined that N-9 has now been proven ineffective against HIV transmission. The possibility of risk, with no benefit, indicates that N-9, a product widely used in spermicides, should not be recommended as an effective means of HIV prevention (Gayle, 2000). Interventions that focus on self-efficacy are most likely to reduce anxiety related to condom use, increase positive perceptions about condoms, and increase the likelihood of adopting condom use behaviors (Dilorio et al, 2000).

WEB SITES FOR EDUCATION

MERLIN See the MERLIN web site for World Wide Web resources for client education.

REFERENCES   Dilorio C et al: A social cognitive-based model for condom use among college students, *Nurs Res* 49(4):208-214, 2000.

Fontaine K: Unlocking sexual issues, *Nurs Clin North Am* 26:737, 1991.

Gayle HD: *Nonoxynol-9 trial: the implications,* Centers for Disease Control and Prevention, CDC Divisions of HIV/AIDS Prevention, Aug 4, 2000 (letter), retrieved from the World Wide Web June 11, 2001. Web site www.cdc.gov/hiv/dhap.htm

Giger JN, Davidhizar RE: *Transcultural nursing,* ed 2, St Louis, 1995, Mosby.

Laurent C: Talking treatment: therapy for cervical cancer has left some women with severe sexual problems, *Nurs Times* 90:14, 1994.

Leininger MM: *Transcultural nursing: theories, research and practices,* ed 2, Hilliard, Ohio, 1996, McGraw-Hill.

Lewis JH: Treatment options for men with sexual dysfunction, *J ET Nurs* 19:131, 1992.

Lundquist G, Ojehagen A: Childhood sexual abuse: an evaluation of a two-year group therapy in adult women, *Eur Psychiatry* 16(1):64-67, 2001.

• = Independent; ▲ = Collaborative

McCoy N: Methodological problems in the study of sexuality and menopause, *Maturitas 1998* 29(1):51-60, 1998.

Noyes D, Mellodey P: *Beauty and cancer,* Los Angeles, 1988, AC Press.

Parish KL et al: Safer sex decision-making among men with haemophilia and HIV and their female partners, *Haemophilia* 7(1):72-81, 2001.

Schover L: *Sexuality and cancer: for the woman who has cancer and her partner,* New York, 1988, American Cancer Society.

Shell J, Smith C: Sexuality and the older person with cancer, *Oncology* 21:553, 1994.

Sprunk E, Alteneder RR: The impact of an ostomy on sexuality, *Clin J Oncol Nurs* 4(2):85-88, 2000.

Steinke E, Patterson-Midgley P: Sexual counseling following acute myocardial infarction, *Clin Nurs Res* 5(4):462-472, 1996.

Steinke EE et al: Sexuality and aging, *J Gerontol Nurs* 12(6):6-10, 1986.

Stuart GW, Laraia MT: Therapeutic nurse-patient relationship. In Stuart GW, Laraia MT, editors: *Principles and practice of psychiatric nursing,* St Louis, 2001, Mosby, p 30.

Taylor P: Beating the taboo, *Nurs Times* 90:51, 1994.

Tucker M et al: *Patient care standards: collaborative practice planning,* ed 6, St Louis, 1996, Mosby.

Impaired Skin integrity

Diane Krasner

NANDA **Definition** Altered epidermis and/or dermis

Defining Characteristics

Invasion of body structures; destruction of skin layers (dermis); disruption of skin surface (epidermis)

Related Factors (r/t)

External   Hyperthermia; hypothermia; chemical substance (e.g., incontinence); mechanical factors (e.g., friction, shearing forces, pressure, restraint); physical immobilization; humidity; extremes in age; moisture; radiation; medications

Internal   Altered metabolic state; altered nutritional state (e.g., obesity, emaciation); altered circulation; altered sensation; altered pigmentation; skeletal prominence; developmental factors; immunological deficit; alterations in skin turgor (change in elasticity); altered fluid status

NOC **Outcomes (Nursing Outcomes Classification)**

Suggested NOC Labels

Tissue Integrity: Skin and Mucous Membranes; Wound Healing: Primary Intention; Wound Healing: Secondary Intention

> **Example NOC Outcome**
>
> Tissue Integrity: Skin and Mucous Membranes will be intact as evidenced by the following indicators: Skin intactness/Tissue lesion-free/Tissue perfusion/Tissue temperature in expected range (Rate each indicator of **Tissue Integrity: Skin and Mucous Membranes:** 1 = extremely compromised, 2 = substantially compromised, 3 = moderately compromised, 4 = mildly compromised, 5 = not compromised [see Section I])

Client Outcomes

- Regains integrity of skin surface
- Reports any altered sensation or pain at site of skin impairment

• = Independent; ▲ = Collaborative

- Demonstrates understanding of plan to heal skin and prevent reinjury
- Describes measures to protect and heal the skin and to care for any skin lesion

NIC **Interventions (Nursing Interventions Classification)**

Suggested NIC Labels

Incision Site Care; Pressure Ulcer Care; Skin Care: Topical Treatments; Skin Surveillance Wound Care

> **Example NIC Interventions—Pressure Ulcer Care**
> - Monitor color, temperature, edema, moisture, and appearance of surrounding skin
> - Note characteristics of any drainage

Nursing Interventions and Rationales

- Assess site of skin impairment and determine etiology (e.g., acute or chronic wound, burn, dermatological lesion, pressure ulcer, skin tear) (Krasner, Sibbald, 1999a, 1999b). *Prior assessment of wound etiology is critical for proper identification of nursing interventions (van Rijswijk, 2001).*
- Determine that skin impairment involves skin damage only (e.g., partial-thickness wound, stage I or stage II pressure ulcer). Classify superficial pressure ulcers in the following manner:
  - Stage I: Observable pressure-related alteration of intact skin with indicators as compared with the adjacent or opposite area on the body that may include changes in one or more of the following: skin temperature (warmth or coolness), tissue consistency (firm or boggy feel), and/or sensation (pain, itching). The ulcer appears as a defined area of persistent redness in lightly pigmented skin, whereas in darker skin tones, the ulcer may appear with persistent red, blue, or purple hues (National Pressure Ulcer Advisory Panel, 1999).
  - Stage II: Partial-thickness skin loss involving epidermis or dermis superficial ulcer that appears as an abrasion, blister, or shallow crater (National Pressure Ulcer Advisory Panel, 1999).

  NOTE: For wounds deeper into subcutaneous tissue, muscle, or bone (stage III or stage IV pressure ulcers), see the care plan for **Impaired Tissue integrity.**
- Monitor site of skin impairment at least once a day for color changes, redness, swelling, warmth, pain, or other signs of infection. Determine whether client is experiencing changes in sensation or pain. Pay special attention to high-risk areas such as bony prominences, skinfolds, the sacrum, and heels. *Systematic inspection can identify impending problems early (Bryant, 1999).*
- Monitor client's skin care practices, noting type of soap or other cleansing agents used, temperature of water, and frequency of skin cleansing.
- Individualize plan according to client's skin condition, needs, and preferences. *Avoid harsh cleansing agents, hot water, extreme friction or force, or cleansing too frequently (Panel for the Prediction and Prevention of Pressure Ulcers in Adults, 1992).*
- Monitor client's continence status, and minimize exposure of skin impairment and other areas to moisture from incontinence, perspiration, or wound drainage.
- ▲ If client is incontinent, implement an incontinence management plan to prevent exposure to chemicals in urine and stool that can strip or erode the skin. Refer to a urologist or gastroenterologist for incontinence assessment (Doughty, 2000; Wound, Ostomy, and Continence Nurses Society, 1992, 1994; Fantl et al, 1996).

- **= Independent; ▲ = Collaborative**

- For clients with limited mobility, use a risk-assessment tool to systematically assess immobility-related risk factors (van Rijswijk, 2001).
  A validated risk-assessment tool such as the Norton or Braden scale should be used to identify clients at risk for immobility-related skin breakdown (Panel for the Prediction and Prevention of Pressure Ulcers in Adults, 1992).
- Do not position client on site of skin impairment. If consistent with overall client management goals, turn and position client at least every 2 hours. Transfer client with care to protect against the adverse effects of external mechanical forces such as pressure, friction, and shear.
- Evaluate for use of specialty mattresses, beds, or devices as appropriate (Fleck, 2001).
  If the goal of care is to keep a client (e.g., a terminally ill client) comfortable, turning and repositioning may not be appropriate. Maintain the head of the bed at the lowest possible degree of elevation to reduce shear and friction, and use lift devices, pillows, foam wedges, and pressure-reducing devices in the bed. Evaluate for the use of specialty mattresses or beds as appropriate (Krasner, Rodeheaver, Sibbald, 2001; Panel for the Prediction and Prevention of Pressure Ulcers in Adults, 1992; Wilson, 1994).
- ▲ Implement a written treatment plan for topical treatment of the site of skin impairment.
  A written plan ensures consistency in care and documentation (Maklebust, Sieggreen, 1996). Topical treatments must be matched to the client, wound, and setting (Krasner, Sibbald 1999a, 1999b).
- ▲ Select a topical treatment that will maintain a moist wound-healing environment and that is balanced with the need to absorb exudate.
  Caution should always be taken not to dry out the wound (Bergstrom et al, 1994).
- Avoid massaging around the site of skin impairment and over bony prominences.
  Research suggests that massage may lead to deep-tissue trauma (Panel for the Prediction and Prevention of Pressure Ulcers in Adults, 1992).
- ▲ Assess client's nutritional status. Refer for a nutritional consult, and/or institute dietary supplements as necessary.
  Inadequate nutritional intake places individuals at risk for skin breakdown and compromises healing (Demling, De Santi, 1998).

Home Care Interventions

- Identify client's phase of wound healing (inflammation, proliferation, maturation) and stage of injury.
  Accurate understanding of tissue status combined with knowledge of underlying diagnoses and product validity provide a basis for determining appropriate treatment objectives (Ovington, 1998). There is no single wound dressing appropriate for all phases of wound healing (Ovington, 1998).
- Instruct and assist client and caregivers to remove or control impediments to wound healing (e.g., management of underlying disease, improved approach to client positioning, improved nutrition).
  Wound healing can be delayed or fail totally if impediments are not controlled (Krasner, Sibbald, 1999a, 1999b).
- ▲ Initiate a consultation in a case assignment with a wound, ostomy, continence nurse (WOC nurse) to establish a comprehensive plan as soon as possible.

• = **Independent;** ▲ = **Collaborative**

Client/Family Teaching

- Teach skin and wound assessment and ways to monitor for signs and symptoms of infection, complications, and healing.

  Early assessment and intervention help prevent serious problems from developing.

▲ Teach client to use a topical treatment that is matched to the client, wound, and setting.

  The topical treatment must be adjusted as the status of the wound changes (van Rijswijk, 2001; Krasner, Sibbald, 1999a, 1999b; Ovington, 1998).

- If consistent with overall client management goals, teach how to turn and reposition at least every 2 hours.

  If the goal of care is to keep a client (e.g., terminally ill client) comfortable, turning and repositioning may not be appropriate (Krasner, Rodeheaver, Sibbald, 2001; Panel for the Prediction and Prevention of Pressure Ulcers in Adults, 1992).

- Teach client to use pillows, foam wedges, and pressure-reducing devices to prevent pressure injury.

WEB SITES FOR EDUCATION

MERLIN See the MERLIN web site for World Wide Web resources for client education.

REFERENCES Bergstrom N et al: *Treatment of pressure ulcers, Clinical Practice Guideline No. 15,* Agency for Health Care Policy and Research, Pub. No. 95-0652, Rockville, Md, 1994, Public Health Service, U.S. Department of Health and Human Services.

Bryant R: *Acute and chronic wounds,* ed 2, St Louis, 1999, Mosby.

Demling R, De Santi, L: Closure of the non-healing wound corresponds with correction of weight loss using the anabolic agent oxandrolone, *Ostomy Wound Manage* 44(10):58-68, 1998.

Doughty D: *Urinary and fecal incontinence: nursing management,* ed 2, St Louis, 2000, Mosby.

Fantl JA et al: *Urinary incontinence in adults: acute and chronic management,* Clinical Practice Guideline, No. 2, 1996 Update, Agency for Health Care Policy and Research, Pub. No. 96-0682, Rockville, Md, 1996, Public Health Service, U.S. Department of Health and Human Services.

Fleck C: Support surfaces: criteria and selection. In Krasner D, Rodeheaver G, Sibbald RG: *Chronic wound care: a clinical source book for healthcare professionals,* ed 2, Wayne, Penn, 2001, HMP Communications.

Krasner D, Rodeheaver G, Sibbald RG: Advanced wound caring for a new millennium. In Krasner D, Rodeheaver G, Sibbald RG: *Chronic wound care: a clinical source book for healthcare professionals,* ed 2, Wayne, Penn, 2001, HMP Communications.

Krasner D, Sibbald RG: Nursing management of chronic wounds: best practices across the continuum of care, *Nurs Clin North Am* 34(4):933-953, 1999a.

Krasner D, Sibbald RG, editors: Moving beyond the AHCPR guidelines: wound care evolution over the last five years, *Ostomy Wound Manage Spec Suppl* 45(1A):15-125, 1999b.

Maklebust J, Sieggreen M: *Pressure ulcers: guidelines for prevention and nursing management,* ed 2, Springhouse, Penn, 1996, Springhouse.

National Pressure Ulcer Advisory Panel, 1999. Web site: www.npuap.org

Ovington LG: The well-dressed wound: an overview of dressing types, *Wounds* 10(suppl)A: IA-IIA, 1998.

Panel for the Prediction and Prevention of Pressure Ulcers in Adults: *Pressure ulcers in adults: prediction and prevention,* Clinical Practice Guideline No. 3, Agency for Health Care Policy and Research, Pub. No. 92-0047, Rockville, Md, 1992, Public Health Service, U.S. Department of Health and Human Services.

van Rijswijk L: Wound assessment and documentation. In Krasner D, Rodeheaver G, Sibbald RG: *Chronic wound care: a clinical source book for healthcare professionals,* ed 2, Wayne, Penn, 2001, HMP Communications.

Wilson S: Mattresses that spell relief, *Am J Nurs* 94:48, 1994.

Wound, Ostomy, and Continence Nurses Society: *Standards of care: patient with urinary incontinence,* Costa Mesa, Calif, 1992, The Society.

Wound, Ostomy, and Continence Nurses Society: *Standards of care: patient with fecal incontinence,* Costa Mesa, Calif, 1994, The Society.

• = **Independent;** ▲ = **Collaborative**

Risk for impaired Skin integrity

Diane Krasner

NANDA **Definition** At risk for skin being adversely altered

Risk Factors
External Hypothermia; hyperthermia; chemical substance; excretions and/or secretions; mechanical factors (e.g., shearing forces, pressure, restraint); radiation; physical immobilization; humidity; moisture; extremes of age

Internal Medication; altered nutritional state (e.g., obesity, emaciation); altered metabolic state; altered circulation; altered sensation; altered pigmentation; skeletal prominence; developmental factors; immunological deficit; alterations in skin turgor (change in elasticity); psychogenetic, immunological factors

NOTE: Risk should be determined by the use of a risk assessment tool (e.g., Norton Scale, Braden Scale).

Related Factors (r/t)
See Risk Factors

NOC **Outcomes (Nursing Outcomes Classification)**

Suggested NOC Labels
Tissue Integrity: Skin and Mucous Membranes; Immobility Consequences: Physiological

> **Example NOC Outcome**
> **Tissue Integrity: Skin and Mucous Membranes** will be intact as evidenced by the following indicators: Skin intactness/Tissue lesion-free/Tissue perfusion/Tissue temperature in expected range (Rate each indicator of **Tissue Integrity: Skin and Mucous Membranes:** 1 = extremely compromised, 2 = substantially compromised, 3 = moderately compromised, 4 = mildly compromised, 5 = not compromised [see Section I])

Client Outcomes
- Reports altered sensation or pain at risk areas
- Demonstrates understanding of personal risk factors for impaired skin integrity
- Verbalizes a personal plan for preventing impaired skin integrity

NIC **Interventions (Nursing Interventions Classification)**

Suggested NIC Labels
Positioning; Pressure Management; Pressure Ulcer Prevention; Skin Surveillance

> **Example NIC Interventions—Pressure Ulcer Care**
> - Monitor color, temperature, edema, moisture, and appearance of surrounding skin
> - Note characteristics of any drainage

Nursing Interventions and Rationales
- Monitor skin condition at least once a day for color or texture changes, dermatological conditions, or lesions. Determine whether client is experiencing loss of sensation or pain.
  Systematic inspection can identify impending problems early (Krasner, Rodeheaver, Sibbald, 2001).

• = Independent; ▲ = Collaborative

- Identify clients at risk for impaired skin integrity as a result of compromised perfusion, immunocompromised status, or chronic medical condition such as diabetes mellitus or renal failure (Colburn, 2001).
  These patient populations are known to be at high risk for impaired skin integrity (Bergstrom et al, 1987; Stotts, Wipke-Tevis, 2001).
- Monitor client's skin care practices, noting type of soap or other cleansing agents used, temperature of water, and frequency of skin cleansing (Doughty, 2000).
  Individualize plan according to client's skin condition, needs, and preferences.
- Avoid harsh cleansing agents, hot water, extreme friction or force, or too-frequent cleansing (Panel for the Prediction and Prevention of Pressure Ulcers in Adults, 1992).
- Monitor client's continence status, and minimize exposure of the site of skin impairment and other areas to moisture from incontinence, perspiration, or wound drainage.
  If client is incontinent, implement an incontinence management plan to prevent exposure to chemicals in urine and stool that can strip or erode the skin; refer to a physician (e.g., urologist, gastroenterologist) for an incontinence assessment (Doughty, 2000; Wound, Ostomy and Continence Nurses Society, 1992, 1994; Fantl et al, 1996).
- For clients with limited mobility, monitor condition of skin covering bony prominences.
  Pressure ulcers usually occur over bony prominences, such as the sacrum, coccyx, trochanter, and heels, as a result of unrelieved pressure between the prominence and support surface (Maklebust, Sieggreen, 1996).
- Use a risk-assessment tool to systematically assess immobility-related risk factors.
  A validated risk-assessment tool such as the Norton or Braden scale should be used to identify clients at risk for immobility-related skin breakdown (Bergstrom et al, 1987; Panel for the Prediction and Prevention of Pressure Ulcers in Adults, 1992; Sussman, Bates-Jensen, 1998).
- Implement a written prevention plan.
  A written plan ensures consistency in care and documentation (Maklebust, Sieggreen, 1996).
- If consistent with overall client management goals, turn and position client at least every 2 hours. Transfer client with care to protect against the adverse effects of external mechanical forces (e.g., pressure, friction, shear).
- ▲ Evaluate for use of specialty mattresses, beds, or devices as appropriate (Fleck, 2001).
  If the goal of care is to keep the client (e.g., a terminally ill client) comfortable, turning and repositioning may not be appropriate. Maintain the head of the bed at the lowest possible degree of elevation to reduce shear and friction and use lift devices, pillows, foam wedges, and pressure-reducing devices in the bed (Krasner, Rodeheaver, Sibbald, 2001; Panel for the Prediction and Prevention of Pressure Ulcers in Adults, 1992).
- Avoid massaging over bony prominences.
  Research suggests that massage may lead to deep-tissue trauma (Panel for the Prediction and Prevention of Pressure Ulcers in Adults, 1992).
- ▲ Assess client's nutritional status; refer for a nutritional consult, and/or institute dietary supplements.
  Inadequate nutritional intake places individuals at risk for skin breakdown and compromises healing (Demling, De Santi, 1998).

• = Independent; ▲ = Collaborative

Geriatric

- Limit number of complete baths to two or three per week, and alternate them with partial baths. Use a tepid water temperature (between 90° and 105° F) for bathing.
  Excessive bathing, especially in hot water, depletes aging skin of moisture and increases dryness.
- Use lotions and moisturizers to prevent skin from drying out, especially in the winter (Sibbald, Cameron, 2001).
  Avoid skin care products that contain allergens such as lanolin, latex, and dyes (Sibbald, Cameron, 2001).
- Increase fluid intake within cardiac and renal limits to a minimum of 1500 ml per day.
  Dry skin is caused by loss of fluid; increasing fluid intake hydrates the skin.
- Increase humidity in the environment, especially during the winter, by using a humidifier or placing a container of water on a warm object.
  Increasing the moisture in the air helps keep moisture in the skin (Sibbald, Cameron, 2001).

Home Care Interventions

- Assess caregiver vigilance and ability.
  In a limited study of the Braden Scale, caregiver vigilance and ability were recognized as potentially significant variables for determining the risk of developing pressure sores (Ramundo, 1995).
- Initiate a consultation in a case assignment with a wound, ostomy, continence nurse (WOC nurse) to establish a comprehensive plan as soon as possible.
- See the care plan for **Impaired Skin integrity.**

Client/Family Teaching

- Teach client skin assessment and ways to monitor for impending skin breakdown.
  Early assessment and intervention help prevent the development of serious problems (Colburn, 2001).
- If consistent with overall client management goals, teach how to turn and reposition client at least every 2 hours.
  If the goal of care is to keep the client (e.g., a terminally ill client) comfortable, turning and repositioning may not be appropriate (Panel for the Prediction and Prevention of Pressure Ulcers in Adults, 1992).
- Teach client to use pillows, foam wedges, and pressure-reducing devices to prevent pressure injury (Bryant, 1999; Krasner, Sibbald, 1999).

WEB SITES FOR EDUCATION

MERLIN See the MERLIN web site for World Wide Web resources for client education.

REFERENCES Bergstrom N et al: The Braden scale for prediction of pressure sore risk, *Nurs Res* 36:205, 1987.
Bryant R: *Acute and chronic wounds,* ed 2, St Louis, 1999, Mosby.
Colburn L: Prevention for chronic wounds. In Krasner D, Rodeheaver G, Sibbald RG: *Chronic wound care: a clinical source book for healthcare professionals,* ed 2, Wayne, Penn, 2001, HMP Communications.
Demling R, De Santi L: Closure of the non-healing wound corresponds with correction of weight loss using the anabolic agent oxandrolone, *Ostomy Wound Manage* 44(10):58-68, 1998.
Doughty D: *Urinary and fecal incontinence: nursing management,* ed 2, St Louis, 2000, Mosby.
Fantl JA et al: *Urinary incontinence in adults: acute and chronic management,* Clinical Practice Guideline No. 2, 1996 Update, Agency for Health Care Policy and Research, Pub. No. 96-0682, Rockville, Md, 1996, Public Health Service, U.S. Department of Health & Human Services.
Fleck C: Support surfaces: criteria and selection. In Krasner D, Rodeheaver G, Sibbald RG: *Chronic wound care: a clinical source book for healthcare professionals,* ed 2, Wayne, Penn, 2001, HMP Communications.

• = **Independent;** ▲ = **Collaborative**

Krasner D, Rodeheaver G, Sibbald RG: Advanced wound caring for a new millennium. In Krasner D, Rodeheaver G, Sibbald RG: *Chronic wound care: a clinical source book for healthcare professionals,* ed 2, Wayne,
Penn, 2001, HMP Communications.

Krasner D, Sibbald RG, editors: Moving beyond the AHCPR guidelines: would care evolution over the last
five years, *Ostomy Wound Manage Spec Suppl* 45(1A):1S-120S, 1999.

Maklebust J, Sieggreen M: *Pressure ulcers: guidelines for prevention and nursing management,* ed 2, Springhouse, Penn, 1996, Springhouse.

Panel for the Prediction and Prevention of Pressure Ulcers in Adults: *Pressure ulcers in adults: prediction
and prevention,* Clinical Practice Guideline No. 3, Agency for Health Care Policy and Research, Pub.
No. 92-0047, Rockville, Md, 1992, Public Health Service, U.S. Department of Health and Human
Services.

Ramundo J: Reliability and validity of the Braden Scale in the home care setting, *J Wound Ostomy Cont Nurs*
22:3, 1995.

Sibbald RG, Cameron J: Dermatological aspects of wound care. In Krasner D, Rodeheaver G, Sibbald RG:
Chronic wound care: a clinical source book for healthcare professionals, ed 2, Wayne, Penn, 2001, HMP Communications.

Stotts NA, Wipke-Tevis: Co-factors in impaired wound healing. In Krasner D, Rodeheaver G, Sibbald RG:
Chronic wound care: a clinical source book for healthcare professionals, ed 2, Wayne, Penn, 2001, HMP
Communications.

Sussman C, Bates-Jensen BM: *Wound care: a collaborative practice manual for physical therapists and nurses,*
Gaithersburg, Md, 1998, Aspen.

Wound, Ostomy, and Continence Nurses Society: *Standards of care: patient with urinary incontinence,* Costa
Mesa, Calif, 1992, The Society.

Wound, Ostomy, and Continence Nurses Society: *Standards of care: patient with fecal incontinence,* Costa
Mesa, Calif, 1994, The Society.

Sleep deprivation

Betty J. Ackley

 Definition Prolonged periods without sleep (sustained natural, periodic suspension of relative unconsciousness)

Defining Characteristics

Daytime drowsiness; decreased ability to function; malaise; tiredness; lethargy; restlessness; irritability; heightened sensitivity to pain; listlessness; apathy; slowed reaction; inability to concentrate; perceptual disorders (e.g., disturbed body sensation, delusions,
feeling afloat); hallucinations; acute confusion; transient paranoia; agitated or combative; anxious; mild, fleeting nystagmus; hand tremors

Related Factors (r/t)

Prolonged physical discomfort; prolonged psychological discomfort; sustained inadequate sleep hygiene; prolonged use of pharmacological or dietary antisoporifics; aging-
related sleep stage shifts; sustained circadian asynchrony; inadequate daytime activity;
sustained environmental stimulation; sustained unfamiliar or uncomfortable sleep environment; nonsleep-inducing parenting practices; sleep apnea; periodic limb movement
(e.g., restless leg syndrome, nocturnal myoclonus); sundowner's syndrome; narcolepsy;
idiopathic central nervous system hypersomnolence; sleep walking; sleep terror; sleep-
related enuresis; nightmares; familiar sleep paralysis; sleep-related painful erections;
dementia

• = Independent; ▲ = Collaborative

Outcomes (Nursing Outcomes Classification)

Suggested NOC Labels

Sleep; Rest; Symptom Severity

> **Example NOC Outcome**
>
> Demonstrates **Sleep** as evidenced by: Hours of sleep/Sleep pattern/Sleep Quality/
> Sleep efficiency/Feelings of rejuvenation after sleep/Napping appropriate for age
> (Rate each indicator of **Sleep:** 1 = extremely compromised, 2 = substantially com-
> promised, 3 = moderately compromised, 4 = mildly compromised, 5 = not com-
> promised [see Section I])

Client Outcomes

- Wakes up less frequently during night
- Awakens refreshed and is less fatigued during day
- Falls asleep without difficulty
- Verbalizes plan to implement bedtime routines
- Identifies actions can take to improve quality of sleep

NIC **Interventions (Nursing Interventions Classification)**

Suggested NIC Labels

Sleep Enhancement

> **Example NIC Interventions—Sleep Enhancement**
> - Monitor/record patient's sleep pattern and number of sleep hours
> - Encourage patient to establish a bedtime routine to facilitate transition from
>   wakefulness to sleep

Nursing Interventions and Rationales

- Assess client's sleep patterns and usual bedtime rituals and incorporate these into the
  plan of care.
  *Usual sleep patterns are individual; data collected through a comprehensive and ho-
  listic assessment are needed to determine the etiology of the disturbance (Spenceley,
  1993).*
- Ask client to keep a sleep diary for several weeks.
  *Often the client can find the cause of the sleep deprivation when the pattern of sleeping is
  examined (Pagel, Zafralotfi, Zammit, 1997).*
- ▲ Observe for underlying physiological illnesses causing insomnia (e.g., cardiovascular,
  pulmonary, gastrointestinal, hyperthyroidism, nocturia occurring with benign hyper-
  trophic prostatitis or pain).
  *Symptomology of disease states can cause insomnia (Evans, Rogers, 1994; Whitney et al,
  1998; Sateia et al, 2000).*
- Determine level of anxiety. If client is anxious, see Nursing Interventions and
  Rationales for **Anxiety.**
  *Anxiety interferes with sleep. Interventions such as relaxation training can help clients
  reduce anxiety (Pagel, Zafralotfi, Zammit, 1997; Sateia et al, 2000).*
- ▲ Assess for signs of depression: depressed mood state, statements of hopelessness,
  poor appetite. Refer for counseling as appropriate.

• = Independent; ▲ = Collaborative

Sleep deprivation in normal subjects did not result in the usual complaints of people with insomnia. Many symptoms associated with sleep deprivation probably arise from central nervous system hyperarousal (Sateia et al, 2000).

▲ Monitor for presence of nocturnal symptoms of restless leg syndrome with uncomfortable restless sensations in legs that occur before sleep onset or during the night. Also monitor for nocturnal panic attacks, presence of headaches, or gastroesophageal reflux disease. Refer for treatment as appropriate.
Numerous nocturnal events and symptoms can contribute to problems with sleep (Sateia et al, 2000).

• Observe client's medication, diet, and caffeine intake. Look for hidden sources of caffeine, such as over-the-counter medications.
Difficulty sleeping can be a side effect of medications such as bronchodilators. Caffeine can also interfere with sleep.

• Provide measures to take before bedtime to assist with sleep (e.g., quiet time to allow the mind to slow down, carbohydrates such as crackers, or a back massage).
Simple measures can increase quality of sleep. Carbohydrates cause release of the neuro-transmitter serotonin, which helps induce and maintain sleep (Somer, 1999). Research has shown back massage to be effective for inducing sleep (Richards, 1994).

▲ Provide pain relief shortly before bedtime, and position client comfortably for sleep.
Clients have reported that uncomfortable positions and pain are common factors in sleep disturbance (Sateia et al, 2000).

▲ Monitor for presence of sleep apnea as evidenced by loud snoring with periods of apnea. Obtain a referral for sleep studies from a physician as needed.
Up to 15% of all chronic insomnia conditions are associated with breathing disturbances (Sateia et al, 2000).

• Keep environment quiet (e.g., avoid use of intercoms, lower the volume on radio and television, keep beepers on nonaudio mode, anticipate alarms on IV pumps, talk quietly on unit).
Excessive noise causes sleep deprivation that can result in ICU psychosis (Barr, 1993). Health volunteers exposed to recorded critical care noise levels experienced poor sleep (Topf, 1992). More than half of the noises in ICUs were caused by human behavior such as talking and TV watching (Kahn, Cook, 1998).

• Use soothing sound generators with sounds of the ocean, rainfall, or waterfall to induce sleep, or use "white noise" such as a fan to block out other sounds.
Ocean sounds promoted sleep for a group of postoperative open-heart surgery clients (Williamson, 1992).

Geriatric

▲ Determine if client has a physiological problem that could result in insomnia such as pain, cardiovascular disease, pulmonary disease, neurological problems such as dementia, or urinary problems.
Sleep disturbances in the elderly may represent a complex interaction of age-related changes and pathological causes (Sateia et al, 2000).

• Observe elimination patterns. Have client decrease fluid intake in the evening, and ensure that diuretics are taken early in the morning.
Many elderly people void during the night. Increasing water intake at night or taking diuretics late in the day increases nocturia, which results in disrupted sleep.

• = Independent; ▲ = Collaborative

- If client is waking frequently during the night, consider the presence of sleep apnea problems and refer to a sleep clinic for evaluation.
  Sleep apnea in the elderly may be caused by changes in the respiratory drive of the central nervous system or may be obstructive and associated with obesity (Foyt, 1992).
- Encourage social activities. Help elderly get outside for increased light exposure and to enjoy nature.
  Exposure to light and social interactions influence the circadian rhythms that control sleep (Elmore, Betrus, Burr, 1994).
- Suggest light reading or TV viewing that does not excite as an evening activity.
  Soothing activities decrease stimulation of the reticular activating system and help sleep come naturally.
- Increase daytime physical activity. Encourage walking as client is able.
- Avoid use of hypnotics and alcohol to sleep.
  Long-term use of hypnotics can induce a drug-related insomnia. Alcohol also disrupts sleep and can exacerbate sleep apnea (Evans, Rogers, 1994).
- Reduce daytime napping in the late afternoon; limit naps to short intervals as early in the day as possible.
  The majority of elderly nap during the day (Evans, Rogers, 1994). Avoiding naps in the late afternoon makes it easier to fall asleep at night.
- ▲ If client continues to have insomnia despite developing good sleep hygiene habits, refer to a sleep clinic for further evaluation (Pagel, Zafralotfi, Zammit, 1997).

Home Care Interventions

- Obtain a full current assessment and history of sleep activity, disturbance, and disturbance-related behaviors.
  A complete assessment promotes accurate determination of the client's needs.
- Assess environment for possible hazards to client during period of deprivation (e.g., appliances, stairs).
  Client safety is a primary goal of care in the home setting.
- Obtain a listing of expected daily behaviors, before and since the onset of deprivation (e.g., mowing lawn, shaving, cooking). Identify tasks that may be delegated. Establish level of client participation in tasks. Use short task periods for client.
  Role changes may be necessary to protect client and family safety. Continued participation in family activities promotes sense of belonging.
- Assess client support system for availability of psychological and task-related support. Refer to chore, homemaker, or home health aide services as necessary.
  Home health aides can assist with activities of daily (ADLs) living; homemakers can do household tasks and shopping to support the family. Chore services can do major household cleaning and yard work.
- ▲ Assess family/caregiver response to client status. Provide nursing support; refer to medical social services or mental health services/support groups as necessary.
  Support of the family/caregiver structure can decrease caregiver burden.
- If client is taking medication, assess for effectiveness and safety in administration. Identify person administering medication if not the client.
  Sleep-deprived persons may not be consistent in self-administration of medications.
- Assist the family to arrange for supervision if the client presents confusion or perceptual dysfunction.

- **• = Independent; ▲ = Collaborative**

Client supervision provides for client safety and may provide additional caregiver respite if obtained from outside the usual support system.

▲ Refer client to medical social services or mental health/group support services such as I Can Cope.

Venting validates feelings of the client. Groups allow the client to recognize the love and caring of others and provide alternative ways of problem-solving.

Client/Family Teaching

• Encourage client to avoid coffee and other caffeinated foods and liquids and to avoid eating large high-protein or high-fat meals close to bedtime.

Caffeine intake increases the time it takes to fall asleep and increases awake time during the night (Evans, Rogers, 1994). A full stomach interferes with sleep.

▲ Advise the client that research on use of melatonin is still equivocal; while it may help the client to fall asleep faster, it does not improve the quality or length of time in the sleep interval, and long-term results are unknown (Hughes, Sack, Lewy, 1998; Defrance, Quera-Salva, 1998).

• Teach relaxation techniques, pain relief measures, or the use of imagery before sleep.

• Teach client need for increased exercise. Encourage to take a daily walk 5 to 6 hours before retiring.

Moderate activity such as walking can increase the quality of sleep (King et al, 1997).

• Encourage client to develop a bedtime ritual that includes quiet activities such as reading, television, or crafts.

• Teach the following guidelines for improving sleep habits:
  ▪ Go to bed only when sleepy.
  ▪ When awake in the middle of the night, go to another room, do quiet activities, and go back to bed only when sleepy.
  ▪ Use the bed only for sleeping—not for reading or snoozing in front of the television.
  ▪ Avoid afternoon and evening naps.
  ▪ Get up at the same time every morning.
  ▪ Recognize that not everyone needs 8 hours of sleep.
  ▪ Do not associate lulls in performance with sleeplessness; sleeplessness should not be blamed for everything that goes wrong during the day.

These guidelines have been effective for improving quality of sleep (Morin, 1999; Pagel, Zafralotfi, Zammit, 1997).

WEB SITES FOR EDUCATION

Merlin See the MERLIN web site for World Wide Web resources for client education.

REFERENCES Barr WJ: Noise notes: working smart, *Am J Nurs* 93:16, 1993.

Defrance R, Quera-Salva MA: Therapeutic applications of melatonin and related compounds, *Horm Res* 49:142-146, 1998.

Elmore SK, Betrus PA, Burr R: Light, social zeitgebers, and the sleep-wake cycle in the entrainment of human circadian rhythms, *Res Nurs Health* 17:471-478, 1994.

Evans BD, Rogers AE: 24-hour sleep/wake patterns in healthy elderly persons, *Appl Nurs Res* 7:75, 1994.

Foyt MM: Impaired gas exchange in the elderly, *Geriatr Nurs* 13:262, 1992.

• = **Independent;** ▲ = **Collaborative**

Hughes RJ, Sack RL, Lewy AJ: The role of melatonin and circadian phase in age-related sleep-maintenance insomnia, *Sleep* 21(1):52-63, 1998.

Kahn EM, Cook TE: Identification of modification of environmental noise in an ICU setting, *Chest* 114(2):535, 1998.

King AC et al: Moderate-intensity exercise and self-rated quality of sleep in older adults, *JAMA* 277(1):32-37, 1997.

Morin C et al: Behavioral and pharmacological therapies for late-life insomnia, *JAMA* 281(11):991-999, 1999.

Pagel JF, Zafralotfi S, Zammit G: How to prescribe a good night's sleep, *Patient Care* 31(4):87-94, 1997.

Reimer M: Sleep pattern disturbance: nursing interventions perceived by patients and their nurses as facilitating nocturnal sleep in hospital. In *Classification of nursing diagnoses: proceedings of the seventh conference,* Philadelphia, 1987, North American Nursing Diagnosis Association.

Richards KC: Sleep promotion in the critical care unit, *AACN Clin Issues* 5(2):152-158, 1994.

Somer E: *Food & mood: the complete guide to eating well and feeling your best,* ed 2, New York, 1999, Henry Holt.

Sateia MJ et al: Evaluation of chronic insomnia, *Sleep* 23(2):243-257, 2000.

Topf M: Effects of personal control over hospital noise on sleep, *Res Nurs Health* 15:19-28, 1992.

Whitney CW et al: Correlates of daytime sleepiness in 4578 elderly persons: the cardiovascular health study, *Sleep* 21(1):27-36, 1998.

Williamson J: The effect of ocean sounds on sleep after coronary artery bypass graft surgery, *Am J Crit Care* 1(1):91-97, 1992.

Disturbed Sleep pattern

Betty J. Ackley

 Definition Time-limited disruption of sleep (natural periodic suspension of consciousness)

Defining Characteristics

Prolonged awakenings; sleep maintenance insomnia; self-induced impairment of normal pattern; sleep onset >30 minutes; early morning insomnia; awakening earlier or later than desired; verbal complaints of difficulty falling asleep; verbal complaints of not feeling well-rested; increased proportion of Stage 1 sleep; dissatisfaction with sleep; less than age-normed total sleep time; three or more nighttime awakenings; decreased proportion of Stages 3 and 4 sleep (e.g., hyporesponsiveness, excess sleepiness, decreased motivation); decreased proportion of REM sleep (e.g., REM rebound, hyperactivity, emotional lability, agitation and impulsivity, atypical polysomnographic features); decreased ability to function

Related Factors (r/t)

Ruminative presleep thoughts; daytime activity pattern; thinking about home; body temperature; temperament; dietary; childhood onset; inadequate sleep hygiene; sustained use of antisleep agents; circadian asynchrony; frequently changing sleep-wake schedule; depression; loneliness; frequent travel across time zones; daylight/darkness exposure; grief; anticipation; shift work; delayed or advanced sleep phase syndrome; loss of sleep partner, life change; preoccupation with trying to sleep; periodic gender-related hormonal shifts; biochemical agents; fear; separation from significant others; social schedule inconsistent with chronotype; aging-related sleep shifts; anxiety; medications; fear of insomnia; maladaptive conditioned wakefulness; fatigue; boredom

• = Independent; ▲ = Collaborative

Environmental Noise; unfamiliar sleep furnishings; ambient temperature, humidity; lighting; other-generated awakening; excessive stimulation; physical restraint; lack of sleep privacy/control; interruptions for therapeutics, monitoring, lab tests; sleep partner; noxious odors

Parental Mother's sleep-wake pattern; parent-infant interaction; mother's emotional support

Physiological Urinary urgency, incontinence; fever; nausea; stasis of secretions; shortness of breath; position; gastroesophageal reflux

NOC **Outcomes (Nursing Outcomes Classification)**

Suggested NOC Labels
Sleep; Rest; Well-Being; Psychosocial Adjustment: Life Change; Quality of Life; Pain Level; Comfort Level

Example NOC Outcome
Demonstrates **Sleep** as evidenced by the following indicators: Hours of sleep/Sleep pattern/Sleep quality/Sleep efficiency/Feelings of rejuvenation after sleep/Napping appropriate for age (Rate each indicator of **Sleep:** 1 = extremely compromised, 2 = substantially compromised, 3 = moderately compromised, 4 = mildly compromised, 5 = not compromised [see Section I])

Client Outcomes

- Wakes up less frequently during night
- Awakens refreshed and is not fatigued during day
- Falls asleep without difficulty
- Verbalizes plan to implement bedtime routines

NIC **Interventions (Nursing Interventions Classification)**

Suggested NIC Labels
Sleep Enhancement

Example NIC Interventions—Sleep Enhancement
- Monitor/record patient's sleep pattern and number of sleep hours
- Encourage patient to establish a bedtime routine to facilitate transition from wakefulness to sleep

Nursing Interventions and Rationales

- Assess client's sleep patterns and usual bedtime rituals and incorporate these into the plan of care.
  Usual sleep patterns are individual; data collected through a comprehensive and holistic assessment are needed to determine the etiology of the disturbance (Spenceley, 1993). Staff nurses' evaluation of client's sleep states are usually valid (Edwards, Schuring, 1993a).
- Determine current level of anxiety, if client is anxious, see Nursing Interventions and Rationales for **Anxiety.**
  Anxiety interferes with sleep. Interventions such as relaxation training can help clients reduce anxiety (Pagel, Zafralotfi, Zammit, 1997). Many clients with insomnia display hyperarousal during the day in addition to the nighttime (Sateia et al, 2000).
- ▲ Assess for signs of new onset of depression: depressed mood state, statements of hopelessness, poor appetite. Refer for counseling as appropriate.

• = Independent; ▲ = Collaborative

Sleep deprivation in normal subjects did not result in the usual complaints of people with insomnia. Many symptoms associated with sleep deprivation probably arise from central nervous system hyperarousal (Sateia et al, 2000).

- Observe client's medication, diet, and caffeine intake. Look for hidden sources of caffeine, such as over-the-counter medications.
  Difficulty sleeping can be a side effect of medications such as bronchodilators; caffeine can also interfere with sleep.
- Provide measures to take before bedtime to assist with sleep (e.g., quiet time to allow the mind to slow down, carbohydrates such as crackers, or a back massage).
  Simple measures can increase quality of sleep. Carbohydrates cause release of the neurotransmitter serotonin, which helps induce and maintain sleep (Somer, 1999). Research has shown back massage to effectively promote sleep (Richards, 1994).
- ▲ Provide pain relief shortly before bedtime and position client comfortably for sleep.
  Clients have reported that uncomfortable positions and pain are common factors of sleep disturbance (Sateia et al, 2000).
- Keep environment quiet (e.g., avoid use of intercoms, lower volume on radio and television, keep beepers on nonaudio mode, anticipate alarms on IV pumps, talk quietly on unit).
  Excessive noise causes sleep deprivation that can result in ICU psychosis (Barr, 1993). Health volunteers exposed to recorded critical care noise levels experienced poor sleep (Topf, 1992). More than half of the noises in ICUs were caused by human behavior such as talking and TV watching (Kahn, Cook, 1998).
- Use soothing sound generators with sounds of the ocean, rainfall, or waterfall to induce sleep, or use "white noise" such as a fan to block out other sounds.
  Ocean sounds promoted sleep for a group of postoperative open-heart surgery clients (Williamson, 1992).
- For hospitalized stable clients, consider instituting the following sleep protocol to foster sleep:
  - ▪ Night shift: Give client the opportunity for uninterrupted sleep from 1 AM to 5 AM. Keep environmental noise to a minimum.
  - ▲ Evening shift: Limit napping between 4 PM and 9 PM. At 10 PM turn lights off, provide sleep medication according to individual assessment, and keep noise and conversation on the unit to a minimum.
  - ▲ Day shift: Encourage short naps before 11 AM. Enforce a physical activity regimen as appropriate. Schedule newly ordered medications to avoid waking client between 1 AM and 5 AM.
  Critical care nurses can take effective actions to promote sleep (Edwards, Schuring, 1993b).

Geriatric

- ▲ Determine if client has a physiological problem that could result in insomnia such as pain, cardiovascular disease, pulmonary disease, neurological problems such as dementia, or urinary problems.
  Sleep disturbances in the elderly may represent a complex interaction of age-related changes and pathological causes (Sateia et al, 2000).
- Observe elimination patterns. Have client decrease fluid intake in the evening, and ensure that diuretics are taken early in the morning.
  Many elderly people void during the night. Increasing water intake at night or taking diuretics late in the day increases nocturia, which results in disrupted sleep.

• = **Independent;** ▲ = **Collaborative**

- Do a careful history of all medications including over-the-counter medications and alcohol intake.
  Alcohol intake and medication effects are common causes of insomnia in the elderly. Rebound insomnia associated with the use of shorter-acting hypnotics may perpetuate a cycle of sleep disturbance and chronic hypnotic use (Sateia et al, 2000).
- ▲ If client is waking frequently during the night, consider the presence of sleep apnea problems and refer to a sleep clinic for evaluation.
  Sleep apnea in the elderly may be caused by changes in the respiratory drive of the central nervous system or may be obstructive and associated with obesity (Foyt, 1992).
- ▲ Evaluate client for presence of depression or anxiety, which can result in insomnia. Refer for treatment as appropriate.
  Anxiety and depression are common in the elderly and can result in insomnia (Sateia et al, 2000).
- Encourage social activities. Help elderly get outside for increased light exposure and to enjoy nature.
  Exposure to light and social interactions influence the circadian rhythms that control sleep (Elmore, Betrus, Burr, 1994; Sateia et al, 2000).
- Suggest light reading or TV viewing that does not excite as an evening activity.
  Soothing activities decrease stimulation of the reticular activating system and help sleep come naturally.
- Increase daytime physical activity. Encourage walking as client is able.
- ▲ Avoid use of hypnotics and alcohol to sleep.
  Long-term use of hypnotics can induce a drug-related insomnia. Alcohol also disrupts sleep and can exacerbate sleep apnea (Evans, Rogers, 1994).
- Reduce daytime napping in the late afternoon; limit naps to short intervals as early in the day as possible.
  The majority of elderly nap during the day (Evans, Rogers, 1994). Avoiding naps in the late afternoon makes it easier to fall asleep at night.
- Help client recognize that there are changes in length of sleep. Client may not be able to sleep for 8 hours as when younger, and more frequent awakening is part of the aging process (Floyd et al, 2000).
- ▲ If client continues to have insomnia despite developing good sleep hygiene habits, refer to a sleep clinic for further evaluation (Pagel, Zafralotfi, Zammit, 1997).

Home Care Interventions

- Provide support to the family of client with chronic sleep pattern disturbance.
  Ongoing sleep pattern disturbances can disrupt family patterns and cause sleep deprivation in the client or family members, which creates increased stress on the family.

Client/Family Teaching

- Encourage client to avoid coffee and other caffeinated foods and liquids and also to avoid eating large high-protein or high-fat meals close to bedtime.
  Caffeine intake increases the time it takes to fall asleep and increases awake time during the night (Evans, Rogers, 1994). A full stomach interferes with sleep.
- Advise the client that research on use of melatonin is still equivocal. While it may help the client to fall asleep faster, it does not improve the quality or length of time in the sleep interval, and long-term results are unknown (Hughes, Sack, Lewy, 1998; Defrance, Quera-Salva, 1998; Walsh et al, 1999).
- Advise client to avoid use of alcohol or hypnotics to induce sleep.

• = **Independent;** ▲ = **Collaborative**

Sleep induced by alcohol is often disrupted later in the night (Walsh et al, 1999). Use of benzodiazapines, while they are effective in inducing and maintaining sleep, have major side effects including daytime drowsiness, dizziness or light-headedness, and memory loss (Holbrook et al, 2000).

- Ask client to keep a sleep diary for several weeks.
  Often the client can find the cause of the sleep deprivation when the pattern of sleeping is examined (Pagel, Zafralotfi, Zammit, 1997).
- Teach relaxation techniques, pain relief measures, or the use of imagery before sleep.
- Teach client need for increased exercise. Encourage to take a daily walk 5 to 6 hours before retiring.
  Moderate activity such as walking can increase the quality of sleep (King et al, 1997).
- Encourage client to develop a bedtime ritual that includes quiet activities such as reading, television, or crafts.
- Teach the following guidelines for good sleep hygiene to improve sleep habits:
  - Go to bed only when sleepy.
  - When awake in the middle of the night, go to another room, do quiet activities, and go back to bed only when sleepy.
  - Use the bed only for sleeping—not for reading or snoozing in front of the television.
  - Avoid afternoon and evening naps.
  - Get up at the same time every morning.
  - Recognize that not everyone needs 8 hours of sleep.
  - Move the alarm clock away from the bed if it is a source of distraction.
  - Do not associate lulls in performance with sleeplessness; sleeplessness should not be blamed for everything that goes wrong during the day.

These guidelines on sleep hygiene have been shown to effectively improve quality of sleep (Morin, 1993; Pagel, Zafralotfi, Zammit, 1997; Walsh et al, 1999).

WEB SITES FOR EDUCATION

REFERENCES   Barr WJ: Noise notes: working smart, *Am J Nurs* 93:16, 1993.

Defrance R, Quera-Salva MA: Therapeutic applications of melatonin and related compounds, *Horm Res* 49:142-146, 1998.

Edward GB, Schuring LM: Pilot study: validating staff nurses' observations of sleep and wake states among critically ill patients using polysomnography, *Am J Crit Care* 2(2):125-132, 1993a.

Edwards GB, Schuring LM: Sleep protocol: a research-based practice change, *Crit Care Nurse* 13:84-88, 1993b.

Elmore SK, Betrus PA, Burr R: Light, social zeitgebers, and the sleep-wake cycle in the entrainment of human circadian rhythms, *Res Nurs Health* 17:471-478, 1994.

Evans BD, Rogers AE: 24-hour sleep/wake patterns in healthy elderly persons, *Appl Nurs Res* 7:75, 1994.

Floyd JA et al: Age-related changes in initiation and maintenance of sleep: a meta-analysis, *Res Nurs Health* 23:106-117, 2000.

Foyt MM: Impaired gas exchange in the elderly, *Geriatr Nurs* 13:262, 1992.

Holbrook AM et al: Meta-analysis of benzodiazepine use in treatment of insomnia, *CMAJ* 162(2):225-233, 2000.

Hughes RJ, Sack RL, Lewy AJ: The role of melatonin and circadian phase in age-related sleep-maintenance insomnia, *Sleep* 21(1):52-63, 1998.

Hyman RB et al: The effects of relaxation training on clinical symptoms: a meta-analysis, *Nurs Res* 38:216, 1989.

Kahn EM, Cook TE: Identification of modification of environmental noise in an ICU setting, *Chest* 114(2):535, 1998.

• = Independent; ▲ = Collaborative

King AC et al: Moderate-intensity exercise and self-rated quality of sleep in older adults, *JAMA* 277(1):32-37, 1997.

Morin C: Cognitive behavior therapy for late-life insomnia, *J Consult Clin Psychol* 61(1):137-145, 1993.

Pagel JF, Zafralotfi S, Zammit G: How to prescribe a good night's sleep, *Patient Care* 31(4):87-94, 1997.

Richards KC: Sleep promotion in the critical care unit, *AACN Clin Issues* 5(2):152-158, 1994.

Sateia MJ et al: Evaluation of chronic insomnia, *Sleep* 23(2):243-257, 2000.

Somer E: *Food & mood: the complete guide to eating well and feeling your best*, ed 2, New York, 1999, Henry Holt.

Spenceley SM: Sleep inquiry: a look with fresh eyes, *Image* 25(3):249-255, 1993.

Topf M: Effects of personal control over hospital noise on sleep, *Res Nurs Health* 15:19-28, 1992.

Walsh J et al: Insomnia: assessment and management in primary care, *Am Fam Phys* 59(11):3029-3037, 1999.

Williamson J: The effect of ocean sounds on sleep after coronary artery bypass graft surgery, *Am J Crit Care* 1(1):91-97, 1992.

Impaired Social interaction

Pam B. Schweitzer and Gail B. Ladwig

NANDA **Definition** Insufficient or excessive quantity or ineffective quality of social exchange

Defining Characteristics

Verbalized or observed inability to receive or communicate a satisfying sense of belonging, caring, interest, or shared history; verbalized or observed discomfort in social situations; observed use of unsuccessful social interaction behaviors; dysfunctional interaction with peers, family and/or others; family report of change of style or pattern of interaction

Related Factors (r/t)

Knowledge/skill deficit regarding ways to enhance mutuality; therapeutic isolation; sociocultural dissonance; limited physical mobility; environmental barriers; communication barriers; altered thought processes; absence of available significant others or peers; self-concept disturbance

NOC Outcomes (Nursing Outcomes Classification)

Suggested NOC Labels

Child Development: 2, Months 4, Months 6, Months, 12 Months, 2 Years, 3 Years, 4 Years, 5 Years, Middle Childhood (6-11 Years), Adolescence (12-17 Years); Play Participation; Role Performance; Social Interaction Skills; Social Involvement

> **Example NOC Outcome**
> Demonstrates **Social Involvement** as evidenced by: Interaction with close friends, neighbors, family members and work groups (Rate each indicator of **Social Involvement:** 1 = none, 2 = limited, 3 = moderate 4 = substantial, 5 = extensive [see Section I])

Client Outcomes

- Identifies barriers that cause impaired social interactions
- Discusses feelings that accompany impaired and successful social interactions
- Uses available opportunities to practice interactions

• = Independent; ▲ = Collaborative

- Uses successful social interaction behaviors
- Reports increased comfort in social situations
- Communicates, states feelings of belonging, demonstrates caring and interest in others
- Reports effective interactions with others

NIC **Interventions (Nursing Interventions Classification)**

Suggested NIC Labels

Socialization Enhancement

> **Example NIC Interventions—Socialization Enhancement**
> - Encourage patience in developing relationships
> - Help client increase awareness of strengths and limitations in communicating with others

Nursing Interventions and Rationales

- Observe for cause of discomfort in social situations; ask client to explain when discomfort began and identify any losses (e.g., loss of health, job, or significant other; aging) and changes (e.g., marriage, birth or adoption of a child, change in body appearance). *Individualized assessment indicates specific interventions (Warren, 1993).*
- Assess client's social support system.
  Use a social support tool or validated assessment tool if possible (e.g., UCLA Loneliness Scale for adolescents [Mahon, Yarcheski, Yarcheski, 1995]).
- Use active listening skills including assessment and clarification of client's verbal and nonverbal responses and interactions.
  Using therapeutic observation and listening skills helps to accurately assess and validate this diagnosis. Clients are often unable to identify the problems or factors that directly contribute to their sense of isolation (O'Brien, Pheiffer, 1993).
- Have client list behaviors that are associated with being disconnected, and discuss alternative responses that may increase comfort.
  Connections occur when a person is actively involved with another person, object, group, or environment; such involvement promotes a sense of comfort, well-being, and anxiety reduction (Hagerty et al, 1993).
- Monitor client's use of defense mechanisms, and support healthy defenses (e.g., client focuses on present and avoids placing blame on others for personal behavior).
  Positive reinforcement of strengths perpetuates them.
- Have client list behaviors that cause discomfort. Discuss alternative ways to alleviate discomfort (e.g., focusing on others and their interests, practicing making caring statements such as, "I understand you are feeling sad").
- Encourage client to express feelings to others (e.g., "I feel sad also").
  Self-expression invites involvement and increases connectedness (Hagerty et al, 1993).
- Identify client strengths. Have client make a list of strengths and refer to it when experiencing negative feelings. He or she may find it helpful to put the list on a note card to carry at all times.
  Extra stress in this study was reduced by positive thinking (Makinen, Suominen, Lauri, 2000). Being aware of strengths when they are needed can increase successful interactions.
- Have group members identify each other's strengths in a group setting.
  This exercise encourages individuals to practice relating to each other on a more intimate level (Drew, 1991).

• = **Independent;** ▲ = **Collaborative**

- Role-play comfortable and uncomfortable social interactions with the client and appropriate responses (e.g., acknowledging a friendly greeting, responding to rude remarks with an "I" statement, such as, "I understand you may feel that way, but this is how I feel"). *Role-plays may help the client develop social interaction skills and identify feelings associated with isolation (Warren, 1993).*
- Model appropriate social interactions. Give positive verbal and nonverbal feedback for appropriate behavior (e.g., make statements such as, "I'm proud that you made it to work on time and did all the tasks assigned to you without saying that your supervisor was picking on you"; make eye contact). If not contraindicated, touch client's arm or hand when speaking.
  One way to learn social skills is to observe the productive interactions of others (Drew, 1991). Shared feelings increased communication with stroke and aphasia clients without words (Sundin, Jansson, Norberg, 2000).
- Use humor as appropriate.
  Humor is important for helping clients cope mentally (Makinen, Suominen, Lauri, 2000).

Geriatric

- Avoid assuming that social isolation is normal for elderly client.
  Caregiver bias and elderly client bias lead to a lack of recognition and treatment of the client's mental health needs (Dellasega, 1991).
- Assess client's potential or actual hearing loss or hearing impairment and make appropriate referrals if a problem is identified.
  Research shows that hearing loss is one of the most prevalent chronic health problems of the elderly in the United States (Christian, Dluhy, O'Neill, 1989). Because of the nature of the sensory deprivation, communication barriers are increased and human intimacy and self-esteem are negatively affected (Chen, 1994). In addition, it is important to note that hearing impairments often go unnoticed and may not be as obvious as more visibly recognized handicaps (Chen, 1994).
- Monitor for depression, a particular risk in the elderly.
  Age and its associated losses may cause formerly socially active people to be alone. Loneliness contributes to depression and social withdrawal (Warren, 1993).
- Provide group situations for client.
  Group settings are necessary for the client to practice new skills.
- Encourage physical activity such as aerobics or stretching and toning in a group.
  These activities decreased loneliness in former sedentary adults ($N = 174$, median age = 65.5 years) (McAuley et al, 2000). Extra stress was reduced for clients in this study (Makinen, Suominen, Lauri, 2000).
- Have clients reminisce.
  Through the process of reminiscence, older adults can actively evaluate life experiences and explore the meaning of memorable events (Harrand, Bollstetter, 2000).

Multicultural

- Acknowledge racial/ethnic differences at the onset of care.
  Acknowledgement of race/ethnicity issues will enhance communication, establish rapport, and promote positive treatment outcomes (D'Avanzo et al, 2001).
- Assess for the influence of cultural beliefs, norms, and values on the client's perception of social activity and relationships.
  What the client considers normal social interaction may be based on cultural perceptions (Leininger, 1996).

• = **Independent;** ▲ = **Collaborative**

- Approach individuals of color with respect, warmth, and professional courtesy.
  Instances of disrespect and lack of caring have special significance for individuals of color and may impede efforts to increase social outlets (D'Avanzo et al, 2001).
- Assess the use of personal space needs, communication styles, acceptable body language, eye contact, perception of touch, and paraverbals when communicating with the client.
  Nurses need to consider these when interpreting verbal and nonverbal messages (Siantz, 1991). Native Americans may consider avoidance of direct eye contact as a sign of respect and asking questions to be rude and intrusive (Seiderman et al, 1996).
- Validate the client's feelings regarding social interaction.
  Validation lets the client know that the nurse has heard and understands what was said, and it promotes the nurse-client relationship (Stuart, Laraia, 2001; Giger, Davidhizar, 1995).

Home Care Interventions

- Assess family and living environment for social dynamics. Refer for medical social services to assist with family dynamics if appropriate.
  The family is a socially significant cultural group that generates behavior, defines roles, and promotes values.
- Suggest that client avoid contact with negative persons.
  Negative interactions reinforce undesired patterns.
- Identify activities that client does alone and assist client with balancing solitary and social activities.
  A healthy balance of social and private time supports positive coping.
- Establish pattern of care and daily activities that involves client socially (e.g., Meals on Wheels, home health aide visits). Give supportive feedback for positive and appropriate interactions.
  The assumption of new patterns of interaction requires practice in safe situations. Feedback reinforces desired behaviors.
- ▲ Refer to or support involvement with supportive groups and counseling.
  Cognitive behavioral group therapy was effective for social phobia in this group of 11 adolescent girls (Hayward et al, 2000). Group settings provide the opportunity to practice new skills. Counseling helps the client to define appropriate actions, and it is a source of support.

Client/Family Teaching

- Help client accept responsibility for own behavior. Have client keep a journal, and review it together at prescheduled intervals. Give client positive feedback for appropriate behaviors, and suggest alternative approaches for behaviors that do not enhance social interaction.
  Positive reinforcement perpetuates appropriate behaviors.
- Teach social interaction skills for use in actual situations the client is faced with daily.
  Through productive connections with others, social skills are learned and a repertoire of roles for many social situations is developed, which leads to an increase in self-esteem and the capacity to interact with others (Drew, 1991).
- Practice social skills one-to-one and, when the client is ready, in group sessions.
  Practice improves performance and comfort level.
- ▲ Refer to appropriate social agencies for assistance (e.g., family therapy, self-help groups, crisis intervention).

- **= Independent; ▲ = Collaborative**

REFERENCES   Chen H: Hearing in the elderly, relation of healing loss, loneliness, and self-esteem, *J Gerontol Nurs* 20:22, 1994.

Christian E, Dluhy E, O'Neill R: Sounds of silence, *J Gerontol Nurs* 15:4, 1989.

D'Avanzo CE et al: Developing culturally informed strategies for substance related interventions. In Naegle MA, D'Avanzo CE, editors: *Addictions and substance abuse, strategies for advanced practice nursing*, St Louis, 2001, Mosby, pp 59-104.

Dellasega C: Meeting the mental health needs of elderly clients, *J Psychosoc Nurs Ment Health Serv* 29:10, 1991.

Drew N: Combating the social isolation of chronic mental illness, *J Psychosoc Nurs Ment Health Serv* 29:14, 1991.

Giger JN, Davidhizar RE: *Transcultural nursing*, ed 2, St Louis, 1995, Mosby.

Hagerty BM et al: An emerging theory of human relatedness, *Image* 25:291, 1993.

Harrand AG, Bollstetter JJ: Developing a community-based reminiscence group for the elderly, *Clin Nurse Spec* 14(1):17-22, 2000.

Hayward C et al: Cognitive-behavioral group therapy for social phobia in female adolescents: results of a pilot study, *J Am Acad Child Adolesc Psychiatry* 39(6):721-726, 2000.

Leininger MM: *Transcultural nursing: theories, research and practices*, ed 2, Hilliard, Ohio, 1996, McGraw-Hill.

Mahon NE, Yarcheski T, Yarcheski A: Validation of the revised UCLA loneliness scale for adolescents, *Res Nurs Health* 18:263, 1995.

Makinen S, Suominen T, Lauri S: Self-care in adults with asthma: how they cope, *J Clin Nurs* 9(4):557, 2000.

McAuley E et al: Social relations, physical activity, and well-being in older adults, *Prev Med* 31(5):608, 2000.

O'Brien ME, Pheiffer W: Physical and psychosocial nursing care for patients with HIV infection, *Nurs Clin North Am* 28:303, 1993.

Seiderman RY et al: Assessing American Indian families, *MCN Am J Matern Child Nurs* 21(6):274-279, 1996.

Siantz ML: How can we be more aware of culturally specific body language and use this awareness therapeutically? *J Psychosoc Nurs* 29(11):38-39, 1991.

Stuart GW, Laraia MT: Therapeutic nurse-patient relationship. In Stuart GW, Laraia MT, editors: *Principles and practice of psychiatric nursing*, St Louis, 2001, Mosby, p 30.

Sundin K, Jansson L, Norberg A: Communicating with people with stroke and aphasia: understanding through sensation without words, *J Clin Nurs* 9(4):481-488, 2000.

Warren BJ: Explaining social isolation through concept analysis, *Arch Psychiatr Nurs* 7:270, 1993.

Social isolation

Gail B. Ladwig

NANDA   **Definition** Aloneness experienced by the individual and perceived as imposed by others and as a negative or threatened state

Defining Characteristics
Objective   Absence of supportive significant others (e.g., family, friends, group); projects hostility in voice, behavior; withdrawn; uncommunicative; shows behavior unaccepted by dominant cultural group; seeks to be alone or exists in a subculture; repetitive and meaningless actions; preoccupation with own thoughts; no eye contact; inappropriate or immature activities for developmental age/stage; evidence of physical/mental handicap or altered state of wellness; sad, dull affect

Subjective   Expresses feelings of aloneness imposed by others; expresses feelings of rejection; inappropriate or immature interests for developmental age/stage; inadequate or absent significant purpose in life; inability to meet expectations of others; expresses values

• = Independent; ▲ = Collaborative

acceptable to the subculture but unacceptable to the dominant cultural group; expresses interest inappropriate to the developmental age/stage; experiences feelings of differences from others; insecurity in public

Related Factors (r/t)
Alterations in mental status; inability to engage in satisfying personal relationships; unacceptable social values; unacceptable social behavior; inadequate personal resources; immature interests; factors contributing to the absence of satisfying personal relationships (e.g., delay in accomplishing developmental tasks); alterations in physical appearance; altered state of wellness

NOC Outcomes (Nursing Outcomes Classification)
Suggested NOC Labels

Loneliness; Mood Equilibrium; Play Participation; Social Interaction Skills; Social Involvement; Social Support; Well-Being

> **Example NOC Outcome**
> Demonstrates **Social Involvement** as evidenced by: Interaction with close friends, neighbors, family members, and work groups (Rate each indicator of **Social Involvement:** 1 = none, 2 = limited, 3 = moderate, 4 = substantial, 5 = extensive [see Section I])

Client Outcomes
- Identifies the reasons for feelings of isolation
- Practices the social and communication skills needed to interact with others
- Initiates interactions with others; sets and meets goals
- Participates in activities and programs at level of ability and desire
- Describes feelings of self-worth

NIC Interventions (Nursing Interventions Classification)
Suggested NIC Labels

Socialization Enhancement

> **Example NIC Interventions**
> - Encourage patience in developing relationships
> - Help client increase awareness of strengths and limitations in communicating with others

Nursing Interventions and Rationales
- Observe for barriers to social interaction (e.g., illness; incontinence; decreasing ability to form relationships; lack of transportation, money, support system, or knowledge).
  Each individual may have different etiologies of social isolation; therefore adequate information must be gathered so that appropriate interventions can be planned (Badger, 1990).
- Note risk factors (e.g., ethnic/cultural minority, chronic physiological or psychological illness or deformities, elderly).
  These clients may be at risk for social isolation (Warren, 1993).
- Discuss causes of perceived or actual isolation.
  The individual's experience of illness; the mediating circumstances of everyday life that influence quality of life; and emotions, fears, and concerns all have a bearing on the way illness is managed (Anderson, 1991).

• = Independent; ▲ = Collaborative

- Promote social interactions. Support grieving and verbalization of feelings.
  Women in one study needed counseling for the management of illness, but some said they would have benefited from psychological counseling as well. They needed help with the emotional aspects of living with a chronic illness (Anderson, 1991).
- Establish trust one-on-one, and then gradually introduce client to others. Allow client opportunities to introduce issues and to describe his or her daily life.
  Individualization of care, or tailoring of care, involves taking into account the client's individuality and allowing that individuality to determine interpersonal approaches and health-illness management actions (Brown, 1994). The first step in reversing social isolation is developing the ability to relate to one person. As this skill is accomplished, the client can gradually learn to relate to others.
- Use active listening skills. Establish a therapeutic relationship and spend time with the client.
  Spending time with the client enhances self-esteem.
- Help client experience success by working together to establish easily attainable goals (e.g., 10 minutes conversing with peer).
  Success encourages repetition of behaviors, and setting small achievable goals can help the client be successful.
- Provide positive reinforcement when client seeks out others.
  Receiving instrumental social support such as practical help, advice, and feedback significantly contributes to positive well-being (White, 1992).
- Help client identify appropriate diversional activities to encourage socialization.
  Active participation by the client is essential for behavioral changes.
- Encourage physical closeness (e.g., use touch) if appropriate.
  Touch can be therapeutic and healing.
- Identify available support systems and involve them in client care.
  Clients cope more successfully with stressful life events if they have support (White, 1992).
- Encourage liberal visitation for clients hospitalized and in extended care facilities.
  Visits from an emotionally close network was associated with perceived support, and this was associated with a decrease in depression (Oxman, Hull, 2001). Frequent contact with support persons decreases feelings of isolation.
- Help client identify role models and others with similar interests.
  Sometimes the client needs someone to model appropriate behavior.
- See the care plan for **Risk for Loneliness.**

Geriatric

- Observe for aggression or other interpersonal problems, poor self-image or signs of powerlessness, confusion of the past with the present, complaints about feeling confined or deserted, or difficulty setting goals and making decisions.
  Social isolation should be considered as a nursing diagnosis when these behaviors are observed (Copel, 1988; Meddaugh, 1991).
- Assess for hearing deficit. Provide aids and use adaptive techniques such as facing the individual when speaking, speaking slowly, lowering the pitch of the voice, and enunciating clearly.
  There is a relationship between hearing acuity and loneliness. Hearing loss is one of the most prevalent chronic health problems of older adults, especially the very old. Adaptive techniques that facilitate communication must be used (Dugan, Kivett, 1994).

• = Independent; ▲ = Collaborative

- If client is in a health care facility, visit him or her for at least 10 minutes every 2 to 3 hours.
  The presence of a trusted individual provides emotional security for the client.
- ▲ Involve nonprofessionals in activities, projects, and goal setting with clients. Practice interdisciplinary management for unit-based activities: arts and crafts, sewing, videos, large-print books, magazines, games, musical instruments, and assistive listening devices.
  Nursing assistants are commonly concerned about the social support of residents; therefore they can be a valuable resource for generating intervention ideas. (Alterations in job descriptions would be required.) Enjoyable interactions between nursing assistants and residents would provide the assistants with diversion and rest from the strenuous aspects of personal care and might have a positive effect on the resident/assistant relationship. Residents with visual, hearing, cognitive, and mobility impairments will participate more readily in events that involve a smaller number of people and in which the staff takes initiative and establishes rapport with each resident (Windriver, 1993).
- Offer client choice of activities and persons with whom to sit and socialize. Introductions to strangers may need to be repeated several times.
  A recognized intervention for loneliness is to provide opportunities and assistance for making choices, setting goals, and making decisions. Cognitively impaired clients may require several repetitions (Windriver, 1993).
- Put clients in groups according to activity preferences, abilities, age, life situations, personal and cultural characteristics, and social networks.
  Positive social interactions are enhanced by the mentioned interventions (Windriver, 1993).
- Develop and display a seating chart for the common areas of each personal care unit, and develop a process for both identifying needed changes and executing them promptly.
  Personality factors that are difficult to predict affect the success of social groupings (Windriver, 1993).
- Consider use of simulated presence therapy (see care plan for **Hopelessness**).
  Simulated presence therapy appears to be the most effective therapy for treating social isolation (Woods, Ashley, 1995).
- ▲ Refer to programs such as Foster Grandparents and Senior Companions.
  Emotional isolation leads to social isolation. Social programs help increase contact with peers and decrease isolation. Programs to alleviate emotional isolation should focus on attachment loss (Dugan, Kivett, 1994).
- Provide physical activity, either aerobic or stretching and toning.
  Physical activity increased social support in this group of older, formerly sedentary adults (McAuley et al, 2000).

Multicultural

- Acknowledge racial/ethnic differences at the onset of care.
  Acknowledgement of race/ethnicity issues will enhance communication, establish rapport, and promote positive treatment outcomes (D'Avanzo et al, 2001).
- Assess for the influence of cultural beliefs, norms, and values on the client's perception of social activity and relationships.
  What the client considers normal social interaction may be based on cultural perceptions (Leininger, 1996).

• = Independent; ▲ = Collaborative

- Approach individuals of color with respect, warmth, and professional courtesy.
  Instances of disrespect and lack of caring have special significance for individuals of color and may impede efforts to increase social outlets (D'Avanzo et al, 2001).
- Assess the use of personal space needs, communication styles, acceptable body language, eye contact, perception of touch, and paraverbals when communicating with the client.
  Nurses need to consider these when interpreting verbal and nonverbal messages (Siantz, 1991). Native Americans may consider avoidance of direct eye contact as a sign of respect and asking questions to be rude and intrusive (Seiderman et al, 1996).
- Use a family centered approach when working with Latino, Asian, African-American, and Native American clients.
  Latinos may perceive family as source of support, solver of problems, and a source of pride. Asian Americans may regard the family as the primary decision maker and influence on individual family members (D'Avanzo et al, 2001).
- Promote sense of ethnic attachment.
  Older Korean clients with strong ethnic attachments had higher levels of social involvement than others (Kim, 1999).
- Validate the client's feelings regarding social isolation.
  Validation lets the client know that the nurse has heard and understands what was said, and it promotes the nurse-client relationship (Stuart, Laraia, 2001; Giger, Davidhizar, 1995).

Home Care Interventions

- Confirm that the home setting has a telephone. Obtain one if necessary for medical safety. If client lives alone, set up a Lifeline safety system that requires the client to answer the telephone.
  The telephone can be used to achieve continuity of care and successful client/family interaction (Skinner, 2001). A Lifeline system can be a safety net for physical and psychological safety.
- Encourage family involvement in daily life in small, nonthreatening activities such as short outings, assistance with shopping, and asking for input from isolated person in decision-making.
  Reversing social isolation is a gradual process.
- Establish pattern of care and daily activities to involve the client socially (e.g., Meals on Wheels, home health aide visits).
  Pattern changes encourage new behaviors.
- Have client keep a diary of social experiences. Discuss diary during visits.
  A review of social experiences helps client identify those that are most comfortable.
- Identify activities that client does alone. Assist client with balancing solitary and social activities, keeping alone time to a minimum.
  A healthy balance of social and private time supports positive coping.
- ▲ Refer for visiting volunteer services.
  Spending time with the client enhances client self-esteem.
- When client is ready, encourage him or her to volunteer for short periods with community agencies in which contact is positive and nonthreatening (e.g., with hospitalized elders for 1 hour per week).
  Contributing to the welfare of others enhances self-esteem.
- Assess options for living that allow client privacy but not isolation (e.g., boarding home, congregate living).
  Group living can provide a safety net for clients predisposed to isolation and depression.

- **= Independent; ▲ = Collaborative**

Client/Family Teaching

- Teach skills related to problem solving, communication, social interaction, activities of daily living (ADLs), and positive self-esteem.
  All of these skills are necessary to change isolating behavior.
- Consider the use of telecommunication and group support via the Internet.
  This study delivered diabetes education and social support to rural women with diabetes. The women expressed the positive effects of the computer-based social support (Smith, Weinert, 2000).
- Teach role-playing (practicing communication skills in specific situations).
  Role-playing may help clients develop social interaction skills and identify feelings associated with their isolation (Warren, 1993).
- Encourage client to initiate contacts with self-help groups, counselors, and therapists.
  If adjustment is to be successful and maintained, management of a chronic illness cannot occur in isolation; it requires a complex interaction of resources (White, 1992).
- Provide information to client about senior citizen services, house sharing, pets, daycare centers, churches, and community resources.
  The well-documented negative effect of social isolation suggests that clients without confidants and supportive others must be referred to alternative sources, such as cardiac rehabilitation programs, support groups, and community agencies (McCauley, 1995).
- ▲ Refer socially isolated caregivers to appropriate support groups as well.
  *Identification and recognition of the overwhelming task of caregiving are needed so that the caregiver does not suffer in silence. Alzheimer's disease support groups offer participants an opportunity to share troubles and triumphs with others who truly understand the turmoil of caregiving (Bergman-Evans, 1994) (see care plan for **Caregiver role strain**).*
- Teach caregivers methods to deal with troublesome behaviors related to memory disturbances, restlessness and agitation, catastrophic reactions, day/night disturbances, delusions, wandering, and physical violence. A general method for clinicians to manage these problems involves the identification of the behavior and its antecedent and consequent events. Stressors that may cause behavioral problems include fatigue, a change of routine, excessive demands, overwhelming stimuli, and acute illness or pain.
  Caregivers can be taught to identify these stressors to prevent or alleviate troublesome behaviors (Alessi, 1991).

WEB SITES FOR EDUCATION

Ⓜ ᴹᴱᴿᴸᴵᴺ See the MERLIN web site for World Wide Web resources for client education.

REFERENCES
Alessi C: Managing the behavioral problems of dementia in the home, *Clin Geriatr Med* 7(4):787-801, 1991.

Anderson JM: Immigrant women speak of chronic illness: the social construction of the devalued self, *J Adv Nurs* 16:710-717, 1991.

Badger VT: Men with cardiovascular diseases and their spouses, coping health and marital adjustment, *Arch Psychiatr Nurs* 4:319-324, 1990.

Bergman-Evans BF: Alzheimer's and related disorders: loneliness, depression, and social support of spousal caregivers, *J Gerontol Nurs* 20:6, 1994.

Brown S: Communication strategies used by an expert nurse, *Clin Nurs Res* 3(1):43-56, 1994.

Copel LC: Loneliness: a conceptual model, *J Psychosoc Nurs Ment Health Serv* 26:14, 1988.

D'Avanzo CE et al: Developing culturally informed strategies for substance related interventions. In Naegle MA, D'Avanzo CE, editors: *Addictions and substance abuse, strategies for advanced practice nursing*, St Louis, 2001, Mosby, pp 59-104.

• = **Independent**; ▲ = **Collaborative**

Dugan E, Kivett V: The importance of emotional and social isolation to loneliness among very old rural adults, *Gerontologist* 34:340, 1994.

Giger JN, Davidhizar RE: *Transcultural nursing,* ed 2, St Louis, 1995, Mosby.

Kim O: Mediation effect of social support between ethnic attachment and loneliness in older Korean immigrants, *Res Nurs Health* 22(2):169-175, 1999.

Leininger MM: *Transcultural nursing: theories, research and practices,* ed 2, Hilliard, Ohio, 1996, McGraw-Hill.

McAuley E et al: Social relations, physical activity, and well-being in older adults, *Prev Med* 31(5):608, 2000.

McCauley K: Assessing social support in patients with cardiac disease, *J Cardiovasc Nurs* 10:73, 1995.

Meddaugh DJ: Before aggression erupts, *Geriatr Nurs* 12:114, 1991. In Windriver W: Social isolation: unit-based activities for impaired elders, *J Gerontol Nurs* 19:15, 1993.

Oxman TE, Hull JG: Social support and treatment response in older depressed primary care patients, *J Gerontol B Psychol Sci Soc Sci* 56(1):P35-P45, 2001.

Seiderman RY et al: Assessing American Indian families, *MCN Am J Matern Child Nurs* 21(6):274-279, 1996.

Siantz ML: How can we be more aware of culturally specific body language and use this awareness therapeutically? *J Psychosoc Nurs* 29(11):38-39, 1991.

Skinner D: Intimacy and the telephone, *Caring* 20(2):28-29, 2001.

Smith L, Weinert C: Telecommunication support for rural women with diabetes, *Diabetes Educ* 26:645-655, 2000.

Stuart GW, Laraia MT: Therapeutic nurse-patient relationship. In Stuart GW, Laraia MT, editors: *Principles and practice of psychiatric nursing,* St Louis, 2001, Mosby, p 30.

Warren B: Explaining social isolation through concept analysis, *Arch Psychiatr Nurs* 7:270, 1993.

White NE: Coping, social support and adaptation to chronic illness, *West J Nurs Res* 14:2, 1992.

Windriver W: Social isolation: unit-based activities for impaired elders, *J Gerontol Nurs* 19:15, 1993.

Woods P, Ashley J: Simulated presence therapy: using selected memories to manage problem behaviors in Alzheimer's disease patients, *Geriatr Nurs* 16:9, 1995.

Chronic Sorrow

Betty J. Ackley and Gail B. Ladwig

NANDA   **Definition** Cyclical, recurring, and potentially progressive pattern of pervasive sadness that is experienced (by a client, parent or caregiver, or individual with chronic illness or disability) in response to continual loss throughout the trajectory of an illness or disability

Defining Characteristics

Feelings that vary in intensity, are periodic, may progress and intensify over time, and may interfere with the client's ability to reach his/her highest level of personal and social well-being; expresses periodic, recurrent feelings of sadness; expresses one or more of the following feelings: anger, being misunderstood, confusion, depression, disappointment, emptiness, fear, frustration, guilt/self-blame, helplessness, hopelessness, loneliness, low self-esteem, recurring loss, overwhelmed

Related Factors (r/t)

Death of a loved one; experiences chronic physical or mental illness or disability such as mental retardation/multiple sclerosis/prematurity, spina bifida, or other birth defects/chronic mental illness/infertility/cancer/Parkinson's disease; experiences one or more trigger events (e.g., crises in management of the illness, crises related to developmental stages and missed opportunities or milestones that bring comparisons with developmental, social, or personal norms); unending caregiving as a constant reminder of loss

  = Independent; ▲ = Collaborative

NOC **Outcomes (Nursing Outcomes Classification)**

Suggested NOC Labels

Grief Resolution; Hope; Mood Equilibrium; Depression Control; Acceptance: Health Status; Depression Level

> **Example NOC Outcome**
>
> Accomplishes **Grief Resolution** with plans for a positive future as evidenced by the following indicators: Expresses feelings about loss/Verbalizes acceptance of loss/ Describes meaning of the loss or death/Reports decreased preoccupation with loss/ Expresses positive expectations about the future (Rate each indicator of **Grief Resolution:** 1 = not at all, 2 = to a slight extent, 3 = to a moderate extent, 4 = to a great extent, 5 = to a very great extent [see Section I])

Client Outcomes

- Expresses appropriate feelings of guilt, fear, anger, or sadness
- Identifies problems associated with sorrow (e.g., changes in appetite, insomnia, nightmares, loss of libido, decreased energy, alteration in activity levels)
- Seeks help in dealing with grief-associated problems
- Plans for future one day at a time
- Functions at a normal developmental level

NIC **Interventions (Nursing Interventions Classification)**

Suggested NIC Labels

Grief work facilitation, Grief Work Facilitation: Perinatal Death

> **Example NIC Interventions**
> - Encourage the patient to verbalizes memories of the loss, both past and current
> - Assist to identify personal coping strategies

Nursing Interventions and Rationales

- Assess client's degree of sorrow. Use the Burke/NCRS Chronic Sorrow Questionnaire (for the individual or caregiver as appropriate) if available.
  This questionnaire is designed to determine the occurrence of chronic sorrow, cues that trigger sorrow, coping strategies, and factors that direct health care personnel to deal with the sorrowful client or caregiver (Hainsworth, Eakes, Burke, 1994).
- Help client to understand that sorrow may be ongoing. Life may be characterized by good times and then bad times when sorrow is triggered by events.
  Studies have demonstrated that feelings of sadness, guilt, anger, frustration, and fear occur periodically throughout the lives of people experiencing chronic loss resulting in chronic sorrow (Eakes, Burke, Hainsworth, 1998).
- Identify problems of eating and sleeping; ensure that basic human needs are being met.
  Losses often interrupt appetite and sleep (Gifford, Cleary, 1990; Bateman et al, 1992).
- Develop a trusting relationship with client by using empathetic therapeutic communication techniques.
  An empathetic presence who takes the time to listen, offers support and reassurance, recognizes and focuses on feelings, and appreciates the uniqueness of each individual and family is helpful to clients experiencing chronic sorrow (Eakes, 1993; Eakes, Burke, Hainsworth, 1998).

• = Independent; ▲ = Collaborative

- Help client recognize that although sadness will occur at intervals for the rest of his or her life, it will become bearable. In time client may develop a relationship with grief that is lifelong, but livable, and as much filled with comfort as it is with sorrow (Moules, 1998).

  The sadness associated with chronic sorrow is permanent, but as the grief resolves there can be times of satisfaction and even happiness (Grainger, 1990; Teel, 1991).

- Encourage use of positive coping techniques:
  - Taking action: Suggested strategies include keeping busy, keeping personal interests, going away, getting out of the house, doing something to gain feeling of control over life.
  - Cognitive coping: Techniques include concentrating on the positive aspects of life, having a "can do" attitude, taking one day at a time, and taking responsibility for quality of own life.
  - Interpersonal coping: Techniques include talking to a close friend, a health care professional, or someone with the same condition. Joining a support group can also help the sorrowful person cope.
  - Emotional coping: Encourage the client to ventilate feelings, cry as desired, give thanks, and pray if desired.

  Clients with chronic sorrow have found these coping techniques helpful. The techniques are arranged in order of effectiveness (Hainsworth, Eakes, Burke, 1994).

- Review past experiences, role changes, and coping skills.

  Help client to identify own strengths for use in dealing with loss; reinforce these strengths.

- Expect client to meet responsibilities; give positive reinforcement.

▲ Refer client to spiritual counseling if desired.

  Spiritual counseling can help the client gain perspective about the loss and give comfort.

- Encourage client to make time to talk to family members about the loss with the help of professional support as needed and without criticizing or belittling each other's feelings about the loss. Once these feelings are shared, family members can better begin to accept the chronic loss, and develop coping strategies.

- Recognize that a stimulus for reactivation of sorrow in women is when a developmentally disabled child develops a health care crisis. In men, reactivation of sorrow is more associated with comparison with social norms (Mallow, Bechtel, 1999).

- Help client determine the best way and where to find social support.

  Social support has been identified as an important predictor of positive bereavement (Cooley, 1992; Herth, 1990).

▲ Identify available community resources, including grief counselors or support groups available for specific losses (e.g., Multiple Sclerosis Society).

  Support groups can serve as helpful ways to improve interpersonal coping strategies to deal with the loss (Hainsworth, Eakes, Burke, 1994).

▲ Encourage the client to become active in interests such as volunteer work, service projects, or church activities.

  When a grieving person can express caring for another, he or she gains a sense of being needed and an increased sense of purpose, which results in increased engagement in the world (Fischer, Hegge, 2000).

• = **Independent**; ▲ = **Collaborative**

▲ Identify whether client is experiencing depression, suicidal tendencies, or other emotional disorders. Refer for counseling as appropriate.

Counseling, including use of relaxation therapy, desensitization, and biofeedback, in addition to traditional psychotherapy, has been shown to be helpful (Arnette, 1996). Depression and the risk of suicide can accompany chronic grieving (Steen, 1998).

Geriatric

• Use reminiscence therapy in conjunction with the expression of emotions.

Reminiscence therapy can help the client look back at past experiences and use coping techniques that have been effective (Puentes, 1998).

• Identify previous losses and assess client for depression.

Losses and changes in older age often occur in rapid succession without adequate recovery time. More than two concurrent losses increases the incidence of unresolved grief (Herth, 1990).

• Evaluate the social support system of elderly client. If support system is minimal, help client determine how to increase available support.

The elderly who have poor grieving outcomes often do not live with family members and have a minimal support system.

Multicultural

• Assess for the influence of cultural beliefs, norms, and values on the client's expressions of sorrow.

Expressions of sorrow may be based on cultural perceptions (Leininger, 1996). African-Americans may be expected to act "strong" and go about with the business of life after a death; Native Americans may not talk about the death because of beliefs that such talk will detract from spirituality and bring bad luck; Latinos may wear black and act subdued during their luto/mourning period; Southeast Asian families may wear white when mourning (McQuay, 1995).

• Identify whether the client had been notified of health status and was able to be present during death and illness.

Not being present during terminal illness and death can disrupt grief process and contribute to chronic sorrow (McQuay, 1995).

• Validate the client's feelings regarding the loss.

Validation lets the client know that the nurse has heard and understands what was said, and it promotes the nurse-client relationship (Stuart, Laraia, 2001; Giger, Davidhizar, 1995).

Home Care Interventions

• Identify causes for and observe client's expression of chronic sorrow.

A clinician's ability to understand a client's perception of the impact of the illness is crucial to the clinician's ability to be therapeutic. Knowledge of a client's perceptions of chronic illness will help nurses intervene sensitively and effectively (Yuen-Juen, 1995).

▲ Refer client to medical social services or mental health services as appropriate.

Counseling services provide an opportunity for ventilation of feelings, increase coping skills, and provide respite for caregivers.

• Encourage client to participate in activities that are diversionary and uplifting as tolerated (e.g., outdoor activities, hobby groups, church-related activities, pet care).

Diversionary activities decrease the time spent in sorrow can give meaning to life and provide a sense of well-being.

• = Independent; ▲ = Collaborative

- Encourage client to participate in support groups appropriate to area of loss or illness (e.g., Crohn's disease support group or Widow to Widow).
  Support groups can increase an individual's sense of belonging. Group activity helps client to identify alternative ways to problem solve and experience feelings.
- Provide psychological support for family/caregivers.
  Family/caregivers who feel supported are often able to provide greater and more consistent support to the affected person.
- See care plans for **Impaired Adjustment, Chronic low Self-esteem, Loneliness,** and **Hopelessness.**

WEB SITES FOR EDUCATION

$\int c_{R_{L}} \int$ See the MERLIN web site for World Wide Web resources for client education.

REFERENCES Arnette JD: Physiological effects of chronic grief: a biofeedback treatment approach, *Death Stud* 20:59, 1996.

Bateman A et al: Dysfunctional grieving, *J Psychosoc Nurs* 30:5, 1992.

Cooley ME: Bereavement care: a role for nurses, *Cancer Nurs* 15:125, 1992.

Eakes GG: Chronic sorrow: a response to living with cancer, *Oncol Nurs Forum* 20:1327, 1993.

Eakes GG, Burke ML, Hainsworth MA: Theory, middle-range theory of chronic sorrow, *Image J Nurs Sch* 30:179, 1998.

Fischer C, Hegge M: The elderly woman at risk, *Am J Nurs* 100(6):54-59, 2000.

Gifford BJ, Cleary BB: Supporting the bereaved, *Am J Nurs* 90:49, 1990.

Giger JN, Davidhizar RE: *Transcultural nursing,* ed 2, St Louis, 1995, Mosby.

Grainger RD: Successful grieving, Am J Nurs 90:12, 1990.

Hainsworth MA, Eakes GG, Burke ML: Coping with chronic sorrow, *Issues Ment Health Nurs* 15:59, 1994.

Herth K: Relationship of hope, coping styles, concurrent losses, and setting to grief resolution in the elderly widow(er), *Res Nurs Health* 13:109, 1990.

Leininger MM: *Transcultural nursing: theories, research and practices,* ed 2, Hilliard, Ohio, 1996, McGraw-Hill.

Mallow GE, Bechtel GA: Chronic sorrow: the experience of parents with children who are developmentally disabled, *J Psychosoc Nurs* 37(7):31-43, 1999.

McQuay JE: Cross-cultural customs and beliefs related to health crises, death, and organ donation/ transplantation: a guide to assist health care professionals understand different responses and provide cross-cultural assistance, *Crit Care Nurs Clin North Am* 7(3):581-594, 1995 (appendix).

Moules NJ: Legitimizing grief: challenging beliefs that constrain, *J Family Nurs* 4(2):142-166, 1998.

Puentes WJ: Incorporating simple reminiscence techniques into acute care nursing practice, *J Gerontol Nurs* 24(2):14-20, 1998.

Steen KF: A comprehensive approach to bereavement, *Nurse Pract* 23(3):54-60, 1998.

Stewart ES: Family-centered care for the bereaved, *Pediatr Nurs* 21:181, 1995.

Stuart GW, Laraia MT: Therapeutic nurse-patient relationship. In Stuart GW, Laraia MT, editors: *Principles and practice of psychiatric nursing,* St Louis, 2001, Mosby, p 30.

Teel CS: Chronic sorrow: analysis of the concept, *J Adv Nurs* 16:1311, 1991.

Yuen-Juen H: The impact of chronic illness on patients, *Rehabil Nurse* 20:221, 1995.

Spiritual distress

Gail B. Ladwig

NANDA **Definition** Disruption in the life principle that pervades a person's entire being and that integrates and transcends one's biological and psychosocial nature

- = **Independent;** ▲ = **Collaborative**

Defining Characteristics

Expresses concern with meaning of life/death and/or belief systems; questions moral/ethical implications of therapeutic regimen; describes nightmares/sleep disturbances; verbalizes inner conflict about beliefs; verbalizes concern about relationship with deity; unable to participate in usual religious practices; seeks spiritual assistance; questions the meaning of suffering; questions meaning of own existence; displacement of anger toward religious representatives; anger toward God; alteration in behavior/mood evidenced by anger, crying, withdrawal, preoccupation, anxiety, hostility, apathy; gallows humor (inappropriate humor in a grave situation)

Related Factors (r/t)

Challenged belief and value system (e.g., due to moral/ethical implications of therapy, intense suffering); separation from religious or cultural ties

NOC ## Outcomes (Nursing Outcomes Classification)

Suggested NOC Labels

Dignified Dying; Hope; Spiritual Well-Being

> **Example NOC Outcome**
>
> Demonstrates **Spiritual Well-Being** as evidenced by: Expression of faith, hope, meaning, and purpose in life/Connectedness with inner-self and with others to share thoughts, feelings, and beliefs (Rate each indicator of **Spiritual Well-Being:** 1 = extremely compromised, 2 = substantially compromised, 3 = moderately compromised, 4 = mildly compromised, 5 = not compromised [see Section I])

Client Outcomes

- States conflicts or disturbances related to practice of belief system
- Discusses beliefs about spiritual issues
- States feelings of trust in self, God, or other belief systems
- Continues spiritual practices not detrimental to health
- Discusses feelings about death
- Displays a mood appropriate for the situation

NIC ## Interventions (Nursing Interventions Classification)

Suggested NIC Labels

Spiritual Support

> **Example NIC Interventions—Spiritual Support**
> - Encourage the use of spiritual resources if desired
> - Be available to listen to the client's feelings

Nursing Interventions and Rationales

- Observe client for self-esteem, self-worth, feelings of futility, or hopelessness. *Verbalization of feelings of low self-esteem, low self-worth, and hopelessness may indicate a spiritual need.*
- Monitor support systems. Be aware of own belief systems and accept client's spirituality. *To effectively help a client with spiritual needs, an understanding of one's own spiritual dimension is essential (Highfield, Carson, 1983).*
- Be physically present and available to help client determine religious and spiritual choices.

• = Independent; ▲ = Collaborative

Physical presence can decrease separation and aloneness, which clients often fear (Dossey et al, 1988). This study showed an overwhelming response that client's faith and trust in nurses produces a positive effect on client and family. Spiritual care interventions promote a sense of well-being (Narayanasamy, Owens, 2001).

- Provide quiet time for meditation, prayer, and relaxation.
Clients need time to be alone during times of health change.
- Help client make a list of important and unimportant values.
The number one need expressed by clients who had been hospitalized, which was expressed by persons of all denominations and faiths, was for their pastor/rabbi/spiritual advisor to not abandon them. For those who did not belong to a religious/spiritual group, their number one need was to at least be asked for some type of religious/spiritual preference (Moller, 1999). Clients are experts on their own paths, and knowing their values helps in exploring their uniqueness (Dossey et al, 1988).
- Ask how to be most helpful, then actively listen, reflect, and seek clarification.
Listening attentively and being physically present can be spiritually nourishing (Berggren-Thomas, Griggs, 1995). Obtain permission from the client to respond to spiritual needs from own spiritual perspective (Smucker, 1996).
- If client is comfortable with touch, hold client's hand or place hand gently on arm.
Touch makes nonverbal communication more personal.
- Help client develop and accomplish short-term goals and tasks.
Accomplishing goals increases self-esteem, which may be related to the client's spiritual well-being.
- Help client find a reason for living and be available for support.
"The need for a positive attitude for optimum healing was by far the most commonly mentioned subtheme by these participants and the strongest area of literature" (Criddle, 1993).
- Listen to client's feelings about death. Be nonjudgmental and allow time for grieving
All grief work takes time and is unique. Acceptance of client differences is essential to open communication.
- Help client develop skills to deal with illness or lifestyle changes. Include client in planning of care.
Clients perceived the experience of healing as an active process and expressed a desire to take conscious control (Criddle, 1993).
- Provide appropriate religious materials, artifacts, or music as requested.
Helping a client incorporate rituals, sacraments, reading, music, imagery, and meditation into daily life can enhance spiritual health (Conrad, 1985).
- Provide privacy for client to pray with others or to be read to by members of own faith.
Privacy shows respect for and sensitivity to the client.
- See care plan for **Readiness for enhanced Spiritual well-being.**

Geriatric

- Assist client with a life review and help client identify noteworthy experiences.
- Discuss personal definitions of spiritual wellness with client.
Listening attentively and helping elderly clients identify past coping strategies is part of helping with life review and finding meaning in life (Berggren-Thomas, Griggs, 1995).
- Identify client's past sources of spirituality. Help client explore his or her life and identify those experiences that are noteworthy. Client may want to read the Bible or have it read to them.
Older adults often identify spirituality as a source of hope (Gaskins, Forte, 1995).

• = **Independent;** ▲ = **Collaborative**

- Discuss the client's perception of God in relation to the illness.
  Different religions view illness from different perspectives.
- Offer to pray with client or caregivers.
  Prayer was described as an important part of spirituality by caregivers (Kaye, Robinson, 1994).
- Offer to read from the Bible or other book chosen by client.
  A religious ritual may comfort the client.

Multicultural

- Assess for the influence of cultural beliefs, norms, and values on the client's ability to cope with spiritual distress
  How the client copes with spiritual distress may be based on cultural perceptions (Leininger, 1996).
- Acknowledge the value conflicts from acculturation stresses that may contribute to spiritual distress.
  Challenges to traditional beliefs are anxiety provoking and can produce distress (Charron, 1998).
- Encourage spirituality as a source of support.
  African-Americans and Latinos may identify spirituality, religiousness, prayer, and church-based approaches as coping resources (Samuel-Hodge et al, 2000; Bourjolly, 1998; Mapp, Hudson, 1997).
- Validate the client's spiritual concerns, and convey respect for his or her beliefs.
  Validation lets the client know the nurse has heard and understands what was said (Stuart, Laraia, 2001; Giger, Davidhizar, 1995).

Home Care Interventions

All of the mentioned nursing interventions apply in the home setting.

Client/Family Teaching

- Teach guided imagery, story telling, meditation, and the use of silence.
  Guided imagery, metaphors, meditative prayer, and prayers of silence are effective spiritual approaches the nurse can implement when caring for the patient with cancer (Brown-Saltzman, 1997).
- Consider using art to express spirituality.
  This author tells a personal story about the activity of drawing flowers with her daughter and how it helped to explore spiritual issues (Toomey, 1999).
- Encourage family and friends to visit and show their concern.
  Social networks support spiritual well-being (Young, Dowling, 1987).
- Encourage family and friends to support client's belief through prayer.
  Positive effects of prayer include rapid recovery and prevention of complications (Byrd, 1988).
- Include directions to hospital chapel when orienting client and family to hospital unit.
  Attendance at services and a visit to the chapel may be important to the client and family.
- ▲ Refer client to spiritual advisor of choice.
  Nurses must collaborate with chaplains and relate to clergy to provide spiritual care for patients and families (VandeCreek, 1997). Caregivers who use religious or spiritual beliefs to cope with caregiving have a better relationship with care recipients, which is associated with lower levels of depression and role submersion (Chang, Noonan, Tennstedt, 1998).
- Prepare for chosen religious rituals.
  Some religions may have ceremonies associated with healing and illness.
- ▲ Refer to counseling, therapy, support groups, or hospice.
  The client may need more support and ongoing spiritual assistance.

• = **Independent**; ▲ = **Collaborative**

REFERENCES   Berggren-Thomas P, Griggs M: Spirituality in aging: spiritual need or spiritual journey? *J Gerontol Nurs* 21:5, 1995.
Bourjolly JN: Differences in religiousness among black and white women with breast cancer, *Soc Work Health Care* 28(1):21-39, 1998.
Brown-Saltzman K: Replenishing the spirit by meditative prayer and guided imagery, *Semin Oncol Nurs* 13(4):255, 1997.
Byrd RC: Positive therapeutic effects of intercessory prayer in a coronary care unit population, *South Med J* 81:826, 1988.
Chang B, Noonan A, Tennstedt S: The role of religion/spirituality in coping with caregiving for disabled elders, *Gerontologist* 38(4):463, 1998.
Charron HS: Anxiety disorders. In Varcarolis EM, editor: *Foundations of psychiatric mental health nursing*, ed 3, Philadelphia, 1998, WB Saunders, pp 447-448.
Conrad NJ: Spiritual support for the dying, *Nurs Clin North Am* 20:415, 1985.
Criddle L: Healing from surgery: a phenomenological study, *Image* 25:208, 1993.
Dossey M et al: *Holistic nursing: a handbook for practice*, Rockville, Md, 1988, Aspen.
Gaskins S, Forte L: The meaning of hope: implications for nursing practice and research, *J Gerontol Nurs* 21:17, 1995.
Giger JN, Davidhizar RE: *Transcultural nursing*, ed 2, St Louis, 1995, Mosby.
Highfield M, Carson C: Spiritual needs of patients: are they recognized? *Cancer Nurs* 6:187-192, 1983.
Kaye J, Robinson K: Spirituality among caregivers, *Image* 26:218, 1994.
Leininger MM: *Transcultural nursing: theories, research and practices*, ed 2, Hilliard, Ohio, 1996, McGraw-Hill.
Mapp I, Hudson R: Stress and coping among African American and Hispanic parents of deaf children, *Am Ann Deaf* 142(1):48-56, 1997.
Moller MD: Meeting spiritual needs on an inpatient unit, *J Psychosoc Nurs Ment Health Serv* 37(11):5, 1999.
Narayanasamy A, Owens J: A critical incident study of nurses' responses to the spiritual needs of their patients, *J Adv Nurs* 33(4):446-455, 2001.
Samuel-Hodge CD et al: Influences on day-to-day self-management of type 2 diabetes among African-American women: spirituality, the multi-caregiver role, and other social context factors, *Diabetes Care* 23(7):928-933, 2000.
Smucker C: A phenomenological description of the experience of spiritual distress, *Nurs Diag* 7:81, 1996.
Stuart GW, Laraia MT: Therapeutic nurse-patient relationship. In Stuart GW, Laraia MT, editors: *Principles and practice of psychiatric nursing*, St Louis, 2001, Mosby, p 30.
Toomey MA: Reflections on the art of observation: reflecting on a spiritual moment, *Can J Occup Ther* 66(4), 1999.
VandeCreek L: Collaboration between nurses and chaplains for spiritual caregiving, *Semin Oncol Nurs* 13(4):279, 1997.
Young G, Dowling W: Dimensions of religiosity in old age: accounting for variation in types of participation, *J Gerontol* 42:376, 1987.

Risk for Spiritual distress

Gail B. Ladwig

   Definition   At risk for an altered sense of harmonious connectedness with all of life and the universe in which dimensions that transcend and empower the self may be disrupted

Risk Factors

Energy-consuming anxiety; low self-esteem; mental illness; physical illness; blocks to self-love; poor relationships; physical or psychological stress; substance abuse; loss of loved one; natural disasters; situation losses; maturational losses; inability to forgive

• = Independent; ▲ = Collaborative

NOC   **Outcomes (Nursing Outcomes Classification)**

Suggested NOC Labels
Dignified Dying; Hope; Spiritual Well-Being

> **Example NOC Outcome**
> Demonstrates **Spiritual Well-Being** as evidenced by: Expression of faith, hope, meaning, and purpose in life/Connectedness with inner-self and with others to share thoughts, feelings, and beliefs (Rate each indicator of **Spiritual Well-Being:** 1 = extremely compromised, 2 = substantially compromised, 3 = moderately compromised, 4 = mildly compromised, 5 = not compromised [see Section I])

Client Outcomes

- States that typical coping during times of stress includes spirituality
- Discusses losses, stressors, and changes in health care status
- States acceptance of suggestions to enhance spirituality
- Practices spirituality by receiving presence from God, nature, family, friends, and community

  Interventions (Nursing Interventions Classification)

Suggested NIC Labels
Spiritual Support

> **Example NIC Interventions—Spiritual Support**
> - Encourage the use of spiritual resources if desired
> - Be available to listen to the client's feelings

Nursing Interventions and Rationales

- Perform a spiritual assessment to determine whether the client's usual means of spirituality are useful during physical or psychosocial stress.
  Results of this study suggest an association between intrinsic spirituality and a patient's experience of health and pain. Assessment of spirituality may be important to consider as a supplement to patient interviews (McBride et al, 1998). Nurses can improve spiritual assessment by eliciting patient accounts of the evolving spiritual journey and prayers that parallel changes in health status (Highfield, 1997).
- Use a spiritual assessment tool such as the Spiritual Involvement and Beliefs Scale.
  A new instrument, called the Spiritual Involvement and Beliefs Scale, designed to be widely applicable across religious traditions, assesses actions and beliefs. It measures the relationship between spirituality and health in the clinical setting (Hatch et al, 1998). Health care professionals are increasingly recognizing the importance of spiritual health as a precursor to physical health (Espeland, 1999).
- Encourage clients who are facing challenges with psychosocial problems to use their usual means of spirituality.
  According to Koenig, Larson, and Weaver (1998), religion plays a largely positive role in mental health. The spiritual dimension has been demonstrated by research to be an important and fundamental aspect of human functioning, one that positively affects healing and health and that should be mobilized as an active part of the health care of individuals (Hamilton, 1998).

• = Independent; ▲ = Collaborative

- Be fully present with each encounter with the client. Provide deliberate focused attention, be receptive to the other person, and have a persistent awareness of the other's shared humanity.

  "Being there" provides comfort for both patient and nurse, providing affirmation, communication of empathy, and availability without words (Zerwekh, 1997).

- Offer to pray with the client or encourage the client to pray; also convey acceptance of the client by actively listening and being fully present.

  Oncology, parish, and hospice nurses in the Midwest state that these are nursing interventions they implement to enhance the spirituality of clients (Sellers, Haag, 1998).

- Encourage clients to be aware of and to receive the transcendent presence of the divine, friends, family, community, and creation (plants, animals, environment) into their hearts.

  In the crisis situation of experiencing a myocardial infarction, participants in this study described spirituality (receiving presence) as having the most positive influence on their recovery (Walton, 1999).

- If the presenting problem involves substance abuse, refer the client to a substance abuse counselor, as well as to pastoral care services or appropriate spiritual counseling.

  Current findings indicate that spiritual/religious involvement may be an important protective factor against alcohol/drug abuse. Spiritual (re)engagement appears to be correlated with recovery (Miller, 1998).

- See care plans for **Spiritual distress,** and **Readiness for enhanced Spiritual well-being.**

Multicultural

- Assess for the influence of cultural beliefs, norms, and values on the client's ability to cope with spiritual distress.

  How the client copes with spiritual distress may be based on cultural perceptions (Leininger, 1996).

- Acknowledge the value conflicts from acculturation stresses that may contribute to spiritual distress.

  Challenges to traditional beliefs are anxiety provoking and can produce distress (Charron, 1998).

- Encourage spirituality as a source of support.

  African-Americans and Latinos may identify spirituality, religiousness, prayer, and church-based approaches as coping resources (Samuel-Hodge et al, 2000; Bourjolly, 1998; Mapp, Hudson, 1997).

- Validate the client's spiritual concerns, and convey respect for his or her beliefs.

  Validation lets the client know the nurse has heard and understands what was said (Stuart, Laraia, 2001; Giger, Davidhizar, 1995).

Home Care Interventions

- Interventions mentioned in other subheadings in this nursing diagnosis also apply to home care.

Client/Family Teaching

- Encourage family to perform caring actions, such as making phone calls and personal visits and sending cards, flowers, gifts, and prayers.

  Caring actions of others were important to the participants in this study. They provided participants with a feeling of wellness and facilitated coping (Walton, 1999).

- Encourage caregivers to seek assistance with caregiving.

  Providing care for a loved one with cancer can be stressful for the family caregiver; yet it can also produce spiritual growth (Carson, 1997).

- = **Independent;** ▲ = **Collaborative**

REFERENCES Bourjolly JN: Differences in religiousness among black and white women with breast cancer, *Soc Work Health Care* 28(1):21-39, 1998.

Carson V: Spiritual care: the needs of the caregiver, *Semin Oncol Nurs* 13(4):271, 1997.

Charron HS: Anxiety disorders. In Varcarolis EM, editor: *Foundations of psychiatric mental health nursing,* ed 3, Philadelphia, 1998, WB Saunders, pp 447-448.

Espeland K: Achieving spiritual wellness: using reflective questions, *J Psychosoc Nurs Ment Health Serv* 37(7), 1999.

Giger JN, Davidhizar RE: *Transcultural nursing,* ed 2, St Louis, 1995, Mosby.

Hamilton DG: Believing in patients' beliefs: physician attunement to the spiritual dimension as a positive factor in patient healing and health, *Am J Hosp Palliat Care* 15(5):276, 1998.

Hatch R et al: The spiritual involvement and beliefs scale, development and testing of a new instrument, *J Fam Pract* 46(6):476, 1998.

Highfield M: Spiritual assessment across the cancer trajectory: methods and reflections, *Semin Oncol Nurs* 13(4):237, 1997.

Koenig HG, Larson DB, Weaver AJ: Research on religion and serious mental illness, *New Dir Ment Health Serv* 80:81, 1998.

Leininger MM: *Transcultural nursing: theories, research and practices,* ed 2, Hilliard, Ohio, 1996, McGraw-Hill.

Mapp I, Hudson R: Stress and coping among African American and Hispanic parents of deaf children, *Am Ann Deaf* 142(1):48-56, 1997.

McBride J et al: The relationship between a patient's spirituality and health experiences, *Fam Med* 30(2):122, 1998.

Miller WR: Researching the spiritual dimensions of alcohol and other drug problems, *Addiction* 93(7):979, 1998.

Samuel-Hodge CD et al: Influences on day-to-day self-management of type 2 diabetes among African-American women: spirituality, the multi-caregiver role, and other social context factors, *Diabetes Care* 23(7):928-933, 2000.

Sellers SC, Haag BA: Spiritual nursing interventions, *J Holist Nurs* 16(3):338, 1998.

Stuart GW, Laraia MT: Therapeutic nurse-patient relationship. In Stuart GW, Laraia MT, editors: *Principles and practice of psychiatric nursing,* St Louis, 2001, Mosby, p 30.

Walton J: Spirituality of patients recovering from an acute myocardial infarction, a grounded theory study, *J Holistic Nurs* 17(1):34, 1999.

Zerwekh J: The practice of presencing, *Semin Oncol Nurs* 13(4):260, 1997.

Readiness for enhanced Spiritual well-being

Gail B. Ladwig

NANDA **Definition** Process of developing/unfolding of mystery though harmonious interconnectedness that springs from inner strengths

Defining Characteristics

- *Inner strengths:* Inner core: transcended; self-consciousness; unifying force; a sense of awareness; sacred source
- *Unfolding mystery:* One's experience about life's purpose and meaning, mystery, uncertainty, and struggles
- *Harmonious interconnectedness:* Harmony with self, others, higher power/God, and the environment; relatedness with self, others, higher power/God, and the environment; connectedness with self, others, higher power/God, and the environment

• = Independent; ▲ = Collaborative

Outcomes (Nursing Outcomes Classification)

Suggested NOC Labels

Hope; Quality of Life; Spiritual Well-Being; Well-Being

> **Example NOC Outcome**
> Demonstrates **Spiritual Well-Being** as evidenced by: Expression of faith, hope, meaning, and purpose in life/Connectedness with inner-self and with others to share thoughts, feelings, and belief (Rate each indicator 1 = extremely compromised, 2 = substantially compromised, 3 = moderately compromised, 4 = mildly compromised, 5 = not compromised [see Section I])

Client Outcomes

- States recognition of inner strengths
- States purpose and meaning for life
- Expresses feelings of hope
- Lists values harmonious with inner core
- States harmony with self, others, higher power/God, and the environment

Interventions (Nursing Interventions Classification)

Suggested NIC Labels

Spiritual Support

> **Example NIC Interventions—Spiritual Support**
> - Encourage the use of spiritual resources if desired
> - Be available to listen to the client's feelings

Nursing Interventions and Rationales

- Perform a spiritual assessment that includes client's relationship with God, purpose and direction in life, religious affiliation, and any other significant beliefs.
  Assessment of spirituality may be important to consider as a supplement to patient interviews (McBride et al, 1998). Nurses can improve spiritual assessment by eliciting patient accounts of the evolving spiritual journey and prayers that parallel changes in health status (Highfield, 1997).
- Assist client with values clarification. Have client list values that are important and on which he or she is willing to consistently act.
  Values clarification is a nursing activity that promotes spiritual health and wellness (Boss, Corbett, 1990). Nurses can facilitate the healing process by helping clients to identify and clarify priority values (Mickley, Cowles, 2001).
- Promote support from family members and significant others by encouraging family visits, phone calls, and involvement in care.
  These strategies help maintain social support networks to foster hope and spiritual well-being (Farran, McCann, 1989).
- Help arrange visits with clergy, and allow private time for prayer and family participation in spiritual reading.
  Adults prefer this type of spiritual care (Reed, 1991). Religious involvement appears to enable the sick, particularly those with serious and disabling medical illness, to cope better (Koenig, Larson, Larson, 2001).

• = Independent; ▲ = Collaborative

- Set mutual times to sit and talk with client; suggest 30 minutes twice a day. If client does not wish to talk, just sit with him or her.
  The nurse's presence and willingness to listen contribute to a sense of hope or well-being (Clark, Heidenreich, 1995). Hope is necessary for life. "Without hope we begin to die" (Simsen, 1988).
- Offer to pray with or for client.
  Spiritual needs can be met by praying with or for the client (Dettmore, 1984).
- Encourage storytelling.
  An intervention nurses can use to promote spiritual health, stories are a medium for assessment and intervention in areas that essentially reflect an individual's spirituality (Taylor, 1997).
- Offer to read to client.
  Some clients cannot read because they are illiterate, have a pathological problem that prevents reading, or are taking medications that cause visual problems or drowsiness. Reading to clients, regardless of whether religious, is an act of care because time is being spent with them (Bolander, 1994).
- Provide listening music to use with stress reduction techniques.
  Participants in this study performed significantly better than the controls on standardized tests of depression, distress, self-esteem, and mood (Hanser, Thompson, 1994).
- See care plan for **Spiritual distress.**

Geriatric

- Provide for spiritual needs, visits from clergy, prayer.
  Preliminary findings indicate that religious belief may have significant influence on the psychological well-being of older adults (Mackenzie et al, 2000).

Multicultural

- Assess for the influence of cultural beliefs, norms, and values on the client's perceptions of spirituality
  The client's expressions of spirituality may be based on cultural perceptions (Leininger, 1996).
- Encourage expressions of spirituality.
  African-American and Latinos may identify spirituality, religiousness, prayer, and church-based approaches as coping resources (Samuel-Hodge et al, 2000; Bourjolly, 1998; Mapp, Hudson, 1997).
- Validate the client's spiritual concerns and convey respect for his or her beliefs.
  Validation lets the client know the nurse has heard and understands what was said (Stuart, Laraia, 2001; Giger, Davidhizar, 1995).

Home Care Interventions

- All of the mentioned nursing interventions apply in the home setting.
- ▲ Refer client to parish nurses.
  Parish nurses are experienced registered nurses committed to helping people meet the health needs of their mind, body, and spirit (Stewart, 2000).

Client/Family Teaching

- Help client obtain religious rites or spiritual guidance.
  Spiritual support (belief in a divine being or God) was identified as a factor that contributed to initiation and maintenance of behavior changes after an illness (McSweeney, 1993). The nurse is rarely the client's primary spiritual caregiver. No single approach to spiritual care is satisfactory for all clients; many kinds of resources are needed (Bolander, 1994).
- Assist client with developing spirituality. List the most valuable qualities he or she can bring from within, circumstances most helpful for unfolding these qualities, and ways of incorporating these circumstances into his or her lifestyle.

• = **Independent;** ▲ = **Collaborative**

Interventions assist clients with bringing forth courage, compassion, inner peace, and creative insight (spirituality) (Macrae, 1995).

WEB SITES FOR EDUCATION

 See the MERLIN web site for World Wide Web resources for client education.

REFERENCES Bolander V: *Sorensen and Luckmann's basic nursing: a psychophysiologic approach,* Philadelphia, 1994, WB Saunders.

Boss JA, Corbett T: The developing practice of the parish nurse: an inner-city experience. In Solari-Twadell PA, Djupe AM, McDermott MA, editors: *Parish nursing: the developing practice,* Park Ridge, Ill, 1990, National Parish Nurse Resource Center.

Bourjolly JN: Differences in religiousness among black and white women with breast cancer, *Soc Work Health Care* 28(1):21-39, 1998.

Clark C, Heidenreich T: Spiritual care for the critically ill, *Am J Crit Care* 4:77, 1995.

Dettmore D: Spiritual care: remembering your patients' forgotten needs, *Nursing* 14:46, 1984.

Farran CJ, McCann J: Longitudinal analysis of hope in community-based older adults, *Psychiatr Arch Nurs* 3:272, 1989.

Giger JN, Davidhizar RE: *Transcultural nursing,* ed 2, St Louis, 1995, Mosby.

Hanser SB, Thompson L: Effects of a music therapy strategy on depressed older adults, *J Gerontol* 49(6):P265, 1994.

Highfield M: Spiritual assessment across the cancer trajectory: methods and reflections, *Semin Oncol Nurs* 13(4):237, 1997.

Koenig HG, Larson DB, Larson SS: Religion and coping with serious medical illness, *Ann Pharmacother* 35(3):352-359, 2001.

Leininger MM: *Transcultural nursing: theories, research and practices,* ed 2, Hilliard, Ohio, 1996, McGraw-Hill.

Mackenzie ER et al: Spiritual support and psychological well-being: older adults' perceptions of the religion and health connection, *Altern Ther Health Med* 6(6):37-45, 2000.

Macrae J: Nightingale's spiritual philosophy and its significance for modern nursing, *Image* 27:8, 1995.

Mapp I, Hudson R: Stress and coping among African American and Hispanic parents of deaf children, *Am Ann Deaf* 142(1):48-56, 1997.

McBride J et al: The relationship between a patient's spirituality and health experiences, *Fam Med* 30(2):122, 1998.

McSweeney J: Making behavior changes after a myocardial infarction, *West J Nurs Res* 15:441, 1993.

Mickley JR, Cowles K: Ameliorating the tension: use of forgiveness for healing, *Oncol Nurs Forum* 28(1):31-37, 2001.

Reed P: Preferences for spiritually related nursing interventions among terminally ill and nonterminally ill hospitalized adults and well adults, *Appl Nurs Res* 4:122, 1991.

Samuel-Hodge CD et al: Influences on day-to-day self-management of type 2 diabetes among African-American women: spirituality, the multi-caregiver role, and other social context factors, *Diabetes Care* 23(7):928-933, 2000.

Stewart LE: Parish nursing: renewing a long tradition of caring, *Gastroenterol Nurs* 23(3):116-120, 2000.

Stuart GW, Laraia MT: Therapeutic nurse-patient relationship. In Stuart GW, Laraia MT, editors: *Principles and practice of psychiatric nursing,* St Louis, 2001, Mosby, p 30.

Taylor E: The story behind the story: the use of storytelling in spiritual caregiving, *Semin Oncol Nurs* 13(4):252, 1997.

Risk for Suffocation

Peggy A. Wetsch and Mary Markle

NANDA **Definition** Accentuated risk of accidental suffocation (inadequate air available for inhalation)

• = **Independent;** ▲ = **Collaborative**

Risk Factors

External   Vehicle warming in closed garage; use of fuel-burning heaters not vented to outside; smoking in bed; children playing with plastic bags or inserting small objects into their mouths or noses; propped bottle placed in an infant's crib; pillow placed in an infant's crib; person who eats large mouthfuls of food; discarded or unused refrigerators or freezers without removed doors; children left unattended in bathtubs or pools; household gas leaks; low-strung clothesline; pacifier hung around infant's neck

Internal   Reduced olfactory sensation; reduced motor abilities; cognitive or emotional difficulties; disease or injury process; lack of safety education; lack of safety precautions

Related Factors (r/t)

See Risk Factors

NOC   Outcomes (Nursing Outcomes Classification)

Suggested NOC Labels

Knowledge: Personal Safety; Risk Detection; Safety Behavior: Home Physical Environment; Substance Addiction Consequences

> **Example NOC Outcome**
> Accomplishes **Risk Control** as evidenced by: Monitors environmental risk factors/ Develops effective risk control strategies (Rate each indicator of **Risk Control:** 1 = never demonstrated, 2 = rarely demonstrated, 3 = sometimes demonstrated, 4 = often demonstrated, 5 = consistently demonstrated [see Section I])

Client Outcomes

- Explains and undertakes appropriate measures to prevent suffocation
- Demonstrates correct techniques for emergency rescue maneuvers (i.e., Heimlich maneuver, rescue breathing, cardiopulmonary resuscitation [CPR]) and describes situations that necessitate them

NIC   Interventions (Nursing Interventions Classification)

Suggested NIC Labels

Environmental Management: Safety

> **Example NIC Interventions—Environmental Management: Safety**
> - Identify safety hazards in the environment (i.e., physical, biological, and chemical)
> - Modify or remove hazards from the environment when possible

Nursing Interventions and Rationales

NOTE: Management of a risk diagnosis necessitates approaches using primary and secondary prevention. Primary prevention interventions, which include such activities as safety instruction, focus on thwarting the development of disease or condition. Secondary prevention is achieved through screening, monitoring, and surveillance (Shirtridge, Valanis, 1992).

- Conduct risk factor identification, noting special circumstances in which preventive or protective measures are indicated. Note presence of environmental hazards including the following:
  - Plastic bags (e.g., dry cleaner's bags, bags used for mattress protection)
  - Cribs with slats wider than $2^3/_8$ inches
  - Ill-fitting crib mattresses that can allow infant to become wedged between mattress and crib

• = Independent; ▲ = Collaborative

- Pillows in cribs
- Abandoned large appliances such as refrigerators, dishwashers, or freezers
- Clothing with cords or hoods that can become entangled
- Bibs, pacifiers on a string, drapery cords, pull-toy strings
- Earth cave-ins
- Food items

Suffocation by airway obstruction is a leading cause of death in children <6 years of age. Cords longer than 12 inches can lead to strangulation. Identification of clients and families at risk signals special teaching and referral needs (Rivara, Bergman, LoGero, 1982; Green, 1993; Jones, 1993; McCloskey, Bulechek, 1992).

- Identify hospitalized clients at particular risk for suffocation, including the following:
  - Clients with altered level of consciousness
  - Infants or young children
  - Clients with developmental delays
- Institute safety measures such as proper positioning and feeding precautions. See care plans for **Risk for Aspiration** and **Impaired Swallowing** for additional interventions.

Vigilance and special protective measures are necessary for clients at greater risk for suffocation (Green, 1993).

Geriatric

- Assess status of swallow reflex and dentition; offer appropriate foods and beverages accordingly.
- Observe client for pocketing of food in side of mouth; remove food as needed.
- Position client in high Fowler's position when eating and for 30 minutes afterward.
  Elderly clients may be at risk for suffocation that results from dysphagia and poor dental health.
- Use care in pillow placement when positioning frail elderly clients who are on bed rest.
  Frail elderly clients are at risk for suffocation if pillows become lodged in the bed and the client cannot reposition because of weakness.

Home Care Interventions

- Assess home for potential safety hazards in systems that are not likely to be fixed (e.g., faulty pilots or gas leaks in gas stoves, carbon monoxide release from heating systems, kerosene fumes from portable heaters). Assist family with having these areas assessed and making appropriate safety arrangements (e.g., installing detectors, making repairs).
  Assessment and correction of system problems prevents accidental suffocation.

Client/Family Teaching

- Counsel families on the following:
  - General safety practices such as not smoking in bed, proper disposal of large appliances, using properly functioning heating systems and ventilation, having functional smoke detectors, and opening garage doors when warming up a car
  - Safety measures appropriate to the functional or developmental age of the client (with emphasis on crib safety in particular)
  - Sleeping precautions such as not sleeping next to small infants, which places them at a greater risk of smothering

  Legislated countermeasures have led to decreased suffocation incidences, with the exception of mechanical crib strangulation. Families and caregivers need to continue to be attentive and aware of potentially dangerous situations (National Safety Council, 1992; Green, 1993).

• = **Independent;** ▲ = **Collaborative**

- Advise parents to avoid food that can be inhaled (e.g., peanuts, popcorn, hard candy, gum, whole or large pieces of hot dog, whole grapes). Nonfood items smaller than 1¼ inches in diameter (e.g., latex balloons, small parts on toys) also present a hazard.

  Rigid items that are of a spherical or cylindrical shape can cause upper airway occlusion. Mechanical suffocation and asphyxia resulting from foreign objects in the respiratory tract are the leading cause of death in children <1 year of age. Children <2 years of age have high level of hands-to-mouth behavior. Combined with a lack of fear, they are at risk even in a child-safe environment (Carson, 1992; Green, 1993; Holida, 1993).

- ▲ Provide information to parents about obtaining the "no-choke test tube" if desired.

  This tube teaches parents about safe sizes of toys and other small objects (Jones, 1993).

- Stress water and pool safety precautions including vigilant, uninterrupted parent supervision.

  An intense drive for exploration combined with a lack of awareness of danger makes drowning a threat to small children. A child's high center of gravity and poor coordination make buckets and toilets a threat because a child looking inside either can fall over and become lodged (Green, 1993; Jones, 1993).

- Underscore the necessity of not allowing children to play with or near electric garage doors and of keeping garage door openers out of reach of young children.

  Children close to the ground may not be large enough to trigger reversal mechanisms on the door and may become trapped.

- ▲ Recommend that families who are seeking day care or in-home care for children, geriatric family members, or at-risk family members with developmental or functional disabilities inspect the environment for hazards and examine the first aid preparation and vigilance of providers.

  Many working families must trust others to care for family members.

- ▲ Involve family members in learning and practicing rescue techniques, including treatment of choking, breathing, and CPR. Initiate referral to formal training classes.

  Family members need adequate preparation to deal with emergency situations (Green, 1993).

WEB SITES FOR EDUCATION

MERLIN See the MERLIN web site for World Wide Web resources for client education.

REFERENCES Carson L: Triage decisions: an 11-month-old with unexplained respiration distress, *J Emerg Nurs* 18:82, 1992.

Green PM: High risk for suffocation. In McFarland GK, McFarlane EA, editors: *Nursing diagnosis and intervention*, St Louis, 1993, Mosby.

Holida DL: Latex balloons: they can take your breath away, *Pediatr Nurs* 19:39, 1993.

Jones NE: Childhood residential injuries, *MCN Am J Matern Child Nurs* 18:168, 1993.

McCloskey JC, Bulechek GM, editors: *Nursing interventions classification*, St Louis, 1992, Mosby.

National Safety Council: *Accident facts*, Itasca, Ill, 1992, The Council.

Rivara FP, Bergman AB, LoGero JP: Epidemiology of childhood injuries II: sex differences in injury rates, *Am J Dis Child* 13:502, 1982.

Shirtridge L, Valanis B: The epidemiological model applied in community health nursing. In Stanhope M, Lancaster J, editors: *Community health nursing: process and practice for promoting health*, ed 3, St Louis, 1992, Mosby.

• = **Independent**; ▲ = **Collaborative**

Risk for Suicide

Gail B. Ladwig

NANDA   **Definition** At risk for self-inflicted, life-threatening injury

Related Factors (r/t)

Behavioral   History of previous suicide attempt; impulsiveness; buying a gun; stockpiling medicines; making or changing a will; giving away possessions; sudden euphoric recovery from major depression; marked changes in behavior, attitude, school performance

Verbal   Threats of killing oneself; states desire to die/end it all

Situational   Living alone; retired; relocation, institutionalization; economic instability; loss of autonomy/independence; presence of gun in home; adolescents living in nontraditional settings (e.g., juvenile detention center, prison, half-way house, group home)

Psychological   Family history of suicide; alcohol and substance use/abuse; psychiatric illness/disorder (e.g., depression, schizophrenia, bipolar disorder); abuse in childhood; guilt; gay or lesbian youth

Demographic   Age: elderly, young adult males, adolescents; race: Caucasian, Native American; gender: male divorced, widowed

Physical   Physical illness; terminal illness; chronic pain

Social   Loss of important relationship; disrupted family life; grief, bereavement; poor support systems; loneliness; hopelessness; helplessness; social isolation; legal or disciplinary problem; cluster suicides

NOC   **Outcomes (Nursing Outcomes Classification)**

Suggested NOC Labels

Cognitive Ability; Depression Control; Distorted Thought Control; Impulse Control; Self-Mutilation Restraint; Suicide Self-Restraint; Will to Live

> **Example NOC Outcome**
> Demonstrates **Suicide Self-Restraint** as evidenced by: Expresses feelings/Seeks help when feeling self-destructive/Verbalizes and controls suicidal ideas and impulses (Rate each indicator of **Suicide Self-Restraint:** 1 = never demonstrated, 2 = rarely demonstrated, 3 = sometimes demonstrated, 4 = often demonstrated, 5 = consistently demonstrated [see Section I])

Client Outcomes

- Does not harm self
- Expresses decreased anxiety and control of hallucinations
- Talks about feelings; expresses anger appropriately
- Obtains no access to harmful objects
- Yields access to harmful objects

NIC   **Interventions (Nursing Interventions Classification)**

Suggested NIC Labels

Anger Control Assistance; Anxiety Reduction; Coping Enhancement; Crisis Intervention; Suicide Prevention; Surveillance

> **Example NIC Interventions—Suicide Prevention**
> - Determine presence and degree of suicide risk
> - Encourage client to seek out care providers to talk as urge to harm self occurs

• = Independent; ▲ = Collaborative

Nursing Interventions and Rationales

- Establish a therapeutic relationship with client

  This study demonstrated the importance of this relationship in identifying and preventing suicide (Rudd et al, 2000).

▲ Monitor, document, and report client's potential for suicide.

  Traits such as impulsivity, poor social adjustment, and mood disorders are associated with adolescent suicide attempts (Brent et al, 1994).

- Be alert for warning signs of suicide:

  - Verbalizations such as, "I can't go on," "Nothing matters anymore," "I wish I were dead"
  - Becoming depressed or withdrawn
  - Behaving recklessly
  - Getting affairs in order and giving away valued possessions
  - Showing a marked change in behavior, attitudes, or appearance
  - Abusing drugs or alcohol
  - Suffering a major loss or life change

  Suicide is rarely a spur-of-the-moment decision. In the days and hours before people kill themselves, there are usually clues and warning signs (Befrienders International, 2001).

- Assess for suicidal ideation when the history reveals:

  - Depression
  - Alcohol or other drug abuse
  - Other psychiatric disorder
  - Attempted suicide
  - Recent divorce and/or separation
  - Recent unemployment
  - Recent bereavement
  - Chronic pain

  Clinicians should be alert for suicide when the above factors are present in asymptomatic persons (National Guideline Clearing House, 2001). This study revealed that clients with chronic pain and depression expressed suicidal ideation (Fisher et al, 2001). The process leading to suicide in young people is often untreated depression (Houston, Hawton, Shepperd, 2001).

▲ Refer to mental health counseling and possible hospitalization if there is evidence of suicidal intent, which may include evidence of preparatory actions (e.g., obtaining a weapon, making a plan, putting affairs in order, giving away prized possession, preparing a suicide note).

▲ Question family members regarding the preparatory actions mentioned.

  Clinicians should be alert for suicide when these factors are present in asymptomatic persons (National Guideline Clearing House, 2001).

▲ Refer family members and friends to local mental health agencies and crisis intervention centers if client has suicidal ideation or there is a suspicion of suicidal thoughts.

  Clients at risk should receive evaluation and help (National Guideline Clearing House, 2001).

▲ Consider outpatient commitment for actively suicidal client.

  Involuntary outpatient commitment can improve treatment, reduce the likelihood of hospital readmission, and reduce episodes of violent behavior in persons with severe psychiatric illnesses (Torrey, Zdanowicz, 2001).

• = Independent; ▲ = Collaborative

- Counsel parents and homeowners to restrict unauthorized access to potentially lethal prescription drugs and firearms within the home.
  Identifying teens at high risk of firearm suicide and limiting access to firearms is a type of public health intervention likely to be successful in preventing firearm suicides (Shah, 2000).
- See care plan for **Risk for self-directed Violence.**

Multicultural

- Assess for the influence of cultural beliefs, norms, and values on the individual's perceptions of suicide.
  What the individual believes about suicide may be based on cultural perceptions (Leininger, 1996).
- With the client's consent, facilitate family-oriented crisis intervention.
  Family-oriented crisis intervention can clarify stresses and allow assessment of family dynamics.
- Facilitate modeling and role-playing for client and family regarding healthy ways to start a discussion about the client's suicide attempt.
  It is helpful for families and the client to practice communication skills in a safe environment before trying them in a real-life situation (Rivera-Andino, Lopez, 2000).
- Identify and acknowledge the stresses unique to culturally diverse individuals.
  Financial difficulties and maintaining cultural values are two of the most common family stressors cited by women of color (Majumdar, Ladak, 1998).
- Encourage the family to demonstrate and offer caring and support to each other.
  The familial characteristics of care and support may be associated with fostering resiliency in African-American families. Resilience is the ability to experience adverse conditions and successfully overcome them (Calvert, 1997).
- Validate the individual's feelings regarding concerns about current crisis and family functioning.
  Validation lets the client know that the nurse has heard and understands what was said, and it promotes the nurse-client relationship (Stuart, Laraia, 2001; Giger, Davidhizar, 1995).

WEB SITES FOR EDUCATION

MERLIN See the MERLIN web site for World Wide Web resources for client education.

REFERENCES   Befrienders International: retrieved from the World Wide Web March 27, 2001. Web site: www.befrienders.org/mainindex.htm

Brent D et al: Personality disorder, personality traits, impulsive violence and completed suicide in adolescents, *J Am Acad Child Adolescent Psychiatry* 33:1080, 1994.

Calvert WJ: Protective factors within the family, and their role in fostering resiliency in African American adolescents, *J Cult Divers* 4(4):110-117, 1997.

Fisher BJ et al: Suicidal intent in patients with chronic pain, *Pain* 89(2-3):199-206, 2001.

Giger JN, Davidhizar RE: *Transcultural nursing*, ed 2, St Louis, 1995, Mosby.

Houston K, Hawton K, Shepperd R: Suicide in young people aged 15-24: a psychological autopsy study, *J Affect Disord* 63(1-3):159-170, 2001.

Leininger MM: *Transcultural nursing: theories, research and practices*, ed 2, Hilliard, Ohio, 1996, McGraw-Hill.

Majumdar B, Ladak S: Management of family and workplace stress experienced by women of color from various cultural backgrounds, *Can J Public Health* 89(1):48-52, 1998.

National Guideline Clearing House: *Screening for suicide risk*, retrieved from the World Wide Web March 27, 2001. Web site: www.ngc.gov/VIEWS/summary.asp?guideline=194&summary_type=brief_summary&view=brief_summary&sSearch_string=

• = **Independent;** ▲ = **Collaborative**

Rivera-Andino J, Lopez L: When culture complicates care, *RN* 63(7):47-49, 2000.

Rudd MD et al: Personality types and suicidal behavior: an exploratory study, *Suicide Life Threat Behav* 30(3):199-212, 2000.

Shah S et al: Adolescent suicide and household access to firearms in Colorado: results of a case-control study, *J Adolesc Health* 26(3):157-163, 2000.

Stuart GW, Laraia MT: Therapeutic nurse-patient relationship. In Stuart GW, Laraia MT, editors: *Principles and practice of psychiatric nursing,* St Louis, 2001, Mosby, p 30.

Torrey EF, Zdanowicz M: Outpatient commitment: what, why, and for whom, *Psychiatr Serv* 52(3):337-341, 2001.

Delayed Surgical recovery

Gail B. Ladwig

NANDA   **Definition** An extension of the number of postoperative days required for individuals to initiate and perform on their own behalf activities that maintain life, health, and well-being

Defining Characteristics

Evidence of interrupted healing of surgical area (e.g., red, indurated, draining, immobile); loss of appetite with or without nausea; difficulty in moving about; requires help to complete self-care; fatigue; report of pain or discomfort; postpones resumption of employment activities; perception that more time is needed to recover

Related Factors (r/t)

To be developed

NOC   **Outcomes (Nursing Outcomes Classification)**

Suggested NOC Labels

Endurance; Infection Status; Mobility Level; Pain Control; Self-Care Activities of Daily Living (ADLs); Wound Healing: Primary Intention; Wound Healing: Secondary Intention

> **Example NOC Outcome**
> Demonstrates **Wound Healing: Primary Intention** as evidenced by the following indicators: Skin approximation/Resolution of signs of infection of wound (Rate each indicator of **Would Healing: Primary Intention:** 1 = none, 2 = limited, 3 = moderate, 4 = substantial, 5 = extensive [see Section I])

Client Outcomes

- Surgical area shows no evidence of healing: no redness, induration, draining, or immobility
- States appetite regained
- States no nausea
- Demonstrates ability to move about
- Demonstrates ability to complete self-care
- States no fatigue
- States pain is controlled or relieved after nursing interventions
- Resumes employment activities

- = **Independent;** ▲ = **Collaborative**

NIC **Interventions (Nursing Interventions Classification)**

Suggested NIC Labels

Incision Site Care; Nutrition Management; Pain Management; Self-Care Assistance

> **Example NIC Interventions—Incision Site Care and Nutrition Management**
> - Teach the client and/or the family how to care for the incision, including how to recognize the signs and symptoms of infection
> - Provide client with high-protein, high-calorie, nutritious finger foods and drinks that can be readily consumed, as appropriate

Nursing Interventions and Rationales

- Perform a thorough assessment of the client, including risk factors.
  Thorough assessment of patients' risk for developing infection allows nurses to act to reduce that risk (Kingsley, 1992). Through a continual holistic assessment of the patient, and the many factors influencing wound healing, interventions can be altered for a more positive outcome (Morales, Andrews, 1993).
- ▲ Assess for presence of medical conditions and treat appropriately before surgery. If the client is diabetic, maintain normal blood glucose levels before surgery.
  Good blood glucose control promotes faster healing (Schemer, 1996). Some of the most commonly encountered and clinically significant impediments to healing include conditions such as diabetes mellitus (Stadelmann, Digenis, Tobin, 1998).
- Provide preoperative teaching by a nurse to decrease postoperative problems of anxiety, pain, nausea, and lack of independence.
  This study showed a significant decrease in anxiety 24 to 72 hours postoperatively for the group who had a preoperative teaching by a nurse. The author recommends that all surgical patients should receive a visit from theatre nurses before their operation (Martin, 1996).
- Provide preoperative information in verbal and written form.
  Preparatory information of various types and in different forms appears to have positive effects on the ability of patients to cope with and recover physically from a total hip replacement. Subjects in the experimental group had significantly less postoperative intramuscular analgesia and mobilized sooner with a Zimmer frame and walking sticks. Additionally, their length of stay was, on average, 2 days shorter than the control group (Gammon, Mulholland, 1996).
- Play music of the client's choice before surgery.
  Music is a simple, inexpensive, aesthetically pleasing means of alleviating the anxiety of surgical candidates during the immediate preoperative period. When allowed to participate in decision-making regarding their care, patients can regain a partial sense of control. Preoperatively, this goal can be achieved by permitting them to choose their own music and to experience the diversionary effect of music (Evans, Rubio, 1994). One study demonstrated that subjects who listened to music while in the surgical holding area had significantly less stress and anxiety than did those who did not listen to music (Winter, Paskin, Baker, 1994).
- For female premenopausal patients, assess the date when their menstrual cycle is most likely to occur and schedule surgery on alternate dates if possible.
  Menstruation at the time of surgery increases the likelihood of vomiting to four times greater than normal (Haynes, Bailey, 1996).

• = **Independent;** ▲ = **Collaborative**

- Do not offer fluids in the immediate postoperative period.

  Early ingestion of fluids in the postoperative period also contributes to emesis. Oral intake before discharge from an ambulatory surgery unit increased the incidence of vomiting to four times that of the control group and prolonged the hospital stay (Haynes, Bailey, 1996).

- ▲ In clients with postoperative nausea and vomiting (PONV), consider multiple antiemetic medications (double or triple combination antiemetic therapy acting at different neuroreceptor sites), less emetogenic anesthesia techniques, and adequate intravenous hydration.

  Combination antiemetic therapy and the other mentioned measures improve efficacy for PONV prevention and treatment (Kovac, 2000).

- Clients should be provided with a complete, balanced therapeutic diet after the immediate postoperative period (24 to 48 hours).

  Suggestive evidence exists that improvement in nutritional status can improve outcomes of wound healing (Thomas, 1996). Good nutrition is important for effective wound healing (Casey, 1998).

- The client should have a nutritious diet with adequate protein intake that restores normal weight for the client.

  In a study that looked at restoration of weight loss and healing of the "nonhealing wound," the rate of wound healing was most prominent after 50% of weight loss had been restored. This finding reflects the key relationship between restoring body weight, body protein stores, and wound healing (Demling, De Santi, 1998).

- Use careful aseptic technique when caring for wounds.

  A significant impediment to wound healing is infection. Treatment of chronic wounds should be directed at the main etiologic factors responsible for the wound. Moreover, factors that may impede healing must be identified and, if possible, for healing to occur (Stadelmann, Digenis, Tobin, 1998).

- ▲ Suggest the use of semipermeable dressing and suction drainage for selected orthopedic clients.

  A new technique in surgical dressing is a combination of a semipermeable dressing and suction drainage. This dressing has been used successfully in 20 orthopedic patients without any wound complication and with satisfactory comfort to the patient. This form of postoperative wound management appears to retain the nursing and hygiene advantages of suction drainage while avoiding the patient discomfort and the possibilities of wound infection associated with deep internal drainage (Strover, Thorpe, 1997).

- ▲ Consider the use of alternative therapy with physician's order, such as aloe vera to promote wound healing.

  In one study, one side of a wound was treated with a polyethylene oxide gel dressing saturated with stabilized aloe vera. Overall, wound healing was approximately 72 hours faster at the aloe site. This acceleration in wound healing is important to reduce bacterial contamination, subsequent keloid formation, and/or pigmentary changes. The exact mechanism of acceleration of wound healing by aloe vera is unknown (Fulton, 1990). In another study the aloe vera gel-treated lesion healed faster than the petroleum jelly gauze-treated area. The average time of healing in the aloe gel area was 11.89 days, compared with 18.19 days for the petroleum jelly gauze-treated wound. This study showed the effectiveness of aloe vera gel on a partial thickness burn wound, and it might be beneficial to do further trials on burn wounds (Visuthikosol et al, 1995).

• = Independent; ▲ = Collaborative

▲ Clients should be allowed to shower after surgery to maintain cleanliness if not contraindicated because of presence of pacemaker wires, etc.

There was no difference in wound healing and no manifest infection in clients undergoing open hernia repair who were allowed to shower and those who were not (Riederer, Inderbitzi, 1997).

• Provide supportive telephone calls from nurses to clients as a means of decreasing anxiety and providing psychosocial support that is necessary for recovery from surgery.

Telephone calls are an effective method of supportive psychosocial care for individuals who may not be able to access this care because of geographic isolation, physical limitations, or discomfort with face-to-face interventions (Gotay, Bottomley, 1998).

• Assess and treat for depression and anxiety in clients complaining of continuing fatigue after surgery.

Fatigue at 30 days after coronary bypass surgery correlated with concurrent levels of depression and anxiety (Pick et al, 1994).

• Consider use of foot massage and orange-scented oils.

This study indicated that postsurgery heart clients who received this treatment experienced less anxiety and tension than a control group massaged with plain oil (Death and Dying, 2001).

• Consider use of alternative therapies: hypnosis, aromatherapy, music, guided imagery, and massage.

Alternative therapies offer high-touch balance when integrated with high-tech surgical treatments and may decrease anxiety (Norred, 2000).

• Encourage client to use prayer as a form of spiritual coping if this is comfortable for him or her.

Results of this study show that most patients pray about their postoperative problems and that private prayer appears to significantly decrease depression and general distress 1 year post-CABG (Ai et al, 1998).

• See care plans for **Anxiety, Acute Pain, Fatigue,** and **Impaired physical Mobility.**

Geriatric

▲ Carefully assess fluid, electrolyte, and glomerular filtration rate (GFR) status of elderly clients before surgery. Provide fluid and electrolyte replacement per physician's order.

In many cases acute renal failure (ARF) can be prevented in older patients (e.g., by correcting any sodium deficit and hypovolemia before a surgical procedure and by considering the true GFR of a given patient before prescribing a potentially nephrotoxic drug). Recovery is delayed in older patients and in those whose oliguric period is prolonged. The high cost of therapy in ARF justifies the use of all current preventive measures in patients at risk. In elderly patients, this incidence is five times higher than that of younger patients (Kleinknecht, Pallot, 1998).

• Carefully evaluate the client's temperature. Know what is normal and abnormal for each client. Check baseline temperature and monitor trends.

Even a normal temperature (98.6° F, 37° C) can indicate an infection because many older adults have subnormal body temperatures (averaging 96.8° F, 36° C) (Faherty, 1994).

▲ To maximize the recovery of walking ability potential for elderly hip fracture patients, a multidisciplinary approach using skilled medical, nursing, and paramedical care appears to be optimal.

• **= Independent;** ▲ **= Collaborative**

In today's cost-cutting environment, caution must be used to prevent short-term cost-saving measures from compromising long-term outcome (Lyons, 1997).

- Offer spiritual support.

Religion and spirituality can help older adults to maintain and recover both physical and mental health (Mackenzie et al, 2000).

Client/Family Teaching

▲ To decrease postoperative nausea and vomiting, the client should be instructed to fast before surgery, the time frame to be determined by the physician.

The patient with a full stomach is also prone to postoperative emesis. Eating and digestion trigger the release of gut hormones that may sensitize the area postrema in the brain stem and facilitate emesis. Gastric emptying is variable, and fasting for 6 to 8 hours before surgery does not guarantee an empty stomach (Haynes, Bailey, 1996).

WEB SITES FOR EDUCATION

⚜ᴹᴱᴿᴸᴵᴺ See the MERLIN web site for World Wide Web resources for client education.

REFERENCES Ai AL et al: The role of private prayer in psychological recovery among midlife and aged patients following cardiac surgery, *Gerontologist* 38(5):591-601, 1998.

Casey G: The importance of nutrition in wound healing, *Nurs Stand* 13(3):51, 1998.

Death and Dying: *Alternative medical forum,* retrieved from the World Wide Web March 27, 2001. Web site: www.death-dying.com/alternative/aroma01.html

Demling R, De Santi L: Closure of the "non-healing wound" corresponds with correction of weight loss using the anabolic agent oxandrolone, *Ostomy Wound Manage* 44(10):58, 1998.

Evans MM, Rubio PAL: Music: a diversionary therapy, *Todays OR Nurse* 16(4):17, 1994.

Faherty B: Myths and facts about older adults, *Nursing 1994* 24(4):75, 1994.

Fulton Jr JE: The stimulation of post dermabrasion wound healing with stabilized aloe vera gel-polyethylene oxide dressing, *J Dermatol Surg Oncol* 16(5):460, 1990.

Gammon J, Mulholland CW: Effect of preparatory information prior to elective total hip replacement on post-operative physical coping outcomes, *Int J Nurs Stud* 33(6):589, 1996.

Gotay CC, Bottomley A: Providing psycho-social support by telephone: what is its potential in cancer patients? *Eur J Cancer Care* 7(4):225, 1998.

Haynes G, Bailey M: Charleston, South Carolina: postoperative nausea and vomiting—review and clinical approaches, *South Med J* 1996, retrieved from the World Wide Web Feb 12, 1999. Web site: www.sma.org/smj/96oct2.htm

Kingsley A: Assessment allows action on risk factors, infection control and surgical wounds, *Prof Nurse* 7(10):644, 1992.

Kleinknecht D, Pallot JL: Epidemiology and prognosis of acute renal insufficiency in 1997, *Nephrologie* 19(2):49, 1998.

Kovac AL: Prevention and treatment of postoperative nausea and vomiting, *Drugs* 59(2):213-243, 2000.

Lyons AR: Clinical outcomes and treatment of hip fractures, *Am J Med* 18:103(2A), 51S (discussion 63S), 1997

Mackenzie ER et al: Spiritual support and psychological well-being: older adults' perceptions of the religion and health connection, *Altern Ther Health Med* 6(6):37-45, 2000.

Martin D: Pre-operative visits to reduce patient anxiety: a study, *Nurs Stand* 10(23):33, 1996.

Morales C, Andrews J: Postoperative wound care: nursing assessment and management, *Semin Perioper Nurs* 2(4):231, 1993.

Norred CL: Minimizing preoperative anxiety with alternative caring-healing therapies, *AORN J* 72(5):838-840, 842-843, 2000.

Pick B et al: Post-operative fatigue following coronary artery bypass surgery: relationship to emotional state and to the catecholamine response to surgery, *J Psychosom Res* 38(6):599, 1994.

Riederer SR, Inderbitzi R: [Does a shower put postoperative wound healing at risk]? *Chirurg* 68(7):715 (discussion 717), 1997.

Schemer N: The best defense may be to have foot surgery now, *Am Diabetes Assoc* 1996, retrieved from the World Wide Web Feb 12, 1999. Web site: www.diabetes.org/diabetesforecast/96nov/foot.htm

• = **Independent;** ▲ = **Collaborative**

Stadelmann WK, Digenis AG, Tobin GR: Impediments to wound healing, *Am J Surg* 176(2A suppl):39S, 1998.

Strover AE, Thorpe R: Suction dressings: a new surgical dressing technique, *J R Coll Surg* 42(2):119, 1997.

Thomas DR: Nutritional factors affecting wound healing, *Ostomy Wound Manage* 42(5):40-42, 44-46, 48-49, 1996.

Visuthikosol V et al: Effect of aloe vera gel to healing of burn wound a clinical and histologic study, *J Med Assoc* 78(8):403, 1995.

Winter MJ, Paskin S, Baker T: Music reduces stress and anxiety of patients in the surgical holding area, *J Post Anesth Nurs* 9(6):340, 1994.

Impaired Swallowing

Roslyn Fine and Betty J. Ackley

 Definition Abnormal functioning of the swallowing mechanism associated with deficits in oral, pharyngeal, or esophageal structure or function

Defining Characteristics

- *Oral phase impairment:* Lack of tongue action to form bolus; weak suck resulting in inefficient nippling; incomplete lip closure; food pushed out of mouth; slow bolus formation; food falls from mouth; premature entry of bolus; nasal reflux; inability to clear oral cavity; long meals with little consumption; coughing, choking, or gagging before a swallow; abnormality in oral phase of swallow study; piecemeal deglutition; lack of chewing; pooling in lateral sulci; sialorrhea or drooling
- *Pharyngeal phase impairment:* Altered head positions; inadequate laryngeal elevation; food refusal; unexplained fevers; delayed swallow; recurrent pulmonary infections; gurgly voice quality; nasal reflux; choking, coughing, or gagging; multiple swallows; abnormality in pharyngeal phase by swallowing study
- *Esophageal phase impairment:* Heartburn or epigastric pain; acidic smelling breath; unexplained irritability surrounding mealtime; vomitous on pillow; repetitive swallowing or ruminating; regurgitation of gastric contents or set burps; bruxism; nighttime coughing or awakening; observed evidence of difficulty in swallowing (e.g., stasis of food in oral cavity, coughing, or choking); hyperextension of head, arching during or after meals; abnormality in esophageal phase by swallow study; odynophagia; food refusal or volume limiting; complaints of "something stuck"; hematemesis; vomiting

Related Factors (r/t)

Congenital deficits; upper airway anomalies; failure to thrive; protein energy malnutrition; conditions with significant hypotonia; respiratory disorders; history of tube feeding; behavioral feeding problems; self-injurious behavior; neuromuscular impairment (e.g., decreased or absent gag reflex, decreased strength or excursion of muscles involved in mastication, perceptual impairment, or facial paralysis); mechanical obstruction (e.g., edema, tracheotomy tube, or tumor); congenital heart disease; cranial nerve involvement; neurological problems; upper airway anomalies; laryngeal abnormalities; achalasia; gastroesophageal reflux disease; acquired anatomic defects; cerebral palsy; internal or external traumas; tracheal, laryngeal, esophageal defects; traumatic head injury; developmental delay; nasal or nasopharyngeal cavity defects; oral cavity or oropharynx abnormalities; premature infants

• = Independent; ▲ = Collaborative

NOC   ## Outcomes (Nursing Outcomes Classification)

Suggested NOC Labels

Swallowing Status; Swallowing Status: Esophageal Phase, Oral Phase, Pharyngeal Phase

Example NOC Outcome

Improves **Swallowing Status** as evidenced by the following indicators: Delivery of bolus to hypopharynx is commensurate with swallow reflex/Ability to clear oral cavity/Number of swallows appropriate for bolus size, texture/Voice quality/Choking, coughing, gagging not present/Normal swallow effort (Rate each indicator of **Swallowing Status:** 1 = extremely compromised, 2 = substantially compromised, 3 = moderately compromised, 4 = mildly compromised, 5 = not compromised [see Section I])

Client Outcomes

- Demonstrates effective swallowing without choking or coughing
- Remains free from aspiration (e.g., lungs clear, temperature within normal range)

NIC   ## Interventions (Nursing Interventions Classification)

Suggested NIC Labels

Aspiration Precautions; Swallowing Therapy

Example NIC Interventions—Swallowing Therapy

- Assist patient to sit in an erect position (as close to 90 degrees as possible) for feeding/exercise
- Instruct patient not to talk during eating, if appropriate

Nursing Interventions and Rationales

- Determine client's readiness to eat. Client needs to be alert, able to follow instructions, hold head erect, and able to move tongue in mouth.
  If one of these factors is missing, it may be advisable to withhold oral feeding and use enteral feeding for nourishment (McHale et al, 1998). Cognitive deficits can result in aspiration even if able to swallow adequately (Poertner, Coleman, 1998).
- If new onset of swallowing impairment, ensure that client receives a diagnostic workup.
  There are multiple causes of swallowing impairment, some of which are treatable (Schechter, 1998).
- Assess ability to swallow by positioning examiner's thumb and index finger on client's laryngeal protuberance. Ask client to swallow; feel larynx elevate. Ask client to cough; test for a gag reflex on both sides of posterior pharyngeal wall (lingual surface) with a tongue blade. Do not rely on presence of gag reflex to determine when to feed.
  Normally the time taken for the bolus to move from the point at which the reflex is triggered to the esophageal entry (pharyngeal transit time) is ≤1 second (Logemann, 1983). Cerebrovascular accident (CVA) clients with prolonged pharyngeal transit times (prolonged swallowing) have a greatly increased chance of developing aspiration pneumonia (Johnson, McKenzie, Sievers, 1993). Clients can aspirate even if they have an intact gag reflex (Baker, 1993; Lugger, 1994).

• = **Independent;** ▲ = **Collaborative**

- Observe for signs associated with swallowing problems (e.g., coughing, choking, spitting of food, drooling, difficulty handling oral secretions, double swallowing or major delay in swallowing, watering eyes, nasal discharge, wet or gurgly voice, decreased ability to move tongue and lips, decreased mastication of food, decreased ability to move food to the back of the pharynx, slow or scanning speech).
  These are all signs of swallowing impairment (Baker, 1993; Lugger, 1994).
- ▲ If client has impaired swallowing, refer to a speech pathologist for bedside evaluation as soon as possible. Ensure that client is seen by a speech pathologist within 72 hours after admission if client has had a CVA.
  Speech pathologists specialize in impaired swallowing. Early referral of CVA clients to a speech pathologist, along with early initiation of nutritional support, results in decreased length of hospital stay, shortened recovery time, and reduced overall health costs (Scott, 1998). Research demonstrates that a program of diagnosis and treatment of dysphagia in acute stroke management decreases the incidence of pneumonia (AHCPR, 1999).
- ▲ For impaired swallowing, use a dysphagia team composed of a rehabilitation nurse, speech pathologist, dietitian, physician, and radiologist who work together.
  The dysphagia team can help the client learn to swallow safely and maintain a good nutritional status (Poertner, Coleman, 1998).
- ▲ If client has impaired swallowing, do not feed until an appropriate diagnostic workup is completed. Ensure proper nutrition by consulting with physician for enteral feedings, preferably a PEG tube in most cases.
  Feeding a client who cannot adequately swallow results in aspiration and possibly death. Enteral feedings via PEG tube are generally preferable to nasogastric tube feedings because studies have demonstrated that there is increased nutritional status and possibly improved survival rates (Bath, Bath, Smithard, 2000).
- If client has an intact swallowing reflex, attempt to feed. Observe the following feeding guidelines:
  - Position client upright at a 90-degree angle with the head flexed forward at a 45-degree angle (Galvan, 2001).
    This position forces the trachea to close and esophagus to open, which makes swallowing easier and reduces the risk of aspiration.
  - Ensure client is awake, alert, and able to follow sequenced directions before attempting to feed.
    As the client becomes less alert the swallowing response decreases, which increases the risk of aspiration.
  - Begin by feeding client one-third teaspoon of applesauce. Provide sufficient time to masticate and swallow.
  - Place food on unaffected side of tongue.
  - During feeding, give client specific directions (e.g., "Open your mouth, chew the food completely, and when you are ready, tuck your chin to your chest and swallow").
  - ▲ Watch for uncoordinated chewing or swallowing; coughing immediately after eating or delayed coughing, which may indicate silent aspiration; pocketing of food; wet-sounding voice; sneezing when eating; delay of more than 1 second in swallowing; or a change in respiratory patterns. If any of these signs are present, put on gloves, remove all food from oral cavity, stop feedings, and consult with a speech and language pathologist and a dysphagia team.

• = **Independent;** ▲ = **Collaborative**

These are signs of impaired swallowing and possible aspiration (Baker, 1993; Galvan, 2001).

▲ If client tolerates single-textured foods such as pudding, hot cereal, or strained baby food, advance to a soft diet with guidance from the dysphagia team. Avoid foods such as hamburgers, corn, and pastas that are difficult to chew. Also avoid sticky foods such as peanut butter and white bread.
The dysphagia team should determine the appropriate diet for the client on the basis of progression in swallowing and ensuring that the client is nourished and hydrated.

• Avoid providing liquids until client is able to swallow effectively. Add a thickening agent to liquids to obtain a soft consistency that is similar to nectar, honey, or pudding, depending on degree of swallowing problems.
Liquids can be easily aspirated; thickened liquids form a cohesive bolus that the client can swallow with increased efficiency (Langmore, Miller, 1994; Poertner, Coleman, 1998).

• Preferably use prepackaged thickened liquids, or use a viscosometer to ensure appropriate thickness.
Often staff members overthicken liquids, resulting in decreased palatability with decreased intake. Using prepackaged thickened liquids can increase intake, which increases hydration and nutrition (Goulding, Bakheit, 2000; Boczko, 2000).

▲ Work with client on swallowing exercises prescribed by dysphagia team (e.g., touching palate with tongue, stimulating tonsillar arch and soft palate with a cold metal examination mirror [thermal stimulation], labial/lingual range of motion exercises).
Swallowing exercises can improve the client's ability to swallow (Langmore, Miller, 1994). Exercises need to be done at intervals necessitating nursing involvement (Poertner, Coleman, 1998).

▲ For many adult clients, avoid using straws if recommended by speech pathologist.
Use of straws can increase the risk of aspiration because straws can result in spilling of a bolus of fluid in the oral cavity as well as decrease control of posterior transit of fluid to the pharynx (Travers, 1999).

• Provide meals in a quiet environment away from excessive stimuli such as a community dining room.
A noisy environment can be an aversive stimulus and can decrease effective mastication and swallowing. Talking and laughing while eating increases the risk of aspiration (Galvan, 2001).

• Ensure that there is adequate time for client to eat.
Clients with swallowing impairments often take two to four times longer than others to eat, if being fed. Often, food is offered rapidly to speed up the task, and this can increase the chance of aspiration (Poertner, Coleman, 1998).

• Have suction equipment available during feeding. If choking occurs and suctioning is necessary, discontinue oral feeding until client is safely assessed with a videofluoroscopic swallow study and fiberoptic endoscopic evaluation of swallowing (FEES), whichever client can safely tolerate.
Suctioning may be necessary if the client is choking on food and could aspirate.

• Check oral cavity for proper emptying after client swallows and after client finishes meal. Provide oral care at end of meal. It may be necessary to manually remove food from client's mouth. If this is the case, use gloves and keep client's teeth apart with a padded tongue blade.

• = Independent; ▲ = Collaborative

Food may become pocketed in the affected side and cause stomatitis, tooth decay, and possible later aspiration.

- Praise client for successfully following directions and swallowing appropriately. *Praise reinforces behavior and sets up a positive atmosphere in which learning takes place.*
- Keep client in an upright position for 30 to 45 minutes after a meal. *An upright position ensures that food stays in the stomach until it has emptied and decreases the chance of aspiration following meals (Galvan, 2001).*
- ▲ Watch for signs of aspiration and pneumonia. Auscultate lung sounds after feeding. Note new crackles or wheezing, and note elevated temperature. Notify physician as needed. *The presence of new crackles or wheezing, an elevated temperature or white blood cell count, and a change in sputum could indicate aspiration of food (Murray, Brzozowski, 1998). It could also indicate the presence of pneumonia (Galvan, 2001). Clients with dysphagia are at serious risk for aspiration pneumonia (Langmore, 1994).*
- Watch for signs of malnutrition and dehydration. Keep a record of food intake. *A food intake record will allow the nurse, speech and language pathologist, and dietician to determine the adequacy of nutritional intake (Beadle, Townsend, Palmer, 1995). Malnutrition is common in dysphagic clients (Galvan, 2001). Clients with dysphagia are at serious risk for malnutrition and dehydration, which can lead to aspiration pneumonia resulting from depressed immune function and weakness, lethargy, and decreased cough (Langmore, 1999).*
- Weigh client weekly to help evaluate nutritional status.
- ▲ Evaluate nutritional status daily. If not adequately nourished, work with dysphagia team to determine whether client needs to avoid oral intake (NPO) with therapeutic feeding only or needs enteral feedings until client can swallow adequately. *Enteral feedings can maintain nutrition if client is unable to swallow adequate amounts of food (Grant, Rivera, 1995).*
- ▲ If client has a tracheotomy, ask for a diagnostic workup before attempting to feed, and ensure all staff members know appropriate feeding technique. *Aspiration is common in clients with tracheotomies, and care must be used in feeding (Murray, Brzozowski, 1998). See care plan for **Risk for Aspiration.***

Pediatric

- ▲ Refer to physician children with difficult swallowing and symptoms such as difficulty manipulating food, delayed swallow response, and pocketing a bolus of food. *Research has indicated that structural deficits should be corrected by surgery (e.g., pyloric stenosis, neurological disorders that involve cranial nerve pathways, and structures resulting in swallowing changes such as brain injury and cerebral palsy [Rosenthal, Sheppard, Lotze, 1995]). Respiratory and gastrointestinal system disorders (GERD) and esophagitis can affect swallowing and nutrition. These systemic disorders are diagnosed by a physician and treated with medications.*
- When feeding and infant or child, place the infant/child in a 90-degree position with head slightly flexed. Change consistency of diet as needed, and use a curly straw for young children to facilitate a chin tuck, which helps improve swallowing ability (Arvedson, Brodsky, 1993).
- Give oral motor stimulation that increases oral-sensory awareness by waking the mouth with exercises that focus on temperature, taste, and texture.

• = Independent; ▲ = Collaborative

Many of these infants require supplemental tube feedings as well as special nipples or bottles to boost oral intake.

- For infants with poor sucking and swallowing:
  - ▪ Support the cheeks and jaw to increase sucking skills. Pace or rhythmically move the bottle, which encourages better coordination of suck-swallow-breath synchrony.
  - ▲ Work with dietitian. Some infants may need a high-calorie formula so that food volume may be decreased (which requires infant to expend less energy) while nutritional requirements are met (Klein, Tracey, 1994). Some infants may also need to have their tongue brushed, which promotes tongue stimulation (tongue tip and tongue lateralization), lip seal, and lip pursing.
  - ▪ Watch for indicators of aspiration: coughing, a change in web vocal quality while feeding, perspiration and color changes during feeding, sneezing, and increased heart rate and breathing.
  - ▪ Watch for warning signs of reflux: sour-smelling breath after eating, sneezing, lack of interest in feeding, crying and fussing extraordinarily when feeding, pained expressions when feeding, and excessive chewing and swallowing after eating (see rationale that follows) (Johnson, McGonigel, Kaufman, 1991).

  Many premature and medically fragile children are surviving as a result of technological advances and sustaining growth and respiratory deficits from an underlying dysphagia diagnosis. They present with limited food intake at a time when extra calories are essential for faster growth and lung repair. Some infants may need to work harder to breathe than others and as a result develop a decreased tolerance for food intake. They also demonstrate inconsistent arousal and poor/uncoordinated suck-swallow-breath synchrony. Many of these infants require supplemental tube feedings, as well as special nipples or bottles to boost oral intake.

Geriatric

- ▲ Evaluate medications client is presently taking, especially if elderly. Consult with the pharmacist for assistance in monitoring for incorrect doses and drug interactions that could result in dysphagia.

  Dysphagia is more prevalent in the elderly than in younger persons because of the coexistence of a variety of neurological, neuromuscular, or oncological conditions (Kosta, Mitchell, 1998). Most elderly clients take numerous medications, which when taken individually can slow motor function, cause anxiety and depression, and reduce salivary flow. When taken together, these medications can interact, resulting in impaired swallowing function. Drugs that reduce muscle tone for swallowing and can cause reflux include calcium channel blockers and nitrates. Drugs that can reduce salivary flow include antidepressants, antiparkinsonism drugs, antihistamines, antispasmodics, antipsychotic agents or major tranquilizers, antiemetics, antihypertensives, and drugs for treating diarrhea and anxiety (Sonies, 1992; Sliwa, Lis, 1993; Schechter, 1998).

Client/Family Teaching

- ▲ Teach client and family exercises prescribed by dysphagia team.
- Teach client a step-by-step method of swallowing effectively.
- Educate client, family, and all caregivers about rationales for food consistency and choices.

  It is common for family members to disregard necessary dietary restrictions and give client inappropriate foods that predispose to aspiration (Poertner, Coleman, 1998).

- Teach family how to monitor client to prevent aspiration during eating.

• = Independent; ▲ = Collaborative

REFERENCES   AHCPR: *Diagnosis and treatment of swallowing disorders (dysphagia) in acute-care stroke patients,* Evidence Report/Technology Assessment No. 8, AHCPR Publication No. 99-E024, 1999.

Arvedson JC, Brodsky L: *Pediatric swallowing and feeding assessment and management,* San Diego, 1993, Singular.

Baker DM: Assessment and management of impairments in swallowing, *Nurs Clin North Am* 28:793, 1993.

Bath PM, Bath FJ, Smithard EG: Interventions for dysphagia in acute stroke, *Cochrane Data Base Syst Rev* (2):CD000323, DJ9, 2000.

Beadle L, Townsend S, Palmer D: The management of dysphagia in stroke, *Nurs Stand* 9:37, 1995.

Boczko T: Increasing liquid consumption in patients with dysphagia, *Advance Speech-Language Pathologists Audiologists* 10(45), 2000.

Galvan TJ: Dysphagia: going down and staying down, *Am J Nurs* 101(1):37-42, 2001.

Goulding R, Bakheit A: Evaluation of the benefits of monitoring fluid thickness in the dietary management of dysphagic stroke patients, *Clin Rehabil* 14:119-124, 2000.

Grant MM, Rivera LM: Anorexia, cachexia, and dysphagia: the symptom experience, *Semin Oncol Nurs* 11:266, 1995.

Johnson BH, McGonigel MJ, Kaufman RK: *Guidelines and recommended practices for the individualized family service plan,* ed 2, Bethesda, Md, 1991, Association for the Care of Children's Health.

Johnson ER, McKenzie SW, Sievers A: Aspiration pneumonia in stroke, *Arch Phys Med Rehabil* 74:973, 1993.

Klein MD, Tracey A: *Feeding and nutrition for the child with special needs,* Tuscon, Ariz, 1994, Therapy Skill Builders.

Kosta JC, Mitchell CA: Current procedures for diagnosing dysphagia in elderly clients, *Geriatr Nurs* 19(4):195, 1998.

Langmore SE, Miller RM: Behavioral treatment for adults with oropharyngeal dysphagia, *Arch Phys Med Rehab* 75:1154, 1994.

Langmore SE: Risk factors for aspiration pneumonia, *Nutr Clin Pract* 14(5):S41-S46, 1999.

Logemann JA: *Evaluation and treatment of swallowing disorders,* San Diego, 1983, College Hill.

Lugger KE: Dysphagia in the elderly stroke patient, *J Neurosci Nurs* 26:78, 1994.

McHale JM et al: Expert nursing knowledge in the care of the patients at risk of impaired swallowing *Image J Nurs Sch* 30(2):237, 1998.

Murray KA, Brzozowski LA: Swallowing in patients with tracheotomies, *AACN Clin Issues* 9(3):416, 1998.

Poertner LC, Coleman RF: Swallowing therapy in adults, *Otolaryngol Clin North Am* 31(3):561, 1998.

Rosenthal WR, Sheppard JJ, Lotze M: *Dysphagia and the child with developmental disabilities,* San Diego, 1995, Singular.

Schechter GL: Systemic causes of dysphagia in adults, *Otolaryngol Clin North Am* 31(3):525-534, 1998.

Scott A: Advances for speech pathologists and audiologists, *Swallowing Stroke* pp 15-17, Oct 26, 1998.

Sliwa JA, Lis S: Drug-induced dysphagia, *Arch Phys Med Rehab* 74:445, 1993.

Sonies BC: Oropharyngeal dysphagia in the elderly. In Baum BJ, editor: *Clinics in geriatric medicine,* Philadelphia, 1992, WB Saunders.

Travers P: Poststroke dysphagia: implications for nurses, *Rehabil Nurs* 24(2):69-73, 1999.

Effective Therapeutic regimen management

Margaret Lunney

NANDA   **Definition** Pattern of regulating and integrating into daily living a program for treatment of illness and its sequelae that is satisfactory for meeting specific health goals

• = **Independent;** ▲ = **Collaborative**

Defining Characteristics

Appropriate choices of daily activities for meeting the goals of a treatment or prevention program; illness symptoms within a normal range of expectation; verbalizes desire to manage the treatment of illness and prevention of sequelae; verbalizes intent to reduce risk factors for progression of illness and sequelae

Related Factors (r/t)

To be developed

NOC   Outcomes (Nursing Outcomes Classification)

Suggested NOC Labels

Knowledge: Treatment Regimen; Participation: Health Care Decisions; Risk Control; Symptom Control

> **Example NOC Outcome**
>
> Demonstrates **Knowledge: Treatment Regimen** as evidenced by: Description of prescribed medication, activity, exercise, and disease process (Rate each indicator of **Knowledge: Treatment Regimen:** 1 = none, 2 = limited, 3 = moderate, 4 = substantial, 5 = extensive [see Section I])

Client Outcomes

- Acknowledges appropriateness of choices for meeting the goals of treatment or prevention programs
- Agrees to continue making appropriate choices
- Verbalizes intent to contact health provider(s) for additional information, support, or resources as needed

NIC   Interventions (Nursing Interventions Classification)

Suggested NIC Labels

Anticipatory Guidance; Health Education; Health Screening; Health System Guidance; Learning Facilitation; Learning Readiness Enhancement; Risk Identification; Self-Modification Assistance

> **Example NIC Interventions—Learning Facilitation**
> - Relate the information in a stimulating manner
> - Encourage the client's active participation

Nursing Interventions and Rationales

- Acknowledge the congruence of activities of daily living (ADLs) with health-related goals.
  Support from health provider(s) in efforts made to manage therapeutic regimens may motivate individuals to continue these efforts despite difficulties (Miller, 1999).
- Support decisions regarding methods of integrating therapeutic regimens with ADLs.
  Support from health providers for previous decisions provides evidence of continued ability to successfully manage therapeutic regimens (Miller, 1999).
- Provide information on possible illness trajectories to plan for future management.
  Knowledge and awareness of illness trajectories enables the individual to plan for future management of therapeutic regimens (Lubkin, 1998).
- Assist to resolve ambivalent feelings about illness and management of therapeutic regimen.

• = **Independent;** ▲ = **Collaborative**

Wide variations may exist in attitudes toward illness and management of the illness regimens. Ambivalence interferes with effective decision-making regarding illness care (Chinn et al, 2000).

▲ Review methods of contacting health provider(s) for changes in therapeutic regimen and/or methods of incorporating therapeutic regimens with ADLs.
Although interventions for problems with managing therapeutic regimens may not be needed at the present time, individuals should know how to obtain such interventions if needed in the future.

• Record the effectiveness of managing therapeutic regimens.
For clients who are at risk of ineffective management of therapeutic regimens, health providers may continue to assess and diagnose this phenomena unnecessarily. It saves the health care system time, effort, and money if the assessment and diagnosis of effective management is communicated to other health providers.

Multicultural

• Assess for the influence of cultural beliefs, norms, and values on the individual's perceptions of the therapeutic regimen.
What the individual considers therapeutic may be based on cultural perceptions (Leininger, 1996).

• Use a family-centered approach when working with Latino, Asian, African-American, and Native American clients.
Latinos may perceive family as a source of support, solver of problems and source of pride. Asian Americans may regard the family as the primary decision maker and influence on individual family members (D'Avanzo et al, 2001). Native American families may be extended structures that exert powerful influences over functioning (Seiderman et al, 1996).

• Discuss with the client those aspects of health and lifestyle that will remain unchanged by his or her health status.
Aspects of the client's life that are meaningful and valuable to him or her should be understood and preserved without change (Leininger, 1996).

• Validate the client's feelings regarding the ability to manage own care and the impact on current lifestyle.
Validation of feelings lets the client know that the nurse has heard and understands what was said, and it promotes the nurse-client relationship (Stuart, Laraia, 2001; Giger, Davidhizar, 1995).

Client/Family Teaching

• Teach about the disease trajectory and ways to manage disease symptoms as the trajectory changes.

WEB SITES FOR EDUCATION

MERLIN See the MERLIN web site for World Wide Web resources for client education.

REFERENCES   Chinn MH et al: Developing a conceptual framework for understanding illness and attitudes in older, African Americans with diabetes, *Diabetes Educ* 26(3):439-449, 2000.
D'Avanzo CE et al: Developing culturally informed strategies for substance-related interventions. In Naegle MA, D'Avanzo CE, editors: *Addictions and substance abuse: strategies for advanced practice nursing*, St Louis, 2001, Mosby, pp 59-104.
Giger JN, Davidhizar RE: *Transcultural nursing*, ed 2, St Louis, 1995, Mosby.

• = **Independent;** ▲ = **Collaborative**

Leininger MM: *Transcultural nursing: theories, research and practices,* ed 2, Hilliard, Ohio, 1996, McGraw-Hill.

Lubkin IM: *Chronic illness: impact and interventions,* ed 4, Boston, 1998, Jones & Bartlett.

Miller JF: *Coping with chronic illness: overcoming powerlessness,* ed 3, Philadelphia, 1999, FA Davis.

Stuart GW, Laraia MT: Therapeutic nurse-patient relationship. In Stuart GW, Laraia MT, editors: *Principles and practice of psychiatric nursing,* St Louis, 2001, Mosby, p 30.

Ineffective Therapeutic regimen management

Margaret Lunney

NANDA   **Definition**   Pattern of regulating and integrating into daily living a program for treatment of illness and the sequelae of illness that is unsatisfactory for meeting specific health goals

Defining Characteristics

Choices of daily living ineffective for meeting the goals of a treatment or prevention program; verbalizes that did not take action to reduce risk factors for progression of illness and sequelae; verbalizes desire to manage the treatment of illness and prevention of sequelae; verbalizes difficulty with regulation of one or more prescribed regimens for prevention of complications and the treatment or illness or its effects; verbalizes that did not take action to include treatment regimens in daily routines

Related Factors (r/t)

Perceived barriers; social support deficits; powerlessness; perceived susceptibility; perceived benefits; mistrust of regimen and/or health care personnel; knowledge deficit; family patterns of health care; family conflict; excessive demands made on individual or family; economic difficulties; decisional conflicts; complexity of therapeutic regimen; complexity of health care system; perceived seriousness; inadequate number and types of cues to action

NOC   **Outcomes (Nursing Outcomes Classification)**

Suggested NOC Labels

Decision Making; Knowledge: Disease Process; Knowledge: Treatment Regimen; Participation: Health Care Decisions; Symptom Severity; Treatment Behavior: Illness or Injury

Example NOC Outcome

Demonstrates **Knowledge: Treatment Regimen** as evidenced by: Description of prescribed medication, activity, exercise, and disease process (Rate each indicator of **Knowledge: Treatment Regimen:** 1 = none, 2 = limited, 3 = moderate, 4 = substantial, 5 = extensive [see Section I])

Client Outcomes

- Describes daily food and fluid intake that meets therapeutic goals
- Describes activity/exercise patterns that meet therapeutic goals
- Describes scheduling of medications to meet therapeutic goals
- Verbalizes ability to manage therapeutic regimens
- Collaborates with health providers to decide on a therapeutic regimen that is congruent with health goals and lifestyle

• = **Independent;** ▲ = **Collaborative**

NIC **Interventions (Nursing Interventions Classification)**

Suggested NIC Labels

Anticipatory Guidance; Health Education; Health Screening; Health System Guidance; Learning Facilitation; Learning Readiness Enhancement; Risk Identification; Self-Modification Assistance

---

Example NIC Interventions—Learning Facilitation
- Relate the information to in a stimulating manner
- Encourage the client's active participation

Nursing Interventions and Rationales

NOTE: This diagnosis does not have the same meaning as the diagnosis **Noncompliance.** This diagnosis is made with the client. If the client does not agree with the diagnosis, it should not be made (Lunney, 1997; Bakker, Kastermans, Dassen, 1995).

- See care plans for **Effective Therapeutic regimen management** and **Ineffective family Therapeutic regimen management.**
- Establish a collaborative partnership with the client for purposes of meeting health-related goals.
  Partnerships with health care consumers are different than traditional roles in health care. Partnerships enable the consumer to take an active role in decision-making regarding the therapeutic regimen (Courtney et al, 1996; Lunney, 1997).
- Discuss all strategies with the client in the context of the client's culture.
  Culture affects all decisions for meeting therapeutic goals (Degazon, 2000).
- Review daily actions that are not therapeutic.
  Client and nurse/provider should agree on which actions are not therapeutic as a basis for interventions.
- Identify the reasons for actions that are not therapeutic (e.g., inaccurate perceptions of risks, fatigue, pain) and discuss alternatives.
  There are many possible reasons for actions that do not meet therapeutic goals. Older women, for example, may not increase their activity levels because they have inaccurate perceptions of the related risks (Cousins, 2000). Fatigue and pain can have profound effects on ability to perform therapeutic actions (Thorne, Paterson, 2000). Perceptions may differ according to diseases (e.g., people with pulmonary diseases are more likely than others to blame themselves for their condition) (Thorne, Paterson, 2000). Substantial numbers of older adults are fatalistic about their diseases (Goodwin, Black, Satish, 1999).
- Explain the rationales for specific therapeutic regimens to meet health-related goals.
  Knowledge of scientific rationales improves client's understanding of and increases responsibility for the therapeutic regimen.
- Provide information about the therapeutic regimen in various formats (e.g., brochure, video, written instructions).
  People learn in various ways (e.g., visual, auditory). Therapeutic regimens that are prescribed by health providers are often harder to learn than providers realize. Adequate resources are needed to enhance learning (Lubkin, 1998).
- Deliberate with the client on changes that are possible to meet therapeutic goals.
  Although decisions about actions to meet therapeutic goals are made by the client, the presence of the nurses and the collaborative nature of a nurse-client relationship can help the client with decision-making.

• = **Independent;** ▲ = **Collaborative**

- Encourage critical thinking to consider strategies for changes in behavior.
  Habits that are unhealthy (e.g., overeating, smoking) are difficult to change. The impetus for change must come from the client, but the nurse can prompt the client to consider alternative strategies.
- Assess temporal orientation and relationship to management of therapeutic regimen.
  Temporal orientation differs among cultures. The client's orientation to the present or the future was shown to affect management of hypertension and may also affect other therapeutic regimens (Brown, Segal, 1996).
- Develop a contract with the client to maintain motivation for changes in behavior.
  Developing a contract between nurse and client, or helping the client to develop a contract with self, provides a concrete means of keeping track of actions to meet health-related goals (Clemen-Stone, McGuire, Eigsti, 1998).
- ▲ Review methods of contacting health provider(s) as needed for changes in therapeutic regimen.
  People with chronic illnesses need to know how to obtain interventions that are needed in the future (Lubkin, 1998).

Multicultural

- Assess for the influence of cultural beliefs, norms, and values on the client's ability to modify health behavior.
  What the client considers normal and abnormal health behavior may be based on cultural perceptions (Leininger, 1996).
- Discuss with the client those aspects of his or her health behavior/lifestyle that will remain unchanged by the therapeutic regimen.
  Aspects of the client's life that are meaningful and valuable to him or her should be understood and preserved without change (Leininger, 1996).
- Negotiate with the client regarding the aspects of health behavior that will need to be modified.
  Give and take with the client will lead to culturally congruent care (Leininger, 1996).
- Assess the role of fatalism on the client's ability to adopt the therapeutic regimen.
  Fatalistic perspectives, which involve the belief that you cannot control your own fate, may influence health behaviors in some African-American and Latino populations (Phillips, Cohen, Moses, 1999; Harmon, Castro, Coe, 1996).
- Validate the client's feelings regarding the impact of therapeutic regimen on current lifestyle.
  Validation lets the client know that the nurse has heard and understands what was said, and it promotes the nurse-client relationship (Stuart, Laraia, 2001; Giger, Davidhizar, 1995).

Client/Family Teaching

- Teach client/family about all aspects of therapeutic regimens; provide as much knowledge as client/family will accept; adjust instruction to account for what family already knows; provide information in a culturally congruent manner.
- Teach ways to adjust daily activities for inclusion of therapeutic regimens.
- ▲ Teach safety in taking medications.
- ▲ Teach client to act as self-advocate with health providers who prescribe therapeutic regimens.

• = **Independent;** ▲ = **Collaborative**

REFERENCES Bakker RH, Kastermans MC, Dassen TWN: An analysis of the nursing diagnosis ineffective management of therapeutic regimen compared to noncompliance and Orem's self-care deficit theory of nursing, *Nurs Diagn* 6:161, 1995.

Brown CM, Segal R: Ethnic differences in temporal orientation and its implications for hypertension management, *J Health Soc Behav* 37:350, 1996.

Clemen-Stone S, McGuire SL, Eigsti DG: *Comprehensive community health nursing: family aggregate and community practice,* ed 5, St Louis, 1998, Mosby.

Courtney R et al: The partnership model: working with individuals, families, and communities toward a new vision of health, *Pub Health Nurs* 13:177, 1996.

Cousins SO: "My heart can't take it": older women's beliefs about exercise benefits and risks, *J Gerontol B Psychol Sci Soc Sci* 55B(5):283-294, 2000.

Degazon C: Cultural diversity and community-oriented nursing practice. In Stanhope M, Lancaster J: *Community and public health nursing,* ed 5, St Louis, 2000, Mosby, pp 138-156.

Giger JN, Davidhizar RE: *Transcultural nursing,* ed 2, St Louis, 1995, Mosby.

Goodwin JS, Black SA, Satish S: Aging versus disease: the opinions of older Black, Hispanic, and non-Hispanic White Americans about the causes and treatment of common medical conditions, *J Am Geriatr Soc* 47(8):973-979, 1999.

Harmon MP, Castro FG, Coe K: Acculturation and cervical cancer: knowledge, beliefs, and behaviors of Hispanic women, *Women Health* 24(3):37-57, 1996.

Leininger MM: *Transcultural nursing: theories, research and practices,* ed 2, Hilliard, Ohio, 1996, McGraw-Hill.

Lubkin IM: *Chronic illness: impact and interventions,* ed 4, Boston, 1998, Jones & Bartlett.

Lunney M: Ineffective management of therapeutic regimen (individuals). In McFarland GK, McFarlane EA: *Nursing diagnosis and intervention: planning for patient care,* ed 3, St Louis, 1997, Mosby.

Phillips JM, Cohen MZ, Moses G: Breast cancer screening and African American women: fear, fatalism, and silence, *Oncol Nurs Forum* 26(3):561-557, 1999.

Stuart GW, Laraia MT: Therapeutic nurse-patient relationship. In Stuart GW, Laraia MT, editors: *Principles and practice of psychiatric nursing,* St Louis, 2001, Mosby, p 30.

Thorne SE, Paterson BL: Two decades of insider research: what we know and don't know about chronic illness experience. In Fitzpatrick JJ, Goeppinger J: *Annual review of nursing research, vol 18,* New York, 2000, Springer, pp 3-25.

Ineffective community Therapeutic regimen management

Margaret Lunney

NANDA **Definition** A pattern of regulating and integrating into community processes programs for the treatment of illness and the sequelae of illness that are unsatisfactory for meeting health-related goals

Defining Characteristics

Illness symptoms above the norm expected for the number and type of population; unexpected acceleration of illness(es); number of health care resources are insufficient for the incidence or prevalence of illness(es); deficits in advocates for aggregates; deficits in people and programs to be accountable for illness care of aggregates; deficits in community activities for secondary and tertiary prevention; unavailable health care resources for illness care

Related Factors (r/t)

To be developed

• = Independent; ▲ = Collaborative

NOC   **Outcomes (Nursing Outcomes Classification)**
Suggested NOC Labels
Decision Making; Knowledge: Disease Process; Knowledge: Treatment Regimen; Participation: Health Care Decisions; Symptom Severity; Treatment Behavior: Illness or Injury

> **Example NOC Outcome**
> Demonstrates **Knowledge: Treatment Regimen** as evidenced by: Description of prescribed medication, activity, exercise, and disease process (Rate each indicator of **Knowledge: Treatment Regimen:** 1 = none, 2 = limited, 3 = moderate, 4 = substantial, 5 = extensive [see Section I])

Community Outcomes
- Obtains for the community persons who are accountable for illness care of specific aggregates
- Remains involved in advocacy for illness care and prevention programs
- Develops health care plans for effective prevention and treatment of illnesses
- Makes resources available for illness care and prevention
- Initiates or improves strategies for prevention of the sequelae of illness

NIC   **Interventions (Nursing Interventions Classification)**
Suggested NIC Labels
Community Health Development; Environmental Management: Community; Health Policy Monitoring; Teaching: Disease Process
   NOTE: NIC interventions that were developed for use with individuals can be adapted for use with communities

> **Example NIC Interventions—Community Health Development**
> - Identify health concerns, strengths, and priorities with community partners
> - Facilitate implementation and revision of community plans

Nursing Interventions and Rationales
NOTE: Nursing interventions are conducted in collaboration with key members of the community, community/public health nurses, and members of other disciplines (Anderson, McFarlane, 2000; Bolton et al, 1998; Courtney et al, 1996; Lowenberg, 1995; Reuter, Neufeld, Harrison, 1995).
- Seek community leaders (e.g., community board members) who are willing to learn about community assessment data and diagnosis and have the potential to work in partnership with nurses and other providers in planning for positive change.
  Communities need to be involved in obtaining the services and resources they need for illness care and prevention. Community boards have been shown to reflect the preferences of community residents (Conway, Hu, Harrington, 1997). Only services that are valued and perceived as needed by community members are used effectively. Community health interventions are complex and often require multidisciplinary strategies (Bolton et al, 1998).
- Advocate for and with the community in multiple arenas (e.g., newspapers, television, legislative activities, community boards).
  The community benefits from the advocacy of nurses and other health providers whose opinions are respected (Anderson, McFarlane, 2000).

• = Independent; ▲ = Collaborative

- Provide information to public and private sources about community assessment, diagnosis, and plans of care.
  The commitment that is needed for improvements in health services can only be obtained when others have adequate information.
- Mobilize support for the community in obtaining the resources necessary for illness care and prevention.
  As with individuals and families, community social supports enable the community to achieve health-related goals (Anderson, McFarlane, 2000).
- ▲ Recruit additional health providers as needed.
  If health providers are aware of inadequate community services, they may be able to contribute the necessary services.
- Determine the cultural appropriateness of all programs.
  The cultural appropriateness of a program is an indicator of the potential success of the program (Degazon, 2000).
- Write grant proposals for funding of new programs or expansion of existing programs. (See Coley, Scheinberg, 2000, for grant writing methods.)
  Public and private sources of funds can often supply the financial bases of health care programs.
- Conduct research studies to convince others of the need for improved services or changes in policy.
  Community assessment and diagnosis may not be sufficient for change. Research findings may be needed to obtain broad support for needed changes.
- With other persons and groups, obtain changes in health policy as indicated.
  Health policies set the stage for effective health programs (Leavitt, Mason, 1998; Milio, 1996). Policy evaluation and development is a core public health function (Turnock, Handler, Miller, 1998; U.S. Public Health Service, 1993).

Multicultural

- Identify what health services and information are currently available in the community.
  This will assist with focusing efforts and promote the wise use of valuable resources. Many communities of color lack access to culturally competent health care providers, pharmacies, and grocery stores (National Institutes of Health, 1998).
- Work with members of the community to prioritize and target health goals specific to the community.
  This will increase feelings of control and sense of ownership of programs and interventions (National Institutes of Health, 1998).
- Approach community leaders and members of color with respect, warmth, and professional courtesy.
  Instances of disrespect and lack of caring have special significance for individuals of color (D'Avanzo et al, 2001).
- Establish and sustain partnerships with key individuals within communities for developing and implementing programs.
  Local leaders are excellent sources of information and will enhance the credibility of programs (National Institutes of Health, 1998).
- Use community church settings as a forum for advocacy, teaching, and program implementation.
  Church-based interventions have been very successful in communities of color (Havas et al, 1994).

- **= Independent; ▲ = Collaborative**

REFERENCES   Anderson ET, McFarlane J: *Community as partner: theory and practice in nursing,* ed. 3, Philadelphia, 2000, JB Lippincott.

Bolton LB et al: Community health collaboration models for the 21st century, *Nurs Admin Q* 22(3):6-17, 1998.

Coley SM, Scheinberg CA: *Proposal Writing,* ed 2, Thousand Oaks, Calif, 2000, Sage.

Conway T, Hu TC, Harrington T: Setting health priorities: community boards accurately reflect the preferences of the community residents, *J Commun Health* 22(1):57-68, 1997.

Courtney R et al: The partnership model: working with individuals, families, and communities toward a new vision of health, *Publ Health Nurs* 13:177-186, 1996.

D'Avanzo CE et al: Developing culturally informed strategies for substance related interventions. In Naegle MA, D'Avanzo CE, editors: *Addictions and substance abuse, strategies for advanced practice nursing,* St Louis, 2001, Mosby, pp 59-104.

Degazon C: Cultural diversity and community-oriented nursing practice. In Stanhope M, Lancaster J: *Community and public health nursing,* ed 5, St Louis, 2000, Mosby, pp 138-156.

Havas S et al: 5 a day for better health: a new research initiative, *J Am Diet Assoc* 94(1):32-36, 1994.

Leavitt JK, Mason DJ: Policy and politics: a framework for action. In Leavitt JK, Mason DJ: *Policy and politics in nursing and health care,* ed 3, Philadelphia, 1998, WB Saunders.

Lowenberg JS: Health promotion and the "ideology of choice," *Publ Health Nurs* 12:319-323, 1995.

Milio N: *Engines of empowerment: using information technology to create healthy communities and challenge public policy,* Ann Arbor, Mich, 1996, Health Administration Press.

National Institutes of Health: *Sauld para su corazon: bringing heart health to Latinos—a guide for building community programs,* DHHS Publication No. 98-3796, Washington, DC, 1998, U.S. Government Printing Office.

Reuter L, Neufeld A, Harrison MJ: Using critical feminist principles to analyze programs for low-income urban women, *Publ Health Nurs* 12:424-431, 1995.

Turnock BJ, Handler AS, Miller CA: Core function-related public health practice effectiveness, *J Public Health Manage Pract* 4(5):26-32, 1998.

U.S. Public Health Service: *The core functions project,* Washington, DC, 1993, Office of Disease Prevention and Health Promotion.

Ineffective family Therapeutic regimen management

Margaret Lunney

 Definition A pattern of regulating and integrating into family processes a program for treatment of illness and its sequelae of illness that is unsatisfactory for meeting specific health goals

Defining Characteristics

Inappropriate family activities for meeting the goals of a treatment or prevention program; acceleration of illness symptoms of a family member; lack of attention to illness and its sequelae; verbalizes difficulty with regulation/integration of one or more effects or prevention of complications; verbalizes desire to manage the treatment of illness and prevention of the sequelae; verbalizes that the family did not take action to reduce risk factors for progression of illness and sequelae

• = Independent; ▲ = Collaborative

Related Factors (r/t)

Complexity of health care system; complexity of therapeutic regimen; decisional conflicts; economic difficulties; excessive demands made on individual or family; family conflict

NOC Outcomes (Nursing Outcomes Classification)

Suggested NOC Labels

Health Orientation; Health-Promoting Behavior; Health-Seeking Behavior; Knowledge: Treatment Regimen; Participation: Health Care Decisions; Treatment Behavior: Illness or Injury

> **Example NOC Outcome**
> Demonstrates **Knowledge: Treatment Regimen** as evidenced by: Description of prescribed medication, activity, exercise, and disease process (Rate each indicator of **Knowledge: Treatment Regimen:** 1 = none, 2 = limited, 3 = moderate, 4 = substantial, 5 = extensive [see Section I])

Client Outcomes

- Make adjustments in usual activities (e.g., diet, activity, stress management to incorporate the therapeutic regimens of its members)
- Reduce illness symptoms of family members
- Desire to manage therapeutic regimens of its members
- Describe a decrease in the difficulties of managing therapeutic regimens
- Describe actions to reduce risk factors

NIC Interventions (Nursing Interventions Classification)

Suggested NIC Labels

Family Involvement Promotion; Family Mobilization; Family Process Maintenance; Teaching: Disease Process

> **Example NIC Interventions—Family Involvement Promotion**
> - Identify and respect family's coping mechanisms
> - Provide information to family members about client in accordance with client preference

Nursing Interventions and Rationales

- Establish open and trusting relationship with the family.
  If trust is established with family members, they are more likely to openly share the real difficulties of integrating therapeutic regimens with family processes (Clemen-Stone, McGuire, Eigsti, 1998).
- Ensure that all strategies for working with the family are congruent with the culture of the family.
  Varying assessments, diagnoses, and interventions are indicated depending on the culture of the family (Clemen-Stone, McGuire, Eigsti, 1998; Degazon, 2000).
- Support religious beliefs and the comfort role of religion.
  Studies have shown that there is a strong relationship between religion and subjective health and that subjective health is predictive of health outcomes. There seems to be a stronger relationship between religion and subjective health for blacks than whites (Musick, 1996).

• = Independent; ▲ = Collaborative

- Review with family members the congruence and incongruence of family behaviors and health-related goals.
  To attain the motivation that is needed for changes in health habits, family members should understand the relationship of daily habits to health-related goals (Miller, 1999). Family goals are stable and take precedence over health-related goals (Stetz, Lewis, Houck, 1994).
- Help family members make decisions regarding ways to integrate therapeutic regimens with daily living. Provide advice or suggestions as solicited and accepted by family.
  Decisions made by the family rather than by health providers or others guide everyday actions (Clemen-Stone, McGuire, Eigsti, 1998). The advice of others, including nurses, will not be followed unless it is valued and respected by the family.
- Demonstrate respect and trust in family decisions.
  People make decisions that they believe are appropriate for them. Family members who are respected and trusted by health providers are more likely to collaborate effectively with them.
- Acknowledge the challenge of integrating therapeutic regimens with family behaviors.
  Therapeutic regimens require modifications of daily activities that have already been established based on family values and beliefs. Acknowledging the difficulty of changing family habits supports families through the process (Clemen-Stone, McGuire, Eigsti, 1998).
- Review symptoms of specific illness(es) and work with the family toward development of greater awareness of symptoms.
  Knowledge and awareness of symptoms improves the ability of family members to adjust behaviors to prevent and manage symptoms (Lubkin, 1998).
- Provide sufficient knowledge to support family decisions regarding therapeutic regimens.
  Knowledge deficits are obstacles to effective management of therapeutic regimens (Fujita, Duncan, 1994).
- Selectively support family decisions to adjust therapeutic regimens as indicated.
  Sometimes families do not have access to health providers and should make independent decisions because of side effects or adverse effects of therapeutic regimens. Family members need to make informed decisions that are in their best interests (Lubkin, 1998). Providing support for appropriate decisions improves the ability of the family to make such decisions.
- Advocate for the family in negotiating therapeutic regimens with health providers.
  Illness regimens generally are neither arbitrary nor absolute; therefore modifications can be discussed as needed to fit with family lifestyle (Lubkin, 1998).
- Help the family to mobilize social supports.
  Increased social support helps families to meet health-related goals (Pender, 1996).
- Help family members to modify perceptions as indicated.
  Individual perceptions of seriousness, susceptibility, and threat of illness may be distorted or inaccurate and, perhaps, can be modified with new information (Pender, 1996).
- Use one or more family theories to describe, explain, or predict family dynamics (e.g., Bowen, Satir, Minuchin).
  Family systems are complex and may not be understood by the nurse without adequate knowledge of family theories (Clemen-Stone, McGuire, Eigsti, 1998).

- **= Independent; ▲ = Collaborative**

▲ Collaborate with nurses or other consultants regarding strategies for working with families.
For some families, the knowledge and skills of nurses with advanced degrees or of other specialists may be needed to design effective interventions (Kang, Barnard, Oshio, 1994).

Multicultural

- Acknowledge racial/ethnic differences at the onset of care.
Acknowledgement of race/ethnicity issues will enhance communication, establish rapport, and promote treatment outcomes (D'Avanzo et al, 2001).
- Approach families of color with respect, warmth, and professional courtesy
Instances of disrespect and lack of caring have special significance for families of color (D'Avanzo et al, 2001).
- Assess for the influence of cultural beliefs, norms, and values on the family's perceptions of the therapeutic regimen.
How the family views the therapeutic regimen may be based on cultural perceptions (Leininger, 1996).
- Give rationale when assessing African-American families about sensitive issues.
Many African-Americans may expect white caregivers to hold negative and preconceived ideas about blacks. Giving a rationale for questions asked will help alleviate this perception (D'Avanzo et al, 2001).
- Use a family-centered approach when working with Latino, Asian, African-American, and Native American clients.
Latinos may perceive family as a source of support, solver of problems and source of pride. Asian Americans may regard the family as the primary decision maker and influence on individual family members (D'Avanzo et al, 2001). Native American families may be extended structures that exert powerful influences over functioning (Seiderman et al, 1996).
- Facilitate modeling and role-playing for family regarding healthy ways to communicate and interact.
It is helpful for families and the client to practice communication skills in a safe environment before trying them in a real-life situation (Rivera-Andino, Lopez, 2000).
- Validate family members' feelings regarding the impact of the therapeutic regimen on family lifestyle.
Validation lets the client know that the nurse has heard and understands what was said, and it promotes the nurse-client relationship (Stuart, Laraia, 2001; Giger, Davidhizar, 1995).

Client/Family Teaching

- Teach about all aspects of therapeutic regimens. Provide as much knowledge as family members will accept, adjust instruction to account for what family already knows, and provide information in a culturally congruent manner.
- Teach ways to adjust family behaviors for inclusion of therapeutic regimens.
▲ Teach safety in taking medications.
▲ Teach family members to act as self-advocates with health providers who prescribe therapeutic regimens.

WEB SITES FOR EDUCATION

$\int_{MERLIN}$ See the MERLIN web site for World Wide Web resources for client education.

• = Independent; ▲ = Collaborative

REFERENCES   Clemen-Stone S, McGuire SL, Eigsti DG: *Comprehensive community health nursing: family aggregate and community practice*, ed 5, St Louis, 1998, Mosby.

D'Avanzo CE et al: Developing culturally informed strategies for substance related interventions. In Naegle MA, D'Avanzo CE, editors: *Addictions and substance abuse, strategies for advanced practice nursing*, St Louis, 2001, Mosby, pp 59-104.

Degazon C: Cultural diversity and community-oriented nursing practice. In Stanhope M, Lancaster J: *Community and public health nursing*, ed 5, St Louis, 2000, Mosby, pp 138-156.

Fujita LJ, Duncan J: High risk for ineffective management of therapeutic regimen: a protocol study, *Rehabil Nurs* 19(2):75, 1994.

Giger JN, Davidhizar RE: *Transcultural nursing*, ed 2, St Louis, 1995, Mosby.

Kang R, Barnard K, Oshio S: Description of the clinical practice of advanced practice nurses in family-centered early intervention in two rural settings, *Pub Health Nurs* 11:376, 1994.

Leininger MM: *Transcultural nursing: theories, research and practices*, ed 2, Hilliard, Ohio, 1996, McGraw-Hill.

Lubkin IM: *Chronic illness: impact and interventions*, ed 4, Boston, 1998, Jones & Bartlett.

Miller JF: *Coping with chronic illness: overcoming powerlessness*, ed 3, Philadelphia, 1999, FA Davis.

Musick MA: Religion and subjective health among black and white elders, *J Health Soc Behav* 37:221, 1996.

Pender NJ: *Health promotion in nursing practice*, ed 3, Stamford, Conn, 1996, Appleton & Lange.

Rivera-Andino J, Lopez L: When culture complicates care, *RN* 63(7):47-49, 2000.

Seiderman RY et al: Assessing American Indian families, *MCN Am J Matern Child Nurs* 21(6):274-279, 1996.

Stetz KM, Lewis FM, Houck GM: Family goals as indicants of adaptation during chronic illness, *Pub Health Nurs* 11:385, 1994.

Stuart GW, Laraia MT: Therapeutic nurse-patient relationship. In Stuart GW, Laraia MT, editors: *Principles and practice of psychiatric nursing*, St Louis, 2001, Mosby, p 30.

Ineffective Thermoregulation

Betty J. Ackley and Sandra K. Cunningham

NANDA   **Definition** Temperature fluctuation between hypothermia and hyperthermia

Defining Characteristics

Fluctuations in body temperature above or below the normal range; cool skin; cyanotic nail beds; flushed skin; hypertension; increased respiratory rate; pallor (moderate); pilo-erection; reduction in body temperature below normal range; seizures/convulsions; shivering (mild); slow capillary refill; tachycardia; warm to touch

Related Factors (r/t)

Trauma; illness; immaturity; aging; fluctuating environmental temperature

NOC   **Outcomes (Nursing Outcomes Classification)**

Suggested NOC Outcomes

Thermoregulation; Thermoregulation: Neonate

> **Example NOC Outcome**
> Accomplishes **Thermoregulation** as evidenced by the following indicators: Body temperature WNL*/Skin temperature IER†/Skin color changes not present/Hydration adequate/Reported thermal comfort (Rate each indicator of **Thermoregulation:** 1 = extremely compromised, 2 = substantially compromised, 3 = moderately compromised, 4 = mildly compromised, 5 = not compromised [see Section I])

*Within Normal Limits
†In Expected Range

• = **Independent**; ▲ = **Collaborative**

Client Outcomes

- Maintains temperature within a normal range
- Explains measures needed to maintain normal temperature
- Explains symptoms of hypothermia or hyperthermia

NIC   Interventions (Nursing Interventions Classification)

Suggested NIC Labels

Temperature Regulation; Temperature Regulation: Inoperative

Example NIC Interventions—Temperature Regulation
- Institute a continuous core temperature monitoring device, as appropriate
- Promote adequate fluid and nutritional intake

Nursing Interventions and Rationales

- Monitor temperature q __ h(rs) or use continuous temperature monitoring as appropriate.
  Normal adult temperature is usually identified as 98.6° F (37° C), but in actuality the normal temperature fluctuates throughout the day. In the early morning it may be as low as 96.4° F (35.8° C) and as high as 99.1° F (37.3° C) in the late afternoon or evening (Bates, Bickley, Hoekelman, 1998). Disease, injury, or pharmacological agents may impair regulation of body temperature (Holtzclaw, 1993; Dennison, 1995).
- Take vital signs q __ h(rs), noting changes associated with hypothermia: first, increased blood pressure, pulse, and respirations, then decreased values as hypthermia progresses (Edwards, 1999).
- Note changes in vital signs associated with hyperthermia: rapid, bounding pulse; increased respiratory rate; and decreased blood pressure with orthostatic hypotension present (Worfolk, 2000).
  Consistency monitoring promotes prevention and early intervention in clients with altered cardiopulmonary status associated with hypothermia or hyperthermia.
- Monitor client for signs of hypothermia (e.g., shivering, cool skin, piloerection, pallor, slow capillary refill, cyanotic nailbeds, decreased mentation, dysrhythmias) (Edwards, 1999).
- Monitor client for signs of hyperthermia (e.g., headache, nausea and vomiting, weakness, absence of sweating, delirium, and coma) (Worfolk, 2000).
  Monitoring for defining characteristics of hypothermia and hyperthermia allows for prevention and/or early intervention.
- Maintain a consistent room temperature (72° F).
  A consistent temperature limits environmental effects on thermoregulation.
- Promote adequate nutrition and hydration.
  These measures help maintain a normal body temperature.
- Adjust clothing to facilitate passive warming or cooling as appropriate.
  This will help maintain a normal body temperature.
- See Nursing Interventions and Rationales for **Hypothermia** or **Hyperthermia** as appropriate.

Geriatric

- Do not allow elderly clients to become chilled. Keep covered when giving a bath, and offer socks to wear in bed. Be aware of factors such as room temperature (heating/air conditioning), clothing (layered/loose), and fluid intake.

• = Independent; ▲ = Collaborative

Older adults have a decreased ability to adapt to temperature extremes and need protection from extreme environmental temperatures. They also have a higher threshold of central temperature for sweating, diminished or absent sweating, impaired warmth or cold perception, an impaired shiver response, diminished thermogenesis, an abnormal peripheral blood flow response to warmth or cold, and a compromised cardiovascular reserve (Robbins, 1989; Florez-Duquet, McDonald, 1998; Ballester, Harchelroad, 1999).

▲ Assess medication profile for potential risk of drug-related altered body temperature.

Anesthetics, barbiturates, salicylates, nonsteroidal antiinflammatory drugs (NSAIDs), diuretics, antihistamines, anticholinergics, beta-blockers, and thyroid hormones have been linked to altered body temperatures (Haskell et al, 1997).

Pediatric

- Recognize that pediatric clients have a decreased ability to adapt to temperature extremes. Take the following actions to maintain body temperature in the infant/child:
  - Keep the head covered
  - Use blankets to keep the client warm
  - Keep client covered during procedures, transport, and diagnostic testing
  - Keep the room temperature at 72° F

These measures can help prevent hypothermia in the child, which is very possible, especially in the pediatric trauma client (Bernardo, Henker, 1999). The combination of a relatively larger body surface area, smaller body-fluid volume, less well-developed temperature control mechanisms, and a smaller amount of protective body fat limits the pediatric client's ability to maintain normal temperatures (Henderson, 1990; Roncoli, Medoff-Cooper, 1992; Noerr, 1997).

Home Care Interventions

- Prevention of Hypothermia in Cold Weather
  - Avoid prolonged exposure outside. Wear gloves and a cap on head. Wool or fleece clothing can help to maintain body heat.
  - Keep room temperature at 68° to 72° F.
  - ▲ Ensure adequate source of heat. Refer to social services if low income and heat could be turned off.
  - Help elderly client determine a warm environment they can go to for safety in cold weather if home environment is no longer warm.
- Prevention of Hyperthermia in Hot Weather
  - Encourage client to wear cotton lightweight clothing. Help elderly client remove usual sweater.
  - Ensure client drinks adequate amounts of fluids—2000 ml/day, avoiding caffeine and alcohol.

    Adequate fluids are needed during hot weather to replace fluids lost from sweating. Fluids containing caffeine and alcohol can serve as a diuretic and decrease fluid volume in the body.
  - Help client obtain a fan or an air conditioner to increase evaporation, as needed.
  - Take the temperature of the elderly in hot weather.

    The elderly may not be able to tell that they are hot because of decreased sensation (Worfolk, 2000).
  - Help elderly client determine a cool environment they can go to for safety in hot weather.

• = **Independent;** ▲ = **Collaborative**

Client/Family Teaching

- Teach client and family signs of hypothermia and hyperthermia and appropriate actions to take if either condition develops.
  Adequate teaching improves compliance and reduces anxiety.
- Teach client and family an age-appropriate method for taking the temperature.
  Optimal placement of the appropriate device is essential for accurate monitoring.
- Teach to avoid alcohol and medications that depress cerebral function.
  When the client is sedated or under the influence of alcohol, mentation is depressed, resulting in decreased activities to maintain an adequate body temperature.

WEB SITES FOR EDUCATION

Merlin See the MERLIN web site for World Wide Web resources for client education.

REFERENCES Ballester JM, Harchelroad FP: Hypothermia: an easy-to-miss, dangerous disorder in winter weather, *Geriatrics* 54(2):51, 1999.

Bates B, Bickley LS, Hoekelman RA: *A guide to physical examination and history taking,* ed 7, Philadelphia, 1998, JB Lippincott.

Bernardo LM, Henker R: Thermoregulation in pediatric trauma: an overview, *Int J Trauma Nurs* 5(3):101-105, 1999.

Dennison D: Thermal regulation of patients during the perioperative period, *AORN J* 61:827, 1995.

Edwards SL: Hypothermia, *Professional Nurse* 14(4): 253-258, 1999.

Florez-Duquet M, McDonald RB: Cold-induced thermoregulation and biological aging, *Physiol Rev* 78(2):339, 1998.

Haskell RM et al: Hypothermia, *AACN Clin Issues Crit Care Nurs* 8(3):368, 1997.

Henderson DP: Pediatric update: hypothermia and the pediatric patient, *J Emerg Nurs* 16:411, 1990.

Holtzclaw BJ: Monitoring body temperature, *AACN Clin Issues Crit Care Nurs* 4:44, 1993.

Noerr B: Keeping the newborn warm: understanding thermoregulation, *Mother Baby J* 2(5):6, 1997.

Robbins AS: Hypothermia and heat stroke: protecting the elderly patient, *Geriatrics* 44, 1989.

Roncoli M, Medoff-Cooper B: Thermoregulation in low-birth-weight infants, *NAACOGS Clin Issu Perinat Womens Health Nurs* 3:25, 1992.

Worfolk JB: Heat waves: their impact on the health of elders, *Geratr Nurs* 21(2):70-77, 2000.

Disturbed Thought processes

Helen Kelley and Judith R. Gentz

NANDA **Definition** Disruption in cognitive operations and activities

Defining Characteristics

Cognitive dissonance; memory deficit/problems; inaccurate interpretation of environment; hypovigilance; hypervigilance; distractibility; egocentricity; inappropriate nonreality-based thinking

Related Factors (r/t)

To be developed

• = Independent; ▲ = Collaborative

NOC Outcomes (Nursing Outcomes Classification)

Suggested NOC Labels

Cognitive Ability; Cognitive Orientation; Concentration; Decision Making; Distorted Thought Control; Identity; Information Processing; Memory; Neurological Status: Consciousness

> **Example NOC Outcome**
>
> Accomplishes **Distorted Thought Control** as evidenced by the following indicators: Recognizes hallucinations or delusions are occurring/Refrains from attending to or responding to hallucinations or delusions/Exhibits reality-based thinking (Rate each indicator of **Distorted Thought Control:** 1 = never demonstrated, 2 = rarely demonstrated, 3 = sometimes demonstrated, 4 = often demonstrated, 5 = consistently demonstrated [see Section I])

Client Outcomes

- Remains oriented to time, place, and person; demonstrates improved cognitive function
- Remains free from physical harm
- Performs activities of daily living (ADLs) appropriately and independently
- Identifies community resources for help after discharge

NIC Interventions (Nursing Interventions Classification)

Suggested NIC Labels

Delusion Management; Dementia Management

> **Example NIC Interventions—Delusion Management**
> - Provide an opportunity for client to discuss delusions with caregivers
> - Focus discussion on the underlying feeling, rather than the content of the delusion ("It appears as if you may be feeling frightened")

Nursing Interventions and Rationales

- Observe for causes of altered thought processes (see Related Factors).
- ▲ Monitor, record, and report changes in client's neurological status (level of consciousness, increased intracranial pressure), mental status (memory, cognition, judgment, concentration), vital signs, laboratory results, and ability to follow commands.
  These examinations help identify pathophysiological symptoms.
- Obtain a medical history to rule out physical illness etiology for mental status changes.
  The characteristics of intellectual and cognitive dysfunction are very similar in Alzheimer's disease and AIDS (as well as other medical entities) (Harvath, 1995).
- Complete a mental status examination of client.
  This examination helps identify psychiatric symptoms (Dellasega, 1998).
- ▲ Report any new onset or sudden increase in confusion.
  A substantial proportion of postsurgical patients suffer an abnormal temporary change in mental status that can have adverse effects on their recovery (Platzer, 1989). Confusion occurs when sensorial cues used to orient oneself are unavailable, increasing anxiety (Neelon, 1990).
- Adjust communication style to client. Speak slowly and calmly; use short phrases and concrete, nontechnical words; use writing if appropriate; allow time for thinking; use face-to-face communication; listen carefully; and seek clarification.
  Effective communication promotes understanding.

• = Independent; ▲ = Collaborative

- Assess pain and promptly provide comfort measures.
  Confused clients cannot accurately report pain; untreated pain increases anxiety and agitation (Foreman, 1989a).
- Identify and remove potentially dangerous items in the environment.
  Alteration of thoughts can lead to misinterpretation of environment and decreased judgment and impulse control. Cognitive impairment can result in a number of problems, such as communication difficulties, compromised safety, self-care deficits, and behavioral problems.
- ▲ Limit use of sedatives and drugs affecting the nervous system.
  Higher medication usage is correlated with more frequent onset of confusion (Foreman, 1989b; Dellasega, Stricklin, 1993).
- ▲ Use soft restraints with discretion and physician order.
  Restraints may exacerbate confusion (Yorker, 1988).
- Orient client and call client by name; introduce self on each contact; frequently mention time, date, and place; prominently display a clock and calendar that are easy to read in room and refer to them; and request family to bring in familiar pictures and articles from home.
  These steps help reinforce reality and provide cues that maintain orientation. External, written reminders are more effective than verbal reinforcement for memory aids (McDougall, 1995).
- Provide validation of thoughts and feelings of client.
  Validation seeks to help the caregiver understand the care receiver, encouraging empathy (Woodrow, 1998).
- Stay with clients if they are agitated and likely to be injured.
  A quiet environment with the presence of another person can calm an agitated client. For some clients, family members (rather than staff) will be more comforting.
- Assess client's assault potential and maintain staff safety.
- Establish predictable care routines and maintain continuity of client's nursing staff.
  Routines promote feelings of security.
- Frequently check on client and have brief interactions to prevent sensory deprivation.
- Avoid an overstimulated or a sensory-deprived environment. Provide adequate lighting that is not too bright. Alternate short, frequent visits with defined rest periods. Monitor noise levels.
  Excessive environmental stimuli can adversely affect client's level of orientation and increase disorganization.
- Assist client with daily hygiene as needed; encourage self-care.
  Good hygiene and self-care increase self-esteem and autonomy.
- Provide support to family during client's period of disorientation. Involve family in current care and in planning of postdischarge care.
  Family involvement promotes continuity of care.
- ▲ Initiate a social service referral to find help for client following discharge.
- Observe for hallucinations as evidenced by behavioral response to internal stimuli, inappropriate laughter, slow verbal responses, lip movements without sound, smiling at inappropriate times, or grimacing.
  Provide reality orientation as tolerated. Assist client with management strategies for hallucinations (Buccheri et al, 1996).
- Ask direct questions such as, "Are you seeing or hearing something now?" or "Do you sometimes hear or see things that other people don't hear or see?"
  Validation of symptoms increases empathy and client's perception of safety.

- **= Independent; ▲ = Collaborative**

- Do not attempt to argue or change the client's beliefs, but do not imply agreement. Without implying agreement, attend to client's reaction or response to beliefs. *Attending to reactions or responses promotes a trusting relationship with the client.*
- Accept that client is seeing or hearing things that are not there, but tactfully tell client that only he or she is hearing or seeing these things. Focus on feelings that accompany hallucinations and delusions rather than content of delusions (e.g., "You look frightened"). *Acceptance promotes trust and understanding.*
- Set limits on delusional conversations (e.g., "We discussed that; let's talk about what is happening now on the unit").
- Ask for clarification when necessary.
- Help client state needs and ask for assistance.
- Involve client in short activities.
- See care plans for **Risk for self- and other-directed Violence** for further nursing interventions and rationales.

Geriatric

- Monitor for dementia, as evidenced by its gradual onset and a progressive deterioration, or for delirium, as evidenced by its acute onset and generally reversible course. *States of confusion require careful assessment (Vermeersch, 1990; Milisen et al, 1998).*
- Focus on feelings associated with hallucinations and delusions rather than content. *Tuning into disoriented clients' feelings is more important than rigidly insisting that they share the nurse's reality. Be comforting and understanding when client has processing difficulties (Bleathman, Morton, 1992).*

Multicultural

- Assess for the influence of cultural beliefs, norms, and values on the family or caregiver's understanding of disturbed thought processes. *What the family considers normal and abnormal health behavior may be based on cultural perceptions (Leininger, 1996).*
- Inform client's family or caregiver of the meaning of and reasons for common behaviors observed in client with disturbed thought processes. *An understanding of behavior will enable the client's family or caregiver to provide the client with a safe environment.*
- Validate the family members' feelings regarding the impact of client behavior on family lifestyle. *Validation lets the client know that the nurse has heard and understands what was said, and it promotes the nurse-client relationship (Stuart, Laraia, 2001; Giger, Davidhizar, 1995).*

Home Care Interventions

- Assess family knowledge of disease process and plan of care; teach as necessary. Encourage participation. *Involving significant others in caregiving often helps them cope with the stress of the client's health problem (Stuart, Sundeen, 1991).*
- Assess home environment for availability of distractions from hallucinations, such as music over headphones. *Distraction can give temporary relief from chronic hallucinations.*
- ▲ If client's condition deteriorates, seek acute medical health intervention immediately.
- Identify an emergency plan and criteria for use with family or caregivers. *An appropriate level of clinical intervention supports client and family well-being.*

- **= Independent; ▲ = Collaborative**

- Identify responsible caregiver for medication administration. Teach purpose, administration, and side effects of medications based on level of knowledge.
  Clients with altered thought process cannot perform health-related care tasks with consistency.
- Identify cultural variables that affect client responses to stimuli. Use cultural information to provide support to client. Avoid reference to threatening cultural values.
  Familiar patterns provide a sense of security for cognitively impaired persons (Stuart, Sundeen, 1991).
- Use a night light.
  Night lights help clients reorient themselves and decrease fear if clients awaken during the night.
- Allow client control over aspects of his or her environment as he or she is able.
  Although sometimes only for a short time, control enhances self-esteem.
- Identify client's interests and skills. Provide an opportunity for client to pursue interests and use skills without taxing client judgment and cognitive ability.
  Diversionary activities decrease anxiety and give meaning to life.

Client/Family Teaching

- Teach family members reorientation techniques and about the need to frequently repeat instructions.
- Teach client distraction techniques to manage hallucinations.
- Teach family members ways to support client without supporting delusional beliefs.
- Help family identify coping skills, environmental supports, and community services for dealing with chronically mentally ill clients.
- Discuss caregiver's need for respite. Offer support, encouragement, and information for meeting those needs.

WEB SITES FOR EDUCATION

MERLIN See the MERLIN web site for World Wide Web resources for client education.

REFERENCES Bleathman C, Morton I: Validation therapy: extracts from 20 groups with dementia sufferers, *J Adv Nurs* 17:658, 1992.

Buccheri R et al: Auditory hallucinations in schizophrenia: group experience in examining symptom management and behavioral strategies, *J Psychosoc Nurs Ment Health Serv* 34:2, 1996.

Dellasega C: Assessment of cognition in the elderly, *Nurs Clin North Am* 33:3, 1998.

Dellasega C, Stricklin ML: Cognitive impairment in elderly home health clients, *Home Health Care Serv Q* 14:81, 1993.

Foreman M: Complexities of acute confusion, *Geriatr Nurs* 3:136, 1989a.

Foreman M: Confusion in the hospitalized elderly: incidence onset and associated factors, *Res Nurs Health* 12:21, 1989b.

Giger JN, Davidhizar RE: *Transcultural nursing*, ed 2, St Louis, 1995, Mosby.

Harvath TA et al: Dementia related behaviors in Alzheimer's disease and AIDS, *J Psychosic Nur Ment Health Serv* 33:1, 1995.

Leininger MM: *Transcultural nursing: theories, research and practices*, ed 2, Hilliard, Ohio, 1996, McGraw-Hill.

McDougall GC: Memory strategies used by cognitively intact and cognitively impaired older adults, *J Am Acad Nurs Pract* 7:369, 1995.

Milisen K et al: Delirium in the hospitalized elderly, *Nurs Clin North Am* 33:3, 1998.

Neelon VJ, Postoperative confusion, *Crit Care Nurs Clin North Am* 2:4, 1990.

Platzer H: Post-operative confusion in the elderly: a literature review, *Int J Nurs Stud* 26:367, 1989.

Stuart GW, Laraia MT: Therapeutic nurse-patient relationship. In Stuart GW, Laraia MT, editors: *Principles and practice of psychiatric nursing*, St Louis, 2001, Mosby, p 30.

• = **Independent**; ▲ = **Collaborative**

Stuart G, Sundeen S: *Pocket guide to psychiatric nursing*, ed 2, St Louis, Mosby, 1991.
Vermeersch PE: The clinical assessment of confusion, *Appl Nurs Res* 3(3):128-133, 1990.
Yorker BC: The nurse's use of restraint with a neurologically impaired patient, *J Neurosci Nurs* 20:390, 1988.
Woodrow P: Interventions for confusion and dementia: alternative approaches, *Br J Nurs* 7:20, 1998.

Impaired Tissue integrity

Diane Krasner

 Definition Damage to mucous membrane, corneal, integumentary, or subcutaneous tissues

Defining Characteristics

Damaged or destroyed tissue (e.g., cornea, mucous membrane, integumentary, or subcutaneous)

Related Factors (r/t)

Mechanical (e.g., pressure, shear, friction); radiation (including therapeutic radiation); nutritional deficit or excess; thermal (temperature extremes); knowledge deficit; irritants, chemical (including body excretions, secretions, medications); impaired physical mobility; altered circulation; fluid deficit or excess

NOC Outcomes (Nursing Outcomes Classification)

Suggested NOC Labels

Tissue Integrity: Skin and Mucous Membranes; Wound Healing: Primary Intention; Wound Healing: Secondary Intention

> **Example NOC Outcome**
> **Tissue Integrity: Skin and Mucous Membranes** will be intact as evidenced by the following indicators: Skin intactness/Tissue lesion-free/Tissue perfusion/Tissue temperature in expected range (Rate each indicator of **Tissue Integrity:** 1 = extremely compromised, 2 = substantially compromised, 3 = moderately compromised, 4 = mildly compromised, 5 = not compromised [see Section I])

Client Outcomes

- Reports any altered sensation or pain at site of tissue impairment
- Demonstrates understanding of plan to heal tissue and prevent injury
- Describes measures to protect and heal the tissue, including wound care
- Wound decreases in size and has increased granulation tissue

NIC Interventions (Nursing Interventions Classification)

Suggested NIC Labels

Incision Site Care; Pressure Ulcer Care; Skin Care: Topical Treatments; Skin Surveillance; Wound Care

> **Example NIC Interventions—Pressure Ulcer Care**
> - Monitor color, temperature, edema, moisture, and appearance of surrounding skin
> - Note characteristics of any drainage

• = Independent; ▲ = Collaborative

Nursing Interventions and Rationales

- Assess site of impaired tissue integrity and determine etiology (e.g., acute or chronic wound, burn, dermatological lesion, pressure ulcer, leg ulcer).
  Prior assessment of wound etiology is critical for proper identification of nursing interventions (van Rijswijk, 2001).
- Determine size and depth of wound (e.g., full-thickness wound, stage III or stage IV pressure ulcer).
  Wound assessment is more reliable when performed by the same caregiver, the client is in the same position, and the same techniques are used (Krasner, Sibbald, 1999; Sussman, Bates-Jensen, 1998).
- Classify pressure ulcers in the following manner:
  - Stage III: Full-thickness skin loss involving damage to or necrosis of subcutaneous tissue that may extend down to but not through underlying fascia; ulcer appears as a deep crater with or without undermining of adjacent tissue (National Pressure Ulcer Advisory Panel, 1989).
  - Stage IV: Full-thickness skin loss with extensive destruction; tissue necrosis; or damage to muscle, bone, or supporting structures (e.g., tendons, joint capsules) (National Pressure Ulcer Advisory Panel, 1989).
- Monitor site of impaired tissue integrity at least once daily for color changes, redness, swelling, warmth, pain, or other signs of infection. Determine whether client is experiencing changes in sensation or pain. Pay special attention to all high-risk areas such as bony prominences, skin folds, sacrum, and heels.
  Systematic inspection can identify impending problems early (Bryant, 1999).
- Monitor status of skin around wound. Monitor client's skin care practices, noting type of soap or other cleansing agents used, temperature of water, and frequency of skin cleansing.
  Individualize plan according to client's skin condition, needs, and preferences. Avoid harsh cleansing agents, hot water, extreme friction or force, or cleansing too frequently (Panel for the Prediction and Prevention of Pressure Ulcers in Adults, 1992; Bergstrom, 1994).
- Monitor client's continence status and minimize exposure of skin impairment site and other areas to moisture from incontinence, perspiration, or wound drainage.
- ▲ If client is incontinent, implement an incontinence management plan to prevent exposure to chemicals in urine and stool that can strip or erode the skin. Refer to a physician (e.g., urologist, gastroenterologist) for an incontinence assessment (Doughty, 2000; Wound, Ostomy, and Continence Nurses Society, 1992, 1994).
- Monitor for correct placement of tubes, catheters, and other devices. Assess skin and tissue affected by the tape that secures these devices (Faller, Beitz, 2001).
  Mechanical damage to skin and tissues as a result of pressure, friction, or shear is often associated with external devices.
- In orthopedic clients, check every 2 hours for correct placement of foot boards, restraints, traction, casts, or other devices, and assess skin and tissue integrity. Be alert for symptoms of compartment syndrome (see care plan for **Risk for Peripheral neurovascular dysfunction**).
  Mechanical damage to skin and tissues (pressure, friction, or shear) is often associated with external devices.
- For clients with limited mobility, use a risk assessment tool to systematically assess immobility-related risk factors.

- • = Independent; ▲ = Collaborative

A validated risk assessment tool such as the Norton or Braden scale should be used to identify clients at risk for immobility-related skin breakdown (Bergstrom et al, 1987; Panel for the Prediction and Prevention of Pressure Ulcers in Adults, 1992; Krasner, Sibbald, 1999).

▲ Implement a written treatment plan for topical treatment of the skin impairment site.
A written treatment plan ensures consistency in care and documentation (Maklebust, Sieggreen, 1996). Topical treatments must be matched to the client, wound, and setting (Krasner, Sibbald, 1999; Ovington, 1998).

▲ Identify a plan for debridement if necrotic tissue (eschar or slough) is present and if consistent with overall client management goals.
Healing does not occur in the presence of necrotic tissue (Panel for the Prediction and Prevention of Pressure Ulcers in Adults, 1992; Bergstrom et al, 1994; Krasner, Sibbald, 1999).

• Select a topical treatment that maintains a moist wound-healing environment that is balanced with the need to absorb exudate and fill dead space.
Caution should always be taken to not dry out the wound (Panel for the Prediction and Prevention of Pressure Ulcers in Adults, 1992; Bergstrom et al, 1994; Ovington, 1998).

• Do not position client on site of impaired tissue integrity. If consistent with overall client management goals, turn and position client at least every 2 hours, and carefully transfer client to avoid adverse effects of external mechanical forces (i.e., pressure, friction, and shear).
Evaluate for use of specialty mattresses, beds, or devices as appropriate (Fleck, 2001). If the goal of care is to keep the client (e.g., a terminally ill client) comfortable, turning and repositioning may not be appropriate. Maintain the head of the bed at the lowest degree of elevation possible to reduce shear and friction, and use lift devices, pillows, foam wedges, and pressure-reducing devices in the bed (Panel for the Prediction and Prevention of Pressure Ulcers in Adults, 1992; Krasner, Rodeheaver, Sibbald, 2001).

• Avoid massaging around site of impaired tissue integrity and over bony prominences.
Research suggests that massage may lead to deep-tissue trauma (Panel for the Prediction and Prevention of Pressure Ulcers in Adults, 1992).

▲ Assess client's nutritional status; refer for a nutritional consultation and/or institute dietary supplements.
Inadequate nutritional intake places the client at risk for skin breakdown and compromises healing (Demling, De Santi, 1998).

Home Care Interventions

• Assess client's current phases of wound healing (inflammation, proliferation, maturation) and stage of injury.
Accurate understanding of tissue status combined with knowledge of underlying diagnoses and product validity provide a basis for determining appropriate treatment objectives (Ovington, 1998). There is no single wound dressing appropriate for all phases of wound healing (Krasner, Sibbald, 1999).

• Instruct and assist client and caregivers with removing or controlling impediments to wound healing (e.g., management of underlying disease, improvement in approach to client positioning, improved nutrition).
Wound healing can be delayed or fail totally if impediments are not controlled (Krasner, Sibbald, 1999).

▲ Initiate a consultation in a case assignment with a wound, ostomy, continence nurse (WOC nurse) to establish a comprehensive plan as soon as possible.

• = **Independent**; ▲ = **Collaborative**

Client/Family Teaching

- Teach skin and wound assessment and ways to monitor for signs and symptoms of infection, complications, and healing.

  Early assessment and intervention helps prevent the development of serious problems (van Rijswijk, 2001).

▲ Teach use of a topical treatment that is matched to client, wound, and setting.

  The topical treatment needs to be adjusted as the status of the wound changes (Krasner, Sibbald, 1999).

- If consistent with overall client management goals, teach how to turn and reposition client at least every 2 hours.

  If the goal of care is to keep the client (e.g., a terminally ill client) comfortable, turning and repositioning may not be appropriate (Krasner, Rodeheaver, Sibbald, 2001; Panel for the Prediction and Prevention of Pressure Ulcers in Adults, 1992).

- Teach use of pillows, foam wedges, and pressure-reducing devices to prevent pressure injury.

WEB SITES FOR EDUCATION

Merlin See the MERLIN web site for World Wide Web resources for client education.

REFERENCES Bergstrom N et al: The Braden scale for prediction of pressure sore risk, *Nurs Res* 36:205, 1987.

Bergstrom N et al: *Treatment of pressure ulcers,* Clinical Practice Guideline No. 15, Agency for Health Care Policy and Research, Pub. No. 95-0652, Rockville, Md, 1994, Public Health Service, U.S. Department of Health and Human Services.

Bryant R: *Acute and chronic wounds,* ed 2, St Louis, 1999, Mosby.

Demling R, De Santi L: Closure of the "non-healing wound" corresponds with correction of weight loss using the anabolic agent oxandrolone, *Ostomy Wound Manage* 44(10):58-62, 64, 66, 1998.

Doughty D: *Urinary and fecal incontinence: nursing management,* St Louis, 2000, Mosby.

Krasner D: Dressing decisions for the twenty-first century: on the cusp of a paradigm shift, *Wounds* 8:16, 1996.

Faller N, Beitz J: When a wound isn't a wound: tubes, drains, fistulas and draining wounds. In Krasner D, Rodeheaver G, Sibbald RG: *Chronic wound care: a clinical source book for healthcare professionals,* ed 2, Wayne, Penn, 2001, HMP Communications.

Fleck D: Support surfaces: criteria and selection. In Krasner D, Rodeheaver G, Sibbald RG: *Chronic wound care: a clinical source book for healthcare professionals,* ed 2, Wayne, Penn, 2001, HMP Communications.

Krasner D, Rodeheaver G, Sibbald RG: Advanced wound caring for a new millennium. In Krasner D, Rodeheaver G, Sibbald RG: *Chronic wound care: a clinical source book for healthcare professionals,* ed 2, Wayne, Penn, 2001, HMP Communications.

Krasner D, Sibbald RG: Moving beyond the AHCPR guidelines: wound care evolution over the last five years, *Ostomy Wound Manage* 45(suppl 1A):1S, 1999.

Maklebust J, Sieggreen M: *Pressure ulcers: guidelines for prevention and nursing management,* ed 2, Springhouse, Penn, 1996, Springhouse.

National Pressure Ulcer Advisory Panel: *Consensus development conference statement,* Buffalo, NY, 1989, The Panel.

Ovington LG: The well-dressed wound: an overview of dressing types, *Wounds* 10(suppl A):1A, 1998.

Panel for the Prediction and Prevention of Pressure Ulcers in Adults: *Pressure ulcers in adults: prediction and prevention,* Clinical Practice Guideline, No 3, Agency for Health Care Policy and Research Pub No 92-0047, Rockville, Md, 1992, U.S. Department of Health and Human Services, Public Health Service.

Sussman C, Bates-Jensen BM: *Wound care: a collaborative practice manual for physical therapists and nurses,* Gaithersburg, Md, 1998, Aspen.

van Rijswijk L: Wound assessment and documentation. In Krasner D, Rodeheaver G, Sibbald RG: *Chronic wound care: a clinical source book for healthcare professionals,* ed 2, Wayne, Penn, 2001, HMP Communications.

• = Independent; ▲ = Collaborative

Wound, Ostomy, and Continence Nurses Society: *Standards of care: dermal wounds: pressure ulcers,* Costa Mesa, Calif, 1992, The Society.

Wound, Ostomy, and Continence Nurses Society: *Standards of care: patient with fecal incontinence,* Costa Mesa, Calif, 1994, The Society.

Ineffective Tissue perfusion (specify type): cerebral, renal, cardiopulmonary, GI, peripheral

Betty J. Ackley

 Definition Decrease in oxygen resulting in failure to nourish tissues at the capillary level

Defining Characteristics

Renal
Altered blood pressure outside of acceptable parameters; hematuria; oliguria or anuria; elevation in BUN/creatinine ratio

Gastrointestinal
Hypoactive or absent bowel sounds; nausea; abdominal distention; abdominal pain or tenderness

Peripheral
Edema; positive Hoeman's sign; altered skin characteristics (hair, nails, moisture); weak or absent pulses; skin discolorations; skin temperature changes; altered sensations; diminished arterial pulsations; skin color pale on elevation, color does not return on lowering the leg; slow healing of lesions; cold extremities; dependent, blue, or purple skin color

Cerebral
Speech abnormalities; changes in pupillary reactions; extremity weakness or paralysis; altered mental status; difficult in swallowing; changes in motor response; behavioral changes

Cardiopulmonary
Altered respiratory rate outside of acceptable parameters; use of accessory muscles; capillary refill >3 seconds; abnormal arterial blood gases; chest pain; sense of "impending doom"; bronchospasms; dyspnea; dysrhythmias; nasal flaring; chest retraction

Related Factors (r/t)
Hypovolemia; interruption of arterial flow; hypervolemia; exchange problems; interruption of venous flow; mechanical reduction of venous and/or arterial blood flow; hypoventilation; impaired transport of oxygen across alveolar and/or capillary membrane; mismatch of ventilation with blood flow; decreased hemoglobin concentration in blood; enzyme poisoning; altered affinity of hemoglobin for oxygen

NOC **Outcomes (Nursing Outcomes Classification)**
Suggested NOC Labels
Circulation Status; Cardiac Pump Effectiveness: Tissue Perfusion: Cardiac; Tissue Perfusion: Cerebral; Tissue Perfusion: Peripheral; Fluid Balance; Hydration; Urinary Elimination

Example NOC Outcome
Demonstrates adequate **Circulation Status** as evidenced by the following indicators: Peripheral pulses strong/Peripheral pulses symmetrical/Peripheral edema not present (Rate each indicator of **Circulation Status:** 1 = extremely compromised, 2 = substantially compromised, 3 = moderately compromised, 4 = mildly compromised, 5 = not compromised [see Section I])

• = **Independent;** ▲ = **Collaborative**

Client Outcomes

- Demonstrates adequate tissue perfusion as evidenced by palpable peripheral pulses, warm and dry skin, adequate urinary output, and the absence of respiratory distress
- Verbalizes knowledge of treatment regimen, including appropriate exercise and medications and their actions and possible side effects
- Identifies changes in lifestyle that are needed to increase tissue perfusion

NIC **Interventions (Nursing Interventions Classification)**

Suggested NIC Labels

Circulatory Care: Arterial Insufficiency

Example NIC Interventions—Circulatory Care: Arterial Insufficiency
- Evaluate peripheral edema and pulses
- Inspect skin for arterial ulcers and tissue breakdown

Nursing Interventions and Rationales

Cerebral perfusion

- If client experiences dizziness because of orthostatic hypotension when getting up, teach methods to decrease dizziness, such as remaining seated for several minutes before standing, flexing feet upward several times while seated, rising slowly, sitting down immediately if feeling dizzy, and trying to have someone present when standing.
  Orthostatic hypotension results in temporary decreased cerebral perfusion.
- ▲ Monitor neurological status; do a neurological examination; and if symptoms of a cerebrovascular accident (CVA) occur (e.g., hemiparesis, hemiplegia, or dysphasia), call 911 and send to the emergency room.
  New onset of these neurological symptoms can signify a stroke. If caused by a thrombus and the client receives treatment within 3 hours, a stroke can often be reversed.
- See care plans for **Decreased Intracranial adaptive capacity, Risk for Injury,** and **Acute Confusion.**

Peripheral perfusion

- ▲ Check dorsalis pedis and posterior tibial pulses bilaterally. If unable to find them, use a Doppler stethoscope and notify physician if pulses not present.
  Diminished or absent peripheral pulses indicate arterial insufficiency (Harris, Brown-Etris, Troyer-Caudle, 1996).
- Note skin color and feel temperature of the skin.
  Skin pallor or mottling, cool or cold skin temperature, or an absent pulse can signal arterial obstruction, which is an emergency that requires immediate intervention. Rubor (reddish-blue color accompanied by dependency) indicates dilated or damaged vessels. Brownish discoloration of skin indicates chronic venous insufficiency (Bright, Georgi, 1992; Feldman, 1998).
- Check capillary refill.
  Nail beds usually return to a pinkish color within 3 seconds after nail bed compression (Dykes, 1993).
- Note skin texture and the presence of hair, ulcers, or gangrenous areas on the legs or feet.
  Thin, shiny, dry skin with hair loss; brittle nails; and gangrene or ulcerations on toes and anterior surfaces of feet are seen in clients with arterial insufficiency. If ulcerations are on the side of the leg, they are usually venous (Bates, Bickley, Hoekelman, 1998).

- = Independent; ▲ = Collaborative

- Note presence of edema in extremities and rate it on a four-point scale. Measure circumference of ankles and calf at the same time each day in the early morning (Cahall, Spence, 1995).
- Assess for pain in extremities, noting severity, quality, timing, and exacerbating and alleviating factors. Differentiate venous from arterial disease.
  In clients with venous insufficiency the pain lessens with elevation of the legs and exercise. In clients with arterial insufficiency the pain increases with elevation of the legs and exercise (Black, 1995). Some clients have both arterial and venous insufficiency. Arterial insufficiency is associated with pain when walking (claudication) that is relieved by rest. Clients with severe arterial disease have foot pain while at rest, which keeps them awake at night. Venous insufficiency is associated with aching, cramping, and discomfort (Bright, Georgi, 1992).

Arterial insufficiency

- ▲ Monitor peripheral pulses. If new onset of loss of pulses with bluish, purple, or black areas and extreme pain, notify physician immediately.
  These are symptoms of arterial obstruction that can result in loss of a limb if not immediately reversed.
- Do not elevate legs above the level of the heart.
  With arterial insufficiency, leg elevation decreases arterial blood supply to the legs.
- For early arterial insufficiency, encourage exercise such as walking or riding an exercise bicycle from 30 to 60 minutes per day.
  Exercise enhances the development of collateral circulation, strengthens muscles, and provides a sense of well-being (Cahall, Spence, 1995). Aerobic exercise training can reverse age-related peripheral circulatory problems in otherwise healthy older men (Beere et al, 1999). Exercise therapy should be the initial intervention in nondisabling claudication (Zafar, Farkouh, Chesebro, 2000).
- Keep client warm, and have client wear socks and shoes or sheepskin-lined slippers when mobile. Do not apply heat.
  Clients with arterial insufficiency complain of being constantly cold; therefore keep extremities warm to maintain vasodilation and blood supply. Heat application can easily damage ischemic tissues (Creamer-Bauer, 1992).
- ▲ Pay meticulous attention to foot care. Refer to podiatrist if client has a foot or nail abnormality.
  Ischemic feet are very vulnerable to injury; meticulous foot care can prevent further injury.
- If client has ischemic arterial ulcers, see care plan for **Impaired Tissue integrity,** but avoid use of occlusive dressings.
  Occlusive dressings should be used with caution in clients with arterial ulceration because of the increased risk for cellulitis (Cahall, Spence, 1995).

Venous insufficiency

- ▲ Elevate edematous legs as ordered and ensure that there is no pressure under the knee.
  Elevation increases venous return and helps decrease edema. Pressure under the knee decreases venous circulation.
- ▲ Apply support hose as ordered.
  Wearing support hose helps to decrease edema. Studies have demonstrated that thigh-high compression stockings can effectively decrease the incidence of deep vein thrombosis (DVT) (Brock, 1994).
- Encourage client to walk with support hose on and perform toe up and point flex exercises.

• = Independent; ▲ = Collaborative

Exercise helps increase venous return, build up collateral circulation, and strengthen the calf muscle pumps (Cahall, Spence, 1995).

- If client is overweight, encourage weight loss to decrease venous disease.
Obesity is a risk factor for development of chronic venous disease (Kunimoto et al, 2001).

- Discuss lifestyle with client to see if occupation requires prolonged standing or sitting, which can result in chronic venous disease (Kunimoto et al, 2001).

▲ If client is mostly immobile, consult with physician regarding use of calf-high pneumatic compression device for prevention of DVT.
Pneumatic compression devices can be effective in preventing deep vein thrombosis in the immobile client (Hyers, 1999).

- Observe for signs of deep vein thrombosis, including pain, tenderness, swelling in the calf and thigh, and redness in the involved extremity. Take serial leg measurements of the thigh and leg circumferences. In some clients there is a palpable, tender venous cord that can be felt in the popliteal fossa. Do not rely on Homans' sign.
Thrombosis with clot formation is usually first detected as swelling of the involved leg and then as pain. Leg measurement discrepancies >2 cm warrant further investigation. Homans' sign is not reliable (Herzog, 1992; Launius, Graham, 1998). Unfortunately, symptoms of already-developed DVT will not be found in 25% to 50% of clients' exams, even though the thrombus is present (Eftychiou, 1996; Launius, Graham, 1998).

▲ Note results of D-Dimer Test.
High levels of D-Dimer, a fibrin degradation fragment, is found in deep vein thrombosis, pulmonary embolism, and disseminated intravascular coagulation (Pagana, Pagana, 2001).

▲ If DVT is present, observe for symptoms of a pulmonary embolism, especially if there is history of trauma.
Based on data from 16 studies, fatal pulmonary embolisms have been reported in one third of trauma clients (Agency for Healthcare Research and Quality, 2000).

Geriatric

- Change positions slowly when getting client out of bed.
The elderly commonly have postural hypotension resulting from age-related losses of cardiovascular reflexes (Matteson, McConnell, Linton, 1997).

▲ Recognize that if elderly develop a pulmonary embolus, the symptoms often mimic those of heart failure or pneumonia (Hyers, 1999).

Home Care Interventions

- Differentiate between arterial and venous insufficiency.
Accurate diagnostic information clarifies clinical assessment and allows for more effective care.

- If arterial disease is present and client smokes, aggressively encourage smoking cessation. See **Health-seeking behaviors.**

- Examine feet carefully at frequent intervals for changes and new ulcerations. Lower Extremity Amputation Prevention Program (LEAP) documentation forms are available at www.bphc.hrsa.gov/leap/ (Feldman, 1998).

▲ Assess client nutritional status, paying special attention to obesity, hyperlipidemia, and malnutrition. Refer to a dietitian if appropriate.
Malnutrition contributes to anemia, which further compounds the lack of oxygenation to tissues. Obese patients encounter poor circulation in adipose tissue, which can create increased hypoxia in tissue (Rolstad, 1990).

- Monitor for development of gangrene, venous ulceration, and symptoms of cellulitis (redness, pain, and increased swelling in an extremity).

• = **Independent;** ▲ = **Collaborative**

Cellulitis often accompanies peripheral vascular disease and is related to poor tissue perfusion (Marrelli, 1994).

Client/Family Teaching

- Explain importance of good foot care. Teach client/family to wash and inspect feet daily. Recommend that diabetic client wear padded socks, special insoles, and jogging shoes.

▲ Teach diabetic client that he or she should have a comprehensive foot examination at least annually, including assessment of sensation with the Semmes-Weinstein monofilaments. If good sensation is not present, refer to a footwear professional for fitting of therapeutic shoes and inserts, the cost of which is covered by Medicare. *Semmes-Weinstein monofilaments are effectively diagnostic of impaired sensation, and early diagnosis enables the nurse to take protective measures to prevent unnecessary amputations (Winslow, Jacobson, 1999). Cushioned footwear can decrease pressure on feet, decrease callus formation, and help save the feet (George, 1993; Feldman, 1998).*

▲ For arterial disease, stress the importance of not smoking, following a weight loss program (if client is obese), carefully controlling diabetic condition, controlling hyperlipidemia and hypertension, and reducing stress. *All of these risk factors for atherosclerosis can be modified (Bright, Georgi, 1992).*

- Teach client to avoid exposure to cold, to limit exposure to brief periods if going out in cold weather, and to wear warm clothing.

▲ For venous disease, teach the importance of wearing support hose as ordered, elevating legs at intervals, and watching for skin breakdown on legs.

▲ Teach client to recognize the signs and symptoms that need to be reported to a physician (e.g., change in skin temperature, color, sensation, or presence of a new lesion on the foot).

NOTE: If client is receiving anticoagulant therapy, see **Ineffective Protection.**

WEB SITES FOR EDUCATION

MERLIN See the MERLIN web site for World Wide Web resources for client education.

REFERENCES Agency for Healthcare Research and Quality: *Prevention of venous thromboembolism after injury,* Summary, Evidence Report/Technology Assessment: Number 22, Rockville, Md, August 2000, The Agency. Web site: www.ahrq.gov/clinic/vtsumm.htm

Bates B, Bickley LS, Hoekelman RA: *A guide to physical examination and history taking,* ed 7, Philadelphia, 1998, JB Lippincott.

Beere PA et al: Aerobic exercise training can reverse age-related peripheral circulatory changes in healthy older men, *Circulation* 100(10):1085-1094, 1999.

Black SB: Venous stasis ulcers: a review, *Ostomy Wound Manage* 41:20, 1995.

Bright LD, Georgi S: Peripheral vascular disease, is it arterial or venous? *Am J Nurs* 92:34, 1992.

Brock JD: Compression stockings: do they prevent DVT? *Am J Nurs* 11:25, 1994.

Cahall E, Spence RK: Practical nursing measures for vascular compromise in the lower leg, *Ostomy Wound Manage* 41:16, 1995.

Creamer-Bauer C: Tissue perfusion, altered peripheral. In Gettrust KV, Brabec PD, editors: *Nursing diagnosis in clinical practice: guidelines for planning care,* Albany, NY, 1992, Delmar.

Dykes PC: Minding the five P's of neurovascular assessment, *Am J Nurs* 93(6):38-39, 1993.

Eftychiou V: Clinical diagnosis and management of the patient with deep venous thromboembolism and acute pulmonary embolism, *Nurse Pract* 21:50, 1996.

Feldman CB: Caring for feet: patients and nurse practitioners working together, *Nurse Pract* Forum 9(2):87, 1998.

George NE: Give em the old soft shoe: working smart, *Am J Nurs* 93:16, 1993.

• = **Independent;** ▲ = **Collaborative**

Harris AH, Brown-Etris M, Troyer-Caudle J: Managing vascular leg ulcers, *Am J Nurs* 1:38, 1996.

Herzog JA: Deep vein thrombosis in the rehabilitation client, *Rehabil Nurs* 17:196, 1992.

Hyers TM: Venous thromboembolism, *Am J Respir Crit Care Med* 159:1, 1999.

Kunimoto B et al: Best practices for the prevention and treatment of venous leg ulcers, *Ostomy Wound Manage* 47(2):34-42, 2001.

Launius BK, Graham BD: Understanding and preventing deep vein thrombosis and pulmonary embolism, *AACN Clin Issues* 9(1):91, 1998.

Marrelli TM: *Handbook of home health standards and documentation guidelines for reimbursement,* ed 2, St Louis, 1994, Mosby.

Matteson MA, McConnell ES, Linton AD: *Gerontological nursing,* Philadelphia, 1997, WB Saunders.

Pagana KD, Pagana TJ: *Mosby's diagnostic and laboratory test reference,* ed 5, St Louis, 2001, Mosby.

Rolstad BS: Treatment objectives in chronic wound care, *Home Healthc Nurse* 9:6, 1990.

Winslow EH, Jacobson AF: Research for practice: saving limbs with the Semmes-Weinstein Monofilament, *Am J Nurs* 99(2):76, 1999.

Zafar MU, Farkouh ME, Chesebro JH: A practical approach to lower-extremity arterial disease, *Patient Care* 30:96-112, 2000.

Impaired Transfer ability

Brenda Emick-Herring

NANDA   **Definition**   Limitation of independent movement between two nearby surfaces

Defining Characteristics
Objective   Impaired ability to transfer: from bed to chair and chair to bed/on or off a toilet or commode/between uneven levels/from chair to car or car to chair/from chair to floor or floor to chair/from standing to floor or floor to standing

Related Factors (r/t)
See Defining Characteristics

NOC   **Outcomes (Nursing Outcomes Classification)**
Suggested NOC Labels
Balance; Body Positioning: Self-Initiated

> **Example NOC Outcome**
> Accomplishes **Body Positioning: Self-Initiated** as evidenced by the following indicators: Transfers from chair to bed and back/Transfers from chair to commode and back/Transfers from chair to car and back (Rate each indicator of **Body Positioning: Self-Initiated:** 1 = dependent—does not participate, 2 = requires assistive person and device, 3 = requires assistive person, 4 = independent with assistive device, 5 = completely independent [see Section I])
> NOTE: This outcome is adapted from the work of NOC.

Client Outcomes
- Transfers from bed to chair and back successfully
- Transfers from chair to chair successfully
- Transfers from chair to toilet and back successfully
- Transfers from chair to car and back successfully

• = **Independent;** ▲ = **Collaborative**

NIC **Interventions (Nursing Interventions Classification)**
Suggested NIC Labels
Exercise Promotion: Strength Training; Exercise Therapy: Muscle Control

> **Example NIC Interventions—Exercise Promotion: Strength Training**
> - Obtain medical clearance for initiating a strength-training program, as appropriate
> - Assist to set realistic short- and long-term goals and to take ownership of the exercise plan

Nursing Interventions and Rationales

▲ Request consult for physical and/or occupational therapists (PT and OT) for upper and lower extremity exercise and strengthening program early in client's progressive mobilization and recovery.
Lower extremity and trunk strengthening will be key for persons doing partial or full weight bearing transfers; upper extremity and trunk strength will be particularly important for sliding board transfers.

▲ Obtain consult for PT, OT, or orthotist to evaluate, prescribe, measure, and fit client with proper orthoses, braces, splints, walking aids, etc.
Assistive devices and walking aids must be individualized to help clients move and function safely, comfortably, effectively, and as independently as possible (Wilson, 1988).

▲ Inquire about and learn the specific techniques and instructions the OT and PT have taught the client to reinforce and assist client as he or she transfers to various surfaces.
Clear communication and a consistent team approach are needed to promote client/family learning, and to monitor client progress so that the approach can be updated as needed (Rehabilitation Nursing Standards Task Force, 2000).

▲ Assess client's size, weight, strength, movement abilities in bed, balance, tolerance to position changes, sensation, behavior, and cognition, as well as staff ratios and experience, to decide whether to do a manual (sitting or standing) or device-assisted transfer. (If PT has already evaluated and identified a specific transfer method and it is compatible with the nursing assessment, use that method).
Data need to be gathered and analyzed to determine a safe type of transfer for clients and staff, once physicians have written out-of-bed orders. Persons who are severely dependent; obese; unmotivated; or who have severe sensorimotor, balance, or postural hypotension problems may benefit from a sitting transfer or a transfer done with an assistive device.

• Do not use the underaxilla method to transfer physically dependent client. Rather, use mechanical devices such as hydraulic or battery-operated mechanical or stand assist lifts.
Underaxilla lifts can cause overexertion back injuries to staff because of the lateral bending, trunk rotation, and full vertical weight lift that it induces. Mechanical devices may be more comfortable physically and psychologically for clients (Owen, Welden, Kane, 1999).

▲ Apply gait belt or walking belt with handles before manually transferring client.
Use of belts decreases staff exertion and back injuries and provides a secure surface to grasp onto if client becomes unsteady or weak or begins to fall (Garg, Owen, 1992; Owen, Garg, 1993).

• Enforce and verbally cue client on how to comply with any weight bearing restrictions ordered.

• = Independent; ▲ = Collaborative

- Assist client to don appropriate orthoses, braces, collars, prostheses, immobilizers, splints, gait belts and binders while in bed (always loosen or remove abdominal binder after client returns to bed).
  These devices stabilize and align necessary body parts during motion. Abdominal binders help prevent postural hypotension.
- Adjust surfaces so that they are as similar in height as possible. For example, lower a hospital bed or use a tub seat or commode that is nearly the same height as the wheelchair.
- Help client put on shoes or socks with nonskid soles before transfers.
  To prevent falls during transfers, have client avoid wearing footwear with a smooth sole, such as antiembolic stockings. Negotiate with diabetics to always wear shoes because their feet heal poorly if injured (Caballero, Habershaw, Pinzur, 2000).
- Remove or swivel a chair's leg rests, armrests, and foot plates off to the side before transferring client.
  This gives client's and nurse's feet more space to maneuver in and provides fewer obstacles to trip over (Ossman, Campbell, 1990; Minor, Minor 1995).
- Place the wheelchair, commode, or shower chair at a 20- to 45-degree angle next to the surface client will transfer onto (e.g., bed, chair, toilet).
  Such an angle gets the two transfer surfaces close to one another yet allows room for client and staff or family to adjust client's movements during the transfer (Wilson 1988; Ossman, Campbell, 1990; Kumagai, 1998).
- Teach client to consistently lock brakes on wheelchairs, commodes, shower chairs, and beds before transfer.
  These devices are often portable and have wheels. If wheels are not locked, they can roll as client transfers into or out of them, thus creating risk for falls.
- Position walking aids logistically so that client can grasp and use them once standing.
  Walking aids provide support and stability to help clients stand and step as safely and functionally as possible (Wilson, 1988).
- ▲ Strongly encourage client to practice transfer techniques in a consistent manner, whether in therapy or during functional activities such as toileting.
  Transfers will be individualized depending on clients' diagnoses, joint range-of-motion, strength, tone, pain, medical restrictions, etc. Repetition promotes motor learning (Carr, Shepherd, 1987).
- Give clear, simple instructions; allow time to process information; and let client do as much of the transfer as possible.
- ▲ Implement and document the interdisciplinary plan of care including the type of transfer (sitting, squat, pivot, etc.), weight-bearing stats (non, partial, full), equipment (lift, sliding board, crutches, etc.), level of assistance (standby, moderate, etc.), and type of assistance to give (manual guidance, balance control, physical levering, verbal cueing, etc.).
  Team collaboration, communication, consistency, and repetitive practice are critical for learning, motor recovery, and safety (Gee, Passarella, 1985; Minor, Minor 1995; Kumagai 1998; Rehabilitation Nursing Standards Task Force, 2000).
- Incorporate set positions before transferring client (i.e., sitting on the edge of the surface/seat with bilateral weight bearing, hips and knees flexed, the front [balls] of the feet aligned under the knees, and the head in midline).

• = **Independent;** ▲ = **Collaborative**

These are the normal movements/postures that prepare humans for weight bearing. These postures permit shifting of weight from the pelvis to the feet as the center of gravity changes during standing (Gee, Passarella, 1985; Kumagai, 1998).

- Recognize the normal sequence of movements for standing (i.e., hips and knees flex; back extends; trunk, head, and finally the knees lean forward over feet; weight shifts to the feet, thus lifting hips and buttocks up; standing occurs as the knees, hips, and trunk extend).

  Realizing normal movements of standing may help nurses identify key points to emphasize and give assistance to client during transfers (Gee, Passarella, 1985; Kumagai, 1998).

- Support or stabilize client's knee(s) with one or both of your knees next to or encircling client's knee(s) rather than "blocking" the client's knee(s).

  This allows client to flex knee(s) and to lean forward during transfers.

- Four methods of transferring clients are described below.

  - Squat transfer: Stand in front of client and guide him or her in the following manner: (1) guide client into the set position for standing, (2) nurse stands with one foot forward as his or her arms lie over client's shoulders with hands on gait belt around client's lower back or on pelvic girdle, (3) nurse shifts weight from his or her front foot to the back foot while reminding the client to lean well forward, (4) client pivots as his or her flexed hips raise from the surface, and (5) nurse rocks forward while lowering the client onto the intended surface.

    These techniques can be used for clients who have sensorimotor disturbances but some muscle control (Ossman, Campbell, 1990; Kumagai, 1998).

  - Seated to standing transfer: Stand in front of client to help unless he or she is using a walker, then stand on the weakest side of the client. Assist client to do the following: (1) attain the set position and lean well forward; (2) slowly stand when instructed to, with nurse placing pressure with his or her hands on client's buttocks to help extend the hips, or on the chest to move the shoulders gently back once erect, or assists with knee extension and stability as client "unfolds" to stand up (a second nurse may be needed if client needs help in all three areas).

    Clients may have difficulty with balance, shifting weight, extension, achieving neutral trunk alignment, or knee buckling or hyperextension. This method is appropriate for clients whose legs and feet are starting to bear weight (Kumagai, 1998).

  - Standing pivot transfer: Stand in front or to the side of client and assist with the following actions: (1) get in the set position; (2) place palms of hands on surface client is transferring from (the chair armrests or mattress), or else on closest surface/armrest client is transferring to; (3) lean forward and flex hips so weight shifts to feet; (4) push with hands; (5) bear weight on both feet while arising to erect position; (6) pivot by shifting and centering weight on the foot next to the chair or surface client is transferring to, which unweights the opposite foot so it can be slid or pivoted; (7) reposition foot back on floor, centering weight on it; (8) unweight the opposite foot; (9) repeat weight shift and pivot maneuver until backside of client touches the desired surface; (10) grasp or place hands on armrest or surface client is transferring to for steadiness; and (11) flex hips, lean forward and sit down. (Using a gait belt, a nurse may need to help client arise, maintain standing balance, and sit back down; a second nurse can help move/control the pelvis from behind the client.)

    This method is appropriate for clients with some weight bearing capability. Unless restricted, it is important for bilateral weight bearing to take place during the sequence of

• = Independent; ▲ = Collaborative

movements, especially in hemiplegics. Pivoting should be done with both feet if possible; if not, with one foot at a time (Kumagai, 1998).

- Sliding board transfer: (1) Ensure client has pants on or put pillow case over board; (2) remove arm and leg rests from chairs and securely lock all brakes; (3) place chair at a 45-degree angle along side the surface the patient is sitting on; (4) assist client to shift weight onto hip opposite the angled chair and place sliding board under the raised buttock; (5) have client shift weight back to normal sitting posture; (6) ensure that board lies angled across both transferring surfaces and that client will miss hitting the wheel of the chair; (7) have client place one hand on sliding board and other hand on surface he or she is sitting on; (8) instruct client to do a series of push ups with the arms, leaning forward slightly to help lift buttocks onto board; (9) move by lifting, not sliding, the body a bit at a time with each push up; (10) nurse(s) may need to stand in front and/or back of client and use a gait belt to help lift client's buttocks with each push up.
Clothing prevents skin from sticking to board. This type of transfer is beneficial for those who can't move their lower extremities or who are extremely weak (Wilson 1988; Borgman-Gainer, 1996).

Home Care Interventions

▲ Obtain referral for OT and/or PT to develop home exercise and transfer regimes, and evaluate home modification and equipment needs such as wheelchairs, tub seats, handrails, and raised toilet seats.
Home evaluation and treatment helps meet the unique mobility needs of clients within their personal environment. Therapists can help families understand, choose, and access needed adaptive equipment to promote independence.

▲ Involve social worker to educate clients and families about equipment cost and financial benefits and regulations associated with Medicare, Medicaid, and third-party payors, as well as local community options for securing durable medical equipment and home care services.
Such information can help families understand the financial implications of desired services and equipment.

▲ Coordinate with therapy services to reinforce client and family education regarding safe and effective transfer methods; application, removal, and care of assistive devices; skin checks and care associated with braces, splints, immobilizers, etc.; and proper fit and use of transfer aids such as canes, walkers, and crutches.
Repetition and a consistent approach reinforce learning and follow through. Over-assisting the client may decrease learning self-esteem and independence.

- For further information see care plans for **Impaired physical Mobility** and **Impaired Walking.**

Client/Family Teaching

- Demonstrate and encourage supervised practice using hydraulic lifts or battery-operated mechanical or stand assist lifts to transfer dependent clients in and out of bed and chairs.
This may help prevent back stress and injuries in family caregivers.

- Teach, model, and monitor client's and family's consistent performance of safety precautions for transfers, including wearing proper shoes, placement of equipment/chairs, locking brakes, applying gait belts, swiveling leg rests out of the way, etc.
Such actions will help prevent falls and injury to clients and caregivers.

- **• = Independent; ▲ = Collaborative**

▲ To reinforce teaching given to family about how to transfer clients left and right, and to/from various surfaces, collaborate with PT and OT if home visits will not be made. Encourage supervised practice before facility discharge and return home.

The basic principles for transfers are constant from surface to surface; however, individuals often need special instruction from a therapist to individualize the approaches for home. Repetitive practice may help habituate these techniques (Gee, Passarella, 1985; Ossman, Campbell, 1990).

• Teach client and family how to check brakes on chairs to make sure they engage. Recommend routine inspection and an annual tune up.

Chronic use may loosen brakes or cause them to slip. The brakes work only if they make sound contact with the tire or wheel; therefore it is important that pneumatic tires are adequately inflated (Minor, Minor, 1995).

WEB SITES FOR EDUCATION

MERLIN See the MERLIN web site for World Wide Web resources for client education.

REFERENCES Borgman-Gainer F: Independent function: movement and mobility. In Hoeman S, editor: *Rehabilitation Nursing: process and application,* ed 2, St Louis, 1996, Mosby, pp 285-269.

Caballero E, Habershaw GM, Pinzur MS: Prevention amputation in patients with diabetes, *Patient Care* May 15, 2000.

Carr JH, Shepherd RB: *A motor relearning program for stroke,* ed 2, London, 1987, William Heinemann.

Garg A, Owen BD: Reducing back stress to nursing personnel: an ergonomic intervention in a nursing home, *Ergonomics* 35:1353-1375, 1992.

Gee AL, Passarella PM: *Nursing care of the stroke patient: a therapeutic approach,* Pittsburgh, 1985, AREN.

Kumagai KAS: Physical management of the neurologically involved client: techniques for bed mobility and transfers. In Chin PA, Finocchiaro D, Rosebrough A, editors: *Rehabilitation nursing practice,* New York, 1998, McGraw-Hill.

Minor MAD, Minor SD: *Patient care skills,* ed 3, Norwalk, Conn, 1995, Appleton & Lange.

Ossman NJH, Campbell M: *Adult positions, transitions, and transfers: reproducible instruction cards for caregivers,* Therapist guide, No. 4166, Tucson, Ariz, 1990, Therapy Skill Builders.

Owen BD, Garg A: Back stress isn't part of the job, *Am J Nurs* 93(2):48-51, 1993.

Owen BD, Welden N, Kane J: What are we teaching about lifting and transferring patients? *Res Nurs Health* 22(1):3-13, 1999.

Rehabilitation Nursing Standards Task Force: *Standards and scope of rehabilitation nursing practice,* ed 2, Glenview, Ill, 2000, Association of Rehabilitation Nurses.

Wilson GB: Progressive mobilization. In Sine RD et al, editors: *Basic rehabilitation techniques: a self-instructional guide,* ed 3, Gaithersburg, Md, 1988, Aspen.

Risk for Trauma

Gail B. Ladwig and Jill M. Barnes

NANDA **Definition** Accentuated risk of accidental tissue injury (e.g., wound, burn, fracture)

Risk Factors
External High-crime neighborhood and vulnerable clients; pot handles facing toward front of stove; knives stored uncovered; inappropriate call-for-aid mechanisms for bed-resting

• = Independent; ▲ = Collaborative

client; inadequately stored combustibles or corrosives (e.g., matches, oily rags, lye); highly flammable children's toys or clothing; obstructed passageways; high beds; large icicles hanging from the roof; nonuse or misuse of seat restraints; overexposure to sun, sun lamps, radiotherapy; overloaded electrical outlets; overloaded fuse boxes; play or work near vehicle pathways (e.g., driveways, lane ways, railroad tracks); playing with fireworks or gunpowder; guns or ammunition stored unlocked; contact with rapidly moving machinery, industrial belts, or pulleys; litter or liquid spills on floors or stairways; defective appliance; bathing in very hot water (e.g., unsupervised bathing of young children); bathtub without hand grip or antislip equipment; children playing with matches, candles, cigarettes, sharp-edged toys; children playing without gates at the top of stairs; children riding in the front seat in car; delayed lighting of gas burner or oven; contact with intense cold; grease waste collected on stove; driving a mechanically unsafe vehicle; driving after partaking of alcoholic beverages or drugs; driving at excessive speeds; entering unlighted rooms; experimenting with chemicals or gasoline; exposure to dangerous machinery; faulty electrical plugs; frayed wires; contact with acids or alkalis; unsturdy or absent stair rails; use of unsteady ladders or chairs; use of cracked dishware or glasses; wearing plastic apron or flowing clothes around open flame; unscreened fires or heaters; unsafe window protection in homes with young children; sliding on coarse bed linen or struggling within bed restraints; use of thin or worn potholders; unanchored electric wires; misuse of necessary headgear for motorized cyclists or young children carried on adult bicycles; potential igniting gas leaks; unsafe road or road-crossing conditions; slippery floors (e.g., wet or highly waxed); smoking in bed or near oxygen; snow or ice collected on stairs or walkways; unanchored rugs; driving without necessary visual aids

Internal   Lack of safety education; insufficient finances to purchase safety equipment or effect repairs; history of trauma; lack of safety precautions; poor vision; reduced temperature and/or tactile sensation; balancing difficulties; cognitive or emotional difficulties; reduced large or small muscle coordination; weakness; reduced hand-eye coordination

Related Factors (r/t)
See Risk Factors

NOC   Outcomes (Nursing Outcomes Classification)
Suggested NOC Labels
Risk Control; Safety Behavior: Fall Prevention

> **Example NOC Outcome**
> Accomplishes **Risk Control** as evidenced by: Monitors environmental risk factors, develops effective risk control strategies, and modifies lifestyle to reduce risk (Rate each indicator of **Risk Control:** 1 = never demonstrated, 2 = rarely demonstrated, 3 = sometimes demonstrated, 4 = often demonstrated, 5 = consistently demonstrated [see Section I])

Client Outcomes
- Remains free from trauma
- Explains actions that can be taken to prevent trauma

NIC   Interventions (Nursing Interventions Classification)
Suggested NIC Labels
Environmental Management; Safety; Skin Surveillance

• = Independent; ▲ = Collaborative

> **Example NIC Interventions—Environmental Management**
> - Provide family/significant other with information about making home environment safe for client
> - Remove harmful objects from the environment

Nursing Interventions and Rationales

▲ Provide vision aids for visually impaired clients.

Vision aids including good lighting, eyeglasses if necessary, and decrease in physical barriers can make it safer for client to participate in activities of daily living (ADLs) (St. Pierre, 1998). A client with a sensory loss must be protected from injury; therefore the visually impaired client must wear vision aids (Potter, Perry, 1993).

• Assist client with ambulation.

Allow client to use assistive devices in ADLs as needed. Assistive devices can augment the client's ability to perform ADLs (Mion, Mercurio, 1992).

• Have family member evaluate water temperature for client.

A client with a tactile sensory impairment resulting from age or psychological or physiological factors needs to be protected from burns.

▲ Assess client for causes of impaired cognition.

Early identification of delirium assists in early intervention, including education and collaboration with other disciplines such as occupational and physical therapy (St. Pierre, 1998).

• Use reality orientation to improve client's cognition.

Clients who are confused lack the insight and judgment to consider physical disabilities and may attempt to walk without assistance (Capezuti et al, 1998).

▲ Make a social service referral for financial assistance.

• Teach safety measures to prevent trauma. Ensure that client can read if using written materials.

The home care nurse can act as advocate, teacher, and caregiver to help patients reach the goals of maintaining function and improving their quality of life (Wright, 1998). Health care professionals have a legal and ethical obligation to provide clients with self-care instructions they can understand (Wong, 1992).

• Keep walkways clear of snow, debris, and household items.

These are personal safety measures to prevent falls (Wright, 1998).

• Provide assistive devices in bathrooms (e.g., handrails, nonslip decals on floor of shower and bathtub).

Assistive devices are personal safety measures to prevent falls (Wright, 1998). These interventions promote mobility, assist to maintain function, and prevent falls (St. Pierre, 1998).

• Ensure that call-light systems are functioning and that client is able to use them.

Hospital injuries often result from a client's attempt to get out of bed and use the bathroom when caregiver cannot be contacted.

• Use a night light after dark.

A night light provides some light in the room to assist with orientation (Hammond, Levine, 1999).

• Never leave young children unsupervised around water or cooking areas.

Young children are at risk for drowning even in small amounts of water. Heat and fire from cooking are a hazard to young children.

• Keep flammable and potentially flammable articles out of the reach of young children.

• Lock up harmful objects such as guns.

• = Independent; ▲ = Collaborative

Accidental discharge of guns is a major cause of trauma.

- Teach to observe safety in high-crime neighborhoods (e.g., lock doors, do not leave home at night without a companion, keep entryways well lighted).
  Adequate lighting helps protect the home and its inhabitants from crime (Potter, Perry, 1993).
- ▲ Instruct clients not to drive under the influence of alcohol or drugs. Assess for substance abuse problem and refer to appropriate resources regarding drug and alcohol education.
  Approximately one out of every sixteen hospitalized patients is admitted because of an injury in which alcohol played a role; therefore a brief intervention for all trauma patients can significantly impact this group of patients (Gentilello et al, 1999). A well-supported relationship exists between alcohol consumption and traumatic deaths from falls, fires, burns, and motor vehicle crashes.
- ▲ Assess all patients for use of alcohol and observe for alcohol withdrawal as appropriate.
  Approximately one out of every sixteen hospitalized patients is admitted because of an injury in which alcohol played a role; therefore a brief intervention for all trauma patients can significantly impact this group of patients (Gentilello et al, 1999). Alcohol withdrawal can be fatal (Mudd et al, 1994).
- ▲ Review drug profile for potential side effects that may inhibit ADLs.
  Drug side effects can alter cognition and gait (St. Pierre, 1998).
- Keep frequently used items in patient's reach.
  This makes manipulating the environment easier for the patient (St. Pierre, 1998).
- See Nursing Interventions and Rationales for **Risk for Injury, Impaired Home maintenance, Risk for Poisoning, Risk for Aspiration,** and **Risk for Suffocation.**

Geriatric

- Assess geriatric patient's level of functioning both at admission and periodically.
  Deconditioning or the physiological changes related to prolonged inactivity are a common problem among hospitalized elderly (Spencer et al, 1999). Admission assessment of the elderly patient's optimal functional status is critical, serving as the goal for functional maintenance and rehabilitation. The key lies in frequent reassessment to detect deviation from the patient's baseline (St. Pierre, 1998).
- Perform a home safety assessment and recommend the following preventive measures: keep electrical cords out of flow of traffic; remove small rugs or make sure they are slip resistant; increase lighting in hallways and other dark areas; place a light in bathroom; keep towels, curtains, and other things that might catch fire away from stove; store harmful products away from food products; provide at least one grab bar in tubs and showers; check prescribed medications for appropriate labels; store medications in original containers or in a dispenser of some type (e.g., egg carton, 7-day plastic dispenser); if the client cannot administer medications according to directions, secure someone to administer medications.
  Home safety assessment and recommendations are personal safety measures to prevent falls. Identifying risks and implementing changes decreases risk of injury (Wright, 1998).
- Mark stove knobs with bright colors (yellow or red), and outline borders of steps.
  Easily visible markings are helpful for clients with decreased depth perception (Potter, Perry, 1993).
- Discourage driving at night.
  A decline in depth perception, slower recovery from glare, and night blindness are common

• = **Independent;** ▲ = **Collaborative**

in the elderly and make night driving a difficult and unsafe task (Ringsven, Bond, 1991).
- Encourage family members to reminisce with agitated client.
  Reminiscence can be used to increase self-esteem, assist in coping, decrease anxiety, and change an altered self-concept (Nugent, 1995). Agitation was the second most common behavior among 1000 residents sampled in 42 skilled nursing homes. Agitated individuals are prone to injury. Reminiscence by a special family member was the only intervention that effectively calmed severely agitated clients observed over a 24-hour period (Woods, Ashley, 1995).
- Encourage client to participate in resistance and impact exercise programs as tolerated.
  These types of exercises have been found to delay bone loss of the total hip (Snow et al, 2000).

Client/Family Teaching

- Educate family regarding age-appropriate child safety, environmental safety precautions, and intervening in an emergency.
  Education in these areas helps to prevent falls and injuries from occurring and enables caregivers to help in an emergency situation (Wright, 1998).
- Teach family to assess day care center's or babysitter's knowledge regarding child safety, environmental safety precautions, and assisting a child in an emergency.
- Discuss various ways an adolescent can protect self from trauma while maintaining peer relationships.
  Most "accidents" are preventable with only a small amount of planning. Motor vehicle crashes and firearm injuries are the two most common causes of traumatic death. Alcohol and drug use are directly or indirectly responsible for 75% to 80% of these injuries (www.rmstewart.uthscsa.edu/Theproblem.html).
- Encourage the regular use of safety belts.
  The risk of fatal injury in motor vehicles is decreased by 45% when wearing a shoulder and lap safety belt (Segui-Gomez, 2000).
- Teach how to plan a safe party.
  Guests can have fun and live to tell about it (MADD, 2001).
- Teach firearm safety. Encourage family to keep firearms and ammunition in locked storage.
  Trauma is a major cause of death in young people. Every day, hundreds of young people die from firearm injuries in inner cities across the country.
- Encourage clients to participate in resistance and impact exercise programs as tolerated.
  These types of exercises have been found to delay bone loss of the total hip (Snow et al, 2000).
- For further information, see care plans for **Risk for Poisoning, Risk for Aspiration, Risk for Suffocation, Risk for Injury,** and **Impaired Home maintenance.**

WEB SITES FOR EDUCATION

MERLIN See the MERLIN web site for World Wide Web resources for client education.

REFERENCES   Capezuti E et al: The relationship between physical restraint removal and falls and injuries among nursing home residents, *J Gerontol* 53(1):M47-M52, 1998.
Gentilello LM et al: Alcohol interventions in a trauma center as a means of reducing the risk of injury recurrence, *Ann Surg* 230(4):473-483, 1999.
Hammond M, Levine JM: Bedrails: choosing the best alternative, *Geriatr Nurs* 20(6):297-301, 1999.

• = **Independent;** ▲ = **Collaborative**

MADD (Mothers Against Drunk Driving): *MADD safe party guide,* retrieved from the World Wide Web June 14, 2001. Web site: www.madd.org/programs/safe_party.shtml

Mion LC, Mercurio AT: Methods to reduce restraints: process, outcomes, and future directions, *J Gerontolog Nurs* 18(11):5, 1992.

Mudd SA et al: Alcohol withdrawal and related nursing care in older adults, *J Gerontolog Nurs* 20(10):17, 1994.

Nugent E: Reminiscence as a nursing intervention, *J Psychosoc Nurs* 33(11):7, 1995.

Potter A, Perry A: *Fundamentals of nursing: concepts, process, and practice,* St Louis, 1993, Mosby.

Ringsven M, Bond D: *Gerontology and leadership skills for nurses,* Albany, NY, 1991, Delmar.

Segui-Gomez M: Evaluating worksite-based interventions that promote safety belt use, *Am J Prev Med* 18(4S):11-22, 2000.

Snow CM et al: Long-term exercise using weighted vests prevents hipbone loss in postmenopausal women, *J Gerontol* 55(9):M489-M491, 2000.

Spencer J et al: Outcomes of protocol-based and adaptation-based occupational therapy interventions for low-income elderly persons on a transitional unit, *Am J Occup Ther* 53(2):159-170, 1999.

St. Pierre J: Functional decline in hospitalized elders: preventive nursing measures, *AACN Clin Issues* 9(1):109, 1998.

Wong M: Self-care instructions: do patients understand educational materials? *Focus Crit Care* 19:47, 1992.

Woods P, Ashley J: Simulated presence therapy: using selected memories to manage problem behaviors in Alzheimer's disease patients, *Geriatr Nurs* 16:9, 1995.

Wright A: Nursing interventions with advanced osteoporosis, *Home Healthc Nurse* 16(3):145, 1998.

Impaired Urinary elimination

Mikel Gray

NANDA   **Definition** Disturbance in urine elimination

NOTE: this broad diagnosis may be used to describe many dysfunctional voiding conditions. The reader is referred to care plans for **Functional urinary Incontinence, Reflex urinary Incontinence, Stress urinary Incontinence, Total urinary Incontinence, Urge urinary Incontinence,** and **Urinary retention** for information on these more specific diagnoses.

Defining Characteristics

The term *lower urinary tract symptoms* (LUTS) is now used to describe the variety of complaints associated with disorders of bladder filling/storage or altered patterns of urine elimination (Jackson, 1999). Bothersome bladder filling/storage symptoms include diurnal frequency (voiding more than once every 2 hours), infrequency urination (voiding less than once every 6 hours), nocturia (arising from sleep more than once or twice to urinate), as well as sensations of excessive urgency or pain associated with bladder filling. Bothersome voiding symptoms include reduced force of the urinary stream, intermittency of the stream, hesitancy, and the need to strain to evacuate the bladder. Other voiding symptoms are postvoid dribbling, feelings of incomplete bladder emptying, and the total inability to urinate (acute urinary retention).

Urinary incontinence is the uncontrolled loss of urine of sufficient magnitude to cause a problem for the patient, family, or caregivers (Hunskaar et al, 1999). Stress urinary incontinence is the loss of urine with physical exertion. Urge incontinence is the loss of urine associated with unstable (hyperactive) detrusor contractions and a precipitous desire to urinate. Reflex incontinence is urine loss associated with hyperreflexic

• = Independent; ▲ = Collaborative

detrusor contractions, diminished or absent sensations of bladder filling, and dyssynergia between detrusor and striated sphincter. Functional incontinence is urine loss associated with deficits of mobility, dexterity, or cognition, or environmental barriers to timely toileting. Urine loss from an extraurethral source can be defined as total incontinence, and urinary retention is the condition in which the patient is unable to completely evacuate urine from the bladder despite micturition. Chronic urinary retention is defined as the inability to completely evacuate urine from the bladder following voiding, while acute urinary retention is the inability to urinate (Gray, 2000).

The term overactive bladder is used to define a cluster of LUTS often associated with urge incontinence (Author unknown, 2000). They include diurnal frequency, excessive episodes of nocturia, and excessive urgency to urinate, with or without the symptom of urge incontinence.

Related Factors (r/t)

- Bothersome lower urinary tract symptoms: urological disorders, neurological lesions, gynecological conditions, dysfunction of bowel elimination
- Incontinence: refer to specific diagnosis
- Urinary retention: refer to specific diagnosis
- Acute urinary retention: refer to care plan for **Urinary retention**

NOC Outcomes (Nursing Outcomes Classification)

Suggested NOC Labels

Urinary Continence; Urinary Elimination; Knowledge: Medication

> **Example NOC Outcome**
> Accomplishes **Urinary Continence** as evidenced by the following indicators:
> Voids >150 ml each time/Empties bladder completely/Absence of postvoid residual
> >100 to 200 ml (Rate each indicator of **Urinary Continence:** 1 = never demonstrated, 2 = rarely demonstrated, 3 = sometimes demonstrated, 4 = often demonstrated, 5 = consistently demonstrated [see Section I])

Client Outcomes

- Diurnal frequency no more than once every 2 hours
- Nocturia 0 to 1 time per night for adults <70 years of age; no more than twice among persons ≥70 years of age
- Able to postpone voiding until toileting facility is accessed, clothing removed
- Able to perceive and recognize cues for toileting, move to toilet or use urinal or portable toileting apparatus, and remove clothing as necessary for toileting
- Postvoiding residual volumes <200 ml or 25% of total bladder capacity
- Absence of pain or excessive urgency with bladder filling and with urination

NIC Interventions (Nursing Interventions Classification)

Suggested NIC Labels

Urinary Elimination Management

> **Example NIC Interventions—Urinary Elimination Management**
> - Monitor urinary elimination including frequency, consistency, odor, volume, and color, as appropriate
> - Teach client signs and symptoms of urinary tract infection

• = Independent; ▲ = Collaborative

Nursing Interventions and Rationales

- Assess bladder function using the following techniques:
  - Focused history including duration of bothersome LUTS, characteristics of symptoms, patterns of diurnal and nocturnal urination, frequency and volume of urine loss, alleviating and aggravating factors, and exploration of possible causative factors
  - ▲ Focused physical assessment of perineal skin integrity and vaginal vault, and evaluation of urethral hypermobility; neurological evaluation including bulbocavernosus reflex and perineal sensations
  - ▲ Review results of urinalysis for presence of urinary infection, polyuria, hematuria, proteinuria, other abnormalities, or obtain urine for analysis

  A history, focused physical assessment, and urinalysis comprise the basic, essential components of evaluation for any patient with dysfunctional voiding complaints (Urinary Incontinence Guideline Panel, 1996; Karlowicz, 1995).
- Complete a more detailed assessment on selected patients, including a bladder log and functional/cognitive assessment. (Refer to care plans for **Functional, Reflex, Stress, Total** and **Urge urinary Incontinence.**)
- Assess the client for urinary retention (refer to care plan for **Urinary retention**).
- Teach the patient general guidelines for bladder health:
  - Avoid dehydration and its irritative effects on the bladder. Fluid consumption for the ambulatory, normally active adult should be approximately 30 ml/kg of body weight (National Academy of Sciences, Food and Nutrition Board, 1980).
  - The patient with irritative voiding symptoms, an overactive bladder, or urinary incontinence should reduce or eliminate bladder irritants from the diet, including caffeine (Gray, 2001) and alcohol (Parazzinni et al, 2000).

    The patient with irritative voiding symptoms or interstitial cystitis should be advised to eliminate a larger variety of bladder irritants including caffeine and alcohol, as well as aspartame, carbonated beverages, alcohol, citrus juices, chocolates, vinegar, and all highly spiced foods such as those flavored with curries or peppers to determine their bothersome LUTS effects (Bade, Peeters, Mensink, 1997; Interstitial Cystitis Association, 1999). To determine the effect of each of these foods, they should be reintroduced into the diet one by one.
  - Avoid constipation via adequate consumption of dietary fluids and fiber, regular exercise, and regular bowel elimination patterns.
  - Avoid or stop smoking.

    Dehydration increases irritative voiding symptoms and may enhance the risk of urinary infection. Constipation predisposes the individual to urinary retention, and it increases the risk of urinary infection. Smoking may increase the severity/risk of stress incontinence, and it is clearly linked with an increased risk for bladder cancer (Pearson, Larson, 1992; Karlowicz, 1995).
- ▲ Consult the physician for culture and sensitivity testing and antibiotic treatment in the individual with evidence of a urinary tract infection.

  The urinary tract infection is a transient, reversible condition that commonly leads to irritative voiding symptoms and urge incontinence in susceptible persons (Urinary Incontinence Guideline Panel, 1996).
- ▲ Refer the individual with irritative symptoms; chronic, burning bladder; and urethral pain to a urologist or specialist in the management of pelvic pain.

- = **Independent;** ▲ = **Collaborative**

Bladder pain and irritative voiding symptoms, in the absence of an acute urinary infection, may indicate the presence of interstitial cystitis, a chronic condition requiring ongoing treatment (Gillenwater, Wein, 1987).

- Teach the client to recognize and manage a urinary tract infection (dysuria, cloudy, odorous urine, suprapubic discomfort with or without fever).
- Teach the client to recognize and to seek help promptly should hematuria occur.
  Hematuria in the presence of irritative voiding symptoms typically indicates urinary infection; however, gross painless hematuria (and bleeding with irritative symptoms) may indicate bladder cancer (Gray, 1992).
- Assist the individual with urinary leakage to select a product that adequately contains urine, avoids soiling clothing, is not apparent when worn under clothing, and protects the underlying skin. (Refer to care plan for **Total urinary Incontinence.**)
- Teach perineal care, including judicious use of soaps and use of vaginal douches only in special circumstances.
  Fastidious grooming or habits in care of the vaginal, rectal, and perineal area may promote dysuria and frequency or may lead to clinically significant urinary tract infection (Maskell, 1986).

Geriatric

- For the elderly client cared for in the home or in acute care, long-term care, or critical care units, provide an environment that encourages toileting.
  Medications, acute or chronic illnesses, insufficient toileting opportunities, and other environmental factors may contribute to functional incontinence or exacerbate other forms of urinary leakage in the elderly client (Morris, Browne, Saltmarche, 1992; Jirovec, Wells, 1990; Gray, Burns, 1996).
- ▲ Perform urinalysis in all elderly clients who demonstrate a sudden change in urine elimination patterns, lower abdominal discomfort, acute confusion, or a fever of unclear origin.
  The common symptoms of a urinary infection, particularly dysuria and suprapubic discomfort, are commonly not apparent in the elderly person (Urinary Incontinence Guideline Panel, 1996).
- Encourage elderly female clients to drink at least 10 ounces of cranberry juice daily and to regularly consume 1 to 2 servings of fresh blueberries, or to supplement the diet with cranberry concentrate capsules (usually taken as 500 mg with each meal).
  Cranberry juice has been reported to exert a bacteriostatic effect on Escherichia coli, *the most common pathogen associated with urinary infection among community-dwelling adult women (Avorn et al, 1994).*

Client/Family Teaching

- Provide all clients with the basic principles for optimal bladder function.
- Teach the community and health care providers that urinary incontinence is not a normal part of aging and that incontinence can be corrected or managed with proper evaluation and care.
- Provide information to health care providers and the community about the signs, symptoms, and management of urinary tract infections and interstitial cystitis.
- Teach all clients the signs and symptoms of urinary tract infection and its management.
- Teach all clients to recognize hematuria and to promptly seek care should this symptom occur.

• = **Independent;** ▲ = **Collaborative**

REFERENCES   Author unknown: Overactive bladder and its treatment consensus conference, *Urology* 55(suppl 5A):1-84, 2000.

Avorn J et al: Reduction of bacteriuria and pyuria after ingestion of cranberry juice, *JAMA* 271:751-754, 1994.

Bade JJ, Peeters JM, Mensink HJ: Is the diet of patients with interstitial cystitis related to their disease? *Eur Urol* 32:179-183, 1997.

Gillenwater JY, Wein AJ: Summary of the National Institute of Arthritis, Diabetes, Digestive and Kidney Diseases workshop on interstitial cystitis, *J Urol* 140:203-206, 1987.

Gray M: Evidence based report card: caffeine and urinary continence, *J Wound Ostomy Continence Nurs* 28(2):66-69, 2001.

Gray M: Urinary retention: management in the acute care setting, part 1, *Am J Nurs* 100:40-48, 2000.

Gray ML, Burns SB: Continence management, *Crit Care Clin North Am* 8:29-38, 1996.

Gray ML: *Genitourinary disorders,* St Louis, 1992, Mosby.

Hunskaar S et al: Epidemiology and natural history of urinary incontinence. In Abrams P, Khoury S, Wein A: *Incontinence,* Plymouth, UK, 1999, Plymbridge Health Publications, pp 198-199.

Interstitial Cystitis Association: *Interstitial cystitis and diet,* Rockville, Md, 1999, The Association.

Jackson S: Lower urinary tract symptoms and nocturia in men and women: prevalence, etiology and diagnosis, *BJU Int* 84(suppl 1):5-8, 1999.

Jirovec MM, Wells TJ: Urinary incontinence in nursing home residents with dementia: the mobility-cognition paradigm, *Appl Nurs Res* 3:11-17, 1990.

Karlowicz KA, editor: *Urologic nursing: principles and practice,* Philadelphia, 1995, WB Saunders.

Maskell R: Are fastidious organisms an important cause of dysuria and frequency? In Asscher AW, Brumfitt W, editors: *Microbial diseases in nephrology,* London, 1986, John Wiley & Sons.

Morris A, Browne G, Saltmarche A: Urinary incontinence among cognitively impaired elderly veterans, *J Gerontol Nurs* 18:33-40, 1992.

National Academy of Sciences, Food and Nutrition Board: *Recommended daily allowances,* ed 9, Washington, DC, 1980, The Academy.

Parazzinni F et al: Risk factors for urinary incontinence in women, *Eur Urol* 37:637-643, 2000.

Pearson BD, Larson J: Improving elder's continence state, *Clin Nurs Res* 1:430-439, 1992.

Urinary Incontinence Guideline Panel: *Urinary incontinence in adults: clinical practice guideline,* ed 2, Rockville, Md, 1996, Agency for Health Care Policy and Research.

Urinary retention

Mikel Gray

NANDA   **Definition**   Incomplete emptying of the bladder

Defining Characteristics

Measured urinary residual >150 to 200 ml or 25% of total bladder capacity; obstructive lower urinary tract symptoms (poor force of stream, intermittency of stream, hesitancy of urination, postvoiding dribbling, feelings of incomplete bladder emptying); irritative lower urinary tract symptoms (urgency to urinate, diurnal frequency of urination, nocturia); overflow incontinence (dribbling urine loss caused when intravesical pressure overwhelms the sphincter mechanism)

Related Factors (r/t)

- Bladder outlet obstruction: benign prostatic hyperplasia, prostate cancer, prostatitis, urethral stricture, bladder neck dyssynergia, bladder neck contracture, detrusor striated sphincter dyssynergia, obstructing cystocele or urethral distortion, urethral tumor, urethral polyp, posterior urethral valves, postoperative complication

- = Independent; ▲ = Collaborative

- Deficient detrusor contraction strength: sacral level spinal lesions, cauda equina syndrome, peripheral polyneuropathies, herpes zoster or simplex affecting sacral nerve roots, injury or extensive surgery causing denervation of pelvic plexus, medication side effect, complication of illicit drug use, impaction of stool

NOC ## Outcomes (Nursing Outcomes Classification)
Suggested NOC Labels
Urinary Elimination; Urinary Continence

> **Example NOC Outcome**
> Accomplishes **Urinary Continence** as evidenced by the following indicators:
> Voids >150 ml each time/Empties bladder completely/Absence of postvoid residual >100 to 200 ml (Rate each indicator of **Urinary Continence:** 1 = never demonstrated, 2 = rarely demonstrated, 3 = sometimes demonstrated, 4 = often demonstrated, 5 = consistently demonstrated [see Section I])

Client Outcomes

- Completely and regularly eliminates urine from the bladder; measured urinary residual volume is <150 to 200 ml or 25% of total bladder capacity (voided volume plus urinary residual volume)
- Correction or relief from obstructive symptoms
- Correction or alleviation of irritative symptoms
- Client is free of upper urinary tract damage (renal function remains sufficient; absence of febrile urinary infections)

NIC ## Interventions (Nursing Interventions Classification)
Suggested NIC Labels
Urinary Retention Care; Urinary Catheterization

> **Example NIC Interventions—Urinary Retention Care**
> - Perform a comprehensive urinary assessment focusing on incontinence (e.g., urinary output, urinary voiding pattern, cognitive function, and preexistent urinary problems)
> - Use the power of suggestion by running water or flushing the toilet

Nursing Interventions and Rationales

- Obtain focused urinary history emphasizing character and duration of lower urinary symptoms, remembering that the presence of obstructive or irritative voiding symptoms is not diagnostic of urinary retention. Query the patient about episodes of acute urinary retention (complete inability to void) or chronic rentention (documented elevated postvoid residual volumes).
  A focused nursing history provides clues to the likely etiology of retention and its management (Gray, 2000a).
- Question the client concerning specific risk factors for urinary retention including:
  - Disorders affecting the sacral spinal cord such as spinal cord injuries of vertebral levels T12 to L2, disk problems, cauda equina syndrome, tabes dorsalis
  - Acute neurological injury causing sudden loss of mobility such as spinal shock
  - Metabolic disorders such as diabetes mellitus, chronic alcoholism, and related conditions associated with polyuria and peripheral polyneuropathies

 = Independent; ▲ = Collaborative

- Heavy metal poisoning (lead, mercury) causing peripheral polyneuropathies
- Advanced stage AIDS
- Medications, including antispasmodics/parasympatholytics, alpha-adrenergics, antidepressants, sedatives, narcotics, psychotropic medications, illicit drugs
- Recent surgery requiring general or spinal anesthesia
- Bowel elimination patterns, history of fecal impaction, encopresis

Urinary retention is related to multiple factors affecting either detrusor contraction strength or urethral (bladder outlet) resistance of flow (Gray, 2000a; Kruse, Bray, deGroat, 1995; Pertek, Haberer, 1995; Anders, Goebel, 1998; Ginsberg et al, 1998).

▲ Perform a focused physical assessment or review the results of a recent physical including perineal skin integrity; neurological examination, inspection, percussion, and palpation of the lower abdomen for obvious bladder distension; neurological examination including perineal skin sensation and the bulbocavernosus reflex; and vaginal vault examination in women/digital rectal examination in men.

The physical assessment provides clues to the likely etiology of urinary retention and its management.

▲ Determine the urinary residual volume by catheterizing the patient immediately after urination, or by obtaining a bladder ultrasound following micturition.

Catheterization provides the most accurate method to determine urinary residual volume, but the procedure is invasive, carries a risk of infection, and may be uncomfortable for the patient. A bladder ultrasound is not as accurate as catheterization; nonetheless it is adequate for clinical judgments and is noninvasive (Bent, Nahhas, Mclennan, 1997; Lewis, 1995).

• Complete a bladder log, including patterns of urine elimination, patterns of urine loss (if present), nocturia, and volume and type of fluids consumed for a period of 3 to 7 days.

The bladder log provides an objective verification of urine elimination patterns and allows comparison between fluids consumed and urinary output in a 24-hour period (Nygaard, Holcomb, 2000).

▲ Consult with the physician concerning eliminating or altering medications suspected of producing or exacerbating urinary retention.

Medication side effects may cause or greatly exacerbate urinary retention in susceptible individuals (Gray, 2000a, 2000b).

• Assess the severity of retention and its impact on quality of life using a symptom score such as the AUA Prostate Symptom Score (BPH Guideline Panel, 1994).

A symptom allows rating of the severity of obstructive and irritative symptoms, providing baseline assessment and evaluation of the efficacy of management.

• Teach the patient with mild to moderate obstructive symptoms to double void by urinating, resting in the rest room for 3 to 5 minutes, then making a second effort to urinate.

Double voiding promotes more efficient bladder evacuation by allowing the detrusor to contract initially, then rest and contract again (Gray, 2000b).

• Teach the patient with urinary retention and infrequent voiding to urinate by the clock.

Timed or scheduled voiding may reduce urinary retention by preventing bladder overdistension (Gray, 2000b).

• = Independent; ▲ = Collaborative

- Advise the male patient with urinary retention related to benign prostatic hyperplasia (BPH) to avoid risk factors associated with acute urinary retention by doing the following:
  - Avoiding over-the-counter cold remedies containing a decongestant (alpha-adrenergic agonist)
  - Avoiding over-the-counter dietary medications (which frequently contain alpha-adrenergic agonists)
  - ▲ Discussing voiding problems with a health care provider before beginning any new prescription medications
  - After prolonged exposure to cool weather, warming the body before attempting to urinate
  - Avoiding overfilling the bladder by adhering to regular urination patterns and refraining from excessive intake of alcohol

  These manageable factors predispose the patient to acute urinary retention by overdistending the bladder and compromising detrusor contraction strength, or by increasing outlet resistance (Gray, 2000b).

- ▲ Teach the elderly male client with BPH to self-administer finasteride or an alpha-adrenergic blocking agent such as doxazosin, terazosin, or tamsulosin as directed. Provide careful instruction concerning the dosage, administration schedule, and side effects of these drugs, including possible adverse effects when multiple doses are inadvertently missed.

  Finasterid is a 5-alpha reductase inhibitor that reduces the risk of acute urinary retention when taken by men with BPH for a prolonged period (McConnell et al, 1998). The magnitude of obstruction associated with BPH is also reduced by routine administration of alpha-adrenergic blocking agents including tamsulosin, terazosin, or doxazosin. However, these agents must be taken regularly to reduce the risk of side effects, including postural hypotension (Narayan, Tewari, 1998; Lepor et al, 1997, 1998).

- Teach the client who is unable to void specific strategies to manage this potential medical emergency including:
  - Drinking a cup of hot tea or coffee
  - Attempting urination in complete privacy
  - Placing the feet solidly on the floor
  - If unable to void using these strategies, taking a warm sitz bath or shower and voiding (if possible) while still in the tub or the shower
  - ▲ If unable to void within 6 hours, or if bladder distension is producing significant pain, seeking urgent or emergency care

  A warm cup of coffee or tea stimulates the bladder and may promote voiding. Attempting urination in complete privacy and placing the feet solidly on the floor help relax the pelvic muscles and may encourage voiding. Warm water also stimulates the bladder and may produce voiding, while the cooling experienced by leaving the tub or shower may again inhibit the bladder (Gray, 2000b).

- ▲ Remove the indwelling urethral catheter at midnight in the hospitalized patient to reduce the risk of acute urinary retention.

  Removal of indwelling catheters offers several advantages to morning removal, including a larger initial voided volume (Crowe et al, 1994) or early hospital discharge with no increased risk for readmission when compared with those undergoing morning removal (McDonald, Thompson, 1999).

• = Independent; ▲ = Collaborative

▲ Consult the physician about bladder stimulation in the patient with urinary retention caused by deficient detrusor contraction strength.
Electrical stimulation of the bladder neck has been reported to provide beneficial results among persons with urinary retention resulting from deficient detrusor contraction strength (Moore et al, 1993).

▲ Teach the client with significant urinary retention to perform self-intermittent catheterization as directed.
Intermittent catheterization allows regular, complete bladder evacuation without serious complications (Horsley, Crane, Reynolds, 1982).

• Advise the person managed by intermittent catheterization that bacteria are likely to colonize the urine but that this condition does not indicate a clinically significant urinary tract infection.
Bacteriuria frequently occurs in the patient managed by intermittent catheterization; only symptoms producing infections warrant treatment (Maynard, Diokno, 1984).

▲ Insert an indwelling catheter for the individual with urinary retention who is not a suitable candidate for intermittent catheterization.
An indwelling catheter provides continuous drainage of urine; however, the risk of serious urinary complications with prolonged use are significant (Anson, Gray, 1993; Stickler, Zimakoff, 1994).

• Advise the person managed by an indwelling catheter that bacteria in the urine is an almost universal finding after the catheter has remained in place for a period of weeks or months and that only symptomatic infections warrant treatment.
The indwelling catheter is associated with frequent bacterial colonization. Most bacteriuria does not produce significant infection and attempts to eradicate bacteriuria often produce subsequent morbidity because resistant bacteria are encouraged to reproduce while more easily managed strains are eradicated (Moore, Rayome, 1995; White, Ragland, 1995).

Geriatric

• Aggressively assess the elderly client for urinary retention, particularly the client with dribbling urinary incontinence, urinary tract infection, or related conditions.
Elderly women (and men) may experience retention of urine of 1500 ml or more with few or no apparent symptoms; a urinary residual volume and related assessments are necessary to determine the presence of retention in this population (Williams, Wallhagen, Dowling, 1993).

• Assess the elderly client for impaction when urinary retention is documented or suspected.
Impaction is a common and reversible factor associated with urine loss and retention among elderly persons (Urinary Incontinence Guideline Panel, 1996).

▲ Assess the elderly male client for retention related to BPH or prostate cancer.
The incidence of urinary retention related to BPH and prostate cancer increase with aging (BPH Guideline Panel, 1994).

Client/Family Teaching

▲ Teach techniques for intermittent catheterization including use of clean rather than sterile technique, washing using soap and water or a microwave technique, and reuse of the catheter.

• Teach the person with an indwelling catheter to assess the tube for patency, maintain the drainage system below the level of the symphysis pubis, and to routinely cleanse the bedside bag.

• = **Independent;** ▲ = **Collaborative**

- Teach the person managed by an indwelling catheter or intermittent catheterization the symptoms of a significant urinary infection, including hematuria, acute onset incontinence, dysuria, flank pain, or fever.

WEB SITES FOR EDUCATION

Merlin See the MERLIN web site for World Wide Web resources for client education.

REFERENCES

Anders HJ, Goebel FD: Cytomegalovirus polyradiculopathy in patients with AIDS, *Clin Infect Dis* 27:345, 1998.

Anson C, Gray M: Secondary complications after spinal cord injury, *Urol Nurs* 13(4):107-112, 1993.

Bent AE, Nahhas DE, McLennan MT: Portable ultrasound determination of urinary residual volume, *Int Urogynecol J Pelvic Floor Dysfunct* 8(4):200-202, 1997.

BPH Guideline Panel: *Benign prostatic hyperplasia: diagnosis and treatment,* Rockville, Md, 1994, Agency for Health Care Policy and Research.

Crowe H et al: Randomized study of the effect of midnight removal of urinary catheter, *Urol Nurs* 14:18-20, 1994.

Ginsberg PC et al: Rare presentation of acute urinary retention secondary to herpes zoster, *J Am Osteo Assoc* 95:508, 1998.

Gray M: Urinary retention: management in the acute care setting, part 1, *Am J Nurs* 100(7):40-48, 2000a.

Gray M: Urinary retention: management in the acute care setting, part 2, *Am J Nurs* 100(8):36-44, 2000b.

Horsley JA, Crane J, Reynolds MA: *Clean intermittent catheterization: conduct and utilization of research in nursing project,* New York, 1982, Grune & Stratton.

Kruse MN, Bray LA, deGroat WC: Influence of spinal cord injury in the morphology of bladder afferent and efferent neurons, *J Auton Nerv Syst* 54(3):215-224, 1995.

Lepor H et al: Doxazosin for benign prostatic hyperplasia: long-term efficacy and safety in hypertensive and normotensive patients, *J Urol* 157:525, 1997.

Lepor H et al: The impact of medical therapy due to symptoms, quality of life and global outcome, and factors predicting response, *J Urol* 160:1358, 1998.

Lewis NA: Implementing a bladder ultrasound program, *Rehabil Nurs* 20:215-217, 1995.

Maynard FM, Diokno AC: Urinary infection and complications during clean intermittent catheterization following spinal cord injury, *J Urol* 132(5):943-946, 1984.

McConnell JD et al: The effect of finasteride on the risk of acute urinary retention and the need for surgical treatment among men with benign prostatic hyperplasia: finasteride long-term efficacy safety study group, *N Engl J Med* 338:557, 1998.

McDonald CE, Thompson JM: A comparison of midnight versus early morning removal of urinary catheters following transurethral resection of the prostate, *J Wound Ostomy Continence Nurs* 26:94-97, 1999.

Moore KN, Rayome RG: Problem solving and trouble shooting: the indwelling catheter, *J Wound Ostomy Continence Nurs* 22:242-246, 1995.

Moore KN et al: Electrostimulation of the bladder neck in acontractile bladder: two case reports, *Urol Nurs* 13(4):113-115, 1993.

Narayan P, Tewari A: A second phase III multicenter placebo study of 2 dosages of modified release tamsulosin in patients with symptoms of benign prostatic hyperplasia: United States 93-01 study group, *J Urol* 160:1701, 1998.

Nygaard I, Holcomb R: Reproducibility of the seven day voiding diary in women with stress urinary incontinence, *Int Urogynecol J Pelvic Floor Dysfunct* 11:15-17, 2000.

Pertek JP, Haberer JP: Effects of anesthesia on postoperative micturition and urinary retention, *Ann Fr Anesth Reanim* 14:340, 1995.

Stickler DJ, Zimakoff J: Complications of urinary tract infections associated with devices used for long term bladder management, *J Hosp Infect* 28:177-194, 1994.

Urinary Incontinence Guideline Panel: *Urinary incontinence in adults: clinical practice guideline,* ed 2, Rockville, Md, 1996, Agency for Health Care Policy and Research.

White MC, Ragland KE: Urinary catheter-related infections among home care patients. *J Wound Ostomy Continence Nurs* 22:286-290, 1995.

Williams MP, Wallhagen M, Dowling G: Urinary retention in elderly hospitalized women, *J Gerontol Nurs* 19:7-14, 1993.

• = Independent; ▲ = Collaborative

Impaired spontaneous Ventilation

Leslie Lysaght

 Definition Decreased energy reserves resulting in an individual's inability to maintain breathing adequate for supporting life

Defining Characteristics

Dyspnea; increased metabolic rate; increased heart rate, decreased PO_2, increased PCO_2; increased restlessness; apprehension; increased use of accessory muscles; decreased tidal volume; decreased cooperation; decreased SAO_2

Related Factors (r/t)

Metabolic factors; respiratory muscle fatigue

NOC **Outcomes (Nursing Outcomes Classification)**

Suggested NOC Labels

Respiratory Status: Ventilation; Respiratory Status: Gas Exchange; Neurological Status; Central Motor Control

> **Example NOC Outcome**
>
> Achieves appropriate **Respiratory Status: Ventilation** as evidenced by the following indicators: Respiratory rate IER*/Respiratory rhythm IER/Depth of inspiration/Chest expansion symmetrical/Ease of breathing/Moves sputum out of airways/Accessory muscle use not present/Adventitious breath sounds not present/Chest retraction not present/Auscultated breath sounds IER/Tidal volume IER/Vital capacity IER (Rate each indicator of **Respiratory Status: Ventilation:** 1 = extremely compromised, 2 = substantially compromised, 3 = moderately compromised, 4 = mildly compromised, 5 = not compromised [see Section I])

*In Expected Range

Client Outcomes

- Maintains arterial blood gases within safe parameters
- Remains free of dyspnea or restlessness
- Effectively maintains airway
- Effectively mobilizes secretions

NIC **Interventions (Nursing Interventions Classification)**

Suggested NIC Labels

Artificial Airway Management; Mechanical Ventilation; Respiratory Monitoring; Resuscitation: Neonate; Ventilation Assistance

> **Example NIC Interventions—Mechanical Ventilation**
> - Monitor for respiratory muscle fatigue
> - Consult with other health care personnel in selection of a ventilator mode

Nursing Interventions and Rationales

▲ Collaborate with client, family, and physician regarding plan and interventions. Ask whether client has advance directive or health care durable power of attorney and integrate those directives into plan of care in conjunction with clinical data regarding overall health and reversibility of medical condition.

• = Independent; ▲ = Collaborative

Many clients and their families make decisions about the level of therapy aggressiveness that they desire. Health care providers have a responsibility to allow the client to participate in care decisions (Campbell, Thill-Baharozian, 1994).

- Assess client's baseline functional status to better understand expectations and the impact of the current clinical condition (Lareau, Meek, Roos, 1998).
- Assess and respond to changes in client's respiratory status. Monitor client for dyspnea, including respiratory rate, use of accessory muscles, intercostal retractions, flaring of nostrils, and subjective complaints.
  It is essential to monitor for these signs of impending respiratory failure (McCord, Cronin-Stubbs, 1992).
- Have client use a numeric scale (0 to 10) to describe dyspnea.
  This allows measurement of the intensity, progression, and resolution of dyspnea (Gift, Narsavage, 1998).
- ▲ Administer indicated diuretics, analgesics, or antianxiety medications. Facilitate position of comfort, and titrate supplemental oxygen as needed (Grossbach, 1994).
  Interventions to decrease heart workload, maintain comfort, minimize anxiety, and increase the available oxygen for gas exchange are necessary interventions in respiratory failure.
- ▲ Assess for chronic respiratory disorder when administering oxygen. With chronic obstructive pulmonary disease (COPD) the respiratory drive is primarily in response to hypoxia, not hypercarbia; oxygenating too aggressively can result in respiratory depression.
  When managing acute respiratory failure in clients with COPD, use caution in administering oxygen because hyperoxygenating can lead to respiratory depression.
- ▲ Collaborate with physician and respiratory therapists in determining appropriateness of noninvasive ventilation. Assist with implementation, client support, and monitoring if noninvasive ventilation is used (Nava et al, 1997).
- Recognize that confusion progressing to somnolence may be an ominous sign of respiratory failure with carbon dioxide narcosis.
- ▲ If client has unresolved dyspnea, deteriorating arterial blood gases, changes in level of consciousness, or panic, prepare client for intubation and placement on ventilator.
  Immediate intervention is necessary for signs and symptoms of acute respiratory failure.
- ▲ Explain intubation intervention to client and family as appropriate and administer sedation for client comfort during procedure per physician order (Kleiber et al, 1994).

Ventilator support

- ▲ Stabilize and tape endotracheal tube securely, auscultate breath sounds, and get a chest x-ray to confirm endotracheal tube placement (Kaplow, Bookbinder, 1994).
  These interventions are necessary to maintain an adequate airway (Hudak, Gallo, 1994).
- ▲ Suction as needed and hyperoxygenate and hyperventilate per policy. Do not routinely instill normal saline (Raymond, 1995). Note frequency, type, and amount of secretions. Communicate any changes to physician.
  These steps ensure adequate oxygenation (Dam, Wild, Baun, 1994).
- Prevent unplanned extubation by maintaining stability of endotracheal tube, suctioning as indicated, ensuring client comfort, and monitoring client ability to understand and follow directions.

- **= Independent; ▲ = Collaborative**

▲ If indicated to prevent extubation, consider relaxation and sedation interventions. Use mitts or wrist restraints if less aggressive interventions are inappropriate or unsuccessful (Grap, Glass, Lindamood, 1995).
Endotracheal tube placement must be maintained to ventilate the client's lungs.

▲ Collaborate with physician in development and implementation of a sedation plan if agitation limits ability to effectively ventilate client's lungs.
Oral intubation and inadequate sedation have been noted to be indicators for unplanned extubation (Chevron et al, 1998).

▲ Analyze and respond to arterial blood gas results.
Ventilatory support must be closely monitored to ensure adequate oxygenation and acid-base balance.

• Support client and family involvement in and awareness of plan of care and treatment goals.

• Assist client in identification and use of an effective alternative communication method, such as using a letter board or paper and pencil or mouthing words.
Alternative strategies of communication prevent isolation and loss (Menzel, 1994).

• Rotate endotracheal tube from side to side every 24 hours. Assess and document skin condition, and note tube placement at lip line. Provide oral care every 4 hours and prn.
These steps prevent skin breakdown at the lip line that results from endotracheal tube pressure (Chang, 1995).

• Assess bilateral anterior and posterior breath sounds every 4 hours and prn; respond to any relevant changes.

• Assess responsiveness to ventilator support; monitor for subjective complaints and sensation of dyspnea (Ferrin, Tino, 1997).

• Monitor respiratory rate and identify ventilator-assisted and independent respiratory efforts.
These methods evaluate the client's respiratory efforts.

• Assess tolerance to ventilatory assistance and monitor for asynchronous chest movement, subjective complaints of breathlessness, and high-pressure alarms.

▲ Collaborate with interdisciplinary team in resolving problems with changes in ventilatory settings, sedation, analgesia, relaxation techniques, or neuromuscular blockers.

▲ Maintain integrity of respiratory circuit. Collaborate with respiratory therapist in response to ventilator alarms; if unable to rapidly locate source of alarm, ambu bag client while waiting for assistance. Common causes of a high-pressure alarm include client resistance and the need for suction. A common cause of a low-pressure alarm is ventilator disconnection.
Bagging the client with an ambu bag connected to oxygen safely supports ventilation until the mechanical problem can be resolved. Ensure that the ambu bag is available, and maintain competence in its use.

▲ Collaborate with interdisciplinary team in treating and responding to cause of underlying acute respiratory failure.
The mechanical ventilator is usually a temporary support until the underlying pathology can be effectively resolved.

• Implement appropriate interventions to maintain client comfort, mobility, nutrition, and skin integrity.
These interventions prevent functional losses (Gift, Austin, 1992).

• = Independent; ▲ = Collaborative

Home Care Interventions

▲ Assist client and family to determine fiscal impact of home care vs. extended care facility with help from medical social worker.

• Assess home setting during the discharge process to ensure home can safely accommodate ventilator support (e.g., space, electricity).

• Have family contact the electric company and place client residence on high risk list in case of power outage (Humphrey, 1994).
Some home-based care requires special conditions for safe home administration.

• Assess the caregivers for commitment to support a ventilator-dependent client in the home.
Commitment to care and valuing home as a healing place provide meaning for participating in caregiving and decrease caregiver role strain (Boland, Sims, 1996).

• Be sure that client and family or caregivers are familiar with operation of all ventilation devices, know how to suction if needed, are competent in doing tracheostomy care, and know schedules for cleaning equipment. Have designated caregiver(s) demonstrate care before discharge.
Some home-based care involves specialized technology and requires specific skills for safe and appropriate care.

• Assess client and caregiver knowledge of disease, client needs, and medications to be administered via ventilation assistive devices. Avoid analgesics. Assess knowledge of how to administer using equipment. Teach as necessary.
Client receiving ventilation support may not be able to articulate needs. Respiratory medications can have side effects that change the client's respiration or level of consciousness.

• Establish an emergency plan and criteria for use. Identify emergency procedures to be used until medical assistance arrives. Teach and role-play emergency care.
A prepared emergency plan reassures the client and family and ensures client safety.

WEB SITES FOR EDUCATION

Merlin See the MERLIN web site for World Wide Web resources for client education.

REFERENCES Boland D, Sims S: Family caregiving at home as a solitary journey, *Image* 28:1, 1996.

Campbell M, Thill-Baharozian M: Impact of the DNR therapeutic plan on patient care requirements, *Am J Crit Care* 3:202, 1994.

Chang V: Protocol for prevention of complications of endotracheal intubation, *Crit Care Nurs* 15:19, 1995.

Chevron V et al: Unplanned extubation risk factors of development and predictive criteria for reintubation, *Crit Care Med* 26(6):1049, 1998.

Dam V, Wild C, Baun B: Effect of oxygen insufflation during endotracheal suctioning on arterial pressure and oxygenation of coronary artery bypass graft patients, *Am J Crit Care* 3:191, 1994.

Ferrin MS, Tino G: Acute dyspnea, *AACN Clin Issues* 8(3):398-410, 1997.

Gift A, Austin D: The effects of a program of systematic movement of COPD patients, *Rehabil Nurs* 17:6, 1992.

Gift A, Narsavage G: Validity of the numeric rating scale as a measure of dyspnea, *Am J Crit Care* 7(3):200, 1998.

Grap M, Glass C, Lindamood M: Factors related to unplanned extubation of endotracheal tubes, *Crit Care Nurs* 15:57, 1995.

Grossbach I: The COPD patient in acute respiratory failure, *Crit Care Nurs* 14:32, 1994.

Hudak C, Gallo B: Management modalities: respiratory system. In *Critical care nursing: a holistic approach,* ed 6, Philadelphia, 1994, JB Lippincott.

• = Independent; ▲ = Collaborative

Humphrey C: *Home care nursing handbook,* ed 2, Gaithersburg, Md, 1994, Aspen.

Kaplow R, Bookbinder M: A comparison of four endotracheal tube holders, *Heart Lung* 23:59, 1994.

Kleiber C et al: Emotional responses of family members during a critical care hospitalization, *Am J Crit Care* 3:70, 1994.

Lareau S, Meek P, Roos P: Development and testing of the modified version of the pulmonary functional status and dyspnea questionnaire, *Heart Lung* 27(3):159, 1998.

McCord M, Cronin-Stubbs D: Operationalizing dyspnea, *Heart Lung* 21:167, 1992.

Menzel L: Need for communication-related research in mechanically ventilated patients, *Am J Crit Care* 3:165, 1994.

Nava S et al: Human and financial costs of noninvasive mechanical ventilation in patients affected by COPD and acute respiratory failure, *Chest* 111(6):1631, 1997.

Raymond S: Normal saline instillation before suctioning: helpful or harmful? a review of the literature, *Am J Crit Care* 4:267, 1995.

Dysfunctional Ventilatory weaning response (DVWR)

Leslie Lysaght

NANDA   **Definition** The state in which a client cannot adjust to lowered levels of mechanical ventilator support, which interrupts and prolongs the weaning process

Defining Characteristics

Severe   Deterioration in arterial blood gases from current baseline; respiratory rate increases significantly from baseline; increase from baseline blood pressure (20 mm Hg); agitation; increase from baseline heart rate (20 beats/min); paradoxical abdominal breathing; adventitious breath sounds, audible airway secretions; cyanosis; decreased level of consciousness; full respiratory accessory muscle use; shallow, gasping breaths; profuse diaphoresis; breathing uncoordinated with the ventilator

Moderate   Slight increase from baseline blood pressure (<20 mm Hg); baseline increase in respiratory rate (<5 breaths/min); slight increase from baseline heart rate (<20 beats/min); pale, slight cyanosis; slight respiratory accessory muscle use; inability to respond to coaching; inability to cooperate; apprehension; color changes; decreased air entry on auscultation; diaphoresis; eye widening, wide-eyed look; hypervigilance to activities

Mild   Warmth; restlessness; slight increase of respiratory rate from baseline; queries about possible machine malfunction; expressed feelings of increased need for oxygen; fatigue; increased concentration on breathing

Related Factors (r/t)

Physiological   Ineffective airway clearance; sleep pattern disturbance; inadequate nutrition; uncontrolled pain or discomfort

Psychological   Knowledge deficit of the weaning process and patient role; perceived inefficacy about the ability to wean; decreased motivation; decreased self-esteem; moderate or severe anxiety or fear; hopelessness; powerlessness; insufficient trust in nurse

Situational   Uncontrolled episodic energy demands or problems; inappropriate pacing of diminished ventilator support; inadequate social support; adverse environment (e.g., noise, activity, negative events in the room); low nurse-client ratio; extended nurse absence from bedside; unfamiliar nursing staff; history of ventilator dependence (>1 week); history of multiple unsuccessful weaning attempts

• = **Independent;** ▲ = **Collaborative**

Outcomes (Nursing Outcomes Classification)
Suggested NOC Labels
Respiratory Status: Gas Exchange; Respiratory Status: Ventilation

> **Example NOC Outcome**
> Achieves appropriate **Respiratory Status: Ventilation** as evidenced by the following indicators: Respiratory rate IER*/Respiratory rhythm IER/Depth of inspiration/ Chest expansion symmetrical/Ease of breathing/Moves sputum out of airways/ Accesory muscle use not present/Adventitious breath sounds not present/Chest retraction not present/Auscultated breath sounds IER/Tidal volume IER/Vital capacity IER (Rate each indicator of **Respiratory Status: Ventilation:** 1 = extremely compromised, 2 = substantially compromised, 3 = moderately compromised, 4 = mildly compromised, 5 = not compromised [see Section I])

*In Expected Range

Client Outcomes
- Remains weaned from ventilator with adequate arterial blood gases
- Maintains blood pressure, pulse, and respiration at baseline
- Remains free of unresolved dyspnea or restlessness
- Effectively clears secretions

Interventions (Nursing Interventions Classification)
Suggested NIC Labels
Mechanical Ventilation; Mechanical Ventilatory Weaning

> **Example NIC Interventions—Mechanical Ventilatory Weaning**
> - Monitor for optimal fluid and electrolyte status
> - Monitor to ensure client is free of significant infection before weaning

Nursing Interventions and Rationales
- While client is on ventilator, coach client to increase overall and respiratory muscle strength. Coach client to strengthen respiratory muscles by differentiating between independent and ventilator breaths.
  Prevent functional losses by setting and maintaining realistic activity goals (Gift, Austin, 1992).
- ▲ Assess client's readiness for weaning as evidenced by the following:
  - Adequate nutritional status with normal serum albumin levels (Grant, 1994)
  - Adequate rest and comfort
  - Resolution of initial medical problem that led to ventilator dependence
  - Stability of any chronic health problems
  - Absence of left ventricular failure
  - Absence of acute hemodynamic event in previous 3 days
  - Psychological readiness, alertness, and stable vital signs
  - Adequate respiratory parameters with a negative inspiratory force >20 cm
  - Ability to clear secretions
  - Fluid balance
  To ensure the best outcome, it is important that the client be in an optimal physiological and psychological state before introducing the stress of weaning (Burns, 1998). Recognize

• = Independent; ▲ = Collaborative

that weaning is both an art and a science. Controlling for known factors that influence weaning success is essential.

▲ Identify any reasons for previous unsuccessful weaning attempts, and include that information in development of weaning plan.
Analyzing client responses after each weaning attempt prevents repeated unsuccessful weanings (Clochesy et al, 1997).

• Support client and family in decision-making regarding placement of tracheostomy tube.
In some cases placement of the tracheostomy tube is associated with a more rapid and successful wean (Koh et al, 1997).

• Promote rest and comfort throughout weaning period (comfortable room temperature, small electric fan if indicated, controlled noise level, comfortable positioning in bed or chair, visitors when desired).
It is important that the client be comfortable during the weaning period.

• Assist client with identifying personal strategies that result in relaxation and comfort (e.g., music, visualization, relaxation techniques, reading, television, family visits). Support implementation of these strategies.
Personal strategies for relaxation are effective (Gift, Moore, Soeken, 1992; Chlan, 1998).

• Support client in setting weaning goals; maximize goal achievement within client's capabilities.
Goals promote client rehabilitation (Weaver, Narsagage, 1992).

• Help client identify the desired amount of information about or participation in the weaning plan; help client identify milestones of progress.
Control of the situation allows clients to participate to their fullest interest and capability.

▲ Collaborate with an interdisciplinary team (physician, respiratory therapist, and nutritionist) to develop a weaning plan with timeline and goals; revise plan throughout weaning period.
Effective interdisciplinary collaboration can positively affect patient outcomes (Baggs et al, 1992).

• Provide a safe and comfortable environment. Make call light button readily available and assure client that needs will be met responsively. Consider timing of other factors in client care environment and impact on ability to provide level of support client may need (e.g., staff off unit, other unit emergencies).
A client who feels safe and trusts the health care providers can focus on the immediate work of weaning.

▲ Do not administer narcotics immediately before weaning; coordinate any pain management routine to effectively offer analgesia with minimal sedative effects (Kollef et al, 1998).

• Schedule weaning periods for time of day that client is most rested. Cluster care activities to promote successful weaning. Avoid other procedures during weaning: keep environment quiet and promote restful activities between weaning periods.
It is important that the client receive adequate rest between weaning periods. The intensive care unit can be a noisy, busy environment. Control of external noises and stimuli can promote restful periods (Cropp et al, 1994).

• Promote normal sleep-wake cycle, allowing uninterrupted periods of nighttime sleep (Higgins, 1998).

• Limit visitors during weaning to close and supportive persons; have visitors leave if they are negatively affecting weaning process.

• = Independent; ▲ = Collaborative

- During weaning, monitor client's physiological and psychological responses; acknowledge and respond to fears and subjective complaints (Logan, 1997).
- ▲ Monitor subjective and objective data (breath sounds, respiratory pattern, respiratory effort, heart rate, blood pressure, oxygen saturation per oximetry, amount and type of secretions, anxiety, energy level) throughout weaning to determine client tolerance and responses.
  Continued assessment and maintenance of airway clearance throughout weaning supports client comfort, safety, and trust (Carroll, Milikowski, 1996).
- Coach client through episodes of increased anxiety. Remain with client or place a supportive and calm significant other in this role. Give positive reinforcement, and with permission use touch to communicate support and concern.
  It is not unusual for a client with lung disease to experience self-limiting episodes of increased shortness of breath. Supporting and coaching a client through such episodes allows weaning to continue.
- Terminate weaning when client demonstrates predetermined criteria or when signs and symptoms of fatigue or intolerance appear as evidenced by a blood pressure increase or decrease of 20 mm Hg, a pulse rate increase or decrease of 20 beats/min, respiration rate of >25 breaths/min or <8 breaths/min, dysrhythmias (especially premature ventricular contractions), decreased oxygen saturation levels, panic, dyspnea, use of accessory muscles, intercostal retraction, flaring of nostrils, changes in level of consciousness, or a subjective inability to continue.
  Immediate response to and intervention in weaning intolerance limits client fatigue and discomfort and promotes the ability for later success.
- ▲ If dysfunctional weaning response is severe, consider slowing down weaning to brief increments of time (e.g., 5 minutes). Continue to collaborate with team to determine if an untreated physiological cause for dysfunctional weaning pattern (e.g., diaphragmatic impairment) remains.
- Consider an alternative care setting (subacute, rehabilitation facility, home) for clients with prolonged ventilator dependence as a strategy that can positively affect outcomes (Rudy et al, 1995).

Home Care Interventions

NOTE: Weaning from a ventilator at home should be based on client stability and comfort of client and caregivers under an intermittent care plan. Client and/or family may be more comfortable having client rehospitalized for the process.

- ▲ Assess comfort and coping ability of client and/or family to wean at home, as well as fiscal implications and home care coverage.
  Compromises in respiratory function are frightening for clients and family who perceive the availability of a high-technology, structured environment as a more appropriate environment for weaning (Sevick et al, 1997).
- Establish an emergency plan and methods of implementation. Include emergency aeration and reestablishment of the ventilation assistive device.
  Having a prepared emergency plan reassures the client and family and provides for client safety.
- ▲ Obtain orders for alternate routes of medication administration when medications have been administered via ventilation device. Instruct client and family in changes.

• = Independent; ▲ = Collaborative

REFERENCES   Baggs J et al: The association between interdisciplinary collaboration and patient outcomes in a medical intensive care unit, *Heart Lung* 21(1):18-24, 1992.

Burns S: The long term mechanically ventilated patient, an outcomes management approach, *Crit Care Nurs Clin North Am* 20(1):87, 1998.

Carroll P, Milikowski K: Getting your patient off a ventilator, *RN* 96(6):42-48, 1996.

Chlan L: Effectiveness of a music therapy intervention on relaxation and anxiety for patients receiving ventilatory assistance, *Heart Lung* 27(3):169, 1998.

Clochesy J et al: Volunteers in participatory sampling of weaning practices: the third national study group on weaning from mechanical ventilation, *Crit Care Nurs* 17(2):72, 1997.

Cropp A et al: Name that tone: the proliferation of noise in the intensive care unit, *Chest* 105:1217, 1994.

Gift A, Austin D: The effects of a program of systemic movement of COPD patients, *Rehabil Nurs* 17:6, 1992.

Gift A, Moore T, Soeken K: Relaxation to reduce dyspnea and anxiety in COPD patients, *Nurs Res* 41:242, 1992.

Grant J: Nutrition care of patients with acute and chronic respiratory failure, *Nutr Clin Prac* 9:11, 1994.

Higgins P: Patient perception of fatigue while undergoing long term mechanical ventilation: incidence and associated factors, *Heart Lung* 27(3):177, 1998.

Koh W et al: Tracheostomy in a neuro intensive care setting: indications and timing, *Anaesth Intensive Care* 25(4):365, 1997.

Kollef M et al: The use of continuous IV sedation is associated with prolongation of mechanical ventilation, *Chest* 114(2):541, 1998.

Logan J: Qualitative analysis of patient's work during mechanical ventilation and weaning, *Heart Lung* 26(2):140, 1997.

Rudy E et al: Patient outcomes for the chronically critically ill: special care unit vs ICU, *Am J Crit Care Nurs* 44:324, 1995.

Sevick M et al: Economic value of caregiver effort in maintaining long term ventilatory assisted individuals, *Heart Lung* 26(2):148, 1997.

Weaver T, Narsagage G: Physiological and psychological variables related to functional status in chronic obstructive pulmonary disease, *Nurs Res* 41:286, 1992.

Risk for other-directed Violence

Gail B. Ladwig and Judith S. Rizzo

NANDA   **Definition**   At risk for behaviors in which an individual demonstrates that he or she can be physically, emotionally, and/or sexually harmful to others

Risk Factors

Body language: rigid posture, clenching of fists and jaw, hyperactivity, pacing, breathlessness, threatening stances; history of violence against others (e.g., hitting someone, kicking someone, spitting at someone, scratching someone, throwing objects at someone, biting someone, attempted rape, rape, sexual molestation, urinating/defecating on a person); history of threats of violence (e.g., verbal threats against property, verbal threats against person, social threats, cursing, threatening notes/letters, threatening gestures, sexual threats); history of violent antisocial behavior (e.g., stealing, insistent borrowing, insistent demands for privileges, insistent interruption of meetings, refusal to

• = Independent; ▲ = Collaborative

eat, refusal to take medication, ignoring instructions); history of violence, indirect (e.g., tearing off clothes, ripping objects off walls, writing on walls, urinating on floor, defecating on floor, stamping feet, temper tantrum, running in corridors, yelling, throwing objects, breaking a window, slamming doors, sexual advances); neurological impairment (e.g., positive EEG, CAT, or MRI; head trauma; positive neurological findings; seizure disorders); cognitive impairment (e.g., learning disabilities, attention deficit disorder, decreased intellectual functioning); history of childhood abuse; history of witnessing family violence; cruelty to animals; fire setting; prenatal/perinatal complications or abnormalities; history of drug or alcohol abuse; pathological intoxication; psychotic symptomatology (e.g., auditory, visual, command hallucinations; paranoid delusions; loose, rambling, or illogical thought processes); motor vehicle offenses (e.g., frequent traffic violations, use of a motor vehicle to release anger); suicidal behavior; impulsivity; availability/possession of weapon(s)

NOC   Outcomes (Nursing Outcomes Classification)

Suggested NOC Labels

Abusive Behavior Self-Control; Aggression Control; Impulse Control; Risk Detection

> **Example NOC Outcome**
> Demonstrates **Aggression Control** as evidenced by: Restrains from harming others/Communicates needs and feelings appropriately/Identifies when angry (Rate each indicator of **Aggression Control:** 1 = never demonstrated, 2 = rarely demonstrated, 3 = sometimes demonstrated, 4 = often demonstrated, 5 = consistently demonstrated [see Section I])

Client Outcomes

- Does not harm others
- Maintains relaxed body language and decreased motor activity
- Displays no aggressive activity
- Demonstrates control or states feelings of control
- Expresses decreased anxiety and control of hallucinations
- Talks about feelings; expresses anger appropriately
- Obtains no access to harmful objects
- Displaces anger to meaningful activities
- Yields access to harmful objects

NIC   Interventions (Nursing Interventions Classification)

Suggested NIC Labels

Anger Control Assistance; Environmental Management: Violence Prevention

> **Example NIC Interventions—Environmental Management: Violence Prevention**
> - Remove other individuals from the vicinity of a violent or potentially violent client
> - Provide ongoing surveillance of all client access areas to maintain client safety; therapeutically intervene as needed

Nursing Interventions and Rationales

▲ Assess for behaviors that indicate impending violence against others: frequent medication change, high use of sedative drugs, past violent behavior, a DSM IV diagnosis of antisocial personality or borderline personality disorder, and long hospitalization.

• = Independent; ▲ = Collaborative

This study indicated that these behaviors and situations are the most powerful predictors of violence (Soliman, Reza, 2001). Knowing, recognizing, and promptly intervening in early precipitating factors prevents violence.

- Assess for presence of hallucinations.
The results of this study support the clinical value of asking about command hallucinations when assessing the risk for violence in clients with major mental disorders (McNeil, Eisner, Binder, 2000).
- Screen for possible abuse in women who have been battered.
Rapid screening tools are needed to identify intimate partner violence. Screening for battering was demonstrated as an effective tool in this study (Coker et al, 2001).
- ▲ Attend to early signs of dangerous interactions with clients; respect boundaries; and talk with colleagues about difficult, uncomfortable situations (Vincent, White, 1994).
Early and appropriate interventions are important to prevent violence. Early warning signs are destruction of objects, thoughts of violence, and aggressive behavior (Vincent, White, 1994). Behavioral warning signs, such as verbal and physical threats, boisterousness, and attacking objects precede violence (Linaker, Bush-Iversen, 1995). Take verbal threats seriously and report them (Linaker, Bush-Iversen, 1995).
- ▲ Allow and encourage client to verbalize anger either one-on-one or in a group setting. Anger is treatable by short-term, cost-effective, structured group programs (Deffenbacher et al, 1994).
- Teach healthy ways to express anger and appropriate gender roles.
A year-long case study at a large university in the south demonstrated the feasibility of meaningfully expanding male students' conceptions of manhood and appropriate gender roles and, thus reducing the likelihood of the men's engaging in sexually or physically violent behavior (Hong, 2000) "Talking replaces action." Talking about anger displaces it and prevents the client from acting on it. Harness anger and use it constructively.
- Help client identify when anger develops. Have client keep an anger diary and discuss alternative responses together.
Creative coping skills and behavioral techniques are helpful for teaching the client (Linaker, Bush-Iversen, 1995).
- Identify stimuli that initiate violence.
Studies found that violence was more likely to take place on inpatient units at shift change, in crowded hallways, at medicine time, and in seclusion rooms during transitional activity time. It occurred less often off the unit in offices when escorted (Holbert, 1995).
- Maintain a calm attitude.
Anxiety is contagious.
- Provide a low level of stimuli in client's environment; place client in a quiet, safe place, and speak slowly and quietly.
A safe, quiet environment decreases the outside stimuli that may be precipitating violent behavior.
- Redirect possible violent behaviors into physical activities (e.g., punching bags, hitting pillows, walking, jogging) if client is physically able.
- ▲ Provide sufficient staff if a show of force is necessary to demonstrate control to client.
When others respond to an escalating or violent situation, it can reassure clients that they will not be allowed to lose control. On the other hand, leave immediately if client becomes violent and you are not trained to handle it.

• = Independent; ▲ = Collaborative

▲ Use chemical restraints as ordered. Obtain an order for medication and administer immediately.
Medications should be offered before physical restraints or seclusion is considered; the medications used most often are haloperidol (Haldol) and lorazepam (Ativan).

▲ Use mechanical restraints if ordered and as necessary.
Physical restraint of children can be therapeutic (Morales, Duphorne, 1995). Clients externalize why restraining occurred ("beyond my control"). Most can verbalize the reason they were restrained (Outlaw, Lowery, 1994).

▲ Follow institution's protocol for releasing restraints. Observe client closely, remain calm, and provide positive feedback as client's behavior becomes controlled.

• If restraints are necessary, provide the client with musical tapes and a headset.
Use of taped music via a headset was an intervention used in hospitalized, restrained patients. Restraints were removed and observable positive behaviors increased from 10 behaviors during the preintervention period to 12 behaviors during the musical intervention. Mr. D. displayed no negative behaviors during the entire study period (Janelli et al, 1995). Listening to music of their own choosing may help produce positive behaviors in previously restrained patients (Janelli, Kanski, 1997).

▲ Know and follow institution's policies and procedures concerning violence.
Being familiar with and following policies and procedures of the department prevents violence. Policies should be developed and training programs provided in proper use and application of restraints (Daum, 1994).

• Protect other clients in the environment from harm. Follow safety protocols of the department.
Proper preparation, training, and implementation of strict protocols can save nurses' and others' lives when violence occurs. Others can be injured during a violent outburst; therefore their safety must be considered.

▲ Always follow up a violent episode with a debriefing of clients and staff.
Debriefing afterward will not only evaluate staff effectiveness but will minimize emotional trauma (Poggenpoel, 1995). Nurses can interact with clients experiencing violence by conducting group or individual debriefing (Poggenpoel, 1995). It is wise to use staff inservicing and debriefing following violence (Morrison, 1989).

Geriatric

• Observe for dementia and depression.

• Observe for signs of fear, anxiety, anger, and agitation and intervene immediately.
Gerontological nurses can prevent the incidence of assault by recognizing the potential risks, preventing patients' fear and anxiety, reducing the outburst of anger, and decreasing patients' agitation (Chou, Kaas, Richie, 1996).

▲ Monitor for paradoxical drug reactions.
Violent behavior can be stimulated by a medication intended to calm the client.

▲ Assess for brain insults such as recent falls or injuries, strokes, or transient ischemic attacks.
Clients with brain injuries need specific interventions such as stimulus control, problem solving, social skills training, relaxation training, and anger management to reduce aggressive behaviors (Teichner, Golden, Giannaris, 1999). Brain injuries, which are related to lowered impulse control and reduced coping, can cause violent reactions to self or others. Brain injury symptoms may be mistaken for mental illness.

• Decrease environmental stimuli if violence is directed at others.

• = **Independent;** ▲ = **Collaborative**

Removal to a quiet area can reduce violent impulses. Use calm voice to "talk down" the client.

▲ If abuse or neglect of the elder is suspected, report the suspicion to local Adult Protective Services (APS) agency. The telephone number for the APS office can be found by checking the blue governmental section of the phone book or by calling directory assistance and asking for the department of social services or aging services. It is essential to call the office with jurisdiction over the geographical area where the elder lives.

This study estimated that a total of 449,924 elderly persons, aged 60 and over, were abused and/or neglected in domestic settings during 1996. More than five times as many of these new incidents of abuse and/or neglect were unreported than those that were reported to and substantiated by APS agencies in 1996 (www.apwa.org/hotnews/neais.htm).

Home Care Interventions

- Assess family members or caregivers for their ability to protect client and themselves.
  Safety of the client between home visits is a nursing priority. Caregivers often need assistance with recognizing or admitting fear of or danger from a loved one.

- Establish an emergency plan including when to use hotlines and 911. Contract with client and family on when to use emergency plan. Role-play access to emergency resources with client and caregivers.
  Having an emergency plan and practicing accessing the plan reassures the client and caregivers. Contracting gives guided control to the client and enhances self-esteem.

- Assess home environment for harmful objects. Have family remove or lock objects as able.
  The safety of the client and caregivers is a nursing priority.

▲ Refer for homemaker services or psychiatric home health aide services for respite and client reassurance.
  Responsibility for a person at high risk for violence creates great caregiver stress. Respite decreases caregiver stress. The presence of caring individuals is reassuring, especially during periods of high client anxiety.

▲ If client is taking psychotropic medications, assess client and family knowledge of medication and its administration and side effects. Teach as necessary.
  Knowledge of the medical regimen supports compliance.

▲ Evaluate effectiveness and side effects of medications.
  Accurate clinical feedback improves physician ability to prescribe an effective medical regimen specific to client needs.

- If client displays mildly intensifying aggressive behavior, attempt to diffuse anger or violence (e.g., ask for a glass of water to distract client). Later in visit explain that aggressive behavior is not acceptable and present consequences of continued aggressive behavior (i.e., right of agency to discontinue services).
  Mild aggression can be diffused safely. Confronting the client before severe aggression is evident places responsibility on the client and family for respectful partnership in care.

- Document all acts or verbalizations of aggression.
  Safety of the staff is a primary responsibility of home health agencies. Law enforcement intervention may be necessary.

- If client verbalizes or displays threatening behavior, notify supervisor and plan to make joint visits with another staff person or a security escort.
  Having a second person at the visit is a show of power and control used to subdue aggressive behavior.

• = Independent; ▲ = Collaborative

▲ Never enter a home or remain in a home if aggression threatens your well-being. Never challenge a show of force such as a gun threat. Leave and notify your supervisor and the appropriate authorities. Document the incident.
Safety of the staff is a primary responsibility of home health agencies. Law enforcement intervention may be necessary.

▲ If client behaviors intensify, refer for immediate mental health intervention.
The degree of disturbance and ability to manage care safely at home determines the level of services needed to protect the client.

Client/Family Teaching

• Teach relaxation and exercise as ways to release anger.

• For religious couples, encourage the use of prayer.
Findings of this study suggest that prayer invokes a couple-God system, which significantly influences couple interaction during conflict. Prayer appears to be a significant "softening" event for religious couples, facilitating reconciliation and problem solving. It deescalates hostile emotions and reduces emotional reactivity (Butler, Gardner, Bird, 1998).

▲ Refer to individual or group therapy.

• Teach the adolescent client violence prevention and encourage him or her to become involved in community service activities.
The results of this study showed that when delivered with sufficient intensity, school programs that couple community service with classroom health instruction can have a measurable impact on violent behaviors of a population of young adolescents at high risk for being both the perpetrators and victims of peer violence. Community service programs may be an effective supplement to curricular interventions and a valuable component of multicomponent violence prevention programs (O'Donnell et al, 1999).

• Teach caregivers and family members of clients with dementia to use expressive physical touch and verbalization (EPT/V) when caring for these clients.
In this study findings are that (1) anxiety is lower immediately following EPT/V and (2) EPT/V causes decreasing episodes of dysfunctional behavior. It is cost-effective, simple to learn and practice, and it is most effective in improving and maintaining a patient's high quality of life (Kim, Buschmann, 1999).

• Teach use of appropriate community resources in emergency situations (e.g., hotline, community mental health agency, emergency room, 911 in most places in the United States, or the toll-free National Domestic Violence Hotline [1-800-799-SAFE]) (National Domestic Violence Hotline).
It is necessary to get immediate help when violence occurs.

▲ Encourage use of self-help groups in nonemergency situations.

▲ Inform client and family about medication actions, side effects, target symptoms, and toxic reactions.

WEB SITES FOR EDUCATION

MERLIN See the MERLIN web site for World Wide Web resources for client education.

REFERENCES   Butler MH, Gardner BC, Bird MH: Not just a time-out: change dynamics of prayer for religious couples in conflict situations, *Fam Process* 37(4):451-478, 1998.
Chou K, Kaas M, Richie M: Assaultive behavior in geriatric patients, *J Gerontol Nurs* 22(11):30, 1996.
Coker AL et al: Assessment of clinical partner violence screening tools, *J Am Med Womens Assoc* 56(1):19-23, 2001.

• = **Independent;** ▲ = **Collaborative**

Daum A: Disruptive antisocial patient: management strategies, *Nurs Manage* 8:46, 1994.

Deffenbacher J et al: Social skills and cognitive relaxation approaches to general anger reduction, *J Counseling Psychol* 41:386, 1994.

Holbert S: *Staff injuries: patient actions*, Canada, 1995 (unpublished manuscript).

Hong L: Toward a transformed approach to prevention: breaking the link between masculinity and violence, *J Am Coll Health* 48(6):269-279, 2000.

Janelli LM, Kanski GW: Music intervention with physically restrained patients, *Rehabil Nurs* 22(1):14, 1997.

Janelli LM et al: Exploring music intervention with restrained patients, *Nurs Forum* 30(4):12, 1995.

Kim EJ, Buschmann MT: The effect of expressive physical touch on patients with dementia, *Int J Nurs Stud* 36(3):235-243, 1999.

Linaker O, Bush-Iversen H: Predictors of imminent violence in psychiatric inpatients, *Acta Psychiatr Scand* 92:250, 1995.

McNeil DE, Eisner JP, Binder RL: The relationship between command hallucinations and violence, *Psychiatr Serv* 51(10):1288-1292, 2000.

Morales E, Duphorne P: Least restrictive measures: alternatives to four-pt. restraints and seclusion, *J Psychosoc Nurs Ment Health Serv* 33:13, 1995.

Morrison E: Theoretical modeling to predict violence in hospitalized psychiatric patients, *Res Nurs Health* 12:31, 1989.

National Domestic Violence Hotline: retrieved from the World Wide Web June 13, 2001. Web site: www.ndvh.org

O'Donnell L et al: Violence prevention and young adolescents' participation in community youth service, *J Adolesc Health* 24(1):28, 1999.

Outlaw F, Lowery B: An attributional study of seclusion and restraint of psychiatric patients, *Arch Psych Nurs* 8:69, 1994.

Poggenpoel M: Role and functions of psychiatric-mental health nurse in care and comfort of individuals, families and communities subject to violence, *Holistic Nurs Pract* 9:91, 1995.

Soliman AE, Reza H: Risk factors and correlates of violence among acutely ill adult psychiatric inpatients, *Psychiatr Serv* 52(1):75-80, 2001.

Teichner G, Golden CJ, Giannaris WJ: A multimodal approach to treatment of aggression in a severely brain-injured adolescent, *Rehabil Nurs* 24(5):207-211, 1999.

Vincent M, White K: Patient violence toward a nurse: predictable and preventable, *J Psychosoc Nurs Ment Health Serv* 32:31, 1994.

Risk for self-directed Violence

Gail B. Ladwig and Judith S. Rizzo

 Definition At risk for behaviors in which an individual demonstrates that he or she can be physically, emotionally, and/or sexually harmful to self

Risk Factors

Body language: rigid posture, clenching of fists and jaw, hyperactivity, pacing, breathlessness, threatening stances; history of violence against others (e.g., hitting someone, kicking someone, spitting at someone, scratching someone, throwing objects at someone, biting someone, attempted rape, rape, sexual molestation, urinating/defecating on a person); history of threats of violence (e.g., verbal threats against property, verbal threats against person, social threats, cursing, threatening notes/letters, threatening gestures, sexual threats); history of violent antisocial behavior (e.g., stealing, insistent borrowing, insistent demands for privileges, insistent interruption of meetings, refusal to eat, refusal to take medication, ignoring instructions); history of violence, indirect (e.g., tearing off clothes, ripping objects off walls, writing on walls, urinating on floor, def-

• = **Independent;** ▲ = **Collaborative**

ecating on floor, stamping feet, temper tantrum, running in corridors, yelling, throwing objects, breaking a window, slamming doors, sexual advances); neurological impairment (e.g., positive EEG, CAT, or MRI; head trauma; positive neurological findings; seizure disorders); cognitive impairment (e.g., learning disabilities, attention deficit disorder, decreased intellectual functioning); history of childhood abuse; history of witnessing family violence; cruelty to animals; fire setting; prenatal/perinatal complications or abnormalities; history of drug or alcohol abuse; pathological intoxication; psychotic symptomatology (e.g., auditory, visual, command hallucinations; paranoid delusions; loose, rambling, or illogical thought processes); motor vehicle offenses (e.g., frequent traffic violations, use of a motor vehicle to release anger); suicidal behavior; impulsivity; availability/possession of weapon(s)

NOC ## Outcomes (Nursing Outcomes Classification)
Suggested NOC Labels
Cognitive Ability, Depression Control, Distorted Thought Control, Impulse Control, Self-Mutilation Restraint, Suicide Self-Restraint, Will to Live

> **Example NOC Outcome**
> Demonstrates **Suicide Self-Restraint** as evidenced by: Expresses feelings and seeks help when feeling self-destructive/Verbalizes and controls suicidal ideas and impulses (Rate each indicator of **Suicide Self-Restraint:** 1 = never demonstrated, 2 = rarely demonstrated, 3 = sometimes demonstrated, 4 = often demonstrated, 5 = consistently demonstrated [see Section I])

Client Outcomes
- Does not harm self
- Maintains relaxed body language and decreased motor activity
- Demonstrates control or states feelings of control
- Expresses decreased anxiety and control of hallucinations
- Talks about feelings; expresses anger appropriately
- Obtains no access to harmful objects
- Displaces anger to meaningful activities
- Yields access to harmful objects

NIC ## Interventions (Nursing Interventions Classification)
Suggested NIC Labels
Anger Control Assistance; Anxiety Reduction; Coping Enhancement; Crisis Intervention; Suicide Prevention; Surveillance

> **Example NIC Interventions—Suicide Prevention**
> - Determine presence and degree of suicide risk
> - Encourage client to seek out care providers to talk as urge to harm self occurs

Nursing Interventions and Rationales
- Refer to care plan for **Risk for Suicide.**
- ▲ Monitor, document, and report client's potential for suicide.
  Traits such as impulsivity, poor social adjustment, and mood disorders are associated with adolescent suicide attempts (Brent et al, 1994).

• = Independent; ▲ = Collaborative

▲ Monitor suicidal behaviors or verbalizations (e.g., giving away possessions, stating "I'm going to kill myself" or "My parents won't have to worry about having me around anymore").
Ideation precedes planning, which may result in an attempt leading to death. If nonfatal, the attempt may increase the likelihood of subsequent ideation, planning, and attempt (Vilhjalmsson, Kristjansdottir, Sveinbjarnardottir, 1998).

▲ Monitor seriousness of intent; ask client, "Do you have a plan?" "How will you do it?" and "Do you have the means?"
Always use a planned intervention model to assess suicide risk and intent.

▲ Observe client's behavior every 15 minutes while the client is actively suicidal; stagger observation times.
Staggering observations ensures that the client does not memorize a pattern.

▲ Remove all dangerous objects from client's environment.
Controlling the environment may be a viable strategy for preventing suicide (Leenaars et al, 2000).

▲ Use suicide precautions if indicated, such as one-to-one staffing (constant attendance) and removal of all dangerous objects.

▲ Make a verbal or written contract with client. Have client state or write, "I will notify staff if I have suicidal or violent thoughts" or "I will not act on my thoughts."
Written contracts are not legal documents and should be used only as an adjunct to other interventions, never as the primary treatment intervention.
NOTE: If suicidal client is demonstrating violent behavior, Nursing Interventions and Rationales for **Risk for other-directed Violence** may be appropriate.

Geriatric

• Monitor for suicidal risk.
The elderly, who experience multiple losses and have fragile support systems, are at greatest risk for suicide. Assess risk, death wishes, and suicidal thoughts. Consider noncompliance with medical treatment a possible means to suicide. Also assess stress, social support, and vulnerability to guide interventions (Valente, 1994).

• Observe for dementia and depression.

• Monitor for paradoxical drug reactions.
Violent behavior can be stimulated by a medication intended to calm the client.

• Assess for brain insults such as recent falls or injuries, strokes, or transient ischemic attacks.
Brain injuries, which are related to lowered impulse control and reduced coping, can cause violent reactions to self or others. Brain injury symptoms may be mistaken for mental illness.

• Decrease environmental stimuli if violence is directed at others.
Removal to a quiet area can reduce violent impulses. Use a calm voice to "talk down" the client.

Home Care Interventions

• Assess family members or caregivers for their ability to protect client and themselves.
Safety of the client between home visits is a nursing priority. Caregivers often need assistance with recognizing or admitting fear of or danger from a loved one.

• Establish an emergency plan including when to use hotlines and 911. Contract with client and family on when to use emergency plan. Role-play access to emergency resources with client and caregivers.

• = **Independent;** ▲ = **Collaborative**

Having an emergency plan and practicing accessing the plan reassures the client and care-givers. Contracting gives guided control to the client and enhances self-esteem.

- Assess home environment for harmful objects. Have family remove or lock objects as able.
Safety of the client and caregivers is a nursing priority.

▲ Refer for homemaker services or psychiatric home health aide services for respite and client reassurance.
Responsibility for a person at high risk for violence creates great caregiver stress. Respite decreases caregiver stress. The presence of caring individuals is reassuring, especially during periods of high client anxiety.

▲ If client is on psychotropic medications, assess client and family knowledge of medication and its administration and side effects. Teach as necessary.
Knowledge of the medical regimen supports compliance.

▲ Evaluate effectiveness and side effects of medications.
Accurate clinical feedback improves physician ability to prescribe an effective medical regimen specific to client needs.

- If client displays mildly intensifying aggressive behavior, attempt to diffuse anger or violence (e.g., ask for a glass of water to distract client). Later in visit explain that aggressive behavior is not acceptable and present consequences of continued aggressive behavior (e.g., right of agency to discontinue services).
Mild aggression can be diffused safely. Confronting the client before severe aggression is evident places responsibility on the client and family for respectful partnership in care.

Client/Family Teaching

- Teach relaxation and exercise as ways to release anger.
▲ Refer to individual or group therapy.
- Teach family how to recognize client is at increased risk for suicide (changes in behavior and verbal and nonverbal communication, withdrawal, depression, or sudden lifting of depression).
A client may be at peace because a suicide plan has been made and the client has the energy to carry it out. Therefore when depression lifts, increased vigilance is necessary.

- Teach use of appropriate community resources in emergency situations (e.g., hotline, community mental health agency, emergency room).
- Encourage use of self-help groups in nonemergency situations.
▲ Inform client and family about medication actions, side effects, target symptoms, and toxic reactions.

WEB SITES FOR EDUCATION

Merlin   See the MERLIN web site for World Wide Web resources for client education.

REFERENCES   Brent D et al: Personality disorder, personality traits, impulsive violence and completed suicide in adolescents, *J Am Acad Child Adolescent Psychiatry* 33:1080, 1994.
Leenaars A et al: Controlling the environment to prevent suicide: international perspectives, *Can J Psychiatry* 45(7):639-644, 2000.
Valente S: Suicide and elderly people: assessment and intervention, *J Death Dying* 28:317, 1994.
Vilhjalmsson R, Kristjansdottir G, Sveinbjarnardottir E: Factors associated with suicide ideation in adults, *Soc Psychiatry Psychiatr Epidemiol* 33(3):97, 1998.

• = **Independent**; ▲ = **Collaborative**

Impaired Walking

Brenda Emick-Herring

NANDA   **Definition** Limitation of independent movement within the environment on foot (or artificial limb)

Defining Characteristics
Unable to climb stairs; unable to walk on uneven surface; unable to walk required distances; unable to walk on even surfaces; unable to walk on an incline or decline; unable to navigate curbs

Related Factors (r/t)
Intolerance to activity; decreased strength and endurance; pain or discomfort; perceptual or cognitive impairment; neuromuscular impairment; musculoskeletal impairment; depression; severe anxiety; and lower extremity amputation

NOTE: These are the same as the etiologies for **Impaired physical Mobility** with the addition of lower extremity amputation.

Suggested functional level classifications follow:

0	Completely independent
1	Requires use of equipment or device
2	Requires help from another person for assistance, supervision, or teaching
3	Requires help from another person and equipment device
4	Dependent—does not participate in activity

NOC   **Outcomes (Nursing Outcomes Classification)**
Suggested NOC Labels
Ambulation: Walking; Mobility Level

> **Example NOC Outcome**
> Accomplishes **Ambulation: Walking** as evidenced by the following indicators: Walks with effective gait/Walks at moderate pace/Walks up and down steps/Walks moderate distance (Rate each indicator of **Ambulation: Walking:** 1 = dependent—does not participate, 2 = requires assistive person and device, 3 = requires assistive person, 4 = independent with assistive device, 5 = completely independent [see Section I])

Client Outcomes/Goals
- Demonstrates optimal independence and safety in walking
- Demonstrates the ability to direct others on how to assist with walking
- Demonstrates the ability to properly and safely use and care for assistive walking devices

NIC   **Interventions (Nursing Interventions Classification)**
Suggested NIC Labels
Exercise Therapy: Ambulation

> **Example NIC Interventions—Exercise Therapy: Ambulation**
> - Assist client to use footwear that facilitates walking and prevents injury
> - Encourage to sit in bed, on side of bed ("dangle"), or in chair, as tolerated

• = Independent; ▲ = Collaborative

Nursing Interventions and Rationales

▲ Reinforce or request physical therapy consult to teach "bridging"; have client use the technique to move side-to-side in bed and to raise buttocks off bed.
This bed activity prepares a person for walking because it involves hip extension with simultaneous weight bearing through the lower extremity. It is particularly helpful for hemiplegics (Bobath, 1978; Gee, Passarella, 1985).

▲ Apply antiembolic stockings and abdominal binders, elevate the head of the bed in small increments to as high a degree as tolerated, and provide adequate hydration to persons who are at risk for or who initially display postural hypotension when standing and walking.
These measures promote circulatory redistribution to prevent blood volume from pooling in the lower extremities (Perdue, 1998).

▲ Remind clients of physician orders regarding weight bearing limitations during walking (e.g., "non–weight bearing on left foot" or "partial weight bearing on right wrist").
Weight bearing may retard bone healing in fractured extremities.

• Encourage frequent weight bearing and walking in persons who have no physician restrictions.
Weight bearing and skeletal muscle contraction stimulates bone growth and calcium resorption thus helping to maintain bone density, prevent disuse osteoporosis, and regulate many physiological processes in the body (Rubin, 1988; Kipnis, 1993).

• Assist clients to properly apply orthoses, immobilizers, splints, and braces before walking.
These devices maintain joint stability, immobilization, and alignment during movement, especially when the wearer is upright (e.g., an ankle foot orthosis maintains the ankle in neutral alignment to prevent ankle twisting, foot drop, and potential falls) (Wilson, 1988).

• Assist clients with lower extremity amputations to correctly don lower extremity sheath, stump socks, liner, and prosthesis before walking.
Prostheses increase a person's functional ability to walk, and they cosmetically look similar to lost lower limbs. A thin nylon sheath is often applied over the residual limb to prevent it from turning in the socket of the prosthesis. Stump socks of varying thickness are used to establish a proper fit between the residual limb and the socket of the prosthesis. A liner is put on last before putting the stump into the socket of the prosthesis. The stump should not touch the bottom of the socket because a pressure ulcer may form (Kipnis 1993; Yeltzer, 1998).

• Collect a baseline pulse rate and rhythm before walking client, then check pulse 5 minutes after walking. Stop walking if the pulse rises 50 beats from baseline, climbs to 122 beats/min, or becomes irregular.
Pulse monitoring indicates cardiac tolerance to walking. If an abnormal pulse occurs, stop walking and let client sit and rest about 5 minutes before taking the pulse again. If pulse is still abnormal, walking may need to be done more slowly, with more help, or for a shorter period. If the pulse rises too high after a few walking trials, it is probably too difficult a task and the physician should be notified (Wilson, 1988; Radwanski, Hoeman, 1996).

▲ Monitor client's tolerance for walking by assessing his or her physical status. Initiate a 5-minute rest period if shortness of breath, use of accessory muscles to breathe, chest pain, nausea, cold sweat, pale or flushed skin, dizziness, syncope, diaphoresis, or mental confusion are noted. If signs persist, notify the physician.
NOTE: For more information on assessing vital sign changes with activity, refer to the care plan for **Activity intolerance.**

• = Independent; ▲ = Collaborative

▲ Use appropriate assistive devices when walking client, including gait (walking) belts, walkers, crutches, wheelchairs, and canes.
Snug gait belts may help prevent staff back injuries and provide a surface for nurses to grasp to steady a client who begins to fall or lose balance (therapists call this "guarding"). Assistive devices help compensate for poor balance, coordination, and strength. They also provide stability and support during walking (Minor, Minor, 1995).

▲ Obtain appropriate number of people to help walk the client. One team member should give simple instructions to the client and assistants (e.g., verbally cue the client to raise the head, straighten the trunk, or lift a foot higher for example, or cue the assistant to help the client lean a certain direction or stabilize a knee while stepping).
Having one spokesperson give directions prevents confusion and mixed messages. Walking takes concentration and thinking, especially if the client is learning to use an assistive device for the first time (Minor, Minor, 1995). Ingvor and Philipson (1977) and Yonekura (1981) found that blood flow increased about 20% when a participant was thinking. Adequate helpers are needed to prevent client falls and injury and to relieve client fear and anxiety. Fear, anxiety, and fatigue can abnormally decrease tone (Gee, Passarella, 1985).

▲ Ask the physical therapist where to stand in relation to client as he or she walks. Assistants commonly stand slightly behind and to the side of the client, holding on to his or her gait belt with one supinated hand. The assistant's other hand then can rest lightly on the client's closest shoulder.
The assistant needs to be nearby and ready to assist in case the client begins to fall, but not so close that the assistant interferes with the client's movements. The forearms have more strength when supinated (Minor, Minor, 1995).

• Limit distractions and environmental clutter while the client walks. Staff should monitor the environment for safety because the client needs to concentrate on walking and often looks at where his or her feet are and where the assistive device is while stepping
Active attending, thinking, and visualization give the client necessary input about where the feet and assistive device are in relation to the body (Minor, Minor, 1995).

• Allow distractions and obstacles as client's balance, gait, coordination, endurance, and concentration improve.
This prepares clients for walking in real life situations.

• Indicate on the care plan how many assistants it takes to walk the client, the level of assistance needed (e.g., maximum, moderate, or minimal assistance or stand-by assist); the type of assistance needed (e.g., physical support, instructional cues [verbal and/or tactile], balance control, or actual lifting), and the specific assistive devices needed to walk.
Clear communication establishes a consistent approach to client care and motor relearning. Consistent practice (repetition and rehearsal) of the motor task promotes learning (Carr, Shepherd, 1987).

Geriatric

• Monitor pulse, respirations, and blood pressure before and 5 minutes after beginning a new activity. Stop activity if any of the following are detected: resting heart rate >100 beats/min; exercise heart rate that is 35% > the resting rate; exercise systolic blood pressure >25 to 35 mm Hg above resting pressure; or a decrease in systolic blood pressure that is >20 mm Hg (Radwanski, Hoeman, 1996).

• = Independent; ▲ = Collaborative

- Employ safety and fall precautions for elderly client such as visual identification (arm bands, etc.) on client at high risk for falling, call system within reach, client education to call for help before standing and walking, bed/chair alarm or one-to-one observation for client with cognitive or memory impairment, obstacle clearance, and assistive devices that are properly chosen and measured specifically for client.
  Assessment and preventative implementation of safety measures are appropriate for elderly clients because many experience impaired balance and unsteadiness when changing positions or walking. Postural control disturbances occur with aging, chronic disease, visual function changes, and medications, all of which place clients at risk for falls (Alexander, 1994; Ulfarsson, Robinson, 1997).
- If client experiences dizziness resulting from orthostatic hypotension when arising, teach methods to decrease dizziness such as rising slowly, remaining seated several minutes before standing, flexing feet upward several times while sitting, sitting down immediately if feeling dizzy, and trying to have someone present when standing.
  The elderly develop decreased baroreceptor sensitivity and decreased ability of compensatory mechanisms to maintain blood pressure when standing up, resulting in postural hypotension (Matteson, McConnell, Linton, 1997).
- Emphasize the importance of wearing firm, low-heeled shoes with nonskid and nonfriction soles.

Home Care Interventions

- ▲ Assess client and obtain complete history with reference to reasons for impairment.
  Complete understanding of the client problem promotes accurate determination of client needs and individualized care.
- Explain the importance of adequate lighting both day and night; tacking carpet edges down, removing throw rugs from traffic flow areas, and having nonskid backing on those that are used; applying nonskid wax on floors; and removing clutter, especially small objects, from the floor.
  Removal of potential environmental hazards is a means of preventing falls in the elderly (Ulfarsson, Robinson, 1997).
- Assess home environment for all barriers to walking.
- If client resides alone, assess support system for emergency and contingency care (e.g., Lifeline).
  Impaired walking mobility may pose a life threat during a crisis (e.g., falls, fire).
- Use safety devices such as a gait belt when assisting the client in ambulation.
  Client safety is a primary goal in home care.
- ▲ Refer to physical and occupational therapists for skills building, strength building, options for restructuring the environment, and present alternative mobility options.
  Referral to specialty services may be a key component of the nursing care plan. A multidisciplinary approach supports total needs assessment and planning.
- ▲ Refer to home health aide services as appropriate for assistance with activities of daily living (ADLs).
  Mobility impairments may serve as a barrier to self-care.
- ▲ Provide support to client and caregivers during long-term impairment. Refer to case manager/medical social services or mental health/support group services as necessary.
  Long-term impairment may necessitate role changes and create anger and frustration. Counseling and support groups provide validation of feelings and alternative methods of problem solving.

• = Independent; ▲ = Collaborative

- Ensure that client has information on advocacy, options for disability access, and related issues (e.g., education, personnel, and equipment availability) under the Americans with Disabilities Act.

  The more informed a person is, the more potential he or she has for being independent.

Client/Family Teaching

- Recommend that clients and family check assistive devices to keep them in safe working order.

  Replace rubber tips if worn and remove dirt in grooves of walkers, crutches, and canes, otherwise they will not grip the floor. Check push button locks on walkers with telescoping legs (Minor, Minor, 1995). Inspect and repair prosthesis for cracks, rough spots inside the socket, and odd noises or movement at the joints or foot (Yeltzer, 1998).

WEB SITES FOR EDUCATION

 See the MERLIN web site for World Wide Web resources for client education.

REFERENCES Alexander NB: Postural control in older adults, *JAGS* 42(1):93-108, 1994.

Bobath B: *Adult hemiplegia: evaluation and treatment*, London, 1978, William Heinemann.

Carr JH, Shepherd RB: *A motor relearning program for stroke*, ed 2, London, 1987, William Heinemann.

Gee ZL, Passarella PM: *Nursing care of the stroke patient: a therapeutic approach*, Pittsburgh, 1985, AREN.

Ingvor DH, Philipson L: Distribution of cerebral blood flow in the dominant hemisphere during motor ideation and motor performance, *Ann Neurol* 2:230, 1977.

Kipnis ND: Musculoskeletal/orthopedic disorders. In McCourt A, editor: *The specialty practice of rehabilitation nursing: a core curriculum*, ed 3, Skokie, Ill, 1993, Rehabilitation Foundation, pp 41-43.

Matteson MA, McConnell ES, Linton AD: *Gerontological nursing*, ed 2, Philadelphia, 1997, WB Saunders.

Minor MAD, Minor SD: *Patient care skills*, ed 3, Norwalk, Conn, 1995, Appleton & Lange.

Perdue C: Treating postural hypotension, *Nurs Times* 94(14):54, 1998.

Radwanski MB, Hoeman SP: Geriatric rehabilitation nursing. In Hoeman SP, editor: *Rehabilitation nursing: process and application*, ed 2, St Louis, 1996, Mosby.

Rubin M: The physiology of bedrest, *Am J Nurs* 88(1):50-57, 1988.

Ulfarsson J, Robinson BE: Falls and falling. In Ham RJ, Sloane PD, editors: *Primary care geriatrics: a case-based approach*, ed 3, St Louis, 1997, Mosby.

Wilson GB: Progressive mobilization. In Sine RD et al, editors: *Basic rehabilitation techniques: a self-instructional guide*, ed 3, Gaithersburg, Md, 1988, Aspen.

Yeltzer EA: Care of the client with an amputation. In Chin PA, Finocchiaro D, Rosebrough A, editors: *Rehabilitation nursing practice*, New York, 1998, McGraw-Hill.

Yonekura M: Evaluation of cerebral blood flow in patients with transient attacks and minor strokes, *J Neurosurg* 15:58, 1981.

Wandering

Donna Algase

NANDA **Definition** Meandering; aimless or repetitive locomotion that exposes the individual to harm; frequently incongruent with boundaries, limits, or obstacles

Defining Characteristics

Frequent or continuous movement from place to place, often revisiting the same destinations; persistent locomotion in search of "missing" or unattainable people or places;

- = **Independent;** ▲ = **Collaborative**

haphazard locomotion; locomotion in unauthorized or private spaces; locomotion resulting in unintended leaving of a premise; long periods of locomotion without an apparent destination; fretful locomotion or pacing; inability to locate significant landmarks in a familiar setting; locomotion that cannot be easily dissuaded or redirected; following behind or shadowing a caregiver's locomotion; trespassing; hyperactivity; scanning, seeking, or searching behaviors; periods of locomotion interspersed with periods of nonlocomotion (e.g., sitting, standing, sleeping); getting lost

Related Factors (r/t)

Cognitive impairment, specifically memory and recall deficits, disorientation, poor visuoconstructive (or visuospatial) ability, and language (primarily expressive) defects; cortical atrophy; premorbid behavior (e.g., outgoing, sociable personality); premorbid dementia; separation from familiar people and places; sedation; emotional state, especially frustration, anxiety, boredom, or depression (agitation); overstimulating/understimulating social or physical environment; physiological state or need (e.g., hunger/thirst, pain, urination, constipation); time of day

NOC Outcomes (Nursing Outcomes Classification)

Suggested NOC Labels

Safety Status: Falls Occurrence; Safety Behavior: Fall Prevention; Caregiver Home Care Readiness

> **Example NOC Outcome**
>
> Accomplishes **Caregiver Home Care Readiness** as evidenced by the following indicators: Knowledge of recommended treatment regimen/Knowledge of prescribed activity/Knowledge of emergency care/Confidence in ability to manage care at home (Rate each indicator of **Caregiver Home Care Readiness:** 1 = none, 2 = limited, 3 = moderate, 4 = substantial, 5 = extensive [see Section I])

Client Outcomes

- Decreased incidence of falls (preferably free of falls)
- Decreased incidence of elopements
- Appropriate body weight maintained
- Caregiver able to explain interventions can use to provide a safe environment for care receiver who displays wandering behavior

NIC Interventions (Nursing Interventions Classification)

Suggested NIC Labels

Dementia Management

> **Example NIC Interventions—Dementia Management**
> - Place identification bracelet on patient
> - Provide space for safe pacing and wandering

Nursing Interventions and Rationales

- Assess and document the amount (frequency and duration), pattern (random, lapping, or pacing), and 24-hour distribution of wandering behavior over a 3-day interval. *Assessment over time provides a baseline against which behavior change can be evaluated (Algase et al, 1997). Such assessment can also reveal the time of day when wandering is greatest and when surveillance or other precautionary measures are most necessary.*

• = **Independent;** ▲ = **Collaborative**

- Obtain a history of personality characteristics and behavioral responses to stress.
  Information about long-standing behavioral tendencies may reveal circumstances under which wandering will occur and can aid in interpreting both positive and negative meanings of wandering behavior of the patient. (Kolanowski, Strand, Whall, 1997; Monsour, Robb, 1982; Thomas, 1997).

▲ Evaluate for neurocognitive strengths and limitations, particularly language, attention, visuospatial skills, and perseveration.
  Wanderers may have expressive language deficits that hamper ability to communicate needs (Algase, 1992; Dawson, Reid, 1987). Knowledge of attentional and visuospatial deficits, which may account for certain patterns of wandering, can lead to identification of appropriate environmental modifications that could enhance functional ambulation, such as elimination of distractions and enhancement of cues marking desired destinations (Fischer, Marterer, Danielczyk, 1990; Henderson, Mack, Williams, 1989; Passini et al, 1995; Passini et al, 2000). The presence of perseveration may indicate that the wanderer is unable to voluntarily stop his or her behavior (Passini et al, 1995; Ryan et al, 1995), thus calling for nursing judgment as to when wandering should be interrupted to enhance the wanderer's safety, comfort, or well-being.

- Assess for physical distress or needs, such as hunger, thirst, pain, discomfort, or elimination.
  While physical needs have not been documented in relation to wandering, the Need-Driven Dementia-Compromised Model hypothesizes this relationship (Algase et al, 1996).

- Assess for emotional or psychological distress, such as anxiety, fear, or feeling lost.
  While emotional needs have not been documented in relation to wandering, the Need-Driven Dementia-Compromised Model hypothesizes this relationship (Algase et al, 1996).

- Observe wandering episodes for antecedents and consequences.
  People, events, or circumstances surrounding the onset or conclusion of wandering may provide cues about triggers or rewards that are stimulating or reinforcing wandering behavior (Hirst, Metcalf, 1989; Hussain, 1981, 1982).

- Assess regularly for the presence of or potential for negative outcomes of wandering, such as weight change, declining social skills, falls, and elopement.
  Wanderers are at greater risk for falls than other cognitively-impaired persons (Kippenbrock, Soja, 1993; Morse, Tylko, Dixon, 1987). Wanderers have also shown greater loss in social skills over time than nonwandering counterparts (Cornbleth, 1977).

- Provide for safe ambulation with comfortable and well-fitting clothes, shoes with nonskid soles and foot support, and any necessary walking aids (such as a cane, walker, or Merry-Walker).
  Falls in persons with advanced dementia (AD) are often related to a decline in vigor in persons who had been previously active (Brody et al, 1984).

- Provide safe and secure surroundings that deter accidental elopements using perimeter control devices or camouflage.
  Eloping can have hazardous outcomes, even death. Perimeter control devices can effectively reduce or prevent exiting behavior (Negley, Molla, Obenchain, 1990). However, in some circumstances, these devices are viewed as unnecessarily restrictive and more passive means, such as camouflage, have been substituted. Camouflage techniques, such as masking the doorknob or creating striped floor patterns in front of exits, have been used with success (Hussain, Brown, 1987; Namazi, Rosner, Calkins, 1989), particularly in subjects with Alzheimer's disease (Hewewasam, 1996), but the effectiveness may be mitigated by other architectural features of the setting (Chafetz, 1990; Hamilton, 1993).

• = Independent; ▲ = Collaborative

- During periods of inactivity, position the wanderer so that desirable destinations, such as the bathroom, are within line of vision and undesirable destinations (such as exits or stairwells) are out of sight.
  Functional, nonwandering ambulation is possible even into late-stage dementia and may be facilitated by keeping appropriate visual cues accessible (Algase, 1999; Martino-Saltzman et al, 1991; Passini et al, 2000).
- If wandering takes a random or haphazard route, reduce environmental distractions and increase relevant environmental cues. Note and eliminate stimuli that distract the wanderer while in route.
  Random pattern wandering may be affected by environmental stimuli (Algase, 1999).
- Provide afternoon rest periods if assessment reveals that random pattern wandering worsens as the day progresses.
  The proportion of wandering that is random increases as the day progresses (Algase et al, 1997; Algase, 1999) and may indicate fatigue.
- Engage wanderers in social interaction and structured activity, especially when wanderers appear distressed or otherwise uncomfortable or their wandering presents a challenge to others in the setting.
  Wandering and social interaction are inversely related. Wanderers often have an outgoing or sociable personality and also have deficits in expressive language skills. Thus while they may prefer social interaction, their ability to initiate it may be compromised (Algase, 1992; Thomas, 1997).
- If wandering has a pacing quality, attempt to identify and address any underlying problems or concerns. Offer stress-reducing approaches, such as music, massage, or rocking. Attempts to distract or redirect the pacing wanderer may worsen wandering.
  Pacing, as a wandering pattern, is not associated with level of cognitive impairment and may reflect anxiety, agitation, pain or another internal process (Algase, Beattie, Therrien, 2001; Gerdner, 2000; Snyder, Olson, 1996).
- If wandering is a new or recently acquired behavior, or if it increases in intensity over previous levels, evaluate for constipation, pneumonia, or acute physical problems.
  Persons who first exhibit wandering within 3 months after admission to a nursing home are more likely than others to have developed physical problems that stimulate wandering (Keily, Morris, Algase, 2000).
- If wandering has a lapping or circuitous pattern, signs or labels may be effective. Substitute another repetitive activity such as folding or rocking if lapping becomes problematic or excessive.
  Not all wanderers display lapping pattern wandering and, when it does occur, it tends to occur early in the day or to follow rest periods. Thus it may be a more functional pattern than random wandering and may indicate a slightly better level of cognitive function for the individual, even if transient. Thus wanderers who lap may be better able to make use of information in the environment (Algase, Beattie, Therrien, 2001). However, this pattern of wandering may also be a form of perseveration and therefore the person may be unable to disengage voluntarily (Passini et al, 1995; Ryan et al, 1995).
- Provide a regularly scheduled and supervised exercise or walking program, particularly if wandering occurs excessively during the night or at times that are inconvenient in the setting.

- **= Independent; ▲ = Collaborative**

While exercise or walking programs do not reduce daytime wandering, they have been shown to reduce or eliminate nighttime wandering (Robb, 1987) and to decrease general agitation levels (Holmberg, 1997).

Multicultural

- Assess for the influence of cultural beliefs, norms, and values on the family's understanding of wandering behavior.
  What the family considers normal and abnormal health behavior may be based on cultural perceptions (Leininger, 1996).
- ▲ Refer family to social services or other supportive services to assist with the impact of caregiving for the wandering client.
  African-American caregivers of dementia clients may evidence less desire than other caregivers to institutionalize their family members and are more likely to report unmet service needs (Hinrichsen, Ramirez, 1992). African-American and white families of dementia clients may report restricted social activity (Haley et al, 1995).
- ▲ Encourage family to use support groups or other service programs.
  Studies indicate that minority families of clients with dementia use few support programs even though these programs could have a positive impact on caregiver well-being (Cox, 1999).
- Validate the family's feelings regarding the impact of client wandering on family lifestyle.
  Validation lets the client know that the nurse has heard and understands what was said (Stuart, Laraia, 2001).

Home Care Interventions

- Help the caregiver set up a plan to deal with wandering behavior using the interventions mentioned in Nursing Interventions and Rationales.
- Help the caregiver develop a plan of action to use if the client elopes.

Client/Family Teaching

- Inform client family of meaning of and reasons for wandering behavior.
  An understanding of wandering behavior will enable the client family to provide the client with a safe environment.
- Teach the caregiver/family methods to deal with wandering behavior using the interventions mentioned in Nursing Interventions and Rationales.

WEB SITES FOR EDUCATION

MERLIN See the MERLIN web site for World Wide Web resources for client education.

REFERENCES Algase DL: Cognitive discriminants of wandering among nursing home residents, *Nurs Res* 41(2):78-81, 1992.
Algase DL: Wandering: a dementia-compromised behavior, *J Gerontolo Nurs* 25(9):10-16, 1999.
Algase DL, Beattie ERA, Therrien B: Impact of cognitive impairment on wandering behavior, *West J Nurs Res* 23:283-295, 2001.
Algase DL et al: Need-driven dementia-compromised behavior: an alternative view of disruptive behavior, *Am J Alzheimers Dis* 11(6):10, 12-19, 1996.
Algase DL et al: Estimates of stability of daily wandering behavior among cognitively impaired long-term care residents, *Nurs Res* 46(3):172-178, 1997.
Brody E et al: Predictors of falls among institutionalized females with Alzheimer's disease, *J Am Geriatr Soc* 32:877-882, 1984.
Chafetz PK: Two dimensional grid is ineffective against demented patients' exiting through glass doors, *Psychol Aging* 5:146-147, 1990.

• = Independent; ▲ = Collaborative

Cornbleth, T: Effects of a protected hospital ward area on wandering and non-wandering geriatric patients, *J Gerentol* 32:573-577, 1977.

Cox C: Race and caregiving: patterns of service use by African American and white caregivers of persons with Alzheimer's, *J Gerontol Soc Work* 32(2):5-19, 1999.

Dawson P, Reid DW: Behavioral dimensions of patients at risk for wandering, *Gerontologist* 27:104-107, 1987.

Fischer P, Marterer A, Danielczyk W: Right-left disorientation in dementia of the Alzheimer's type, *Neurology* 40:1619-1620, 1990.

Gerdner LA: Effects of individualized versus classical "relaxation" music on the frequency of agitation in elderly persons with Alzheimer's disease and related disorders, *Int Psychogeriatr* 12(1):49-65, 2000.

Haley WE et al: Psychological, social, and health impact of caregiving: a comparison of black and white dementia family caregivers and noncaregivers, *Psychol Aging* 10(4):540-552, 1995.

Hamilton C: *The use of tape patterns as an alternative method for controlling wanderers' exiting behavior in a dementia care unit,* Unpublished master's thesis, 1993, Virginia Polytechnic Institute and State University.

Henderson V, Mack W, Williams BW: Spatial disorientation in Alzheimer's disease, *Arch Neurol* 46:391-394, 1989.

Hewewasam L: Floor patterns limit wandering of people with Alzheimer's, *Nurs Times* 92:41-44, 1996.

Hinrichsen GA, Ramirez M: Black and white dementia caregivers: a comparison of their adaptation, *Gerontologist* 32(3):375-381, 1992.

Hirst ST, Metcalf BJ: Whys and whats of wandering, *Geriatr Nurs Am J Care Aging* 10(5):237-238, 1989.

Holmberg SK: Evaluation of a clinical intervention for wanderers on a geriatric nursing unit, *Arch Psychiatr Nurs* 11:21-28, 1997.

Hussain RA: Psychotherapeutic intervention: organic mental disorders. In *Geriatric psychology: a behavioral perspective,* New York, 1981, Van Nostrand Reinhold, pp 123-151.

Hussain RA: Stimulus control in the modification of problematic behavior in elderly institutionalized patients, *Int J Behavior Geriatr* 1:33-40, 1982.

Hussain RA, Brown DC: Use of two dimensional grid patterns to limit hazardous ambulation in demented patients, *J Gerentol* 42:558-560, 1987.

Keily DK, Morris JN, Algase DL: Resident characteristics associated with wandering in nursing homes, *Int J Geriatr Psychiatry* 15:1013-1020, 2000.

Kippenbrock T, Soja M: Preventing falls in the elderly: interviewing patients who have fallen, *Geriatr Nurs* 14:205-209, 1993.

Kolanowski AM, Strand G, Whall A: A pilot study of the relation in premorbid characteristics to behavior in dementia, *J Gerontol Nurs* 23:21-30, 1997.

Leininger MM: *Transcultural nursing: theories, research and practices,* ed 2, Hilliard, Ohio, 1996, McGraw-Hill.

Martino-Saltzman D et al: Travel behavior of nursing home residents perceived as wanderers and nonwanderers, *The Gerontologist* 31:666-672, 1991.

Monsour N, Robb S: Wandering behavior in old age: a psychosocial study, *Soc Work* 27:411-416, 1982.

Morse J, Tylko S, Dixon H: Characteristics of the fall-prone patient, *The Gerontologist* 27:516-522, 1987.

Namazi KH, Rosner TT, Calkins MP: Visual barriers to prevent ambulatory Alzheimer's patients from exiting through an emergency door, *The Gerontologist* 29:699-702, 1989.

Negley E, Molla PM, Obenchain J: No exit: the effects of an electronic security system on confused patients, *J Gerontol Nurs* 16:21-25, 1990.

Passini R et al: Wayfinding in dementia of the Alzheimer's type: planning abilities, *J Clin Exper Neuropsychol* 17:820-832, 1995.

Passini R et al: Wayfinding in a nursing home for advanced dementia of the Alzheimer's type, *Environment Behavior* 32(5):684-710, 2000.

Robb SS: Exercise treatment for wandering. In Altman HJ, editor: *Alzheimer's disease: problems, prospects, and perspectives,* New York, 1987, Plenum, pp 213-218.

Ryan JP et al: Graphomotor perseveration and wandering in Alzheimer's disease, *J Geriatr Psychiatry Neurol* 8:209-212, 1995.

Snyder M, Olson J: Music and hand massage interventions to produce relaxation and reduce aggressive behaviors in cognitively impaired elders: a pilot study: *Clin Gerontol* 17(1):64-69, 1996.

Stuart GW, Laraia MT: Therapeutic nurse-patient relationship. In Stuart GW, Laraia MT, editors: *Principles and practice of psychiatric nursing,* St Louis, 2001, Mosby, p 30.

Thomas DW: Understanding the wandering patient: a continuity of personality perspective, *J Gerontol Nurs* 23(1):16-24, 1997.

• = **Independent**; ▲ = **Collaborative**

Appendix A

Nursing Diagnoses Arranged by Maslow's Hierarchy of Needs

Because human beings adapt in many ways to establish and maintain the self, health problems are much more than simple physical matters. Maslow's Hierarchy of Needs (see diagram below) is a system of classifying human needs. Maslow's hierarchy is based on the idea that lower-level physiological needs must be met before higher-level abstract needs can be met.

For nurses, Maslow's hierarchy has special significance in decision-making and planning for care. By considering need categories as you identify client problems, you will be able to provide more holistic care. For example, a client who demands frequent attention for a seemingly trivial matter may require help with self-esteem needs. Need levels vary from client to client. If a client is short of breath, the client is probably not interested in or capable of discussing spirituality. In addition, a client's need level may change throughout planning and intervention, so you will need to be vigilant in your assessment.

Read the descriptions of each category in the diagram, and see how you would relate them to nursing diagnoses. Compare your evaluation with how the authors categorized the nursing diagnoses according to this hierarchy. Be sure to assess clients for potential problems at all levels of the pyramid, regardless of their initial complaint.

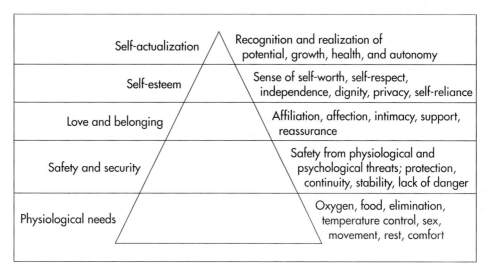

Reprinted with permission from *Nursing diagnosis reference manual,* copyright 1991, Springhouse Corp. All rights reserved.

Physiological needs

Activity intolerance
Activity intolerance, risk for
Airway clearance, ineffective
Aspiration, risk for
Body temperature, risk for imbalanced
Bowel incontinence
Breastfeeding, effective
Breastfeeding, ineffective
Breastfeeding, interrupted
Breathing pattern, ineffective
Cardiac output, decreased
Confusion, acute
Confusion, chronic
Constipation
Constipation, perceived
Constipation, risk for
Dentition, impaired
Diarrhea
Environmental interpretation syndrome, impaired
Fatigue
Fluid volume, deficient
Fluid volume, excess
Fluid volume, risk for deficient
Fluid volume, risk for imbalanced
Gas exchange, impaired
Hyperthermia
Hypothermia
Incontinence, functional urinary
Incontinence, reflex urinary
Incontinence, risk for urge urinary
Incontinence, stress urinary
Incontinence, total urinary
Incontinence, urge urinary
Infant behavior, disorganized
Infant behavior, readiness for enhanced organized
Infant behavior, risk for disorganized
Infant feeding pattern, ineffective
Intracranial adaptive capacity, decreased
Memory, impaired
Mobility, impaired bed
Mobility, impaired physical
Mobility, impaired wheelchair
Nausea
Nutrition, imbalanced: less than body requirements
Nutrition, imbalanced: more than body requirements
Nutrition, imbalanced: risk for more than body requirements
Oral mucous membrane, impaired

Pain, acute
Pain, chronic
Protection, ineffective
Self-care deficit, bathing/hygiene
Self-care deficit, dressing/grooming
Self-care deficit, feeding
Self-care deficit, toileting
Sensory perception, disturbed (specify): visual, auditory, kinesthetic, gustatory, tactile, olfactory
Sexual dysfunction
Sexuality patterns, ineffective
Skin integrity, impaired
Skin integrity, risk for impaired
Sleep deprivation
Sleep pattern, disturbed
Surgical recovery, delayed
Swallowing, impaired
Thermoregulation, ineffective
Thought processes, disturbed
Tissue integrity, impaired
Tissue perfusion, ineffective (specify): renal, cerebral, cardiopulmonary, gastrointestinal, peripheral
Transfer ability, impaired
Urinary elimination, impaired
Urinary retention
Ventilation, impaired spontaneous
Ventilatory weaning response, dysfunctional
Walking, impaired

Safety and security needs

Allergy response, latex
Allergy response, risk for latex
Anxiety, death
Autonomic dysreflexia
Autonomic dysreflexia, risk for
Communication, impaired verbal
Disuse syndrome, risk for
Falls, risk for
Fear
Grieving, anticipatory
Grieving, dysfunctional
Growth, risk for disproportionate
Health maintenance, ineffective
Home maintenance, impaired
Infection, risk for
Injury, risk for
Injury, risk for perioperative-positioning
Knowledge, deficient
Peripheral neurovascular dysfunction, risk for
Poisoning, risk for
Sorrow, chronic
Suffocation, risk for

Therapeutic regimen management, ineffective
Therapeutic regimen management, ineffective community
Therapeutic regimen management, ineffective family
Trauma, risk for
Neglect, unilateral
Wandering

Love and belonging needs

Failure to thrive, adult
Anxiety
Attachment, risk for impaired parent/infant/child
Caregiver role strain
Caregiver role strain, risk for
Coping, compromised family
Coping, disabled family
Coping, readiness for enhanced family
Family processes, interrupted
Loneliness, risk for
Parental role conflict
Parenting, impaired
Parenting, risk for impaired
Relocation stress syndrome
Relocation stress syndrome, risk for
Social interaction, impaired
Social isolation

Self-esteem needs

Adjustment, impaired
Body image, disturbed
Conflict, decisional
Coping, defensive

Coping, ineffective
Coping, ineffective community
Coping, readiness for enhanced community
Denial, ineffective
Diversional activity, deficient
Family processes, dysfunctional: alcoholism
Hopelessness
Noncompliance
Identity, disturbed personal
Post-trauma syndrome
Post-trauma syndrome, risk for
Powerlessness
Powerlessness, risk for
Rape-trauma syndrome
Rape-trauma syndrome: compound reaction
Rape-trauma syndrome: silent reaction
Role performance, ineffective
Self-esteem, chronic low
Self-esteem, situational low
Self-mutilation
Self-mutilation, risk for
Suicide, risk for
Violence, risk for other-directed
Violence, risk for self-directed

Self-actualization needs

Development, risk for delayed
Energy field, disturbed
Growth and development, delayed
Health-seeking behaviors
Spiritual distress
Spiritual distress, risk for
Spiritual well-being, readiness for enhanced
Therapeutic regimen management, effective

Appendix B

Taxonomy II: NANDA's Domains, Classes, Diagnostic Concepts, and Diagnoses*

Domain	Class	Diagnostic Concept	Diagnoses
1. Health promotion	1. Health awareness		
	2. Health management	Therapeutic regimen management	Effective Therapeutic regimen management
			Ineffective Therapeutic regimen management
			Ineffective family Therapeutic regimen management
			Ineffective community Therapeutic management
2. Nutrition	1. Ingestion	Infant feeding pattern	Ineffective Infant feeding pattern
		Swallowing	Impaired Swallowing
		Nutrition	Imbalanced Nutrition: less than body requirements
			Imbalanced Nutrition: more than body requirements
			Risk for imbalanced Nutrition: more than body requirements
	2. Digestion		
	3. Absorption		
	4. Metabolism		
	5. Hydration	Fluid volume	Deficient Fluid volume
			Risk for deficient Fluid volume
			Excess Fluid volume
			Risk for Fluid volume imbalance
3. Elimination	1. Urinary system	Urinary elimination	Impaired Urinary elimination
		Urinary retention	Urinary retention
		Urinary incontinence	Total urinary Incontinence
			Functional urinary Incontinence
			Stress urinary Incontinence
			Urge urinary Incontinence

*From North American Nursing Diagnosis Association: *Nursing diagnoses: definitions and classification 2001-2002,* Philadelphia, 2001, The Association.

Taxonomy II: NANDA's Domains, Classes, Diagnostic Concepts, and Diagnoses*

Domain	Class	Diagnostic Concept	Diagnoses
	2. Gastrointestinal system	Bowel incontinence	Reflex urinary Incontinence Risk for urge urinary Incontinence Bowel incontinence
		Diarrhea Constipation	Diarrhea Constipation Risk for Constipation Perceived Constipation
	3. Integumentary system		
	4. Pulmonary system	Gas exchange	Impaired Gas exchange
4. Activity/rest	1. Sleep/rest	Sleep pattern	Disturbed Sleep pattern Sleep deprivation
	2. Activity/exercise	Disuse syndrome	Risk for Disuse syndrome
		Mobility	Impaired physical Mobility Impaired bed Mobility Impaired wheelchair Mobility
		Transfer ability	Impaired Transfer ability
		Walking	Impaired Walking
		Diversional activity	Deficient Diversional activity
		Wandering	Wandering
		Self-care deficit	Dressing/grooming deficit Bathing/hygiene deficit Feeding self-care deficit Toileting self-care deficit
		Surgical recovery	Delayed Surgical recovery
	3. Energy balances	Energy field	Disturbed Energy field
		Fatigue	Fatigue
	4. Cardiovascular/pulmonary responses	Cardiac output	Decreased Cardiac output
		Spontaneous ventilation	Impaired spontaneous Ventilation
		Breathing pattern	Ineffective Breathing pattern
		Activity tolerance	Activity intolerance Risk for Activity intolerance

Continued

Taxonomy II: NANDA's Domains, Classes, Diagnostic Concepts, and Diagnoses*

Domain	Class	Diagnostic Concept	Diagnoses
		Ventilatory weaning	Dysfunctional Ventilatory weaning response
		Tissue perfusion	Ineffective Tissue perfusion (specify type: renal, cerebral, cardiopulmonary, gastrointestinal, peripheral)
5. Perception/ cognition	1. Attention	Unilateral neglect	Unilateral Neglect
	2. Orientation	Environmental interpretation	Impaired Environmental interpretation syndrome
	3. Sensation/ perception	Sensory perception	Disturbed Sensory perception (specify: visual, auditory, kinesthetic, gustatory, tactile, olfactory)
	4. Cognition	Knowledge	Deficient Knowledge (specify)
		Confusion	Acute Confusion
			Chronic Confusion
		Memory	Impaired Memory
		Thought processes	Disturbed Thought processes
	5. Communication	Verbal communication	Impaired verbal Communication
6. Self-perception	1. Self-concept	Identity	Disturbed personal Identity
			Powerlessness
			Risk for Powerlessness
			Hopelessness
		Loneliness	Risk for Loneliness
	2. Self-esteem	Self-esteem	Chronic low Self-esteem
			Situational low Self-esteem
			Risk for situational low Self-esteem
	3. Body image	Body image	Disturbed Body image
7. Role relationships	1. Caregiving roles	Caregiver role strain	Caregiver role strain
			Risk for Caregiver role strain
		Parenting	Impaired Parenting
			Risk for impaired Parenting
	2. Family relationships	Family processes	Interrupted Family processes
			Dysfunctional Family processes: alcoholism
		Attachment	Risk for impaired parent/infant/child Attachment
	3. Role performance	Breastfeeding	Effective Breastfeeding

Taxonomy II: NANDA's Domains, Classes, Diagnostic Concepts, and Diagnoses*

Domain	Class	Diagnostic Concept	Diagnoses
		Role performance	Ineffective Breastfeedng
			Interrupted Breastfeeding
			Ineffective Role performance
			Parental Role conflict
		Social interaction	Impaired Social interaction
8. Sexuality	1. Sexual identity		
	2. Sexual function	Sexual function	Sexual dysfunction
		Sexual patterns	Ineffective Sexuality patterns
	3. Reproduction		
9. Coping/stress tolerance	1. Post-trauma responses	Relocation stress	Relocation stress syndrome
			Risk for Relocation stress syndrome
		Rape-trauma	Rape-trauma syndrome
			Rape-trauma syndrome: silent reaction
			Rape-trauma syndrome: compound reaction
		Post-trauma response	Post-trauma syndrome
			Risk for Post-trauma syndrome
	2. Coping responses	Fear	Fear
		Anxiety	Anxiety
			Death Anxiety
		Sorrow	Chronic Sorrow
		Denial	Ineffective Denial
			Anticipatory Grieving
			Dysfunctional Grieving
		Adjustment	Impaired Adjustment
		Coping	Ineffective Coping
			Disabled family Coping
			Compromised family Coping
			Defensive Coping
			Ineffective community Coping
			Readiness for enhanced family Coping
			Readiness for enhanced community Coping
		Dysreflexia	Autonomic dysreflexia
			Risk for Autonomic dysreflexia
		Infant behavior	Disorganized Infant behavior
			Risk for disorganized Infant behavior
			Readiness for enhanced organized Infant behavior

continued

Taxonomy II: NANDA's Domains, Classes, Diagnostic Concepts, and Diagnoses*

Domain	Class	Diagnostic Concept	Diagnoses
		Adaptive capacity	Decreased Intracranial adaptive capacity
10. Life principles	1. Values		
	2. Beliefs	Spiritual well-being	Readiness for enhanced Spiritual well-being
	3. Value/belief/action congruence	Spiritual distress	Spiritual distress
			Risk for Spiritual distress
		Decisional conflict	Decisional Conflict (specify)
		Noncompliance	Noncompliance (specify)
11. Safety/protection	1. Infection	Infection	Risk for Infection
	2. Physical Injury	Oral mucous membrane	Impaired Oral mucous membrane
		Injury	Risk for Injury
			Risk for perioperative-positioning Injury
			Risk for Falls
		Trauma	Risk for Trauma
		Skin integrity	Impaired Skin integrity
			Risk for impaired Skin integrity
		Tissue integrity	Impaired Tissue integrity
		Dentition	Impaired Dentition
		Suffocation	Risk for Suffocation
		Aspiration	Risk for Aspiration
		Airway clearance	Ineffective Airway clearance
		Neurovascular function	Risk for Peripheral neurovascular dysfunction
	3. Violence	Self-mutilation	Risk for Self-mutilation
			Self-mutilation
		Violence	Risk for other-directed Violence
			Risk for self-directed Violence
			Risk for Suicide
	4. Environmental hazards	Poisoning	Risk for Poisoning
	5. Defensive process	Latex allergy response	Latex Allergy response
			Risk for latex Allergy response
	6. Thermoregulation	Body temperature	Risk for imbalanced Body temperature
		Thermoregulation	Ineffective Thermoregulation

Taxonomy II: NANDA's Domains, Classes, Diagnostic Concepts, and Diagnoses*

Domain	Class	Diagnostic Concept	Diagnoses
			Hypothermia
			Hyperthermia
12. Comfort	1. Physical comfort	Pain	Acute Pain
			Chronic Pain
		Nausea	Nausea
	2. Environmental comfort		
	3. Social comfort	Social isolation	Social isolation
13. Growth/ develop- ment	1. Growth	Growth	Risk for disproportionate Growth
		Failure to thrive	Adult Failure to thrive
	2. Development	Development	Delayed Growth and development
			Risk for delayed Development

Appendix C

Nursing Outcomes Classification (NOC) Outcome Labels*

Abuse Cessation
Abuse Protection
Abuse Recovery: Emotional
Abuse Recovery: Financial
Abuse Recovery: Physical
Abuse Recovery: Sexual
Abusive Behavior Self-Control
Acceptance: Health Status
Activity Tolerance
Adherence Behavior
Aggression Control
Ambulation: Walking
Ambulation: Wheelchair
Anxiety Control
Aspiration Control
Asthma Control
Balance
Blood Glucose Control
Blood Transfusion Reaction Control
Body Image
Body Positioning: Self-Initiated
Bone Healing
Bowel Continence
Bowel Elimination
Breastfeeding Establishment: Infant
Breastfeeding Establishment: Maternal
Breastfeeding Maintenance
Breastfeeding Weaning
Cardiac Pump Effectiveness
Caregiver Adaptation to Patient Institutional-
   ization
Caregiver Emotional Health
Caregiver Home Care Readiness
Caregiver Lifestyle Disruption
Caregiver-Patient Relationship
Caregiver Performance: Direct Care
Caregiver Performance: Indirect Care
Caregiver Physical Health
Caregiver Stressors
Caregiver Well-Being
Caregiving Endurance Potential
Child Adaptation to Hospitalization
Child Development: 2 Months

Child Development: 4 Months
Child Development: 6 Months
Child Development: 12 Months
Child Development: 2 Years
Child Development: 3 Years
Child Development: 4 Years
Child Development: 5 Years
Child Development: Middle Childhood (6-11
   years)
Child Development: Adolescence (12-17 years)
Circulation Status
Coagulation Status
Cognitive Ability
Cognitive Orientation
Comfort Level
Communication Ability
Communication: Expressive Ability
Communication: Receptive Ability
Community Competence
Community Health Status
Community Health: Immunity
Community Risk Control: Chronic Disease
Community Risk Control: Communicable Dis-
   ease
Community Risk Control: Lead Exposure
Compliance Behavior
Concentration
Coping
Decision Making
Depression Control
Depression Level
Dialysis Access Integrity
Dignified Dying
Distorted Thought Control
Electrolyte & Acid/Base Balance
Endurance
Energy Conservation
Family Coping
Family Environment: Internal
Family Functioning
Family Health Status
Family Integrity
Family Normalization

*From Johnson M, Maas M: *Nursing outcomes classification (NOC)*, ed 2, St Louis, 2000, Mosby.

Family Participation in Professional Care
Fear Control
Fetal Status: Antepartum
Fetal Status: Intrapartum
Fluid Balance
Grief Resolution
Growth
Health Beliefs
Health Beliefs: Perceived Ability to Perform
Health Beliefs: Perceived Control
Health Beliefs: Perceived Resources
Health Beliefs: Perceived Threat
Health Orientation
Health Promoting Behavior
Health Seeking Behavior
Hearing Compensation Behavior
Hope
Hydration
Identity
Immobility Consequences: Physiological
Immobility Consequences: Psycho-Cognitive
Immune Hypersensitivity Control
Immune Status
Immunization Behavior
Impulse Control
Infection Status
Information Processing
Joint Movement: Active
Joint Movement: Passive
Knowledge: Breastfeeding
Knowledge: Child Safety
Knowledge: Conception Prevention
Knowledge: Diabetes Management
Knowledge: Diet
Knowledge: Disease Process
Knowledge: Energy Conservation
Knowledge: Fertility Promotion
Knowledge: Health Behaviors
Knowledge: Health Promotion
Knowledge: Health Resources
Knowledge: Illness Care
Knowledge: Infant Care
Knowledge: Infection Control
Knowledge: Labor and Delivery
Knowledge: Maternal-Child Health
Knowledge: Medication
Knowledge: Personal Safety
Knowledge: Postpartum
Knowledge: Preconception
Knowledge: Pregnancy
Knowledge: Prescribed Activity
Knowledge: Sexual Functioning
Knowledge: Substance Use Control
Knowledge: Treatment Procedure(s)

Knowledge: Treatment Regimen
Leisure Participation
Loneliness
Maternal Status: Antepartum
Maternal Status: Intrapartum
Maternal Status: Postpartum
Medication Response
Memory
Mobility Level
Mood Equilibrium
Muscle Function
Neglect Recovery
Neurological Status
Neurological Status: Autonomic
Neurological Status: Central Motor Control
Neurological Status: Consciousness
Neurological Status: Cranial Sensory/Motor
  Function
Neurological Status: Spinal Sensory/Motor
  Function
Newborn Adaptation
Nutritional Status
Nutritional Status: Biochemical Measures
Nutritional Status: Body Mass
Nutritional Status: Energy
Nutritional Status: Food & Fluid Intake
Nutritional Status: Nutrient Intake
Oral Health
Pain Control
Pain: Disruptive Effects
Pain Level
Pain: Psychological Response
Parent-Infant Attachment
Parenting
Parenting: Social Safety
Participation: Health Care Decisions
Physical Aging Status
Physical Fitness
Physical Maturation: Female
Physical Maturation: Male
Play Participation
Prenatal Health Behavior
Preterm Infant Organization
Psychomotor Energy
Psychosocial Adjustment: Life Change
Quality of Life
Respiratory Status: Airway Patency
Respiratory Status: Gas Exchange
Respiratory Status: Ventilation
Rest
Risk Control
Risk Control: Alcohol Use
Risk Control: Cancer
Risk Control: Cardiovascular Health

Risk Control: Drug Use
Risk Control: Hearing Impairment
Risk Control: Sexually Transmitted Diseases (STD)
Risk Control: Tobacco Use
Risk Control: Unintended Pregnancy
Risk Control: Visual Impairment
Risk Detection
Role Performance
Safety Behavior: Fall Prevention
Safety Behavior: Home Physical Environment
Safety Behavior: Personal
Safety Status: Falls Occurrence
Safety Status: Physical Injury
Self-Care: Activities of Daily Living (ADL)
Self-Care: Bathing
Self-Care: Dressing
Self-Care: Eating
Self-Care: Grooming
Self-Care: Hygiene
Self-Care: Instrumental Activities of Daily Living (IADL)
Self-Care: Non-Parenteral Medication
Self-Care: Oral Hygiene
Self-Care: Parenteral Medication
Self-Care: Toileting
Self-Direction of Care
Self-Esteem
Self-Mutilation Restraint
Sensory Function: Cutaneous
Sensory Function: Hearing
Sensory Function: Proprioception
Sensory Function: Taste & Smell
Sensory Function: Vision
Sexual Functioning
Sexual Identity: Acceptance
Skeletal Function

Sleep
Social Interaction Skills
Social Involvement
Social Support
Spiritual Well-Being
Substance Addiction Consequences
Suffering Level
Suicide Self-Restraint
Swallowing Status
Swallowing Status: Esophageal Phase
Swallowing Status: Oral Phase
Swallowing Status: Pharyngeal Phase
Symptom Control
Symptom Severity
Symptom Severity: Perimenopause
Symptom Severity: Premenstrual Syndrome (PMS)
Systemic Toxin Clearance: Dialysis
Thermoregulation
Thermoregulation: Neonate
Tissue Integrity: Skin & Mucous Membranes
Tissue Perfusion: Abdominal Organs
Tissue Perfusion: Cardiac
Tissue Perfusion: Cerebral
Tissue Perfusion: Peripheral
Tissue Perfusion: Pulmonary
Transfer Performance
Treatment Behavior: Illness or Injury
Urinary Continence
Urinary Elimination
Vision Compensation Behavior
Vital Signs Status
Weight Control
Well-Being
Will to Live
Wound Healing: Primary Intention
Wound Healing: Secondary Intention

Appendix D

Nursing Interventions Classification (NIC) Intervention Labels*

Abuse Protection Support
Abuse Protection Support: Child
Abuse Protection Support: Domestic Partner
Abuse Protection Support: Elder
Abuse Protection Support: Religious
Acid-Base Management
Acid-Base Management: Metabolic Acidosis
Acid-Base Management: Metabolic Alkalosis
Acid-Base Management: Respiratory Acidosis
Acid-Base Management: Respiratory Alkalosis
Acid-Base Monitoring
Active Listening
Activity Therapy
Acupressure
Admission Care
Airway Insertion and Stabilization
Airway Management
Airway Suctioning
Allergy Management
Amnioinfusion
Amputation Care
Analgesic Administration
Analgesic Administration: Intraspinal
Anaphylaxis Management
Anesthesia Administration
Anger Control Assistance
Animal-Assisted Therapy
Anticipatory Guidance
Anxiety Reduction
Area Restriction
Art Therapy
Artificial Airway Management
Aspiration Precautions
Assertiveness Training
Attachment Promotion
Autogenic Training
Autotransfusion
Bathing
Bed Rest Care
Bedside Laboratory Testing
Behavior Management
Behavior Management: Overactivity/Inattention

Behavior Management: Self-Harm
Behavior Management: Sexual
Behavior Modification
Behavior Modification: Social Skills
Bibliotherapy
Biofeedback
Birthing
Bladder Irrigation
Bleeding Precautions
Bleeding Reduction
Bleeding Reduction: Antepartum Uterus
Bleeding Reduction: Gastrointestinal
Bleeding Reduction: Nasal
Bleeding Reduction: Postpartum Uterus
Bleeding Reduction: Wound
Blood Products Administration
Body Image Enhancement
Body Mechanics Promotion
Bottle Feeding
Bowel Incontinence Care
Bowel Incontinence Care: Encopresis
Bowel Irrigation
Bowel Management
Bowel Training
Breast Examination
Breastfeeding Assistance
Calming Technique
Cardiac Care
Cardiac Care: Acute
Cardiac Care: Rehabilitative
Cardiac Precautions
Caregiver Support
Case Management
Cast Care: Maintenance
Cast Care: Wet
Cerebral Edema Management
Cerebral Perfusion Promotion
Cesarean Section Care
Chemotherapy Management
Chest Physiotherapy
Childbirth Preparation
Circulatory Care: Arterial Insufficiency
Circulatory Care: Mechanical Assist Device

*From McCloskey JC, Bulechek GM, editors: *Nursing interventions classification (NIC),* ed 3, St Louis, 2000, Mosby.

Circulatory Care: Venous Insufficiency
Circulatory Precautions
Code Management
Cognitive Restructuring
Cognitive Stimulation
Communicable Disease Management
Communication Enhancement: Hearing Deficit
Communication Enhancement: Speech Deficit
Communication Enhancement: Visual Deficit
Community Disaster Preparedness
Community Health Development
Complex Relationship Building
Conflict Mediation
Conscious Sedation
Constipation/Impaction Management
Consultation
Contact Lens Care
Controlled Substance Checking
Coping Enhancement
Cost Containment
Cough Enhancement
Counseling
Crisis Intervention
Critical Path Development
Culture Brokerage
Cutaneous Stimulation
Decision-Making Support
Delegation
Delirium Management
Delusion Management
Dementia Management
Developmental Care
Developmental Enhancement: Adolescent
Developmental Enhancement: Child
Diarrhea Management
Diet Staging
Discharge Planning
Distraction
Documentation
Dressing
Dying Care
Dysreflexia Management
Dysrhythmia Management
Ear Care
Eating Disorders Management
Electrolyte Management
Electrolyte Management: Hypercalcemia
Electrolyte Management: Hyperkalemia
Electrolyte Management: Hypermagnesemia
Electrolyte Management: Hypernatremia
Electrolyte Management: Hyperphosphatemia
Electrolyte Management: Hypocalcemia
Electrolyte Management: Hypokalemia

Electrolyte Management: Hypomagnesemia
Electrolyte Management: Hyponatremia
Electrolyte Management: Hypophosphatemia
Electrolyte Monitoring
Electronic Fetal Monitoring: Antepartum
Electronic Fetal Monitoring: Intrapartum
Elopement Precautions
Embolus Care: Peripheral
Embolus Care: Pulmonary
Embolus Precautions
Emergency Care
Emergency Cart Checking
Emotional Support
Endotracheal Extubation
Energy Management
Enteral Tube Feeding
Environmental Management
Environmental Management: Attachment Process
Environmental Management: Comfort
Environmental Management: Community
Environmental Management: Home Preparation
Environmental Management: Safety
Environmental Management: Violence Prevention
Environmental Management: Worker Safety
Environmental Risk Protection
Examination Assistance
Exercise Promotion
Exercise Promotion: Strength Training
Exercise Promotion: Stretching
Exercise Therapy: Ambulation
Exercise Therapy: Balance
Exercise Therapy: Joint Mobility
Exercise Therapy: Muscle Control
Eye Care
Fall Prevention
Family Integrity Promotion
Family Integrity Promotion: Childbearing Family
Family Involvement Promotion
Family Mobilization
Family Planning: Contraception
Family Planning: Infertility
Family Planning: Unplanned Pregnancy
Family Process Maintenance
Family Support
Family Therapy
Feeding
Fertility Preservation
Fever Treatment
Financial Resource Assistance
Fire-Setting Precautions

First Aid
Fiscal Resource Management
Flatulence Reduction
Fluid Management
Fluid Monitoring
Fluid Resuscitation
Fluid/Electrolyte Management
Foot Care
Forgiveness Facilitation
Gastrointestinal Intubation
Genetic Counseling
Grief Work Facilitation
Grief Work Facilitation: Perinatal Death
Guilt Work Facilitation
Hair Care
Hallucination Management
Health Care Information Exchange
Health Education
Health Policy Monitoring
Health Screening
Health System Guidance
Heat Exposure Treatment
Heat/Cold Application
Hemodialysis Therapy
Hemodynamic Regulation
Hemofiltration Therapy
Hemorrhage Control
High-Risk Pregnancy Care
Home Maintenance Assistance
Hope Instillation
Humor
Hyperglycemia Management
Hypervolemia Management
Hypnosis
Hypoglycemia Management
Hypothermia Treatment
Hypovolemia Management
Immunization/Vaccination Management
Impulse Control Training
Incident Reporting
Incision Site Care
Infant Care
Infection Control
Infection Control: Intraoperative
Infection Protection
Insurance Authorization
Intracranial Pressure (ICP) Monitoring
Intrapartal Care
Intrapartal Care: High-Risk Delivery
Intravenous (IV) Insertion
Intravenous (IV) Therapy
Invasive Hemodynamic Monitoring
Kangaroo Care
Labor Induction

Labor Suppression
Laboratory Data Interpretation
Lactation Counseling
Lactation Suppression
Laser Precautions
Latex Precautions
Learning Facilitation
Learning Readiness Enhancement
Leech Therapy
Limit Setting
Malignant Hyperthermia Precautions
Mechanical Ventilation
Mechanical Ventilatory Weaning
Medication Administration
Medication Administration: Ear
Medication Administration: Enteral
Medication Administration: Epidural
Medication Administration: Eye
Medication Administration: Inhalation
Medication Administration: Interpleural
Medication Administration: Intradermal
Medication Administration: Intramuscular
   (IM)
Medication Administration: Intraosseous
Medication Administration: Intravenous (IV)
Medication Administration: Oral
Medication Administration: Rectal
Medication Administration: Skin
Medication Administration: Subcutaneous
Medication Administration: Vaginal
Medication Administration: Ventricular Reser-
   voir
Medication Management
Medication Prescribing
Meditation Facilitation
Memory Training
Milieu Therapy
Mood Management
Multidisciplinary Care Conference
Music Therapy
Mutual Goal Setting
Nail Care
Nausea Management
Neurologic Monitoring
Newborn Care
Newborn Monitoring
Nonnutritive Sucking
Normalization Promotion
Nutrition Management
Nutrition Therapy
Nutritional Counseling
Nutritional Monitoring
Oral Health Maintenance
Oral Health Promotion

Oral Health Restoration
Order Transcription
Organ Procurement
Ostomy Care
Oxygen Therapy
Pain Management
Parent Education: Adolescent
Parent Education: Childrearing Family
Parent Education: Infant
Parenting Promotion
Pass Facilitation
Patient Contracting
Patient-Controlled Analgesia (PCA) Assistance
Patient Rights Protection
Peer Review
Pelvic Muscle Exercise
Perineal Care
Peripheral Sensation Management
Peripherally Inserted Central (PIC) Catheter Care
Peritoneal Dialysis Therapy
Pessary Management
Phlebotomy: Arterial Blood Sample
Phlebotomy: Blood Unit Acquisition
Phlebotomy: Venous Blood Sample
Phototherapy: Neonate
Physical Restraint
Physician Support
Pneumatic Tourniquet Precautions
Positioning
Positioning: Intraoperative
Positioning: Neurologic
Positioning: Wheelchair
Postanesthesia Care
Postmortem Care
Postpartal Care
Preceptor: Employee
Preceptor: Student
Preconception Counseling
Pregnancy Termination Care
Prenatal Care
Preoperative Coordination
Preparatory Sensory Information
Presence
Pressure Management
Pressure Ulcer Care
Pressure Ulcer Prevention
Product Evaluation
Program Development
Progressive Muscle Relaxation
Prompted Voiding
Prosthesis Care
Pruritis Management

Quality Monitoring
Radiation Therapy Management
Rape-Trauma Treatment
Reality Orientation
Recreation Therapy
Rectal Prolapse Management
Referral
Religious Addiction Prevention
Religious Ritual Enhancement
Reminiscence Therapy
Reproductive Technology Management
Research Data Collection
Resiliency Promotion
Respiratory Monitoring
Respite Care
Resuscitation
Resuscitation: Fetus
Resuscitation: Neonate
Risk Identification
Risk Identification: Childbearing Family
Risk Identification: Genetic
Role Enhancement
Seclusion
Security Enhancement
Seizure Management
Seizure Precautions
Self-Awareness Enhancement
Self-Care Assistance
Self-Care Assistance: Bathing/Hygiene
Self-Care Assistance: Dressing/Grooming
Self-Care Assistance: Feeding
Self-Care Assistance: Toileting
Self-Esteem Enhancement
Self-Modification Assistance
Self-Responsibility Facilitation
Sexual Counseling
Shift Report
Shock Management
Shock Management: Cardiac
Shock Management: Vasogenic
Shock Management: Volume
Shock Prevention
Sibling Support
Simple Guided Imagery
Simple Massage
Simple Relaxation Therapy
Skin Care: Topical Treatments
Skin Surveillance
Sleep Enhancement
Smoking Cessation Assistance
Socialization Enhancement
Specimen Management
Spiritual Growth Facilitation
Spiritual Support

Splinting
Sports-Injury Prevention: Youth
Staff Development
Staff Supervision
Subarachnoid Hemorrhage Precautions
Substance Use Prevention
Substance Use Treatment
Substance Use Treatment: Alcohol Withdrawal
Substance Use Treatment: Drug Withdrawal
Substance Use Treatment: Overdose
Suicide Prevention
Supply Management
Support Group
Support System Enhancement
Surgical Assistance
Surgical Precautions
Surgical Preparation
Surveillance
Surveillance: Community
Surveillance: Late Pregnancy
Surveillance: Remote Electronic
Surveillance: Safety
Sustenance Support
Suturing
Swallowing Therapy
Teaching: Disease Process
Teaching: Group
Teaching: Individual
Teaching: Infant Nutrition
Teaching: Infant Safety
Teaching: Preoperative
Teaching: Prescribed Activity/Exercise
Teaching: Prescribed Diet
Teaching: Prescribed Medication
Teaching: Procedure/Treatment
Teaching: Psychomotor Skill
Teaching: Safe Sex
Teaching: Sexuality
Teaching: Toddler Nutrition
Teaching: Toddler Safety
Technology Management
Telephone Consultation
Telephone Follow-up
Temperature Regulation

Temperature Regulation: Intraoperative
Therapeutic Play
Therapeutic Touch
Therapy Group
Total Parenteral Nutrition (TPN) Administration
Touch
Traction/Immobilization Care
Transcutaneous Electrical Nerve Stimulation (TENS)
Transport
Triage: Disaster
Triage: Emergency Center
Triage: Telephone
Truth Telling
Tube Care
Tube Care: Chest
Tube Care: Gastrointestinal
Tube Care: Umbilical Line
Tube Care: Urinary
Tube Care: Ventriculostomy/Lumbar Drain
Ultrasonography: Limited Obstetric
Unilateral Neglect Management
Urinary Bladder Training
Urinary Catheterization
Urinary Catheterization: Intermittent
Urinary Elimination Management
Urinary Habit Training
Urinary Incontinence Care
Urinary Incontinence Care: Enuresis
Urinary Retention Care
Values Clarification
Vehicle Safety Promotion
Venous Access Devices (VAD) Maintenance
Ventilation Assistance
Visitation Facilitation
Vital Signs Monitoring
Vomiting Management
Weight Gain Assistance
Weight Management
Weight Reduction Assistance
Wound Care
Wound Care: Closed Drainage
Wound Irrigation

Appendix E

Pain: Assessment Guide and Equianalgesic Chart

Margo McCaffery

ASSESSMENT: USE OF PAIN RATING SCALES

Nursing Assessment/Diagnosis of Pain Sensation. Ask the client about the current level of pain if at all possible. The client's self-report of pain is the single most reliable indicator of how much pain the client is experiencing. The rating given by the client is always what is recorded in the patient's record.

Basic Measures of Pain. The hierarchy of importance of basic measures of pain are as follows (Agency for Health Care Policy and Research: *Quick Reference on Acute Pain in Childhood,* 1992; Schechter, Altman, Weisman, editors: Report of the Consensus Conference on the Management of Pain in Childhood Cancer, *Pediatrics* 86:813, 1990):

1. Client's self-report
2. Report of parent, family, or others close to client
3. Behaviors (e.g., facial expressions, body movements, crying)
4. Physiological measures, "neither sensitive nor specific as indicators of pain" (Agency for Health Policy and Research: *Quick Ref. Acute Pain in Children,* 1992, p 7)

Client/Family Teaching

NOTE: When it is obvious that pain is severe (e.g., following trauma or major surgery), a pain rating scale need not be used initially. Give an analgesic and wait until the client is better able to cooperate.

1. Explain the primary purposes of a pain rating scale. Show the client and family the scale.
   a. This step allows quick, consistent communication between client and caregiver/nurse/physician. Emphasize that the client must volunteer information because the caregivers may not know when the client has pain.
   b. This step also helps establish a pain relief goal that is satisfactory to the client.
2. Explain the specific pain rating scale (e.g., 0 to 10; 0 = no pain and 10 = worst possible pain). When a numerical scale is used, verify that the client can count up to the number used. If the client does not understand whatever scale is standard in that clinical setting, use another scale.
3. Discuss the word *pain.* Explain that pain is discomfort that may occur anywhere in the body; may have various characteristics such as aching, hurting, pulling, tightness, burning, or pricking; and may be mild to severe. If the client prefers some other term such as *hurt,* use that word.
4. To verify that client understands how the word *pain* (or other word preferred by client) is used, ask client to give two examples of pain he or she has now or has experienced.
5. Ask client to practice using the pain rating scale by rating the current pain or past painful experiences.
6. Ask the client what pain rating would be acceptable or satisfactory while at rest and active. This helps set a realistic, initial goal. Zero pain is not always possible. Once

the initial goal is achieved, the possibility of better pain relief can be considered. Emphasize to the client that satisfactory pain relief is a level of pain that is noticeable but not distressing and enables the client to sleep, eat, and perform other required or desired physical activities.

0-10 Numerical Descriptive Pain Intensity Scale

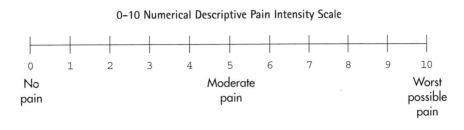

Wong-Baker FACES Pain Rating Scale

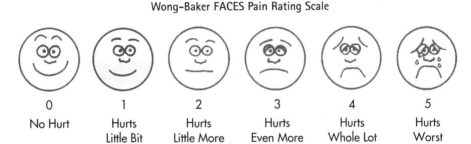

0	1	2	3	4	5
No Hurt	Hurts Little Bit	Hurts Little More	Hurts Even More	Hurts Whole Lot	Hurts Worst

Original instructions: Explain to the person that each face is for a person who feels happy because he has no pain (hurt) or sad because he has some or a lot of pain. **Face 0** is very happy because he doesn't hurt at all. **Face 1** hurts just a little bit. **Face 2** hurts a little more. **Face 3** hurts even more. **Face 4** hurts a whole lot. **Face 5** hurts as much as you can imagine, although you don't have to be crying to feel this bad. Ask the person to choose the face that best describes how he is feeling.

Rating scale is recommended for persons age 3 years and older.

Brief word instructions: Point to each face using the words to describe the pain intensity. Ask the child to choose face that best describes his own pain and record the appropriate number. *Note:* In a study of 148 children ages 4 to 5 years, there were no differences in pain scores when children used the original or brief word instructions. (From Wong DH, Hockenberry-Eaton M, Wilson D, Winkelstein ML, Schwartz P: *Wong's essentials of pediatric nursing,* ed 6, St Louis, 2001, p 1301. Copyrighted by Mosby, Inc. Reprinted by permission.)

Dose Equivalents for Opioid analgesics in Opioid-Naïve Adults and Children ≥50 kg Body Weight[1]

Drug	Approximate Equianalgesic Dosage		Usual Starting Dosage for Moderate to Severe Pain	
	Oral	Parenteral	Oral	Parenteral
Opioid Agonist[2]				
Morphine[3]	30 mg q3-4h (repeat around-the-clock dosing) 60 mg q3-4h (single dose or intermittent dosing)	10 mg q3-4h	30 mg q3-4h	10 mg q3-4h
Morphine, controlled release[3,4] (MS Contin, Oramorph)	90-120 mg q12h	N/A	90-120 mg q12h	N/A
Hydromorphone[3] (Dilaudid)	7.5 mg q3-4h	1.5 mg q3-4h	6 mg q3-4h	1.5 mg q3-4h
Levorphanol (Levo-Dromoran)	4 mg q6-8h	2 mg q6-8h	4 mg q6-8h	2 mg q6-8h
Meperidine (Demerol)	300 mg q2-3h	100 mg q3h	N/R	100 mg q3h
Methadone (Dolophine, other)	20 mg q6-8h	10 mg q6-8h	20 mg q6-8h	10 mg q6-8h
Oxymorphone[3] (Numorphan)	N/A	1 mg q3-4h	N/A	1 mg q3-4h
Combination Opioid/NSAID Preparations[5]				
Codeine[6] (with aspirin or acetaminophen)	180-200 mg q3-4h	130 mg q3-4h	60 mg q3-4h	60 mg q2h (IM/SC)
Hydrocodone (in Lorcet, Lortab, Vicodin, others)	30 mg q3-4h	N/A	10 mg q3-4h	N/A
Oxycodone (Roxicodone, also in Percocet, Percodan, Tylox, others)	20 mg q3-4h	N/A	10 mg q3-4h	N/A

Data from Jacox H et al: *Management of cancer pain*, Clinical Practice Guideline No 9, Agency for Health Care Policy and Research, Pub No 94-0529, 1994, U.S. Department of Health and Human Services, Public Health Services. From Pasero C, Portenoy RK, McCaffery M: Opioid analgesics. In McCaffery M, Pasero C: *Pain: clinical manual*, ed 2, St Louis, 1999, Mosby.

q, Every; *N/A,* not available; *N/R,* not recommended; *NSAID,* nonsteroidal antiinflammatory drug; *IM,* intramuscular; *SC,* subcutaneous.

[1]Caution: Recommended doses do not apply for adult patients with body weight <50 kg.

[2]Caution: Recommended doses do not apply to patients with renal or hepatic insufficiency or other conditions affecting drug metabolism and kinetics.

[3]Caution: For morphine, hydromorphone, and oxymorphone, rectal administration is an alternative route for patients unable to take oral medications. Equianalgesic doses may differ from oral and parenteral doses because of pharmacokinetic differences.

[4]Transdermal fentanyl (Duragesic) is an alternative option. Transdermal fentanyl dosage is not calculated as equianalgesic to a single morphine dose. See the package insert for dosing calculations. Dosages >25 μg/h should not be used in opioid-naive patients.

[5]Caution: Doses of aspirin and acetaminophen in combination opioid/NSAID preparations must also be adjusted to the patient's body weight. Aspirin is contraindicated in children in the presence of fever or other viral disease because of its association with Reye's syndrome.

[6]Caution: Codeine doses >65 mg often are not appropriate because of diminishing incremental analgesia with increasing doses but continually increasing nausea, constipation, and other side effects.

(NOTE: Published tables vary in the suggested doses that are equianalgesic to morphine. Clinical response is the criterion that must be applied for each patient; titration to clinical responses is necessary. Because there is not complete cross-tolerance among these drugs, it is usually necessary to use a lower-than-equianalgesic dose when changing drugs and to retitrate to response.)

Index